LAW AND THE MENTAL HEALTH SYSTEM

CIVIL AND CRIMINAL ASPECTS

Second Edition

By

Ralph Reisner
Professor of Law
University of Illinois-Champaign

and

Christopher Slobogin
Professor of Law
University of Florida-Gainesville

AMERICAN CASEBOOK SERIES®

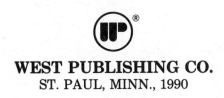

WEST PUBLISHING CO.
ST. PAUL, MINN., 1990

COPYRIGHT © 1985 By WEST PUBLISHING CO.
COPYRIGHT © 1990 By WEST PUBLISHING CO.
                     50 West Kellogg Boulevard
                     P.O. Box 64526
                     St. Paul, MN 55164–0526

Library of Congress Cataloging-in-Publication Data

Reisner, Ralph, 1931–
    Law and the mental health system : civil and criminal aspects / by Ralph Reisner and Christopher Slobogin. — 2nd ed.
      p.   cm. — (American casebook series)
    ISBN 0–314–73302–7
    1. Mental health laws—United States—Cases. 2. Mental health personnel—Legal status, laws, etc.—United States—Cases.
3. Insanity—Jurisprudence—United States—Cases. 4. Insane—Commitment and detention—United States—Cases. I. Slobogin, Christopher, 1951– . II. Title III. Series.
KF3828.A7R44 1990
344.73′044—dc20
[347.30444]   90–12262
                                          CIP

ISBN 0–314–73302–7

To Danute
– Ralph Reisner

―――――――

To Cindy
– Christopher Slobogin

*

American Casebook Series
Hornbook Series and Basic Legal Texts
Black Letter Series and Nutshell Series

of

WEST PUBLISHING COMPANY
P.O. Box 64526
St. Paul, Minnesota 55164–0526

Accounting

FARIS' ACCOUNTING AND LAW IN A NUT-SHELL, 377 pages, 1984. Softcover. (Text)

FIFLIS, KRIPKE AND FOSTER'S TEACHING MATERIALS ON ACCOUNTING FOR BUSINESS LAWYERS, Third Edition, 838 pages, 1984. (Casebook)

SIEGEL AND SIEGEL'S ACCOUNTING AND FINANCIAL DISCLOSURE: A GUIDE TO BASIC CONCEPTS, 259 pages, 1983. Softcover. (Text)

Administrative Law

BONFIELD AND ASIMOW'S STATE AND FEDERAL ADMINISTRATIVE LAW, 826 pages, 1989. Teacher's Manual available. (Casebook)

GELLHORN AND LEVIN'S ADMINISTRATIVE LAW AND PROCESS IN A NUTSHELL, Third Edition, approximately 420 pages, 1990. Softcover. (Text)

MASHAW AND MERRILL'S CASES AND MATERIALS ON ADMINISTRATIVE LAW—THE AMERICAN PUBLIC LAW SYSTEM, Second Edition, 976 pages, 1985. (Casebook) 1989 Supplement.

ROBINSON, GELLHORN AND BRUFF'S THE ADMINISTRATIVE PROCESS, Third Edition, 978 pages, 1986. (Casebook)

Admiralty

HEALY AND SHARPE'S CASES AND MATERIALS ON ADMIRALTY, Second Edition, 876 pages, 1986. (Casebook)

MARAIST'S ADMIRALTY IN A NUTSHELL, Second Edition, 379 pages, 1988. Softcover.

(Text)

SCHOENBAUM'S HORNBOOK ON ADMIRALTY AND MARITIME LAW, Student Edition, 692 pages, 1987 with 1989 pocket part. (Text)

Agency—Partnership

FESSLER'S ALTERNATIVES TO INCORPORATION FOR PERSONS IN QUEST OF PROFIT, Second Edition, 326 pages, 1986. Softcover. Teacher's Manual available. (Casebook)

HENN'S CASES AND MATERIALS ON AGENCY, PARTNERSHIP AND OTHER UNINCORPORATED BUSINESS ENTERPRISES, Second Edition, 733 pages, 1985. Teacher's Manual available. (Casebook)

REUSCHLEIN AND GREGORY'S HORNBOOK ON THE LAW OF AGENCY AND PARTNERSHIP, Second Edition, 683 pages, 1990. (Text)

SELECTED CORPORATION AND PARTNERSHIP STATUTES, RULES AND FORMS. Softcover. 727 pages, 1989.

STEFFEN AND KERR'S CASES ON AGENCY-PARTNERSHIP, Fourth Edition, 859 pages, 1980. (Casebook)

STEFFEN'S AGENCY-PARTNERSHIP IN A NUTSHELL, 364 pages, 1977. Softcover. (Text)

Agricultural Law

MEYER, PEDERSEN, THORSON AND DAVIDSON'S AGRICULTURAL LAW: CASES AND MATERIALS, 931 pages, 1985. Teacher's Manual available. (Casebook)

Alternative Dispute Resolution

KANOWITZ' CASES AND MATERIALS ON ALTERNATIVE DISPUTE RESOLUTION, 1024 pages,

Alternative Dispute Resolution—Cont'd

1986. Teacher's Manual available. (Casebook) 1990 Supplement.

RISKIN AND WESTBROOK'S DISPUTE RESOLUTION AND LAWYERS, 468 pages, 1987. Teacher's Manual available. (Casebook)

RISKIN AND WESTBROOK'S DISPUTE RESOLUTION AND LAWYERS, Abridged Edition, 223 pages, 1987. Softcover. Teacher's Manual available. (Casebook)

American Indian Law

CANBY'S AMERICAN INDIAN LAW IN A NUTSHELL, Second Edition, 336 pages, 1988. Softcover. (Text)

GETCHES AND WILKINSON'S CASES AND MATERIALS ON FEDERAL INDIAN LAW, Second Edition, 880 pages, 1986. (Casebook)

Antitrust—see also Regulated Industries, Trade Regulation

FOX AND SULLIVAN'S CASES AND MATERIALS ON ANTITRUST, 935 pages, 1989. Teacher's Manual available. (Casebook)

GELLHORN'S ANTITRUST LAW AND ECONOMICS IN A NUTSHELL, Third Edition, 472 pages, 1986. Softcover. (Text)

HOVENKAMP'S BLACK LETTER ON ANTITRUST, 323 pages, 1986. Softcover. (Review)

HOVENKAMP'S HORNBOOK ON ECONOMICS AND FEDERAL ANTITRUST LAW, Student Edition, 414 pages, 1985. (Text)

OPPENHEIM, WESTON AND MCCARTHY'S CASES AND COMMENTS ON FEDERAL ANTITRUST LAWS, Fourth Edition, 1168 pages, 1981. (Casebook) 1985 Supplement.

POSNER AND EASTERBROOK'S CASES AND ECONOMIC NOTES ON ANTITRUST, Second Edition, 1077 pages, 1981. (Casebook) 1984–85 Supplement.

SULLIVAN'S HORNBOOK OF THE LAW OF ANTITRUST, 886 pages, 1977. (Text)

Appellate Advocacy—see Trial and Appellate Advocacy

Architecture and Engineering Law

SWEET'S LEGAL ASPECTS OF ARCHITECTURE, ENGINEERING AND THE CONSTRUCTION PROCESS, Fourth Edition, 889 pages, 1989. Teacher's Manual available. (Casebook)

Art Law

DUBOFF'S ART LAW IN A NUTSHELL, 335 pages, 1984. Softcover. (Text)

Banking Law

LOVETT'S BANKING AND FINANCIAL INSTITUTIONS LAW IN A NUTSHELL, Second Edition, 464 pages, 1988. Softcover. (Text)

SYMONS AND WHITE'S TEACHING MATERIALS ON BANKING LAW, Second Edition, 993 pages, 1984. Teacher's Manual available. (Casebook) 1987 Supplement.

Business Planning—see also Corporate Finance

PAINTER'S PROBLEMS AND MATERIALS IN BUSINESS PLANNING, Second Edition, 1008 pages, 1984. (Casebook) 1990 Supplement.

Statutory Supplement. *See Selected Corporation and Partnership*

SELECTED CORPORATION AND PARTNERSHIP STATUTES, RULES AND FORMS. 727 pages, 1989. Softcover.

Civil Procedure—see also Federal Jurisdiction and Procedure

AMERICAN BAR ASSOCIATION SECTION OF LITIGATION—READINGS ON ADVERSARIAL JUSTICE: THE AMERICAN APPROACH TO ADJUDICATION, 217 pages, 1988. Softcover. (Coursebook)

CLERMONT'S BLACK LETTER ON CIVIL PROCEDURE, Second Edition, 332 pages, 1988. Softcover. (Review)

COUND, FRIEDENTHAL, MILLER AND SEXTON'S CASES AND MATERIALS ON CIVIL PROCEDURE, Fifth Edition, 1284 pages, 1989. Teacher's Manual available. (Casebook)

COUND, FRIEDENTHAL, MILLER AND SEXTON'S CIVIL PROCEDURE SUPPLEMENT. Approximately 450 pages, 1990. Softcover. (Casebook Supplement)

FEDERAL RULES OF CIVIL PROCEDURE—EDUCATIONAL EDITION. Softcover. Approximately 635 pages, 1990.

FRIEDENTHAL, KANE AND MILLER'S HORNBOOK ON CIVIL PROCEDURE, 876 pages, 1985. (Text)

KANE AND LEVINE'S CIVIL PROCEDURE IN CALIFORNIA: STATE AND FEDERAL 498 pages, 1989. Softcover. (Casebook Supplement)

Civil Procedure—Cont'd

KANE'S CIVIL PROCEDURE IN A NUTSHELL, Second Edition, 306 pages, 1986. Softcover. (Text)

KOFFLER AND REPPY'S HORNBOOK ON COMMON LAW PLEADING, 663 pages, 1969. (Text)

MARCUS, REDISH AND SHERMAN'S CIVIL PROCEDURE: A MODERN APPROACH, 1027 pages, 1989. Teacher's Manual available. (Casebook)

MARCUS AND SHERMAN'S COMPLEX LITIGATION–CASES AND MATERIALS ON ADVANCED CIVIL PROCEDURE, 846 pages, 1985. Teacher's Manual available. (Casebook) 1989 Supplement.

PARK'S COMPUTER-AIDED EXERCISES ON CIVIL PROCEDURE, Second Edition, 167 pages, 1983. Softcover. (Coursebook)

SIEGEL'S HORNBOOK ON NEW YORK PRACTICE, 1011 pages, 1978, with 1987 pocket part. (Text)

Commercial Law

BAILEY AND HAGEDORN'S SECURED TRANSACTIONS IN A NUTSHELL, Third Edition, 390 pages, 1988. Softcover. (Text)

EPSTEIN, MARTIN, HENNING AND NICKLES' BASIC UNIFORM COMMERCIAL CODE TEACHING MATERIALS, Third Edition, 704 pages, 1988. Teacher's Manual available. (Casebook)

HENSON'S HORNBOOK ON SECURED TRANSACTIONS UNDER THE U.C.C., Second Edition, 504 pages, 1979, with 1979 pocket part. (Text)

MURRAY'S COMMERCIAL LAW, PROBLEMS AND MATERIALS, 366 pages, 1975. Teacher's Manual available. Softcover. (Coursebook)

NICKLES' BLACK LETTER ON COMMERCIAL PAPER, 450 pages, 1988. Softcover. (Review)

NICKLES, MATHESON AND DOLAN'S MATERIALS FOR UNDERSTANDING CREDIT AND PAYMENT SYSTEMS, 923 pages, 1987. Teacher's Manual available. (Casebook)

NORDSTROM, MURRAY AND CLOVIS' PROBLEMS AND MATERIALS ON SALES, 515 pages, 1982. (Casebook)

NORDSTROM, MURRAY AND CLOVIS' PROBLEMS AND MATERIALS ON SECURED TRANSACTIONS, 594 pages, 1987. (Casebook)

RUBIN AND COOTER'S THE PAYMENT SYSTEM: CASES, MATERIALS AND ISSUES, 885 pages, 1989. (Casebook)

SELECTED COMMERCIAL STATUTES. Softcover. Approximately 1650 pages, 1990.

SPEIDEL'S BLACK LETTER ON SALES AND SALES FINANCING, 363 pages, 1984. Softcover. (Review)

SPEIDEL, SUMMERS AND WHITE'S COMMERCIAL LAW: TEACHING MATERIALS, Fourth Edition, 1448 pages, 1987. Teacher's Manual available. (Casebook)

SPEIDEL, SUMMERS AND WHITE'S COMMERCIAL PAPER: TEACHING MATERIALS, Fourth Edition, 578 pages, 1987. Reprint from Speidel et al., Commercial Law, Fourth Edition. Teacher's Manual available. (Casebook)

SPEIDEL, SUMMERS AND WHITE'S SALES: TEACHING MATERIALS, Fourth Edition, 804 pages, 1987. Reprint from Speidel et al., Commercial Law, Fourth Edition. Teacher's Manual available. (Casebook)

SPEIDEL, SUMMERS AND WHITE'S SECURED TRANSACTIONS: TEACHING MATERIALS, Fourth Edition, 485 pages, 1987. Reprint from Speidel et al., Commercial Law, Fourth Edition. Teacher's Manual available. (Casebook)

STOCKTON'S SALES IN A NUTSHELL, Second Edition, 370 pages, 1981. Softcover. (Text)

STONE'S UNIFORM COMMERCIAL CODE IN A NUTSHELL, Third Edition, 580 pages, 1989. Softcover. (Text)

WEBER AND SPEIDEL'S COMMERCIAL PAPER IN A NUTSHELL, Third Edition, 404 pages, 1982. Softcover. (Text)

WHITE AND SUMMERS' HORNBOOK ON THE UNIFORM COMMERCIAL CODE, Third Edition, Student Edition, 1386 pages, 1988. (Text)

Community Property

MENNELL AND BOYKOFF'S COMMUNITY PROPERTY IN A NUTSHELL, Second Edition, 432 pages, 1988. Softcover. (Text)

VERRALL AND BIRD'S CASES AND MATERIALS

Community Property—Cont'd

ON CALIFORNIA COMMUNITY PROPERTY, Fifth Edition, 604 pages, 1988. (Casebook)

Comparative Law

BARTON, GIBBS, LI AND MERRYMAN'S LAW IN RADICALLY DIFFERENT CULTURES, 960 pages, 1983. (Casebook)

GLENDON, GORDON AND OSAKWE'S COMPARATIVE LEGAL TRADITIONS: TEXT, MATERIALS AND CASES ON THE CIVIL LAW, COMMON LAW AND SOCIALIST LAW TRADITIONS, 1091 pages, 1985. (Casebook)

GLENDON, GORDON AND OSAKWE'S COMPARATIVE LEGAL TRADITIONS IN A NUTSHELL. 402 pages, 1982. Softcover. (Text)

LANGBEIN'S COMPARATIVE CRIMINAL PROCEDURE: GERMANY, 172 pages, 1977. Softcover. (Casebook)

Computers and Law

MAGGS AND SPROWL'S COMPUTER APPLICATIONS IN THE LAW, 316 pages, 1987. (Coursebook)

MASON'S USING COMPUTERS IN THE LAW: AN INTRODUCTION AND PRACTICAL GUIDE, Second Edition, 288 pages, 1988. Softcover. (Coursebook)

Conflict of Laws

CRAMTON, CURRIE AND KAY'S CASES–COMMENTS–QUESTIONS ON CONFLICT OF LAWS, Fourth Edition, 876 pages, 1987. (Casebook)

HAY'S BLACK LETTER ON CONFLICT OF LAWS, 330 pages, 1989. Softcover. (Review)

SCOLES AND HAY'S HORNBOOK ON CONFLICT OF LAWS, Student Edition, 1085 pages, 1982, with 1988–89 pocket part. (Text)

SEIGEL'S CONFLICTS IN A NUTSHELL, 470 pages, 1982. Softcover. (Text)

Constitutional Law—Civil Rights—see also Foreign Relations and National Security Law

ABERNATHY'S CASES AND MATERIALS ON CIVIL RIGHTS, 660 pages, 1980. (Casebook)

BARRON AND DIENES' BLACK LETTER ON CONSTITUTIONAL LAW, Second Edition, 310 pages, 1987. Softcover. (Review)

BARRON AND DIENES' CONSTITUTIONAL LAW

IN A NUTSHELL, 389 pages, 1986. Softcover. (Text)

ENGDAHL'S CONSTITUTIONAL FEDERALISM IN A NUTSHELL, Second Edition, 411 pages, 1987. Softcover. (Text)

FARBER AND SHERRY'S HISTORY OF THE AMERICAN CONSTITUTION,   458 pages, 1990. Softcover.   Teacher's Manual available. (Text)

GARVEY AND ALEINIKOFF'S MODERN CONSTITUTIONAL THEORY: A READER,   494 pages, 1989. Softcover. (Reader)

LOCKHART, KAMISAR, CHOPER AND SHIFFRIN'S CONSTITUTIONAL LAW: CASES–COMMENTS–QUESTIONS, Sixth Edition, 1601 pages, 1986. (Casebook) 1990 Supplement.

LOCKHART, KAMISAR, CHOPER AND SHIFFRIN'S THE AMERICAN CONSTITUTION: CASES AND MATERIALS, Sixth Edition, 1260 pages, 1986. Abridged version of Lockhart, et al., Constitutional Law: Cases–Comments–Questions, Sixth Edition. (Casebook) 1990 Supplement.

LOCKHART, KAMISAR, CHOPER AND SHIFFRIN'S CONSTITUTIONAL RIGHTS AND LIBERTIES: CASES AND MATERIALS, Sixth Edition, 1266 pages, 1986. Reprint from Lockhart, et al., Constitutional Law: Cases–Comments–Questions, Sixth Edition. (Casebook) 1990 Supplement.

MARKS AND COOPER'S STATE CONSTITUTIONAL LAW IN A NUTSHELL, 329 pages, 1988. Softcover. (Text)

NOWAK, ROTUNDA AND YOUNG'S HORNBOOK ON CONSTITUTIONAL LAW, Third Edition, 1191 pages, 1986 with 1988 pocket part. (Text)

ROTUNDA'S MODERN CONSTITUTIONAL LAW: CASES AND NOTES, Third Edition, 1085 pages, 1989. (Casebook) 1990 Supplement.

VIEIRA'S CONSTITUTIONAL CIVIL RIGHTS IN A NUTSHELL, Second Edition, 322 pages, 1990. Softcover. (Text)

WILLIAMS' CONSTITUTIONAL ANALYSIS IN A NUTSHELL, 388 pages, 1979. Softcover. (Text)

Consumer Law—see also Commercial Law

EPSTEIN AND NICKLES' CONSUMER LAW IN A NUTSHELL, Second Edition, 418 pages,

Consumer Law—Cont'd

1981. Softcover. (Text)

SELECTED COMMERCIAL STATUTES. Softcover. Approximately 1650 pages, 1990.

SPANOGLE AND ROHNER'S CASES AND MATERIALS ON CONSUMER LAW, 693 pages, 1979. Teacher's Manual available. (Casebook) 1982 Supplement.

Contracts

CALAMARI AND PERILLO'S BLACK LETTER ON CONTRACTS, Second Edition, approximately 450 pages, 1990. Softcover. (Review)

CALAMARI AND PERILLO'S HORNBOOK ON CONTRACTS, Third Edition, 1049 pages, 1987. (Text)

CALAMARI, PERILLO AND BENDER'S CASES AND PROBLEMS ON CONTRACTS, Second Edition, 905 pages, 1989. Teacher's Manual Available. (Casebook)

CORBIN'S TEXT ON CONTRACTS, One Volume Student Edition, 1224 pages, 1952. (Text)

FESSLER AND LOISEAUX'S CASES AND MATERIALS ON CONTRACTS—MORALITY, ECONOMICS AND THE MARKET PLACE, 837 pages, 1982. Teacher's Manual available. (Casebook)

FRIEDMAN'S CONTRACT REMEDIES IN A NUTSHELL, 323 pages, 1981. Softcover. (Text)

FULLER AND EISENBERG'S CASES ON BASIC CONTRACT LAW, Fifth Edition, approximately 1100 pages, 1990. (Casebook)

HAMILTON, RAU AND WEINTRAUB'S CASES AND MATERIALS ON CONTRACTS, 830 pages, 1984. (Casebook)

JACKSON AND BOLLINGER'S CASES ON CONTRACT LAW IN MODERN SOCIETY, Second Edition, 1329 pages, 1980. Teacher's Manual available. (Casebook)

KEYES' GOVERNMENT CONTRACTS IN A NUTSHELL, Second Edition, approximately 530 pages, 1990. Softcover. (Text)

SCHABER AND ROHWER'S CONTRACTS IN A NUTSHELL, Third Edition, approximately 438 pages, 1990. Softcover. (Text)

SUMMERS AND HILLMAN'S CONTRACT AND RELATED OBLIGATION: THEORY, DOCTRINE AND PRACTICE, 1074 pages, 1987. Teacher's Manual available. (Casebook)

Copyright—see Patent and Copyright Law

Corporate Finance

HAMILTON'S CASES AND MATERIALS ON CORPORATION FINANCE, Second Edition, 1221 pages, 1989. (Casebook)

Corporations

HAMILTON'S BLACK LETTER ON CORPORATIONS, Second Edition, 513 pages, 1986. Softcover. (Review)

HAMILTON'S CASES AND MATERIALS ON CORPORATIONS—INCLUDING PARTNERSHIPS AND LIMITED PARTNERSHIPS, Fourth Edition, approximately 1250 pages, 1990. (Casebook) 1990 Statutory Supplement.

HAMILTON'S THE LAW OF CORPORATIONS IN A NUTSHELL, Second Edition, 515 pages, 1987. Softcover. (Text)

HENN'S TEACHING MATERIALS ON THE LAW OF CORPORATIONS, Second Edition, 1204 pages, 1986. Teacher's Manual available. (Casebook)

    Statutory Supplement. *See Selected Corporation and Partnership*

HENN AND ALEXANDER'S HORNBOOK ON LAWS OF CORPORATIONS, Third Edition, Student Edition, 1371 pages, 1983, with 1986 pocket part. (Text)

SELECTED CORPORATION AND PARTNERSHIP STATUTES, RULES AND FORMS. Softcover. 727 pages, 1989.

SOLOMON, SCHWARTZ AND BAUMAN'S MATERIALS AND PROBLEMS ON CORPORATIONS: LAW AND POLICY, Second Edition, 1391 pages, 1988. Teacher's Manual available. (Casebook) 1990 Supplement.

    Statutory Supplement. *See Selected Corporation and Partnership*

Corrections

KRANTZ' CASES AND MATERIALS ON THE LAW OF CORRECTIONS AND PRISONERS' RIGHTS, Third Edition, 855 pages, 1986. (Casebook) 1988 Supplement.

KRANTZ' THE LAW OF CORRECTIONS AND PRISONERS' RIGHTS IN A NUTSHELL, Third Edition, 407 pages, 1988. Softcover. (Text)

ROBBINS' CASES AND MATERIALS ON POST-CONVICTION REMEDIES, 506 pages, 1982. (Casebook)

Creditors' Rights

BANKRUPTCY CODE, RULES AND OFFICIAL FORMS, LAW SCHOOL EDITION. Approximately 875 pages, 1990. Softcover.

EPSTEIN'S DEBTOR-CREDITOR RELATIONS IN A NUTSHELL, Third Edition, 383 pages, 1986. Softcover. (Text)

EPSTEIN, LANDERS AND NICKLES' CASES AND MATERIALS ON DEBTORS AND CREDITORS, Third Edition, 1059 pages, 1987. Teacher's Manual available. (Casebook)

LOPUCKI'S PLAYER'S MANUAL FOR THE DEBTOR-CREDITOR GAME, 123 pages, 1985. Softcover. (Coursebook)

NICKLES AND EPSTEIN'S BLACK LETTER ON CREDITORS' RIGHTS AND BANKRUPTCY, 576 pages, 1989. (Review)

RIESENFELD'S CASES AND MATERIALS ON CREDITORS' REMEDIES AND DEBTORS' PROTECTION, Fourth Edition, 914 pages, 1987. (Casebook) 1990 Supplement.

WHITE'S CASES AND MATERIALS ON BANKRUPTCY AND CREDITORS' RIGHTS, 812 pages, 1985. Teacher's Manual available. (Casebook) 1987 Supplement.

Criminal Law and Criminal Procedure—see also Corrections, Juvenile Justice

ABRAMS' FEDERAL CRIMINAL LAW AND ITS ENFORCEMENT, 866 pages, 1986. (Casebook) 1988 Supplement.

AMERICAN CRIMINAL JUSTICE PROCESS: SELECTED RULES, STATUTES AND GUIDELINES. 723 pages, 1989. Softcover.

CARLSON'S ADJUDICATION OF CRIMINAL JUSTICE: PROBLEMS AND REFERENCES, 130 pages, 1986. Softcover. (Casebook)

DIX AND SHARLOT'S CASES AND MATERIALS ON CRIMINAL LAW, Third Edition, 846 pages, 1987. (Casebook)

GRANO'S PROBLEMS IN CRIMINAL PROCEDURE, Second Edition, 176 pages, 1981. Teacher's Manual available. Softcover. (Coursebook)

HEYMANN AND KENETY'S THE MURDER TRIAL OF WILBUR JACKSON: A HOMICIDE IN THE FAMILY, Second Edition, 347 pages, 1985. (Coursebook)

ISRAEL, KAMISAR AND LAFAVE'S CRIMINAL

PROCEDURE AND THE CONSTITUTION: LEADING SUPREME COURT CASES AND INTRODUCTORY TEXT. Approximately 725 pages, 1990 Edition. Softcover. (Casebook)

ISRAEL AND LAFAVE'S CRIMINAL PROCEDURE—CONSTITUTIONAL LIMITATIONS IN A NUTSHELL, Fourth Edition, 461 pages, 1988. Softcover. (Text)

JOHNSON'S CASES, MATERIALS AND TEXT ON CRIMINAL LAW, Fourth Edition, approximately 790 pages, 1990. Teacher's Manual available. (Casebook)

JOHNSON'S CASES AND MATERIALS ON CRIMINAL PROCEDURE, 859 pages, 1988. (Casebook) 1990 Supplement.

KAMISAR, LAFAVE AND ISRAEL'S MODERN CRIMINAL PROCEDURE: CASES, COMMENTS AND QUESTIONS, Seventh Edition, 1593 pages, 1990. (Casebook) 1990 Supplement.

KAMISAR, LAFAVE AND ISRAEL'S BASIC CRIMINAL PROCEDURE: CASES, COMMENTS AND QUESTIONS, Seventh Edition, 792 pages, 1990. Softcover reprint from Kamisar, et al., Modern Criminal Procedure: Cases, Comments and Questions, Seventh Edition. (Casebook) 1990 Supplement.

LAFAVE'S MODERN CRIMINAL LAW: CASES, COMMENTS AND QUESTIONS, Second Edition, 903 pages, 1988. (Casebook)

LAFAVE AND ISRAEL'S HORNBOOK ON CRIMINAL PROCEDURE, Student Edition, 1142 pages, 1985, with 1989 pocket part. (Text)

LAFAVE AND SCOTT'S HORNBOOK ON CRIMINAL LAW, Second Edition, 918 pages, 1986. (Text)

LANGBEIN'S COMPARATIVE CRIMINAL PROCEDURE: GERMANY, 172 pages, 1977. Softcover. (Casebook)

LOEWY'S CRIMINAL LAW IN A NUTSHELL, Second Edition, 321 pages, 1987. Softcover. (Text)

LOW'S BLACK LETTER ON CRIMINAL LAW, Revised First Edition, approximately 430 pages, 1990. Softcover. (Review)

SALTZBURG'S CASES AND COMMENTARY ON AMERICAN CRIMINAL PROCEDURE, Third Edition, 1302 pages, 1988. Teacher's Manual available. (Casebook) 1990 Supplement.

Criminal Law and Criminal Procedure—Cont'd

UVILLER'S THE PROCESSES OF CRIMINAL JUSTICE: INVESTIGATION AND ADJUDICATION, Second Edition, 1384 pages, 1979. (Casebook) 1979 Statutory Supplement. 1986 Update.

VORENBERG'S CASES ON CRIMINAL LAW AND PROCEDURE, Second Edition, 1088 pages, 1981. Teacher's Manual available. (Casebook) 1990 Supplement.

Decedents' Estates—see Trusts and Estates

Domestic Relations

CLARK'S HORNBOOK ON DOMESTIC RELATIONS, Second Edition, Student Edition, 1050 pages, 1988. (Text)

CLARK AND GLOWINSKY'S CASES AND PROBLEMS ON DOMESTIC RELATIONS, Fourth Edition. Approximately 1125 pages, 1990. Teacher's Manual available. (Casebook)

KRAUSE'S BLACK LETTER ON FAMILY LAW, 314 pages, 1988. Softcover. (Review)

KRAUSE'S CASES, COMMENTS AND QUESTIONS ON FAMILY LAW, Third Edition, 1433 pages, 1990. (Casebook)

KRAUSE'S FAMILY LAW IN A NUTSHELL, Second Edition, 444 pages, 1986. Softcover. (Text)

KRAUSKOPF'S CASES ON PROPERTY DIVISION AT MARRIAGE DISSOLUTION, 250 pages, 1984. Softcover. (Casebook)

Economics, Law and—see also Antitrust, Regulated Industries

GOETZ' CASES AND MATERIALS ON LAW AND ECONOMICS, 547 pages, 1984. (Casebook)

MALLOY'S LAW AND ECONOMICS: A COMPARATIVE APPROACH TO THEORY AND PRACTICE, Approximately 152 pages, 1990. Softcover. (Text)

Education Law

ALEXANDER AND ALEXANDER'S THE LAW OF SCHOOLS, STUDENTS AND TEACHERS IN A NUTSHELL, 409 pages, 1984. Softcover. (Text)

Employment Discrimination—see also Women and the Law

ESTREICHER AND HARPER'S CASES AND

MATERIALS ON THE LAW GOVERNING THE EMPLOYMENT RELATIONSHIP, 962 pages, 1990. Teacher's Manual available. (Casebook) Statutory Supplement.

JONES, MURPHY AND BELTON'S CASES AND MATERIALS ON DISCRIMINATION IN EMPLOYMENT, (The Labor Law Group). Fifth Edition, 1116 pages, 1987. (Casebook) 1990 Supplement.

PLAYER'S FEDERAL LAW OF EMPLOYMENT DISCRIMINATION IN A NUTSHELL, Second Edition, 402 pages, 1981. Softcover. (Text)

PLAYER'S HORNBOOK ON EMPLOYMENT DISCRIMINATION LAW, Student Edition, 708 pages, 1988. (Text)

PLAYER, SHOBEN AND LIEBERWITZ' CASES AND MATERIALS ON EMPLOYMENT DISCRIMINATION LAW, Approximately 810 pages, 1990. (Casebook)

Energy and Natural Resources Law—see also Oil and Gas

LAITOS' CASES AND MATERIALS ON NATURAL RESOURCES LAW, 938 pages, 1985. Teacher's Manual available. (Casebook)

SELECTED ENVIRONMENTAL LAW STATUTES—EDUCATIONAL EDITION. Softcover. Approximately 1040 pages, 1990.

Environmental Law—see also Energy and Natural Resources Law; Sea, Law of

BONINE AND MCGARITY'S THE LAW OF ENVIRONMENTAL PROTECTION: CASES—LEGISLATION—POLICIES, 1076 pages, 1984. Teacher's Manual available. (Casebook)

FINDLEY AND FARBER'S CASES AND MATERIALS ON ENVIRONMENTAL LAW, Second Edition, 813 pages, 1985. (Casebook) 1988 Supplement.

FINDLEY AND FARBER'S ENVIRONMENTAL LAW IN A NUTSHELL, Second Edition, 367 pages, 1988. Softcover. (Text)

RODGERS' HORNBOOK ON ENVIRONMENTAL LAW, 956 pages, 1977, with 1984 pocket part. (Text)

SELECTED ENVIRONMENTAL LAW STATUTES—EDUCATIONAL EDITION. Softcover. Approximately 1040 pages, 1990.

Equity—see Remedies

Estate Planning—see also Trusts and Estates; Taxation—Estate and Gift

LYNN'S AN INTRODUCTION TO ESTATE PLANNING IN A NUTSHELL, Third Edition, 370 pages, 1983. Softcover. (Text)

Evidence

BROUN AND BLAKEY'S BLACK LETTER ON EVIDENCE, 269 pages, 1984. Softcover. (Review)

BROUN, MEISENHOLDER, STRONG AND MOSTELLER'S PROBLEMS IN EVIDENCE, Third Edition, 238 pages, 1988. Teacher's Manual available. Softcover. (Coursebook)

CLEARY, STRONG, BROUN AND MOSTELLER'S CASES AND MATERIALS ON EVIDENCE, Fourth Edition, 1060 pages, 1988. (Casebook)

FEDERAL RULES OF EVIDENCE FOR UNITED STATES COURTS AND MAGISTRATES. Softcover. Approximately 380 pages, 1990.

GRAHAM'S FEDERAL RULES OF EVIDENCE IN A NUTSHELL, Second Edition, 473 pages, 1987. Softcover. (Text)

LEMPERT AND SALTZBURG'S A MODERN APPROACH TO EVIDENCE: TEXT, PROBLEMS, TRANSCRIPTS AND CASES, Second Edition, 1232 pages, 1983. Teacher's Manual available. (Casebook)

LILLY'S AN INTRODUCTION TO THE LAW OF EVIDENCE, Second Edition, 585 pages, 1987. (Text)

MCCORMICK, SUTTON AND WELLBORN'S CASES AND MATERIALS ON EVIDENCE, Sixth Edition, 1067 pages, 1987. (Casebook)

MCCORMICK'S HORNBOOK ON EVIDENCE, Third Edition, Student Edition, 1156 pages, 1984, with 1987 pocket part. (Text)

ROTHSTEIN'S EVIDENCE IN A NUTSHELL: STATE AND FEDERAL RULES, Second Edition, 514 pages, 1981. Softcover. (Text)

Federal Jurisdiction and Procedure

CURRIE'S CASES AND MATERIALS ON FEDERAL COURTS, Fourth Edition, approximately 1125 pages, 1990. (Casebook)

CURRIE'S FEDERAL JURISDICTION IN A NUTSHELL, Third Edition, approximately 260 pages, 1990. Softcover. (Text)

FEDERAL RULES OF CIVIL PROCEDURE—EDUCATIONAL EDITION. Softcover. Approxi-

mately 635 pages, 1990.

REDISH'S BLACK LETTER ON FEDERAL JURISDICTION, 219 pages, 1985. Softcover. (Review)

REDISH'S CASES, COMMENTS AND QUESTIONS ON FEDERAL COURTS, Second Edition, 1122 pages, 1989. (Casebook) 1990 Supplement.

VETRI AND MERRILL'S FEDERAL COURTS PROBLEMS AND MATERIALS, Second Edition, 232 pages, 1984. Softcover. (Coursebook)

WRIGHT'S HORNBOOK ON FEDERAL COURTS, Fourth Edition, Student Edition, 870 pages, 1983. (Text)

Foreign Relations and National Security Law

FRANCK AND GLENNON'S FOREIGN RELATIONS AND NATIONAL SECURITY LAW, 941 pages, 1987. (Casebook)

Future Interests—see Trusts and Estates

Health Law—see Medicine, Law and

Human Rights—see International Law

Immigration Law

ALEINIKOFF AND MARTIN'S IMMIGRATION PROCESS AND POLICY, Second Edition, approximately 1100 pages, October, 1990 (Casebook)

　　Statutory Supplement. *See Immigration and Nationality Laws*

IMMIGRATION AND NATIONALITY LAWS OF THE UNITED STATES: SELECTED STATUTES, REGULATIONS AND FORMS. Softcover. Approximately 400 pages, 1990.

WEISSBRODT'S IMMIGRATION LAW AND PROCEDURE IN A NUTSHELL, Second Edition, 438 pages, 1989, Softcover. (Text)

Indian Law—see American Indian Law

Insurance Law

DEVINE AND TERRY'S PROBLEMS IN INSURANCE LAW, 240 pages, 1989. Softcover. Teacher's Manual available. (Coursebook)

DOBBYN'S INSURANCE LAW IN A NUTSHELL, Second Edition, 316 pages, 1989. Softcover. (Text)

KEETON'S CASES ON BASIC INSURANCE LAW,

Insurance Law—Cont'd

Second Edition, 1086 pages, 1977. Teacher's Manual available. (Casebook)

KEETON'S COMPUTER-AIDED AND WORKBOOK EXERCISES ON INSURANCE LAW, 255 pages, 1990. Softcover. (Coursebook)

KEETON AND WIDISS' INSURANCE LAW, Student Edition, 1359 pages, 1988. (Text)

WIDISS AND KEETON'S COURSE SUPPLEMENT TO KEETON AND WIDISS' INSURANCE LAW, 502 pages, 1988. Softcover. (Casebook)

WIDISS' INSURANCE: MATERIALS ON FUNDAMENTAL PRINCIPLES, LEGAL DOCTRINES AND REGULATORY ACTS, 1186 pages, 1989. (Casebook)

YORK AND WHELAN'S CASES, MATERIALS AND PROBLEMS ON GENERAL PRACTICE INSURANCE LAW, Second Edition, 787 pages, 1988. Teacher's Manual available. (Casebook)

International Law—see also Sea, Law of

BUERGENTHAL'S INTERNATIONAL HUMAN RIGHTS IN A NUTSHELL, 283 pages, 1988. Softcover. (Text)

BUERGENTHAL AND MAIER'S PUBLIC INTERNATIONAL LAW IN A NUTSHELL, Second Edition, 275 pages, 1990. Softcover. (Text)

FOLSOM, GORDON AND SPANOGLE'S INTERNATIONAL BUSINESS TRANSACTIONS—A PROBLEM-ORIENTED COURSEBOOK, 1160 pages, 1986. Teacher's Manual available. (Casebook) 1989 Documents Supplement.

FOLSOM, GORDON AND SPANOGLE'S INTERNATIONAL BUSINESS TRANSACTIONS IN A NUTSHELL, Third Edition, 509 pages, 1988. Softcover. (Text)

HENKIN, PUGH, SCHACHTER AND SMIT'S CASES AND MATERIALS ON INTERNATIONAL LAW, Second Edition, 1517 pages, 1987. (Casebook) Documents Supplement.

JACKSON AND DAVEY'S CASES, MATERIALS AND TEXT ON LEGAL PROBLEMS OF INTERNATIONAL ECONOMIC RELATIONS, Second Edition, 1269 pages, 1986. (Casebook) 1989 Documents Supplement.

KIRGIS' INTERNATIONAL ORGANIZATIONS IN THEIR LEGAL SETTING, 1016 pages, 1977. Teacher's Manual available. (Casebook) 1981 Supplement.

WESTON, FALK AND D'AMATO'S INTERNATIONAL LAW AND WORLD ORDER—A PROBLEM-ORIENTED COURSEBOOK, Second Edition, approximately 1305 pages, 1990. Teacher's Manual available. (Casebook) Documents Supplement.

Interviewing and Counseling

BINDER AND PRICE'S LEGAL INTERVIEWING AND COUNSELING, 232 pages, 1977. Teacher's Manual available. Softcover. (Coursebook)

BINDER, BERGMAN AND PRICE'S LAWYERS AS COUNSELORS: A CLIENT CENTERED APPROACH, Approximately 400 pages, October, 1990 Pub. Softcover. (Coursebook)

SHAFFER AND ELKINS' LEGAL INTERVIEWING AND COUNSELING IN A NUTSHELL, Second Edition, 487 pages, 1987. Softcover. (Text)

Introduction to Law—see Legal Method and Legal System

Introduction to Law Study

HEGLAND'S INTRODUCTION TO THE STUDY AND PRACTICE OF LAW IN A NUTSHELL, 418 pages, 1983. Softcover. (Text)

KINYON'S INTRODUCTION TO LAW STUDY AND LAW EXAMINATIONS IN A NUTSHELL, 389 pages, 1971. Softcover. (Text)

Judicial Process—see Legal Method and Legal System

Jurisprudence

CHRISTIE'S JURISPRUDENCE—TEXT AND READINGS ON THE PHILOSOPHY OF LAW, 1056 pages, 1973. (Casebook)

Juvenile Justice

FOX'S CASES AND MATERIALS ON MODERN JUVENILE JUSTICE, Second Edition, 960 pages, 1981. (Casebook)

FOX'S JUVENILE COURTS IN A NUTSHELL, Third Edition, 291 pages, 1984. Softcover. (Text)

Labor and Employment Law—see also Employment Discrimination, Social Legislation

FINKIN, GOLDMAN AND SUMMERS' LEGAL PROTECTION OF INDIVIDUAL EMPLOYEES, (The La-

Labor and Employment Law—Cont'd

bor Law Group). 1164 pages, 1989. (Casebook)

GORMAN'S BASIC TEXT ON LABOR LAW—UNIONIZATION AND COLLECTIVE BARGAINING, 914 pages, 1976. (Text)

LESLIE'S LABOR LAW IN A NUTSHELL, Second Edition, 397 pages, 1986. Softcover. (Text)

NOLAN'S LABOR ARBITRATION LAW AND PRACTICE IN A NUTSHELL, 358 pages, 1979. Softcover. (Text)

OBERER, HANSLOWE, ANDERSEN AND HEINSZ' CASES AND MATERIALS ON LABOR LAW—COLLECTIVE BARGAINING IN A FREE SOCIETY, Third Edition, 1163 pages, 1986. (Casebook) Statutory Supplement.

RABIN, SILVERSTEIN AND SCHATZKI'S LABOR AND EMPLOYMENT LAW: PROBLEMS, CASES AND MATERIALS IN THE LAW OF WORK, (The Labor Law Group). 1014 pages, 1988. Teacher's Manual available. (Casebook) 1988 Statutory Supplement.

Land Finance—Property Security—see Real Estate Transactions

Land Use

CALLIES AND FREILICH'S CASES AND MATERIALS ON LAND USE, 1233 pages, 1986. (Casebook) 1988 Supplement.

HAGMAN AND JUERGENSMEYER'S HORNBOOK ON URBAN PLANNING AND LAND DEVELOPMENT CONTROL LAW, Second Edition, Student Edition, 680 pages, 1986. (Text)

WRIGHT AND GITELMAN'S CASES AND MATERIALS ON LAND USE, Third Edition, 1300 pages, 1982. Teacher's Manual available. (Casebook) 1987 Supplement.

WRIGHT AND WRIGHT'S LAND USE IN A NUTSHELL, Second Edition, 356 pages, 1985. Softcover. (Text)

Legal History—see also Legal Method and Legal System

PRESSER AND ZAINALDIN'S CASES AND MATERIALS ON LAW AND JURISPRUDENCE IN AMERICAN HISTORY, Second Edition, 1092 pages, 1989. Teacher's Manual available. (Casebook)

Legal Method and Legal System—see also Legal Research, Legal Writing

ALDISERT'S READINGS, MATERIALS AND CASES IN THE JUDICIAL PROCESS, 948 pages, 1976. (Casebook)

BERCH AND BERCH'S INTRODUCTION TO LEGAL METHOD AND PROCESS, 550 pages, 1985. Teacher's Manual available. (Casebook)

BODENHEIMER, OAKLEY AND LOVE'S READINGS AND CASES ON AN INTRODUCTION TO THE ANGLO-AMERICAN LEGAL SYSTEM, Second Edition, 166 pages, 1988. Softcover. (Casebook)

DAVIES AND LAWRY'S INSTITUTIONS AND METHODS OF THE LAW—INTRODUCTORY TEACHING MATERIALS, 547 pages, 1982. Teacher's Manual available. (Casebook)

DVORKIN, HIMMELSTEIN AND LESNICK'S BECOMING A LAWYER: A HUMANISTIC PERSPECTIVE ON LEGAL EDUCATION AND PROFESSIONALISM, 211 pages, 1981. Softcover. (Text)

KEETON'S JUDGING, 842 pages, 1990. Softcover. (Coursebook)

KELSO AND KELSO'S STUDYING LAW: AN INTRODUCTION, 587 pages, 1984. (Coursebook)

KEMPIN'S HISTORICAL INTRODUCTION TO ANGLO-AMERICAN LAW IN A NUTSHELL, Third Edition, approximately 302 pages, 1990. Softcover. (Text)

REYNOLDS' JUDICIAL PROCESS IN A NUTSHELL, 292 pages, 1980. Softcover. (Text)

Legal Research

COHEN'S LEGAL RESEARCH IN A NUTSHELL, Fourth Edition, 452 pages, 1985. Softcover. (Text)

COHEN, BERRING AND OLSON'S HOW TO FIND THE LAW, Ninth Edition, 716 pages, 1989. (Text)

COHEN, BERRING AND OLSON'S FINDING THE LAW, 570 pages, 1989. Softcover reprint from Cohen, Berring and Olson's How to Find the Law, Ninth Edition. (Coursebook)

Legal Research Exercises, 3rd Ed., for use with Cohen, Berring and Olson, 229 pages, 1989. Teacher's Manual available.

ROMBAUER'S LEGAL PROBLEM SOLVING—

Legal Research—Cont'd

ANALYSIS, RESEARCH AND WRITING, Fourth Edition, 424 pages, 1983. Teacher's Manual with problems available. (Coursebook)

STATSKY'S LEGAL RESEARCH AND WRITING, Third Edition, 257 pages, 1986. Softcover. (Coursebook)

TEPLY'S LEGAL RESEARCH AND CITATION, Third Edition, 472 pages, 1989. Softcover. (Coursebook)

Student Library Exercises, 3rd ed., 391 pages, 1989. Answer Key available.

Legal Writing

CHILD'S DRAFTING LEGAL DOCUMENTS: MATERIALS AND PROBLEMS, 286 pages, 1988. Softcover. Teacher's Manual available. (Coursebook)

DICKERSON'S MATERIALS ON LEGAL DRAFTING, 425 pages, 1981. Teacher's Manual available. (Coursebook)

FELSENFELD AND SIEGEL'S WRITING CONTRACTS IN PLAIN ENGLISH, 290 pages, 1981. Softcover. (Text)

GOPEN'S WRITING FROM A LEGAL PERSPECTIVE, 225 pages, 1981. (Text)

MELLINKOFF'S LEGAL WRITING—SENSE AND NONSENSE, 242 pages, 1982. Softcover. Teacher's Manual available. (Text)

PRATT'S LEGAL WRITING: A SYSTEMATIC APPROACH, 422 pages, 1989. Teacher's Manual available. (Coursebook)

RAY AND RAMSFIELD'S LEGAL WRITING: GETTING IT RIGHT AND GETTING IT WRITTEN, 250 pages, 1987. Softcover. (Text)

SQUIRES AND ROMBAUER'S LEGAL WRITING IN A NUTSHELL, 294 pages, 1982. Softcover. (Text)

STATSKY AND WERNET'S CASE ANALYSIS AND FUNDAMENTALS OF LEGAL WRITING, Third Edition, 424 pages, 1989. Teacher's Manual available. (Text)

TEPLY'S LEGAL WRITING, ANALYSIS AND ORAL ARGUMENT, 576 pages, 1990. Softcover. Teacher's Manual available. (Coursebook)

WEIHOFEN'S LEGAL WRITING STYLE, Second Edition, 332 pages, 1980. (Text)

Legislation

DAVIES' LEGISLATIVE LAW AND PROCESS IN A NUTSHELL, Second Edition, 346 pages, 1986. Softcover. (Text)

ESKRIDGE AND FRICKEY'S CASES AND MATERIALS ON LEGISLATION: STATUTES AND THE CREATION OF PUBLIC POLICY, 937 pages, 1988. Teacher's Manual available. (Casebook) 1990 Supplement.

NUTTING AND DICKERSON'S CASES AND MATERIALS ON LEGISLATION, Fifth Edition, 744 pages, 1978. (Casebook)

STATSKY'S LEGISLATIVE ANALYSIS AND DRAFTING, Second Edition, 217 pages, 1984. Teacher's Manual available. (Text)

Local Government

FRUG'S CASES AND MATERIALS ON LOCAL GOVERNMENT LAW, 1005 pages, 1988. (Casebook)

McCARTHY'S LOCAL GOVERNMENT LAW IN A NUTSHELL, Third Edition, approximately 400 pages, 1990. Softcover. (Text)

REYNOLDS' HORNBOOK ON LOCAL GOVERNMENT LAW, 860 pages, 1982, with 1990 pocket part. (Text)

VALENTE'S CASES AND MATERIALS ON LOCAL GOVERNMENT LAW, Third Edition, 1010 pages, 1987. Teacher's Manual available. (Casebook) 1989 Supplement.

Mass Communication Law

GILLMOR, BARRON, SIMON AND TERRY'S CASES AND COMMENT ON MASS COMMUNICATION LAW, Fifth Edition, 947 pages, 1990. (Casebook)

GINSBURG'S REGULATION OF BROADCASTING: LAW AND POLICY TOWARDS RADIO, TELEVISION AND CABLE COMMUNICATIONS, 741 pages, 1979 (Casebook) 1983 Supplement.

ZUCKMAN, GAYNES, CARTER AND DEE'S MASS COMMUNICATIONS LAW IN A NUTSHELL, Third Edition, 538 pages, 1988. Softcover. (Text)

Medicine, Law and

FURROW, JOHNSON, JOST AND SCHWARTZ' HEALTH LAW: CASES, MATERIALS AND PROBLEMS, 1005 pages, 1987. Teacher's Manual available. (Casebook) 1989 Supplement.

HALL AND ELLMAN'S HEALTH CARE LAW AND

Professional Responsibility—Cont'd

GAL ETHICS, Second Edition, 341 pages, 1988. (Coursebook)

SELECTED STATUTES, RULES AND STANDARDS ON THE LEGAL PROFESSION. Softcover. Approximately 600 pages, 1990.

SMITH AND MALLEN'S PREVENTING LEGAL MALPRACTICE, 264 pages, 1989. Reprint from Mallen and Smith's Legal Malpractice, Third Edition. (Text)

SUTTON AND DZIENKOWSKI'S CASES AND MATERIALS ON THE PROFESSIONAL RESPONSIBILITY FOR LAWYERS, 839 pages, 1989. Teacher's Manual available. (Casebook)

WOLFRAM'S HORNBOOK ON MODERN LEGAL ETHICS, Student Edition, 1120 pages, 1986. (Text)

Property—see also Real Estate Transactions, Land Use, Trusts and Estates

BERNHARDT'S BLACK LETTER ON PROPERTY, 318 pages, 1983. Softcover. (Review)

BERNHARDT'S REAL PROPERTY IN A NUTSHELL, Second Edition, 448 pages, 1981. Softcover. (Text)

BOYER'S SURVEY OF THE LAW OF PROPERTY, Third Edition, 766 pages, 1981. (Text)

BROWDER, CUNNINGHAM, NELSON, STOEBUCK AND WHITMAN'S CASES ON BASIC PROPERTY LAW, Fifth Edition, 1386 pages, 1989. Teacher's Manual available. (Casebook)

BRUCE, ELY AND BOSTICK'S CASES AND MATERIALS ON MODERN PROPERTY LAW, Second Edition, 953 pages, 1989. Teacher's Manual available. (Casebook)

BURKE'S PERSONAL PROPERTY IN A NUTSHELL, 322 pages, 1983. Softcover. (Text)

CUNNINGHAM, STOEBUCK AND WHITMAN'S HORNBOOK ON THE LAW OF PROPERTY, Student Edition, 916 pages, 1984, with 1987 pocket part. (Text)

DONAHUE, KAUPER AND MARTIN'S CASES ON PROPERTY, Second Edition, 1362 pages, 1983. Teacher's Manual available. (Casebook)

HILL'S LANDLORD AND TENANT LAW IN A NUTSHELL, Second Edition, 311 pages, 1986. Softcover. (Text)

KURTZ AND HOVENKAMP'S CASES AND

MATERIALS ON AMERICAN PROPERTY LAW, 1296 pages, 1987. Teacher's Manual available. (Casebook) 1988 Supplement.

MOYNIHAN'S INTRODUCTION TO REAL PROPERTY, Second Edition, 239 pages, 1988. (Text)

Psychiatry, Law and

REISNER AND SLOBOGIN'S LAW AND THE MENTAL HEALTH SYSTEM, CIVIL AND CRIMINAL ASPECTS, Second Edition, approximately 1127 pages, 1990. (Casebook)

Real Estate Transactions

BRUCE'S REAL ESTATE FINANCE IN A NUTSHELL, Second Edition, 262 pages, 1985. Softcover. (Text)

MAXWELL, RIESENFELD, HETLAND AND WARREN'S CASES ON CALIFORNIA SECURITY TRANSACTIONS IN LAND, Third Edition, 728 pages, 1984. (Casebook)

NELSON AND WHITMAN'S BLACK LETTER ON LAND TRANSACTIONS AND FINANCE, Second Edition, 466 pages, 1988. Softcover. (Review)

NELSON AND WHITMAN'S CASES ON REAL ESTATE TRANSFER, FINANCE AND DEVELOPMENT, Third Edition, 1184 pages, 1987. (Casebook)

NELSON AND WHITMAN'S HORNBOOK ON REAL ESTATE FINANCE LAW, Second Edition, 941 pages, 1985 with 1989 pocket part. (Text)

Regulated Industries—see also Mass Communication Law, Banking Law

GELLHORN AND PIERCE'S REGULATED INDUSTRIES IN A NUTSHELL, Second Edition, 389 pages, 1987. Softcover. (Text)

MORGAN, HARRISON AND VERKUIL'S CASES AND MATERIALS ON ECONOMIC REGULATION OF BUSINESS, Second Edition, 666 pages, 1985. (Casebook)

Remedies

DOBBS' HORNBOOK ON REMEDIES, 1067 pages, 1973. (Text)

DOBBS' PROBLEMS IN REMEDIES. 137 pages, 1974. Teacher's Manual available. Softcover. (Coursebook)

DOBBYN'S INJUNCTIONS IN A NUTSHELL, 264 pages, 1974. Softcover. (Text)

Remedies—Cont'd

FRIEDMAN'S CONTRACT REMEDIES IN A NUT-SHELL, 323 pages, 1981. Softcover. (Text)

LEAVELL, LOVE AND NELSON'S CASES AND MATERIALS ON EQUITABLE REMEDIES, RESTITUTION AND DAMAGES, Fourth Edition, 1111 pages, 1986. Teacher's Manual available. (Casebook)

McCORMICK'S HORNBOOK ON DAMAGES, 811 pages, 1935. (Text)

O'CONNELL'S REMEDIES IN A NUTSHELL, Second Edition, 320 pages, 1985. Softcover. (Text)

SCHOENBROD, MACBETH, LEVINE AND JUNG'S CASES AND MATERIALS ON REMEDIES: PUBLIC AND PRIVATE, Approximately 807 pages, 1990. Teacher's Manual available. (Casebook)

YORK, BAUMAN AND RENDLEMAN'S CASES AND MATERIALS ON REMEDIES, Fourth Edition, 1029 pages, 1985. Teacher's Manual available. (Casebook)

Sea, Law of

SOHN AND GUSTAFSON'S THE LAW OF THE SEA IN A NUTSHELL, 264 pages, 1984. Softcover. (Text)

Securities Regulation

HAZEN'S HORNBOOK ON THE LAW OF SECURITIES REGULATION, Second Edition, Student Edition, approximately 1000 pages, 1990. (Text)

RATNER'S MATERIALS ON SECURITIES REGULATION, Third Edition, 1000 pages, 1986. Teacher's Manual available. (Casebook) 1989 Supplement.

Statutory Supplement. *See Selected Securities Regulation*

RATNER'S SECURITIES REGULATION IN A NUT-SHELL, Third Edition, 316 pages, 1988. Softcover. (Text)

SELECTED STATUTES, REGULATIONS, RULES, DOCUMENTS AND FORMS ON SECURITIES REGULATION. Softcover. 1272 pages, 1990.

Social Legislation

HOOD, HARDY AND LEWIS' WORKERS' COMPENSATION AND EMPLOYEE PROTECTION LAWS IN A NUTSHELL, Second Edition, 361 pages, 1990. Softcover. (Text)

LAFRANCE'S WELFARE LAW: STRUCTURE AND ENTITLEMENT IN A NUTSHELL, 455 pages, 1979. Softcover. (Text)

MALONE, PLANT AND LITTLE'S CASES ON WORKERS' COMPENSATION AND EMPLOYMENT RIGHTS, Second Edition, 951 pages, 1980. Teacher's Manual available. (Casebook)

Sports Law

SCHUBERT, SMITH AND TRENTADUE'S SPORTS LAW, 395 pages, 1986. (Text)

Tax Practice and Procedure

GARBIS, STRUNTZ AND RUBIN'S CASES AND MATERIALS ON TAX PROCEDURE AND TAX FRAUD, Second Edition, 687 pages, 1987. (Casebook)

MORGAN'S TAX PROCEDURE AND TAX FRAUD IN A NUTSHELL, Approximately 382 pages, 1990. Softcover. (Text)

Taxation—Corporate

KAHN AND GANN'S CORPORATE TAXATION, Third Edition, 980 pages, 1989. Teacher's Manual available. (Casebook)

WEIDENBRUCH AND BURKE'S FEDERAL INCOME TAXATION OF CORPORATIONS AND STOCKHOLDERS IN A NUTSHELL, Third Edition, 309 pages, 1989. Softcover. (Text)

Taxation—Estate & Gift—see also Estate Planning, Trusts and Estates

McNULTY'S FEDERAL ESTATE AND GIFT TAXATION IN A NUTSHELL, Fourth Edition, 496 pages, 1989. Softcover. (Text)

PENNELL'S CASES AND MATERIALS ON INCOME TAXATION OF TRUSTS, ESTATES, GRANTORS AND BENEFICIARIES, 460 pages, 1987. Teacher's Manual available. (Casebook)

Taxation—Individual

DODGE'S THE LOGIC OF TAX, 343 pages, 1989. Softcover. (Text)

GUNN AND WARD'S CASES, TEXT AND PROBLEMS ON FEDERAL INCOME TAXATION, Second Edition, 835 pages, 1988. Teacher's Manual available. (Casebook) 1990 Supplement.

HUDSON AND LIND'S BLACK LETTER ON FEDERAL INCOME TAXATION, Third Edition, approximately 390 pages, 1990. Softcover. (Review)

Taxation—Individual—Cont'd

KRAGEN AND MCNULTY'S CASES AND MATERIALS ON FEDERAL INCOME TAXATION—INDIVIDUALS, CORPORATIONS, PARTNERSHIPS, Fourth Edition, 1287 pages, 1985. (Casebook)

MCNULTY'S FEDERAL INCOME TAXATION OF INDIVIDUALS IN A NUTSHELL, Fourth Edition, 503 pages, 1988. Softcover. (Text)

POSIN'S HORNBOOK ON FEDERAL INCOME TAXATION, Student Edition, 491 pages, 1983, with 1989 pocket part. (Text)

ROSE AND CHOMMIE'S HORNBOOK ON FEDERAL INCOME TAXATION, Third Edition, 923 pages, 1988, with 1989 pocket part. (Text)

SELECTED FEDERAL TAXATION STATUTES AND REGULATIONS. Softcover. Approximately 1650 pages, 1991.

SOLOMON AND HESCH'S PROBLEMS, CASES AND MATERIALS ON FEDERAL INCOME TAXATION OF INDIVIDUALS, 1068 pages, 1987. Teacher's Manual available. (Casebook)

Taxation—International

DOERNBERG'S INTERNATIONAL TAXATION IN A NUTSHELL, 325 pages, 1989. Softcover. (Text)

KAPLAN'S FEDERAL TAXATION OF INTERNATIONAL TRANSACTIONS: PRINCIPLES, PLANNING AND POLICY, 635 pages, 1988. (Casebook)

Taxation—Partnership

BERGER AND WIEDENBECK'S CASES AND MATERIALS ON PARTNERSHIP TAXATION, 788 pages, 1989. Teacher's Manual available. (Casebook)

Taxation—State & Local

GELFAND AND SALSICH'S STATE AND LOCAL TAXATION AND FINANCE IN A NUTSHELL, 309 pages, 1986. Softcover. (Text)

HELLERSTEIN AND HELLERSTEIN'S CASES AND MATERIALS ON STATE AND LOCAL TAXATION, Fifth Edition, 1071 pages, 1988. (Casebook)

Torts—see also Products Liability

CHRISTIE AND MEEKS' CASES AND MATERIALS ON THE LAW OF TORTS, Second Edition, 1264 pages, 1990. (Casebook)

DOBBS' TORTS AND COMPENSATION—PERSONAL ACCOUNTABILITY AND SOCIAL RESPONSIBILITY FOR INJURY, 955 pages, 1985. Teacher's Manual available. (Casebook) 1990 Supplement.

KEETON, KEETON, SARGENTICH AND STEINER'S CASES AND MATERIALS ON TORT AND ACCIDENT LAW, Second Edition, 1318 pages, 1989. (Casebook)

KIONKA'S BLACK LETTER ON TORTS, 339 pages, 1988. Softcover. (Review)

KIONKA'S TORTS IN A NUTSHELL: INJURIES TO PERSONS AND PROPERTY, 434 pages, 1977. Softcover. (Text)

MALONE'S TORTS IN A NUTSHELL: INJURIES TO FAMILY, SOCIAL AND TRADE RELATIONS, 358 pages, 1979. Softcover. (Text)

PROSSER AND KEETON'S HORNBOOK ON TORTS, Fifth Edition, Student Edition, 1286 pages, 1984 with 1988 pocket part. (Text)

ROBERTSON, POWERS AND ANDERSON'S CASES AND MATERIALS ON TORTS, 932 pages, 1989. Teacher's Manual available. (Casebook)

Trade Regulation—see also Antitrust, Regulated Industries

MCMANIS' UNFAIR TRADE PRACTICES IN A NUTSHELL, Second Edition, 464 pages, 1988. Softcover. (Text)

OPPENHEIM, WESTON, MAGGS AND SCHECHTER'S CASES AND MATERIALS ON UNFAIR TRADE PRACTICES AND CONSUMER PROTECTION, Fourth Edition, 1038 pages, 1983. Teacher's Manual available. (Casebook) 1986 Supplement.

SCHECHTER'S BLACK LETTER ON UNFAIR TRADE PRACTICES, 272 pages, 1986. Softcover. (Review)

Trial and Appellate Advocacy—see also Civil Procedure

APPELLATE ADVOCACY, HANDBOOK OF, Second Edition, 182 pages, 1986. Softcover. (Text)

BERGMAN'S TRIAL ADVOCACY IN A NUTSHELL, Second Edition, 354 pages, 1989. Softcover. (Text)

BINDER AND BERGMAN'S FACT INVESTIGATION: FROM HYPOTHESIS TO PROOF, 354 pages, 1984. Teacher's Manual available. (Coursebook)

Trial and Appellate Advocacy—Cont'd

CARLSON AND IMWINKELRIED'S DYNAMICS OF TRIAL PRACTICE: PROBLEMS AND MATERIALS, 414 pages, 1989. Teacher's Manual available. (Coursebook)

GOLDBERG'S THE FIRST TRIAL (WHERE DO I SIT? WHAT DO I SAY?) IN A NUTSHELL, 396 pages, 1982. Softcover. (Text)

HAYDOCK, HERR, AND STEMPEL'S FUNDAMENTALS OF PRE-TRIAL LITIGATION, 768 pages, 1985. Softcover. Teacher's Manual available. (Coursebook)

HEGLAND'S TRIAL AND PRACTICE SKILLS IN A NUTSHELL, 346 pages, 1978. Softcover. (Text)

HORNSTEIN'S APPELLATE ADVOCACY IN A NUTSHELL, 325 pages, 1984. Softcover. (Text)

JEANS' HANDBOOK ON TRIAL ADVOCACY, Student Edition, 473 pages, 1975. Softcover. (Text)

LISNEK AND KAUFMAN'S DEPOSITIONS: PROCEDURE, STRATEGY AND TECHNIQUE, Law School and CLE Edition. 250 pages, 1990. Softcover. (Text)

MARTINEAU'S CASES AND MATERIALS ON APPELLATE PRACTICE AND PROCEDURE, 565 pages, 1987. (Casebook)

NOLAN'S CASES AND MATERIALS ON TRIAL PRACTICE, 518 pages, 1981. (Casebook)

SONSTENG AND HAYDOCK'S TRIAL: THEORIES, TACTICS, TECHNIQUE, Approximately 650 pages, 1990. Softcover. (Text)

SONSTENG, HAYDOCK AND BOYD'S THE TRIALBOOK: A TOTAL SYSTEM FOR PREPARATION AND PRESENTATION OF A CASE, 404 pages, 1984. Softcover. (Coursebook)

WHARTON, HAYDOCK AND SONSTENG'S CALIFORNIA CIVIL TRIALBOOK, Law School and CLE Edition. Approximately 300 pages, 1990. Softcover. (Text)

Trusts and Estates

ATKINSON'S HORNBOOK ON WILLS, Second Edition, 975 pages, 1953. (Text)

AVERILL'S UNIFORM PROBATE CODE IN A NUTSHELL, Second Edition, 454 pages, 1987. Softcover. (Text)

BOGERT'S HORNBOOK ON TRUSTS, Sixth Edition, Student Edition, 794 pages, 1987. (Text)

CLARK, LUSKY AND MURPHY'S CASES AND MATERIALS ON GRATUITOUS TRANSFERS, Third Edition, 970 pages, 1985. (Casebook)

DODGE'S WILLS, TRUSTS AND ESTATE PLANNING–LAW AND TAXATION, CASES AND MATERIALS, 665 pages, 1988. (Casebook)

KURTZ' PROBLEMS, CASES AND OTHER MATERIALS ON FAMILY ESTATE PLANNING, 853 pages, 1983. Teacher's Manual available. (Casebook)

MCGOVERN'S CASES AND MATERIALS ON WILLS, TRUSTS AND FUTURE INTERESTS: AN INTRODUCTION TO ESTATE PLANNING, 750 pages, 1983. (Casebook)

MCGOVERN, KURTZ AND REIN'S HORNBOOK ON WILLS, TRUSTS AND ESTATES–INCLUDING TAXATION AND FUTURE INTERESTS, 996 pages, 1988. (Text)

MENNELL'S WILLS AND TRUSTS IN A NUTSHELL, 392 pages, 1979. Softcover. (Text)

SIMES' HORNBOOK ON FUTURE INTERESTS, Second Edition, 355 pages, 1966. (Text)

TURANO AND RADIGAN'S HORNBOOK ON NEW YORK ESTATE ADMINISTRATION, 676 pages, 1986. (Text)

UNIFORM PROBATE CODE, OFFICIAL TEXT WITH COMMENTS. 615 pages, 1989. Softcover.

WAGGONER'S FUTURE INTERESTS IN A NUTSHELL, 361 pages, 1981. Softcover. (Text)

WATERBURY'S MATERIALS ON TRUSTS AND ESTATES, 1039 pages, 1986. Teacher's Manual available. (Casebook)

Water Law—see also Energy and Natural Resources Law, Environmental Law

GETCHES' WATER LAW IN A NUTSHELL, Second Edition, approximately 441 pages, 1990. Softcover. (Text)

SAX AND ABRAMS' LEGAL CONTROL OF WATER RESOURCES: CASES AND MATERIALS, 941 pages, 1986. (Casebook)

TRELEASE AND GOULD'S CASES AND MATERIALS ON WATER LAW, Fourth Edition, 816 pages, 1986. (Casebook)

Wills—see Trusts and Estates

Women and the Law—see also Employment Discrimination

KAY'S TEXT, CASES AND MATERIALS ON SEX-BASED DISCRIMINATION, Third Edition, 1001 pages, 1988. (Casebook) 1990 Supplement.

THOMAS' SEX DISCRIMINATION IN A NUT-SHELL, 399 pages, 1982. Softcover. (Text)

Workers' Compensation—see Social Legislation

Medicine, Law and—Cont'd

ETHICS IN A NUTSHELL, 401 pages, 1990. Softcover (Text)

KING'S THE LAW OF MEDICAL MALPRACTICE IN A NUTSHELL, Second Edition, 342 pages, 1986. Softcover. (Text)

SHAPIRO AND SPECE'S CASES, MATERIALS AND PROBLEMS ON BIOETHICS AND LAW, 892 pages, 1981. (Casebook)

SHARPE, BOUMIL, FISCINA AND HEAD'S CASES AND MATERIALS ON MEDICAL LIABILITY, Approximately 500 pages, September, 1990 Pub. (Casebook)

Military Law

SHANOR AND TERRELL'S MILITARY LAW IN A NUTSHELL, 378 pages, 1980. Softcover. (Text)

Mortgages—see Real Estate Transactions

Natural Resources Law—see Energy and Natural Resources Law, Environmental Law

Negotiation

GIFFORD'S LEGAL NEGOTIATION: THEORY AND APPLICATIONS, 225 pages, 1989. Softcover. (Text)

WILLIAMS' LEGAL NEGOTIATION AND SETTLEMENT, 207 pages, 1983. Softcover. Teacher's Manual available. (Coursebook)

Office Practice—see also Computers and Law, Interviewing and Counseling, Negotiation

HEGLAND'S TRIAL AND PRACTICE SKILLS IN A NUTSHELL, 346 pages, 1978. Softcover (Text)

STRONG AND CLARK'S LAW OFFICE MANAGEMENT, 424 pages, 1974. (Casebook)

Oil and Gas—see also Energy and Natural Resources Law

HEMINGWAY'S HORNBOOK ON OIL AND GAS, Second Edition, Student Edition, 543 pages, 1983, with 1989 pocket part. (Text)

KUNTZ, LOWE, ANDERSON AND SMITH'S CASES AND MATERIALS ON OIL AND GAS LAW, 857 pages, 1986. Teacher's Manual available. (Casebook) Forms Manual. Revised.

LOWE'S OIL AND GAS LAW IN A NUTSHELL,

Second Edition, 465 pages, 1988. Softcover. (Text)

Partnership—see Agency—Partnership

Patent and Copyright Law

CHOATE, FRANCIS AND COLLINS' CASES AND MATERIALS ON PATENT LAW, INCLUDING TRADE SECRETS, COPYRIGHTS, TRADEMARKS, Third Edition, 1009 pages, 1987. (Casebook)

MILLER AND DAVIS' INTELLECTUAL PROPERTY—PATENTS, TRADEMARKS AND COPYRIGHT IN A NUTSHELL, Second Edition, approximately 440 pages, 1990. Softcover. (Text)

NIMMER'S CASES AND MATERIALS ON COPYRIGHT AND OTHER ASPECTS OF ENTERTAINMENT LITIGATION ILLUSTRATED—INCLUDING UNFAIR COMPETITION, DEFAMATION AND PRIVACY, Third Edition, 1025 pages, 1985. (Casebook) 1989 Supplement.

Products Liability

FISCHER AND POWERS' CASES AND MATERIALS ON PRODUCTS LIABILITY, 685 pages, 1988. Teacher's Manual available. (Casebook)

NOEL AND PHILLIPS' CASES ON PRODUCTS LIABILITY, Second Edition, 821 pages, 1982. (Casebook)

PHILLIPS' PRODUCTS LIABILITY IN A NUTSHELL, Third Edition, 307 pages, 1988. Softcover. (Text)

Professional Responsibility

ARONSON, DEVINE AND FISCH'S PROBLEMS, CASES AND MATERIALS IN PROFESSIONAL RESPONSIBILITY, 745 pages, 1985. Teacher's Manual available. (Casebook)

ARONSON AND WECKSTEIN'S PROFESSIONAL RESPONSIBILITY IN A NUTSHELL, 399 pages, 1980. Softcover. (Text)

MELLINKOFF'S THE CONSCIENCE OF A LAWYER, 304 pages, 1973. (Text)

PIRSIG AND KIRWIN'S CASES AND MATERIALS ON PROFESSIONAL RESPONSIBILITY, Fourth Edition, 603 pages, 1984. Teacher's Manual available. (Casebook)

ROTUNDA'S BLACK LETTER ON PROFESSIONAL RESPONSIBILITY, Second Edition, 414 pages, 1988. Softcover. (Review)

SCHWARTZ AND WYDICK'S PROBLEMS IN LE-

Preface

In choosing the subjects covered in this book and organizing their presentation, we have tried to achieve a number of objectives. First, we want to give the student a clear picture of past, present and possible future legal doctrine, as well as some feel for the most significant clinical and empirical literature, relating to two major topics: the regulation of the mental health professions and the relationship between society and the mentally disabled. Second, we try to provide insights into how and to what degree the legal system can be used to implement desired social objectives connected with these topics. Third, this book should sensitize lawyers and mental health professionals to each other's perspective on the issues involved.

To further these ends, this book is divided into three parts. Part I, "The Mental Health Professions and the Law" deals with the various ways in which the legal system shapes and monitors the activities of mental health professionals. After describing the structure of the mental health professions, Chapter One explores administrative licensing. The remaining chapters in Part One look at legislative and judicial regulatory approaches in the areas of negligence law (Chapter Two), informed consent (Chapter Three) and confidentiality (Chapter Four).

Part II, "Deprivations of Liberty and Property," switches the focus to the mentally disabled and state intervention in their lives. By way of introduction to this subject, Chapter Five looks at the concept of mental disability and Chapter Six examines the ability of the mental health professions to identify disability and its consequences. The next three chapters provide materials on laws affecting mentally disabled individuals who are charged with or convicted of crime (Chapter Six), thought to be in need of hospitalization (Chapter Eight) and thought to be incompetent to make decisions (Chapter Nine). Chapter Ten ends Part II with an exploration of issues which arise in treating mentally disabled persons who have been the subject of state intervention.

Part III "Benefits Eligibility and Other Protective Legislation," examines a number of laws, most of them statutory in origin, meant to benefit all mentally disabled persons, whether or not the state has acted to deprive them of liberty or property. Chapter Eleven looks at federal benefit programs for the mentally disabled connected with education and social security. Chapter Twelve discusses laws which deal with discrimination against the mentally disabled.

It would probably be impossible to teach this entire book in one semester. We think the materials could be presented in several different packages. A teacher wishing to focus on the mentally disabled would teach Part II, or Parts II and III.* A teacher more interested in legal regulation of the mental health professions would teach Part I and the first two chapters of Part II. A traditional "civil" mental health law course might focus on Part I and Chapters Five, Eight, Nine (sections I through III), and Ten. A more modern version would include Part III, or at least Chapter Eleven. A course on "criminal" mental health law could cover Chapters Five through Seven, Eight (sections V–A, V–B and V–C), Nine (section IV), and Ten. Undoubtedly, there are other combinations.

The subject matter of this book has undergone rapid and substantial change during the past two decades. We anticipate that trend to continue; in particular, Part III of this book, which is new with this edition, is likely to expand significantly through supplementation in the near future. As both law and the behavioral sciences have become more sophisticated, the interaction of the two fields has become greater and more complex. This book will hopefully facilitate and sharpen that interaction.

Some comments concerning the citation form and editing of the cases may be in order. Citation form conforms closely to the Uniform System of Citation, but some modifications were made for ease of printing. Most cases have been edited substantially. The deletion of *textual* portions is indicated by three asterisks or three dots. The deletion of *citations* or *footnotes* is not indicated by any signal. When case footnotes have been included they are numbered as in the original text; our footnotes are lettered.

Professor Reisner acknowledges the encouragement, counsel and assistance of numerous individuals who furthered this endeavor. In particular he is indebted to Ms. Sherry Cibelli whose extraordinary skill, patience, and ability to decipher his scrawl made the book possible. Special thanks is also due to Ms. Mimi Jordan for her invaluable research and editing assistance throughout the preparation of the book. Thanks are also due to Ms. Elizabeth Caddick for the research assistance she rendered in the past semester. It has also been his good fortune over twenty-five years to have as a colleague, Wayne R. LaFave. His advice and encouragement on this and other writing projects has been signally valuable. Acknowledgements are also due to Professors Kit Kinports and Debbie Merritt for their helpful suggestions.

For their comments on the part of the book for which he was primarily responsible (Part II), Professor Slobogin is indebted to a

---

* One of the authors has comfortably taught Part II in a two-hour seminar format over a 14-week semester. A three-hour course could probably cover both Parts II and III.

number of individuals: Professor David Wexler of Arizona Law School, Professor Nancy Ehrenreich of Denver Law School, Professor Garv Melton of the University of Nebraska Law School, Professor Michael Perlin of New York Law School, Professor Elyn Saks of the University of Southern California Law School, and Professors Richard Bonnie, John Monahan, and Elizabeth Scott of the University of Virginia Law School. Professor Slobogin would also like to acknowledge the assistance of the law library staffs at the University of Virginia and the University of Florida, and of Diane Cronk and Laura Hayes of the secretarial staffs at the University of Virginia and the University of Florida, respectively.

RALPH REISNER
CHRISTOPHER SLOBOGIN

April 15, 1990

*

Acknowledgments

The authors wish to acknowledge, with gratitude, permission to reprint the following copyrighted materials.

Social Workers Vault Into Leading Role in Psychotherapy, by Daniel Goleman, from THE NEW YORK TIMES, April 30, 1985, p. 17. Copyright © 1985 by The New York Times Company. Reprinted by permission.

From THE PSYCHIATRISTS, by Arnold A. Rogow. Copyright © 1970 by Arnold A. Rogow. Reprinted by permission of G.P. Putnam's Sons.

From SOCIAL CLASS AND MENTAL ILLNESS: A COMMUNITY STUDY, by August B. Hollingshead and Fredrick C. Redlich. Copyright © 1958 by John Wiley & Sons, Inc.

From THE PROFESSION OF PSYCHOLOGY, by Wilse B. Webb. Copyright © 1962 by Holt, Rinehart and Winston, Inc. Reprinted by permission of Holt, Rinehart and Winston, CBS College Publishing.

From READINGS IN LAW AND PSYCHIATRY, by Richard C. Allen, Elyce Z. Ferster and Jesse G. Rubin. Copyright © 1975 by The Johns Hopkins Press. Reprinted by permission.

From THE MENTALLY DISABLED AND THE LAW, 3rd Ed., by Samuel J. Brakel, John Parry and Barbara A. Weiner. Copyright © 1985 by The American Bar Foundation. Reprinted by permission.

From THE PSYCHIATRIC THERAPIES, T.B. Karasu, Ed. Copyright © 1984 by the American Psychiatric Association. Reprinted by permission.

Sex Therapy: As Popularity Grows, Critics Question Whether it Works, by Dava Sobel, from THE NEW YORK TIMES, November 14, 1980, p. 17. Copyright © 1980 by The New York Times Company. Reprinted by permission.

From THE POWERS OF PSYCHIATRY, by Jonas Robitscher. Copyright © 1980 by Jonas Robitscher. Published by Houghton Mifflin Company. Reprinted by permission of Jean Robitscher.

Psychotherapy Has Measurable Effect on Depression in Closely Watched Test, by Jerry E. Bishop, from THE WALL STREET JOURNAL, November 13, 1989, p. B4. Copyright © 1989 by the Wall Street Journal. Reprinted by permission.

Occupational Licensing: A Framework For Analysis, by Jonathan Rose, 1979 ARIZONA STATE LAW JOURNAL 189 (1979). Copyright © 1979 by Arizona State University College of Law. Reprinted by permission of the Arizona State Law Journal and the author.

Slobogin, from 66 VIRGINIA LAW REVIEW, 427 (1980). Reprinted with permission from the Virginia Law Review Association.

Demographic Evidence in Capital Sentencing, by Daniel Goodman, from 39 STANFORD LAW REVIEW 499 (1987). Copyright © 1987 by the Board of Trustees of the Leland Stanford Junior University. Reprinted with permission from the Stanford Law Review.

From COMPETENCY TO STAND TRIAL, by Ronald Roesch and Stephen Golding (1980). Reprinted with permission from Ronald Roesch.

From PSYCHOLOGICAL EVALUATIONS FOR THE COURTS: A HANDBOOK FOR MENTAL HEALTH PROFESSIONALS AND LAWYERS, by Gary Melton, John Petrila, Norman Poythress, Christopher Slobogin (1987). Reprinted with permission granted by Guilford Press.

Insanity Defense in Criminal Trials and Limitations of Psychiatric Testimony: Report of the Board of Trustees, June 8, 1984, p. 2967–2981. Copyright © 1984, American Medical Association. Reprinted with permission.

Psychiatry and the Dangerous Criminal, by Norval Morris, from 41 SOUTHERN CALIFORNIA LAW REVIEW 514 (1968). Reprinted with the permission of the Southern California Law Review.

Book review of Abraham Goldstein's THE INSANITY DEFENSE, by Lady Wooton (1968). Reprinted by permission of the Yale Law Journal Company and Fred B. Rothman & Company, Vol. 77, pp. 1019–1051.*

From THE INSANITY DEFENSE, by David Hermann (1983). Courtesy of Charles C. Thomas, Publisher, Springfield, Illinois.

Acute Psychiatric Hospitalization of the Mentally Ill in the Metropolis: An Empirical Study, by George Dix, from 1968 WASHINGTON UNIVERSITY LAW QUARTERLY 485 (1968). Reprinted with permission from the Washington University Law Quarterly.

Developments in the Law—Civil Commitment of the Mentally Ill, from 87 HARVARD LAW REVIEW 1190 (1974). Reprinted with permission from the Harvard Law Review.

A Preference for Liberty: The Case Against Involuntary Commitment of The Mentally Disordered, by Stephen Morse, from 70 CALIFORNIA LAW REVIEW 54 (1982). Copyright © 1982 by California Law Review, Inc. Reprinted by permission of California Law Review, Inc. and the author.

Assessing and Predicting Violence: Research, Law, and Applications, by T. Litwack and L. Schlesinger, in HANDBOOK OF FORENSIC PSYCHOLOGY 205 (Weiner, Hess, eds. 1987). Copyright © 1987 by John Wiley & Sons, Inc.

Dangerousness Defined, from LAW, PSYCHIATRY & MENTAL HEALTH SYSTEMS, by Alexander Brooks. Copyright © 1974 by Little, Brown. Reprinted with permission of Little, Brown and author.

Dangerousness as a Criterion for Confinement, by Alan Dershowitz, from 11 BULLETIN OF AMERICAN ACADEMY OF PSYCHIATRY AND LAW 172 (1974). Copyright © 1974 by American Academy of Psychiatry and Law. Reprinted by permission.

From OFFENSE TO OTHERS, by Joel Feinberg (1985). Reprinted by permission of Oxford University Press.

Involuntary Psychiatric Commitments to Prevent Suicide, by David Greenberg. 49 N.Y.U.L.Rev. 227, 257–58 (1974). Reprinted with permission granted from the New York University Law Review.

From MENTAL HEALTH LAW, by David Wexler. Copyright © 1981. Reprinted with permission granted by Plenum Publishing Corporation and the author.

Least Restrictive Treatment of the Mentally Ill: A Doctrine in Search of Its Senses, by Browning Hoffman and Larry Foust, from 14 SAN DIEGO LAW REVIEW 1100 (1977). Reprinted with permission from the San Diego Law Review.

The Therapeutic Significance of the Civil Commitment Hearing: An Unexplored Potential, by John Ensminger and Thomas Liguori, from 6 JOURNAL OF PSYCHIATRY AND LAW 5 (1978). Reprint permission granted by the Federal Legal Publications.

Guidelines for Involuntary Civil Commitment, by the National Center for State Courts, from 10 MENTAL DISABILITY LAW RE-PORTER 409 (1986). Reprint permission granted by Ingo Keilitz, Director, Institute of Mental Disability and Law, National Center for State Courts.

Institutionalization, Deinstitutionalization, and the Adversary Process, by Judge David Bazelon, from 75 COLUMBIA LAW REVIEW 897 (1975). Copyright © 1975 by the Directors of the Columbia Law Review Association, Inc. All rights reserved. Reprinted by permission.

A Model State Law on Civil Commitment of the Mentally Ill, by Clifford Stromberg and Alan Stone, from 20 HARVARD JOURNAL OF LEGISLATION 274 (1983). Copyright © 1983 by the President and Fellows of Harvard College. Reprinted by permission of the Harvard Journal of Legislation.

The Waivability of Recommitment Hearings, by David Wexler, from 20 ARIZONA LAW REVIEW 175 (1978). Copyright © 1978 by the Arizona Board of Regents. Reprinted by permission of the Arizona Law Review and the author.

Voluntary Hospitalization of the Mentally Ill, by Janet Gilboy and John Schmidt, from 66 NORTHWESTERN LAW REVIEW 429 (1971). Reprinted with permission.

The Consequences of the Insanity Defense: Proposals to Reform Post-Acquittal Commitment Law, by James Ellis, from 35 CATHOLIC UNIVERSITY LAW REVIEW 961 (1986). Reprinted by permission of Catholic University Law Review.

Distributive and Paternalist Motives in Contract and Tort Law, With Special Reference to Compulsory Terms and Unequal Bargaining Power, by Duncan Kennedy, from 41 MARYLAND LAW REVIEW 563 (1982). Reprinted with permission from the Maryland Law Review.

Competency to Consent to Research: A Psychiatric Overview, by Paul Appelbaum and Loren Roth, from 39 ARCHIVES OF GENERAL PSYCHIATRY 951 (1982). Copyright © 1982 by American Medical Association. Reprinted by permission.

Sterilization of Mentally Retarded Persons: Reproductive Rights and Family Privacy, by Elizabeth Scott, from 1986 DUKE LAW JOURNAL 806 (1986). Reprinted with permission from the Duke Law Journal.

The Right to Refuse Antipsychotic Medications: Law and Policy, by Alexander Brooks, from 39 RUTGERS LAW REVIEW 339 (1987). Reprinted with permission of the author.

Regulation of Electroconvulsive Therapy, by Carol Sanger, from 75 MICHIGAN LAW REVIEW 363 (1976). Reprinted with permission of Michigan Law Review and the author.

Limiting the Therapeutic Orgy: Mental Patients' Right To Refuse Treatment, by Robert Plotkin, from 72 NORTHWESTERN LAW REVIEW 479 (1977). Reprinted by special permission of Northwestern University, School of Law.

Psychosurgery: National Commission Issues Surprisingly Favorable Report, by R. Culliton, from 194 SCIENCE 299 (1976). Copyright © by American Association for the Advancement of Science. Reprinted by permission.

Legal Regulation of Applied Behavior Analysis in Mental Institutions and Prisons, by Paul Friedman, from 17 ARIZONA LAW REVIEW 61 (1975). Copyright © 1975 by Arizona Board of Regents. Reprinted by permission.

The Role of the Criminal Defense Lawyer in Representing the Mentally Impaired Defendant: Zealous Advocate or Office of the Court?, by Rodney Uphoff, from 1988 WISCONSIN LAW REVIEW 65. Copyright © by Wisconsin Law Review. Reprinted by permission.

Incompetency to Stand Trial: As Assessment of Costs and Benefits, and a Proposal for Reform, by Bruce Winick, from 39 RUTGERS LAW REVIEW 243 (1987). Reprinted with permission of Rutgers Law Review and the author.

Voluntariness, Free Will and the Law of Confessions, by Joseph Grano, from 65 VIRGINIA LAW REVIEW 859 (1979). Reprinted with permission from the Virginia Law Review Association and Fred B. Rothman & Co.

The Long Lonesome Road, by Joseph Nocera, from THE TEXAS MONTHLY, November, 1986. Copyright © 1987 by Texas Monthly. Reprinted with permission.

Note: The Supreme Court: 1981 Term, from 96 HARVARD LAW REVIEW 62 (1982). Copyright © 1982 by the Harvard Law Review Association. Reprinted with permission.

Mental Hospitals and the Civil Liberties Dilemma, by H. Davidson, from 31 MENTAL HYGIENE 371 (1967). Reprinted with permission of the National Mental Health Association, Alexandria, Va.

Note: The *Wyatt* Case: Implementation of a Judicial Decree Ordering Institutional Change, from 84 YALE LAW JOURNAL 1338 (1975). Reprinted by permission of The Yale Law Journal Company and Fred B. Rothman & Company.

Beyond Least Restrictive Alternative Doctrine: A Constitutional Right to Treatment for Mentally Disabled Persons in the Community, by Jan Costello and James Preis, from 20 LOYOLA LOS ANGELES LAW REVIEW 1527 (1987). Reprinted with permission of the Loyola L.A. Law Review.

Abroad at home; Enough was Enough, by Anthony Lewis, from THE NEW YORK TIMES, September 20, 1984, p. 25. Copyright © 1984 by The New York Times Company. Reprinted by permission.

Mentally Disabled May Gain Thousands in Back Benefits, by Jesus Rangel, from THE NEW YORK TIMES, January 15, 1988, p. 1. Copyright © 1988 by The New York Times Company. Reprinted by permission.

Suburb Sued For Unfair Zoning, by Jacqueline Lee, from the AMERICAN BAR ASSOCIATION JOURNAL, September 1989l, p. 40. Copyright © by the American Bar Association. Reprinted by permission.

Summary of Contents

Table of Contents

PART II. DEPRIVATIONS OF LIBERTY AND PROPERTY

*

Table of Cases

The principal cases are in bold type. Cases cited or discussed in the text are roman type. References are to pages. Cases cited in principal cases and within other quoted materials are not included.

LAW AND THE MENTAL HEALTH SYSTEM

CIVIL AND CRIMINAL ASPECTS

Second Edition

*

Part I

THE MENTAL HEALTH PROFESSIONS AND THE LAW

Chapter One

REGULATION OF THE MENTAL HEALTH PROFESSIONS

I. PERSPECTIVES ON THE MENTAL HEALTH PROFESSIONS

A. DEVELOPMENT, EDUCATION, TRAINING AND FUNCTIONS

The purveyors of mental health treatment can be classified into three major groups—psychiatrists (including psychoanalysts), psychologists, and psychiatric social workers. Recent years have witnessed a dramatic shift in the role played by each of these professions as

2

providers of mental health treatment. Psychotherapy increasingly has become the domain of non-medically trained professionals such as psychologists and social workers. According to one report:

> "Psychiatry, which once accounted for the largest single group of psychotherapists, has seen a sharp decrease in those joining its ranks in recent years. In the last 10 years it grew only by a third while other groups were doubling or growing even faster. While in 1975 there were 26,000 psychiatrists, there are now 38,000, according to estimates by the American Psychiatric Association.

> "Clinical psychologists have doubled their ranks over the same period. While there were an estimated 15,000 clinical psychologists in 1975, today they number approximately 33,000, the association says.

> "The growth in numbers of social workers who offer psychotherapy is even greater. A decade ago, according to the National Association of Social Workers, 25,000 were engaged in therapy; this year there are 60,000. While many of them work in mental health clinics, a growing number are in private practice. The proportion of clinical social workers receiving $20,000 a year or more from private practice, according to one survey, is 82 percent. Fifteen percent earn $60,000 or more from private practice."

See, *Social Workers Vault Into a Leading Role in Psychotherapy*, New York Times, April 30, 1985, p. 17, col. 5.

The reasons for these changes in the respective roles of the various professions are complex. In part, they are economically driven, representing a shift of consumers from the more highly priced service provided by medically trained psychiatrists to lower priced service providers. At the same time, as detailed in section III "Emerging Issues in the Allocation of Function Among the Mental Health Professions," infra, these changes also have been effected by court decisions and legislation which have reduced the medical profession's control over the provision of mental health services. Before turning to issues facing legislatures and courts, it is relevant to examine the development, characteristics and functions of each of the professions.

1. Psychiatrists

a. Development of the Profession

The origins of psychiatry lie in the practice of medicine within asylums for the insane where, during the 19th century, physicians attributed the deviant behavior of inmates to diseases of the mind. However, as the following excerpt indicates, psychiatric practice as we know it today is a more recent phenomenon:

> Psychiatry, unlike psychoanalysis, did not begin in the twentieth century, but its influence and eminence are of relatively recent origin. If we view 1844, the founding year of what later became the American Psychiatric Association, as the official birthdate of American psychiatry, it is possible to suggest that psychiatry did not come of age until World War II, when, quite apart from its usefulness in the war,

psychiatry became an accepted part of the American scene and even achieved a certain fashionableness. Since this development owes so much to the impact upon psychiatry of Freudian psychoanalysis—one is tempted to credit Freud with both the birth of psychoanalysis and the rebirth of psychiatry—it is conceivable that psychiatry without psychoanalysis would have taken quite a different direction, perhaps back toward the mental hospital from which it emerged more than a century ago, or toward an easier synthesis with other behavioral sciences. For it is clear that the broad acceptance of psychiatry relates not only to a rising incidence of mental distress but to the prestige of psychoanalysis, the principles of which transformed the nature of psychiatric training, practice, and research. Whatever the future holds, the growth patterns of psychiatry and psychoanalysis have been remarkably similar, and they face somewhat similar problems with respect to orientation and direction.

Arnold A. Rogow, *The Psychiatrists* (New York: G.P. Putnam's Sons, 1970), pp. 31–32.

b. Education, Training & Function

It is important to note at the outset that the definition of who is a psychiatrist or, more important, who is qualified to practice psychiatry is determined at least on a formal level by state law. Under the law of most states *any licensed physician* can practice and render psychiatric services. As a practical matter, however, norms imposed by the medical profession itself serve to ensure that the practice of psychiatry is restricted to those physicians who have completed a psychiatric residency program which is a requirement for membership in the American Psychiatric Association. These informal methods of control are normally exercised at the local level. Thus, only physicians who have completed the residency program and are members of the American Psychiatric Association will receive referrals from other physicians in the community. Similarly, only physicians who are members of the American Psychiatric Association will be accorded hospital privileges which enable them to function as psychiatrists in a hospital setting.

Since only licensed physicians are qualified to become psychiatrists, the training of a psychiatrist necessarily begins with medical school. The psychiatric residency which follows the completion of medical school is normally of three years duration. Residency programs may be either of a generalized nature or specialized in such fields as child or juvenile psychiatry. Whatever the specialty, the programs vary in their academic orientation; some emphasize psychoanalysis, others behavior therapy while some stress psychopharmacological approaches to the treatment of mental illness. In spite of some differences in the orientation of particular programs all will normally have a curriculum which includes formal courses and seminars combined with clinical training. As noted by one observer:

> The central core of the curriculum, however, usually consists of a didactic program focused on the principles and techniques of psycho-

therapy and somato-therapy (shock treatment and drug therapy). Residents generally are involved with patients from the start of training and in addition take courses and seminars concerned with the psychopathology of neuroses and psychoses, clinical neurology, personality development, personality assessment, child psychiatry, psychopharmacology, research problems, and other topics. Much attention is given to interviewing techniques and the skills involved in probing a patient's history and accurately diagnosing his problems * * *. Depending on staff interests, residents may also take work in hypnosis, group psychotherapy, family therapy, law and psychiatry, the psychology of sleeping and dreaming, and community or social psychiatry. Psychoanalytic theories are subsumed under various labels in the didactic program or taught in special courses and seminars.

Arnold A. Rogow, *The Psychiatrists* (New York: G.P. Putnam's Sons, 1970), p. 48.

As in the cases of other medical specialties psychiatry is subject to an accreditation procedure established under the auspices of relevant medical professional groups. In the case of psychiatry it is the American Board of Psychiatry and Neurology, whose membership is drawn from the American Medical Association, which certifies candidates in either general psychiatry, child psychiatry or neurology. Certification in one of these fields is available to any candidate who passes a rather rigorous examination and has completed a psychiatry residence. Significantly, most practicing psychiatrists are not board certified (the percentage of "board certified" psychiatrists has been variously estimated at between 33 and 48 percent). In fact, certification is only a necessity for those psychiatrists who frequently serve as expert witnesses or act as consultants to agencies which require board certification.

In the common parlance psychiatrists are frequently confused with psychoanalysts. While these two professional groups overlap in many ways, they are distinct professional categories. Basically, psychoanalysts are psychiatrists who have additional specialized training provided by one of the institutes of the American Psychoanalytical Association. The present structure of the American Psychoanalytic Institute was established in 1933 and is at present a federation of 29 societies and 20 training institutions. Each of these institutes operates its own training program, which is of six to ten years duration. Admission into a training program is decided by an institute committee. Admission usually requires a medical background, though decisions as to admissibility also take into account the personality characteristics of the applicant in terms of his or her suitability for analytic training. The following excerpt describes a typical training program.

Once admitted for training, the candidate must undergo the preparatory analysis previously noted "four or more times a week" and also carry through a program of assigned reading, lectures, and supervised clinical experience, all of which is designed to provide him with a thorough knowledge of Freud's theories and other relevant psychoanalytic contributions. He is further required to analyze under supervision at least two adult cases, devoting to each a minimum of 150 hours of analysis and "carrying at least one of them through the terminal phase of analysis." It is expected that material from these analyses will be presented by him "in no less than three extended presentations" at clinical conferences, of which he is required to attend at least fifty during his training. At each stage of training his progress is determined by the institute's educational committee. * * * If the candidate successfully completes the training program, he is given a written statement to that effect by the institute, and he may then apply for membership in the American Psychoanalytic Association.

Arnold A. Rogow, *The Psychiatrists* (New York: G.P. Putnam's Sons 1970), p. 49.

The settings in which psychiatrists practice, as well as the types of disorders they deal with, vary widely. Some may practice full time on the staff of a public or private hospital, generally treating patients with severe psychiatric disorders. Others may be attached, either full or part time, to community outpatient clinics. Still others may be established in private practice, either exclusively or in conjunction with other employment with an inpatient or outpatient facility. The disorders treated by psychiatrists range from conditions which are clearly psychotic to those which are not disabling but nonetheless impede the individual's adaptation to life's stresses. The conditions subsumed within the latter category could include anxiety reactions, phobias, sexual dysfunction, or substance abuse.

Sociological studies of the psychiatric profession suggests that psychiatrists can be divided into two groups: those who have an analytical (Freudian) and psychological orientation (the A–P group) and those who have a directive and organic orientation (the D–O group). The following excerpt describes the distinctions between the treatment approaches of these two groups:

The analytic approach consists essentially of analyzing behavior, relationships, and conscious and unconscious motivations according to psychoanalytic theories. The classical psychoanalytic approach consists of analyzing symptoms and defenses, transference and resistance, with the purpose of strengthening the ego through insight into unconscious forces, particularly into those which are apt to produce psychopathology. The so-called dynamic psychotherapeutic approach follows this general line with less rigor and greater flexibility. The emphasis is on gaining insight and applying insight and not on manipulation or direction, unless this is absolutely necessary because of a weak ego; whenever directions are given they must at least be based on analytic insights of the therapists. The approach is almost entirely psychological; organic methods of diagnosis and treatment are extraneous to it and are rarely employed by its practitioners.

The directive approach consists of changing attitudes, opinions, and behavior of the patient by means of directive and supportive methods such as assertion, suggestion, reassurance, advice, manipulation, and even coercion. It is usually not based on analytic insight, but on the therapist's judgment and what is called clinical experience and evaluation of the patient's problems and situation. Depending on the therapist and the patient, the therapist may try to buck-up the patient's low esteem, convert him to the therapist's own philosophy of life, give him a stern lecture or friendly advice, tell him to go to a resort, to take it easy or work harder, to treat his wife kindly or get a divorce. The success of any of these maneuvers, and they can be quite successful, depends on the wisdom and strength of the therapist rather than on his technical knowledge, and also on the suggestibility and the ego strength of the patient. The directive approach requires, besides clinical experience, and even more urgently than technical knowledge, broad human experience and a willingness to assume authority.

Directive techniques are often combined with organic medical techniques [e.g., psychotropic medication], both diagnostic and therapeutic. D–O practitioners are likely to do medical and neurological examinations, to carry out laboratory tests, prescribe drugs, administer shock treatments, and refer their patients to neurosurgeons or even carry out, themselves, "minor" neurosurgical procedures, like transorbital lobotomies. Many of their explanations, to themselves and to their patients, are couched in medical or pseudomedical terms.

A. Hollingshead and F. Redlich, *Social Class and Mental Illness*: A Community Study (New York: John Wiley & Sons, Inc., 1958), pp. 155–156.*

2. *Psychologists*

a. *Development of the Profession*

The emergence of psychology as one of the treating professions is a relatively recent phenomenon. In fact, from the mid-nineteenth century to the middle 1940's, psychology essentially was an academically based discipline. The following excerpt traces the developments leading to the field's eventual emergence as a major player in the psychotherapy field:

[T]he bulk of psychologists were employed in institutions of higher learning where they engaged in teaching and conducting research in animal learning behavior and brain behavior relations. It was in the mid–1940s that the psychologist practitioner role within the health field began to emerge in a significant manner. The large-scale employment of clinical and counseling psychologists by the Veterans Administration during the World War II era is widely accepted as providing a significant impetus to the emergence of psychologists as practitioners in the health area (Wolman, 1965). In the mental health area, the initial functioning of the psychologist was within the framework of the mental health team. This was particularly the case within health service delivery systems such as hospitals and mental health clinics. Such teams usually were comprised of a psychiatrist (who was frequently the team leader), a social worker, a nurse (whose special interest and training were in psychiatric nursing), and usually a clinical psychologist.

Francis R.J. Fields and Rudy J. Horwitz, *Psychology and Professional Practice* (Westport, Connecticut: Quorum Books, 1982), p. xi.

b. Education, Training and Function

Any description of the educational background of clinical psychologists is complicated, since there are no uniform nationwide standards as to who in any particular jurisdiction is qualified to practice as a psychologist. However, as a practical matter, norms imposed by the profession itself, through the American Psychological Association, have served to establish national standards as to education and training.

"As early as 1947, the American Psychological Association established professional standards for guaranteeing the level of services provided by the psychologist practitioner. In that year, the American Board of Examiners in Professional Psychology was formed. This approach, modeled after the medical profession, established the requirements of the Ph.D. degree and five years' experience in one of three specialty areas, clinical psychology, counseling psychology, and industrial psychology."

Francis R.J. Fields and Rudy J. Horwitz, *Psychology and Professional Practice* (Westport, Connecticut: Quorum Books, 1982), pp. xii-xiii.

The standards of the American Psychological Association have been adopted by various state licensing and certification agencies. In these states practicing psychologists will generally possess a Ph.D. in clinical psychology. In other states there are either no formal educational requirements or lower educational requirements than those imposed by the American Psychological Association.

Thus, the educational standards or requirements for entry vary from state to state. Nevertheless, some generalizations are possible. A master's or Ph.D. degree in clinical psychology is the general rule. These degrees typically have been earned at one of the more than 130 universities in the U.S. which offer doctoral programs in clinical psychology. In some cases the degree will have been awarded not by universities but by specialized training centers which have developed in recent years. These non-university programs are by and large comparable to the Ph.D. programs offered by universities, though they differ in emphasis by stressing practical training and field work rather than academic research. Most of the university-centered programs as well as some of the special training programs have been accredited by the American Psychological Association, which serves as the profession's educational review and accrediting arm.

As in most fields of study there are significant variations in the length of time that it takes for a student to qualify for a Ph.D. degree. The excerpt below describes some common elements of most Ph.D. programs.

Three years of full-time study beyond the baccalaureate degree is the minimum requirement, with the four-year program much more frequent, and five years not unusual. Most graduate departments prefer to emphasize the qualitative requirements rather than the number of credits, but 90 hours of graduate course work is fairly typical of catalog statements, with one third of these representing research credits. The graduate program sometimes includes a few courses, or even a "minor," in other departments: mathematics and mathematical statistics, philosophy, neurology, physiology, anthropology, chemistry, or others. There is usually some comprehensive examination ("prelims") covering the subject matter of certain fields of psychology, given after two or three years of work. The requirement of language examinations (or completion of language courses) is justified on the grounds that much research requires an acquaintance with some foreign literature in psychology, and, perhaps implicitly, that all doctors of philosophy should share a common mark of cultural distinction. The Ph.D. is traditionally a research degree, and the conclusion of a major piece of original work is almost universally required. (Many departments expect the student to take as an intermediate step a master's degree, frequently including the requirement of a less formidable research project.) There is usually a final oral examination of this dissertation research and relevant areas. Most curricula in clinical psychology involve some practical experience, including a year's closely supervised internship in a mental health installation.

Wilse B. Webb, *The Profession of Psychology* (New York: Holt, Rinehart and Winston, 1962), pp. 40–41.

Like psychiatrists, psychologists are employed by institutions or clinics, or are established in private practice. A 1976 survey indicated that about one third of psychologists were employed in institutions; another one third were employed by universities; and almost one quarter were engaged in private practice. However, almost half of the psychologists surveyed indicated they engaged in some part time private practice. See Francis R.J. Fields, and Rudy J. Horwitz, *Psychology and Professional Practice* (Westport, Connecticut: Quorum Books, 1982), p. 35.

While a primary function of psychologists in earlier years was psychological assessment and diagnosis, psychologists today are increasingly engaged in psychotherapy rather than diagnosis. Even today, however, an important part of the work of psychologists involves psychological assessment. The assessment process typically involves the administration and interpretation of standardized tests as well as diagnosis based on more subjective impressions. Frequently, the assessment or diagnosis of patients is the result of team efforts involving input by psychologists as well as other mental health professionals.

As noted above, the traditional function of psychologists as diagnosticians is giving way to a greater role in the provision of psychotherapy. As in the case of psychiatrists, there are different treatment approaches. Basically, these can be divided into two approaches—one behaviorally oriented, the other more Freudian or psychoanalytic. Psychologists that are behaviorally oriented tend to focus on specific abnormal behavior patterns and use learning theory to "decondition" maladaptive behavior. Because of legal limitations, psychologists are prohibited from prescribing psychotropic medication or other medically based treatments such as electro-convulsive therapy.

3. Psychiatric Social Workers

Social work as a profession may be divided into a number of specialty areas, one of which is psychiatric social work. Licensing requirements, where they exist, vary from state to state. Nevertheless, certain common denominators characterize the profession.

The psychiatric social worker will have obtained a Master of Social Work (M.S.W.) degree from an accredited school of social work. This takes a minimum of two years of full-time graduate study. A portion of each of the two years of graduate study is spent in a field placement in the community. During this time, the psychiatric social worker attains a beginning competence in the areas of knowledge of individual development and behavior, dynamics of interpersonal interaction, skill in dealing with disturbed patients and their families, techniques of individual, group, and family therapy, and use of community resources for psychiatrically disturbed patients. Certification is by the Academy of Certified Social Workers (ACSW) and is obtained after two years of full-time practice beyond the Master's degree, during which the applicant must be supervised by a member of the Academy.

* * *

The psychiatric social worker often engages in duties far removed from those traditionally associated with social work. Psychiatric social workers generally are not "welfare workers," but are concerned with the relationship of the emotionally disturbed individual to his community and with the best use of community and family resources in helping him. Work within this field is quite varied and may include social evaluation of patients, liaison with patients' families, work with hospitalized patients, work in child guidance clinics, private diagnostic and treatment work, and work in community mental health centers. Although some psychiatric social workers function independently in private practice, the vast majority work as a part of a mental health team.

R. Allen, E. Ferster and J. Rubin, *Readings in Law and Psychiatry* (Baltimore: The Johns Hopkins University Press, 1975), pp. 25–26.

Significantly, not only are psychiatrists being displaced by other professionals as the principal providers of mental health treatment services but social workers rather than psychologists are beginning to dominate the field. According to one recent report:

A quiet revolution is going on in psychotherapy. As a result, by far the largest portion of the nation's therapy is now done by nonmedical professionals.

* * *

The three major groups offering psychotherapy are psychiatrists, psychologists and social workers. They are joined by a mix of other professions such as clergymen and a significant number of nonpsychiatric doctors who also deal with emotional problems.

But the new shift is most pronounced in the comparison between psychiatrists and social workers. Ten years ago, for example, there were about as many psychiatrists as social workers offering psychotherapy, while today social workers outnumber psychiatrists two to one. Moreover, although social workers provide the bulk of therapy in institutions, growing numbers are treating more affluent, private clients, thus moving into the traditional preserve of the elite psychiatrists and clinical psychologists, as well.

The social workers, in turn, are being challenged by a new category of therapist specializing in the treatment of troubled family and marital relationships. This new category of therapists may be the fastest-growing of all: in California, for example, there are now close to 16,000 of these marriage and family counselors, as they are called there—almost a threefold increase in the last decade.

See, *Social Workers Vault Into a Leading Role in Psychotherapy,* New York Times, April 30, 1985, p. 17, 20, col. 4.

Comments

1. *Patient's choice of professional.* The discussion in the preceding section is based upon the premise that the mental health field is made up of different professional categories and that the consumer need only elect the one that most closely fits his needs. In reality, however, prospective patients may have their choice circumscribed by economic or related factors. For instance, state licensing laws have had a significant influence on the public's use of one rather than another category of professional. There has been an increasing tendency on the part of the disfavored professions to seek relief through legislative or judicial channels. The nature of these initiatives are considered in section III "Emerging Issues in the Allocation of Function Among the Mental Health Professions," infra. Further, if the patient has medical insurance that covers outpatient mental health treatment, the terms of the insurance policy may dictate the choice. It is not uncommon, for instance, for health care insurance policies to require that outpatient mental health treatment be provided by a psychiatrist or alternatively, that psychologists can only be used if there has been a medical referral and the fees are billed through a physician. While numerous states have enacted freedom of choice laws which prevent insurance companies from imposing such limitations on the use of psychologists, in some states these types of restrictions remain in effect and consequently serve to channel patients towards psychiatrists and away from other mental health professionals. Dujovne, *Third Party Recognition of Psychological Services,* Professional Psychology, 574, 575, 1980.

Similar restrictions as to choice may be imposed on those covered by public insurance plans such as Medicare or Medicaid. For instance, under Medicare the *therapeutic* services of psychologists in private practice are not covered. Programs Operation Manual Systems, § 00610.140, 1981. Moreover, payment for *diagnostic* services performed by psychologists who are in private practice will be reimbursed only when "a physician orders such testing." *Id.* While Medicaid programs for the "medically needy" differ somewhat from state to state, most programs provide only limited reimbursement for outpatient psychiatric services. Mitchell and Cromwell, *Medicaid Participation by Psychiatrists in Private Practice,* 139 Am.J. Psychiatry, 810, 813 (1982). Even when outpatient mental health services are covered, some jurisdictions "will reimburse outpatient mental health services only within a clinic setting: office-based psychologists must obtain prior authorization to treat Medicaid patients." Id.

2. *Cost of mental health services.* Aside from insurance considerations, the choice of a therapist will be influenced by the overall economic circumstances of the patient. Those of limited means are likely to be more sensitive to differences in the fee structure of the respective professions and consequently are more likely to seek the services of auxiliary mental health professionals rather than psychiatrists or certified psychologists. *See, generally,* Mitchell and Cromwell, *Medicaid Participation by Psychiatrists in Private Practice,* 139 Am.J. Psychiatry, 810 (1982).

There are significant variations in the fee structure of the respective professions. According to one report:

> "[t]he national median fee for psychiatrists in private practice is estimated to be $90 a session. In contrast, clinical psychologists average $65 a session and social workers average $50. Some social workers or marriage and family counselors will see clients for as little as $25 or $30 a session." See, *Social Workers Vault Into a Leading Role in Psychotherapy,* New York Times, April 30, 1985, p. 17, 20, col. 4.

Those who do not qualify under any insurance program may need to rely on the subsidized services provided by community mental health centers. Here, the patients' opportunity to select a particular professional category to provide treatment may be restricted by staff availability or by the assignment practices of the center.

B. PERSPECTIVES ON DIAGNOSIS AND TREATMENT

1. *Defining Psychiatric Disorders*

As noted, practitioners of psychotherapy come from different educational backgrounds and are likely to be differentiated in terms of the parent professional organizations to which they belong and by state law which licenses each profession separately.

Overlapping these variations in educational background and professional affiliations are differences in treatment methodology. Significantly, neither licensing laws nor other forms of regulation controls treatment modalities used by the different professions. The only legal restriction is on the use of pharmaceutical agents or other invasive therapies, which are the sole prerogative of therapists who are *medically* trained and licensed. Thus, the only effective determinant of an individual practitioner's treatment method is his or her orientation which, in turn, is likely to be the product of the training background of the therapist. For instance, psychologists, psychiatrists or psychiatric social workers whose training was psychoanalytically oriented are likely to practice in this mode. Similarly, those whose training emphasized behavior modification tend to adopt a treatment approach utilizing these techniques in their practice.

A particular therapist's perspective as to the preferred mode of psychotherapy is also likely to be influenced by his or her perception of what constitutes "illness" or a "disorder" calling for treatment. For instance, adherence to a medical model, which presupposes a specific disease characterized by clearly defined symptomatology, is likely to influence the therapist's orientation as to choice of therapies. On the other hand is the view that therapeutic intervention is appropriate for any adjustment problems even if the causation is of a social nature.

The following excerpt describes some of a number of views on the nature and basic characteristics of psychiatric disorders:

> There are multiple models and criteria that can be applied to the diagnostic enterprise, but the reference to some normative standard cannot be avoided. Whether the approach is statistical/general or clinical/individual, the designation of someone as mentally ill or healthy presupposes some adaptive norm. Under the former, it may be social or cultural expectation. Under the latter, mental health or illness may be measured against a whole host of more personal criteria: living up to one's functioning potential, the dominance of conscious over unconscious motivation for one's actions, the presence or absence of stress or pain in one's chosen lifestyle or living decisions, the ability to handle conflict "maturely," the presence or absence of symptoms of maladaptation, and various other standards of greater or lesser circularity and subjectivity. Is mental health simply the absence of mental illness or disease? Or is it more productive, as some theorists have suggested, to view mental health and mental illness as noncorrelative concepts, as functional states represented by distinct continua rather than different points on the same continuum? Does that mean mental health and illness are mutually exclusive, or is everyone in a state of less than full mental health and no one wholly ill?

> The organized psychiatric profession does not pretend to have dispositive answers to these questions, and many individual psychiatrists conduct their practice in full awareness of the conflicts and ambiguities inherent in the various theories about the nature of mental illness. Progress in diagnostic theory and clinical practice is not thereby foreclosed. The American Psychiatric Association recently produced the third edition of its *Diagnostic and Statistical Manual of Mental Disorders* (DSM–III),[a] giving ample recognition to the continuing uncertainties that are part of such an effort. The editors of the document emphasize the objective of maximizing its usefulness to clinicians of various theoretical orientations practicing in a variety of clinical settings. They acknowledge the element of compromise and

a. The APA revised the manual again in 1987 (DSM-III-Revised).

trial and error in settling on a broad-ranging classification scheme. Finally, the need for continual revision and refinement of the document is made explicit in its characterization by the editors as "only one still frame in the ongoing process of attempting to better understand mental disorders."

Similarly, much of the tremendous progress in the chemical treatment of mental illnesses—the so-called psychopharmacological revolution—has occurred despite major gaps in understanding the precise remedial processes: why the treatment works, what works, what is at work. Beyond the basic knowledge that certain mental disorders are associated with certain chemical imbalances in the affected persons and that certain drugs work toward restoring a balance, there still lies a vast unknown. And much of what is accomplished with drug treatment—including the development of new drugs or the specification of type and dosage by illness—continues to be based on ad hoc clinical experience and experimentation.

Brakel, Parry and Weiner, *The Mentally Disabled and the Law,* 3rd Ed., (Chicago: American Bar Foundation, 1985), pp. 19–20.

2. Treatment Modalities

Psychiatric treatment modalities may include both somatic and nonsomatic therapies. The former includes the administration of psychotropic drugs and electro-convulsive therapy (ECT). The latter includes psychoanalysis and other communicative therapies which do not involve invasive medical procedures, and which are employed by both medically and non-medically trained mental health professionals. The somatic treatment modalities are discussed in greater detail in Chapter Nine. The following excerpt describes the principal characteristics of the major nonsomatic psychotherapies, the so-called "psychosocial" therapies:

CLASSICAL PSYCHOANALYSIS

When Freud gave up the use of hypnosis and turned to free association as the basic technique for eliciting psychological information from his patients, he effected a change in the nature of the therapeutic relationship which enabled him to observe the manifestations of resistance and the transference neurosis. The analysis of these phenomena rapidly became a central element in the psychoanalytic process and provided the basis for the later development of the analysis of the ego that characterizes modern analytic procedures.

* * *

The primary aim of psychoanalysis is to help the patient to achieve structural psychological changes through emotional insight into the unconscious dynamic and psychogenetic aspects of his mental life which are manifested in symptoms, characterological distortions, and disturbances in personal relationships. This change is achieved by techniques that promote a regressive transference in which id, ego, and superego forces dominate the doctor-patient relationship in the form of the transference neurosis, which recapitulates the infantile neurosis first appearing during the early years of the patient's psychological development. As the transference neurosis develops, the patient gradually becomes consciously aware of previously hidden primitive forms of psychic functioning, which become the central focus of analysis. The resolution of the transference neurosis is the primary task during the terminal phase of analysis, although it is generally not finally resolved until a significant time has elapsed after the last analytic session.

The development of the transference neurosis is enhanced by the following specific technical procedures:

A. The basic method of analysis is *free association,* i.e., the patient is asked to report, without editing or withholding, all that comes to mind, no matter how painful, frightening, distasteful, shameful, or humiliating. A special aspect of free association is the reporting of dreams and the associations stemming from the elements of the manifest content of the dream.

B. Free association is promoted through the use of the couch. The horizontal position of the patient, with the analyst out of sight behind him, exerts pressure on the patient's conscious and unconscious internal autistic processes to influence the flow and content of the associations.

C. This pressure is further augmented by the regularity and frequency of the analytic hours. In Freud's Vienna the usual practice was a daily hour six days a week. * * * For a variety of reasons, economic and otherwise, the tendency in this country has been to drop the number of hours to four per week, and certainly any less than three would not entitle the procedure to be called analysis even if other technical procedures were maintained.

D. The analyst maintains a position of neutrality with respect to the patient's associations (without, however, losing his empathic concern) and often may remain silent for greater or lesser periods of time as he listens to the patient's productions. This technique encourages the flow and freedom of the patient's speech and avoids the possibility of contaminating his thoughts with those of the analyst.

* * *

Although he is neutral and often apparently inactive, it is the analyst's task to become active in two ways: in making *clarifications* and in offering *interpretations.* Many of the patient's patterns of behavior and relationships are ego syntonic, and he does not initially see the pathological elements that may color them. The analyst, however, in the course of applying his free-floating attention, gradually becomes aware of the distortions in these complex patterns. As he does so, he proceeds to help the patient to gain distance from them and to perceive them more objectively. Initially *confronting* the patient with the nature of his behavior, he guides the patient, often by direct and focused questions, to an amplification and *clarification* of the details and circumstances of his behavior and relationships.

* * *

In *interpretation* the analyst introduces to the patient his, the analyst's, perceptions and understanding of the *unconscious* elements beneath the patient's surface behavior. If the proper groundwork has been laid through adequate clarification, the analyst's interpretation will strike a resonant note in his patient, who at that point becomes conscious of feelings, memories, attitudes, and fantasies previously hidden in the unconscious.

*   *   *

PSYCHOANALYTIC PSYCHOTHERAPY

Two major factors underlie the modern practice of psychoanalytic psychotherapy: (a) the widespread dissemination of psychodynamic concepts and techniques and (b) the development of object-relations theory.

The rapid expansion of training in psychotherapy which followed World War II coincided with the rise of interest in psychoanalytic ideas, which, particularly in the United States, soon dominated psychotherapists' thinking and teaching. Influenced by the precepts of their supervisors, many of whom were formally trained in psychoanalysis, thousands of young psychotherapists were imbued with a psychodynamic approach to the diagnostic understanding and treatment of patients with emotional disorders. Though relatively few of this new generation of therapists underwent the rigorous psychoanalytic training that would allow them to practice psychoanalysis proper, the majority adapted psychoanalytic theories and techniques to their clinical activities and, in so doing, introduced numerous modifications that have transformed classical psychoanalysis into modern psychoanalytic psychotherapy.

Simultaneously with this huge increase in clinicians practicing psychodynamic psychiatry, the psychoanalytic approach was applied to a wider variety of clinical psychiatric conditions. Initially restricted to patients with psychoneuroses, the use of psychoanalytic techniques was gradually extended to patients with psychotic illness and complicated characterological disorders.

*   *   * It is not possible to give hard and fast criteria that sharply distinguish classical psychoanalysis from psychoanalytic psychotherapy. Like analysis, psychoanalytic therapy aims, when possible, to bring about structural psychological changes through insights arrived at by the use of free association, clarification, interpretation, and analysis of the transference. At the same time, psychoanalytic therapy allows the therapist to use a variety of supportive measures when these are required by the patient's clinical condition. Unlike analysis, psychoanalytic therapy is carried out with the patient sitting face-to-face with the therapist. The frequency of hours is usually once or twice a week, but (like analysis) therapy may continue for a number of years. The therapist is generally more active than the analyst in seeking information and focusing on specific areas of conflict.

In its uncovering mode, psychoanalytic psychotherapy is similar to classical psychoanalysis in its basic approach and therapeutic goals.

The therapist aims to help his patient to resolve psychic conflict through an analysis of defenses and the underlying impulses. Such analysis, however, is more circumscribed than classical psychoanalysis. The therapist does not seek to resolve *all* areas of psychic conflict but limits his activities to effecting those changes in psychic structure which will be sufficient to enable the patient to overcome his major problems. Although the therapist may deal with transference issues, this area is balanced with equal attention to disturbances in current relationships and their genesis in early life experiences, without the emphasis that is central to classical psychoanalytic treatment on encouraging and analyzing a regressive transference.

As noted earlier, the flexibility of psychoanalytic psychotherapy permits the therapist to use a variety of supportive measures when indicated. Such measures are particularly useful and appropriate for patients with narcissistic and borderline character disorders—in strengthening unstable defenses and ego functions, in curtailing acting out, and in providing the "holding environment" in which patients may safely express primitive affects and attitudes to an empathic and containing therapist.

*   *   *

BRIEF PSYCHOTHERAPIES

*   *   * Like classical psychoanalysis and psychoanalytic psychotherapy in its uncovering mode, the brief psychotherapies are aimed at bringing about internal psychological changes through engendering emotional insight into underlying psychodynamic conflicts. The techniques are applied to patients specifically selected for their capacity to respond positively in a relatively few treatment hours over a limited period of time.

Although they share with other analytic psychotherapies the basic orientation of change through the development of emotional insight, brief dynamic psychotherapies have several characteristics that set them apart:

A. As the adjective "brief" implies, these therapies limit the number of hours devoted to the therapeutic work, a limitation that is made explicit to the patient before treatment begins.

B. Brief dynamic psychotherapies are focused on specific areas of conflict and do not attempt to bring about the more extensive psychological reconstructions aimed at by psychoanalysis and psychoanalytic psychotherapy.

C. Brief dynamic psychotherapies are confrontative—that is, the patient's attention is directed repeatedly to significant areas of psychic conflict, often with the arousal of painful anxiety and depression.

D. As is implied in the characteristics already listed, the therapist is far more active in carrying out brief dynamic therapy than when he is engaged in analysis or long-term psychoanalytic psychotherapy. As in other forms of insight-oriented therapy, he must, of course, listen to the patient's associations and reach an intuitive understanding of his conflicts. At the same time, he must actively direct the patient's attention to specific areas of conflict and solicit the related free associations.

E. Within the areas selected for observation and psychological analysis, emphasis is placed on systematically defining and examining the patient's conflicts in three areas: transference, current, and past relationships. In this regard, too, the therapist actively focuses the patient's attention on each of these areas and their interrelationships.

* * *

SUPPORTIVE PSYCHOTHERAPY

* * * The modern era of supportive psychotherapy goes back to the period of "moral therapy" and the subsequent "nonrestraint" movement in the mid-nineteenth century treatment of psychotic patients, which was based on the use of human relationships rather than mechanical restraints to control psychotic symptoms and behavior. Since that time, the human milieu has been an important component of the management of patients with psychopathology resulting from serious disorders of ego functioning.

The therapist-patient relationship is central to the process of supportive psychotherapy. The opportunity to be in the presence of and to reveal one's conflicts and suffering to a calm, attentive, concerned, and understanding therapist often has a beneficial effect on human anxiety, depression, and despair. This is particularly so in the face of acute emotional turmoil or crisis, but a longer-term relationship can be similarly supportive to individuals with chronic emotional problems. Such a stable, supportive relationship is central to the "holding environment" currently recommended for patients with severe narcissistic and borderline character disorders.

In addition to the central relationship itself, patients may be helped by several specific maneuvers that, in part at least, derive their effectiveness from the authoritarian role the supportive psychotherapist plays with the patient.

* * *

One important aspect of this kind of therapeutic activity is limit-setting, aimed at preventing the patient from indulging in destructive behavior toward himself or others and at avoiding damaging regressive reactions. It should, furthermore, be noted that quite apart from what the therapist does, he lends himself as a model for identification, enabling the patient to acquire new and useful patterns of behavior based on his internalization of the therapist's image, attitudes, and strengths. And, finally, it should be emphasized that the therapist's dynamic understanding of the patient's conflicts, character structure, and needs forms an essential component of his ability to supply the appropriate supportive measures.

* * *

BEHAVIOR THERAPY

Behavior therapy is inextricably related to learning; its main intent is the development of effective psychological treatment. The role of behavioral science in changing human behavior is a central concern. Wherever possible, clinical phenomena are operationally defined, and those variables that are amenable to experimental investigation are given priority. Thus, constructs such as "the unconscious" and inferences derived from "psychodynamics" are avoided.

Behavior, instead of being viewed as necessarily symptomatic or reflective of deeper processes within the psyche, is often regarded as significant in its own right. It is held that any psychopathological syndrome, when analyzed in terms of antecedents and consequences, may be dissected into a series of target behaviors that require augmentation or elimination. This assessment would include cognitive processes. Even behavior with major biological determinants such as occurs in schizophrenia and primary affective disorders may be evaluated and often modified in accordance with this formulation. * * * Treatment interventions are aimed directly at altering unwanted behavior, establishing its incompatible alternatives, or promoting desired behavior. Thus, behavior therapists attend to a range of specified behaviors on the assumption that behavior change often precedes rather than follows attitude and affect change.

* * *

Most behavior therapists are opposed to descriptive or diagnostic labels. Instead of referring to a patient as having a "passive-aggressive personality," the behavioral clinician seeks operational ingredients. What behaviors do patients demonstrate which lead others to label them as passive-aggressive? In what specific situations, as the result of which stimuli, does the patient respond maladaptively? The crucial focus is on observable behaviors and the selection of appropriate interventions.

* * *

Basically, from a behavioral standpoint, problems fall into one or more of the following three categories: (a) behavioral excesses (e.g., compulsive rituals, substance abuse), (b) behavioral deficits (e.g., memory impairment, limited social skills), and (c) behavioral inappropriateness, (e.g., intimate disclosures to uninterested strangers). To effect constructive changes, behavior therapists draw primarily from the principles of extinction, positive and negative reinforcement, stimulus control, modeling, generalization, and other components of operant and respondent (classical) conditioning.

The Psychiatric Therapies, T.B. Karasu, Ed. (Washington: American Psychiatric Association, 1984).

Questions and Comments

1. *Behavioral therapy techniques.* Behavior therapy incorporates a number of techniques. Among those commonly utilized are the following:

a. *Relaxation training.* The patient is instructed in muscle relaxation techniques as a method of reducing anxiety.

b. *Flooding.* The patient is given intense exposure to anxiety-evoking stimuli; he initially experiences stress, then relief when the expected adverse consequences do not occur.

c. *Implosion therapy.* Used to treat obsessive-compulsive disorders, implosion therapy involves both exposure to a feared or anxiety producing object or situation and prevention of the patient's typical response to it. If successful, the patient's anxiety and his ritualistic behavior will be ameliorated.

d. *Behavioral rehearsal.* The goal of this form of behavior therapy is to replace the patient's inappropriate social responses with effective behavior patterns. In the course of therapy, the therapist and patient act out social encounters to develop more effective social skills and reduce social anxiety.

e. *Modeling.* The patient learns appropriate behaviors and responses by observing desired behavior and imitating that behavior. This therapy is effective in treating phobias, obsessive-compulsive disorders and anxiety.

f. *Aversion therapy.* Used to eliminate undesirable behaviors such as substance abuse and exhibitionism, this technique involves the pairing of the target behavior with an unpleasant event such as an electric shock or drug-induced nausea. A more humane and less controversial variation of this treatment is aversive imagery, whereby the patient vividly imagines the behavior followed by unpleasant consequences.

g. *Behavior control.* The goal of this technique is to teach the patient to modify and control his own behavior. The process generally involves three stages: self-monitoring (observing and noting the target behavior); self-evaluation (comparing the adequacy or appropriateness of the behavior to an internal or external standard); and self-reinforcement (administering consequences or rewards according to the appropriateness of the behavior as performed).

For a more detailed discussion of these and other behavior therapy techniques, see *The Psychiatric Therapies,* T.B. Karasu, Ed. (Washington: American Psychiatric Association, 1984), pp. 494–505.

2. *Sex therapy.* The development of specialized techniques for the treatment of sexual dysfunction represents the most important movement in the field over the past twenty years. Current development in this field of specialization and some of the issues which have come to the forefront as a result of its growing popularity are described in a *New York Times* article:

Sex Therapy: As Popularity Grows, Critics Question Whether It Works

"Sex," they said, and the world responded with anger, titillation, relief and respect.

That was 15 years ago. Today again, Dr. William H. Masters and Virginia E. Johnson are under attack for the rapid form of psychotherapy they devised to treat marriages burdened by sexual dysfunction. The widely asked question is: Does this treatment, or others like it, really work?

The complaints come from detractors who reject the concept of sexual dysfunction as a "disorder" and sex therapy as a treatment, and from psychiatrists and psychologists who believe they have improved on the original approach, or who question how many people are actually helped by such treatment.

They also come from moralists opposed to the role of prostitutes and surrogate wives in the technique's development and practice, as well as from consumers who have been the victims of unscrupulous practitioners.

For better or worse, the Masters and Johnson therapeutic technique came to be known as sex therapy.

* * *

[T]he therapy is now well established. Riding a swell of social change atop advances in birth control, women's liberation and the 1960's thirst for freedom and spontaneity, sex therapy quickly took hold as a specialty field with thousands of licensed and unlicensed practitioners and hundreds of thousands of patients worldwide clamoring after the cure.

The Masters and Johnson treatment, widely discussed but often distorted, is a two-week assault on the couple's complaint, requiring daily meetings between them and a male-and-female team of cotherapists. Since all but 10 percent of the 175 to 200 couples seen annually at the Masters & Johnson Institute in St. Louis come from out of town or even out of the country, patients find their own local hotel accommodations where they carry out the prescribed "sensate exercises" in private.

* * *

The cost of the treatment is $3,000 per couple, and only couples need apply.

* * *

Approximately 30,000 physicians, therapists and other professionals have taken courses in treating sexual problems from Masters and Johnson, but only a handful of practitioners apply the teachings in the two-week, co-therapist, couples-only model.

* * *

Dr. Helen Singer Kaplan of the New York Hospital–Cornell Medical Center . . . routinely accepts single patients, out of her observation that many people have sexual disorders before they ever meet their partner.

Dr. Kaplan usually sees patients once a week, instead of every day, over a period of 12 to 25 weeks, depending on the nature of the problem: Her rates are within the $65–to–$150–per–hour range typical of privately practicing sex therapists, although patients at hospital clinics may be seen without charge.

* * *

Dr. Kaplan insists on a thorough physical examination of her patients, as do Masters and Johnson, before accepting anyone for treatment, since impotence, for example, can be caused by hidden medical problems ranging from a subtle circulatory disorder of the penis to hormonal imbalances, severe diabetes, the use of anti-hypertensive medications or the abuse of alcohol, heroin or other drugs.

USE OF DRUGS WITH THERAPY

As a psychiatrist, Dr. Kaplan also uses medicine as part of sex therapy, where indicated. (Masters and Johnson do not.) With sexual phobias and sexual problems secondary to depression, she said, treatment is often ineffective without appropriate psychotropic drugs, notably tricyclic antidepressants.

* * *

And for the case where a partner is needed and none exists, there is what Dr. Kaplan calls "the surrogate solution."

Sex surrogates may work freelance or in collaboration with a therapist. They are paid for their services, in the range of $40 to $50 per two-hour session, and are thus technically prostitutes. However, their medical affiliation evidently protects them from prosecution in most states.

New York Times, November 14, 1980, p. 17.

3. Capacity of Professions to Diagnose and Treat

As suggested by the preceding materials, treatment modalities can roughly be divided into two categories: the invasive forms which include psychotropic medication, ECT and aversive conditioning techniques, and the "psychosocial therapies," which rely essentially on verbal communications between the therapist and the patient. Also as has been noted, the invasive therapies tend to be the domain of psychiatrists who are medically trained. On the other hand, both psychiatrists and non-medically trained mental health professionals utilize various psychotherapies to treat "functional" disorders, i.e., those not having any known organic medical basis. In fact, the application of various psychotherapuetic techniques constitutes the principal mode of intervention by all categories of mental health professionals.

The section which follows focuses on the role of government in regulating mental health professionals. One form of regulation gives certain licensed professionals an exclusive right to perform a given function such as psychotherapy. This form of regulation is ostensibly predicated on the *special* capacity of certain professions to provide a particular treatment function. In addressing the issues of regulation it is therefore relevant as an initial matter to inquire as to the capacity of the mental health professions to both diagnose the disorder and thereafter apply psychotherapeutic techniques to ameliorate or cure such disorder or dysfunction.   Some perspectives on these basic questions are provided by the materials which follow.

In spite of the fact that the nomenclature has evolved over centuries and has gone through many revisions, it lacks the precision of diagnostic classifications in other branches of medicine. In addition, in recent years psychiatrists have adopted new names for conditions that do not seem to be covered by the nosology. A large percentage of patients are being given these new labels—pseudoneurotic schizophrenia, borderline state, narcissistic personality. There has been a tendency to blame the classification scheme for what is perhaps an ambiguity inherent in psychiatry, for psychiatry deals with behavior rather than with more definite disease symptoms and the causes of psychiatric upset are multifactoral. Mental patients are square pegs and psychiatry provides round holes to accommodate them.

*   *   *

Few psychiatrists have been willing to delve to the bottom of the problem [of classifying mental disorders], to admit that psychiatric diagnoses are and have always been far less exact than diagnoses in the rest of medicine, that in many cases they describe processes or cover conditions bearing no resemblance to traditional medical disease, and that, in the interest of buttressing up their authority, psychiatrists have been content to live with their diagnostic classification schemes— and now are proposing to expand them—without a thorough discussion of either their scientific basis or their social-legal consequences. Very few psychiatrists are willing to say, as has Victor Adebimpe of Pittsburgh's Western Psychiatric Institute and Clinic, that in some psychiatric situations "you have no way of knowing whether your diagnosis is better than anyone else's . . . until you see if the treatment works."

Jonas Robitscher, *The Powers of Psychiatry* (Boston: Houghton Mifflin Company, 1980), pp. 163–181.

(The following excerpt from *The Psychiatric Therapies,* T.B. Karasu, Ed. (Washington: American Psychiatric Association, 1984), pp. 834–836, discusses the inconclusive results of research on the efficacy of various psychotherapeutic techniques):

EFFICACY ISSUES

Many people identify the beginning of the critical evaluation of psychotherapy outcome research with the review by Eysenck (1952), which was based on 24 reports that he collected from various sources, most of which did not describe any controlled investigations of psychotherapy. The arguments were indirect and inferential, and statistics were uncritically pooled. Instead of being ignored, the review, which threw doubt on the efficacy of psychotherapy, stimulated despair, anger, criticism, and rebuttals. Despite the belief of some that Eysenck's arguments have been undermined and defeated, it is interesting to note that a paper published in 1980 in a prestigious psychological journal has essentially resurrected Eysenck's critique and argued that his claims have never been adequately dealt with.

To illustrate some of the diversity of opinion resulting from the various reviews of the literature, a number of authors may be quoted or cited. In 1964, Cross stated that the "efficacy [of psychotherapy] has not been scientifically demonstrated beyond a reasonable doubt." In 1966, after reviewing 14 controlled studies of psychotherapy, Dittman stated that his own "conclusions are modest, and are, moreover, diluted by confusion." On a more optimistic note, Meltzoff and Kornreich (1970) concluded that "controlled research has been notably successful in demonstrating more behavioral change in treated patients than in untreated controls." More cautiously, Bergin (1971) stated that "psychotherapy, as practiced over the last 40 years, has had an average effect that is modestly positive." Malen (1973) arrived at a mixed conclusion after his review of the literature. He stated that "there is considerable evidence that dynamic psychotherapy is effective in psychosomatic conditions; but, that the evidence in favor of dynamic psychotherapy * * * [for] neurosis and character disorders * * * is weak * * *."

The review by Luborsky et al. (1975) concludes that "everyone has won and all must have prizes," meaning that no one psychotherapy is more effective than any other. Frank (1979) concludes from his review of the literature that "psychotherapy * * * [is] more effective than informal, unplanned help."

That these conclusions do not apply only to individual therapy may be illustrated by citing several reviews of other modalities. In a survey covering 42 years (1921–1963) of group psychotherapy with psychotic patients, Stotsky and Zolik (1965) concluded: "The results of controlled experimental studies do not give clear endorsement for the use of group therapy as an independent modality." In 1971, a review by Bednar and Lawlis came to the same conclusion. More recently, Parloff and Dies (1977) reviewed the group psychotherapy outcome literature for the period 1966 to 1975. Because they were particularly concerned with "real" patients rather than volunteer college students or growth potential groups, their analysis covered group therapy as used with schizophrenics, psychoneurotics, offenders, and addicts. They concluded that the research evidence indicated that group therapy had little or no effect on schizophrenics or addicts and that the evidence was too limited or irrelevant to make any decisions about its effects on delinquents or psychoneurotics. They wrote: "Very little can be concluded regarding the efficacy of group psychotherapy." Essentially similar conclusions of little or no *proven* efficacy have been reached in reviews of the literature on family and marital therapy and social and milieu treatments. The only recent reviewers of the literature who present their conclusions in positive and stronger terms are Smith et al. (1980).

Controlled Studies

Over the years, the general trend has been for the recent and more comprehensive reviews to conclude that psychotherapy is effective for a variety of symptomatic and behavioral problems, i.e., chronic moderate anxiety states, simple phobias, depressive symptoms, sexual dysfunctions, adjustment disorders, family conflicts, and communication difficulties.

A large number of studies have been concerned with combined treatment for various diagnostic conditions. Research on schizophrenia has not shown that traditional psychotherapies significantly enhance the benefit of pharmacotherapy, but the effects of the psychotherapy are much more difficult to quantify than are the drug effects. However, token economy therapies and psychosocial rehabilitation are valuable as an adjunct treatment for schizophrenics. Studies of drug/psychotherapy interactions for major affective disorders reveal that psychotherapy for some depressed patients produced better results and that the effects of psychotherapy plus drugs are basically additive in treating depression. Studies of psychotherapy for medically ill patients suggest that psychotherapy plus a medical regimen is more effective in influencing some of the target symptoms for certain medical illnesses than is medical treatment alone. Psychotherapy is especially useful for post-illness psychosocial rehabilitation. A general conclusion about interaction effects is that drugs affect symptoms relatively early whereas psychotherapy has an influence on interpersonal relations and social adjustment, especially at a later stage of treatment.

* * *

Although a number of papers have proposed the possibility of deterioration effects due to psychotherapy and anecdotes on this topic have been reported by clinicians, research data on the subject are limited. In addition, the idea of negative effects is fraught with conceptual as well as research problems. The most extensive review of this literature comes to the conclusion that about five percent of patients in psychotherapy get worse (Sloane et al., 1975).

* * *

Controversy still reigns over the question of whether certain types of therapy are more effective than other types for certain kinds of problems. Another issue that also has not been adequately studied is what aspects or elements of the complex therapeutic interaction are relatively the most effective. Then there is the question of spontaneous remission, which may be high in certain conditions.

In addition, the comparability of therapies bearing the same generic labels has been challenged, and many investigators have noted that relatively little is known about the actual process of psychotherapy and about the degree of variation that exists in the way it is carried out. Attempts are now being made to create manuals designed to provide guidelines for the therapist on the conduct of different modes of therapy. Such guidelines may be useful in controlled research settings but are believed by many clinicians to be largely unsuitable to the operation of their day-to-day practice. It is unclear at the present time whether this apparent conflict between the research demands of reproducibility and standardization will ever be reconciled with the clinicians' need for flexibility, creativity, and sensitivity to the uniqueness of individual patients.

Comments

1. The preceding discussion focuses on the capacity of *psychiatrists* to accurately diagnosis and treat mental disorders. There is no reason to believe that mental health professionals such as psychologists or psychiatric social workers have any greater capacity to diagnose and treat functional disorders.

2. *The DSM classification system.* The American Psychiatric Association first adopted a system of nomenclature for mental disorders in 1917. Published as the *Diagnostic and Statistical Manual of Mental Disorders of the APA,* this scheme has been revised several times, the most recent in 1987 (DSM–III–Revised). According to some commentators the evolution of the DSM system has not necessarily reflected a move toward precision in diagnostic classifications, but rather, changes in attitude on the part of society and the profession. Illustrative of the APA's reaction to societal changes is the DSM system's treatment of homosexuality. Prior to the 1960's, homosexual activity was a crime in most states. Beginning in the early 1960's, many states either repealed such laws or stopped enforcing them. The psychiatric community long had considered homosexuality a "disease", and it was classified as such in the DSM system. With the decriminalization of homosexual activity, however, the disease label became less useful to homosexuals as a mechanism to escape criminal sanctions. In response to widespread criticism on the part of various lobbying groups, in 1973 the APA "delisted" homosexuality as a disease classification. See, Jonas Robitscher, *The Powers of Psychiatry* (Boston: Houghton Mifflin Company, 1980), pp. 170–177.

3. *Treatment outcome studies.* The federal Food and Drug Administration tests and approves psychotropic drugs, thereby ensuring some oversight of the efficacy of specific pharmaceutical agents used in treatment. There exist no similar governmental constraints on the use of non-somatic therapies. Recently, however, the National Institute of Mental Health conducted a study of the efficacy of psychotherapy. While the significance of the study is limited by the fact that it dealt only with the treatment of depression, it is nonetheless of interest as representing the first comprehensive federally funded effort to investigate the efficacy of various mental health treatment modalities. The results of that study are reported as follows:

> Weekly sessions with a psychologist or psychiatrist have a measurable effect on mental distress, according to the final report of a landmark federal experiment.

> The experiment measured the effects of short-term psychotherapy on patients suffering mild to severe depression. It found that depressed patients undergoing as many as 20 sessions with a trained psychotherapist were better off 18 months later than depressed patients who saw a doctor every week but didn't receive psychotherapy. The treated patients, however, didn't improve as much as another group given standard anti-depressant drug treatment.

The experiment, begun more than five years ago, has been watched carefully by mental health experts, health insurers and employee benefit managers who have been demanding evidence that the psychotherapy has an effect. Health insurers and employers, in particular, are growing increasingly disturbed about the sums they are spending on psychotherapy for employees and their families under health insurance plans.

Individuals covered by health insurance may spend six months to two years in weekly sessions with a therapist at a cost of $50 to $100 a session. Insurers and employers complain they haven't any evidence their money is being well spent other than therapists' and patients' subjective judgment that patients are better off than they would have been otherwise.

*   *   *

The experiment with depressed patients was an attempt by the National Institute of Mental Health to see if it could test the effects of psychotherapy in the same way the effects of drugs and operations are tested—that is, with a controlled clinical trial. If it worked, the agency believed, the experiment could become a model for testing psychotherapy's effects in other areas of mental and emotional distress besides depression.

In the experiment, the control group consisted of patients given the anti-depressant drug, imipramine, which has been proven over the years to be effective for straightforward depression. The control patients also saw a doctor weekly who offered support and encouragement but didn't attempt any formal psychotherapy. To make sure the effects of imipramine were being gauged correctly, a second control group of patients received a placebo plus the weekly supportive sessions.

The treatment groups consisted of depressed patients, half of whom received "cognitive behavior therapy" and half of whom received "interpersonal psychotherapy"—the two major competing types of psychotherapy. Cognitive therapy attempts to get the depressed patient to recognize his or her depression stems from a distorted and negative view of the world. Interpersonal therapy is aimed at getting the patient to understand the internal unconscious conflicts underlying depression.

The 18 psychotherapists who gave the 16 to 20 weekly sessions were guided by standardized manuals for their respective types of psychotherapy. The degree of depression in the 239 patients was measured before and after the experiment by several standard psychological tests.

Jerry E. Bishop, *Psychotherapy Has Measurable Effect On Depression in Closely Watched Test,* Wall Street Journal, November 13, 1989, p. B4.

4. *Capacity to predict.* The problem of lack of precision in the diagnosis of mental disorders is compounded by the problem of prediction, which comes into play in the application of civil commitment laws and in the doctrine of a therapist's liability to third parties, where the cause of action is predicated on the psychiatrist's failure to take steps to warn a potential victim or prevent a patient's dangerous behavior. The capacity to

predict in these two contexts is discussed in Chapters Two (liability to third parties) and Eight (civil commitment), infra.

II.   ADMINISTRATIVE REGULATION AND REMEDIATION

A.   INTRODUCTION

As previously indicated, mental health treatment is provided by several categories of professionals utilizing a wide range of treatment techniques.   Except for somatic therapies, which are reserved to psychiatrists and other physicians, the efficacy of the various forms of psychotherapy has not been conclusively determined.   In the treatment of some disorders, such as depression, psychotherapy merely has been shown more effective than no treatment at all, but substantially less effective than pharmaceutical agents.   Given the current state of knowledge in this area, what should be the role of government in regulating the mental health professions?   The following materials describe the basic forms of current regulation and the purposes they are intended to serve.

B.   REGULATION OF ENTRY

Regulation usually takes one of two basic forms—licensing or certification.   A license grants a special privilege, by allowing the holder to engage in activities otherwise proscribed by law.   Licensing statutes contain two essential aspects: (1) they limit the performance of certain activities or the rendition of specified services to a designated class of persons; and (2) they restrict the acquisition of a license to those who meet established qualifications and follow certain procedures.   For instance, the practice of medicine is restricted to those holding a medical license.

Certification, in contrast, does not seek to reserve certain functions or activities to a specifically designated class of individuals, i.e., those holding a license, but rather limits the use of a designated *title* to those who meet specified training and experience requirements.   This form of regulation is also sometimes referred to as "title licensing."   A certification or title licensing statute may provide, for example, that only those who have completed a Ph.D. in psychology may describe themselves as "certified psychologists" or "psychologists," or use any other title incorporating the term "psychology" or similar phraseology.

The practice of psychiatry is, in effect, always regulated by way of licensing.   This is because under state law the practice of psychiatry is in all states conditioned on the holding of a medical license.   However, the completion of a residency in psychiatry is likely to be a practical necessity for any physician functioning as a psychiatrist.   For instance, most hospitals accord admission privileges to the psychiatric wing of the hospital only to those physicians who have completed a psychiatric residency.

In about three-quarters of the states, the practice of psychology is subject to a licensing requirement. Technically, this means that anyone not licensed may not practice and perform the services normally rendered by a psychologist.

California employs fairly typical language in its licensing statutes. It stipulates that anyone who is not a licensed psychologist cannot render "psychological services" for a fee. The key phrase, "psychological services," is in turn defined as "the application of psychological principles, methods, and procedures of understanding, predicting, and influencing behavior, such as the principles pertaining to learning, perception, motivation, emotions, and interpersonal relationships; and the methods and procedures of interviewing, counseling, psychotherapy, behavior modification, and hypnosis; and of constructing, administering, and interpreting tests of mental abilities, aptitudes, interests, attitudes, personality characteristics, emotions, and motivations" (California Business and Professions Code § 2903 [1978]).

The remaining states which regulate psychological practice adhere to the certification model. Certification laws typically provide that an individual may not hold himself out as a "psychologist" or as rendering "psychological services" unless he has achieved certain educational requirements (usually a Ph.D. or, in some cases, a master's degree) and has successfully passed a state-administered examination.

As is apparent from the above materials, licensing enables the state to exercise greater control over certain functions than does certification or title licensing. However, outright licensing schemes frequently encounter problems of definition that may hamper their enforcement.

A common adjunct of state regulation is the establishment of a disciplinary system designed to ensure adherence to a professional code of conduct. This function is usually undertaken by an administrative body which has the authority to both promulgate rules of conduct and to conduct disciplinary proceedings where there has been a breach of professional conduct. The agency's governing board and staff usually are composed of members of the regulated profession. This aspect of state regulation is treated in the subsection which follows.

Regulation, whatever its form, is presumably designed to promote some legitimate governmental purpose. The following excerpt summarizes the rationale for occupational regulation noting particularly the ostensible justification for such regulation in the health field:

> Consumer protection is the rationale most commonly advanced as a justification for occupational licensing. In particular it is believed that control of entry and regulation of the practice are necessary to protect consumers from incompetent, dishonest, financially irresponsible, unsafe, and unsanitary provision of various services.
>
> Such a broad consumer protection rationale is incomplete and deficient. First and foremost, government intervention to protect consumers is only necessary when the market fails to perform that

function. A market solution is preferable to an administrative solution unless the latter facilitates the transaction more efficiently than the market. While the market may fail to produce competitive results because the firms engage in anticompetitive conduct or because an industry is not competitively structured, the type of market failure that is particularly relevant here involves that caused by transaction costs. * * * [T]he question is whether consumers of a particular service are able to make informed and intelligent selections of various service providers, free from undue exploitation by the latter. If the market failure is significant, [e.g., because of failure by the industry to provide adequate information or inability of the consumer to comprehend available information], consumers will not be able to make such a selection. Consequently they will have difficulty determining their needs, evaluating the quality of the alternatives or the services rendered, and judging the price and other characteristics of the transaction. Thus the market will not permit consumers quickly to detect and avoid incompetent, fraudulent, or financially irresponsible providers. On the other hand, if there is no significant market failure, a consumer will be able to choose those service providers who, in the mind of the consumer, represent the best combination of high quality service and cost. Such a process will adequately protect consumers from incompetency, dishonesty, and the other problems mentioned above.

Thus in examining occupational licensing the critical question is which types of service transactions are likely to be characterized by sufficient market failure to warrant governmental intervention. In many situations an administrative solution seems unnecessary. For example, in the case of barbers, cosmetologists, funeral homes, taxidermists, driver training schools, private investigators, and probably contractors, architects, and engineers, to name a few, a priori reasoning suggests that the market functions adequately. In fact in such areas it is doubtful that consumers of the services know or care whether the provider is licensed. * * * In some areas it is difficult to generalize, particularly since the nature and sophistication of all consumers are not equivalent. The health field, and perhaps lawyers, present the most difficult questions. Market failure may be more likely in these areas. * * * Moreover one may be influenced by the fact that the potential for serious harm from an incorrect decision is greater in these areas, and by a fear that consumers of these services may be insufficiently risk-adverse. In any event, some licensing seems warranted with doctors, dentists, other providers of health services, and lawyers.

J. Rose, *Occupational Licensing: A Framework For Analysis,* 1979 Arizona State Law Journal 189, 190–192.

While licensing seems to be an established part of the regulatory landscape, a vocal minority contends that licensing is contrary to the public interest. In this connection, consider the merits of the arguments against licensing advanced by one commentator:

* * * Invariably, the rationale advanced for restricting the right to practice is protection of the public. But a strong case can be made

that the only ones really being protected are the professionals themselves. First, psychotherapy is nearly incapable of definition, and regulations invariably encroach on such related fields as education. Second, academic credentials and written examinations are worthless as measures of therapeutic effectiveness. After reviewing the research in this area, David McClelland, a Harvard professor of psychology, has concluded that neither criteria predicts anything but future grades and test scores, no matter what the profession. (Interestingly, by existing prerequisites, giants in the field such as Erik Erikson would never be licensed.)

So licensing does not insure that those practicing are any more competent than those who are not licensed. Not only that, but once licensed, a practitioner need not worry about being disciplined. In 1969, 33 states did not revoke a single physician's license. Fewer than 0.1 percent of all practicing lawyers were disbarred in 1972. When discipline does take place, a study of the New York City Bar found, publicized offenses tend to be punished much more severely than similar, but unpublicized ones, indicating that the professions are more concerned with public image than public protection. Moreover, there are so many negative side effects to licensing that it is hard to imagine when it would be a useful means of regulation: Evidence is accumulating that licensing significantly increases the cost of professional services, decreases the supply of practitioners, inhibits improvements in the organization and delivery of services, stifles innovative training programs, and is discriminatory.

It should be no surprise, then, that many economists and political scientists see in licensing the return of the medieval guilds. The question is whether alternatives exist. Major improvements could obviously be gained by small changes in existing laws. For instance, statutes might only restrict the right to use certain titles while basing the requirements for licensing on competency, not credentials. Such changes, however, don't go far enough. Since we know so little about therapeutic effectiveness, we need regulations that encourage responsible experimentation and diversity, but also protect the public from incompetence and unethical conduct.

All practitioners should be required to register with the state but not to make academic or other credentials a prerequisite to practice. Laws should, however, require therapists to disclose their training and techniques to all clients. An active, powerful and well-financed disciplinary board, a variety of nongovernment certification organizations, and a comprehensive campaign to educate the public are necessary, if this system is to work properly. There are certainly risks involved in this approach, but I believe they are fewer than if we continue on our current path. The fact is that the only sure losers in today's continuing war among the mental-health professions will ultimately be their patients.

Daniel B. Hogan, *Licensing Mental Therapists,* New York Times, July 18, 1979, p. A–23.

Questions and Comments

1. *Questions.* What are the relative advantages and disadvantages of certification and licensing schemes? Which is superior for the regulation of the mental health professions? Why?

2. *Effectiveness of state regulation.* How effective are state licensing and certification laws in protecting the public from non-qualified mental health service providers? Consider in this connection the excerpt from the obituary of L. Ron Hubbard, founder of the Church of Scientology:

> Clients paid Scientology up to $300 an hour for a one-on-one counseling process, known as auditing. To monitor a client's responses to questions, church staff members use an electrical instrument on the client's skin.
>
> The goal of "auditing," which can go on for years and cost clients hundreds of thousands of dollars, is to increase control over thought processes in a portion of the mind where, Scientologists assert, emotional problems and psychosomatic illnesses are born.

New York Times, January 29, 1986, p. 22.

Could licensing laws be applied to prevent the rendering of counseling services by the Church of Scientology? Would there be any First Amendment problems in such regulation?

Despite the fact that approximately three-quarters of states license psychologists, and a violation of the licensing act is usually generally a criminal misdemeanor, very few cases charging unauthorized practice of psychology are ever brought.

3. *Retroactive effect of regulation.* Can newly enacted state licensing and certification statutes operate to exclude established therapists from continuing to provide mental health services? Frequently newly enacted statutes and regulations will include "grandfather clauses," under which persons who do not meet the statutory criteria but who had practiced before the statute took effect nonetheless may be licensed. If grandfather clauses are not provided, does the practitioner have any legal remedies? In *Berger v. Board of Psychologist Examiners,* 521 F.2d 1056 (D.C.Cir.1975), the court found a rather restrictive grandfather clause to be unconstitutional. The clause in question permitted the substitution of a master's degree or 24 credit hours of psychology taken subsequent to a bachelor's degree and seven years practice for a doctorate degree and passage of an examination. Berger, a practicing psychologist for 14 years, received his training through apprenticeships with several psychiatrists. The court found that the statute's irrebuttable presumption of appellant's incompetence to practice psychology violated the Due Process Clause of the Fifth Amendment. The court remanded to the licensing board to determine whether Berger's experience was commensurate with that of licensed psychologists.

4. *Indirect effects of licensing.* State licensing serves not only to provide an imprimatur of competency, but may be a pre-condition to qualifying services rendered by that profession for reimbursement under private health insurance plans. See, *Social Workers Vault Into a Leading Role in Psychotherapy,* New York Times, April 30, 1985, p. 17.

5. *Self regulation by the professions.* In addition to state regulation, each of the major mental health professions has adopted an internal regulatory system which supervises the ethical standards of its members. Most professional organizations, in addition to the educational qualifications required for membership (see section I, supra), have developed and promulgated their own codes of ethics, which frequently influence, at least indirectly, the development of standards applicable to the whole profession. For instance, while psychiatrists, as physicians, must adhere to the ethical standards of the medical profession, the American Psychiatric Association in addition has adopted the American Medical Association *Principles of Medical Ethics With Annotations Especially Applicable to Psychiatry.* Promulgated by the APA Ethics Committee, the annotations are intended to assist psychiatrists in dealing with the "special ethical problems in psychiatric practice that differ in coloring and degrees from ethical problems in other branches of medical practice, even though the basic principles are the same." Forward, *APA Principles of Medical Ethics With Annotations Especially Applicable to Psychiatry* (1986 ed.). Similarly, ethical standards for psychologists and social workers are provided, respectively, by the American Psychological Association's Ethical Principles of Psychologists and the Code of Ethics of the National Association of Social Workers.

The professional organizations also perform a policing function in that they may investigate allegations of a member's misconduct or malpractice. The organization's peer group review committees may censure a member or even withdraw membership upon a finding of misconduct. In addition to individual disciplinary action, these organizations have attempted to take more pervasive measures to solve profession-wide problems. For example, in the face of growing evidence of sexual exploitation of patients by therapists, both the American Psychological Association and the American Psychiatric Association recently have directly addressed the problem. Their efforts are discussed in the following report:

Amid growing concern about psychologists, psychiatrists and social workers who have sex with patients, therapists around the country are devising new strategies to confront a problem they say has been neglected for too long.

Among the efforts is one by a group in Massachusetts, where therapists were jolted into action this spring after a series of reports about colleagues who were disciplined for sexually abusing patients. At the annual meeting of the American Psychological Association in New Orleans last week, the group called for better training and public education, stricter monitoring and harsher punishments. The goal is to end "a conspiracy of silence so we can face the reality of the problem," said Dr. Rina Z. Folman, chairwoman of a panel set up by the Massachusetts Psychological Association to deal with the issue.

* * *

At the psychologists' meeting in New Orleans, Dr. Folman called for the association to require that accredited training programs include a one-year ethics course. Included would be lessons on why even voluntary sexual contact harms patients, how to recognize patients who were abused by another therapist, and how to treat victims and help those who wish to file complaints.

The association's ethics code, which forbids sex between patients and therapists, was recently amended to include a prohibition against teachers' having sex with therapy students. Research shows that therapists who abuse patients often had sexual contact with their teachers.

* * *

In May, the American Psychiatric Association revised its ethics code to bar teacher-student sex. "We had a lot of nasty criticism that we did not have a strong stand," said Dr. McDevitt, the chairman of the association's ethics committee. Although the psychiatrists' association said statistics are not available on how many members it has disciplined, it has started a program to train ethics committees in the state associations to better assist patients and therapists with complaints about abuse.

Susan Diesenhouse, *Therapists Start to Address Damage Done by Therapists,* New York Times, August 20, 1989, p. E5.

6. *Role of professional organizations in the establishment of regulatory standards.* Licensing and certification statutes operate parallel to and independently of the informal, self-disciplinary policies of professional organizations such as the American Psychiatric Association, the American Psychological Association or the Association of Psychiatric Social Workers. In practice, however, governmental regulation is heavily influenced, if not controlled, by members of the regulated professions. The process begins at the state legislature with the drafting of regulatory statutes. State legislators, themselves laymen, are likely to rely on the recommendations of professional organizations concerning the nature and extent of regulation and the type of training and experience prerequisite to professional practice. Often statutes merely establish broadly worded requirements and delegate to an administrative board the duty to develop more specific criteria for licensing or certification. (See, e.g., *Mississippi State Board of Psychological Examiners v. Hosford,* infra, where the state licensing board incorporated in its regulatory standards the ethical standards of the APA). These administrative boards may consist partially or entirely of respected members of the profession in question, and any lay members are likely to defer to the opinions of the professional experts.

Members of the regulated profession are also influential in enforcement. The laws allocate to state administrative agencies the responsibility of reviewing individual applications for licenses or certification, the investigation of charges of professional misconduct, and the conduct of hearings for license revocation or other disciplinary action. These functions are also generally entrusted to special panels or boards operating under the control of the agency. And again, most positions are filled by members of the professions. An agency is likely to judge allegations of professional misconduct in the light of standards of practice and codes of ethics promulgated by professional organizations. Additionally, agencies rely upon the testimony of respected professionals at disciplinary hearings. As a result, the influence of a professional organization may reach well beyond its immediate membership. Because of the active participation and significant influence of the profession's own members, critics contend that government regulation is not an external control, but a form of state-approved self-regulation.

7. *Conflicts of interest.* What problems exist when members of the regulated profession exert influence upon government regulation? Is this the best method to insure protection of the public, or does it tend to pervert a consumer protection scheme into a device to insulate and protect professionals?

C. DISCIPLINE AND SANCTIONS: THE MECHANICS OF REMEDIATION

Although some state legislatures do not delegate the task of defining precise criteria for initial entry into the mental health field, nearly all state laws charge an administrative agency with the task of providing ongoing supervision of members of the regulated profession. For example, a legislature may authorize an agency to investigate complaints of professional misconduct and to impose appropriate sanctions on wrongdoers. Permissible sanctions include license revocation or suspension or the imposition of a fine. In a case of alleged professional misconduct, the accused practitioner is entitled to a hearing on the charges. The primary purpose of that hearing is to provide the accused an opportunity to be heard, to present evidence, and to challenge the testimony of adverse witnesses. The hearing need not be a formal trial before a judge or jury; rather, it is usually relatively informal, conducted by an individual member of a panel or by the full board of the regulatory agency. An accused practitioner has various procedural rights, including the right to prior notice of and to be present at the hearing. While the assistance of legal counsel is usually permitted, it has not been viewed as a constitutional right of an individual facing a disciplinary board. Witnesses may present testimony in an informal narrative fashion, rather than in accordance with rules of evidence at trials.

Despite its informality, a disciplinary hearing must, as a matter of constitutional doctrine, comport with basic notions of fairness. The tribunal must reach a decision of guilt or innocence on the basis of probative evidence, and not on the basis of unsupported allegations or prejudice. Normally, an accused practitioner may obtain judicial review of an adverse agency decision. The scope of review is, however, limited. Typically, a court will confine its inquiry to determining whether the accused received a fair hearing, and whether the tribunal based its decision upon substantial probative evidence and not upon speculation, bias, or other arbitrary factors.

The case set forth below illustrates both the legal issues that are commonly raised in these types of proceedings and the role of courts in reviewing the administrative decisions.

MISSISSIPPI STATE BOARD OF PSYCHOLOGICAL EXAMINERS v. HOSFORD

Supreme Court of Mississippi, 1987.
508 So.2d 1049.

ROBERTSON, JUSTICE, for the Court:

I.

This case presents sensitive questions regarding the authority of a state-created board, charged with the governance of a learned profession, to interpret the canons of ethics of that profession and in accordance therewith to discipline a member of that profession. The case also presents questions regarding the scope of appellate judicial review of such disciplinary action.

Substantially, the case involves a charge that a psychologist disclosed patient confidences without the patient's consent and in violation of his profession's confidentiality principles. The state board found that the violation had occurred and suspended the psychologist's license for ninety days. The Chancery Court reversed. As we regard the action taken within the authority and discretion of the Board, we reverse and reinstate the order of suspension.

II.

A.

Robert L. Hosford, Ph.D., holds a license issued by the Mississippi State Board of Psychological Examiners to engage in the professional practice of psychology in this state. Dr. Hosford maintains his offices in Jackson, Mississippi, and exercises his license by practicing in the field of clinical psychology. Dr. Hosford was the Respondent below and is the Appellee here.

The Mississippi State Board of Psychological Examiners (the Board) has been organized and exists via statutory enactment. Miss.Code Ann. §§ 73–31–5, et seq. (Supp.1980). At all times relevant hereto the Board was authorized and empowered to conduct hearings upon complaints seeking the disciplining of psychologists it has licensed and, where violation be found, to revoke or suspend such license. Miss.Code Ann. §§ 73–31–7(b)(4), (5) and 73–31–21 (1982). The Board is the Appellant here.

This case has its genesis in the psychologist-patient relationship between Dr. Hosford and Patricia F. Lindsey and her former husband, Jimmy G. Lindsey. That relationship came into being on December 31, 1981, when the Lindseys, then husband and wife, consulted Dr. Hosford in his professional capacity and sought counseling and advice regarding difficulties they were experiencing in their marital relationship. These consultations continued for a little over two months. During their course, from time to time Patricia Lindsey would meet with Dr. Hosford privately, at other times Jimmy Lindsey would meet with Dr. Hosford privately, and on still other occasions the Lindseys would jointly consult with Dr. Hosford.

In March of 1982 the Lindseys' marriage was clearly on the rocks as Patricia filed in the Chancery Court of Madison County, Mississippi, an action for divorce. Of immediate concern was the temporary custody of the parties' six-year-old son, Jon D. Lindsey. A temporary custody hearing was scheduled in Chancery Court for March 19, 1982. At that hearing Jimmy Hosford [sic] submitted an affidavit made by Dr. Hosford, dated March 18, 1982, setting forth the background of his professional relationship with the Lindseys and giving his opinion that temporary custody of the child should be placed with his father, Jimmy G. Lindsey. The giving of this affidavit has given rise to the present proceedings.

At some time prior to the temporary hearing Dr. Hosford talked with the attorney representing Jimmy G. Lindsey and furnished certain information to the attorney who then prepared a draft of the proposed affidavit. Dr. Hosford then reviewed the affidavit and made editing changes and corrections. The affidavit was then retyped in final form and was executed by Dr. Hosford on March 18, 1982, in the presence of a notary public.

In relevant part the affidavit states that Dr. Hosford counseled with Patricia Lindsey and Jimmy Lindsey both together and separately concerning their personal relationship as well as their respective relationships with their son; that during the course of these consultations Dr. Hosford reached conclusions regarding the "psychological traits of the parties including those which have a bearing on or relate to their respective concepts of parenthood in general and their respective responsibilities and roles as parents to their child in particular." The affidavit continued, making clear that the opinion to be given was "based upon his [Dr. Hosford's] counseling with the parties, his observations of them. . . ." In the affidavit Dr. Hosford then gave rather specific opinions regarding the parenting skills of the two parties, the details of which need not be recounted, except to say that the opinion of Patricia F. Lindsey was quite unfavorable. In the final analysis, Dr. Hosford gave his "professional opinion that the interest and welfare of the child will be best served and promoted by placing his care, custody and control with Jimmy G. Lindsey,. . . ."

Patricia Lindsey did not consent to the giving of this affidavit. As the point is of some moment, we note the following colloquy between Dr. Hosford and counsel at the hearing before the Board.

Q. Did you ever at any time call Mrs. Lindsey and ask her whether or not it was all right for you to give this affidavit?

A. I did not.

Q. Did Mrs. Lindsey ever authorize you to give this affidavit?

A. She did not.

In the course of her testimony before the Board, Patricia Lindsey read the affidavit and stated that it was based upon information she had given Dr. Hosford in the course of her professional relationship with him and that she had not authorized him to release this information. If we understand the record correctly, Dr. Hosford stipulated before the Board that he "did not receive a signed waiver of the psychologist-patient privilege." [1]

B.

On March 9, 1983, Patricia F. Lindsey filed with the Mississippi State Board of Psychological Examiners a complaint against Dr. Robert L. Hosford wherein she charged Dr. Hosford with unauthorized, unprofessional and illegal disclosure of matters communicated to him and protected from disclosure by the psychologist-patient privilege. The matter came on for hearing before the Board on November 30, 1984. At that hearing Patricia and Dr. Hosford appeared personally and testified. Patricia established her prima facie case as recited above. Dr. Hosford defended on the alternative grounds that he disclosed no matters the confidentiality of which was protected or, in the alternative, that there was a "clear danger" to the child which created an exception to his profession's confidentiality principle and necessitated disclosure.

In due course on January 22, 1985, the Board rendered its final decision finding that Dr. Hosford had violated Principle 5 of the American Psychological Association's Ethical Principles of Psychologists [2] and further that this violation could not be excused under the

---

1. On May 10, 1985, some three and a half months *after* the Board decision suspending his license, Dr. Hosford filed with the Chancery Court a motion to dismiss his appeal and the complaint against him, asserting that "Patricia Lindsey gave her consent for disclosure of any and all communications which may or may not have appeared in the affidavit." This motion was joined by Patricia Lindsey who "affirms all things therein set forth." More will be said of this *post-hearing* consent below.

2. Principle 5, considered by the Board under the authority of Miss.Code Ann. § 73–31–21(a)(1) (1972), reads as follows:

CONFIDENTIALITY

Psychologists have a primary obligation to respect the confidentiality of information obtained from persons in the course of their work as psychologists. They reveal such information to others only with the consent of the person or the person's legal representative, except in those unusual circumstances in which not to do so would result in clear danger to the person or to others. Where appropriate, *psychologists inform their clients of the legal limits of confidentiality.*

a. Information obtained in clinical or consulting relationships, or evaluative data concerning children, students, employees, and others, is discussed only for professional purposes and only with persons clearly concerned with the case. Written and oral reports present only data germane to the purposes of the evaluation, and every effort is made to avoid undue invasion of privacy.

b. Psychologists who present personal information obtained during the course of professional work in writings, lectures, or other public forums either obtain adequate prior consent to do so or adequately disguise all identifying information.

c. Psychologists make provisions for maintaining confidentiality in the storage and disposal of records.

d. When working with minors or other persons who are unable to give voluntary, informed consent, psychologists take special care to protect these persons' best interests. *See* Ethical Princi-

clear danger principle, the Board finding "that the clear danger exception to Principle 5 pertains to only life and death situations." The Board exonerated Dr. Hosford from violation of the Mississippi statutory psychologist-patient privilege. Miss.Code Ann. § 73–31–29 (1972). By reason of Dr. Hosford's violation of APA Principle 5, the Board ordered Dr. Hosford's license to practice psychology in the State of Mississippi suspended for a period of ninety days.

Thereafter Dr. Hosford perfected his appeal to the Chancery Court of the First Judicial District of Hinds County, Mississippi. On the date of the hearing thereof, May 10, 1985, Dr. Hosford presented a motion to dismiss joined by Patricia Lindsey and claimed that the decision of the Board had become moot by virtue of Patricia's withdrawal of her claim. On the same day, apparently on the authority of the aforesaid motion and without examination of the record of proceedings before the Board, [the Chancery Court reversed the Board's decision] and ordered Dr. Hosford's license reinstated and all proceedings pertaining to the matter expunged.

The Board now appeals to this Court and asks reinstatement of its order of suspension.

III.

Dr. Hosford raises a number of premerits points in support of affirmance. First, he argues that the Board, as a quasi-judicial body, has no standing to prosecute this appeal. The point is without merit. A statutorily created board governing the practice of members of a profession in this state, when faced with an adverse decision of a Chancery Court via appellate review of the Board's action regarding one subject to the Board's authority, has clear standing to prosecute a further appeal to this Court. *State Board of Psychological Examiners v. Coxe,* 355 So.2d 669 (Miss.1978) (implicitly recognizing the point); *Mississippi Real Estate Commission v. Ryan,* 241 So.2d 667, 668 (Miss.1970); *Mississippi State Board of Dental Examiners v. Mandell,* 198 Miss. 49, 64, 21 So.2d 405, 498 (1945).

Dr. Hosford next argues that this matter is moot in that Patricia Lindsey has withdrawn her complaint against Dr. Hosford. She couples this with her argument that the Board has no standing to proceed. Patricia sought to withdraw her complaint after final decision by the Board, after that decision had been appealed to the Chancery Court, after she had settled her civil action [3] against Dr. Hosford and after she had recanted her testimony before the Board. In these circumstances, we consider her withdrawal ineffective to preclude the Board from proceeding further.

ples of Psychologists, as printed in *American Psychologist,* Vol. 36, No. 6, pp. 633, 635–36 (June 1981).

3. Although the record is sketchy on this point, apparently Ms. Lindsey had filed suit against Dr. Hosford in Circuit Court. Pursuant to a private settlement in consideration of $9,000.00, Ms. Lindsey executed a release of all claims against Hosford.

The Board's authority in such a context is analogous to that of the State of Mississippi when complaint is made by a citizen that someone has committed a crime. It may well be that as time goes by the complaining party loses interest in the matter or for other reason wishes to withdraw the charge. The State nevertheless has an interest in the prosecution of the accused independent of that of the prosecuting witness, and this interest is reflected in a right vested in the State to go forward with the prosecution notwithstanding the desire or wishes of the complaining party. Even more so where, after conviction and pending appeal, the original complainant wants to "drop the charges."

By the same token the Board of Psychological Examiners has a responsibility that the ethical principles of the psychology profession be respected and, where violations are called to its attention by one such as Patricia Lindsey, the Board has the authority to proceed, notwithstanding the subsequent contrary wishes of the complaining party. The Board's interest and authority are independent of those of the complaining patient. The Board's interest is in the integrity of the profession it regulates and vindication of the ethical principles thereof, to the end that the long range best interests of the consuming public may most effectively be protected. These interests transcend the wishes of a private citizen who may for whatever reason desire that the matter be dropped.

IV.

Another preliminary note. Proceedings seeking suspension or termination of the license of a professional are serious matters. Quite literally one's ability to earn a living is at stake. Balanced against the professional's legitimate self-interest is the interest of the profession and the consumers of its services in honesty, competency and the observance of reasonable ethical principles.

In a variety of contexts we have held that disciplinary charges against a professional must be proved by clear and convincing evidence. [T]his burden of proof rule applies as well to disciplinary proceedings before the State Board of Psychological Examiners.

Board decisions affecting the license of a psychologist are appealable. In such case the Chancery Court sits as an appellate court, as do we. The Chancery Court has no authority to proceed de novo. Rather, review is limited to the record which has been made before the Board. The decision of a professional board in a matter regarding the discipline of one of its members may not be overturned where the decision is supported by substantial evidence. Put otherwise, only where the decision is arbitrary and capricious may a court on appeal intervene.

The Chancery Court violated this premise with regard to the issue of consent. The record before the Board reflects that Patricia Lindsey gave no consent or otherwise waived her right to confidentiality. The Chancery Court, however, found consent, apparently basing this on the post-hearing motion filed by Dr. Hosford. The record before the Board, however, was never supplemented or corrected. Moreover, it appears that the motion joined by Patricia Lindsey withdrawing her complaint was made as a part of a "settlement" with Dr. Hosford. It was made three and a half months after the Board had made its findings that Principle 5 had been violated and after the Board had entered its order of suspension. Such a post-hearing, post-decision consent should not have been considered by the Chancery Court.

We emphasize further the role of the Board. It consisted at the time of six members, five of whom were licensed psychologists. One Board member was a person not a psychologist but who has expressed a continuing interest in the field of psychology. Its members are selected by the governor from a list of nominees submitted by the Mississippi Psychological Association. Ordained by statute, the Board is the keeper of the conscience of those who engage in the professional practice of psychology in this state. From this it follows that the Board be the primary interpretor of the ethical principles to which psychologists in this state are subject.

V.

At all times relevant hereto, the Board had authority to suspend the license of one subject to its jurisdiction where that individual "has violated the current code of ethics of the American Psychological Association." Miss.Code Ann. § 73–31–21(a)(1) (1972). One provision of that code regards patient confidences. Principle 5 of the Ethical Principles of Psychologists requires respect for "the confidentiality of information obtained from persons in the course of their work as psychologists." Only two exceptions to the principle of confidentiality are found. The first, of course, is where the patient consents to the disclosure. In the second, even though no consent be given, the psychologist may disclose otherwise confidential information where "not to do so would result in clear danger to the person or to others."

Having well in mind our limited scope of review in matters such as this, there can be little doubt but that the matters disclosed in Dr. Hosford's affidavit [5] were protected from disclosure by the confidentiality strictures of Principle 5. Indeed, we perceive nothing in this appeal which turns upon disputed facts. All agree what happened. At issue is the Board's authority and the propriety of the sanction it has imposed.

* * *

We are not concerned with the situation where in a court of law there has been a judicial determination that a psychologist should

---

5. The record is not clear whether the Board considered Dr. Hosford's transgression to have been at the point of disclosure of the affidavit to the Chancery Court or at the earlier point of disclosure to Jimmy Lindsey's attorney of the information necessary for preparation of the affidavit. We will proceed here on the assumption that the violation of Principle 5 occurred when the affidavit was filed with the court. Because Dr. Hosford also had a professional relationship with Jimmy Lindsey, he was to some extent empowered to communicate otherwise confidential information to Jimmy's attorney. The ultimate dimensions of this "some extent" need not be addressed as the point was not directly presented below nor is it before us this day.

disclose information and give opinions otherwise privileged. We say this to say that at the very least Dr. Hosford should have refused to make the disclosures until ordered to do so by the Chancery Court of Madison County.

If the disclosure had been made pursuant to a court order—even one that may subsequently have been reversed on appeal—we would not afford judicial sanction to the Board's imposition of a license suspension or other form of discipline. But where, as here, the psychologist proceeded unilaterally, voluntarily, without notice to or consent from his patient, and without prior authorization or direction from the Chancery Court, we hold that on this record the Board was well within its authority in finding there has been a violation of Principle 5.

VI.

By way of defense Dr. Hosford claimed before the Board that the information he disclosed and the opinion he rendered were excluded from Principle 5 by the "clear danger" exception. He renews that claim here. He argues that the welfare and best interest of the Lindseys' six-year-old son overrode the confidentiality principle.

The Board does not have carte blanche authority to say that Principle 5 means anything it wishes. Yet we do not consider it appropriate that we interject ourselves between the Board and Dr. Hosford regarding its interpretation of the clear danger exception. The Board construes the exception narrowly to apply only to cases where "life and limb" were in danger. Dr. Hosford would have us read it more broadly, to cover situations where the best interest[s] of the child are at stake. In the context of this case, the danger at issue is that without the disclosure temporary custody of the child may not be placed with the parent better suited to exercise such custody in the child's best interest. The Board has considered this danger as one not within the scope of the ethical principle.

While today's opinion should not be read as suggesting that we will sanction any reading the Board may give to the language of the APA Ethical Principles, the reading the Board has given these principles in the case at bar is not one that is so arbitrary or unreasonable that we should intervene. It may be true that placement of temporary custody within the wrong parent may result in some emotional or psychological damage to the child. And, indeed, where that issue is presented to a Chancery Court and the issue and facts fully fleshed out, we are by no means prepared to say that the psychologist's lips will be forever sealed by the privilege (although we do not decide that point today as the matter is not before us).[6]

In the context of this record we recognize the Board's authority, in the construction of the clear danger exception to Principle 5, to deter-

---

6. We are aware that there is authority in other jurisdictions that the best interest of the child does override the psychologist- patient privilege in a child custody proceeding. * * *

mine that the requirement of confidentiality is paramount to the danger that temporary custody of the child might be placed with the wrong parent. Put otherwise, it is within the Board's authority, as the keeper of the conscience of the psychologists of this state, to consider the requirement of confidentiality of sufficient strength and importance that the clear danger exception should be read narrowly and limited to cases involving imminent danger to life and limb.

Reversed and Rendered.

Questions and Comments

1. *Questions.* How explicit must ethical standards be before sanctions are applied? Was the ethical principle which the Board found Dr. Hosford had violated drawn clearly enough for Dr. Hosford to know whether or not he could disclose the information be obtained from Mrs. Lindsey? Did he have adequate notice that "the clear danger exception * * * pertains to only life and death situations"?

2. *Hypothetical.* How would you, as an attorney, advise your client, a psychologist, who tells you that one of his patients, while not an abusive parent, fantasizes abusing her child because she does not like the child and does not like parenthood? Would disclosure in the course of a custody proceeding violate Principle 5 of the APA's Ethical Principles of Psychologists? Could such information be subpoenaed by a court under most state laws? For further discussion of confidentiality between patient and therapist, see Chapter 4.

3. *Effectiveness of administrative remediation.* How effective are disciplinary hearings as a remedial device? Is the public interest likely to be adequately protected by hearings conducted and controlled by members of the profession of the accused? Is there any significant risk that leaving the control of discipline to representatives of the profession will lead to policies that are overly protective of the profession and individual practitioners? Any definite answer to these questions is difficult to come by since there have been no systematic studies gauging the efficiency of state disciplinary boards. However, occasionally reported cases suggest that administrative panels controlled by the professions are sometime unduly lax in carrying out their assigned duties. A series of articles in a Florida newspaper, for instance, reported on two cases that received considerable notoriety in the 1970's. One was the case of Dr. Louis Tsavaris, who was charged with the murder of a female patient. Three years later, with the first degree murder charges still pending, Dr. Tsavaris was free on bond and continuing his practice of psychiatry.

The same series also reported the case of Dr. Eduardo Russario, a Florida psychiatrist, who had reportedly impregnated a patient. He later settled a malpractice suit brought by her for $45,000. Subsequently, charges seeking the revocation of Dr. Russario's license were brought before the Florida Board of Medical Examiners. The only sanction imposed by the board was to place Dr. Russario on probation for three years and require that he undergo therapy. Gene Miller, *Sex and the Psychiatrists,* Miami Herald, June 4–7, 1978. According to one commentator, "[t]he series documents the ineffectuality of the state licensing board in enforcing professional standards." Jonas B. Robitscher, *The Powers of Psychiatry* (Boston: Houghton Mifflin, 1980), p. 532.

More recently, however, greater publicity of sexual abuse of patients by physicians and therapists has resulted in more effective action by state disciplinary boards. In Massachusetts, for instance, "[s]ince 1988, the state licensing board has disciplined 25 physicians for sexual misconduct, including at least three psychotherapists, and at least one other has handed in his license." Susan Diesenhouse, *Therapists Start to Address Damage Done by Therapists,* New York Times, August 20, 1989, p. E5.

4. *Regulation of sexual misconduct.* There exists a broad-based professional consensus that sexual relations between a psychotherapist and the patient are likely to be damaging to the patient. Support for this view is provided by studies showing that such "intimacy is damaging to at least 90 percent of the patients involved, sometimes resulting in despondency, loss of motivation, exacerbation of the patient's alcoholism or other drug dependency, hospitalization, and even suicide." *Sex With Therapists Said to Harm Clients,* New York Times, August 29, 1981, p. 7. *See also, Study Examines Adverse Effects of Psychotherapist–Patient Affairs,* New York Times, February 4, 1985, p. 9, col. 1.

Professional recognition of the harms flowing from sexual encounters between therapist and patients finds expression in the canons of ethics of both the American Psychiatric Association and the American Psychologist Association which proscribe intimate relations between therapist and patient. Notwithstanding these injunctions, various studies suggest that sexual misconduct by mental health professionals remains a significant problem. The findings of one study suggests that between five and six percent of male psychotherapists (including psychiatrists, psychologists, and psychiatric social workers) become sexually involved with their patients. In some cases, the therapists were found to have been involved with 20 to 30 patients at a time. *Sex With Therapists Said to Harm Clients,* New York Times, August 29, 1981, p. 7. The magnitude of the problem is also suggested by the incidence of legal actions brought by patients charging their therapist with sexual misconduct. Such actions presently constitute 17 percent of the malpractice actions filed throughout the country. *Study Examines Adverse Effects of Psychotherapist–Patient Affairs,* New York Times, February 4, 1985, p. 9, col. 1. A 1986 survey of psychiatrists found that, of 1,423 respondents, 7 percent of male and 3 percent of female psychiatrists reported having sexual contact with patients. See, *Therapists Start to Address Damage Done by Therapists,* New York Times, August 20, 1989, p. E5.

A variety of legal mechanisms exist which have the potential of discouraging sexual relations between therapist and patient. In states where mental health professionals are licensed, licensing agencies are typically empowered to establish professional standards and impose sanctions in the event that these standards are violated. The effectiveness of this regulatory mode, however, depends very much on the extent to which state licensing agencies are willing to vigorously investigate complaints and impose meaningful legal sanctions. There are seemingly significant differences in the capacity or willingness of different state licensing agencies to deal with this particular problem. (In this connection, compare the reports cited in note 3, supra, with the outcome of some recent disciplinary proceedings in North Carolina. See, *Seven Doctors Disciplined in Sexual Allegations,* Raleigh, N.C., News and Observer, September 8, 1986, p. 18c (license suspensions of psychiatrists who became sexually involved with patients)). In at least one state, California, psychologists who engage in sexual relations with patients may also confront the possibility of criminal sanctions. See, West's Ann.Cal.Bus. & Prof.Code §§ 2960(n) and 2970, which on their face make sexual relations between a psychologist and the patient a criminal offense punishable by imprisonment for up to six months or a fine not exceeding $2,000. However, there is no reported decision applying criminal sanctions to any therapist for having violated this particular provision. But see, *Peer v. Municipal Court of South Bay Jud. Dist.,* 128 Cal.App.3d 733, 180 Cal.Rptr. 137 (1982), where the court found it unnecessary to decide whether such conduct stated a criminal offense under the Business and Professions Code.

The tort system may also deter sexual relations between therapist and patient by exposing the therapist to civil liability for damages. As noted, sexual misconduct accounts for 17 percent of the malpractice actions brought by patients. A number of problems, however, limit the effectiveness of the tort system as a deterrent. For one thing, some patients are deterred from suing by the publicity and exposure of confidential matters that may accompany a law suit. Any patient who sues must disclose not only the details of the sexual relations but also the fact that he or she had been undergoing treatment from a therapist. Beyond this are the costs of a law suit and the uncertainty of damages that will be recovered even if the plaintiff prevails.

The deterrent potential of the tort system may also be limited by the availability of malpractice insurance which tends to shield the therapist from economic loss. However, some insurance programs such as that managed by the American Psychiatric Association have recently eliminated coverage for sexual misconduct, thereby presumably enhancing the deterrent value of the tort system. See, *Study Examines Adverse Effects of Psychotherapist–Patient Affairs,* New York Times, February 4, 1985, p. 9, col. 1.

5. *Regulation and self interest.* Are regulatory boards controlled by the professions they are mandated to regulate capable of formulating policies that would be injurious to the economic interests of the profession in question? In this connection, consider the history of state regulation of professional advertising. The codes of ethics of many professions, including lawyers, pharmacists, physicians, and dentists, at one time prohibited advertising. The restrictions began as the policies of private voluntary professional organizations and found their way into state law or administrative agency regulations. In this way, state agencies with the power of law behind them began to enforce the prohibition on advertising which was previously only imbedded in the professions code of ethics. In 1976, however, the Supreme Court held that these broad restrictions on professional advertising violated the First Amendment. See *Virginia Pharmacy*

Board v. Virginia Consumer Council, 425 U.S. 748, 96 S.Ct. 1817, 48 L.Ed.2d 346 (1976).

6. *Administrative remediation versus the tort system.* What are the advantages, if any, of administratively conducted disciplinary hearings over other remedial actions such as private suits for malpractice or criminal prosecution? To what extent will the monetary costs and other burdens of litigation discourage an injured or aggrieved patient from pursuing his or her private remedies? Are administrative disciplinary proceedings a good substitute? Does the patient obtain relief in this system, even if the disciplinary proceeding results in a sanction against the practitioner?

Note in this connection that one of the possible advantages of disciplinary proceedings is that the patient or witnesses can frequently avoid the publicity that is invariably connected with a public law suit. Under the law of some states, a disciplinary hearing may be closed to the public and the press. Could this be a significant advantage to a complaining witness? To what extent is the accused practitioner prejudiced by a closed hearing if he is represented by counsel?

7. *Limits of regulation.* Are there any limits on the power of a state licensing agency to proscribe certain conduct? For instance, does the First Amendment limit such state authority, and, if so, what is the scope of the limitation? In this connection, consider the following report:

BOSTON, Nov. 21—Four psychologists here are facing the possibility of state disciplinary action because they speculated about the reasons for Kitty Dukakis's depression and alcohol abuse in newspaper interviews.

The State Board of Registration of Psychologists last week sent letters of inquiry to the four raising "questions about the possible violation of the ethical principles of psychologists," the board's chairwoman, Dr. Jessica H. Daniel, said today. The inquiry was first reported today in The Boston Globe.

Dr. Daniel said the board's nine members had decided to open the inquiry "after a lengthy and thorough discussion" of an article published Nov. 10 in The Globe. The article, under the headline "Therapists Speculate About Kitty Dukakis," appeared two days after Mrs. Dukakis's doctor said she had been hospitalized for drinking a small amount of rubbing alcohol at a time when she was depressed, exhausted and showing symptoms of the flu.

The Globe article specified in its third paragraph that the psychologists had "stressed that they could only speculate about the private personalities and interpersonal dynamics of Michael and Kitty Dukakis." The article then quoted them as conjecturing about the Dukakises' relationship as a factor that might have aggravated Mrs. Dukakis's depression.

*   *   *

Dr. Daniel would not say which ethical principles might have been violated when the four offered their conjecture to The Globe.

New York Times, November 22, 1989, p. 11.

Principles 4 and 5 of the APA's Ethical Principles of Psychologists are set forth below:

Principle 4. PUBLIC STATEMENTS. Public statements, announcements of services, advertising, and promotional activities of psychologists serve the purpose of helping the public make informed judgments and choices. Psychologists represent accurately and objectively their professional qualifications, affiliations, and functions, as well as those of the institutions or organizations with which they or the statements may be associated. In public statements providing psychological information or professional opinions or providing information about the availability of psychological products, publications, and services, psychologists base their statements on scientifically acceptable psychological findings and techniques with full recognition of the limits and uncertainties of such evidence.

Principle 5. CONFIDENTIALITY. Psychologists have a primary obligation to respect the confidentiality of information obtained from persons in the course of their work as psychologists. They reveal such information to others only with the consent of the person or the person's legal representative, except in those unusual circumstances in which not to do so would result in clear danger to the person or to others. Where appropriate, psychologists inform their clients of the legal limits of confidentiality.

Is it clear that the conduct being questioned is a violation of these principles? Are there any First Amendment problems in applying these principles to the four psychologists?

8. *Right to counsel.* State law inevitably allows professionals facing disciplinary proceedings before a regulatory agency to have legal representation. The right to have the assistance of counsel is generally discretionary where the disciplinary hearings are conducted through the self-regulation mechanisms of the professional organizations. For example, the American Psychiatric Association's *Recommended Procedures for District Branch Ethics Committee Hearings* provide for notice of the complaint, legal counsel at the discretion of the hearing panel, informal hearing at which both the complainant and the accused may present evidence, non-adversarial questioning by the hearing panel, and a decision based upon a preponderance of the evidence. In addition to creating an atmosphere of fairness to the accused, such procedures may help to reduce the risk of erroneous disciplinary action by the hearing panel, for which the accused may choose to file a civil suit for damages. See, *APA Ethics Newsletter,* Vol. I, No. 3, September 1985.

9. *Violations under federal law.* A psychotherapist's breach of duty may also violate a federal law or regulation. In a somewhat unusual case, the Securities and Exchange Commission charged a psychiatrist who had traded shares based on insider information. The information had been acquired by the therapist in the course of treating a patient who was a senior executive of a company involved in a merger. The psychiatrist, who had been charged under the fraud provisions of the federal securities law, agreed to pay a civil penalty of $27,000 plus any illegal profits he had

earned as a result of the insider training. See, *Insider Trading By Psychiatrist Is Charged By SEC,* Wall Street Journal, March 4, 1986, p. 10.

III. EMERGING ISSUES IN THE ALLOCATION OF FUNCTION AMONG THE MENTAL HEALTH PROFESSIONS

As the Congress moves closer to enacting national health insurance, watch for a conspicuously uncivil war to break out among psychiatrists, psychologists and social workers. At issue is who will be certified and entitled to reimbursement for professional services. Billions of dollars in fees are at stake. So is the quality and range of mental-health care available to the public.

The dispute among the professionals has been warming for more than 25 years, ever since psychologists first began to view themselves as psychotherapists. Sensing a threat, in 1954 the American Psychiatric Association, the American Psychoanalytic Association and the American Medical Association issued a joint resolution opposing any laws that would allow other professional groups to practice psychotherapy independently. They lost. By 1977, having lobbied the state legislatures with remarkable success, psychologists were licensed in all 50 states and the District of Columbia.

Psychiatrists are now attempting to block "freedom-of-choice" laws that allow professionals other than psychiatrists to be reimbursed directly by insurance companies for providing mental-health services. The psychiatrists lost the first few rounds of this skirmish also, but the tide may be turning. In Virginia, for instance, the American Psychiatric Association and two of its district branches successfully defeated a freedom-of-choice bill for social workers. * * *

Daniel B. Hogan, *Licensing Mental Therapists,* New York Times, July 18, 1979, p. A–23.

As indicated by the above excerpt, professional groups are actively attempting to shape state and federal health legislation to protect their own interests. The following cases illustrate the use of federal antitrust laws and state laws regulating hospitals to remove barriers which had traditionally served to restrict the provisioning of mental health treatment services by non-medically trained professionals.

VIRGINIA ACADEMY OF CLINICAL PSYCHOLOGISTS v. BLUE SHIELD OF VIRGINIA

United States Court of Appeals, Fourth Circuit, 1980.
624 F.2d 476.

K.K. HALL, CIRCUIT JUDGE:

This controversy arises over the refusal by defendants Blue Shield of Virginia and Blue Shield of Southwestern Virginia to pay for services rendered by clinical psychologists unless such services are billed through a physician. Plaintiffs Virginia Academy of Clinical Psychologists and Dr. Robert J. Resnick, a practicing clinical psychologist, claim that this policy violates Section 1 of the Sherman Act. 15 U.S.C. § 1. The district court found no violation.

We affirm in part and reverse in part.

Since 1962, Blue Shield of Virginia [BSV or the Richmond Plan] and Blue Shield of Southwestern Virginia [BSSV or the Roanoke Plan] have included outpatient coverage for mental and nervous disorders and for psychotherapy as a method of treating those disorders. Between 1962 and 1972, Richmond Plan coverage included direct payment to psychologists for psychotherapy rendered to subscribers. In 1972, this policy was revised to allow payment only when the services were billed through a physician.

The revised policy of the Richmond Plan was announced after consultation with various provider groups, including the American Psychological Association and the defendant Neuropsychiatric Society of Virginia [NSV]. Contact between the Richmond Plan and NSV, however, was particularly close.

Beginning in 1971, Dr. Levi Hulley, M.D., the head of the Plan's professional relations committee, met several times with NSV's president, Dr. Terrell Wingfield, M.D., over the question of payment for psychotherapy. Cooperation between the two groups followed: NSV, at the Plan's request, conducted a survey of Virginia psychiatrists on various aspects of psychiatric practice and later passed a resolution recommending, inter alia, that the Richmond Plan terminate direct payment to clinical psychologists. Immediately prior to adopting its policy, Richmond Plan officials met with a special NSV committee to discuss the scope of mental health coverage. The Plan adopted some of NSV's recommendations, including that of refusing to cover services rendered by psychologists unless billed by a physician.

* * *

[The court first reversed the district court's holding that the challenged activity was entitled to First Amendment protection. It then rejected the district court's alternative holding that the defendant's agreement was protected by the McCarran–Ferguson Act, which exempts from antitrust liability all state regulated "business of insurance." 15 U.S.C. § 1913(b) (1976)].

The final, critical issue is whether these combinations were "in restraint of trade." 15 U.S.C. § 1. The district court held that under the rule of reason, no violation was established. We disagree.

The district court began: "[t]he starting point in deciding the proper factual context for this case is deciding what sector of the economy is affected. * * * In other words, the court looks to see who is competing with whom." 469 F.Supp. at 560. The court found that clinical psychologists are not equal providers of therapy with psychiatrists because they do not render medical treatment and are not qualified to diagnose nervous and mental disorders or ascertain their source. The court further found that medical necessity in most, if not all cases requires regular contact between the psychologist's patient and a medical doctor.

The district court concluded that the clinical psychologist is not competitive with the psychiatrist unless the clinical psychologist is working under the "supervision" of a medical doctor. A psychologist working with a physician, the court continued, is paid by the Plans on an equal basis with a psychiatrist, except that the psychologist must bill through a physician.

> The court can well understand that plaintiffs do not like to bill through a physician as a matter of professional pride. The evidence shows that billing through a medical doctor is a requirement of the Blue Shield plan as a means of ascertaining that the treatment given and billed for was medically necessary. This procedure also tends to promote contact between the clinical psychologists and the physicians at all stages of treatment, and thus enhances the supervisory process.

469 F.Supp. at 561.

Appellants assert that the evidence establishes a boycott and therefore their exclusion from direct Blue Shield coverage is illegal *per se*. We agree that the challenged policy closely resembles that alleged in *Ballard v. Blue Shield of Southern West Virginia,* 543 F.2d 1075 (4th Cir.1976), which we found to be a boycott. Nor does the comparison necessarily fail because the concerted refusal to deal is conditional, rather than absolute.

The "boycott" characterization, however, avails us little in determining whether an agreement such as this is *per se* illegal. Because of the special considerations involved in the delivery of health services, we are not prepared to apply a *per se* rule of illegality to medical plans which refuse or condition payments to competing or potentially competing providers.

While we agree with the district court's rejection of a *per se* rule in this case, we think the court's analysis was misdirected. The rule of reason looks to the impact of the challenged practice upon competitive conditions.

The district court's finding that "the clinical psychologist is not competitive with the psychiatrist in treating nervous and mental disorders unless the clinical psychologist is working under the supervision of a medical doctor" reflects a value judgment, rather than an evaluation of anticompetitive effects.

The record demonstrates that psychologists and psychiatrists do compete; indeed it is susceptible to judicial notice. Both provide psychotherapy, 469 F.Supp. at 560, and are licensed to do so by State law. Competition in the health care market between psychologist and M.D. providers of psychotherapy is encouraged by the legislature, and its existence is well documented.

The Blue Shield Plans are a dominant source of health care coverage in Virginia. Their decisions as to who will be paid for psychotherapy necessarily dictate, to some extent, which practitioners will be chosen from among those competent under the law to provide such services.

Whether the "medical necessity" of referral and close contact between the therapist and a physician satisfies the rule of reason, as a cost control measure, is a matter not before us. The Plan's requirement that the psychologists' fee be billed through a physician, however, cannot stand.

The issue is more than one of professional pride. State law recognizes the psychologist as an independent economic entity as it does the physician. The Blue Shield policy forces the two independent economic entities to act as one, with the necessary result of diminished competition in the health care field. The subscriber who has a need for psychotherapy must choose a psychologist who will work as an employee of a physician; a psychologist who maintains his economic independence may well lose his patient. In either case, the psychologist ceases to be a competitor.

* * * [W]e are not inclined to condone anticompetitive conduct upon an incantation of "good medical practice." Moreover, we fail to see how the policy in question fulfills that goal. Any assertion that a physician must actually *supervise* the psychologist to assure the quality of the psychotherapy treatment administered is refuted by the policy itself. The Blue Shield policy provides for payment to psychologists for psychotherapy if billed through *any* physician—not just those who regularly treat mental and nervous disorders. It defies logic to assume that the average family practitioner can supervise a licensed psychologist in psychotherapy, and there is no basis in the record for such an assumption.

There are, of course, procompetitive reasons for requiring examination and consultation by a physician in order to assure that psychotherapy is not needlessly performed to treat a problem with physical etiology, but such safeguards must be accomplished in ways which do not sacrifice the economic independence of the psychologist.

The elimination of the bill-through provision does not preclude a variety of other cost control and quality control measures by Blue Shield. It does, however, expand consumer and provider alternatives. In addition, competition from licensed non-M.D. providers is likely to result in lower costs and the elimination of needless duplication of administrative costs created by the bill-through requirement.

Affirmed in Part, Vacated and Remanded in Part.

Comments

1. *Comment.* The *Blue Shield of Virginia* case illustrates the use of the federal antitrust laws to prevent insurance companies from limiting coverage and reimbursement for psychotherapy unless the services were rendered under the aegis of a licensed physician. However, because the rule applied in the *Blue Shield of Virginia* case stems from the antitrust laws, a violation occurs only when the insurance carrier's policy is the product of an agreement by the carrier with another entity. Thus, the decision would not preclude an individual company from unilaterally

adopting a policy limiting reimbursement for clinical services performed under the supervision of a psychiatrist unless such restrictions are prohibited by state law (*See,* Note 2 infra.)

2. *Freedom of choice laws.* A number of states have adopted what are known as freedom of choice laws [FOC]. These laws limit the authority of private insurance companies to condition reimbursement for psychotherapy to services that are prescribed and billed through a physician. A recent report summarizes current trends:

> 40 states now have "freedom of choice" laws that require insurance companies to reimburse psychologists for therapy if patients prefer them to psychiatrists. The psychological association is lobbying for similar laws in those states that do not have such laws.

> Social workers are following in the psychologists' footsteps, but are meeting with more opposition, both from insurance companies and psychiatrists. Social work associations have managed to get laws passed in 35 states licensing social workers, but have persuaded only 14 to pass laws requiring insurers to reimburse social workers for psychotherapy.

> New York is one place that recently passed a law requiring insurance companies to reimburse social workers for therapy; psychiatrists opposed the law. "One reason the New York State Psychiatric Association opposed the law," said Edward Hanin, vice president of the association, "is that there is only a limited pool of insurance money available for treating people with mental disorders. Insurance coverage for treating mental illness is generally horrendous, relative to other disorders. In expanding coverage to groups like social workers, who treat patients who are less seriously ill, it would dilute what is available to those who have more serious need for treatment."

> Marriage and family counselors have managed to get state licensing or certification in only nine states, including New Jersey and Connecticut. Just one of these states, California, requires insurance companies to reimburse them for therapy. "Similar laws in other states have been opposed by both psychiatrists and psychologists," said Richard Leslie, legal counsel for the California association of marriage and family counselors.

Social Workers Vault Into a Leading Role in Psychotherapy, New York Times, April 30, 1985, p. 17, col. 5.

CALIFORNIA ASSOCIATION OF PSYCHOLOGY PROVIDERS v. RANK

201 Cal.App.3d 987, 247 Cal.Rptr. 641, 1988.
Court of Appeal, Second District, 1988.

DANIELSON, ASSOCIATE JUSTICE.

California Hospital Association, California Medical Association, California Psychiatric Association, Barton J. Blinder, M.D., William H. Boyd, M.D., Thomas K. Ciesla, M.D., Edward H. Liston, M.D., and Charles W. Portney, M.D., ("movants") appeal from:

(1) the summary judgment dated January 17, 1986, in favor of plaintiffs the California Association of Psychology Providers, Stuart Wilson, Ph.D., Stephen Edward Berger, Ph.D., Lawrence N. Blum, Ph. D., Gary E. Bodner, Ph.D., Corey Douglas Fox, Ph.D., A. Steven Frankel, Ph.D., Lisa Pomeroy, Ph.D., Carlton W. Purviance, Ph.D. ("the plaintiffs"), and against defendants Peter Rank, Director of the California Department of Health Services, the Department of Health Services ("DHS"), Jesse Huff, Acting Director of the California Department of Finance, and the Department of Finance ("the defendants"); and

(2) an order dated April 11, 1986, in favor of plaintiffs and against movants.

QUESTION PRESENTED

Does Health and Safety Code section 1316.5 ("section 1316.5") compel health facilities to allow their appointed clinical psychologists to render services without physician supervision?

FACTUAL AND PROCEDURAL STATEMENT

On June 20, 1984, plaintiffs filed a "Complaint For Writ Of Mandate, Injunctive Relief, And Declaratory Relief" pleading seven causes of action.

* * *

They challenged those regulations, which required a psychiatrist to be responsible for the diagnosis and treatment of all patients, on the ground such requirement unlawfully discriminated against clinical psychologists in violation of section 1316.5, which empowers a clinical psychologist to provide psychological services within the scope of their licensure without discrimination.

* * *

Following a hearing on July 30, 1985, the court granted plaintiffs' motion for summary judgment on the seventh cause of action.

In the summary judgment filed January 17, 1986, the court declared: The provision of psychological services by a psychologist referred to in section 1316.5 "includes ultimate responsibility for the psychological care of hospitalized patients and authority to admit and discharge patients provided that a physician shall be responsible for the necessary medical care of patients including completion of a physical examination upon admission of each patient."

The court further declared that sections 70577(d)(1) and 71203(a)(1) (A), as written and in effect on July 30, 1985, were invalid, as conflicting with section 1316.5, for the reasons that those regulations prohibited psychologists from independently (1) admitting patients to health facilities and (2) diagnosing and treating patients within the scope of psychology licensure.

The court ordered DHS to amend sections 70577(d)(1) and 71203(a) (1)(A) to provide: "Psychiatrists or clinical psychologists within the scope of their licensure and subject to the rules of the facility shall be responsible for the diagnostic formulation for their patients and the development and implementation of each patient's treatment plan."

On March 21, 1986, the movants, as aggrieved parties, filed a motion to set aside and vacate the judgment filed on January 17, 1986, and to enter another and different judgment, i.e., that sections 70577(d) (1) and 71203(a)(1)(A), as written and in effect on July 30, 1985, were valid and did not conflict with section 1316.5.

* * *

DISCUSSION

I. Does Section 1316.5 Compel Health Facilities To Allow Their Clinical Psychologists To Render Services Without Physician Supervision?

Movants argue that nothing in section 1316.5 requires a health facility, specifically, a general acute care hospital or an acute psychiatric hospital, to allow clinical psychologists to admit patients or to diagnose and treat patients without the supervision of a physician. They further urge that the trial court erred in construing section 1316.5 to mandate that requirement.

From our review of the applicable law and legislative history of section 1316.5, we conclude that movants are partially correct. The thrust of section 1316.5 is to ensure to clinical psychologists having patients in health facilities the right to practice their profession without discrimination. On the other hand, section 1316.5 does not authorize clinical psychologists to perform health services which are beyond "the scope of their licensure".

Pursuant to section 1316.5 clinical psychologists [7] are authorized to "hold membership and serve on committees of the medical staff and carry professional responsibilities consistent with the scope of their licensure and their competence, subject to the rules of the health facilities." The key phrase is "consistent with the scope of their licensure". Section 1316.5 further provides: "If a health service is offered by a health facility with both licensed physicians and surgeons ['physicians'] and clinical psychologists on the medical staff, which both licensed physicians . . . and clinical psychologists are authorized by law to perform, such service may be performed by either, without discrimination." The key phrase here is "which [service] both . . . are authorized by law to perform."

In order to determine the parameters of section 1316.5 we ascertain the meaning of those phrases. To accomplish this we must first define

---

7. " 'Clinical psychologist,' as used in this section, means a psychologist licensed by this state and (1) who possesses an earned doctorate degree in psychology from an educational institution meeting the criteria of subdivision (c) of Section 2914 of the Business and Professions Code and (2) has not less than two years clinical experience in a multidisciplinary facility licensed or operated by this or another state or by the United States to provide health care, or, is listed in the latest edition of the National Register of Health Service Providers in Psychology, as adopted by the Council for the National Register of Health Service Providers in Psychology." (§ 1316.5, subd. (c).)

certain operative words, i.e., "psychologist", "psychology", "psychiatrist", "psychiatry", "diagnose" and "diagnosis".

A "psychologist", which term includes a "clinical psychologist", is an individual who holds a license to practice psychology pursuant to the "Psychology Licensing Law" (Bus. & Prof.Code, § 2900 et seq.).

"The practice of psychology is defined as rendering or offering to render . . . any psychological service involving the application of psychological principles, methods, and procedures of understanding, predicting, and influencing behavior, such as the principles pertaining to learning, perception, motivation, emotions, and interpersonal relationships; and the methods and procedures of interviewing, counseling, psychotherapy, behavior modification, and hypnosis; and of constructing, administering, and interpreting tests of mental abilities, aptitudes, interests, attitudes, personality characteristics, emotions, and motivations. [¶] The application of such principles and methods includes, but is not restricted to: diagnosis, prevention, treatment, and amelioration of psychological problems and emotional and mental disorders of individuals and groups. [¶] Psychotherapy . . . means the use of psychological methods in a professional relationship to assist a person or persons to acquire greater human effectiveness or to modify feelings, conditions, attitudes and behavior which are emotionally, intellectually, or socially ineffectual or maladjustive." (§ 2903.)

The above definition of the practice of psychology controls despite any existing statute to the contrary. (§ 2905.)

On the other hand, "[t]he practice of psychology shall not include prescribing drugs, performing surgery or administering electro-convulsive therapy." (§ 2904.)

Psychologists must be distinguished from psychiatrists. (See *California State Psychological Assn. v. County of San Diego* (1983) 148 Cal. App.3d 849, 853, 198 Cal.Rptr. 1.) A "psychiatrist" is "[a] physician especially learned in psychiatry". (3 Schmidt, Attorney's Dictionary of Medicine and Word Finder (1988) p. P–361; see also, 22 CAC, § 71053, subd. (16).) "Psychiatry" is "[t]he branch of medicine dealing with disorders of the mind, emotions, and mental life, including conscious, subconscious, and unconscious manifestations." (3 Schmidt, Attorney's Dictionary of Medicine and Word Finder (1988) p. P–361.) Unlike psychologists, psychiatrists are authorized "to use drugs or devices in or upon human beings and to sever or penetrate the tissues of human beings and to use any and all methods in the treatment of diseases, injuries, deformities, and other physical and mental conditions." (§ 2051.)

Although section 2903 authorizes a psychologist to diagnose psychological problems and emotional and mental disorders, the words "diagnose" and "diagnosis" are not statutorily defined in that context. With regard to physicians, however, section 2038 defines the words "diagnose" and "diagnosis" to "include any undertaking by any method, device, or procedure whatsoever, . . . to ascertain or establish whether a person is suffering from any physical or mental disorder. . . ."

Given the broader scope of authority accorded physicians, we conclude that the above definition cannot be applied to a psychologist. We hold, instead, that the words "diagnose" and "diagnosis" when referring to a psychologist mean any undertaking to ascertain or establish whether a person is suffering from a mental disorder discoverable by any method or procedure consistent with a psychologist's licensure.

From the above it is clear that while a physician's function may encompass the practice of psychology (see § 2908), the converse is not true, i.e., a psychologist may not practice medicine. It is this distinction and difference which lies at the heart of the issue.

Only a physician is authorized to render a diagnosis concerning a mental disorder organic in origin or nature. Similarly, to the extent that a mental disorder is susceptible to treatment by drugs, surgery, or electro-convulsive therapy only a physician is authorized to create and implement such a treatment plan therefor. Psychologists cannot make a medical diagnosis or devise and implement a treatment plan utilizing such means since those matters are not "consistent with the scope of their licensure". A gap in patient care arises if a physician does not have the initial and ultimate responsibility for a patient suffering from a mental disorder under those circumstances. If the psychologist were accorded unfettered discretion to admit his or her patient to the health facility and to implement a nonmedical treatment based on a nonmedical diagnosis without the supervision of a physician, then the patient's health may be at risk. Such was not the Legislature's intent.

We further hold the Legislature intended to require health facilities to allow their appointed clinical psychologists the right to diagnose and treat their patients without interference or hindrance from a physician only in those instances where a physician has initially ruled out a medical basis for the patient's mental disorder and determined that it is not subject to medical treatment, and where the patient's mental disorder does not subsequently become susceptible to medical treatment after admission to the health facility. Under such circumstances the functions of the psychologist and physician become coextensive in that either would be authorized to practice psychology. In the words of section 1316.5 this would be a service "which both [physicians] and clinical psychologists are authorized by law to perform, [which] service may be performed by either without discrimination." On the other hand, to require the patient to be diagnosed and treated by a psychiatrist, or the psychologist to be supervised by a psychiatrist, after a medical diagnosis and medical treatment have been ruled out, would constitute the discrimination against the psychologist as proscribed by the Legislature.

II. *Order Denying Motion to Vacate the Judgment*

* * *

Based on our above analysis on the merits of movants' position we remand this cause with directions to the trial court to reverse the summary judgment and enter a new judgment embodying the views set forth in this opinion.

This disposition obviates the need to address movants' contentions concerning the judgment itself.

Questions and Comments

1. *Restrictive practices in education.* Challenges to the dominance of the medically trained therapist have also been pressed in the field of education. For instance, psychoanalytic institutes which are the primary training base for psychoanalysts had traditionally excluded non-medically trained applicants. Thus, training institutes would normally only accept applicants who had already had a psychiatric residency. In 1985 a group of non-physician mental health professionals brought suit against the American Psychoanalytic Association [APA], challenging on antitrust grounds their exclusion from affiliated training institutes. *Bryant Welch, Ph.D. et al. v. American Psychoanalytic Association* et al., No. 85–1651 (S.D.N.Y. filed 3/1/85). The case was settled before trial under an agreement reached by the parties in which the APA agreed to admit non-physicians into the association's training institutes. As noted in the commentary which follows, the result in *Welch v. APA* was applauded not only by psychologists but also by other non-medical mental health professionals.

To the Editor:

Millions of Americans have undergone, or will undergo, psychoanalysis. All of us, therefore, should applaud the legal settlement of a lawsuit brought by four psychologists against the American Psychoanalytic Association and the International Psychoanalytical Association to get them to open the doors of their major training institutes to therapists who do not hold medical degrees (Health pages, Oct. 20).

Before this case, the American Psychoanalytic Association and the International Psychoanalytical Association restricted admission to their training institutes to psychiatrists, barring clinical social workers, psychologists and other mental-health professionals who are not psychiatrists. This policy disregarded the basic reality that nonmedical therapists now perform most of this country's therapy.

That this is so was documented in a May 1, 1985 article, according to which the number of social workers offering psychotherapy in the United States more than doubled between 1975 and 1985, rising from 25,000 to 60,000. During the same period, the number of clinical psychologists doubled from 15,000 to slightly more than 30,000. In comparison, the total number of psychiatrists increased by only one-third, from 26,000 to 38,000.

In addition, as your report on the successful suit noted, competent provision of psychotherapy and psychoanalysis does not require medical training. In the event that a client needs drug therapy or other medical care, he or she can be referred to a psychiatrist or other physician for treatment.

That clinical social workers and psychologists can now attend American Psychoanalytic and International Psychoanalytical Association institutes is not a crucial victory. They have long studied side by side with psychiatrists in the many psychoanalytical institutes that are not affiliated with those organizations. It is, however, a gain for simple fairness. The majority of this country's therapists will no longer be subject to arbitrary restrictions on their training.

ROBERT J. EVANS
New York, Oct. 28, 1988

The writer is president of the New York State Society of Clinical Social Work Psychotherapists.

New York Times, November 12, 1988, p. 14.

2. *Perspectives on the allocation of responsibility in out-patient settings.* The result of the *Welch* case settlement discussed in Note 1 is to legitimize non-medically trained professionals as independent providers of mental health treatment service. To what extent are the concerns which caused the court in *California Association of Psychology Providers v. Rank,* supra, to grant physicians or psychiatrists rather than psychologists the exclusive authority to hospitalize and diagnose patients relevant in allocating diagnostic and treatment responsibility in an outpatient setting?

Should the answer turn on the frequency with which mental disorders are associated with *organic* causes? Similarly, is the fact that non-medical therapists cannot prescribe psychotropic medication a relevant factor in allocating diagnostic or treatment responsibility?

In connection with these questions consider the following commentaries:

To the Editor:

The growth of lay psychotherapy in the United States ("Social Workers Vault Into a Leading Role in Psychotherapy" by Daniel Goleman, Science Times, April 30) threatens to denude the country of its only wholly qualified line of defense against mental and emotional illness: the physician trained both in biological and psychodynamic psychiatry. Behind this growth are historical, economic and social reasons.

For decades, social workers, psychologists, nurses and others were brought into the herculean task of dealing with mental illness in hospitals and outpatient clinics. All originally had other tasks, but were permitted, under supervision, to assume some treatment with certain patients. They were essentially "barefoot doctors" in this struggle.

The development of Medicaid and Medicare furthered the process. It became very profitable for hospitals and clinics to use salaried nonmedical personnel to treat patients, since the hourly rates for reimbursement were identical whether treatment was by physician-psychiatrists or others.

Many of these barefoot doctors jumped to the erroneous conclusion that they were fully competent to do what they had been encouraged to do in an emergency, and now present themselves as independent practitioners capable of treating all patients for all conditions. They left salaried positions, where there was at least a semblance of medical and psychiatric supervision, for the marketplace.

They are often either unaware, or will deny, that they lack the essential medical and psychiatric training that is the only basis for diagnosis and treatment. The result is malpractice.

Depression, for instance, is not diagnosed or is misdiagnosed, and the wrong kind of treatment is then prescribed; a patient is given psychotherapy for a type of phobia that responds well to other treatment; physical symptoms are misinterpreted as "psychosomatic." Since patients rarely complain or sue, this has not caught the public attention.

A preliminary physical examination by a physician; getting a psychiatrist or general physician who will agree to "cover" by prescribing antianxiety or antidepressant medication; "supervision" of cases by a psychiatrist—none of these suffice to prevent serious errors of diagnosis and treatment by a lay therapist in independent private practice. Every patient is, in effect, unwittingly playing Russian roulette. And fees by all who entered the market have risen quickly to a common level.

Psychiatrists are not blameless. Heads of department are reluctant to antagonize professional blocs within their administrations. * * * Absence of criticism has emboldened lay therapists.

The extent to which they are emboldened is indicated by lawsuits entered or pending against the American Psychoanalytic Association and the American Academy of Psychoanalysis, major educational bodies that train physician-psychiatrists. The suits seek to force these organizations to train nonphysicians. The suits will not be won because these organizations have the right to set the standards they consider proper for the public health, but the suits will affect public opinion and serve to harass those organizations.

Will the barefoot doctors drive out the doctors? Will treatment of mental and emotional illness sink to the lowest common denominator? Since anyone can claim competence, is it likely, by a Gresham's Law, that there will be no truly competent medical specialists to treat mental or emotional illness? The implication for the public health is not good.

SEYMOUR C. POST, M.D.
Assoc. Clinical Professor of
Psychiatry
College of Physicians and
Surgeons of Columbia University
New York, May 15, 1985

New York Times, May 19, 1985, p. 20, col. 3.

To the Editor:

Dr. Seymour C. Post's letter ("And Now the Age of the Barefoot Psychotherapist," May 19), in response to Daniel Goleman's article on the growing psychotherapeutic role of social workers (Science Times, April 30) was, sadly, further evidence of the elitist attitude American psychiatry has toward the treatment of mental illness. One need only look at the shrinking therapy dollar in terms of third-party unwillingness to underwrite lengthy treatment to understand American Psychiatric Association rationalizations for its "closed-shop" attitude.

Dr. Post's choice of the "barefoot doctor" metaphor is interesting in light of differences in medical versus graduate training within psychology. While most medical schools offer a four- to six-week course in behavioral science in addition to several weeks' rotation through a psychiatric unit, graduate programs in clinical and service-oriented psychology provide four years of academic and specialized training in psychopathology and its treatment in addition to a year's internship, usually in a hospital or an outpatient setting.

While a newly graduated physician entering a psychiatric residency knows little about psychopathology, a newly graduated psychologist already possesses specialized graduate training. It is common practice in many medical centers for psychologists to participate in the training of psychiatry residents.

Dr. Post does, however, have a valid point in emphasizing that a medical background is necessary in dealing with specific psychiatric disorders. Most psychologists would agree that there are subgroups of psychiatric disorders that require medication. Despite this, there are psychological disorders that do not require medication and that respond favorably to drug-free psychotherapy. Since most hospital-based staff psychiatrists rarely carry regular therapy cases within the hospital, a task usually relegated to psychologists, it is difficult not to wonder who the most experienced and specialized individual is.

Let us propose a truce, with medication issues and medically oriented diagnoses within the purview of psychiatry and behavioral psychodiagnostics and psychotherapy as the domain of psychologists and others licensed to practice. "The implication for the public health," of which Dr. Post speaks, is certainly "not good," given the unfortunate animosity these fields have toward one another, and taking potshots at each other is not conducive to the cooperation necessary to provide quality mental-health care.

PAUL MICHAEL RAMIREZ
Clinical Neuropsychologist
Bronx Psychiatric Center
Bronx, May 21, 1985

New York Times, May 29, 1985, p. 20, col. 3.

Chapter Two

NEGLIGENCE AND ALTERNATIVE THEORIES

I. INTRODUCTION

As noted in Chapter One, the public interest in protecting the mental health service consumers has led to a system of state regulation that seeks to ensure the quality of services by limiting entry into the various mental health fields to those who meet certain minimum qualifications. The emphasis of this approach is prospective in the sense that prevention of injury is the main objective. In contrast, the legal system has established a regulatory scheme which is remedial in nature. Its emphasis is on furnishing those injured by substandard professional care with opportunities for obtaining judicial relief. All claims of this nature fall within the general rubric of malpractice suits. The term "malpractice" is something of a catchall, and encompasses all

61

actions for substandard professional care regardless of the specific doctrinal basis of the claim.   Private actions for malpractice may be based on any of several legal grounds.   Most actions are grounded in the negligence doctrine, but some malpractice claims rest on the intentional tort doctrines of assault and battery, invasion of privacy, or breach of confidentiality.   Additionally, occasional malpractice suits are based entirely on principles of contract law.

Malpractice suits against mental health professionals are still fairly uncommon.   As a group, psychiatrists are involved in significantly less litigation than other groups of medical specialists.   Indeed, psychiatric claims accounted for only 0.3% of the malpractice claims filed with California malpractice insurers between 1974 and 1978. Slawson and Guggenheim, *Psychiatric Malpractice: A Review of the National Loss Experience,* 141 Am.J.Psychiatry, 979 (1984).

A number of factors account for the relative paucity of malpractice actions against mental health professionals.   A major reason may be the lack of professional consensus as to the limits of proper mental health treatment.   Additionally, even when psychotherapy is improperly rendered, it is unlikely to result in visible physical injuries.   Thus, in some jurisdictions, particularly those restricting recovery for mental suffering to physical contact situations, the potential claimant may face substantial difficulties in proving that injury did in fact occur.   In addition, when the alleged injury is psychological in nature, claimants may find it difficult to prove that the therapist's malfeasance, or nonfeasance, and not their pre-existing mental condition, was the cause of their injuries.   Moreover, many former psychiatric patients undoubtedly choose to avoid litigation rather than face public disclosure of the fact that they have undergone treatment.

While these factors appear to have deterred lawsuits in the past, there are indications that the relative immunity enjoyed by mental health professionals over the years may be ending.   For instance, a review of recent case law reveals that psychiatrists are no longer the only mental health professionals being charged with malpractice.   The majority of malpractice suits involve psychiatrists, but patients and clients are suing their former psychologists and social workers with increasing frequency.   For instance, courts and juries have become more willing to assign liability when therapists have breached their duty of trust by engaging in sexual intimacies with patients.   These cases have significantly broadened the bases of malpractice liability to allow recovery in cases involving only psychological injury.   Additionally, changes in legal doctrines in some jurisdictions have expanded the class of persons to whom a therapist owes a duty of care.   Recent cases have imposed on the therapist a duty of care to persons other than those with whom he has established a professional relationship.   The scope of this doctrine and its impact on the mental health profession will be explored more fully in section II of this chapter.

The materials which follow explore the various theories available to injured patients. Part A focuses on the doctrine of negligence as a basis for recovery by a patient who has received substandard professional care. Recovery of damages based on contractual theories is considered in Part B. Malpractice cases alleging invasion of privacy or breach of confidentiality are considered in the chapter dealing with confidentiality and the testimonial privilege, and the doctrine of informed consent, which has developed as a separate theory of recovery, is dealt with in Chapter Three.

Comments

1. *Drugs and psychiatric malpractice.* The three most common claims in psychiatric malpractice suits have been mistakes in diagnosis, improper treatment, and drug reactions. Perr, *Psychiatric Malpractice Issues,* in S. Rabkin (Ed.) Legal Encroachment on Psychiatric Practice, New Dimensions for Mental Health Services, no. 25, (San Francisco: Jossey–Bass, March 1985) p. 47. The rising use of drugs which affect mood or behavior makes increasingly likely suits related to adverse drug reactions. The serious side effects associated with the prolonged use of anti-psychotic medication can be expected to lead to an increasing number of malpractice actions against psychiatrists and psychiatric institutions. This trend may, in fact, have already begun.

For instance, in *Clites v. Iowa,* 322 N.W.2d 917 (Iowa App.1982), the appeals court affirmed an award of $760,000 where a mentally retarded patient had developed tardive dyskinesia following six years of the administration of anti-psychotic medication; "Tardive dyskinesia is a mild to severe disorder consequent to the long term use of certain medications. Its occurrence does not reflect negligence, because it frequently occurs without negligence. * * * Therefore, from the standpoint of negligence law, its presence should generally not be a successful basis for a lawsuit." Perr, *Psychiatric Malpractice Issues* at 55. For an intensive discussion of tardive dyskinesia, see Taub, *Tardive Dyskinesia: Medical Facts and Legal Fiction,* 30 St. Louis U.L.J. 833, 839–843 (1982).

2. *Effects on insurance costs.* The increase in psychiatric malpractice claims in recent years has been accompanied by increased malpractice insurance costs. In 1972 when the American Psychiatric Association initiated its insurance program, a policy with limits of $1,000,000 cost $744 in California and $64 in New Hampshire. In 1976 the same coverage had risen to $228 in New Hampshire and an average of $3,000 in California. Trent, *Psychiatric Malpractice and Its Problems: An Overview* in Barton and Sanborn, Law and the Mental Health Professions (New York: International Universities Press, 1978), p. 101. Since psychiatrists are generally grouped together with general practitioners as a risk category, the increase in premiums over the four year period does not necessarily reflect the actual claims experience of the psychiatric profession. Id. at 111.

II. CLAIMS BASED ON NEGLIGENCE

A. THE DOCTRINE: AN OVERVIEW

The unique characteristics of a therapist's work pose a particular challenge to legal institutions when the quality of the services rendered must be judged. For one thing, psychiatry has been described as both a science, requiring technical skills, and an art, dependent upon the personal relationship between the psychiatrist and his patient. In addition, even experts frequently have difficulty in assessing whether the therapy has been successful. The changes in the patient may be so subtle as to be imperceptible. Moreover, it is sometimes difficult to attribute a particular outcome, be it negative or positive, to the therapeutic intervention.

In spite of these complications, decisions as to the quality of care which was rendered in a particular instance cannot be avoided. The doctrinal framework under which these claims are measured is the law of negligence. In general terms this means that any professional who renders services has a legal duty to perform his professional functions in a manner comporting with the skill and technical proficiency normally exercised by other professionals in the same field. A professional's failure to meet this legal standard when rendering services establishes the key element of a claim of negligence. But to be successful in a law suit a patient-plaintiff must be able to prove more than that the services were of substandard quality. In fact, negligence has at least four distinct elements, each of which must be established by the plaintiff. These elements have been described in the following terms by one noted commentator:

1. A duty, or obligation, recognized by the law, requiring the person to conform to a certain standard of conduct, for the protection of others against unreasonable risks.

2. A failure on the person's part to conform to the standard required: a breach of the duty. * * *

3. A reasonably close causal connection between the conduct and the resulting injury. * * *

4. Actual loss or damage resulting to the interests of another. Prosser and Keeton, On the Law of Torts, § 30 (5th ed., 1984).

The application of these elements to real cases in the face of a technologically changing society remains one of the major challenges faced by the legal system. In the mental health field it is not only the availability of new technologies, e.g., psychotropic medication, but changes in public policy, such as the emphasis on institutionalization, that complicates the development of coherent legal standards. Nevertheless, it is in this context that courts are being called upon to shape and apply the professional negligence standards. The following materials explore the special problem raised in the adjudication of malpractice claims against mental health professionals.

Comments

1. *Liability to third parties.* A threshold question in any case alleging professional negligence is whether the injured party is a member of the class of persons legally protected under the law of negligence. Traditionally, the answer to this question was relatively clear cut. No duty of care was owed except to those with whom the professional had established a contractual relationship. Thus, if the plaintiff had not been the professional's client, the case was dismissed, unless the plaintiff alleged more than mere negligence. However, the existence of a professional relationship, establishing what is called privity between the patient-claimant and therapist-defendant, is no longer the dispositive factor in professional negligence cases. An increasing number of jurisdictions have modified or repudiated the privity doctrine. The circumstances under which a therapist may be held liable to persons with whom he has no professional relationship are elaborated in subsection C, infra. Even under the contemporary expansive view, the presence of a contractual relationship may make it easier for a plaintiff to prevail in his claim. Thus, privity continues to be a significant factor in any action that alleges professional negligence.

2. *Third party liability for diagnostic functions carried out at request of third party.* A related question concerns the liability of a therapist for negligence when he or she is performing a diagnostic service at the request of a third party. Here the individual being evaluated is not technically a patient for purposes of treatment and is not in contractual privity with the therapist. This situation arises most commonly in the employment context when an employer requires an employee or an applicant for employment to submit to a psychological evaluation. May the clinician or physician be held liable to the employee if he is negligent in carrying out the diagnostic evaluation and, consequently, misdiagnoses the employee's condition? See, *Hoesl v. United States of America and Dr. David Allen Kasuboski,* 629 F.2d 586 (9th Cir.1980) (where the court did not reach the claim of negligence but held that misdiagnosis was actionable as defamation). But, see *Hammer v. Polsky,* 36 Misc.2d 482, 233 N.Y.S.2d 110 (1962) (traditional view that action for malpractice for misdiagnosis will only lie where complaint alleges that defendant was plaintiff's physician).

1. Defining the Standard

STEPAKOFF v. KANTAR

Supreme Judicial Court of Massachusetts, 1985.
393 Mass. 836, 473 N.E.2d 1131.

O'CONNOR, JUSTICE.

Helen J. Stepakoff, widow of Gerald Stepakoff (Stepakoff) and executrix of his estate, brought this action in the Superior Court against William G. Kantar, Stepakoff's psychiatrist. The plaintiff alleged that, although the defendant either knew or reasonably should have known that Stepakoff was suicidal, he negligently failed to inform her of that fact or to make appropriate arrangements for Stepakoff's protection, as a result of which Stepakoff committed suicide. The plaintiff seeks damages for Stepakoff's conscious suffering and wrongful death.

The case was tried to a jury. The trial judge directed a verdict for the defendant on the claim for conscious suffering, and the jury found for the defendant on the claim for wrongful death. Judgment was entered, and the plaintiff appealed. We transferred the appeal to this court on our own motion.

The plaintiff argues that the judge erred by refusing to instruct the jury that a psychiatrist who knows or reasonably should know that his patient is likely to harm himself has a duty to take reasonable precautions to prevent such harm, and by refusing to instruct the jury regarding a psychiatrist's statutory authority to hospitalize a patient involuntarily. The plaintiff also claims that the judge improperly instructed the jury concerning the burden of proof, and that he erroneously directed a verdict for the defendant on the claim for conscious suffering. We conclude that the judge did not commit reversible error, and we affirm the judgment for the defendant.

The jury could have found the following facts. Stepakoff began to see the defendant in November of 1973, and the two established a relationship as psychiatrist and patient that lasted until Stepakoff's death on or about February 16, 1975. The defendant diagnosed Stepakoff as a manic-depressive psychotic, and he formed the opinion that Stepakoff was "potentially suicidal." The defendant thought, however, that Stepakoff had a defense mechanism that rendered him less able to take decisive action as his predicament worsened. Furthermore, the defendant thought that he had a "solid pact" with Stepakoff that Stepakoff would contact him if Stepakoff felt suicidal.

During 1974 and early 1975, the plaintiff and Stepakoff had marital difficulties. On February 13, 1975, the plaintiff went to Florida. Before going, she told Stepakoff to be out of the house when she returned. She telephoned the defendant to express her concern about the situation, but he assured her that she should feel free to go.

The defendant planned to spend the weekend that began on Saturday, February 15, in Maine. Before his departure, he prepared Stepakoff for his absence. He gave Stepakoff the name and telephone number of another psychiatrist who had agreed to cover for him. He developed with Stepakoff a plan for the weekend, and he told Stepakoff that he would call him each night that he remained away. On Friday, February 14, the defendant and Stepakoff had an "emergency" meeting. During that meeting, the defendant considered involuntarily hospitalizing Stepakoff, but decided against it. After the meeting, he dictated a note for his files that included the following sentence: "There is a question of whether he will make it over the weekend." [1]

---

1. At trial, the defendant testified that when he used those words he meant: "Whether he would be able to carry out the activities that he and I outlined, or whether the type of thing that happened to him just preceding his psychiatric admission to Newton–Wellesley [in 1974] would occur, in which he seemed to be paralyzed

The defendant also called the covering psychiatrist and described Stepakoff's situation.

On Saturday, February 15, Stepakoff called the covering psychiatrist, and the two met. Stepakoff reassured the doctor that he did not intend to commit suicide. That night, as planned, the defendant called Stepakoff. Based on that conversation, the defendant formed a favorable diagnostic impression of Stepakoff's condition. The defendant hung up after agreeing with Stepakoff that they would talk again the next night, but on Sunday, February 16, the police found Stepakoff in his garage, dead from carbon monoxide inhalation.

The jury heard the testimony of two psychiatrists. One of them expressed the opinion that the defendant's treatment of Stepakoff did not conform to good medical practice. He testified that the defendant should have involuntarily hospitalized Stepakoff. The other disagreed. In his opinion, Stepakoff did not meet the requirements for involuntary hospitalization set forth in G.L. c. 123, § 12. Over the plaintiff's objection, the judge allowed the witness to testify as to what those requirements were.

1. *Instructions as to the Defendant's Duty.*

The plaintiff argues that the trial judge committed reversible error by failing to give the jury her requested instructions, numbered 10, 11, and 12, regarding a psychiatrist's duty to his patient. We reprint those requested instructions in the margin.[2] After the judge's charge, the plaintiff objected, by number, to the judge's failure to give those instructions.

* * *

The plaintiff concedes that the judge correctly instructed the jury concerning the defendant's "general medical malpractice duty to exercise the care and skill of the average psychiatrist," but she contends that the judge should *also* have instructed the jury that if, under that general malpractice standard, the defendant knew or should have known that Stepakoff presented a serious danger to himself, the defendant owed Stepakoff a specific legal duty to safeguard him from that danger, or at least to use reasonable care to do so. We will assume that requests 10, 11, and 12 fairly presented that instruction to the judge, but we conclude that the judge correctly refused to give it.

in his capacities to function, to—at that time, he couldn't get up out of the chair in my office and drive his car home. And it was that type of regression and inability to function that I was questioning."

2. "10. A treating psychiatrist owes to his patient a duty to safeguard the patient from danger due to mental incapacity where that incapacity is known, or ought to have been known, to the psychiatrist through the exercise of ordinary care. . . .

"11. If Dr. Kantar knew of facts from which he could have reasonably thought that the patient was likely to harm himself in the absence of protective measures, then Dr. Kantar had a duty to use reasonable care under the circumstances to prevent such harm and to safeguard the patient from self-inflicted injury or death. . . .

"12. This duty is proportionate to the patient's needs, that is, such reasonable care and attention as the patient's known mental condition requires. . . ." (Citations omitted.)

"Negligence, without qualification and in its ordinary sense, is the failure of a responsible person, either by omission or by action, to exercise that degree of care, vigilance and forethought which, in the discharge of the duty then resting on him, the person of ordinary caution and prudence ought to exercise under the particular circumstances." *Altman v. Aronson*, 231 Mass. 588, 591, 121 N.E. 505 (1919). Negligence of a physician who practices a specialty consists of a failure to exercise the degree of care and skill of the average qualified physician practicing that specialty, taking into account the advances in the profession and the resources available to the physician. *Brune v. Belinkoff*, 354 Mass. 102, 109, 235 N.E.2d 793 (1968). The rule with respect to the physician-patient relationship is an adaption of the broader negligence principle. In the context of that relationship, the law views the care and skill commonly exercised by the average qualified physician as the equivalent of the "care, vigilance and forethought which . . . the person of ordinary caution and prudence ought to exercise under the particular circumstances." *Altman v. Aronson, supra.*

The judge instructed the jury: "[I]f you find that the care and treatment given by Dr. Kantar to Gerald Stepakoff from December of 1973 to February of 1975 was not in accordance with good medical practice and in violation or breach of the standard of care and skill of the average member of the medical profession practicing his specialty of psychiatry between December '73 and February of 1975, and that, if as a direct and proximate result of that negligence, Gerald Stepakoff died, the plaintiff, Helen Stepakoff, would be entitled to recover. . . . ." That instruction fully and accurately stated the law. The plaintiff was not entitled to further instructions relative to the reasonableness of the defendant's acts or failures to act. The plaintiff has not directed our attention to any case in which a court has bifurcated the duty owed by a psychiatrist to a suicidal patient by declaring that, when diagnosing a patient, the psychiatrist must exercise the care and skill customarily exercised by an average qualified psychiatrist, while, after diagnosing a patient as suicidal, the psychiatrist's duty to take preventive measures becomes one of "reasonableness." We are unwilling to disturb our longstanding rule that a physician, practicing a specialty, owes to his or her patient a duty to comply in all respects with the standard set by the average physician practicing that specialty.

We are not moved to a different conclusion * * * by cases from other jurisdictions cited by the plaintiff in support of the proposition that a hospital and its staff must exercise reasonable care for the safety of confined patients likely to harm themselves. Even if those cases support the proposition that hospitals must meet an ordinary negligence standard, as distinguished from a good medical practice standard, they do not persuade us that the duty owed by a psychiatrist to a suicidal outpatient should differ from that imposed by this court on physicians to other patients.

* * *

Judgment affirmed.

Questions and Comments

1. *Some examples of failure to exercise ordinary care.* *Stepakoff v. Kantar* suggests that a failure to act may constitute negligence if such failure can be shown to be a departure from the exercise of ordinary or due care.

A departure from the standard of due care may also result from either the election of an inappropriate therapy or improper *implementation* of the therapy. The improper use of a treatment modality might involve either its use when no beneficial result could reasonably be expected or its use when one could reasonably anticipate exacerbation of the condition or some other side effect. Because, for example, the administration of thorazine is contraindicated in the case of an individual suffering from depression, its administration to a depressed patient who subsequently commits suicide might result in liability. See, e.g., *Brandt v. Grubin*, 131 N.J.Super. 182, 329 A.2d 82 (1974). An example of improper implementation of a customary therapeutic modality would be the administration of ECT without the administration of the muscle relaxant. It might also include the uninterrupted and prolonged administration of psychotropic medication coupled with a failure to terminate treatment upon the appearance of symptoms of tardive dyskinesia. See, e.g. *Clites v. State*, 322 N.W.2d 917 (Iowa App. 1982).

2. *The instruction in* Kantar. What was the basis of the appellate court's affirmance of the trial court's denial of instructions requested by plaintiff set out in note 2 of the opinion? Was it because they were legally incorrect or was it because they were redundant?

3. *Which standard applies?* The liability of a therapist for negligence may turn on the expertise and knowledge of those in a particular profession. Thus, a psychologist, unlike a medically trained psychiatrist, would generally not be liable for a failure to diagnose an *organic* disorder presented by the patient. On the other hand, a therapist who holds himself out as having the expertise of another specialized profession may be held to have the knowledge and expertise of that profession.

2. Defenses and Limitations on Liability

a. *Professional Judgment Rule*

SCHREMPF v. STATE

Court of Appeals of New York, 1985.
66 N.Y.2d 289, 496 N.Y.S.2d 973, 487 N.E.2d 883.

OPINION OF THE COURT

WACHTLER, CHIEF JUDGE.

Claimant's husband was stabbed and killed by Joseph Evans, a mental patient who had been released from a State institution and was still receiving outpatient care from that facility. In a suit for wrongful death the Court of Claims found the State liable for negligently failing to have the assailant committed as an inpatient sometime prior to the assault. The Appellate Division affirmed, with one justice dissenting.

On this appeal, the State of New York urges that the claim be dismissed for two reasons. First, it argues that the State cannot be held liable for failure to prevent a criminal act unless it had a special relationship with the victim, which concededly was not proven in this case. Second, it is urged that the decisions of the State psychiatrist fell within the area of professional medical judgment and thus cannot serve as a basis for a negligence or malpractice award. For the reasons that follow, we agree with the State's second contention and reverse the Appellate Division's order.

In December 1981 claimant's husband, Albert Schrempf, was employed at Consolidated Industries of Greater Syracuse, Inc., a private nonprofit organization which provides vocational rehabilitation for out-patients from mental institutions. On December 9, 1981 he was stabbed to death at his place of employment by Joseph Evans, a 27–year–old outpatient from Hutchings Psychiatric Institute, a State mental facility.

Evans had been admitted for treatment at Hutchings on six occasions beginning in May 1979. The admissions usually followed violent altercations with members of his family and involved some property damage and attempted assaults, but not the infliction of personal injury. On these occasions he claimed that he was prompted by inner voices commanding him to act. He was generally diagnosed as a manic depressive hypomanic type or, more rarely, as a paranoid schizophrenic, which were described at trial as degrees of the same general condition. Three of the admissions involved commitments as an inpatient; three were on outpatient status. Several of the admissions were voluntary. Evans generally resented the involuntary commitments and sometimes responded with threats against staff members or resorted to violent resistance. On one occasion, he broke the jaw of another patient.

Evans' condition was generally improved or stabilized by psycho-therapy and medication which could be provided on an outpatient basis. However, he was a difficult outpatient because he had an erratic attendance record and did not regularly take prescribed medications. He was sensitive to, and had an adverse reaction to, certain drugs and sometimes stated that he would not take his medication because it was against his religion.

Evans' last involuntary commitment as an inpatient ended in January of 1981. In the summer of that year, he broke windows in his mother's house and subsequently pleaded guilty to criminal mischief. He was sentenced to probation and his probation officer suggested that he seek psychiatric treatment.

On September 28, 1981 he returned to Hutchings and was voluntarily admitted. He was examined on that occasion by the psychiatrist who had first admitted him in 1979 and who had also treated him on most of his subsequent admissions. She found that he was experiencing "persecutory delusions" that he was possessed and might be changing into a homosexual. However, she noted that he was calm and remained cooperative. Based on the examination and her knowledge of his psychiatric history, she determined that he was again suffering from manic depression and that at that time he did not pose a risk to himself or others. She placed him on outpatient status but assigned him to a special clinic for recalcitrant outpatients so that his use of the medication could be monitored.

In October Evans worked at a part-time job, without apparent incident. In November he was referred by his probation officer to Consolidated Industries for vocational rehabilitation. He participated in that program on a trial basis for approximately 10 days over the next three or four weeks.

Throughout this period his participation in the outpatient program diminished. In October he said he did not want to come any more because he had a job. He rarely met with his psychiatrist in October and did not see her after November 1. He did not regularly go to the clinic for his medication in October, and in November only appeared on two dates, November 9 and November 30.

His psychiatrist encouraged him to continue in the outpatient program and to take his medication. When he complained that the drugs made him drowsy at work, she reduced the dosage and directed him to take the medicine at night. On November 17 she informed his probation officer that he was not taking his medication. She also monitored his behavior through the probation officer and others and found no evidence that his condition was deteriorating. On the contrary, she was informed that he appeared to be polite and cooperative by all who observed him at the clinic, the probation office and Consolidated Industries. Indeed he was being considered for permanent membership at Consolidated at the time of the assault on December 9, 1981.

At the trial, the claimant urged that the State had been negligent in the care and treatment of Evans by releasing him and permitting him to remain on outpatient status in 1981, particularly after his psychiatrist had reason to believe he was not taking his medication as prescribed. The Court of Claims held that the decision to release Evans in January 1981 involved a medical judgment for which the State could not be held liable. However, the court concluded that the State was negligent in admitting Evans to outpatient care, instead of confining him as an inpatient in September 1981. The court also held that the State psychiatrist should have done "something more" when it became evident that the patient was not taking his prescribed medication.

The Appellate Division affirmed, without opinion. * * *

As noted, the State's first contention on this appeal is that the claim should have been dismissed because the claimant failed to establish a special relationship between the State and the injured party.

* * *

[The court held that under established New York doctrine the state may be liable to third parties for the consequence of its negligence].

A physician's duty is to provide the level of care acceptable in the professional community in which he practices (*Toth v. Community Hosp.*, 22 N.Y.2d 255, 292 N.Y.S.2d 440, 239 N.E.2d 368). He is not required to achieve success in every case and cannot be held liable for mere errors of professional judgment. * * * The "line between medical judgment and deviation from good medical practice is not easy to draw" particularly in cases involving psychiatric treatment. * * *

Although in the past, the care of those suffering from mental infirmities was generally limited to confinement, the modern and more humane policy of the medical profession and the law contemplates returning the mental patient to society, if he does not pose an immediate risk of harm to himself or others. * * * This [decision], we have noted, requires a sensitive appraisal of competing interests: "(1) the State's duty to treat and care for its mental defective wards, with an eye toward returning them to society more useful citizens, and (2) the State's concern that the inmates in its institutions cause no injury or damage to the property of those in the vicinity." * * * Because psychiatry is not an exact science, decisions with respect to the proper course of treatment often involve a calculated risk and disagreement among experts as to whether the risk was warranted or in accord with accepted procedures. * * * These circumstances necessarily broaden the area of professional judgment to include treatments tailored to the particular case, where the "accepted procedure" does not take into account factors which the treating physician could reasonably consider significant. * * *

The only remaining question is whether the treating physician was negligent in failing to intervene in some manner once she had reason to believe that Evans was not taking his medication as prescribed. In view of the fact that Evans was a voluntary outpatient, the State's control over him, and consequent duty to prevent him from harming others, is more limited than in cases involving persons confined to mental institutions. Even the claimant's experts did not agree as to what should and could be done with such a patient. They variously proposed compelling or coercing him to resume medication, changing the medication to a drug with longer lasting effects, conducting a full reexamination of him, initiating involuntary commitment proceedings or threatening him with commitment if he did not cooperate. The court held that the treating psychiatrist should have done "something more", and suggested that "at the very least, an in-depth psychiatric evaluation should have been conducted to determine Evans' level of functioning." The court did not indicate what should have been done had Evans refused to cooperate.

One point on which all the experts agreed was that the patient's failure to take his medication did not necessarily mean that his condition was deteriorating or that he would become dangerous. That would largely depend on his behavior and, again, there was agreement that his outward appearance and behavior did not show any "warning signs" indicative of this kind of change. Although claimant's experts ignored or discounted these factors, they played a significant role in the attending physician's assessment. They indicated to her that there was a chance that his condition was improving as it appeared to be, and suggested a corresponding risk that intervention by resort to aggressive measures might disrupt the process. As noted, she knew from past experience that he resented involuntary treatment and often responded violently in that setting. Thus, there were risks either way. The treating physician, as she testified at trial, simply attached greater significance to those factors which seemed most promising and chose the course which appeared to offer the best opportunity for long-term rehabilitation. We know with hindsight that it was a mistaken impression. However, under the circumstances, it must be recognized as an exercise of professional judgment for which the State cannot be held responsible.

Accordingly, the order of the Appellate Division should be reversed and the claim dismissed.

JASEN, MEYER, KAYE, ALEXANDER and TITONE, JJ., concur.

SIMONS, J., taking no part.

Order reversed, with costs, and claim dismissed.

Questions and Comments

1. *Recognition of doctrine in other jurisdictions.* The professional judgment rule which, when applicable, calls for appropriate instructions to the jury, has not been universally adopted. In fact, to date, it has been expressly recognized by only a minority of jurisdictions and has been rejected by at least one state. See, *Ouellette v. Subak,* 391 N.W.2d 810 (Minn.1986). The rule seems to have had its origins in New York where it has been applied to all phases of malpractice, including psychiatry. See, *Littleton v. Good Samaritan Hospital,* 39 Ohio St.3d 86, 529 N.E.2d 449 (1988). The "best judgment rule" shields a physician from liability "for mere errors of judgment provided he does what he thinks best after careful examination." *Littleton v. Good Samaritan Hospital,* 39 St.3d 86, 529 N.E. 2d 449, 457 (1988).

In the mental health context it has most commonly been applied to exculpate psychiatrists for their decision to not seek a patient's involuntary hospitalization. As explained by the Supreme Court of Ohio:

"Under such a 'psychotherapist judgment rule,' the court would not allow liability to be imposed on therapists for simple errors in judgment. Instead, the court would examine the 'good faith, indepen- dence and thoroughness' of a psychotherapist's decision not to commit a patient. * * * Factors in reviewing such good faith include the competence and training of the reviewing psychotherapists, whether the relevant documents and evidence were adequately, promptly and independently reviewed, whether the advice or opinion of another therapist was obtained, whether the evaluation was made in light of the proper legal standards for commitment, and whether other evidence of good faith exists." (Citation omitted).

The court derived its psychotherapist judgment rule from the business judgment rule used to review decisions of corporate directors:

"In the business judgment rule, courts defer to the decisions of disinterested directors absent bad faith or self-interest. Many of the considerations cited as justifications for the business judgment rule are applicable to the present case. For example, as with business decisions, the court is not particularly qualified to review commitment decisions involving mental health and dangerousness. In addition, these types of commitment procedures require quick action, and 'after-the-fact litigation is a most imperfect device to evaluate' those decisions, as in the corporate setting. * * * Finally, policy considerations favor giving psychotherapists, as well as corporate directors, significant discretion to use their best judgment, recognizing that '[a] rule which penalizes the choice of seemingly riskier alternatives * * * may not be in the interest' of the parties or society." (Citations omitted).

Id. at 458.

2. *Subsilentio adoption.* The courts of some jurisdictions have without expressly relying on the professional judgment doctrine refused to assign liability where the psychiatrist failed to commit and the patient subsequently injured a third party. For instance, in *Soutear v. United States,* 646 F.Supp. 524 (E.D.Mich.1986) in holding against a claimant who asserted that the facility's failure to psychiatrically commit the patient constituted negligence, the court observed:

"Psychiatry * * * is not an exact science. Medical doctors cannot predict with perfect accuracy whether or not an individual will do violence to himself or to someone else. Thus, we hold a psychiatrist to only the standard of care of his profession. That standard "must take into consideration the uncertainty which accompanies psychiatric analysis * * *. The concept of 'due care' in appraising psychiatric problems, assuming proper procedures are followed, must take account of the difficulty often inevitable in definitive diagnosis." *Lipari v. Sears, Roebuck & Co.,* [497 F.Supp. 185, 192 (D.Neb.1980)] quoting *Hicks v. United States,* * * * 511 F.2d 407, 417 (D.C.Cir.1975). *Thus, a psychiatrist will not be held liable for his patient's violent behavior simply because he failed to predict it accurately.*

Id. at 536, quoting *Davis v. Lhim,* 124 Mich.App. 291, 301, 335 N.W.2d 481 (1983) (emphasis added by the court).

Cases such as *Soutear v. United States* undoubtedly reflect an unwillingness on the part of courts to adopt the professional judgment rule outside a narrow gauge of situations and particularly those involving psychiatric predictions of aberrant behavior.

3. *Limitations on the professional judgment rule.* Note that the professional judgment rule only applies where the decision taken has been preceded by a "careful examination" of the patient. *Littleton,* 529 N.E.2d

at 457. If this is true, should the court in *Schrempf* have applied the rule as a matter of law? Was there any evidence in *Schrempf* that the psychiatrist did not conduct a thorough examination before reaching a judgment on the question of commitment?

---

b. Respectable Minority Doctrine

A patient who has received treatment involving the use of a particular technique may, if the outcome is not satisfactory, claim that the physician or therapist was negligent in not utilizing a more effective treatment modality. Such claim of negligence in the selection of treatment may be advanced, moreover, even where the physician or therapist has obtained the informed consent of the patient. (The doctrine of informed consent is treated in Chapter Three).

Generally, claims that physicians or therapists utilized the wrong therapeutic technique or failed to use the most effective one will, as with all other aspects of performance, be measured by the standard of due care, i.e., what members of the profession would customarily do under the circumstances. While a finding that the therapeutic approach used was not "customary" does not necessarily lead to liability, proof of conformity to custom generally precludes a finding of liability. Thus, whether a particular treatment is "customary" or "accepted" by the profession may well be dispositive of the issue of liability.

Proof that a particular procedure is customary does not, however, require that it be used by a majority of practitioners. In fact, in a number of jurisdictions, a defense is established by a showing that a particular treatment approach is supported by a "respectable minority" of those in the field. See *McHugh v. Audet*, 72 F.Supp. 394 (M.D.Pa. 1947). As described by one court the "respectable minority" rule means that "[W]here two or more schools of thought exist among competent members of the medical profession concerning proper medical treatment for a given ailment, each of which is supported by responsible medical authority, it is not malpractice to be among the minority * * * [of those following] one of the accepted schools." *Chumbler v. McClure*, 505 F.2d 489, 492 (6th Cir.1974). There remain, however, some unresolved questions as to the scope of the doctrine. For instance, does the doctrine immunize a practitioner from liability upon a showing that a particular treatment technique is used by a "respectable minority", even though the therapy used is on the average likely to be less effective than an alternate treatment modality? In the treatment of mental disorders, this question is likely to arise with increasing frequency as new treatment techniques compete with traditional forms of psychotherapy. The case of *Osheroff v. Chestnut Lodge* which follows is illustrative of the context in which cases of this type are likely to arise.

OSHEROFF v. CHESTNUT LODGE, INC.

[Since the action was initially brought in 1982 as an arbitration proceeding before the Maryland Health Care Arbitration Panel, no official report of the case exists. The facts set out below are based on several secondary sources.]

SUMMARY OF LEGAL PROCEEDINGS

In 1982, Dr. Rafael Osheroff initiated a lawsuit against Chestnut Lodge, Inc. claiming that Chestnut Lodge negligently misdiagnosed his condition and negligently failed to utilize psychopharmacological treatment. This, he alleged, prevented him from returning promptly to normal functioning, with the consequential loss of a lucrative medical practice, and his standing in the medical community.

As required under Maryland law, Dr. Osheroff's suit was submitted to the Maryland Health Care Arbitration Panel (HCAP) which held extended hearings at which numerous experts were called to testify. In his review of the case, Professor Gerald L. Klerman summarized the events leading up to the settlement:

> The Arbitration Panel found for the plaintiff and awarded him financial damages [in the amount of $250,000]. This was not a majority decision, however, and the director of the Arbitration Panel sent the panel back for an amended decision, which reduced the award. Under Maryland statute, once an arbitration process is concluded, any party to the proceedings may reject the panel's arbitration and call for court review. Both sides appealed. The claimant, Dr. Osheroff, requested a jury trial, which was to have taken place in October, 1987. However, before any action was taken by the court, a settlement was agreed upon by both parties.

Klerman, *The Psychiatric Patient's Right to Effective Treatment: Implications of Osheroff vs. Chestnut Lodge,* 147 American Journal of Psychiatry 409, 410–411 (April 1990)* [hereinafter Klerman]. See also, *Osheroff v. Chestnut Lodge,* 62 Md.App. 519, 490 A.2d 720 (Md.App.1985) (challenge to procedures followed by the Maryland Health Claims Arbitration office).

FACTUAL BACKGROUND

Dr. Klerman in his study summarized the medical social history of Dr. Osheroff prior to his hospitalization:

> "The patient, Dr. Rafael Osheroff, a 42-year-old, white male physician, was admitted to Chestnut Lodge in Maryland . . . on Jan. 2, 1979. His history included brief periods of depressive and anxious symptoms as an adult; these had been treated on an outpatient basis. He had completed medical school and residency training, was certified as an internist and became a sub-specialist in nephrology.

---

* American Journal of Psychiatry, vol. 147, pp. 409–418 (1990). Copyright © 1990 by The American Psychiatric Association. All excerpts from Dr. Klerman's article have been reprinted by permission of the American Psychiatric Association.

Before his 1979 hospitalization, Dr. Osheroff had been suffering from anxious and depressive symptoms for approximately two years, and had been treated as an outpatient with individual psychotherapy and tricyclic antidepressant medications. Dr. Nathan Kline, a prominent psychopharmacologist in New York, had initiated outpatient treament with tricyclic medication, which, according to Dr. Kline's notes, produced moderate improvement. The patient, however, did not maintain the recommended dose, his clinical condition gradually worsened and hospitalization was recommended."
Klerman, p. 410.

In January 1979, Dr. Osheroff admitted himself into Chestnut Lodge which, for over forty years, had been one of the major centers devoted to "a clinical practice in intensive individual psychotherapy based on psychoanalytic and interpersonal paradigms". Klerman, p. 411. A number of prominent American psychiatrists had been trained at Chestnut Lodge, many of whom subsequently became leaders in psychoanalytically oriented clinical psychiatry.

Upon admission, Dr. Osheroff was diagnosed as suffering from "psychotic reaction, agitated type and narcissistic personality disorder". Malcolm, *Treatment Choices and Informed Consent in Psychiatry: Implications of the Osheroff Case for the Profession,* 14 J. Psychiatry & Law, 9, 16 (1986). [hereinafter Malcolm]. Both following his admission and throughout his stay in Chestnut Lodge, the treatment program for Dr. Osheroff consisted of four sessions of individual psychotherapy per week and group therapy. Malcolm, pp. 19–20. At no time was he given antidepressive medication because of the facility's decision to "attempt a 'more ambitious treatment goal' of dealing with the long range difficulties of the underlying personality disorder." Malcolm, p. 19.

Although the hospital records indicate that at various times the staff felt that Dr. Osheroff was making progress, it seems evident that Dr. Osheroff did not noticeably improve during his seven months stay at Chestnut Lodge. As reported by Dr. Klerman, "He lost 40 pounds, experienced severe insomnia, and had marked psychomotor agitation. His agitation, manifested by incessant pacing, was so extreme that his feet became swollen and blistered, requiring medical attention." Klerman, p. 410.

The circumstances leading to Dr. Osheroff's release and admission into another facility are also described in Professor Klerman's study:

"The patient's family became distressed by the length of the hospitalization and by his lack of improvement. They consulted a psychiatrist in the Washington, D.C., area, who spoke to the hospital leadership on the patient's behalf. In response, the staff at Chestnut Lodge held a clinical case conference to review the patient's treatment. They decided not to make any major changes—specifically not to institute any medication regimen but to continue the intensive individual psychotherapy. Dr. Osheroff's clinical condition continued to worsen. At the end of 7 months, his family had him discharged from Chestnut Lodge and admitted to Silver Hill Foundation in Connecticut.

On admission to Silver Hill Foundation, Dr. Osheroff was diagnosed as having a psychotic depressive reaction. His treating physician began treatment with a combination of phenothiazines and tricyclic antidepressants. Dr. Osheroff showed improvement within 3 weeks and was discharged from Silver Hill Foundation within 3 months.

* * *

Following his discharge from Silver Hill Foundation in the summer of 1979, the patient resumed his medical practice. He has been in outpatient treatment, receiving psychotherapy and medication. He has not been hospitalized and has not experienced any episodes of depressive symptoms severe enough to interfere with his professional or social functioning. He has resumed contact with his children and has also become active socially."

Klerman, p. 410.

IMPACT OF PRACTITIONER ORIENTATION ON DIAGNOSIS AND TREATMENT

A useful starting point in considering the diagnostic and treatment issues raised by the Osheroff case are the observations of Professor Klerman as to the theoretical divisions which characterize psychiatry in the country:

"Resolution of both the clinical and scientific issues is made difficult by the divisions within psychiatry in the United States, where psychiatry is divided theoretically and clinically into different schools—biological, psychoanalytic, and behavioral. * * * Various terms have been used to describe these divisions and splits—schools, movements, ideologies, and paradigms. * * * Whatever term is used, there is agreement that these differences in theory and practice involve controversies over the nature of mental illness [and] the appropriateness of different forms of treatment * * *".

Klerman, p. 411.

Chestnut Lodge, where Dr. Osheroff was initially admitted is, as noted previously, one of the leading psychoanalytically oriented inpatient treatment centers in the country. There is a general consensus that the theoretical orientation of the treating therapist is likely to significantly influence both the diagnostic process and the choice of treatment. In the case of Dr. Osheroff, the admitting psychiatrist at Chestnut Lodge made a *primary* diagnosis of "major narcissistic personality disorder". A diagnosis of "manic-depressive illness, depressed type" was entered as a secondary diagnosis. Malcolm, p. 16. While the existence of "personality disorder"[a] as a diagnostic category is not

---

a. "The essential feature is a Personality Disorder in which there are a grandiose sense of self-importance or uniqueness; preoccupation with fantasies of unlimited success; exhibitionistic need for constant attention and admiration; characteristic responses to threats to self-esteem; and characteristic disturbances in interpersonal relationships, such as feelings of entitlement, interpersonal exploitativeness, relationships that alternate between the extremes of overidealization and devaluation, and lack of empathy.

The exaggerated sense of self-importance may be manifested as extreme self-centeredness and self-absorption. Abilities and achievements tend to be unrealistically overestimated. Frequently the sense of self-importance alternates with feelings of

necessarily rejected by biologically oriented psychiatrists, it is far more central to the psychoanalytic paradigm. As in the case of other similar psychopathologies a "narcissistic personality disorder" is seen as derivative of an early childhood development crisis. Malcolm, pp. 17–18. Thus, under one prevalent hypothesis the disorder results because during childhood the affected individual "failed to internalize an idealized parental image because he either lost or was traumatically disappointed in idealized objects. This idealized image is a forerunner of the superego. Because this idealized image is missing, certain superego functions are missing." Malcolm, pp. 17.

Not only is the diagnostic approach likely to be influenced by the theoretical orientation of the therapist, but so is the choice of treatment. Adherence to the psychoanalytic model is likely to influence the therapeutic approach in three ways. First, there is a general consensus on the part of those adhering to the psychoanalytic model that many disorders can only be treated through long term psychoanalysis. Second, and of equal significance, certain forms of depression are perceived as being derived from, and associated with a psychopathology whose origin is in early childhood development. Klerman, p. 412. As a consequence whatever treatment program is undertaken must address the underlying root causes of the disorder rather than the surface symptomatology. In the case under consideration this meant that the staff of Chestnut Lodge placed emphasis on the treatment of the narcissistic personality disorder rather than the depression which was seen as a derivative symptom. Finally, a psychoanalytic orientation leads many therapists to avoid the use of psychotropic medication during the course of therapy, "because of the possible adverse effects of the pharmacotherapy". Klerman, p. 413.

The Silver Hill Foundation where Dr. Osheroff was admitted following his release from Chestnut Lodge, entered a diagnosis of severe depressive reaction. In this respect, the diagnosis of the two institutions were in accord. However, unlike Chestnut Lodge, the psychiatrist at Silver Hill did not diagnose the patient as suffering from a narcissistic personality disorder.[b]

Silver Hill's diagnosis of "psychotic depression" led to a treatment program of psychotropic medication combined with "supportive therapy" rather than analytical therapy. This choice of treatment would be regarded as standard by those in the biologically oriented schools of psychiatry. Klerman, p. 412.

THE EFFICACY OF ALTERNATE TREATMENT MODALITIES

A court hearing on an Osheroff type of claim could be expected to admit evidence relevant to the efficacy of the treatment modalities that

special unworthiness * * *." Diagnostic and Statistical Manual of Mental Disorders, 3rd ed., American Psychiatric Association, 1980, pp. 315–316.

b. In subsequent testimony the admitting psychiatrist at Silver Hill stated that while she considered a diagnosis of personality disorder, she did not enter the diagnosis because it was "not preeminent" at the time. Malcolm at 22.

were used or could have been used. The state of evidence relevant to this issue has been summarized by Professor Klerman:

> With regard to all kinds of therapeutics—pharmacotherapy, surgery, radiation, psychotherapy—the most scientifically valid evidence as to the safety and efficacy of a treatment comes from randomized controlled trials when these are available. Although there may be other methods of generating evidence, such as naturalistic and follow-up studies, the most convincing evidence comes from randomized controlled trials.

> There have been many controlled clinical trials of psychiatric treatments; most have been conducted to evaluate psychopharmacological agents.

> *   *   *

> Research on the efficacy of psychotherapy has lagged behind that of psychopharmacology, but has, nevertheless, been extensive. *   *   * Specific reviews of the evidence have appeared with regard to psychotherapy of neurosis, schizophrenia, depression, and obsessive-compulsive disorders.

> *   *   *

> With regard to the treatment of the patient's diagnosis of *narcissistic personality* [emphasis added] disorder, there were no reports of controlled trials of any pharmacological or psychotherapeutic treatment for this condition at the time of his hospitalization. The doctors at Chestnut Lodge decided to treat Dr. Osheroff's personality disorder with intensive individual psychotherapy based on psychodynamic theory.

> With regard to the treatment of the patient's DSM–II diagnosis of psychotic depressive reaction, there was very good evidence at the time of his hospitalization for the efficacy of two biological treatments—ECT and the combination of phenothiazines and tricyclic antidepressants. The combination pharmacotherapy was the treatment later prescribed at Silver Hill Foundation.

> There are no reports of controlled trials supporting the claims for efficacy of psychoanlytically-oriented intensive individual psychotherapy of the type advocated and practiced at Chestnut Lodge and administered to Dr. Osheroff.

> *   *   *

> It should not be concluded there is no evidence for the value of any psychotherapy in the treatment of depressive states. Depressive states are heterogeneous and there are many forms of psychotherapy. There is very good evidence from controlled clinical trials for the value of a number of brief psychotherapies for nonpsychotic and nonbipolar forms of depression in ambulatory patients. The psychotherapies for which there is evidence include cognitive-behavioral therapy, interpersonal psychotherapy, and behavioral therapy. However, no clinical trials have been reported to support the claims for efficacy of psychoanalysis of intensive individual psychotherapy based on psychoanalytic theory for any form of depression.

> *   *   *

Even if we assume that the personality disorder was correctly diagnosed in Dr. Osheroff's case, there is no evidence to support the premise that the presence of a narcissistic personality disorder militates against the use of antidepressant medication.

* * *

A related therapeutic issue raised by the case has to do with the possible negative interactions between psychotherapy and pharmacotherapy for depression. Many psychoanalytically oriented psychotherapists have argued against the use of medication in patients receiving psychotherapy because of the possible adverse effects of the pharmacotherapy on the conduct of the psychotherapy, although there is evidence that the combination of drugs and psychotherapy does not interfere with the psychotherapy of depression. Moreover, findings from controlled trials suggest the combination of drugs and psychotherapy may have beneficial additive effects in the treatment of depression.

Klerman, pp. 412–413.

Questions and Comments

1. *The relationship of diagnosis to treatment.* In his complaint, Dr. Osheroff alleged negligence both as to diagnosis, i.e., narcissistic personality disorder, and as to choice of treatment. To what extent is a decision of the second issue dependent on the resolution of the first?

2. *Application of the respectable minority doctrine.* Should disposition of an Osheroff type of case take into account the existence of a minority view made up of traditional psychoanalytically oriented psychiatrists who tend to avoid the use of psychotropic medication on the grounds that it interferes with the classical analytic course of treatment? Should the question of liability be at all influenced by the fact that classical psychoanalytic treatment envisions a course of treatment lasting from three to four years compared to the standard treatment of depressive symptomatology which involves a course of treatment utilizing psychopharmacology of six to twelve weeks?

3. *Effect of informed consent.* Should it be relevant in assessing liability whether the patient was informed of the relative lengths of treatment and the conceivable advantages under each? If so, does this suggest that the doctrine of informed consent, which will be treated in Chapter Three, may have some relevance in assessing liability for alleged negligence in selection of a course of treatment? In other words, why should a patient who has made an informed choice after being presented with all the relevant facts, be allowed to pursue a claim for negligence if the outcome is disappointing? Doesn't the answer here depend on whether a patient can, at the outset, contractually exempt the therapist from liability? The enforceability of covenants not to sue in the context of medical treatment is in some doubt. In some instances, particularly as to standardized treatment, such contractual limitations from liability have been held to violate public policy. However, where the procedure is experimental and the patient has been informed of the alternatives and risks, such provisions are usually enforced. See, *Schneider v. Revici,* 817 F.2d 987 (2d Cir.1987).

4. *Defining one standard.* Is there any danger that diversity in treatment would be stifled if the immunity normally provided by the respectable minority rule could be overridden by evidence that the challenged treatment is demonstratively less effective on the average than an alternative form? What degree of proof as to superiority in efficacy should be required? Would this standard have been met in the instant case?

5. *Question.* Could a case with facts identical to those of Osheroff be decided on a narrower ground than negligence in the *initial* choice of therapy? Could it be argued that the Chestnut Lodge facility was not necessarily negligent in its initial use of intensive individual psychotherapy but that it became negligent when it persisted in the use of this technique over the period of several months even though the patient's condition did not improve but, in fact, deteriorated?

6. *Duty to refer.* What would be the implications for mental health professionals who are not psychiatrists of a holding that the staff of Chestnut Lodge was negligent in not using antidepressants to treat Dr. Osheroff. Recall, in this connection, that non-psychiatrists do not have the legal authority to prescribe psychotropic medication. Would a finding that Chestnut Lodge was negligent in not using psychotropic medication suggest that a non-psychiatrist dealing with a depressed patient has a duty to refer the patient to a psychiatrist so that the patient may receive psychopharmacological treatment?

7. *Treatment "beyond the pale".* Treatment techniques may be used which do not meet the respectable minority level. This may occur either where the treatment is explicitly experimental, or where it is simply the product of an idiosyncratic treatment approach. Sometimes it may be a combination of the two. There are two reported cases imposing liability on mental health professionals who used non-biologically based "innovative" therapy. One such case is *Hammer v. Rosen*, 7 N.Y.2d 376, 198 N.Y.S.2d 65, 165 N.E.2d 756 (1960), where the psychiatrist, Dr. John Nathaniel Rosen, "had developed immediately after World War II a reputation for dramatic success in treatment and cure of schizophrenic patients (those suffering from a serious mental disorder marked by a loss of contact with reality). * * *

Dr. Rosen treated schizophrenics rather than neurotics. To bridge the communication gap which treating persons of this much lower mental level posed, Dr. Rosen, after ascertaining his patient's mental level and before attempting to raise the mental level of his patient, attempted to project himself on the communicable mental plateau of his patient in order to establish mental contact and eventually rapport and trust. In executing this technique, which of course was highly personalized, but which was consented to by the spouse, next of kin, or legal guardian of each patient, it would certainly be presumed that Dr. Rosen might touch certain patients from time to time with differing degrees of force, depending upon the mental condition and needs of the patient, in order to effectively and fully explore and utilize the possibilities and potentialities which his method offered." Morse, *The Tort Liability of the Psychiatrist*, 18 Syracuse L.R. 691, 704–707 (1967). In reversing the trial court's dismissal of the plaintiff's claim for malpractice, the appellate court held that the plaintiff's case could, in view of the "fantastic" nature of the treatment, be submitted to the jury without any expert testimony that the treatment constituted malpractice. Significantly, at the trial neither the plaintiff nor the defense introduced any evidence either as to the reasonableness or acceptability to the psychiatric profession of the experimental therapy developed by Dr. Rosen. It is unclear how the case might ultimately have been decided had Dr. Rosen introduced testimony attesting to the efficacy of his therapeutic approach or introduced evidence that the therapy was viewed as promising by some accepted segment of the psychiatric profession.

The only reported similar case imposing liability on a psychologist using innovative therapy is *Abraham v. Zaslow* (San Francisco, Cy.Sup.Ct. 1972) reported in *New York Times,* July 5, 1972, p. 27 and APA *Monitor,* March 1973. The therapy in question was called "Rage Reduction Therapy or Z–Process." This involved breaking down the patient's resistance, by applying extensive physical stimulation to an immobilized patient in order to reduce the repressed compulsion to escape. The process was originally developed for use on autistic children, but Dr. Zaslow expanded it for use with disturbed adults. At trial the plaintiff testified, "I was tortured, including choking, beating, holding and tying me down and sticking fingers in my mouth." Ralph Slovenko, *Psychiatry and Law* (Boston: Little, Brown, 1973), p. 428, n. 39.

8. *Standards governing innovative therapy.* The standards governing the liability of physicians undertaking experimental or innovative therapy have undergone a marked change in recent years. As one commentator notes, "The rule to be extracted from the early cases involving human experimentation is that physicians vary from established treatment at their own peril." Michael H. Shapiro and Roy G. Spence, *Bioethics and Law* (St. Paul, Minn.: West Pub. Co., 1981), p. 871. "The more modern courts take a less restrictive view of untried medical treatment and surgical procedures; and several decisions establish the right of the general field of medicine and surgery to progress and advance to some experimentation." Id.

9. *Standards governing liability for experimentation.* The development of the present legal standards of assessing liability for experimentation results from an attempt to promote the advancement of medical science while protecting society from reckless innovation. *See, Carpenter v. Blake,* 60 Barb. 488 (N.Y.1871), *rev'd on other grounds,* 50 N.Y. 696 (1872). Has the proper balance been struck? How confident must a physician, breaking new ground, be that his techniques are "reasonable" before he exposes his patients and himself to the attendant risks? Will the patient about to undergo experimental treatment have more or less reason to trust his doctor's judgment if he knows the standard to which he will be held?

10. *Hypothetical.* How should the legal system respond to claims challenging the experimental use of hemodialysis to treat schizophrenia? Some researchers have suggested the "possibility that schizophrenia may be caused by a mysterious substance in the blood and cured by removing it with hemodialysis techniques used for kidney disease." *Dialysis for Schizophrenia? Doctors Debate Effects,* New York Times, March 7, 1981, pg. 1, col. 1. Dialysis, however, may be "so stressful that it often produces

unpleasant psychological effects," including a high incidence of depression and suicide among renal dialysis recipients. Id.

"Dialysis is presently considered by most psychiatric researchers to represent only an experimental approach and treatment modality." Id. Some studies have cast substantial doubt on the efficacy of dialysis as an acceptable treatment for schizophrenia. For instance, researchers at the National Institute of Mental Health recently issued a report finding hemodialysis to be totally ineffective in relieving schizophrenic patients of their hallucinations or other psychiatric symptoms. Nevertheless, some families of schizophrenic patients "desperately seeking a new promise of help are pursuing dialysis despite its great expense and grave dangers." Id. While actual statistics are not known, some researchers have estimated the number of schizophrenics receiving hemodialysis in the hundreds. Id.

Given the present state of knowledge, what should be the liability of a psychiatrist who prescribes dialysis treatment for a schizophrenic patient who subsequently manifests depression which results in suicide? Should the fact that a small minority of professionals believe that hemodialysis can effectively treat schizophrenia be relevant in determining whether the use of this procedure establishes a *prima facie* case of negligence? Would a holding that the use of the procedure constitutes a lack of due care as a matter of law stifle legitimate medical experimentation? Should the result perhaps rest on whether the treatment was offered as customary therapy as distinct from closely controlled experimentation?

c.   The "Non-therapist" Counselor

NALLY v. GRACE COMMUNITY CHURCH OF THE VALLEY

Supreme Court of California, 1988.
47 Cal.3d 278, 253 Cal.Rptr. 97, 763 P.2d 948.

LUCAS, CHIEF JUSTICE.

I.   INTRODUCTION

On April 1, 1979, 24–year–old Kenneth Nally (hereafter Nally) committed suicide by shooting himself in the head with a shotgun. His parents (hereafter plaintiffs) filed a wrongful death action against Grace Community Church of the Valley (hereafter Church), a Protestant Christian congregation located in Sun Valley, California, and four Church pastors: MacArthur, Thomson, Cory and Rea (hereafter collectively referred to as defendants), alleging "clergyman malpractice," i.e., negligence and outrageous conduct in failing to prevent the suicide. (See Code Civ.Proc., § 377.) Nally, a member of the Church since 1974, had participated in defendants' pastoral counseling programs prior to his death.

This case was previously before us in 1984 after the Court of Appeal reversed summary judgment for defendants and remanded to the trial court (hereafter *Nally I*). After we denied a hearing and depublished the *Nally I* Court of Appeal opinion, the matter was sent back to the trial court. At the close of plaintiffs' evidence at the trial on remand, the court granted defendants' motion for nonsuit on all counts on the basis of insufficiency of the evidence.

The Court of Appeal again reversed and we granted review to address: (i) whether we should impose a duty on defendants and other "nontherapist counselors" (i.e., persons other than licensed psychotherapists, who counsel others concerning their emotional and spiritual problems) to refer persons to licensed mental health professionals once suicide becomes a foreseeable risk, and (ii) whether the evidence presented at trial supports plaintiffs' cause of action for wrongful death based on defendants' alleged "intentional infliction of emotional distress" on Nally.

II. FACTS

A. Background

In 1973, while attending University of California at Los Angeles (hereafter UCLA), Nally became depressed after breaking up with his girlfriend. He often talked about the absurdity of life, the problems he had with women and his family, and he occasionally mentioned suicide to his friends. Though Nally had been raised in a Roman Catholic household, he converted to Protestantism while he was a student at UCLA, and in 1974 he began attending the Church, the largest Protestant church in Los Angeles County. Nally's conversion became a source of controversy between him and his family. During this time, Nally developed a close friendship with defendant Pastor Cory, who was responsible for overseeing the ministry to the collegians attending the Church. On occasion, Nally discussed his problems with Cory, but the two never established a formal counseling relationship. Between 1974 and 1979, Nally was active in defendants' various Church programs and ministries.

Defendants offered pastoral counseling to church members in matters of faith, doctrine and the application of Christian principles. During 1979, defendant Church had approximately 30 counselors on its staff, serving a congregation of more than 10,000 persons. Defendants taught that the Bible is the fundamental Word of God containing truths that must govern Christians in their relationship with God and the world at large, and in their own personal lives. Defendant Church had no professional or clinical counseling ministry, and its pastoral counseling was essentially religious in nature. Such counseling was often received through instruction, study, prayer and guidance, and through mentoring relationships called "discipleships."

* * *

In essence, defendants held themselves out as *pastoral* counselors able to deal with a variety of problems—not as professional, medical or psychiatric counselors.

In 1975, Nally was seeing a secular psychologist to discuss problems he was having with his girlfriend. After graduating from UCLA in 1976, he spent one semester at Biola College in La Mirada and was enrolled in the Talbot Theological Seminary's extension on defendants' church grounds. During this time, Nally became involved in a relationship with a girlfriend who was a fellow Bible student. In January 1978, he established a "discipling relationship" with Pastor Rea with whom he often discussed girlfriend and family problems. They met five times in early 1978, but when Nally lost interest in "discipling," the meetings were discontinued.

Following the breakup with his girlfriend in December 1978, Nally became increasingly despondent. Pastor Cory encouraged him to seek the counsel of either Pastor Thomson or Rea. The friendship with Cory and the five discipling sessions with Rea in early 1978, constituted the full extent of the "counseling" Nally received from defendants before the spring of 1979.

In February 1979, Nally told his mother he could not "cope." She arranged for him to see Dr. Milestone, a general practitioner, who prescribed Elavil, a strong anti-depressant drug, to relieve his depression. Milestone also recommended Nally undergo a series of blood and chemical tests. The record reveals that Milestone never referred Nally to a psychiatrist.

* * *

B. The Events Preceding Nally's Suicide

On March 11, 1979, Nally took an overdose of the antidepressant prescribed by Dr. Milestone. Plaintiffs found him the following day and rushed him to a hospital. At the hospital, Dr. Evelyn, Nally's attending physician, advised plaintiffs that because their son "was actually suicidal," she could not authorize his release from the hospital until he had seen a psychiatrist. The record indicates that plaintiffs, concerned about their friends' reactions to their son's suicide attempt, asked Dr. Evelyn to inform other persons that Nally had been hospitalized only for the aspiration pneumonia he suffered after the drug overdose rendered him unconscious.

On the afternoon of March 12, Pastors MacArthur and Rea visited Nally at the hospital. Nally, who was still drowsy from the drug overdose, separately told both pastors that he was sorry he did not succeed in committing suicide. Apparently, MacArthur and Rea assumed the entire hospital staff was aware of Nally's unstable mental condition, and they did not discuss Nally's death-wish comment with anyone else.

Four days later, Dr. Hall, a staff psychiatrist at the hospital, examined Nally and recommended he commit himself to a psychiatric hospital. When both Nally and his father expressed reluctance at the thought of formal commitment, Hall agreed to release Nally for outpatient treatment, but warned Nally's father that it would not be unusual for a suicidal patient to repeat his suicide attempt. Nally was released from the hospital by Drs. Hall and Evelyn the next day.

On his release from the hospital on March 17, 1979, Nally arranged to stay with Pastor MacArthur, because he did not want to return home. MacArthur encouraged Nally to keep his appointments with Dr. Hall, and arranged for him to see Dr. John Parker, a physician and Church deacon, for a physical examination.

* * *

Eleven days before his suicide, Nally met with Pastor Thomson for spiritual counseling. According to the record, Nally asked Thomson whether Christians who commit suicide would nonetheless be "saved." Thomson referred Nally to his training as a seminary student and acknowledged "a person who is once saved is always saved," but told Nally that "it would be wrong to be thinking in such terms." Following their discussion, Thomson made an appointment for Nally to see Dr. Bullock for a physical examination but did not refer Nally to a psychiatrist.

* * *

The day after his visit with Bullock, Nally encountered Pastor Thomson in the Church parking lot. Nally told Thomson that he was thinking of seeing a psychologist. Thomson recommended Nally contact Dr. Mohline, Director of the Rosemead Graduate School of Professional Psychology. The following day, Nally spent approximately 90 minutes with Mohline, who in turn referred him to the Fullerton Psychological Clinic. Nally and his father went to the clinic the next day, and Nally discussed possible therapy with Mr. Raup, a registered psychologist's assistant. Raup testified he believed that Nally was "shopping for a therapist or counselor or psychologist" and that he was not going to return to the clinic. At the end of the week, Nally met with a former girlfriend. She turned down an apparent marriage proposal by telling Nally, "I can't marry you when you are like this. You have got to pull yourself together. You have got to put God first in your life." The next day, Nally left plaintiffs' home following a family disagreement. Two days later, he was found in a friend's apartment, dead of a self-inflicted gunshot wound.

III. PROCEDURAL BACKGROUND

A. *Allegations of the Complaint*

As stated above, the *Nally I* Court of Appeal reversed, in a published opinion, a summary judgment for defendants. In the first two counts of the complaint, alleging wrongful death based on "clergyman malpractice" and negligence, plaintiffs asserted that defendant Church was negligent in the training, selection and hiring of its spiritual counselors. Plaintiffs also claimed that following Nally's suicide attempt by drug overdose, defendants failed to make themselves available to Nally for counseling and "actively and affirmatively dissuaded and discouraged [Nally] from seeking further professional psychological and/or psychiatric care."

* * *

Following the Court of Appeal's decision in Nally I, [reversing the grant of defendant's motion for summary judgment], defendants petitioned this court for review. We denied review and depublished the opinion. The case was returned to the trial court.

* * *

Plaintiffs introduced several counseling manuals that were apparently sold in the Church bookstore as supporting an inference that defendants advertised that its counselors were competent to treat a myriad of emotional problems, and as evidence of defendants' inadequate training as counselors. The manuals, however, while advocating "If a problem is not organically caused . . . the counselor can, with full assurance look to God's Word for its proper solution," do not appear to have presented defendants as anything other than pastoral counselors.

In ruling on the nonsuit motion, the trial court noted that Nally voluntarily sought defendants' counsel and that the court had no compelling reason to interfere in defendants' pastoral activities.

* * *

The Court of Appeal again reversed, holding that although the "clergyman malpractice" count failed to state a cause of action separate from the "negligence" count, both could be construed as stating a cause of action for the "negligent failure to prevent suicide" by "nontherapist counselors." In this context, the Court of Appeal held that nontherapist counselors—*both religious and secular*—have a duty to refer suicidal persons to psychiatrists or psychotherapists qualified to prevent suicides. Moreover, the court held, imposition of a negligence standard of care on pastoral counselors does not impinge on the free exercise of religion guaranteed by the First Amendment, because the state's compelling interest in the preservation of life justifies the narrowly tailored burden on religious expression imposed by such tort liability.

* * *

Our review of the record reveals the trial court correctly granted a nonsuit as to plaintiffs' causes of action. Neither the evidence adduced at trial nor well-established principles of tort law support the Court of Appeal's reversal of nonsuit in this case. As we explain below, we need not address the constitutional issues posed by defendants.

* * *

1. *Legal Requirements for Imposing a Duty of Care*

a) *Creation of a Duty*

"A tort, whether intentional or negligent, involves a violation of a *legal duty,* imposed by statute, contract or otherwise, owed by the defendant to the person injured. Without such a duty, any injury is 'damnum absque injuria'—injury without wrong. [Citations.]" (5 Witkin, Summary of Cal.Law (10th ed. 1988) Torts, § 6, p. 61, italics in original.) Thus, in order to prove facts sufficient to support a finding of negligence, a plaintiff must show that defendant had a duty to use due care, that he breached that duty, and that the breach was the proximate or legal cause of the resulting injury.

* * *

b) Special Relationship

Although we have not previously addressed the issue presently before us, we have imposed a duty to prevent a foreseeable suicide only when a special relationship existed between the suicidal individual and the defendant or its agents. For example, two cases imposed such a duty in wrongful death actions after plaintiffs proved that the deceased committed suicide in a hospital or other in-patient facility that had accepted the responsibility to care for and attend to the needs of the suicidal patient. * * * In *Meier,* a cause of action for negligence was held to exist against both the treating psychiatrist and the hospital, and in *Vistica,* liability was imposed on the hospital alone, the only named defendant in the case.

The Court of Appeal here would extend the previously carefully limited precedent, relying initially for the creation of a duty of care (on defendants and other nontherapist counselors) in the foregoing *Meier* and *Vistica* cases. Indeed, the Court of Appeal specifically stated that "Logic and policy both dictate the duty announced in those cases applies to non-therapist counselors as well." We disagree. As defendants and amici curiae point out, *Meier* and *Vistica* are readily distinguishable from the facts of the present case and, as we explain, severely circumscribe the duty they create.

Both *Meier* and *Vistica* address the issue of a special relationship, giving rise to a duty to take precautions to prevent suicide, in the limited context of hospital-patient relationships where the suicidal person died while under the care and custody of hospital physicians who were aware of the patient's unstable mental condition. In both cases, the patient committed suicide while confined in a hospital psychiatric ward. Liability was imposed because defendants failed to take precautions to prevent the patient's suicide even though the medical staff in charge of the patient's care knew that the patient was likely to attempt to take his own life.

Neither case suggested extending the duty of care to personal or religious counseling relationships in which one person provided nonprofessional guidance to another seeking advice and the counselor had no control over the environment of the individual being counseled. In sharp contrast, Nally was not involved in a supervised medical relationship with defendants, and he committed suicide well over two weeks after he was released from the hospital against the advice of his attending psychiatrist and physician.

Plaintiffs and the Court of Appeal also rely on *Bellah v. Greenson* (1978) 81 Cal.App.3d 614, 620–623, 146 Cal.Rptr. 535, as supporting the existence of a special relationship sufficient to impose a duty of care on nontherapist counselors to refer a counselee to a licensed mental health professional once the potential suicide becomes foreseeable. As we explain, the Court of Appeal would unduly extend the *Bellah* holding.

In *Bellah,* two years after their daughter's suicide, plaintiffs brought a wrongful death action against a psychiatrist who had been treating the daughter on an out-patient basis. Plaintiffs alleged the existence of a psychiatrist-patient relationship between defendant and their daughter, knowledge on the part of the defendant that their daughter was likely to attempt suicide, and a failure by defendant to take appropriate preventative measures "consonant with good medical practice in the community." (*Bellah,* supra, 81 Cal.App.3d at p. 620, 146 Cal.Rptr. 535.) The Court of Appeal affirmed the trial court's order sustaining defendant's demurrer after concluding that the action was barred by the one-year statute of limitations contained in Code of Civil Procedure section 340.5.

In dictum, the *Bellah* court recognized that although plaintiffs' action was time barred, they had stated a traditional medical malpractice cause of action for the breach of a psychiatrist's duty of care to his patient. *Bellah* stated that this duty may be imposed on the treating psychiatrist even though his patient committed suicide outside the confines of a hospital. (Id., at p. 620, 146 Cal.Rptr. 535.) It is important to recognize, however, that rather than creating a broad duty to refer, the *Bellah* court simply recognized that plaintiffs had stated a "cause of action for the breach by a medical practitioner of the duty of care owed to his patient [which] has long existed in this state."

* * *

Thus, contrary to the Court of Appeal's interpretation of *Bellah,* *Vistica,* and *Meier,* none of these cases supports the finding of a special relationship between Nally and defendants, or the imposition of a duty to refer a suicidal person to a professional therapist as urged in the present case. Indeed, on their limited facts, *Bellah, Vistica* and *Meier* weigh against creating such a duty. With the foregoing in mind, we now turn to other considerations articulated in *Rowland v. Christian,* supra, 69 Cal.2d 108, 112–113, 70 Cal.Rptr. 97, 443 P.2d 561, and explain further why we should not impose a duty to prevent suicide on defendants and other nontherapist counselors.

c) The Connection Between Defendants' Conduct and Nally's Suicide and the Foreseeability of Harm

Other factors to consider in determining whether to impose a duty of care on defendants include the closeness of the causal connection between defendants' conduct and the injury suffered, and the foreseeability of the particular harm to the injured party. * * *

Plaintiffs argue that Nally's statement to Pastors Rea and MacArthur (while he was recovering from his suicide attempt at the hospital), "that he was sorry he wasn't successful and that he would attempt suicide after his release from the hospital," were "hidden dangers" that would have affected his prognosis and treatment. Accordingly, plaintiffs reason that Rea and MacArthur should have warned the hospital staff and plaintiffs that Nally was still contemplating suicide after his initial attempt. We disagree.

The closeness of connection between defendants['] conduct and Nally's suicide was tenuous at best. As defendants observe, Nally was examined by five physicians and a psychiatrist during the weeks following his suicide attempt. Defendants correctly assert that they "arranged or encouraged many of these visits and encouraged Nally to continue to cooperate with all doctors." In addition, as stated above, following Nally's overdose attempt Dr. Evelyn warned plaintiffs that Nally remained suicidal and that they should encourage him to see a psychiatrist on his release from the hospital. Plaintiffs also rejected both Dr. Hall's and Dr. Parker's suggestion that Nally be institutionalized because, according to plaintiffs, their son was "not crazy."

Nevertheless, we are urged that mere knowledge on the part of the defendants that Nally may have been suicidal at various stages in his life should give rise to a duty to refer. Imposition of a duty to refer Nally necessarily would imply a general duty on all nontherapists to refer all potentially suicidal persons to licensed medical practitioners.

One can argue that it is foreseeable that if a nontherapist counselor fails to refer a potentially suicidal individual to professional, licensed therapeutic care, the individual may commit suicide. While under some circumstances counselors may conclude that referring a client to a psychiatrist is prudent and necessary, our past decisions teach that it is inappropriate to impose a duty to refer—which may stifle all gratuitous or religious counseling—based on foreseeability alone. Mere foreseeability of the harm or knowledge of the danger, is insufficient to create a legally cognizable special relationship giving rise to a legal duty to prevent harm.

d) *Public Policy Considerations*

Imposing a duty on defendants or other nontherapist counselors to, in the Court of Appeal's words, "insure their counselees [are also] under the care of psychotherapists, psychiatric facilities, or others authorized and equipped to forestall imminent suicide," could have a deleterious effect on counseling in general. Although both plaintiffs and the present Court of Appeal, in dictum, exempt services such as "teen hotlines" which offer only "band aid counseling," from a newly formulated standard of care that would impose a "duty to refer," the indeterminate nature of liability the Court of Appeal imposes on nontherapist counselors could deter those most in need of help from seeking treatment out of fear that their private disclosures could subject them to involuntary commitment to psychiatric facilities.

As defendants, amici curiae, and the Court of Appeal dissenter observe, neither the Legislature nor the courts have ever imposed a legal obligation on persons to take affirmative steps to prevent the suicide of one who is not under the care of a physician in a hospital. * * * Indeed, for all practical purposes, a doctor to whom a nontherapist counselor refers a suicidal person may refuse to take the patient.

Furthermore, under the Lanterman–Petris–Short Act (Welf. & Inst. Code, §§ 5200, 5201), "[a]ny individual may" but is not required to institute involuntary commitment proceedings.

We also note that the Legislature has exempted the clergy from the licensing requirements applicable to marriage, family, child and domestic counselors (Bus. & Prof.Code, § 4980 et seq.) and from the operation of statutes regulating psychologists (id., § 2908 et seq.). In so doing, the Legislature has recognized that access to the clergy for counseling should be free from state imposed counseling standards, and that "the secular state is not equipped to ascertain the competence of counseling when performed by those affiliated with religious organizations." (Ericsson, *Clergyman Malpractice: Ramifications of a New Theory* (1981) 16 Val.U.L.Rev. 163, 176.)

Furthermore, extending liability to voluntary, noncommercial and noncustodial relationships is contrary to the trend in the Legislature to encourage private assistance efforts. This public policy goal is expressed in the acts of the Legislature abrogating the "Good Samaritan" rule. Statutes barring the imposition of ordinary negligence liability on one who aids another now embrace numerous scenarios. (See, e.g., Gov.Code, § 50086 [exempting from liability first aid volunteers summoned by authorities to assist in search or rescue operations]; Health & Saf.Code, §§ 1799.100, 1799.102 [exempting from liability nonprofessional persons giving cardiopulmonary resuscitation].)

* * *

Even assuming that workable standards of care could be established in the present case, an additional difficulty arises in attempting to identify with precision those to whom the duty should apply. Because of the differing theological views espoused by the myriad of religions in our state and practiced by church members, it would certainly be impractical, and quite possibly unconstitutional, to impose a duty of care on pastoral counselors. Such a duty would necessarily be intertwined with the religious philosophy of the particular denomination or ecclesiastical teachings of the religious entity. * * * We have previously refused to impose a duty when to do so would involve complex policy decisions, and we are unpersuaded by plaintiffs that we should depart from this policy in the present case. * * *

e) Availability of Insurance

As several commentators observe, although lawsuits stemming from spiritual counseling are few, a new type of "clergyman malpractice" insurance has been offered to religious organizations to protect against potential liability for spiritual counseling that causes injury. (See, e.g., Note, *Intentional Infliction of Emotional Distress by Spiritual Counselors: Can Outrageous Conduct Be "Free Exercise"?* (1986) 84 Mich.L.Rev. 1296, 1300, fn. 12.) Apparently, such insurance provides coverage to religious congregations and their pastors for damages caused by the counseling activities of the pastors while acting within the scope of their duties. (Ibid.) The value of such insurance, however, is unknown and difficult to determine because few cases have been filed against the clergy.

f) Conclusion

For the foregoing reasons, we conclude that plaintiffs have not met the threshold requirements for imposing on defendants a duty to prevent suicide. Plaintiffs failed to persuade us that the duty to prevent suicide (heretofore imposed only on psychiatrists and hospitals while caring for a suicidal patient) or the general professional duty of care (heretofore imposed only on psychiatrists when treating a mentally disturbed patient) should be extended to a nontherapist counselor who offers counseling to a potentially suicidal person on secular or spiritual matters.

In the present case, the Court of Appeal erroneously created a broad duty to refer, and to hold defendants potentially accountable for Nally's death based on their counseling activities would place blame unreasonably and contravene existing public policy. Accordingly, we conclude the trial court correctly granted defendants' nonsuit motion as to the "clergyman malpractice" or negligence causes of action.

* * *

The judgment of the Court of Appeal is reversed and the Court of Appeal is directed to enter judgment affirming the judgment of nonsuit and dismissing the action.

MOSK, PANELLI, ARGUELLES and EAGLESON, JJ., concur.

KAUFMAN, JUSTICE, concurring.

I concur in the judgment that nonsuit was properly granted, but disagree with the majority's holding that defendants owed no duty of care to the plaintiffs.

The majority appears to reject the proposition that defendants in this matter, or "nontherapist counselors in general," have a duty to advise potentially suicidal counselees to seek competent medical care. (Maj. opn. at p. 105 of 253 Cal.Rptr., at p. 956 of 763 P.2d.) Yet the majority does not purport to "foreclose imposing liability on nontherapist counselors, who hold themselves out as professionals, for injuries related to their counseling activities." (Maj. opn. at p. 110, fn. 8 of 253 Cal.Rptr., at p. 961, fn. 8 of 763 P.2d.)

In view of the majority's suggestion that a nontherapist counselor who holds himself out as competent to treat a suicidal person owes a duty of care to that person, I am baffled as to the basis or the *necessity* of the majority's broad conclusion that "nontherapist counselors in general" do *not* owe such a duty. The evidence in the record, viewed—as the law requires—in *plaintiffs'* favor, demonstrates that defendants (1) expressly held themselves out as fully competent to deal with the most severe psychological disorders, including major depression with suicidal symptoms, (2) developed a close counseling relationship with Kenneth Nally for that very purpose, and (3) realized that Nally's suicide was at least a possibility. Thus, the evidence was more than sufficient, in my view, to trigger a minimal duty of care to Nally. What was fatally *absent* from plaintiffs' case was not evidence of duty, but proof that defendants breached that duty, and that such breach constituted a proximate cause of Nally's suicide. Therefore, while I concur in the decision to reverse the judgment of the Court of Appeal and to reinstate the judgment of nonsuit and dismissal of the action, I strongly disagree with the conclusion that defendants owed no duty of care in this matter.

* * *

BROUSSARD, J., concurs.

Questions and Comments

1. *Questions.* Which view is more compelling, that of the majority or that of Justice Kaufman, who would not foreclose the imposition of liability on non-therapist counselors if they "hold themselves out as professionals, for injuries related to their counseling activities"? What might be the negative consequences of adopting the dissent's position? Would it necessarily cut down on religious counselors or would it tend to encourage religious counselors to make referrals where they are in doubt as to the condition or prognosis of the person they are counseling?

If liability were imposed on religious counselors who purport to deal with mentally distressed parishioners, is there any way of distinguishing "teen hotlines" or other telephone hotlines which offer only "band aid counseling"? Does the majority opinion speak to this?

2. *Liability of unlicensed therapists.* Persons who hold themselves out as mental health professionals, even though they are not licensed under state law, will generally be held to the standard of care of the profession that they are purporting to practice. For instance, in *Horak v. Biris*, the defendant, a certified social worker who operated a "center for psychotherapy", was charged with malpractice (having engaged in sexual relations with a patient) and defended on the grounds that he should not be held to a standard of care of a psychologist. In rejecting this defense, the court made the following observation:

> The field of practice engaged in by defendant here more closely resembles the practice of psychology rather than social work, as those two practices are currently defined in the Illinois Revised Statutes. (See Ill.Rev.Stat.1979, ch. 111, pars. 5304 and 6302.) Because of the apparent overlapping of these two fields, we think the proofs may well reveal that defendant possessed or should have possessed a basic knowledge of fundamental psychological principles which routinely come into play during marriage and family counseling. The "transference phenomenon" is apparently one such principle, and has been defined in psychiatric practice as "a phenomenon * * * by which the patient transfers feelings towards everyone else to the doctor, who then must react with a proper response, the counter transference, in order to avoid emotional involvement and assist the patient in overcoming problems." (*Aetna Life & Casualty Co. v. McCabe* (E.D.Pa.1983), 556 F.Supp. 1342, 1346.) The mishandling of this phenomenon, which

generally results in sexual relations or involvement between the psychiatrist or therapist and the patient, has uniformly been considered as malpractice or gross negligence in other jurisdictions, whether the sexual relations were prescribed by the doctor as part of the therapy, or occurred outside the scope of treatment.

Horak v. Biris, 130 Ill.App.3d 140, 85 Ill.Dec. 599, 474 N.E.2d 13, 18 (2 Dist.1985). See also, *Corgan v. Muehling,* 167 Ill.App.3d 1093, 118 Ill. Dec. 698, 522 N.E.2d 153 (1 Dist.1988) (non-licensed psychologist was held to the standard of care of licensed professional psychologists).

d. Sovereign Immunity

As the preceding section makes clear, a mental health professional who provides substandard care or fails to conform to legal requirements such as informed consent may be liable for damages. The employing agency also may be liable for damages caused by the mental health professional. However, when the employing agency is a governmental one, such as a Veterans Administration hospital, or the professional is a public employee, special rules often apply to limit liability. These rules stem from the doctrines of sovereign immunity and official immunity.

The doctrine of sovereign immunity is largely historical in nature. When the United States was created from the former colonies of Great Britain, the new government inherited the sovereign immunity that had been enjoyed by the king. The doctrine was based on a monarchical semi-religious tenet that "the king can do no wrong," and its effect was to prevent the government from being sued without its consent. Justice Holmes stated the proposition in a more pragmatic way when he wrote in *Kawanankoa v. Polyblank,* 205 U.S. 349, 353, 27 S.Ct. 526, 527, 51 L.Ed. 834 (1907):

> A sovereign is exempt from suit, not because of any formal conception or obsolete theory, but on the logical and practical ground that there can be no legal right as against the authority that makes the law on which the right depends.

Sovereign immunity is rooted in social policy as well as in history. It is seen as preserving government's control over its funds, property, and instrumentalities. Without immunity, it is argued, the government would be hampered in its essential functions. In addition, some argue that a democratic society needs sovereign immunity to prevent individuals from depleting the treasury at the expense of the majority of the population.

The immunity doctrine has come under increasing criticism, however, as government has become larger and more pervasive. It is argued that injuries caused by the government should be born by the entire society as a cost of government rather than by the particular individual injured.

Originally the federal government alleviated this burden upon individuals on a case by case basis, with Congress adopting private acts allowing certain individuals to sue the government. In 1946, however,

Congress passed the Federal Tort Claims Act [FTCA], which waived the federal government's immunity from suit in a broad range of circumstances. Through the FTCA, Congress intended to compensate victims of the negligent conduct of government activities in circumstances in which a victim could collect damages from a private tort feasor.

The FTCA, however, excludes some torts from coverage, and thus the immunity doctrine remains in effect for those causes of action. For example, the federal government remains immune from suit for damages resulting from combat activities in time of war. A section of the FTCA provides that the United States will not be liable for "any claim arising out of arrest, battery, false imprisonment, false arrest, malicious prosecution, abuse of process, libel, slander, misrepresentation, deceit, or interference with contract rights" except in law enforcement cases. 28 U.S.C. § 2680(b). This provision has sometimes been broadly construed to preclude recovery from the government for medical malpractice. Thus, a claim of battery for an operation performed in a Veterans Administration hospital on the wrong leg of the plaintiff was denied in *Moos v. United States,* 118 F.Supp. 275 (D.Minn.1954), *affirmed* 225 F.2d 705 (8th Cir.1955).

The FTCA also excludes the federal government from liability for acts or omissions that are within the "discretionary function or duty" of any federal agency or employee. 28 U.S.C. § 2680(a). The distinction between discretionary and non-discretionary duties is often difficult. Almost every act performed by a government official includes some discretion in the manner in which it is performed. Therefore, the discretionary function exclusion has been construed by courts to involve a planning/operational distinction. *Dalehite v. United States,* 346 U.S. 15, 73 S.Ct. 956, 97 L.Ed. 1427 (1953). Under this test, the federal government has been held to be immune from suit based on negligence in making top-level planning decisions such as whether to export fertilizer. *Dalehite, id.* In contrast, the federal government may be held liable for the negligence of federal employees in the "operational" level of government in carrying out the plans even though such actions may involve a certain amount of discretion. For example, the Supreme Court in *Indian Towing Co. v. United States,* 350 U.S. 61, 76 S.Ct. 122, 100 L.Ed. 48 (1955), found that checking the electrical system of a lighthouse was at the "operational level" and did not involve discretion within the meaning of the FTCA. The government was therefore not immune from suit to recover damages suffered by a barge that ran aground while a Coast Guard lighthouse was not operating.

The FTCA additionally places various procedural requirements on persons with claims against the government. The most important is the requirement of exhaustion of administrative remedies. The injured party must have been denied relief from the agency from which recovery is sought before suit may be brought in court. In this way Congress sought to encourage compromise and to minimize the burden added to the courts when immunity was waived.

The principle that the sovereign cannot be sued without its consent applies with full force to the various states of the United States. Absent waiver, states, state agencies, and state officers in their official capacities are generally immune from suit. The doctrine has been criticized by some state courts, however, and appears to be in disfavor. See e.g., *Crowder v. Department of State Parks,* 228 Ga. 436, 185 S.E.2d 908 (1971), *cert. denied,* 406 U.S. 914, 92 S.Ct. 1768, 32 L.Ed.2d 113 (1972); *Muskopf v. Corning Hospital District,* 55 Cal.2d 211, 11 Cal. Rptr. 89, 359 P.2d 457 (1961). The Supreme Court of Colorado totally abandoned the doctrine in *Evans v. Board of County Commissioners,* 174 Colo. 97, 482 P.2d 968 (1971). Every state has, to at least some extent, consented to be sued by adopting legislation waiving sovereign immunity in some circumstances. These statutes, although generally not as comprehensive as the FTCA, serve much the same purpose. Immunity is waived only for those circumstances explicitly set forth in the statute and only if the prescribed procedures are followed. There are some circumstances, however, in which a state or state agency may be sued even though it has not waived its immunity. Such a circumstance arises when the state is acting not in its governmental capacity, but in a "proprietary" capacity, as when the state creates an agency to engage in a primarily commercial venture.

There is no uniform rule declaring whether state and municipal hospitals exist under the proprietary or governmental function of the state. The maintenance of a hospital for the service of the public health and to treat indigent patients is generally held to be a governmental function, and thus the hospital is immune from suit absent waiver of immunity. In contrast, the operation of a hospital for the purpose of obtaining a pecuniary profit is generally considered to be a proprietary function not immune from suit. Unfortunately, the majority of state hospitals fall within a middle category for which generalizations are impossible. *See* generally Annot. 25 A.L.R.2d 203, 228 (1952) and Supp. (1981).

Some cases arise in which the governmental agency is immune from suit, but the employee who actually committed the wrong is amenable to suit in his individual capacity. Such an action may be possible when its result will not affect the state's actions. Additionally, a plaintiff may wish to seek recovery from both the government agency and the individual employee. However, in any suit against a government employee one must consider the doctrine of official immunity.

Government employees are not, of course, absolved from their private and personal tort liabilities merely because of their employment. When, however, a person is injured as a result of government (federal, state, or local) action, the employee causing the injury may be immune from liability under the doctrine of official immunity.

Official immunity has been recognized by the courts as a means of relieving the burden that would otherwise fall upon government officials if they were held accountable in private tort suits for every action taken or decision made. The immunity allows government employees to execute their duties without unreasonable fear of liability and prevents qualified persons from being discouraged from entering government employment out of such fear. Courts have, however, recognized that not every government employee requires the same type of protection. The scope of the immunity therefore varies among government employees.

In essence there are two types of immunity: absolute and qualified. Judges have long been granted absolute immunity for their judicial acts, even when their conduct is corrupt or malicious. Such an immunity was recognized in order to preserve an independent judiciary by eliminating the possibility of vexatious suits. Because the immunity extends to all members of the judicial branch, such mental health professionals as hearing officers in commitment proceedings and psychiatrists appointed by the court benefit from the doctrine. A doctor who signs papers in a commitment process or who testifies at a commitment hearing has "absolute immunity" from liability for actions taken in his capacity as an officer of the court. *Duzynski v. Nosal,* 324 F.2d 924 (7th Cir.1963); *Williams v. Westbrook Psychiatric Hospital,* 420 F.Supp. 322 (E.D.Va.1976).

Generally, when a defamatory statement is made during the course of a judicial proceeding it is absolutely privileged, even if made maliciously and with knowledge that it was false. So long as the act was required or permitted by law, the privilege bars a civil cause of action for libel or slander. In some jurisdictions, the privilege exists during preliminary proceedings involving pleadings, affidavits, or other papers, whereas in other jurisdictions the privilege exists only after the action has begun. The privilege also extends to post-trial motions and final judgment enforcement proceedings.

An additional requirement for the immunity to attach is that the statement be made with the honest belief that it was relevant or material to the litigation. It does not protect slanderous statements which were plainly irrelevant, were voluntarily made, and which the declarant could not reasonably have believed were relevant.

In the mental health context, physicians are immune from suit regarding their diagnostic statements which would include testimony as to the presence of mental illness in a commitment proceeding, or reports and recommendations to a court in child custody proceedings. See, *Rogers v. Janzen,* 711 F.Supp. 306 (E.D.La.1989).

The policy supporting this absolute privilege is that society will benefit if witnesses are not deterred by the fear of civil liability from speaking the truth. This societal interest is thought to outweigh the risk that a witness will make false and malicious statements in a judicial proceeding.

In some jurisdictions, the absolute privilege also applies to quasi-judicial administrative proceedings, which include hearings before tribunals that perform judicial functions whether ex parte or not, and whether public or not. See *Petyan v. Ellis,* 200 Conn. 243, 510 A.2d 1337 (1986). The privilege has also been held to extend to social workers. See *Creamer v. Danks,* 700 F.Supp. 1169 (D.Me.1988).

Additionally, federal courts have tended to extend absolute immunity to lower level executive branch officers. Courts have recognized that many officers in federal administrative agencies (e.g., administrative law judges) perform functions similar to those traditionally performed by the judiciary. Thus those officers performing "quasi-judicial" functions may also qualify for absolute immunity.

In general, however, lower administrative officers are afforded only a qualified immunity, and this qualified immunity is only applied to those officers whose duties are regarded as "discretionary" as opposed to "ministerial." When performing ministerial duties, government employees or officers are held to the normal negligence standard.

Ministerial acts are those constituting mere obedience to orders or performance of a duty in which one has little or no choice. Discretionary acts, on the other hand, are those requiring personal deliberation, decision and judgment. One who decides to engage in a particular activity and decides how best to implement it, performs a discretionary act. The policy behind qualified immunity for discretionary acts is that the decision making process is benefitted when the decision maker is not threatened with the fear of future litigation by the few who may be harmed by the decision.

Generally, decisions relating to diagnosis, care and treatment require judgment and choice and are, therefore, considered discretionary. Specifically, a decision to detain a mentally ill patient or to release on a temporary or permanent basis requires the exercise of judgment and is, therefore, discretionary. See, *Porter v. Maunnangi,* 764 S.W.2d 699 (Mo.App.1988). Similarly, an evaluation of the suitability of a mentally ill patient to participate in an outpatient versus an inpatient program is discretionary. See *Canon v. Thumudo,* 430 Mich. 326, 422 N.W.2d 688 (1988).

If qualified immunity does apply, the officer cannot be held liable for any act within his governmental duties that was performed in good faith. Thus, for example, a psychiatrist employed by a state mental hospital who negligently determines that a civilly committed patient remains mentally ill and denies the patient release would be immune from liability for false imprisonment. If, however, the psychiatrist makes his report knowing that the patient is qualified for release, his report is probably in bad faith, and qualified immunity will not protect him from liability. *See e.g., Hoffman v. Halden,* 268 F.2d 280 (9th Cir. 1959); *Mierop v. State,* 22 Misc.2d 216, 201 N.Y.S.2d 2 (1960).

Actions that are wholly outside of the authority of the official, however, are not protected by the doctrine of official immunity. This limitation of the doctrine applies whether the immunity is absolute or qualified and may even allow plaintiffs to recover for discretionary acts of the official. However, courts will often extend the immunity to the officer if determination of the scope of his authority would have required a determination of legal questions that could perplex a court. Thus, if an officer acted under authority of a statute later determined to be unconstitutional, he is protected by the same immunity he would have if the statute had been valid. The immunity of public officials in actions brought under the federal Civil Rights Acts is discussed in section III. B. infra.

The various types of immunity recognized for governments and government employees have come under increasing attack as the role of government has increased in this country. Many have argued that liability should be borne by all as a cost of government and that government employees should not enjoy more privileges than they would have if employed in a similar function in the private sector. Certainly many of the original justifications for the immunities have changed. Courts and legislatures have therefore adjusted the immunity doctrines to try to deal with these changes by waiving or eroding immunity in some areas and extending it into others. That process continues today. Whatever the ultimate outcome, government and official immunity will undoubtedly continue to have an important place in litigation involving the mental health professions.

B. SELECTED ISSUES IN THE APPLICATION OF THE DOCTRINE OF NEGLIGENCE

1. *Proximate Cause and Suicide*

WEATHERS v. PILKINTON

Court of Appeals of Tennessee, 1988.
754 S.W.2d 75.

OPINION

CANTRELL, JUDGE.

In this action for wrongful death against a doctor who allegedly failed to take the proper steps to prevent his patient from taking his own life, the trial judge held that the suicide of the [decedent] was an independent intervening cause and directed a verdict for the defendant. We affirm, on a related, although slightly different, ground.

The decedent, Michael Weathers, was born on November 6, 1955 and married the plaintiff, Ellen Weathers, on March 5, 1982. Mrs. Weathers gave birth to a son, Michael Houston, who was born on July 27, 1983. At Christmas of 1983 the decedent made his first overt reference to his death when, during an argument with the plaintiff, he pulled a gun from the drawer and invited the plaintiff to shoot him. In March of 1984, when his wife was out of town, the decedent called her long distance to tell her he had just taken an overdose of codeine. Fortunately, he regurgitated the codeine and when the plaintiff arrived home the next day he was all right. On Easter Sunday of 1984 the decedent got into an argument with the plaintiff and again invited her to kill him with a knife. Following that event he entered the Vanderbilt Hospital where he stayed for two weeks under the care of Dr. Robert Jack, a psychiatrist. Dr. Jack dismissed the decedent from the hospital and prescribed Elavil for his depression and referred him to the Luton Mental Health Center for outpatient consultation. For a time Mr. Weathers' condition improved but he cut back on his medicine and his depression and paranoia returned.

Mr. and Mrs. Weathers separated in late August of 1984, after arguing about an incident in which the decedent had gone to scout a field for dove hunting and left the plaintiff and their sick child at home without any transportation. On September 14, 1984 Mr. Weathers took an overdose of Elavil and was admitted to Memorial Hospital in Nashville under the care of the defendant, Dr. Robert D. Pilkinton. Mr. Weathers had apparently attempted to commit suicide since he had left a suicide note behind. Dr. Pilkinton stated to members of the family that he could treat Mr. Weathers' medical condition but that psychological problems were out of his (Dr. Pilkinton's) field.

After a period in intensive care and a total of eight days in the hospital Mr. Weathers was discharged. On November 7, 1984 he apparently took another overdose of drugs and left a suicide note. Mrs. Weathers and his sister were able to rouse him but for a time he had hallucinations and appeared disoriented.

On November 10, 1984 Mr. Weathers again took an overdose of drugs and was taken unconscious to Memorial Hospital. He stayed overnight in Dr. Pilkinton's care but demanded to be released the next morning. Although Mrs. Weathers and other members of the family requested Dr. Pilkinton to commit Mr. Weathers involuntarily, the doctor released him and urged him to return to the Luton Mental Health Clinic for treatment.

After his release from the hospital on November 11, 1984 Mr. Weathers begged his wife to return to live with him, and he returned to his mother's home where he lived for the next seventeen days in an apparently normal manner. He went back to work, he drove a car, he went hunting once or twice, and he attended a family gathering with his son at Thanksgiving. He was in a good mood, appearing to be more friendly and talkative than he had been in the recent past.

On November 16, 1984 the plaintiff, Ellen Weathers, consulted an attorney and signed a complaint for a divorce. On November 17 she told Mr. Weathers that she had commenced the divorce action but that if he would seek help they could be remarried.

On November 28 Mr. Weathers went to work as usual. After work he expected the plaintiff to bring the family car over to his mother's house for him to do some work on it. Mrs. Weathers did not keep the appointment because their child was upset, but the parties had several telephone conversations. In one of the conversations Mr. Weathers told Mrs. Weathers that he intended to shoot himself. Mrs. Weathers tried to keep him on the telephone but Mr. Weathers apparently carried out his threat before the members of the family or the police arrived.

The plaintiff, Ellen Weathers, brought this action against Dr. Pilkinton. The complaint contains two counts. The first count is for the wrongful death of Michael Weathers under our wrongful death statute, Tenn.Code Ann. § 20–5–110. The second count is for the tort of outrageous conduct and is brought on behalf of Mrs. Weathers personally. Under the first count the plaintiff alleged that the negligence of Dr. Pilkinton was the proximate cause of Mr. Weathers' death.

At the trial the plaintiff presented two expert witnesses. They testified that to fulfill the standard of care in effect in the Nashville area, Dr. Pilkinton should have committed Mr. Weathers involuntarily on November 11, 1984 and should have ordered a psychiatric evaluation of Mr. Weathers after the three recent suicide attempts. In addition the experts testified that it was a mistake for Dr. Pilkinton to order Mr. Weathers to return to Luton Mental Health Center for outpatient care since his previous experience there had proved unsuccessful. Finally, each expert testified that in his opinion Dr. Pilkinton's negligence was the proximate cause of Mr. Weathers' death.

At the close of the plaintiff's proof the trial judge directed a verdict in favor of Dr. Pilkinton on both counts. On the negligence count the trial judge held that Mr. Weathers' suicide was an intervening intentional act that proximately caused his death. (Therefore, assuming that Dr. Pilkinton deviated from the standard of care, his negligence could not constitute the proximate cause of the death of Mr. Weathers.) On the second count, the trial judge held that there was simply no evidence of an intentional infliction of emotional distress on Mrs. Weathers which is a necessary element of the tort of outrageous conduct.

The Outrageous Conduct Action

We affirm the directed verdict on the outrageous conduct count.

*   *   *

The facts of this case simply do not warrant a finding that Dr. Pilkinton's conduct was outrageous nor a finding that as a result of his conduct Mrs. Weathers suffered the type of severe emotional distress that is a necessary element of the tort.

The Wrongful Death Action

*   *   *

There is evidence in the record from which the jury might find that Dr. Pilkinton was negligent in treating Mr. Weathers. *   *   *

If there is evidence from which the jury could have concluded that Dr. Pilkinton was negligent, the sole remaining question is whether there is evidence from which the jury could have concluded that the alleged negligence of Dr. Pilkinton was the proximate cause of the death of the decedent. As our Supreme Court said in *Lancaster v.*

Montesi, 216 Tenn. 50, 390 S.W.2d 217 (1965), the cases in this jurisdiction and elsewhere have generally held that an act of suicide breaks the chain of causation unless the decedent's reason and memory were so far obscured that he did not know and understand what he was doing and was not therefore a responsible human agency. *Id.* at 60, 390 S.W.2d at 222. * * *

In *Jones v. Stewart,* 183 Tenn. 176, 191 S.W.2d 439 (1946), a young man committed suicide after being accused of burglarizing a neighbor's home. The declaration alleged that the accusation was made without probable cause and that as a consequence the young man was so shocked and frightened that he was unable to endure the shame. Nevertheless, the court held that the intervening act of the deceased and not the tort of the defendant was the sole proximate cause of death. *Id.* at 181, 191 S.W.2d at 441. The court quoted the following excerpt from *Daniels v. New York N.H. & H.R. Co.,* 183 Mass. 393, 67 N.E. 424 (1903): "An act of suicide resulting from a moderately intelligent power of choice, even though the choice is determined by a disordered mind, should be deemed a new and independent, efficient cause of the death that immediately ensues." 67 N.E. at 426.

From this line of cases we conclude that where a defendant injures another either wilfully or negligently and as a result of the injury, the injured person commits suicide the act of suicide is, as a matter of law, an intervening independent cause if the decedent knew and understood the nature of his or her act or the act resulted from a moderately intelligent power of choice.

The appellant does not contest the rule established in *Jones* and *Lancaster,* but instead argues that there is a different rule where the decedent is under the care of a health care provider and consequently the health care provider has a specific duty of care to the patient. We acknowledge that there is a difference and—since proximate cause is based on forseeability—that the fact that mentally ill persons might take their lives if adequate precautions are not taken to protect them from themselves is more forseeable than the fact that a person injured by an ordinary act of negligence might become so depressed that suicide would result.

However, we must recognize that this is still an action for wrongful death and the right that survives to the widow is the same cause of action the decedent would have had had he survived. Thus, if the decedent could not have sued no right survives. *McCreary v. Nashville C. & St.L. Ry.,* 161 Tenn. 691, 696, 34 S.W.2d 210, 211 (1931).

Can we say that an action for wrongful death may be maintained where the decedent himself ended his life in a deliberate, calculated, and voluntary act of suicide; where he had "an understanding of the physical nature and effect of his act, and . . . a wilful and intelligent purpose to accomplish it"? In such a case the decedent himself would not have had a cause of action against his doctor for his own (the decedent's) voluntary act. Consequently, no cause of action would pass to the surviving spouse.

The rule is otherwise, of course, where the decedent did not know the nature or consequences of his act, or his reason and memory [were], at the time, so far obscured that he did not know and understand what he was doing and was therefore not a responsible human agency. Under those circumstances the act of suicide would not be a wilful, calculated, deliberate act that would defeat an action for wrongful death.

Therefore, we are of the opinion that the result in this case turns on the question of whether there is evidence in the record from which the jury might conclude that on the date of his death Mr. Weathers did not know and understand the nature of his suicidal act and, therefore, did not have a wilful and intelligent purpose to accomplish it. The only evidence in the record tending to show that Mr. Weathers did not know and understand the nature of his acts on November 28, 1984 is the circumstantial evidence of his history of depression, his treatment, and his prior suicide attempts. Neither of the medical experts who testified on behalf of the plaintiff testified that Mr. Weathers was bereft of reason or that he did not know and understand what he was doing.

On the other hand, the overwhelming evidence shows that from November 11 until November 28, 1984, Mr. Weathers functioned normally and lived an unremarkable life. Viewing the evidence in the light most favorable to the plaintiff, we are of the opinion that there is no evidence from which the jury could conclude that Mr. Weathers was, on November 28, 1984, in such a state of anxiety or depression that he did not know what he was doing. Therefore, the trial judge was correct in directing a verdict for the defendant.

The judgment of the court below is affirmed.   *   *   *

TODD, P.J., concurs.

TATUM, SPECIAL JUDGE, dissenting:

I agree with the majority in the dismissal of the outrageous conduct action, but must respectfully dissent from the majority opinion affirming the action of the Trial Court in directing a verdict for the defendant in the negligence action. In my view, a jury question was presented.

I agree with the majority that there was evidence of negligence on the part of the defendant. I disagree that such negligence could not be found by a jury to be the proximate cause of the death of the decedent.

The history of the previous attempts of the decedent to commit suicide is strong evidence that he was afflicted with a mental illness that caused suicidal compulsions. It was for this reason that the decedent was placed in the care of the defendant, a health provider. It was the duty of the defendant to attempt to prevent the decedent from committing suicide.

In *Adams v. Carter County Memorial Hospital*, 548 S.W.2d 307 (Tenn.1977), our Supreme Court cited, with apparent approval, a treatise in 24 Vanderbilt Law Review, 217 (1971) entitled "Civil Liability for Causing Suicide: A Synthesis of Law and Psychiatry." I quote from this treatise:

> "Hospitals and psychiatrists may be charged with an affirmative duty to prevent their patients from committing suicide. . . .

> First, it seems clear that liability could be imposed upon a psychiatrist for a gross error in judgment with respect to whether a patient should be confined. Giving full ambit to psychological justifications for not confining patients unless absolutely necessary, suicidal symptoms may be so apparent that confinement would be ordered by a psychiatrist of ordinary skill. For example, if an individual has made serious suicidal attempts, has been deeply depressed, has suffered loss of sleep, appetite, and in effect is almost unable to function in society, but his psychiatrist has declined to have him placed in a hospital, the psychiatrist might be held liable for the individual's subsequent suicide.

*   *   *

I agree with the New Jersey Superior Court in *Cowan v. Doering*, 215 N.J.Super. 484, 522 A.2d 444 (1987). In that case, a physician admitted a depressed patient to intensive care, who had taken an overdose of sleeping pills. The physician failed to take suicidal precautions. The patient subsequently attempted suicide by jumping from the hospital window. At trial, the physician took the position that the patient understood and appreciated the consequences of her acts and therefore her suicidal attempt was an independent intervening cause. In rejecting this defense and upholding a jury verdict, the New Jersey court stated:

> "Observation has particular efficacy where, as here, the duty of the physician and the hospital encompasses the responsibility to safeguard the patient from the reasonably foreseeable risk of self-inflicted harm.

> We find no sound reason to adopt the sterile and unrealistic approach that if a disabled plaintiff is not totally incompetent, he is fully legally accountable for his own negligence. In view of the present state of medical knowledge, it is possible and practical to evaluate the degrees of mental acuity and correlate them with legal responsibility. In our view, a patient known to harbor suicidal tendencies whose judgment has been blunted by a mental disability should not have his conduct measured by external standards applicable to a normal adult. Where it is reasonably foreseeable that a patient by reason of his mental or emotional illness may attempt to injure himself, those in charge of his care owe a duty to safeguard him from his self-damaging potential. This duty contemplates the reasonably foreseeable occurrence of self-inflicted injury regardless of whether it is the product of the patient's volitional or negligent act."

*   *   *

In my view, suicide is not an intervening independent cause that will relieve a physician of liability or negligence when the patient had no power of choice. There was evidence in this case that the decedent acted with compulsion and not through a power of choice. Even in criminal cases, a defense of insanity is good even when the accused has substantial capacity to appreciate the wrongfulness of his conduct when, due to mental illness, he does not have the capacity to "conform his conduct to the requirements of law." *Graham v. State*, 547 S.W.2d 531 (Tenn.1977). By analogy, I would hold that even if the decedent knew and understood the nature of the suicidal act, the physician would not be relieved of liability if decedent acted through compulsion and not by an "intelligent power of choice." As stated, the history of the decedent's previous attempts to commit suicide is circumstantial evidence sufficient to make a jury question as to whether the suicide was committed by "intelligent power of choice" or by compulsion due to mental illness. I repeat that this suicidal tendency or compulsion was specifically the ailment which the defendant was entrusted to treat.

* * *

I have a high respect for the opinions of my colleagues. However, I would reverse the judgment of the trial court and remand the case for trial on the negligence issue.

Questions and Comments

1. *Questions.* The majority in *Weathers v. Pilkinton* holds that suicide is an independent intervening cause unless the patient "did not know and understand the nature of his suicidal act and, therefore, did not have willful and intelligent purpose to accomplish this." Would this include or exclude an individual suffering from psychotic depression whose basic motivation for suicide is a feeling of worthlessness and a pessimism as to the future? If such individual would be held to "understand the nature of his suicidal act" wouldn't it result in nonliability even where the patient is being treated specifically to minimize the risk of suicide?

2. *Professional judgment rule.* Is the Pilkinton case really a disguised application of the professional judgment rule? While the opinion focuses on the issue of proximate cause, isn't the underlying rationale of the case based on the difficulties of suicide prediction?

3. *Standards applicable to hospitalized patients.* When an individual commits or attempts suicide while a resident of a hospital or psychiatric facility, courts have been less willing to exonerate the hospital and the professional staff for liability. In this situation, the therapist will be held to the ordinary standard of care and must take reasonable precautions to protect a patient from the possibility of suicide where the circumstances suggest that the patient is at risk of attempting suicide. See, for instance, *Farrow v. Health Services Corp.*, 604 P.2d 474 (Utah 1979).

4. *Proximate cause in other contexts.* The issue of proximate cause has also arisen in a different context. For instance, hospitalized psychiatric patients will sometimes wander away from the facility and die from exposure. While it was not negligent to permit the patient to be on the grounds unaccompanied, the question that may need to be resolved is whether the death could have been prevented by an earlier or more

diligent search of the surrounding grounds. This was the basic fact situation in *Lando v. State,* 47 A.D.2d 972, 366 N.Y.S.2d 679 (1975), modified, 39 N.Y.2d 803, 385 N.Y.S.2d 759, 351 N.E.2d 426 (1976), involving a suit against a state psychiatric hospital by the administrator of the estate of a deceased mental patient. The suit alleged negligence for failure on the part of the hospital to promptly conduct a search for the patient after she disappeared from the hospital grounds. The body was not found until eleven days after her disappearance. At the trial the extent and thoroughness of the search were seriously questioned, and the testimony as to the measures taken by the hospital was sharply disputed. Reversing an award for the plaintiff administrator, the court concluded that the element of proximate cause had not been adequately proved:

> To demonstrate entitlement to an award in this situation, the claimant must establish the existence of a duty; that the duty was breached and that the breach was the proximate cause of death. Even if we assume the existence of a duty and assume but do not concede its breach, the claim here must *fail because of a lack of proof that the breach was the proximate cause of the result.* Without this connection between the duty and the result, there can be no recovery * * *. The deceased may have been the victim of foul play or she may have died from natural causes and the time of death is uncertain. There is no proof as to when Miss Lando's body fell or was placed or thrown into the obscuring foliage. Hence, several possibilities as to what occurred exist and, since the State would not be responsible for one or more of these possibilities, the claimant cannot recover without proving that the death was sustained wholly or in part by a cause for which the State was responsible * * *. To conclude here that the failure to make an adequate search was the proximate cause requires speculation of the rankest sort.

Id. at 973, 366 N.Y.S.2d at 680. On review by New York's highest court the decision of the appellate division denying the claim for decedent's wrongful death was affirmed. However, the father's claim for damages for mental anguish resulting from his being "denied access and control over the body of his deceased daughter for a period of 11 days" was reinstated. 39 N.Y.2d 803, 385 N.Y.S.2d 759, 351 N.E.2d 426 (1976). See also, *Castillo v. United States of America,* 552 F.2d 1385 (10th Cir.1977).

2. Damages for Sexual Misconduct

CORGAN v. MUEHLING

Appellate Court of Illinois, First District, 1988.
167 Ill.App.3d 1093, 118 Ill.Dec. 698, 522 N.E.2d 153.

JUSTICE SCARIANO delivered the opinion of the court:

In March of 1979, Penelope Corgan came under the psychological care of Conrad Muehling. She alleges in count I of her complaint that he conducted her treatment negligently, was negligent in having sexual relations with her during this treatment, and "negligently failed either to recognize the evolution of the psychotherapeutic phenomenon of transference and countertransference or deal appropriately with such evolving phenomenon," all of which caused her emotional trauma.

*   *   *

This appeal is taken from those orders of the trial court which dismissed counts II and IV of the plaintiff's third amended complaint * * *. [In addition] the trial judge certified the related questions of whether *Rickey v. Chicago Transit Authority* (1983), 98 Ill.2d 546, 75 Ill. Dec. 211, 457 N.E.2d 1, bars Corgan from recovering for emotional damages under counts I and III. *   *   *

COUNTS I, III

A. Introduction.

In count I, Corgan charges Muehling with malpractice. Malpractice is a form of negligence *   *   * thus the first count is in essence for negligence. *   *   *

Furthermore, the parties agree that count III, wherein Corgan alleges willful and wanton misconduct, also is basically an action for negligence, since this court has held that willful and wanton misconduct is an aggravated form of negligence. *   *   * Count III is *not* for the intentional infliction of emotional distress; indeed, Corgan does not contend otherwise. While we must accept all well-pleaded facts as true *   *   * Corgan does not plead the elements that constitute intentional infliction of emotional distress. *   *   * She does not allege that Muehling's actions were calculated to cause severe emotional distress; rather, among other allegations, she claims that he was acting solely for his own sexual gratification. *   *   *

B. The Rickey Case.

Simply and briefly, the questions certified by the circuit court in this case are whether counts I and III of Corgan's third amended complaint are barred by *Rickey v. Chicago Transit Authority* (1983), 98 Ill.2d 546, 75 Ill.Dec. 211, 457 N.E.2d 1. In *Rickey,* the plaintiff was attempting to recover damages for the emotional distress he allegedly suffered as a result of the CTA's negligence when he saw his brother being injured on an escalator. (*Rickey,* 98 Ill.2d at 548, 75 Ill.Dec. 211, 457 N.E.2d 1.) The Illinois supreme court, in a unanimous opinion, framed the issue in the following manner: "The underlying question is, of course, whether any person who suffers emotional distress can recover, but the question here specifically is whether a bystander at the injury of another who, generally under the decisions, is a close relative of the bystander can recover." *Rickey,* 98 Ill.2d at 553, 75 Ill.Dec. 211, 457 N.E.2d 1.

The court then discussed the "impact rule," the governing law in Illinois at that time, which required physical impact or injury in order for a plaintiff to recover in an action for the negligent infliction of emotional distress. The *Rickey* court noted that this requirement had been frequently satisfied by trivial contacts, and that consequently the impact rule had fallen into disfavor. * * * The court also recognized that although recovery for emotional distress should not be determined solely on the basis of whether there was any physical impact visited upon the plaintiff, the appellate court went too far in adopting a standard which "would permit recovery for emotional disturbance alone." (*Rickey,* 98 Ill.2d at 554, 75 Ill.Dec. 211, 457 N.E.2d 1, citing approvingly Restatement (Second) of Torts § 436A (1965).) Our supreme court acknowledged that courts were hesitant in allowing recovery for purely emotional injuries and explained such unwillingness as follows: "courts have given as reasons for this reluctance apprehensions that the door would be opened for fraudulent claims, that damages would be difficult to ascertain and measure, that emotional injuries are hardly foreseeable and that frivolous litigation would be encouraged." *Rickey,* 98 Ill.2d at 555, 75 Ill.Dec. 211, 457 N.E.2d 1.

The court then proceeded to announce its holding:

> "The standard that we substitute for the one requiring contemporaneous injury or impact is the standard which has been adopted in the majority of jurisdictions where this question of *recovery by a bystander* for emotional distress has been examined. [Citations.] That standard has been described as the zone-of-physical-danger rule. Basically, under it a *bystander who is in a zone of physical danger* and who, because of the defendant's negligence, has reasonable fear for his own safety is given a right of action for physical injury or illness resulting from emotional distress. * * * *The bystander,* as stated, must show physical injury or illness as a result of the emotional distress caused by the defendant's negligence." (Emphasis added.) (*Rickey,* 98 Ill.2d at 555, 75 Ill.Dec. 211, 457 N.E.2d 1.)

Accordingly, the supreme court remanded the cause because the complaint did allege physical manifestations, and it was unclear whether the plaintiff was endangered by the alleged negligence and had a reasonable fear for his own safety. *Rickey,* 98 Ill.2d at 556, 75 Ill.Dec. 211, 457 N.E.2d 1.

C. Therapist–Patient Sexual Contact.

We have long been aware that plaintiffs in other states have successfully maintained malpractice actions against their psychologist, psychiatrist, or social worker, predicated primarily on the therapist's alleged sexual contact with his patient. The leading case is from the State of New York, wherein the plaintiff alleged that she "was induced to have sexual intercourse with the defendant as part of her prescribed therapy," and was as a result "so emotionally and mentally injured that she was required to seek hospitalization on two occasions during 1971." (*Roy v. Hartogs* (1976) 85 Misc.2d 891, 381 N.Y.S.2d 587, 588.) The court in *Roy* upheld the trial court's award of damages to the plaintiff, justifying its holding as follows: "By alleging his client's mental and emotional status was adversely affected by this deceptive and damaging treatment, plaintiff's counsel asserted a viable cause of action * * *." *Roy,* 381 N.Y.S.2d at 588.

The court of appeals in our sister state of Michigan, relying on *Roy*, held that allegations analogous to those in *Roy* were sufficient to state a cause of action for psychiatrist malpractice. (*Cotton v. Kambly* (1980), 101 Mich.App. 537, 300 N.W.2d 627.) * * *

The United States court of appeals has upheld an award for a plaintiff who alleged that the individual treating her psychiatric problems had committed malpractice by having sexual intercourse with her. (*Simmons v. United States* (9th Cir.1986), 805 F.2d 1363.) The plaintiff contended that her therapist, employed by the United States as a social worker in the Indian Health Service, was guilty of malpractice which had caused her to attempt suicide. A doctor who gave psychiatric counseling to Simmons subsequent to her having terminated consultation with the social worker "stated that her counselor's misconduct was the cause of her psychological problems and that her problems were due essentially to his inappropriate response to the normal 'transference phenomenon' in therapy." *Simmons*, 805 F.2d at 1364.

The court, in a unanimous opinion, proceeded to analyze the plaintiff's malpractice claim. It said that "[t]ransference is the term used by psychiatrists and psychologists to denote a patient's emotional reaction to a therapist * * *." (*Simmons*, 805 F.2d at 1364.) The court went on to explain that transference is crucial to the therapeutic process and that "[t]he proper therapeutic response is countertransference, a reaction which avoids emotional involvement and assists the patient in overcoming problems." (*Simmons*, 805 F.2d at 1365.) The court described as follows the legal consequences of a counselor's failure to properly manage the transference phenomenon: "When the therapist mishandles transference and becomes sexually involved with a patient, medical authorities are nearly unanimous in considering such conduct to be malpractice. [Citations.]" (*Simmons*, 805 F.2d at 1365.) Moreover, it recognized that "[c]ourts have uniformly regarded mishandling of transference as malpractice or gross negligence. [Citations.]" *Simmons*, 805 F.2d at 1365–66.

In a malpractice action in the State of Washington, the plaintiff alleged that she had a sexual relationship with her psychiatrist which "was the direct and proximate cause of damages to the plaintiff, including humiliation, mental anguish, shock, outrage, depression, inconvenience, medical expenses, loss of wages, marital difficulties and general deterioration of emotional well being." (*Omer v. Edgren* (1984), 38 Wash.App. 376, 685 P.2d 635, 636.) The trial court granted summary judgment to the therapist, but the appellate court reversed, holding that there was sufficient evidence for a finder of fact to determine that the defendant had committed malpractice.

The court concluded by addressing the doctor's contention that his patient had not been damaged. It noted that the plaintiff "testified in her deposition she suffered no loss with respect to medical expenses, lost earnings, or marital difficulties," but that she "claimed general as well as special damages." (*Omer*, 685 P.2d at 638.) The court, although cognizant of the difficulty articulated in *Rickey* of proving damages of this nature, nevertheless held that this problem in itself was not enough to bar the plaintiff from recovery because "[i]njury flowing from the alleged relationship, though difficult to prove, may be as real as that type of injury which can be proven with mathematical certainty." *Omer,* 685 P.2d at 638.

D. The Application of Rickey

* * *

* * * [T]here is considerable controversy and confusion over whether the zone of danger test should be used in cases involving direct victims of negligence. It is clear, however, that *Rickey* does not become inapplicable solely because a case involves a malpractice claim.

* * *

We believe that the application of the *Rickey* test in cases involving direct victims of malpractice is inappropriate. * * * Our conclusion is supported by the decisions of courts in other jurisdictions which have awarded damages to plaintiffs who have had sexual relations with their therapists, although these plaintiffs have not alleged that they were physically injured. As we have seen, the Washington court in *Omer* directly addressed this concern, concluding that the plaintiff nevertheless deserved compensation. Moreover, were we to hold to the contrary, it would be hopelessly difficult for individuals to plead an action for psychologist malpractice which results only in emotional distress, for it seems incongruous to the point of absurdity that in cases involving malpractice by psychologists a victim should be required to demonstrate that he or she was put in fear of *physical* injury. Nor can there be any rational justification for our courts to mandate that in order to qualify for damages in a psychologist or social worker malpractice case a patient exhibit physical manifestations of his or her emotional trauma suffered at the hand of therapists who are qualified to minister to their needs only in cases of mental or emotional malaise, especially since, as the *Omer* court points out, such an injury, "though difficult to prove, may be as real as that type of injury which can be proven with mathematical certainty." (*Omer,* 685 P.2d at 638.) We do not glean from *Rickey* any overarching unitary theory that would apply to the case at bar.

Therefore, in the absence of a decision by our supreme court which mandates a clearly different result, and supported by the law of our own appellate court and other jurisdictions, we hold that the zone of danger rule enunciated in *Rickey* has no application in this case, which involves a direct victim of negligence.

* * *

In conclusion, we hold that counts I, III, and IV of the complaint state * * * valid causes of action.

HARTMAN, P.J., and BILANDIC, J., concur.

Questions and Comments

1. *Requirement of intentional infliction or physical impact.* Some jurisdictions continue to adhere to the rule that recovery for mental suffering will not be allowed unless: a) the distress was inflicted intentionally, or b) the mental suffering is accompanied by a physical manifestation of the injury. Prosser & Keeton on Torts, 5th edition, West Publishing (1984), § 12. Since the emotional harm resulting from the sexual misconduct of the therapist cannot be said to have been *intentionally* inflicted, the plaintiff has at least a theoretical barrier to overcome in those jurisdictions which require either a physical impact or that the harms have been inflicted intentionally. *Corgan v. Muehling* is illustrative of the approach of courts in jurisdictions which require a physical impact or injury. On what basis was the court able to hold that the plaintiff had a cause of action, in spite of the fact that there was neither a physical impact or injury?

2. *Historical perspective.* Litigation charging malpractice for sexual misconduct is of fairly recent origin. Until the 1970's such conduct rarely led to litigation. In fact, a fringe element of the psychiatric profession had, at one point, openly advocated patient/therapist sexual relations as a legitimate form of therapy. Robertson, *Psychiatric Malpractice: Liability of Mental Health Professionals,* John Wiley & Sons, New York, 1988, pp. 325–326. The case of *Roy v. Hartogs,* 85 Misc.2d 891, 381 N.Y.S.2d 587 (1976), signaled a decided turn of attitude on the part of courts and the psychiatric profession. In *Hartogs,* the defendant was charged with having "induced" the plaintiff "to have sexual intercourse as a part of her prescribed therapy." The plaintiff alleged, as a result of the improper treatment, she had become "so emotionally and mentally injured that she was required to seek hospitalization on two occasions," 381 N.Y.S.2d at 588. *Roy v. Hartogs,* which resulted in a judgment for the plaintiff, received considerable publicity particularly as a result of a subsequent book, *Betrayal,* co-authored by the plaintiff and Lucy Freeman (New York: Stein & Day, 1976).

3. *Proof of damages.* What is the character of proof that must be shown by a plaintiff seeking recovery of damages for the sexual misconduct of the therapist? Must the patient/claimant submit proof that the sexual relations with the therapist either actually delayed his or her recovery or caused a further deterioration? Are there likely to be proximate cause problems in meeting such a requirement?

Would it make sense for courts to adopt a *per se* rule that sexual misconduct is actionable as negligence even in the absence of proof of actual damages? Some cases have suggested that difficulties of proof in cases of sexual misconduct should not bar a recovery. In *Omer v. Edgren,* 38 Wash.App. 376, 685 P.2d 635 (1984), the therapist defended on the grounds that the patient had not been damaged by the affair. As noted by the court:

> "The most elementary conceptions of justice and public policy require that the wrongdoer shall bear the risk of the uncertainty [of actual damages] which his own wrong has created. * * *

" 'The constant tendency of the courts is to find some way in which damages can be awarded where a wrong has been done. Difficulty of ascertainment is no longer confused with right of recovery' for a proven invasion of the plaintiff's rights. * * *"

Id. at 638.

4. *Other theories for recovery.* In jurisdictions which do not recognize a cause of action for *negligent* infliction of emotional distress the patient who has been sexually involved with the therapist may be able to rely on other theories to recover damages. Washington state courts, for instance, have allowed an action for assault against the offending therapist, even though the patient technically consented to the act of intercourse. As reasoned by the court, the fiduciary relationship that a therapist has to his patient serves to vitiate any consent that may have been given.

Aside from negligence and assault, what other theories might be used to obtain a recovery against a therapist who becomes sexually involved with his patient during the course of treatment?

5. *Punitive damages.* Punitive damages may be awarded when there are "circumstances of aggravation or outrage, such as spite or 'malice,' or a fraudulent or evil motive on the part of the defendant, or such a conscious and deliberate disregard of the interests of others that his conduct may be called willful or wanton." W. Prosser, *Handbook of the Law of Torts,* § 2, pp. 9–10 (4th ed. 1971), Prosser & Keeton On Torts, 5th edition, West Publishing (1984), § 2. Surprisingly, cases of sexual misconduct have not awarded punitive damages. For instance, in *Roy v. Hartogs,* discussed in note 2, supra, the trial judge had allowed $100,000 in punitive damages on the grounds that a "patient must not be fair game for a lecherous doctor." However, the Court of Appeals, while sustaining general damages, eliminated punitive damages altogether on the basis that actions constituting malpractice were not "wanton or reckless". Punitive damages have, however, been sustained in a few sexual misconduct cases. See, e.g., *Greenberg v. McCabe,* 454 F.Supp. 765 (E.D.Pa.1978).

6. *Non-patient claims.* Does a patient have a cause of action when the therapist has sexual relations with the patient's spouse? A recovery has been allowed to a non-participating party where both spouses were patients of the offending therapists. *Mazza v. Huffaker,* 61 N.C.App. 170, 300 S.E.2d 833 (1983), review denied, 309 N.C. 192, 305 S.E.2d 734 (1983). In sustaining a judgment in favor of a patient who discovered the therapist and the plaintiff's wife (who was also a patient) together in bed, the court relied on the theory of *de facto* abandonment. In its conventional form a cause of action for abandonment lies for the "failure by a physician to continue to provide services to a patient when it is needed in a case for which the physician has assumed responsibility and from which he has not been properly relieved." *Brandt v. Grubin,* 131 N.J.Super. 182, 329 A.2d 82 (1974) (finding no abandonment of a psychiatric patient). Aside from abandonment, could it be argued that the therapist's relations with the patient's wife also constituted negligent treatment of the husband?

7. *Damages for procedural irregularities in hospitalization.* Should damages be allowed where the plaintiff is found to have been in need of hospitalization but the hospitalization was accomplished by the use of irregular or illegal procedures? In *Di Giovanni v. Pessel,* 104 N.J.Super. 550, 250 A.2d 756 (1969), the defendant doctor who certified that the plaintiff was insane for purposes of commitment disregarded his statutory duty to examine the plaintiff within ten days of the commitment. The court held that while the examining psychiatrist deviated from his statutory duty, a dismissal of the malpractice claim was proper since there was uncontradicted evidence that she was in need of the hospitalization and treatment and so suffered no actual damage.

Note, however, that if the professional who deviated from a statutory duty which results in a deprivation of the patient's federal rights was acting "under color" of law, the plaintiff may be able to recover damages under 42 U.S.C. § 1983. See section III. B., "Claims Based on Federal Civil Rights Laws".

C. NEW DIRECTIONS IN THE DUTY OF CARE: LIABILITY TO THIRD PARTIES

As mentioned in a previous section of this chapter the traditional limit on professional liability was the contractual relationship, usually called privity of contract, between the professional and his client. Thus, the threshold question in a negligence suit was always whether the plaintiff had been the defendant's client. Unless a professional relationship had existed between the two parties, the court would usually dismiss the plaintiff's negligence suit. The privity doctrine is no longer the dispositive factor in professional negligence cases. An increasing number of jurisdictions have modified or repudiated this doctrine, concluding that while the privity limit on liability provides certainty in the law, it may not promote justice or deter negligent conduct. A move away from traditional limitations on a professional's liability to third parties (those with whom no contractual relationship exists) is traceable to a 1928 decision rendered by one of the most influential state courts of the time.

In the landmark case of *Palsgraf v. Long Island Railroad,* 248 N.Y. 339, 162 N.E. 99 (1928), the New York Court of Appeals established a test of foreseeability to determine whether the actor had a duty of care to the injured party.[a] Under this test, the court asked whether the

---

a. In *Palsgraf* a passenger was attempting to board one of the defendant's trains while carrying a bulky and apparently fragile package. The defendant railroad's employees while attempting to help the passenger board the train, jostled him, and the package fell to the ground. The unmarked package contained fireworks, which exploded upon impact. The force of the explosion knocked over a platform scale thirty feet away, which in turn fell upon and injured another passenger, the plaintiff in the case. At trial the jury found the defendant's employees negligent and entered an award for the plaintiff. New York's highest court, however, reversed that decision, concluding that although the trainmen might have been negligent toward the passenger boarding the train, those trainmen could not have foreseen that their negligent actions would injure the plaintiff, who had been standing

defendant actor should have reasonably foreseen that his actions would injure the plaintiff. If that question was answered affirmatively, the defendant would be found liable.

The court characterized this limitation on the extent of liability for negligence as follows:

> [T]he risk reasonably to be perceived defines the duty to be obeyed, and risk imports relation; it is risk to another or to others within the range of apprehension.

248 N.Y. at 344, 162 N.E. at 100.

Foreseeability of injury to a third person, therefore, may constitute an alternative basis of professional malpractice liability, imposing liability on a defendant-therapist who had no contractual relationship with the injured party. This foreseeability criterion, though a convenient benchmark of liability, is decidedly imprecise of measurement and extends professional liability beyond the limits set by the privity doctrine.

While foreseeability became a basis for tort liability under *Palsgraf*, malpractice cases against physicians continued to be governed by notions of privity for most circumstances. However, extension of a physician's liability to third parties was seen in the early 20's in cases involving contagious diseases. In 1919, the Supreme Court of Minnesota found a valid cause of action against a physician treating a patient for scarlet fever for failing to advise her parents that the disease was infectious and for advising them that it was safe to visit her, and even to remove her to her home without risk of the disease being communicated. *Skillings v. Allen*, 143 Minn. 323, 173 N.W. 663 (1919). The court found that the physician owed a duty of care to those who were "naturally exposed to infection to a greater degree than anyone else". Id. at 664.

In 1928, the Ohio Supreme Court held that a physician has a duty to warn persons in dangerous proximity to a smallpox patient of the infectiousness of the disease. *Jones v. Stanko*, 118 Ohio St. 147, 160 N.E. 456 (1928). The court upheld an award for the wrongful death of a man who visited the doctor's patient after being assured that the patient was not contagious. The patient died of black smallpox, as did the decedent in the case. The following materials trace the development of the third-person liability doctrine in the context of mental health treatment.

thirty feet away. The relationship between the parties, Chief Justice Cardozo said, would determine whether the defendant's actions constituted negligence toward the plaintiff.

MERCHANTS NATIONAL BANK & TRUST CO. OF FARGO v. UNITED STATES

United States District Court, District of North Dakota, 1967.
272 F.Supp. 409.

RONALD N. DAVIES, DISTRICT JUDGE.

This is an action brought by the Merchants National Bank and Trust Company of Fargo, a corporation, as Administrator and Personal Representative of the Estate of Eloise A. Newgard, deceased, against the United States of America, to recover damages by reason of the alleged negligent conduct of the defendant's agents and employees which resulted in the killing of Eloise A. Newgard by her husband, William Bry Newgard, in Detroit Lakes, Minnesota, July 31, 1965. Jurisdiction is predicated upon Title 28, U.S.C.A. § 1346 et seq., commonly described as the Federal Tort Claims Act. The suit is brought on behalf of the three minor children of the decedent. * * *

Early in the morning of January 17, 1965, Dr. Mack V. Traynor, a Fargo physician, was called to the Newgard apartment in Fargo, North Dakota, by Newgard's wife, Eloise. She was frantic-voiced and said she needed help. The doctor, promptly responding to the call, found Newgard glassy-eyed and making senseless talk about horses, cattle "and God most of the time." Dr. Traynor felt Newgard was completely psychotic. * * *

Dr. Albert C. Kohlmeyer, a well qualified psychiatrist, saw Newgard the same day in the Neuropsychiatric Institute section of the hospital. He found him very agitated, "carrying on" about religious ideas and testified that Newgard thought "he was Christ or some representative of Christ." Because of his delusional ideas, the psychiatrist thought Newgard was psychotic and although he saw Newgard only a couple of days, it was his belief that Newgard's illness had been coming on for a long time. Dr. Kohlmeyer felt Newgard was a schizophrenic, chronic, with acute exacerbation, paranoid type.

On January 19, 1965, the Cass County, North Dakota, Mental Health Board after a hearing, ordered Newgard committed to the State Hospital at Jamestown, North Dakota. Later because he was a veteran, an amended order was issued by the board, making the commitment a dual one so that Newgard could eventually be transferred to the Veterans Administration Hospital at Fort Meade, South Dakota. Effective March 23, 1965, Newgard was transferred to Meade where he was admitted to a ward and placed under the direct supervision of Dr. Leonard S. Linnell, a medical doctor and psychiatrist. * * *

For a number of weeks Newgard was treated with tranquilizers and saw a clinical psychologist, Dr. Jesse H. Craft, weekly, for psychotherapy and examinations. During the course of Newgard's treatment and care he was interviewed by Dr. Linnell about once a week. The psychiatrist also sent Newgard to Dr. Truman M. Cheney, a vocational psychologist, for testing and reporting his job aptitudes. Newgard was given various jobs around the hospital, a procedure followed by Meade in the treatment of hospital patients and which is followed in hospitals of a similar nature. * * *

Sometime before July 18, 1965, Dr. Truman M. Cheney, Counseling Psychologist at Meade, had made arrangements to put Newgard on leave at the ranch owned by Mr. and Mrs. Clarence A. Davis located some ten miles north of Belle Fourche, South Dakota. Dr. Cheney told Mr. Davis that Newgard had had "a mental disturbance, a nervous breakdown" and that Newgard wanted hard work to forget some of his troubles and for rehabilitation purposes. Mr. Davis had never before had a Meade patient working on his ranch.

On July 18, 1865, Newgard was released by Dr. Linnell on work leave to rancher Davis. * * *

It develops that on July 24, 1965, Newgard left the ranch for the weekend. He was to have returned Monday, July 26th, but Newgard went to his parents' home at Mayville, North Dakota. His wife Eloise had no idea he was in Mayville and was there herself only for a brief visit. Newgard wanted his wife to return with him to Fargo but she declined. Newgard got possession of a car and ultimately drove to his mother-in-law's home in Detroit Lakes, Minnesota, where on July 31, 1965, he first attempted to run Eloise Newgard down with the car and failing that, got out of the vehicle, shot and killed her.

* * *

[The court reviewed evidence which showed that in arranging for Newgard's placement on the ranch, no one at Meade took any steps to inform Rancher Davis of Newgard's condition or the conditions governing his release. It was also shown that the Meade staff made no attempt to monitor Newgard from the time he was placed on the ranch up to the time he shot his wife.]

Dr. Linnell ignored and rejected every warning signal that Newgard was delusional at Meade and every warning signal that Eloise A. Newgard had every reason to be in mortal fear of her husband because of his prior conduct and the nature of some of the letters he wrote her while a patient at Meade.

The plaintiff alleges that the Government, acting through its duly authorized agents employed by the Veterans Administration, undertook the custody, care and treatment of Newgard, knowing him to be an insane and incompetent person with homicidal tendencies, and that the Government's inexcusable negligence was the proximate cause of Eloise A. Newgard's death on July 31, 1965, at the hands of her husband.

The plaintiff's burden in this type of case is not an easy one, but it has successfully borne it, in proving, by a preponderance of the relevant, material and credible evidence, that the negligence of the defendant acting by and through its duly authorized agents and employees was indeed the sole and proximate cause of the death of Eloise A.

Newgard, and the damages sustained by the plaintiff as a result of her slaying.

The Government argued that modern psychiatry was on trial in this lawsuit. I reject that argument. It is not overstatement to suggest, however, that the *modi operandi* of some of its practitioners are. And that of some psychologists as well.

* * *

Considering the circumstances under which Newgard was placed on leave of absence at the Davis ranch, as disclosed by the credible evidence, the Government's agents and employees not only did not exercise due care; in the view of this Court they exercised no care at all. * * *

This Court is of the opinion that in the case of Newgard the defendant's agents were tortiously negligent both in the matter of substandard professional conduct on the part of Dr. Linnell, and because of gross negligence on the part of Dr. Linnell and Dr. Cheney in the careless custodial care of Newgard. * * *

It is difficult indeed to place a monetary value on the loving care and the advice and guidance of which the Newgard children will be forever deprived through the loss of their mother. It must be included, dispassionately, with the other factors set out herein in reaching the complex and always vexing question of compensatory loss in this type of case, and the declining value of the dollar has been taken into account.

The Court concludes that plaintiff is entitled to recover the sum of Two Hundred Thousand Dollars ($200,000.00) from the defendant, as compensatory damages, arising out of and from the gross negligence of the defendant, acting by and through its agents and employees, which was the sole and proximate cause of the death of Eloise A. Newgard, * * *.

Questions and Comments

1. *Restatement of Torts.* While the court in *Merchants National Bank* did not rely on the Second Restatement of Torts, § 319 of the Restatement does provide a basis for the imposition of liability on institutions:

> § 319 One who takes charge of a third person whom he knows or should know to be likely to cause bodily harm to others if not controlled is under a duty to exercise reasonable care to control the third person to prevent him from doing such harm.

The commentaries to this section of the Restatement make clear that the institution may be liable to a third party who is injured by a patient if:

> 1. A patient is released when the facility knew or had reason to know of the patient's dangerous proclivities;

2. The institution fails to conduct an adequate predischarge examination of a patient with a history of violent behavior; or

3. The institution's failure to take adequate precautions allows a patient to escape.

2. *Liability for release of dangerous patients.* A number of recent cases have imposed liability on psychiatric facilities for the release of patients that the institution knew or should have known to be dangerous. See, *Estate of Mathes v. Ireland,* 419 N.E.2d 782 (Ind.App.1981); *Semler v. Psychiatric Institute of Washington, D.C.,* 538 F.2d 121 (4th Cir.1976). In *Semler* the psychiatric facility had custody of a convicted felon, who, without court authorization, was placed on outpatient status. The patient killed an individual, and in a subsequent wrongful death suit the institution was found liable to the victim's parents.

While liability may attach where the institution releases a patient that it should have known was dangerous, the standard, as the materials which follow indicate, may be different when the individual who inflicted the injury was being treated on an outpatient basis by the therapist being sued.

3. *Voluntary patients.* Does it make a difference in terms of liability if the patient is voluntary, rather than involuntarily committed? Voluntary patients have the right to be released upon their request unless civilly committed. Some courts have adopted the position that a different standard will apply where the patient who causes the injury was in the institution on a voluntary status. See e.g., *Sellers v. United States,* 870 F.2d 1098 (6th Cir.1989), infra at 139, in which the court stated:

[T]here are additional reasons why Sellers cannot succeed on his claim of negligent discharge.

Firestine was admitted to the VAH voluntarily. A review of the case law will demonstrate that this fact is central to a determination of the VAH's duty regarding the length of Firestine's commitment. An analysis of this issue centers on the question of whether a "special relationship" exists between the patient and the hospital.

In *Hinkelman v. Borgess Medical Center,* 157 Mich.App. 314, 403 N.W.2d 547 (1987), the court specifically addressed the issue of when a special relationship should be found to exist. The court explained that the existence of a special relationship, such as that between a physician and patient, is premised on the notion of control over the patient. *Id.* at 550. In *Hinkelman,* the court found that there was no special relationship between the patient and the hospital when the patient had been admitted voluntarily, had not stayed more than a few days, and had left before he could be treated. *Id.* at 551. The court placed great weight on the fact that the duty imposed on mental hospitals is "based on the control vested by *involuntary* commitment." *Id.* at 552 (emphasis added). "In contrast, where a patient's hospitalization was voluntary, no duty has been imposed due to the facility's inability to compel patient confinement."

At 1104.

See also, Hinkelman v. Borgess Medical Center, 157 Mich.App. 314, 403 N.W.2d 547 (1987) (lack of control over voluntary patient precludes imposition of liability).

4. *Statutory immunity.* Some states have enacted laws that specifically grant immunity to institutions that improvidently release a patient or prisoner who subsequently injures a third party. In *Beauchene v. Synanon Foundation, Inc.,* 88 Cal.App.3d 342, 151 Cal.Rptr. 796 (1979), the court construed a state immunity statute, which on its face applied only to state correctional facilities, to protect private institutions that provide inpatient treatment to convicted criminals placed on probation. In denying relief to the plaintiff, who had been shot by a former patient of the institution, the court observed:

> [O]f paramount concern is the detrimental effect a finding of liability would have on prisoner release and rehabilitation programs. Were we to find a cause of action stated we would in effect be encouraging the detention of prisoners in disregard of their rights and society's needs.

At 348.

TARASOFF v. REGENTS OF UNIVERSITY OF CALIFORNIA

Supreme Court of California, 1976.
17 Cal.3d 425, 131 Cal.Rptr. 14, 551 P.2d 334.

TOBRINER, JUSTICE.

On October 27, 1969, Prosenjit Poddar killed Tatiana Tarasoff. Plaintiffs, Tatiana's parents, allege that two months earlier Poddar confided his intention to kill Tatiana to Dr. Lawrence Moore, a psychologist employed by the Cowell Memorial Hospital at the University of California at Berkeley. They allege that on Moore's request, the campus police briefly detained Poddar, but released him when he appeared rational. They further claim that Dr. Harvey Powelson, Moore's superior, then directed that no further action be taken to detain Poddar. No one warned plaintiffs of Tatiana's peril.

Concluding that these facts set forth causes of action against neither therapists and policemen involved, nor against the Regents of the University of California as their employer, the superior court sustained defendants' demurrers to plaintiffs' second amended complaints without leave to amend.[2] This appeal ensued.

Plaintiffs' complaints predicate liability on two grounds: defendants' failure to warn plaintiffs of the impending danger and their failure to bring about Poddar's confinement pursuant to the Lanterman–Petris–Short Act.

---

2. The therapist defendants include Dr. Moore, the psychologist who examined Poddar and decided that Poddar should be committed; Dr. Gold and Dr. Yandell, psychiatrists at Cowell Memorial Hospital who concurred in Moore's decision; and Dr. Powelson, chief of the department of psychiatry, who countermanded Moore's decision and directed that the staff take no action to confine Poddar.

* * *

Defendants, in turn, assert that they owed no duty of reasonable care to Tatiana * * *

We shall explain that defendant therapists cannot escape liability merely because Tatiana herself was not their patient. When a therapist determines, or pursuant to the standards of his profession should determine, that his patient presents a serious danger of violence to another, he incurs an obligation to use reasonable care to protect the intended victim against such danger. The discharge of this duty may require the therapist to take one or more of various steps, depending upon the nature of the case. Thus it may call for him to warn the intended victim or others likely to apprise the victim of the danger, to notify the police, or to take whatever other steps are reasonably necessary under the circumstances.

In the case at bar, plaintiffs admit that defendant therapists notified the police, but argue on appeal that the therapists failed to exercise reasonable care to protect Tatiana in that they did not confine Poddar and did not warn Tatiana or others likely to apprise her of the danger.

* * *

1. PLAINTIFFS' COMPLAINTS

Plaintiffs, Tatiana's mother and father, filed separate but virtually identical second amended complaints. The issue before us on this appeal is whether those complaints now state, or can be amended to state, causes of action against defendants. We therefore begin by setting forth the pertinent allegations of the complaints.

Plaintiffs' first cause of action, entitled "Failure to Detain a Dangerous Patient," alleges that on August 20, 1969, Poddar was a voluntary outpatient receiving therapy at Cowell Memorial Hospital. Poddar informed Moore, his therapist, that he was going to kill an unnamed girl, readily identifiable as Tatiana, when she returned home from spending the summer in Brazil. Moore, with the concurrence of Dr. Gold, who had initially examined Poddar, and Dr. Yandell, assistant to the director of the department of psychiatry, decided that Poddar should be committed for observation in a mental hospital. Moore orally notified Officers Atkinson and Teel of the campus police that he would request commitment. He then sent a letter to Police Chief William Beall requesting the assistance of the police department in securing Poddar's confinement.

Officers Atkinson, Brownrigg, and Halleran took Poddar into custody, but, satisfied that Poddar was rational, released him on his promise to stay away from Tatiana. Powelson, director of the department of psychiatry at Cowell Memorial Hospital, then asked the police to return Moore's letter, directed that all copies of the letter and notes that Moore had taken as therapist be destroyed, and "ordered no action to place Prosenjit Poddar in 72–hour treatment and evaluation facility."

Plaintiffs' second cause of action, entitled "Failure to Warn Of a Dangerous Patient," incorporates the allegations of the first cause of action, but adds the assertion that defendants negligently permitted Poddar to be released from police custody without "notifying the parents of Tatiana Tarasoff that their daughter was in grave danger from Posenjit Poddar." Poddar persuaded Tatiana's brother to share an apartment with him near Tatiana's residence; shortly after her return from Brazil, Poddar went to her residence and killed her.

* * *

2. PLAINTIFFS CAN STATE A CAUSE OF ACTION AGAINST DEFENDANT THERAPISTS FOR NEGLIGENT FAILURE TO PROTECT TATIANA

The second cause of action can be amended to allege that Tatiana's death proximately resulted from defendants' negligent failure to warn Tatiana or others likely to apprise her of her danger. Plaintiffs contend that as amended, such allegations of negligence and proximate causation, with resulting damages, establish a cause of action. Defendants, however, contend that in the circumstances of the present case they owed no duty of care to Tatiana or her parents and that, in the absence of such duty, they were free to act in careless disregard of Tatiana's life and safety.

In analyzing this issue, we bear in mind that legal duties are not discoverable facts of nature, but merely conclusory expressions that, in cases of a particular type, liability should be imposed for damage done.

* * *

* * * [Duty] is not sacrosanct in itself, but only an expression of the sum total of those considerations of policy which lead the law to say that the particular plaintiff is entitled to protection.

* * *

We depart from "this fundamental principle" only upon the "balancing of a number of considerations"; major ones "are the foreseeability of harm to the plaintiff, the degree of certainty that the plaintiff suffered injury, the closeness of the connection between the defendant's conduct and the injury suffered, the moral blame attached to the defendant's conduct, the policy of preventing future harm, the extent of the burden to the defendant and consequences to the community of imposing a duty to exercise care with resulting liability for breach, and the availability, cost and prevalence of insurance for the risk involved."

The most important of these considerations in establishing duty is foreseeability. As a general principle, a "defendant owes a duty of care to all persons who are foreseeably endangered by his conduct, with respect to all risks which make the conduct unreasonably dangerous." As we shall explain, however, when the avoidance of foreseeable harm requires a defendant to control the conduct of another person, or to warn of such conduct, the common law has traditionally imposed liability only if the defendant bears some special relationship to the dangerous person or to the potential victim. Since the relationship between a therapist and his patient satisfies this requirement, we need not here decide whether foreseeability alone is sufficient to create a duty to exercise reasonable care to protect a potential victim of another's conduct.

Although, as we have stated above, under the common law, as a general rule, one person owed no duty to control the conduct of another nor to warn those endangered by such conduct, the courts have carved out an exception to this rule in cases in which the defendant stands in some special relationship to either the person whose conduct needs to be controlled or in a relationship to the foreseeable victim of that conduct (see Rest.2d Torts, supra, §§ 315–320). Applying this exception to the present case, we note that a relationship of defendant therapists to either Tatiana or Poddar will suffice to establish a duty of care; as explained in section 315 of the Restatement Second of Torts, a duty of care may arise from either "(a) a special relation * * * between the actor and the third person which imposes a duty upon the actor to control the third person's conduct, or (b) a special relation * * * between the actor and the other which gives to the other a right of protection."

Although plaintiffs' pleadings assert no special relation between Tatiana and defendant therapists, they establish as between Poddar and defendant therapists the special relation that arises between a patient and his doctor or psychotherapist. Such a relationship may support affirmative duties for the benefit of third persons. Thus, for example, a hospital must exercise reasonable care to control the behavior of a patient which may endanger other persons. A doctor must also warn a patient if the patient's condition or medication renders certain conduct, such as driving a car, dangerous to others.

Although the California decisions that recognize this duty have involved cases in which the defendant stood in a special relationship *both* to the victim and to the person whose conduct created the danger, we do not think that the duty should logically be constricted to such situations. Decisions of other jurisdictions hold that the single relationship of a doctor to his patient is sufficient to support the duty to exercise reasonable care to protect others against dangers emanating from the patient's illness. The courts hold that a doctor is liable to persons infected by his patient if he negligently fails to diagnose a contagious disease or, having diagnosed the illness, fails to warn members of the patient's family.

Since it involved a dangerous mental patient, the decision in *Merchants Nat. Bank & Trust Co. of Fargo v. United States* comes closer to the issue. The Veterans Administration arranged for the patient to work on a local farm, but did not inform the farmer of the man's background. The farmer consequently permitted the patient to come and go freely during nonworking hours; the patient borrowed a car, drove to his wife's residence and killed her. Notwithstanding the lack of any "special relationship" between the Veterans Administration and the wife, the court found the Veterans Administration liable for the wrongful death of the wife.

*   *   *

Defendants contend, however, that imposition of a duty to exercise reasonable care to protect third persons is unworkable because therapists cannot accurately predict whether or not a patient will resort to violence. In support of this argument amicus representing the American Psychiatric Association and other professional societies cites numerous articles which indicate that therapists, in the present state of the art, are unable reliably to predict violent acts; their forecasts, amicus claims, tend consistently to overpredict violence, and indeed are more often wrong than right. Since predictions of violence are often erroneous, amicus concludes, the courts should not render rulings that predicate the liability of therapists upon the validity of such predictions.

The role of the psychiatrist, who is indeed a practitioner of medicine, and that of the psychologist who performs an allied function, are like that of the physician who must conform to the standards of the profession and who must often make diagnoses and predictions based upon such evaluations. Thus the judgment of the therapist in diagnosing emotional disorders and in predicting whether a patient presents a serious danger of violence is comparable to the judgment which doctors and professionals must regularly render under accepted rules of responsibility.

We recognize the difficulty that a therapist encounters in attempting to forecast whether a patient presents a serious danger of violence. Obviously we do not require that the therapist, in making that determination, render a perfect performance; the therapist need only exercise "that reasonable degree of skill, knowledge, and care ordinarily possessed and exercised by members of [that professional specialty] under similar circumstances."

Within the broad range of reasonable practice and treatment in which professional opinion and judgment may differ the therapist is free to exercise his or her own best judgment without liability; proof, aided by hindsight, that he or she judged wrongly is insufficient to establish negligence.

In the instant case, however, the pleadings do not raise any question as to failure of defendant therapists to predict that Poddar presented a serious danger of violence. On the contrary, the present complaints allege that defendant therapists did in fact predict that Poddar would kill, but were negligent in failing to warn.

Amicus contends, however, that even when a therapist does in fact predict that a patient poses a serious danger of violence to others, the therapist should be absolved of any responsibility for failing to act to protect the potential victim. In our view, however, once a therapist does in fact determine, or under applicable professional standards reasonably should have determined that a patient poses a serious danger of violence to others, he bears a duty to exercise reasonable care to protect the foreseeable victim of that danger. While the discharge of this duty of due care will necessarily vary with the facts of each case, in each instance the adequacy of the therapist's conduct must be measured against the traditional negligence standard of the rendition of reasonable care under the circumstances.

*   *   *

*   *   * In sum, the therapist owes a legal duty not only to his patient, but also to his patient's would-be victim and is subject in both respects to scrutiny by judge and jury.

The risk that unnecessary warnings may be given is a reasonable price to pay for the lives of possible victims that may be saved. We would hesitate to hold that the therapist who is aware that his patient expects to attempt to assassinate the President of the United States would not be obligated to warn the authorities because the therapist cannot predict with accuracy that his patient will commit the crime.

Defendants further argue that free and open communication is essential to psychotherapy that "Unless a patient *   *   * is assured that *   *   * information [revealed by him] can and will be held in utmost confidence, he will be reluctant to make the full disclosure upon which diagnosis and treatment *   *   * depends." The giving of a warning, defendants contend, constitutes a breach of trust which entails the revelation of confidential communications.

We recognize the public interest in supporting effective treatment of mental illness and in protecting the rights of patients to privacy and the consequent public importance of safeguarding the confidential character of psychotherapeutic communication. Against this interest, however, we must weigh the public interest in safety from violent assault. The Legislature has undertaken the difficult task of balancing the countervailing concerns. In Evidence Code section 1014, it established a broad rule of privilege to protect confidential communications between patient and psychotherapist. In Evidence Code section 1024, the Legislature created a specific and limited exception to the psychotherapist-patient privilege: "There is no privilege *   *   * if the psychotherapist has reasonable cause to believe that the patient is in such mental or emotional condition as to be dangerous to himself or to the person or property of another and that disclosure of the communication is necessary to prevent the threatened danger."

We realize that the open and confidential character of psychotherapeutic dialogue encourages patients to express threats of violence, few of which are ever executed. Certainly a therapist should not be encouraged routinely to reveal such threats; such disclosures could seriously disrupt the patient's relationship with his therapist and with the persons threatened. To the contrary, the therapist's obligations to his patient require that he not disclose a confidence unless such disclosure is necessary to avert danger to others, and even then that he do so discreetly, and in a fashion that would preserve the privacy of his patient to the fullest extent compatible with the prevention of the threatened danger.

The revelation of a communication under the above circumstances is not a breach of trust or a violation of professional ethics; as stated in the Principles of Medical Ethics of the American Medical Association (1957), section 9: "A physician may not reveal the confidence entrusted to him in the course of medical attendance * * * *unless he is required to do so by law or unless it becomes necessary in order to protect the welfare of the individual or of the community.*" (Emphasis added.) We conclude that the public policy favoring protection of the confidential character of patient-psychotherapist communications must yield to the extent to which disclosure is essential to avert danger to others. The protective privilege ends where the public peril begins.

Our current crowded and computerized society compels the interdependence of its members. In this risk-infested society we can hardly tolerate the further exposure to danger that would result from a concealed knowledge of the therapist that his patient was lethal. If the exercise of reasonable care to protect the threatened victim requires the therapist to warn the endangered party or those who can reasonably be expected to notify him, we see no sufficient societal interest that would protect and justify concealment. The containment of such risks lies in the public interest. For the foregoing reasons, we find that plaintiffs' complaints can be amended to state a cause of action against defendants Moore, Powelson, Gold, and Yandell, and against the Regents as their employer, for breach of a duty to exercise reasonable care to protect Tatiana.

[The court went on to reject a claim by the defendants that release of information obtained from Poddar would violate a state statute governing the disclosure of confidential information in the possession of state officials. The court also held that the plaintiffs' claim was not barred by the state's governmental immunity statute in so far as it related to the psychiatrist's failure to warn third persons.]

WRIGHT, C.J., and SULLIVAN and RICHARDSON, JJ., concur.

MOSK, JUSTICE (concurring and dissenting).

I concur in the result in this instance only because the complaints allege that defendant therapists did in fact predict that Poddar would kill and were therefore negligent in failing to warn of that danger. Thus the issue here is very narrow: we are not concerned with whether the therapists, pursuant to the standards of their profession, "should have" predicted potential violence; they allegedly did so in actuality. Under these limited circumstances I agree that a cause of action can be stated.

* * *

I would restructure the rule designed by the majority to eliminate all reference to conformity to standards of the profession in predicting violence. If a psychiatrist does in fact predict violence, then a duty to warn arises. The majority's expansion of that rule will take us from the world of reality into the wonderland of clairvoyance.

CLARK, JUSTICE (dissenting).

Until today's majority opinion, both legal and medical authorities have agreed that confidentiality is essential to effectively treat the mentally ill, and that imposing a duty on doctors to disclose patient threats to potential victims would greatly impair treatment. Further, recognizing that effective treatment and society's safety are necessarily intertwined, the Legislature has already decided effective and confidential treatment is preferred over imposition of a duty to warn.

The issue whether effective treatment for the mentally ill should be sacrificed to a system of warnings is, in my opinion, properly one for the Legislature, and we are bound by its judgment. Moreover, even in the absence of clear legislative direction, we must reach the same conclusion because imposing the majority's new duty is certain to result in a net increase in violence.

The majority rejects the balance achieved by the Legislature's Lanterman–Petris–Short Act. (Welf. & Inst.Code, § 5000 et seq., hereafter the act.) In addition, the majority fails to recognize that, even absent the act, overwhelming policy considerations mandate against sacrificing fundamental patient interests without gaining a corresponding increase in public benefit.

* * *

COMMON LAW ANALYSIS

Entirely apart from the statutory provisions, the same result must be reached upon considering both general tort principles and the public policies favoring effective treatment, reduction of violence, and justified commitment.

Generally, a person owes no duty to control the conduct of another. Exceptions are recognized only in limited situations where (1) a special relationship exists between the defendant and injured party, or (2) a special relationship exists between defendant and the active wrongdoer, imposing a duty on defendant to control the wrongdoer's conduct. The majority does not contend the first exception is appropriate to this case.

* * *

Overwhelming policy considerations weigh against imposing a duty on psychotherapists to warn a potential victim against harm. While offering virtually no benefit to society, such a duty will frustrate psychiatric treatment, invade fundamental patient rights and increase violence.

The importance of psychiatric treatment and its need for confidentiality have been recognized by this court.

"It is clearly recognized that the very practice of psychiatry vitally depends upon the reputation in the community that the psychiatrist will not tell." (Slovenko, *Psychiatry and a Second Look at the Medical Privilege* (1960) 6 Wayne L.Rev. 175, 188.)

Assurance of confidentiality is important for three reasons.

DETERRENCE FROM TREATMENT

First, without substantial assurance of confidentiality, those requiring treatment will be deterred from seeking assistance. It remains an unfortunate fact in our society that people seeking psychiatric guidance tend to become stigmatized. Apprehension of such stigma—apparently increased by the propensity of people considering treatment to see themselves in the worst possible light—creates a well-recognized reluctance to seek aid. This reluctance is alleviated by the psychiatrist's assurance of confidentiality.

FULL DISCLOSURE

Second, the guarantee of confidentiality is essential in eliciting the full disclosure necessary for effective treatment. The psychiatric patient approaches treatment with conscious and unconscious inhibitions against revealing his innermost thoughts. "Every person, however well-motivated, has to overcome resistances to therapeutic exploration. These resistances seek support from every possible source and the possibility of disclosure would easily be employed in the service of resistance."

Until a patient can trust his psychiatrist not to violate their confidential relationship, "the unconscious psychological control mechanism of repression will prevent the recall of past experiences."

SUCCESSFUL TREATMENT

Third, even if the patient fully discloses his thoughts, assurance that the confidential relationship will not be breached is necessary to maintain his trust in his psychiatrist—the very means by which treatment is effected.

* * * All authorities appear to agree that if the trust relationship cannot be developed because of collusive communication between the psychiatrist and others, treatment will be frustrated.

Given the importance of confidentiality to the practice of psychiatry, it becomes clear the duty to warn imposed by the majority will cripple the use and effectiveness of psychiatry. Many people, potentially violent—yet susceptible to treatment—will be deterred from seeking it; those seeking it will be inhibited from making revelations necessary to effective treatment; and, forcing the psychiatrist to violate the patient's trust will destroy the interpersonal relationship by which treatment is effected.

VIOLENCE AND CIVIL COMMITMENT

By imposing a duty to warn the majority contributes to the danger to society of violence by the mentally ill and greatly increases the risk of civil commitment—the total deprivation of liberty—of those who should not be confined. The impairment of treatment and risk of improper commitment resulting from the new duty to warn will not be limited to a few patients but will extend to a large number of the mentally ill. Although under existing psychiatric procedures only a relatively few receiving treatment will ever present a risk of violence, the number making threats is huge, and it is the latter group—not just the former—whose treatment will be impaired and whose risk of commitment will be increased.

Both the legal and psychiatric communities recognize that the process of determining potential violence in a patient is far from exact, being fraught with complexity and uncertainty. In fact precision has not even been attained in predicting who of those having already committed violent acts will again become violent, a task recognized to be of much simpler proportions.

This predictive uncertainty means that the number of disclosures will necessarily be large. As noted above, psychiatric patients are encouraged to discuss all thoughts of violence, and they often express such thoughts. However, unlike this court, the psychiatrist does not enjoy the benefit of overwhelming hindsight in seeing which few, if any, of his patients will ultimately become violent. Now, confronted by the majority's new duty, the psychiatrist must instantaneously calculate potential violence from each patient on each visit. The difficulties researchers have encountered in accurately predicting violence will be heightened for the practicing psychiatrist dealing for brief periods in his office with heretofore nonviolent patients. And, given the decision not to warn or commit must always be made at the psychiatrist's civil peril, one can expect most doubts will be resolved in favor of the psychiatrist protecting himself.

Neither alternative open to the psychiatrist seeking to protect himself is in the public interest. The warning itself is an impairment of the psychiatrist's ability to treat, depriving many patients of adequate treatment. It is to be expected that after disclosing their threats, a significant number of patients, who would not become violent if treated according to existing practices, will engage in violent conduct as a result of unsuccessful treatment. In short, the majority's duty to warn will not only impair treatment of many who would never become violent but worse, will result in a net increase in violence.

The second alternative open to the psychiatrist is to commit his patient rather than to warn. Even in the absence of threat of civil liability, the doubts of psychiatrists as to the seriousness of patient threats have led psychiatrists to overcommit to mental institutions. This overcommitment has been authoritatively documented in both legal and psychiatric studies.

Given the incentive to commit created by the majority's duty, this already serious situation will be worsened, contrary to Chief Justice Wright's admonition "that liberty is no less precious because forfeited in a civil proceeding than when taken as a consequence of a criminal conviction."

CONCLUSION

*   *   *

The tragedy of Tatiana Tarasoff has led the majority to disregard the clear legislative mandate of the Lanterman–Petris–Short Act. Worse, the majority impedes medical treatment, resulting in increased violence from—and deprivation of liberty to—the mentally ill.

We should accept legislative and medical judgment, relying upon effective treatment rather than on indiscriminate warning.

The judgment should be affirmed.

McCOMB, J., concurs.

Questions and Comments

1. *Impact of Tarasoff.* Although "the vast majority of courts that have considered the issue have accepted the *Tarasoff* analysis", the doctrine has been rejected by several states. *Currie v. United States,* 644 F.Supp. 1074, 1078 (M.D.N.C.1986). South Carolina has declined to decide on the *Tarasoff* doctrine. *Sharpe v. South Carolina Dept. of Mental Health,* 292 S.C. 11, 354 S.E.2d 778 (1987). Maryland courts have found that their statutorily enacted law of privileged communications bars any disclosure to third persons by a psychotherapist. *Shaw v. Glickman,* 45 Md.App. 718, 415 A.2d 625 (1980). (See also Chapter Four, section II. D. "Judicial Proceedings and the Testimonial Privilege"). A number of states have privilege laws similar to Maryland's.

2. *Scope of holding.* Note that the *Tarasoff* opinion does not decide whether Dr. Moore or the University of California outpatient clinic was negligent. The case merely holds that the plaintiff has stated a cause of action that, if proved at trial, would entitle the plaintiff to relief. On remand to the lower court, the trier of fact would have had to decide whether Dr. Moore's failure to notify the victim or her family did in fact constitute a breach of his duty to the third-party victim. A jury might also have found that by notifying the police Dr. Moore had exercised due care and thus was not negligent. (The *Tarasoff* case was settled by the parties out of court prior to retrial.)

3. *Comment on* Tarasoff. The majority decision in *Tarasoff* strives to make the formulation of new doctrine appear as a natural and logical extension of existing doctrine. In reaching its conclusion that the therapist has a duty to third parties, the majority pursues three lines of analysis. First, it cites earlier medical cases from other jurisdictions that imposed a duty on physicians to notify third parties who are likely to come into contact with a patient suffering from a contagious disease. The majority opinion, however, fails to distinguish imposing a duty when there is a clearly diagnosable and invariably contagious disease from the facts of *Tarasoff,* where the duty was triggered not by a clearly diagnosible condition, but by a clinical prediction of probable future conduct on the part of the patient.

Second, the majority opinion looks to Section 315 of the Restatement of Torts Second, which provides:

There is no duty so to control the conduct of a third person as to prevent him from causing physical harm to another unless

(a) a special relation exists between the actor and the third person which imposes a duty upon the actor to control the third person's conduct, or

(b) a special relation exists between the actor and the other which gives to the other a right to protection.

Although the wording of Section 315 seems compatible with the majority's holding in *Tarasoff,* the commentaries to this section should not be overlooked. They emphasize that the duty attaches only in certain enumerated "special relations," when, for example, the defendant is an innkeeper, common carrier, or landowner. Presumably, therefore, the drafters of the Restatement Second did not intend to include the psychiatrist-patient relationship in Section 315.

The third part of the court's opinion was a policy analysis. Here the court addressed the competing interests of affording protection to persons who may be endangered by a patient against the interest of protecting the integrity of the therapist-patient relationship. The court concluded as a matter of policy that the need to protect persons from serious harm outweighed the possibly destructive effects on the patient-therapist relationship that might be caused from a rule requiring disclosure to third parties.

4. *Tarasoff and the ability to predict.* To what extent are the divergent conclusions of the majority as expressed by Justice Tobriner's opinion and the dissenting opinion of Justice Clark founded on different perceptions as to the ability of clinicians to predict dangerous or abnormal behavior? Do any policy considerations support the imposition of a duty to warn if, in fact, the ability of the therapist to predict dangerous behavior correctly is very limited? In this context, see the discussion in Chapter Six on the problem of predicting dangerous behavior.

Regarding clinicians' abilities to predict dangerousness, consider Givelber, Bowers & Blitch, *Tarasoff, Myth and Reality: An Empirical Study of Private Law in Action,* 1984 Wis.L.Rev. 443 (1984). The authors asked a group of psychiatrists, psychologists, and social workers to gauge their own ability to predict dangerous behavior. Over seventy-five percent of the clinicians responded that they could make firm predictions ranging from probable violence to certain violence. Only five percent suggested that violence is impossible to predict.

5. *An alternative approach.* In his concurring opinion Justice Mosk would limit the duty to warn to those cases in which the "psychiatrist does in fact predict violence." Presumably this means that liability cannot be imposed unless the psychiatrist has actually concluded that the patient is likely to be violent. One commentator has praised this approach:

Making the legal duty dependent on the therapist's subjective determination of the patient's dangerousness would of course extremely limit the number of instances in which suit could successfully be brought. In the usual case, once the therapist has convinced himself that a patient is certainly dangerous, he will take some action. Only where he has reached this conclusion—and made it clear in records or consultation—and then failed to act would liability be imposed. Unlike the *Tarasoff* standard, then, this formulation would provide no incentive to the therapist to overpredict dangerousness early in the treatment process and to act to warn potential victims who might or might not be in serious danger. It seems to me quite clear that both the public interest and the patient's needs are better served by a legal standard which does not serve to discourage or undermine the effective treatment of potentially dangerous individuals. Moreover, the safety of the potential victims may well be more successfully promoted by such a standard, since premature action by the therapist is likely to terminate the therapeutic relationship, with the result that patients whose illnesses might have been successfully treated would remain a source of danger to those they originally threatened.

Stone, *The Tarasoff Decisions: Suing Psychotherapists to Safeguard Society,* 90 Harv.L.Rev. 358, 375–376 (1976).

How practical is Justice Mosk's standard? Are the arguments in favor of it convincing? What evidence would a plaintiff have to introduce to establish the existence of a duty? Would this approach in effect permit the psychiatrist to insulate himself from liability? In other words, would not any psychiatrist be able to avoid liability for failure to warn by merely refusing to formulate predictions?

6. *Hypothetical.* If Dr. Moore had initiated commitment proceedings rather than merely notifying the university police, would his potential liability have been any different? In connection with that question, consider the following hypothetical situation. Assume that the dangerous patient was admitted as an involuntary emergency admission (the nature of emergency admissions are considered in Chapter Six). The psychiatric facility released him after several days, and shortly thereafter the patient murdered an acquaintance. Assume further that the therapist who had originally initiated the commitment proceedings had not warned either the victim or the victim's family; the therapist, however, knew of the patient's violent intentions. Could the therapist still be held liable under these circumstances? In answering this question consider the subsection on proximate cause, infra.

7. *Expansion of the third party liability doctrine.* The expanding concept of the duty of care to third persons has not been confined to the psychiatric setting. The *Tarasoff* court cited three California decisions that had imposed third-party liability for the actions of another. In *Ellis v. D'Angelo,* 116 Cal.App.2d 310, 253 P.2d 675 (1953), the court recognized a cause of action against the parents of a child who failed to warn a babysitter of the violent proclivities of their child. *Johnson v. State of California,* 69 Cal.2d 782, 73 Cal.Rptr. 240, 447 P.2d 352 (1968), sustained a cause of action against the state for its failure to warn foster parents of the dangerous personality traits of their ward. And in *Morgan v. Yuba County,* 230 Cal.App.2d 938, 41 Cal.Rptr. 508 (1964), a cause of action was similarly upheld when the sheriff failed to carry out his promise to warn the

decedent before releasing a dangerous prisoner. Implicit in these cases is judicial recognition that victims of violent crimes should have a remedy for their injuries. Of course, victims can sue the person who committed the offense, but in most cases the offender is penniless. As a result, victims must search for a "deep pocket" and seek compensation from someone who stands in a special relationship to the person who caused the injury. It is in determining both whether this special relationship exists, and, if so, what actions should be taken to avoid similar future injuries that have caused the greatest difficulty.

In *Grimm v. Arizona Board of Pardons and Paroles*, 115 Ariz. 260, 564 P.2d 1227 (1977), the Arizona Supreme Court held that the state parole board had a duty to individual members of the general public to avoid the grossly negligent or reckless release of a highly dangerous prisoner. The court also concluded that the parole board members could claim only qualified immunity for their administrative acts. The doctrine of immunity of the state and officials and employees of the state is governed largely by statute. Thus, the liability of state-run hospitals and the therapists working there depends upon the scope of the immunity which may have been granted by the legislature.

8. *Statutory limitations on Tarasoff.* Several states have enacted statutes which restrict psychotherapists' liability to third parties. Colorado has restricted the duty to warn to situations where the patient has made specific threats. Colo.Rev.Stat. 13–21–117. Louisiana has created a specific duty to warn third parties who have been specifically threatened. La. Stat.Ann.–R.S. 2800.2. In some states the duty to warn is not expressly imposed by statute but may be implied by specific limitations in their requirements of confidentiality. (See, e.g., West's Fla.Stat. § 455.2415).

California now exempts psychiatrists from liability under certain involuntary treatment situations. For example, psychiatrists cannot be held liable for "any action by a person released" from a facility offering 72–hour treatment and evaluation at or before the end of 72 hours. (West's Ann. Cal.Welf & Inst.Code § 5173). Other statutes address facilities specifically treating suicidal patients (§ 5267) and facilities offering 90–day involuntary treatments of "imminently dangerous persons" (§ 5306).

California modified the *Tarasoff* duty in 1985 by adopting Section 43.92 of the Civil Code, West's Ann.Cal.Civ.Code § 43.92. Section 43.92 immunizes therapists from liability except where the patient "has communicated to the psychotherapist a serious threat of physical violence against a reasonably identifiable victim or victims." Governor Deukemejian had vetoed a similar measure in 1984, claiming that the bill increased the danger to the public by limiting the *Tarasoff* duty. Does Section 43.92 embrace a standard even narrower than that advocated by Justice Mosk? Suppose that in *Tarasoff*, Poddar, during therapy sessions, made numerous statements exhibiting extreme hostility toward Tatiana but never explicitly threatened to kill her. If the defendants nevertheless concluded that Poddar evinced a threat to Tatiana, would the *Tarasoff* majority find a duty to warn? Would there be a duty under Justice Mosk's formulation? How explicit must the communication be before liability will be found under Section 43.92?

BRADY v. HOPPER

United States District Court, District of Colorado, 1983.
570 F.Supp. 1333.

I.

ALLEGATIONS OF THE COMPLAINT

Plaintiffs James Scott Brady, Timothy John McCarthy, and Thomas K. Delahanty were all shot and seriously injured by John W. Hinckley, Jr. ("Hinckley") in his attempt to assassinate President Reagan on March 30, 1981, in Washington, D.C. The defendant, Dr. John J. Hopper, Jr., is the psychiatrist who had been treating Hinckley from late October, 1980, until March, 1981.

Plaintiffs' complaint alleges that Dr. Hopper was negligent in examining, diagnosing, and treating Hinckley in conformity with reasonable standards of psychiatric care. According to the complaint, Hinckley was brought to Dr. Hopper in late October, 1980, by Hinckley's parents because the parents were concerned about their son's behavior, including a purported suicide attempt by drug overdose. Plaintiffs allege despite Hinckley's attempted suicide on at least one if not several occasions, Dr. Hopper negligently formed the opinion that Hinckley was not seriously ill. (Complaint ¶ 15). Dr. Hopper proceeded to treat Hinckley and and prescribed valium and biofeedback therapy. Dr. Hopper also recommended to Hinckley's parents that Hinckley be on his own by the end of March, 1981. Plaintiffs assert that Dr. Hopper's treatment was not only ineffective, but that it actually aggravated Hinckley's mental condition, and made him more aggressive and dangerous, thereby creating an unreasonable risk of harm to others. (Complaint ¶¶ 16–29).

The complaint alleges that Dr. Hopper knew or should have known that Hinckley was a danger to himself or others, and that Dr. Hopper either possessed or had access to, information which would have indicated that Hinckley identified with the assassin in the movie "Taxi Driver"; that he was collecting books and articles on political assassination; and that Hinckley possessed guns and ammunition. (Complaint ¶ 28). According to the complaint, Hinckley's parents were aware of and concerned about their son's worsening condition, and contacted Dr. Hopper and recommended that their son be hospitalized. Despite the possibility Hinckley might have been amenable to that idea, Dr. Hopper recommended that Hinckley not be hospitalized, and that treatment continue on an outpatient basis.

The rest of Hinckley's strange story is well known. In March, 1981, Hinckley left Denver and traveled across the country to Washington, D.C. On March 30, 1981, he attempted to assassinate President Reagan, and, in the process, shot and injured plaintiffs. Hinckley was subsequently tried for these crimes and found not guilty by reason of insanity. He is currently confined to St. Elizabeth's Hospital where he is receiving medical and psychiatric care.

The gravamen of plaintiffs' complaint is that if Dr. Hopper had properly performed his professional duties, he would have controlled Hinckley's behavior; therefore, Hinckley would not have made the presidential assassination attempt. Specifically, plaintiffs assert that the prescription of valium and biofeedback therapy, coupled with the advice that Hinckley's parents "cut him off", aggravated Hinckley's condition and actually contributed to his dangerous propensity. Further, plaintiffs assert that Dr. Hopper should have consulted with another psychiatrist regarding his form of treatment, and that Dr. Hopper should have taken steps to have Hinckley confined. Finally, plaintiffs allege that Dr. Hopper should have warned Hinckley's parents of their son's extremely dangerous condition, and that he should have warned law enforcement officials of Hinckley's potential for political assassination. (Complaint ¶¶ 22–28).

II.

SUMMARY OF THE ARGUMENTS

The primary issue raised by defendant's motion is whether the relationship between therapist and patient gives rise to a legal duty such that Dr. Hopper can be held liable for the injuries caused to plaintiffs by Hinckley. The Restatement (Second) of Torts § 315 states as follows:

> There is no duty so to control the conduct of a third person as to prevent him from causing physical harm to another unless
>
> (a) a special relation exists between the actor and the third person which imposes a duty upon the actor to control the third person's conduct, or
>
> (b) a special relation exists between the actor and the other which gives to the other a right to protection.

The thrust of defendant's argument is that the relationship between Dr. Hopper and Hinckley, that of a therapist and outpatient, is not a "special relationship" which gives rise to a duty on the part of the therapist to control the actions of the patient. In other words, defendant asserts that the therapist-outpatient relationship lacks sufficient elements of control required to bring the therapist within the language of § 315.

* * *

Defendant next argues that the duty to control the violent acts of another does not arise absent specific threats directed to a reasonably identifiable victim. The leading case on a therapist's liability for the violent actions of a patient is *Tarasoff v. Regents of University of California*, 17 Cal.3d 425, 131 Cal.Rptr. 14, 551 P.2d 334 (1976).

(R. & S.) Mental Health, 2d Ed. ACB—7   * * *

In *Thompson v. County of Alameda,* 27 Cal.3d 741, 167 Cal.Rptr. 70, 614 P.2d 728 (1980), the California Supreme Court again faced the question of the extent of liability to a third party for the dangerous acts of another. In *Thompson,* a juvenile offender known to have dangerous propensities was confined in a county institution. This patient had made generalized threats regarding his intention to kill, but had made no specific threats regarding any identifiable person. The county institution released the patient on temporary leave, and, within a day, the patient killed a young boy in his neighborhood. The court refused to extend *Tarasoff* to a setting where there was no identifiable victim. Instead, it took a more limited approach to the duty to warn, and concluded that even in the case of a person with a history of violence, no duty existed when the person had made only nonspecific threats of harm directed at nonspecific victims. *Id.* at 614 P.2d 735. *See also, Doyle v. United States,* 530 F.Supp. 1278 (C.D.Cal.1982); *Furr v. Spring Grove State Hospital,* 53 Md.App. 474, 454 A.2d 414 (1983).

* * *

III.

DISCUSSION

In my opinion, the main issue raised by the pleadings and briefs is not simply whether the therapist-outpatient relationship is a "special relationship" which gives rise to a legal duty on the part of the therapist; rather the key issue is to what extent was Dr. Hopper obligated to protect these particular plaintiffs from this particular harm?[8] It is implicit in the majority of cases in this area that the therapist-patient relationship is one which under certain circumstances will give rise to a duty on the part of the therapist to protect third persons from harm. *Tarasoff v. Regents of University of California, supra.* However, the existence of a special relationship does not necessarily mean that the duties created by that relationship are owed to the world at large. It is fundamental that the duty owed be measured by the foreseeability of the risk and whether the danger created is sufficiently large to embrace the specific harm. *Palsgraf v. Long Island R. Co.,* 248 N.Y. 339, 162 N.E. 99 (1928).

It is this requirement of foreseeability which has led numerous courts to conclude that a therapist or others cannot be held liable for injuries inflicted upon third persons absent specific threats to a readily identifiable victim. *Thompson v. County of Alameda, supra; Doyle v. United States,* 530 F.Supp. 1278 (C.D.Cal.1982); *Furr v. Spring Grove Hospital, supra; Megeff v. Doland, supra; see also Hasenei v. United States, supra* at 1012, n. 22; *c.f. Jablonski v. United States,* 712 F.2d 391 (9th Cir.1983) (hospital liable for acts of outpatient where victim was foreseeable object of patient's violence). Unless a patient makes specific threats, the possibility that he may inflict injury on another is vague,

---

8. Definition of the scope of the defendant's duty is a question of law for the court. *Metropolitan Gas Repair Serv., Inc.* *v. Kulick,* Colo., 621 P.2d 313 (1980). *See also, Sanchez v. United States,* 506 F.2d 702 (10th Cir.1974).

speculative, and a matter of conjecture. However, once the patient verbalizes his intentions and directs his threats to identifiable victims, then the possibility of harm to third persons becomes foreseeable, and the therapist has a duty to protect those third persons from the threatened harm.

For purposes of this motion only, it must be assumed that Dr. Hopper's treatment and diagnosis of Hinckley fell below the applicable standard of care. Moreover, the doctor-patient relationship between Dr. Hopper and Hinckley was one which gave rise to certain duties on the part of Dr. Hopper. The real question, however, is whether that duty encompasses the injuries of which plaintiffs complain. In other words, was there a foreseeable risk that Hinckley would inflict the harm that he did?

Accepting as true the facts alleged in the complaint and viewing them in a light most favorable to plaintiffs, it is my conclusion that plaintiffs' injuries were not foreseeable; therefore, the plaintiffs fall outside of the scope of defendant's duty. Nowhere in the complaint are there allegations that Hinckley made any threats regarding President Reagan, or indeed that he ever threatened anyone. At most, the complaint states that if Dr. Hopper had interviewed Hinckley more carefully, he would have discovered that Hinckley was obsessed with Jody Foster and the movie "Taxi Driver", that he collected books on Ronald Reagan and political assassination, and that he practiced with guns. According to plaintiffs, if Dr. Hopper had properly performed his professional duties, he would have learned that Hinckley suffered from delusions and severe mental illness, as opposed to being merely maladjusted. Even assuming all of these facts and many of plaintiffs' conclusions to be true, the allegations are still insufficient to create a legal duty on the part of Dr. Hopper to protect these plaintiffs from the specific harm.

The parties have for the most part cast their arguments in terms of whether the relationship between Dr. Hopper and *Hinckley* gave rise to a particular duty on the part of Dr. Hopper. However, the legal obstacle to the maintenance of this suit is that there is no relationship between Dr. Hopper and *plaintiffs* which creates any legal obligation from Dr. Hopper to these plaintiffs. As explained by Justice Cardozo, negligence is a matter of relation between the parties, and must be founded upon the foreseeability of harm to the person in fact injured. *Palsgraf v. Long Island R. Co.*, 162 N.E. at 101. *See also, Taitt v. United States of America*, Civil Action No. 82–M–1731 (D.Colo.1983) (Matsch, J.).

In essence, defendant argues that the instant case presents an even clearer basis than *Thompson* for a finding of no duty. It is argued that even according to the allegations in the complaint, Hinckley had no history of violence directed to persons other than himself; he had no history of arrests; no previous hospitalizations arising from any violent episodes; and in fact, he did not appear to be a danger to others. Thus, defendant asserts, this case involves, and plaintiffs have pled, none of the "warning signs" by which Hinckley's conduct or mental state would give rise to a duty on the part of Dr. Hopper.

The question of whether a legal duty should be imposed necessarily involves social policy considerations. See *Prosser, Law of Torts* § 43, 257 (4th Ed. 1971). In the present case, there are cogent policy reasons for limiting the scope of the therapist's liability. To impose upon those in the counseling professions an ill-defined "duty to control" would require therapists to be ultimately responsible for the actions of their patients. Such a rule would closely approximate a strict liability standard of care, and therapists would be potentially liable for all harm inflicted by persons presently or formerly under psychiatric treatment. Human behavior is simply too unpredictable, and the field of psychotherapy presently too inexact, to so greatly expand the scope of therapists' liability. In my opinion, the "specific threats to specific victims" rule states a workable, reasonable, and fair boundary upon the sphere of a therapist's liability to third persons for the acts of their patients.

The present case is one which makes application of the previously stated rules and policy considerations particularly difficult. Plaintiffs' injuries are severe and their damages extensive. Their plight as innocent bystanders to a bizarre and sensational assassination attempt is tragic and evokes great sympathy. Nevertheless, the question before the Court is whether Dr. Hopper can be subjected to liability as a matter of law for the injuries inflicted upon plaintiffs by Hinckley. I conclude that under the facts pleaded in the complaint, the question must be answered in the negative.

Accordingly, it is

ORDERED that defendant's motion to dismiss is granted.

Questions and Comments

1. Brady's *impact.* At least one jurisdiction has adopted *Brady's* rule. In *Eckhardt v. Kirts,* 179 Ill.App.3d 863, 128 Ill.Dec. 734, 534 N.E.2d 1339 (1989), the court held:

Based upon the prior discussion of the law, we believe the plaintiff must establish the following elements relating to the alleged duty owed in order to sustain her cause of action. First, the patient must make specific threat(s) of violence; second, the threat(s) must be directed at a specific and identified victim; and, third, a direct physician-patient relationship between the doctor and the plaintiff or a special relationship between the patient and the plaintiff. *Brady v. Hopper,* 570 F.Supp. at 1338–39; *Kirk,* 117 Ill.2d at 531, 111 Ill.Dec. at 955, 513 N.E.2d at 399.

SELLERS v. UNITED STATES

United States Court of Appeals, Sixth Circuit, 1989.
870 F.2d 1098.

Before KRUPANSKY and BOGGS, CIRCUIT JUDGES, and EDWARDS, SENIOR CIRCUIT JUDGE.

PER CURIAM.

Sellers appeals the decision of the district court finding that, as a matter of law, the government owed no duty to Sellers's ward for the conduct of Allen Firestine, who was treated for manic depression at the Veteran's Administration Hospital (VAH) in Battle Creek, Michigan. Sellers's ward, Terrance Sellers, was severely beaten by Firestine on February 17, 1985. Firestine had been an inpatient and was still receiving outpatient treatment at the time of the incident. Sellers filed suit against the VAH under the Federal Tort Claims Acts (FTCA), 28 U.S.C. § 2671 *et seq.*, for negligent discharge of Firestine from the VAH, negligent outpatient treatment, and negligent failure to warn the public of Firestine's potentially violent behavior. We affirm the district court's decision on the grounds that a psychiatrist has no duty to warn the general public in such situations, but has only a relatively narrow duty to warn readily identifiable potential victims.

Firestine was voluntarily admitted to the VAH on October 1, 1984, stating "I cannot handle myself without proper medications, I have mood swings and I need help." * * * The discharge summary shows that Firestine was described as hyperactive and labile (unstable). He was diagnosed as having a bipolar disorder, commonly known as manic depression, and was initially placed on Thorazine. * * * While in the VAH, Firestine exhibited aggressive or assaultive behavior a number of times. Notes in his files indicate that he was variously hyperactive, threatening * * * and extremely aggressive. * * * He was discharged on December 19, 1984 and was to continue to receive outpatient treatment. He was prescribed lithium carbonate.

Sellers alleges that the dosage of lithium was too small during the outpatient stage of treatment. Indeed, tests showed that Firestine's lithium blood level dropped from 1.00 mEq (milli-equivalent) while an inpatient * * *. He was seen again about a month later, on February 13, 1985, at which time his blood lithium level was 0.52 mEq. At the time of that visit, he was cheerful and complained of poor sleep, both symptoms of relapse. Dr. Nagler, Sellers's expert, stated that "[f]alling lithium levels and sleep disturbances are sirens that should alert one to potential difficulties in patients with bipolar disorders and require further blood tests and immediate followup and monitoring."

Early on February 17, 1985, Firestine confronted Terrance Sellers and beat him over the head with a baseball bat. A witness to the beating, Frank Wagner, testified that Sellers was not armed nor was he angry or intruding. The altercation took place in a motor home of Sellers's former girlfriend, Colleen Savage, who had become Firestine's girlfriend and is now his wife. * * * Kenneth Dubois, the taxi-driver who drove Sellers to Savage's home, stated that Sellers was not belligerent when he got out of the cab.

[Expert testimony established that the therapeutic or maintenance blood lithium level lies somewhere between 0.4 mEq and 1.0 mEq, with some discrepancy between the witnesses as to what levels are associated with clinical efficacy.]

* * *

The Physician's Desk Reference states that "desirable serum lithium levels are 0.6 to 1.2." Dr. Inumerable testified that a psychiatrist would worry about a person with bipolar disorder becoming violent if he had a relapse.

It is undisputed that Firestine never mentioned Terrance Sellers to any of the personnel at the VAH, nor did he voice any threats towards Sellers prior to the incidents. In fact, there is nothing in the record to indicate that Firestine knew Sellers at all until after his release.

* * *

Sellers argues that the VAH *did* owe a duty to Sellers's ward as a member of the public. He argues that it was entirely foreseeable that Firestine would exhibit aggressive behavior, and that he might act violently. In addition, because of decreased lithium blood levels and increased symptoms associated with manic depression, Sellers argues that the VAH knew or should have known that Firestine was in need of greater doses of medication, and that he was heading towards a relapse. The government argues that the psychiatrist's duty is only to readily identifiable persons, and that Sellers was in no sense readily identifiable.

* * *

The Michigan courts have followed *Tarasoff,* holding that "a psychiatrist owes a duty of reasonable care to a person who is foreseeably endangered by his patient." *Davis.* However, this duty is a limited one because of the inexact nature of the science of psychiatry, and the burden a more expansive duty might impose on psychiatrists. Not only is the duty limited to the standard of care of the profession, but the class of persons to whom a duty is owed is limited "to only those persons readily identifiable as foreseeably endangered."

* * *

[Michigan has accepted the policy considerations set forth in *Thompson v. County of Alameda,* 27 Cal.3d 741, 752, 167 Cal.Rptr. 70, 76, 614 P.2d 728, 734 (1980) where] the court explained how damaging it could be to the therapeutic relationship if a patient were inhibited from voicing threats, and how complacent the public might get were every threat made in the presence of a psychiatrist reported.

[Following this rationale, the Michigan court has adopted the following rule:]

[W]hen a psychiatrist determines or, pursuant to the standard of care of his profession, should determine that his patient poses a *serious danger of violence to a readily identifiable person,* the psychiatrist has as a duty to use reasonable care to protect that individual against such danger.

Davis, 335 N.W.2d at 489 (emphasis added). The Michigan Supreme Court reversed the judgment against the psychiatrist in *Davis* because it found that he was protected by immunity. *Canon,* 700. However, the court did not undermine or challenge the lower court's statement of the general rule as to when a duty attaches; in fact, statements such as "the decision whether to warn a third party . . . requires highly professional judgment . . .," and "reaching such a determination . . . requires . . . professional evaluation . . .," *ibid.,* imply the court's acceptance of the rule announced in *Davis.* The rule in *Davis* has been employed consistently by the Michigan Courts of Appeals.

* * *

Although this question of whether a duty exists is a question of law, and so is appropriate for resolution on a motion for summary judgment, *Welke,* the question of whether a third person was "readily identifiable" "requires review of the evidence." *Davis.* In the instant case, Firestine had never mentioned Sellers to anyone at the VAH. In fact, as the trial judge noted, Firestine did not even know Sellers at the time of his release. As regards the claim of post-release negligence, although medical testimony regarding appropriate blood lithium levels and Firestine's state of mind indicate that, in the opinion of the experts, the VAH should have been concerned, Sellers *never* became a readily identifiable potential target of Firestine's violent tendencies. In *Davis,* the court noted that there was general expert testimony as there was in this case; however, that testimony was not enough to resolve the question of whether injury to the particular victim was foreseeable, and so the court focused on the question of whether the victim was readily identifiable prior to the incident. Here, the evidence is undisputed that the VAH had no reason to know that Sellers was in any danger from Firestine.

There have been exceptions to the "readily identifiable" rule in Michigan in the case of physicians. In *Welke,* in which the defendant driver hit and killed the plaintiff's deceased, the court stated that a doctor who had injected a patient-driver with an "unknown substance" had a special relationship with the patient; unlike in the instant case, "the doctor's malpractice is the proximate cause of a plaintiff's injuries and . . . the doctor himself is in the best position to prevent the harm." This is vastly different from the instant case in that, there, the doctor alone knew what he was injecting and its side-effects, including whether it could impair driving ability; the likelihood that an injury would occur was foreseeable to the doctor and only the doctor. In the present case, it is clear that nobody at the VAH was in the best position—or any position—to have foreseen the specific harm. Sellers went to the home of his former girlfriend, found Firestine there, and subsequent events regarding the reason and mode of initiation of the struggle between the two men can only be conjectured.

* * *

We agree with the Michigan Court of Appeals regarding the validity of the distinction between a physician's duty and a psychiatrist's duty to the public at large. The science of psychiatry is relatively inexact as compared with the physical sciences. The behavior of psychiatric patients, and their reactions to psychoactive drugs, is much more difficult to predict, and thus to foresee, than the behavior and reactions of patients who are treated for purely physical conditions. Thus, we find cases like *Duvall* and *Welke*, involving the duty of physicians, to be distinguishable.

This case is more like *Jackson v. New Center Community Mental Health Services*, in which a psychiatric patient went on a "random shooting spree." The court found that, because the victims were not readily identifiable, their representatives' claims of negligence in treatment and supervision could not be maintained, thus granting summary judgment. In *Bardoni v. Kim*, the patient was a paranoid schizophrenic, which illness may produce violent behavior. Upon his release from a mental institution, the patient killed his mother and brother. The court held that the duty of the doctor to have warned the patient's family members that the patient was dangerous was entirely dependent on whether the family members were readily identifiable.

* * *

Therefore, we hold that the VAH was not negligent in failing to warn the general public, including Sellers, of Firestine's possible behavior; nor was the VAH negligent in Firestine's outpatient treatment as it may have affected Sellers. Negligence cannot be found absent a duty to the complaining party. *Bardoni.* Thus, we affirm the decision of the district court on these two issues.

IV

The claim of negligent discharge of a patient requires a slightly different analysis, although the above discussion regarding an absence of a duty towards Sellers applies here as well. However, there are additional reasons why Sellers cannot succeed on his claim of negligent discharge.

Firestine was admitted to the VAH voluntarily. A review of the case law will demonstrate that this fact is central to a determination of the VAH's duty regarding the length of Firestine's commitment. An analysis of this issue centers on the question of whether a "special relationship" exists between the patient and the hospital.

* * *

In *Soutear v. United States*, 646 F.Supp. 524 (E.D.Mich.1986), a VA hospital was sued for failing to try to commit involuntarily a patient who later killed his parents. The court stated that, although in hindsight it was clear that commitment and medication would have been appropriate, the VA doctors had not fallen below the standard of their profession by failing to commit him involuntarily. The court was very adamant about the rule that " 'a psychiatrist will not be held liable for his patient's violent behavior simply because he failed to predict it accurately.'" (quoting *Davis.*) Thus, the court concluded that the VA doctors could not be held liable under Michigan law for failing to commit and treat a patient whose violence, and the subject of that violence, were not easily predictable.

* * *

V

Although it is easy in hindsight to point to the falling blood lithium levels and cheerfulness as signs of an oncoming relapse, it is clear that Sellers was not a readily identifiable victim, nor was Firestine symptomatic enough to have excited the fears of the VA doctors. Thus, although we sympathize with the plight of victims such as Sellers, we cannot place the blame on the VAH and its doctors. Therefore, the district court's judgment is AFFIRMED.

Questions and Comments

1. *Application of the "identifiable victim" standard.* The manner in which the "identifiable victim" standard is applied will materially influence the ultimate scope of the *Tarasoff* doctrine. Strict construction will limit the circumstances under which liability may be found; an expansive interpretation will enlarge them.

Several recent decisions indicate that the identifiable victim requirement is likely to be broadly construed. For instance, in *Jablonski v. United States,* 712 F.2d 391 (9th Cir.1983), the patient who had served a five year prison term for raping his wife subsequently killed his girlfriend after attempting to rape her mother. In holding the psychiatrist liable, the court ruled that although the patient had not made a *specific* threat "[h]is psychological profile indicated that his violence was likely to be directed against women very close to him." Id. at 398. Similarly, in *Davis v. Lhim,* 124 Mich.App. 291, 335 N.W.2d 481 (1983), where the patient shot and killed his mother during a scuffle, the psychiatrist was found liable. The mother was found to be a foreseeable victim on the basis of evidence that two years before the homicide the patient had acted "strangely" and had threatened her for money. This together with the fact that the therapist had knowledge that the patient was a drug addict and would need money to obtain drugs was "sufficient to support a jury finding that defendant [the psychiatrist] should have known * * * that [the patient] posed a serious threat to his mother." Id. at 490. *See also, Hedlund v. Superior Court of Orange County,* 34 Cal.3d 695, 194 Cal.Rptr. 805, 669 P.2d 41 (1983).

The requirement of a clearly foreseeable victim does not apply in an action against an institution for negligently releasing an individual where the facility's staff knew or should have known that the patient was likely to impose harm on others. Where the patient is improperly released, the institution may be held liable even where the specific victim was not foreseeable. See note 2. following *Merchants Nat'l Bank v. United States,* supra at p. 116.

2. *Non-professionals and the duty to warn.* Should the duty to warn apply to a non-professional? In *Rozycki v. Peley,* 199 N.J.Super. 571, 489

A.2d 1272 (1984), a group of neighborhood children were sexually assaulted by Arthur Peley in 1981. Their parents sued on the children's behalf, naming Peley's wife, Catherine, as a defendant. Peley had been previously arrested in 1977 on a morals charge involving a minor. At that time he was placed in a diversion program in which he, accompanied by Catherine, received psychiatric treatment. The plaintiffs alleged that Catherine knew of her husband's pedophilia and thus had a duty to warn the children of the potential danger. The New Jersey court declined to extend its prior holding in *McIntosh v. Milano,* 168 N.J.Super. 466, 403 A.2d 500 (1979) (adopting the *Tarosoff* doctrine), to include non-professionals. The court reasoned that lay persons are not experts and could not be expected to assess another person's dangerousness. The court added that in this particular case the public interest in protecting the marital relationship also counseled against imposing such a duty on the defendant.

If liability is limited only to psychotherapists, which professions should fall into the category of "therapists"? A licensed marriage counselor? An unlicensed marriage counselor? A marriage counselor in a state which does not require a license?

HAMMAN v. COUNTY OF MARICOPA

Supreme Court of Arizona, 1989.
161 Ariz. 58, 775 P.2d 1122.

HOLOHAN, JUSTICE (Retired).

We granted the plaintiffs' petition for review to determine the nature and extent of a psychiatrist's duty to third parties injured by the psychiatrist's patient. The plaintiffs filed a tort action against the defendants for injuries inflicted on Robert Hamman by John Carter, a patient of the defendant, Dr. Manuel Suguitan. The superior court granted the defendants' motion for summary judgment, and the Court of Appeals affirmed the judgment of the lower court in part and reversed in part. 161 Ariz. 53, 775 P.2d 1117 (App.1987).

* * *

John Carter is the son of plaintiff Alice Hamman, and stepson of plaintiff Robert Hamman. On January 5, 1982, the Hammans brought Carter to the Maricopa County Hospital emergency psychiatric center because Carter had been exhibiting strange behavior. Dr. Suguitan, a psychiatrist who had previously admitted Carter to the hospital in August, 1981, interviewed Carter for about five minutes and noted the following symptoms: (1) anxious but cooperative, (2) fear and apprehension about a place to live, (3) loose associations and blocking,[1] (4) inappropriate affect,[2] (5) tries to conceal depression by grimacing, and

---

[1]. " 'Loose associations' occur when a person starts talking on one subject and going on a tangent and continues on another subject unrelated to the first topic. . . ."

" 'Blocking' is when a person starts to say something and in midsentence he stops and he is unable to proceed to complete that sentence or statement that he intended to make." (Deposition of Manuel G. Suguitan, M.D., March 7, 1984, at 21).

[2]. "Affect" is "a freudian term for the feeling of pleasantness or unpleasantness evoked by a stimulus; also the emotional complex associated with a mental

(6) employs denial [3] and projection.[4]   Dr. Suguitan did not review the medical records of Carter's 1981 hospitalization.

After interviewing Carter, Dr. Suguitan had a discussion with Mrs. Hamman, the specifics of which are disputed by the parties. Mrs. Hamman stated in her deposition that she told Dr. Suguitan the details of Carter's abnormal behavior since his hospitalization in August 1981. She described various incidents of strange behavior, a few instances of violent conduct, and a recent incident in which Carter was discovered to be carrying photos of animals with their heads cut off. Mrs. Hamman also testified in her deposition that she told Dr. Suguitan that she and Mr. Hamman feared that Carter would either be killed or kill somebody and that they never turned their backs on Carter. Mrs. Hamman further testified that Dr. Suguitan told her that Carter was schizophrenic and psychotic, but that he was "harmless." Dr. Suguitan denied in his deposition that Mrs. Hamman told him about the specific details of the patient's conduct, and he denied that he ever told her that Carter was "harmless."

Dr. Suguitan did not refer to Carter's medical records from his previous hospitalization at Maricopa County. Those records would have shown among other things that Carter expressed jealousy of his stepfather and that the treatment plan had been to "seclude and restrain" the patient from agitation, assaultive, or dangerous behavior. Carter had also been examined and treated in the past at Desert Samaritan Hospital. Dr. Suguitan did not review the patient's medical records from that hospital. Those records would have revealed that Carter had a history of drug abuse and violent behavior, and he had made statements that he wanted to punish someone.

On January 5, 1982, as Mrs. Hamman discussed Carter's behavior and the Hammans' fear of him, she repeatedly begged Dr. Suguitan to admit Carter to the hospital. Dr. Suguitan refused to admit Carter. Instead, he wrote a prescription for Navane, gave it to Mrs. Hamman, and instructed her to give Carter 10 milligrams of Navane each morning and night. Dr. Suguitan admits he ordered this treatment knowing that Carter had not been taking the Navane which had been previously prescribed for him in August, 1981. Mrs. Hamman stated that Dr. Suguitan then told her to call him again in one week. Dr. Suguitan states that he advised Mrs. Hamman to take Carter to Tri–City Medical Center for follow-up care.

Upon being denied admission, Carter fled down the street brushing his teeth. The Hammans eventually persuaded him to get in their truck and go home. They gave him the medication as prescribed that night and again the following morning and night on January 6.

state. . . ." Dorland's Illustrated Medical Dictionary 44 (25th ed. 1974).

3. " 'Denial' is manifestations when the patient does not want to talk about what is bothering them." (Deposition of Manuel G. Suguitan, M.D. at 34).

4. "Projection" is "a mental mechanism by which a repressed complex is disguised by being regarded as belonging to the external world or to someone else." Dorland's Illustrated Medical Dictionary at 1262.

Although Mrs. Hamman tried to give Carter his medication on the morning of January 7, Carter refused to take it. At approximately 11:00 a.m. that day, Mr. Hamman while working on a home project with an electric drill, was attacked without warning by Carter. He repeatedly beat Hamman over the head with wooden dowels. Mr. Hamman suffered a heart attack during the beating as well as severe brain damage from the blows to his head. Carter later stated he believed Mr. Hamman was going to physically attack Mrs. Hamman with the drill, and that he (Carter) reacted as he did to protect his mother. Carter was later criminally charged for the beating, but found not guilty by reason of insanity.

The Hammans subsequently filed this civil action. The complaint contained three counts charging medical malpractice by Dr. Suguitan while employed by Maricopa County, general negligence, and a claim against Maricopa County for negligent training and supervision of psychiatric personnel.

The defendants filed a motion for summary judgment, essentially contending Dr. Suguitan owed no duty to the Hammans because Carter had never communicated to Suguitan any specific threat against the Hammans. The trial court granted the defendants' motion, and entered judgment against the plaintiffs dismissing all their claims for relief.

On appeal, the Court of Appeals divided the plaintiffs' claims into two separate theories of liability: (1) that Dr. Suguitan owed them a duty not to negligently diagnose and treat Carter's condition, and (2) that they reasonably relied upon Dr. Suguitan's advice that Carter was harmless. Regarding the first theory, the majority of the Court of Appeals followed the "specific threats to specific victims" approach. *See Brady v. Hopper*, 570 F.Supp. 1333 (D.Colo.1983), *aff'd*, 751 F.2d 329 (10th Cir.1984). Under this view, a psychiatrist incurs no duty to any third party unless his patient communicates to the psychiatrist a specific threat against a specific person.

* * *

We approve of the ruling of the Court of Appeals that the alleged negligent representation by Dr. Suguitan that Carter was "harmless" stated a valid claim. The issue taken for review is whether Dr. Suguitan and Maricopa County owed a duty to the Hammans, absent a specific threat by the patient against them, properly to diagnose, treat or control the patient.

ANALYSIS

A negligence action may be maintained only if there is a duty or obligation, recognized by law, which requires the defendant to conform to a particular standard of conduct in order to protect others from unreasonable risks of harm. The issue of duty is usually one for the court as a matter of law. The danger reasonably to be perceived defines the duty to be obeyed.

* * *

Tarasoff and its progeny

The landmark case regarding the duty of a psychiatrist to protect others against the conduct of a patient is *Tarasoff v. Regents of Univ. of Cal.,* * * * The *Tarasoff* court held that the psychiatrist-patient relationship was sufficient under [Restatement of Torts, Second] § 315 to support the imposition of an affirmative duty on the defendant for the benefit of third persons. * * * The court ruled that when a psychiatrist determines or, pursuant to the standards of the profession, should determine that a patient presents a serious danger of violence to another, the psychiatrist incurs an obligation to use reasonable care to protect the intended victim against such danger. According to the *Tarasoff* court, discharge of that duty may require the psychiatrist to warn the intended victim or others reasonably likely to notify the victim, to notify the police, *"or to take whatever other steps are reasonably necessary under the circumstances."* (Emphasis added).

Although the *Tarasoff* decision did not state that a psychiatrist's duty to third parties arises only when his patient communicates a specific threat concerning a specific individual, numerous subsequent decisions interpret *Tarasoff.* For example, in *Brady, supra,* John W. Hinckley, Jr. injured the plaintiffs in his attempt to assassinate President Reagan. The suit alleged, in part, that Hinckley's psychiatrist had negligently diagnosed and treated him. The *Brady* court held that the psychiatrist owed no duty to the plaintiffs because Hinckley had not made specific threats against a readily identifiable victim. 570 F.Supp. at 1339.

Similarly, in *Thompson v. County of Alameda,* 27 Cal.3d 741, 614 P.2d 728, 167 Cal.Rptr. 70 (1980), the parents of a young child sued the county for the wrongful death of their son. The juvenile offender, James F., killed the child within 24 hours of his release from confinement into the temporary custody of his mother. James stated he would kill a child in the community at random, and the county knew it. Nonetheless, county officials released him without warning local police, parents, or James' mother. Distinguishing *Thompson* from *Tarasoff,* the majority of the California Supreme Court refused to impose "blanket liability." The court stated that liability may be imposed only in those instances in which the released offender posed a predictable threat of harm to a named or readily identifiable victim. James made a generalized threat to a segment of the population. Consequently, the majority refused to impose upon the psychiatrist a duty to protect such a large group in the community.

Other courts, however, have not required a specific threat as a prerequisite for liability. Instead, they require that the psychiatrist reasonably foresee that the risk engendered by the patient's condition would endanger others. For example, in *Petersen v. State,* 100 Wash.2d 421, 671 P.2d 230 (1983), a patient was hospitalized for several weeks and treated with Navane after his psychiatrist diagnosed him as having schizophrenic and hallucinogenic symptoms. The hospital allowed the patient to go home for Mother's Day, but required him to return that night. Upon his return, hospital personnel observed the patient driving recklessly and spinning his car in circles on hospital grounds. The psychiatrist nevertheless released the patient the following morning and continued to prescribe Navane even though he knew of the patient's reluctance to take such medication. Five days later, the patient drove through a red light at 50–60 miles per hour, striking plaintiff's car and injuring her. The *Petersen* court emphasized the importance of foreseeability in defining the scope of a person's duty to exercise due care. In affirming plaintiff's claim based on negligent treatment of the patient, the court ruled that the psychiatrist had a duty to protect any person foreseeably endangered by the patient. at 237.

* * *

In the present case, the Court of Appeals would limit a psychiatrist's duty and liability to cases in which there are specific threats against third parties, *i.e.,* the *Brady* approach. The plaintiffs concede that Carter never made any specific threats against Mr. Hamman.

STANDARD

We believe the *Brady* approach is too narrow. *Tarasoff* envisioned a broader scope of a psychiatrist's duty when the court stated: "[O]nce a therapist does in fact determine, or under applicable professional standards reasonably should have determined, that a patient poses a serious danger of violence to others, he bears a duty to exercise reasonable care to protect the foreseeable victim of that danger." Additionally, we agree with those cases interpreting *Tarasoff* which state that a psychiatrist should not be relieved of this duty merely because his patient never verbalized any specific threat. We recognize the concern about adopting a rule which would be too inclusive, subjecting psychiatrists to an unreasonably wide range of potential liability. However, we believe that the approach used by the Ninth Circuit in *Jablonski*, 712 F.2d 891 (9th Cir.1983) allays such fears and represents a sound analytical foundation for the facts before us. In holding that Jablonski's girlfriend (Kimball) was a foreseeable victim, the court stated:

> Unlike the killer in *Tarasoff*, Jablonski made no specific threats concerning any specific individuals. Nevertheless, Jablonski's previous history indicated that he would likely direct his violence against Kimball. He had raped and committed other acts of violence against his wife. His psychological profile indicated that his violence was likely to be directed against women very close to him. This, in turn, was borne out by his attack on Pahls. Thus, Kimball was specifically identified or "targeted" to a much greater extent than were the neighborhood children in *Thompson*.

712 F.2d at 398.

Dr. Suguitan was aware that schizophrenic-psychotic patients such as Carter are prone to unexpected episodes of violence. He knew that Carter was living with and being cared for by the Hammans. Dr.

Suguitan, in denying Carter's admission to the hospital, released the patient into the care of the Hammans. If indeed Dr. Suguitan negligently diagnosed Carter as harmless, the most likely affected victims would be the Hammans. Their constant physical proximity to Carter placed them in an obvious zone of danger. The Hammans were readily identifiable persons who might suffer harm if the psychiatrist was negligent in the diagnosis or treatment of the patient. The fact that Carter never verbalized any specific threats against the Hammans does not change the circumstances that, even without such threats, the most likely victims of the patient's violent reaction would be the Hammans. We reject the notion that the psychiatrist's duty to third persons is limited to those against whom a specific threat has been made. We hold that the standard originally suggested in *Tarasoff* is properly applicable to psychiatrists. When a psychiatrist determines, or under applicable professional standards reasonably should have determined, that a patient poses a serious danger of violence to others, the psychiatrist has a duty to exercise reasonable care to protect the *foreseeable victim* of that danger. The foreseeable victim is one who is said to be within the zone of danger, that is, subject to probable risk of the patient's violent conduct.

CONTROL

The defendants contend that Dr. Suguitan did not fail in any obligation to protect the Hammans. They point out that any duty by the psychiatrist to control his patient is limited by statute. Unless a patient meets the statutory criteria, the psychiatrist cannot involuntarily admit a patient into the hospital.

The defendants argue if the patient was not dangerous, there could be no involuntary commitment. Dr. Suguitan found Carter not dangerous, therefore, he could not be committed and the defendant could not control him.

The plaintiffs, however, submitted evidence from two psychiatrists in opposition to the defendants' motion for summary judgment. The plaintiffs' psychiatrists, in their affidavits, stated that a competent examination and proper diagnosis would have disclosed that Carter was a person suffering from a mental illness which made him dangerous to others. He was, therefore, admittable to the hospital on an involuntary basis under the statutes. They further stated that the defendant's examination of the patient fell below the acceptable standard for psychiatrists. The issue of ability to control is one which must be decided at trial.

The plaintiffs' experts in their affidavits also stated that even if Carter was not admittable as an emergency patient, there were numerous other acceptable medical procedures and precautions which Dr. Suguitan should have taken to lessen the danger posed to the Hammans. Some of these other steps include not only warning the Hammans of Carter's potential for danger, but also providing detailed instructions to follow should Carter's condition deteriorate. The doctor should have provided for outpatient follow-up care which would take into consideration the risk inherent in Carter's medical condition. Thus, the discharge of the defendant psychiatrist's duty is not limited to instances when the psychiatrist can control a patient by commitment to a hospital. The psychiatrist to fulfill his duty to those within the zone of risk must take the action reasonable under the circumstances.

CONCLUSION

The rule which we adopt does not impose upon psychiatrists a duty to protect the public from all harm caused by their patients. We do not, however, limit the duty of the psychiatrist to third parties only in those instances in which a specific threat is made against them. We hold that the duty extends to third persons whose circumstances place them within the reasonably foreseeable area of danger where the violent conduct of the patient is a threat.

That part of the Court of Appeals' opinion which is inconsistent with views expressed herein is vacated. The judgment of the trial court is reversed, and the case is remanded for further proceedings consistent with this opinion.

Questions and Comments

1. *Scope of holding.* Is *Hamman* an expansion of *Tarasoff* and, if so, in which way? In holding that the plaintiff in *Hamman* stated a cause of action, does the court indicate what action(s) on the part of the treating psychiatrist would have met the duty of care to third parties? Was it reasonably possible for the psychotherapist to warn the potential victim? To whom should the warning have been directed? Was it a matter of informing everyone in the household that he was potentially dangerous? Would neighbors of the Carters also have been within the "zone of danger" and, therefore, entitled to be warned?

Should the *Hamman* case be read as expanding the duty of care beyond the need to warn a potential victim? Is the court in fact imposing a duty to commit when a patient is or should have been found to be potentially dangerous? If this is the basis of the court's holding, how is the imposition of this duty to be balanced against the public policy of encouraging the deinstitutionalization and outpatient treatment of those suffering from mental disorder?

2. *Other cases involving liability.* Should the situation in *Hamman* be distinguished from a case brought by a party who is inadvertently injured because he was in close proximity to an ascertainable victim? In this connection, consider *Hedlund v. Superior Court of Orange County,* 34 Cal.3d 695, 194 Cal.Rptr. 805, 669 P.2d 41 (1983), involving an action by a mother and her three-year-old son, the latter of whom was inadvertently injured when the patient assaulted the child's mother. Significantly in *Hedlund,* the plaintiffs did not allege that the psychotherapist had *actual* knowledge of the danger posed by the patient but rather that the therapist "*should* have known" that the patient "presented a serious danger of

violence to her." (Emphasis added). In finding that both complaints stated a cause of action, the court observed:

"Diagnosis of psychological problems and emotional and mental disorders is a professional service for which a psychologist is licensed, and a negligent failure in this regard is therefore "professional negligence". This diagnosis and prediction is an essential element of a cause of action for failure to warn. It is the basis upon which the duty to the third party victim is found. A negligent failure to diagnose dangerousness in a *Tarasoff* action is as much a basis for liability as is a negligent failure to warn a known victim once such diagnosis has been made."

669 P.2d 41, 45 (1983).

3. *A dissenting view.* With reference to the *Hedlund* case, consider the dissenting opinion of Justice Mosk:

The majority opinion unfortunately perpetuates the myth that psychiatrists and psychologists inherently possess powers of clairvoyance to predict violence. There is no evidence to support this remarkable belief, and, indeed, all the credible literature in the field discounts the existence of any such mystical attribute in those who practice the mind-care professions.

The serious flaw in the majority opinion is its acceptance of the claim that a failure to diagnose "dangerousness" may be a basis for liability. In its text, the opinion employs such terms as failure to "predict" behavior, and flatly declares that a negligent act occurs "when the therapist has, or *should have* diagnosed dangerousness" (italics added), as if that subjective characteristic would be revealed through a stethoscope or by an X-ray.

In *People v. Burnick* (1975) 14 Cal.3d 306, 121 Cal.Rptr. 488, 535 P.2d 352, we discussed at considerable length the virtually unanimous authorities in the field of psychiatry who concede their inability to predict violence. "In light of recent studies it is no longer heresy to question the reliability of psychiatric predictions. Psychiatrists themselves would be the first to admit that however desirable an infallible crystal ball might be, it is not among the tools of their profession. It must be conceded that psychiatrists still experience considerable difficulty in confidently and accurately *diagnosing* mental illness. Yet those difficulties are multiplied manyfold when psychiatrists venture from diagnosis to prognosis and undertake to predict the consequences of such illness: ' "A diagnosis of mental illness tells us nothing about whether the person so diagnosed is or is not dangerous. Some mental patients are dangerous, some are not. Perhaps the psychiatrist is an expert at deciding whether a person is mentally ill, but is he an expert at predicting which of the persons so diagnosed are dangerous? Sane people, too, are dangerous, and it may legitimately be inquired whether there is anything in the education, training or experience of psychiatrists which renders them particularly adept at predicting dangerous behavior. Predictions of dangerous behavior, no matter who makes them, are incredibly inaccurate, and there is a growing consensus that psychiatrists are not uniquely qualified to predict dangerous behavior and are, in fact, less accurate in their predictions than other professionals." '

"During the past several years further empirical studies have transformed the earlier trend of opinion into an impressive unanimity: 'The evidence, as well as the consensus of opinion by responsible scientific authorities, is now unequivocal.' (Diamond, *The Psychiatric Prediction of Dangerousness* (1975) 123 U.Pa.L.Rev. 439, 451.) In the words of spokesmen for the psychiatric profession itself, 'Unfortunately, this is the state of the art. Neither psychiatrists nor anyone else have reliably demonstrated an ability to predict future violence or "dangerousness." Neither has any special psychiatric "expertise" in this area been established.' And the same studies which proved the inaccuracy of psychiatric predictions have demonstrated beyond dispute the no less disturbing manner in which such prophecies consistently err: they predict acts of violence which will not in fact take place ('false positives'), thus branding as 'dangerous' many persons who are in reality totally harmless."

Because of the inherent undependability of such predictions, we adopted in *Burnick* the beyond-a-reasonable-doubt standard for commitment to mental facilities.

Unfortunately a year later in *Tarasoff v. Regents of University of California* a thin majority of this court employed a loose and ill-conceived dictum that encourages a dilution of *Burnick*. Although the case involved *actual* knowledge of planned violence, the four-to-three majority spoke expansively in terms of what the doctor "knew or should have known." My separate opinion pointed out that there are no professional standards for forecasting violence and concluded that any rule should "eliminate all reference to conformity to standards of the profession in predicting violence. If a psychiatrist does in fact predict violence, then a duty to warn arises. The majority's expansion of that rule will take us from the world of reality into the wonderland of clairvoyance."

* * *

Id. at 48–49.

Are the arguments by Justice Mosk against imposing liability in a case such as *Hedlund* convincing? Does adoption of the majority opinion subject psychotherapists to an unreasonable risk of being found liable given their current abilities to predict behavior and particularly violence?

4. *Contributory negligence.* Should liability attach to the psychotherapist when the victim was aware of the danger posed by the patient? At least one court has held that knowledge by the victim forecloses liability on the part of the psychotherapist to warn. In *Votteler,* a psychiatric patient seriously injured plaintiff by intentionally running over her with a car. Although the patient had attempted to run her down twice before, plaintiff nevertheless argued that the defendant psychiatrist had a duty to warn her about his patient's violent nature. Plaintiff insisted that she would have appreciated the seriousness of the danger only if warned by a professional. Without deciding whether it would embrace the *Tarasoff* doctrine, the Iowa Supreme Court held that in any case the duty would not extend to

situations where the foreseeable victim knew of the danger. See also, *Connolly v. Ramsey County Welfare Dept.,* 323 N.W.2d 20 (Mn.1982). But see, Hedlund v. Superior Court of Orange County, 34 Cal.3d 695, 194 Cal. Rptr. 805, 669 P.2d 41 (1983), holding a psychologist liable for having failed to warn the victim in spite of evidence that the victim had actual knowledge that the patient intended to inflict serious bodily harm on her.

III. RECOVERY AND DAMAGES UNDER ALTERNATIVE THEORIES

A. MISCELLANEOUS NON–NEGLIGENCE THEORIES

A deviation from professional standards may give rise to a cause of action based on theories other than negligence. Some of these special theories, such as an action for failure to obtain the patient's informed consent or for a breach of confidentiality are treated in Chapters Three and Four, respectively. Depending on the circumstances the patient may also be able to resort to various intentional tort theories to vindicate his rights (e.g., an action for assault where the therapist has engaged in sexual relations with a patient who because of the nature of the relationship lacks effective capacity to give consent). See, *Omer v. Edgren,* 38 Wash.App. 376, 685 P.2d 635 (1984).

A therapist's failure to meet professional standards may also lead to an action for breach of contract. The reason why a patient's claim will be grounded in contract will vary. At times, it may be to take advantage of a longer statute of limitations. In other instances, the plaintiff may use the contract theory to avoid problems of proof of negligence. For instance, as noted in the subsection Damages for Sexual Misconduct, supra, in some jurisdictions recovery under a negligence theory for mental distress will only be allowed where the infliction was intentional or where the mental suffering was accompanied by physical harm or injury. In these jurisdictions, a plaintiff may be more successful under a breach of contract theory which will allow at least a recovery of all fees paid to the therapist. See *Anclote Manor Foundation v. Wilkinson,* 263 So.2d 256 (Fla.App.1972).

Some courts have, however, imposed limitations on the patient's freedom to select a contractual theory of recovery over standard negligence. In *Dennis v. Allison,* 698 S.W.2d 94 (Tex.1985), for instance, the Texas Supreme Court, in holding that the plaintiff who had been sexually assaulted by her therapist could not maintain an action in breach of implied warranty, stated:

> "It is not necessary to impose an implied warranty theory as a matter of public policy because the plaintiff/patient has adequate remedies [in tort] to redress wrongs committed during treatment." Id. at 96.

B. CLAIMS BASED ON FEDERAL CIVIL RIGHTS LAWS

Certain federal statutes, collectively known as the Civil Rights Statutes, allow patients to sue mental health professionals for deprivations of their civil rights. The most widely used of these statutes provides that:

> Every person who, under color of any statute, ordinance, regulation, custom, or usage, of any State or Territory, subjects, or causes to be subjected, any citizen of the United States or other person within the jurisdiction thereof to the deprivation of any rights, privileges, or immunities secured by the Constitution and laws, shall be liable to the party injured in an action at law, suit in equity, or other proper proceeding for redress.

42 U.S.C. § 1983 (1970).

Although these statutes were originally passed after the Civil War to assure the rights of the newly emancipated slaves, since the civil rights movements of the 1960's and 70's the scope of their application has continuously expanded beyond racial discrimination. Accordingly, the number of civil rights actions filed each year has increased from 296 in 1960 to 3,985 in 1970, and to 16,332 in 1981 (Director, Administrative Office of the United States Courts, Annual Report [1982]). Today a mental health patient can bring a civil rights action against a mental health professional under the following circumstances: (1) the conduct complained of was committed by a person acting under color of state law; (2) this conduct deprived the patient of rights, privileges, or immunities secured by the Constitution or laws of the United States; and (3) the conduct complained of was not protected by the professional's qualified immunity.

While meeting these three requirements will often be somewhat burdensome, the advantages of the civil rights action over the traditional state tort action will often justify this effort. The most obvious advantage in seeking a federal forum is that the plaintiff-patient will be able to remove his case from the state court, which may have subtle political ties to the state agency involved. Additionally, a successful plaintiff may qualify for attorney's fees under 42 U.S.C. § 1988. Also, resort to the Civil Rights statutes allows a plaintiff to avoid state exhaustion of remedies requirements. The federal forum may also be necessary to avoid state created limitations on liability, whether it be the creation of a fixed ceiling of liability or the nonrecognition of punitive damages for particular actions. However, certain immunities may still operate to bar recovery of damages (though not necessarily injunctive relief). Where the patient seeks only relief that is equally available under state tort law, the advantages of a federal action may be outweighed by the additional elements of proof which confront a plaintiff in a federal civil rights action.

A major hurdle in every claim based on section 1983 [set out above] is the requirement that the conduct forming the basis of the action be that of one acting under color of state law. The case which follows highlights the difficult issues involved in the application of this criterion.

SPENCER v. LEE

United States Court of Appeals, Seventh Circuit, 1989.
864 F.2d 1376.

POSNER, CIRCUIT JUDGE.

Do a private physician and a private hospital act under color of state law, and therefore lay themselves open to suit under 42 U.S.C. § 1983, when they commit a mentally disturbed person? Adhering to *Byrne v. Kysar,* 347 F.2d 734 (7th Cir.1965), and *Duzynski v. Nosal,* 324 F.2d 924, 929–31 (7th Cir.1963), we hold they do not. The other courts that have addressed this issue agree with our position, see *Hall v. Quillen,* 631 F.2d 1154 (4th Cir.1980), and cases cited there, with the exception of the plurality opinion in *Burch v. Apalachee Community Mental Health Services, Inc.,* 840 F.2d 797, 803 (11th Cir.1988) (en banc), which however devoted only three sentences to the issue and cited no authority for its conclusion.

The plaintiff, William Spencer, appeals from the dismissal of his complaint for failure to state a claim, so we must proceed on the assumption that the facts alleged in the complaint are true. In 1982 and 1984, Spencer's physician, defendant Bumyong Lee, authorized Spencer to be involuntarily committed to St. Elizabeth Hospital. On the second of these occasions the police were called in to take Spencer to the hospital against his will, and on the fourth day of his five days of hospitalization Dr. Lee directed a nurse to inject Spencer with a drug. Spencer protested that he was allergic to the drug, but he was injected anyway and sustained bodily injury. Spencer seeks damages under 42 U.S.C. § 1983 for the deprivation of his liberty without due process of law and for the reckless infliction of injury during his second confinement. Pendent counts seek damages under the common law of Illinois for false imprisonment and malpractice. Spencer had no lawyer in the district court, and his complaint is barely coherent. The district court ordered him to furnish a more definite statement of his claim. In response, Spencer submitted medical records * * * These documents depict Spencer as a schizophrenic with suicidal tendencies who has been in and out of mental institutions many times. Among his delusions are that "all winter he was sick until this time when the police starting a kind of prostitution operation also near motel where he is staying, they have been running a chain saw, the chain saw produced hormones in his testes and he couldn't sit still." * * * However, the district judge did not rely on any of the medical records—which Spencer did not vouch for (he just produced them in response to the judge's order) and has had no chance to explain (away)—and we won't rely on them either.

The casting of this lawsuit as one for the redress of a violation of the Fourteenth Amendment's due process clause, which forbids *states* to deprive persons of life, liberty, or property without due process of law, would certainly strike the innocent eye as puzzling. The due process clause is directed to action by state government; 42 U.S.C. § 1983 creates a remedy against persons acting under color of state law, such as police officers. The defendants in this case are not public employees. They provide no services under contract to the state government or any of its subdivisions. They do not participate (so far as is relevant to this case) in any state or other governmental programs. A purely private physician and a purely private hospital are alleged to have confined the plaintiff against his will and to have injured him by improper medical treatment. These are classic allegations of false imprisonment and malpractice—torts for which the common law of Illinois provides remedies that the plaintiff does not suggest are inadequate.

In arguing that the defendants are nonetheless state actors for purposes of the Fourteenth Amendment and section 1983, the plaintiff relies on the Illinois Mental Health and Developmental Disabilities Code, which provides that "when a person is asserted to be subject to involuntary admission and in such a condition that immediate hospitalization is necessary for the protection of such person or others from physical harm, any person 18 years of age or older may present a [commitment] petition to the facility director of a mental health facility in the county where the respondent resides or is present." Ill.Rev.Stat. ch. 91½, § 3–601(a). The petition must include much factual detail and be accompanied by a certificate, signed by a physician or other qualified professional, stating that the respondent requires immediate hospitalization and that the physician has examined the respondent within the previous 72 hours, and setting forth the factual basis for the physician's opinion that immediate hospitalization is required. §§ 3–601(b), 3–602. Within 24 hours of the respondent's admission to the mental health facility, the facility must forward the relevant papers to the local state court, which must in turn hold a hearing within 5 days (exclusive of weekends and holidays—so the longest possible prehearing commitment is 8 days) on whether there are grounds for continuing to hold the respondent. § 3–611.

This complex of provisions, Spencer argues, operates to "deputize" private physicians such as Dr. Lee and private hospitals such as St. Elizabeth to carry out the exclusive state function of committing the mentally ill. * * * For a maximum of eight days these ostensibly private actors are empowered by the Mental Health Code to hold and treat people against their will. This power, Spencer concludes, is a state power that does not cease to be such merely because delegated to private persons.

If the State of Illinois ordered or encouraged private persons to commit the mentally ill, they would indeed be state actors, for they would be doing the state's business. * * * It would make no difference that they were not technically employees of the state. Or if the state decided to contract out the provision of state highway police or the administration of state prisons to private entrepreneurs of security and correctional services, the entrepreneurs and their employees would (we may assume) be state actors. The details of the contractual relationship between state agencies and the persons who actually implement state policy—whether those persons are state employees or independent contractors or the employees of independent contractors— are of no moment. In accordance with *Marsh v. Alabama,* 326 U.S. 501, 66 S.Ct. 276, 90 L.Ed. 265 (1946), we may further assume that if the state allowed a residential subdivision or high-rise apartment building to form its own de facto municipal government, that government would be an arm of the state for purposes of the Fourteenth Amendment, just as de jure municipal governments are; again the technicality of govern- mental employment would not control the case. * * * Who does the state's business is the state's actor.

At the opposite extreme is the situation where the state decides to reduce the scope of government. Suppose the state owned a railroad, and decided to sell it to a private person. Would the new owner be deemed a state actor under the Constitution, on the ground that the state had "deputized" him to operate "its" railroad? He would not. The scope of government is not fixed; deregulation does not create a host of state actors in the private sector, like the moraine that marks the farthest advance of a glacier. Certain powers, however, are "tradi- tionally the exclusive prerogative of the State," and their exercise by private persons is state action. * * * *Marsh* can be understood in this light—as a case not of deregulation, but of the delegation of public powers to private actors.

We have to situate the present case in this grid. It is not a case of governmental encouragement or direction of private persons; and "a State normally can be held responsible for a private decision only when it has exercised coercive power or has provided such significant encour- agement, either overt or covert, that the choice must in law be deemed to be that of the State." *Blum v. Yaretsky, supra,* 457 U.S. at 1004, 102 S.Ct. at 2786. * * * [The plaintiff's] argument is that the commit- ment of the mentally ill, like the arrest of criminal suspects, is so central and traditional a function of government that the state cannot limit its responsibility for performing the function. Any private indi- vidual who is empowered to commit a person to an institution against the person's will *is* government, just as the "company town" in *Marsh* was a part of the government of Alabama, although a part that had been handed over to a private entity to administer.

Spencer is thus appealing—with support in the language of cases like *Blum* and in the outcome of *Marsh*—to the idea that governmental functions that have traditionally been the *exclusive* prerogative of government, usually because they involved a high degree of coercion, can be delegated but not abandoned. The treatment of the mentally disabled, however, as of the sick and infirm generally, is not such a function. * * * The issue here, it is true, is involuntary commitment rather than treatment. But the analogy that Spencer seeks to draw to arrest is inapt, since a citizen's arrest is not subject to challenge under section 1983. * * * There have been citizen arrests for as long as there have been public police—indeed much longer. In ancient Greece and Rome, and in England until the nineteenth century, most arrests and prosecutions were by private individuals. (Some crimes, e.g., shoplifting, are still privately prosecuted in England.) Arrest has never been an exclusively governmental function. Not all state-authorized coercion is government action.

* * *

The question we are trying to answer is whether a private person is doing the state's business and should be treated as an employee or other formal agent of the state. So we ask, is there a tradition of treating civil commitment of the mentally disturbed as a governmental function and, if so, how well established is it? * * *

The specific provisions of the Mental Health Code dealing with emergency commitment by private physicians to private hospitals are not 200 years old; they are less than 50 years old. See Revised Mental Health Act, art. 5, 1945 Ill.Laws 1011. But commitment has long been a private remedy, albeit one subject (like repossession, self-defense, citizen's arrest, and other infringements on rights of liberty or property) to rigorous safeguards. Even public commitment in Illinois is private in a sense, because the state requires relatives of voluntarily and involuntarily committed mental patients alike to pay the cost of their upkeep in the state's institutions, and it allows the involuntarily committed to be placed in private homes as well as public and private hospitals. * * * And long before the passage of the 1945 statute, the law of Illinois authorized the confinement of an insane person by private persons, for up to ten days, if he was a danger to himself or others. * * *

Private commitment was not novel in 1893; nor was it invented in Illinois. According to Blackstone, writing in 1765, "On the first attack of lunacy, or other occasional insanity, while there may be hope of a speedy restitution of reason, it is usual to confine the unhappy objects in private custody under the direction of their nearest friends and relations." 1 Commentaries on the Laws of England 305. Histories of the treatment of the insane focus on public institutions, but involuntary extrajudicial commitment to private institutions has long been commonplace. London's notorious lunatic asylum, nicknamed "Bedlam," was originally private; it was representative of private medieval institutions to which the insane were committed to have their demons exorcised. See Albert Deutsch, The Mentally Ill in America 15, 40, 62, 418–24 (2d ed. 1949). * * *

The reasons for private commitment, as for self-defense, citizen's arrests, and other private remedies, are intensely practical. If a person displays symptoms of acute and violent mental illness, his family or physician—in an appropriate case a passerby or other stranger—may have to act immediately to restrain him from harming himself or others, and there may be no public institution at hand. That is why the Illinois Mental Health Code allows private persons to commit to private (as well as to public) institutions. We do not know the circumstances in which Mr. Spencer was committed, but it appears that the first commitment was because he had tried to commit suicide, and let us assume this was indeed the reason. If his father and Dr. Lee and St. Elizabeth had had to initiate a judicial proceeding before committing him, he might have killed himself before they could obtain the necessary order. When family members commit a person who has just tried to kill himself, they do not, by virtue of this action, become state actors subject to suit under section 1983.

To allow family members, physicians, and other private persons to exercise the commitment power without safeguards, however, including a provision for a hearing eventually—and sooner rather than later— would be monstrous. If Spencer thinks the eight days allowed by Illinois law for confinement prior to hearing is too much, he can challenge the constitutionality of the statute, * * * He has not done so. Indeed, he relies on the statute to make the defendants state actors. But a private commitment is no more state action than a citizen's arrest, the repossession of chattels, or the ejection of trespassers is. The statutes authorizing or constraining these private activities may or may not be constitutional; the activities themselves remain private * * *.

We are given some pause by the allegation in Spencer's complaint of involvement by the local police: * * * It is possible that the police were called in to assist with one of Spencer's commitments, though this does not seem to be what he is alleging. At all events, police assistance in the lawful exercise of self-help does not create a conspiracy with the private person exercising that self-help. * * * The citizen who makes a citizen's arrest is not transformed into a state actor by handing over the arrested person to the police—indeed, if he fails to do so, the arrest is invalid and he is liable for false imprisonment.

The pressure to transform state common law torts into federal constitutional torts comes from the immunities and the damage ceilings that states frequently impose on suits against their public officials (see, e.g., *Archie v. City of Racine,* 847 F.2d 1211, 1227 (7th Cir.1988) (concurring opinion)), from a sense that state judges are sometimes unsympathetic to suits against the state, and from the availability of attorney's fee awards in civil rights suits under 42 U.S.C. § 1988. Only the last of these considerations is present in a case such as this where the only defendants are private persons (or private institutions) not acting pursuant to formal judicial order. * * * There is neither practical nor legal basis for this suit.

Affirmed.

RIPPLE, CIRCUIT JUDGE, with whom FLAUM, CIRCUIT JUDGE, joins, concurring in part and dissenting in part.

* * *

CUMMINGS, CIRCUIT JUDGE, with whom CUDAHY, CIRCUIT JUDGE, joins, dissenting.

Disagreeing with the majority's conclusion that the actions of the defendants in committing Spencer to St. Elizabeth Hospital necessarily cannot constitute state action, I respectfully dissent from the majority's holding.

* * *

Spencer has clearly articulated a sufficient liberty interest in his allegations of involuntary commitment and treatment during his detention at St. Elizabeth Hospital. * * * The only issue remaining is whether the actions of Dr. Lee and St. Elizabeth Hospital implicate state action.

I. INVOLUNTARY COMMITMENT

A. *Function of the State*

The involuntary commitment of an individual believed to be a danger to himself or others without a judicial hearing is no doubt one of the most severe infringements of personal liberty. However, the state has power to cause such a deprivation acting pursuant to its *parens patriae* power to protect and provide care for the mentally ill. *Addington v. Texas,* 441 U.S. at 426, 99 S.Ct. at 1809. Although neither Dr. Lee nor St. Elizabeth Hospital is a state employee, the state action component may be fulfilled if their actions may be "fairly attributable to the state." *Lugar,* 457 U.S. at 939, 102 S.Ct. at 2755. The test of "fair attribution" involves two elements where a private party is alleged to be a state actor: First, the deprivation must be caused by the exercise of some right or privilege created by the State or by a rule of conduct imposed by the State or by a person for whom the State is responsible. . . . Second, the party charged with the deprivation must be a person who may fairly be said to be a state actor.

Lugar at 937, 102 S.Ct. at 2753–2754. The Supreme Court explained further that mere action by a private party pursuant to a statute without "something more" will not transform the private party into a state actor. The "something more" necessary to convert the private activity into state action varies with the factual circumstances, resulting in correspondingly varied tests: the "public function" test, the "state compulsion" test, the "nexus" test, and the "joint action" test. *Lugar* at 939, 102 S.Ct. at 2754–2755.

* * *

As support for its decision, the majority traces the historical roots of involuntary commitment, concluding that since the commitment of the mentally ill has never been the exclusive prerogative or traditional function of the state, it is not state action when performed by a private entity. However interesting this history lesson may be, the more relevant question for determining whether state action exists is not whether private citizens were capable of unilaterally committing the mentally ill in the days when Bedlam existed in England, but whether under the present law private citizens are capable of depriving individuals of their liberty to the same extent as may the state or whether the state has a superior, unique authority to deprive individuals of liberty in this manner, an authority not inured in the general citizenry. Indeed, as the majority readily concedes, every public function has an analogous private function in history. The majority's opinion, nonetheless, assumes as a premise of its argument that what constitutes a public function is relatively stagnant over time. It may have been the case that in the time of Bedlam the rights of the mentally ill were not recognized and protected to the same extent they are today, as were the rights of minorities prior to the Thirteenth and Fourteenth Amendments. Illinois has altered the course of history by affirmatively recognizing the rights of the mentally ill through its enactment of Chapter II of the Illinois Mental Health and Developmental Disabilities Code.

The majority finds further support for its conclusion that confinement of the mentally ill does not constitute state action by analogy to citizen's arrest. The argument is that since citizens are capable of depriving individuals of personal liberty when they have a reasonable belief that an offense is being committed without becoming state actors, then the deprivation of liberty is not an exclusive state function. The analogy is faulty. Although the citizen may use reasonable force to prevent the commission of an offense, the citizen's right to make an arrest, now codified in Ill.Rev.Stat. ch. 38, § 107-3, is not coextensive with that of the state. The citizen's role in such an arrest involves that minimal amount of restraint on the suspect's liberty necessary to prevent the commission of an offense or escape of an offender. The line is one of degree. A citizen performing an arrest may only detain a suspect until law enforcement agents are available, while a physician may detain and treat an involuntarily committed patient for up to eight days without a hearing.

The analogy to citizen's arrest is further inappropriate because prior to taking a suspect into custody based on the citizen's complaint, a police officer must make an independent determination of reasonable grounds to believe the suspect has committed or is committing an offense. A private citizen could not cause an individual to be confined for up to eight days, as may a physician pursuant to Illinois law, unless the police had also found reasonable grounds for the arrest and detention of the individual. Ill.Rev.Stat. ch. 38, § 107-2(c). Under the mental health code, the sheriff is under a duty to take custody of and transport the patient based solely upon presentation of the petition and certificate, obviating the need for an independent determination of mental illness by the sheriff.

* * *

It is clear from the statutory framework that no private individual may commit a patient to a mental health institution for treatment on an emergency basis without a prior determination by a qualified physician or mental health facility that the patient warrants confinement. In the commitment procedure, the physician's certificate serves a quasi-judicial function correlative to an arrest warrant issued by a judge authorizing the seizure of a suspect. This Court recognized the nature of the physician's function in the commitment process in *Byrne,* 347 F.2d at 736, where doctors, who were members of a court-appointed committee, were held to have performed a quasi-judicial function in examining and recommending commitment of the patient. Under the Illinois mental health code, the state has delegated its adjudicatory determination in the emergency context to the physician, empowering the physician to use the force of state law enforcement agencies to confine any individual the physician determines to be in need of emergency commitment.

* * *

B. Participation of State Officials

* * *

In his *pro se* complaint, as indicated by the majority opinion, Spencer does not specifically allege a "conspiracy" with police officers in his emergency involuntary commitment at St. Elizabeth Hospital. Indeed, it would be surprising if a *pro se* plaintiff with a history of mental illness had sufficient working knowledge of the law to plead the legal phrases which compose the elements of a Section 1983 action. The Court should not penalize Spencer for his inartfully pleaded complaints and subsequent motions. Nonetheless, the majority summarily disposes of this claim due to Spencer's inability to name police officers as defendants or mention the involvement of the police with sufficient frequency. Given the Court's obligation to construe Spencer's complaint liberally and dismiss the complaint only if he can prove no set of facts which would entitle him to relief, Spencer has sufficiently alleged the involvement of the Danville Police Department to sustain defendants' motion to dismiss.

* * *

[T]he mere presence of the police while Spencer was detained at St. Elizabeth Hospital is sufficient participation to constitute state action.

* * *

In my opinion, the judgment should be reversed and the cause remanded for further proceedings.

Questions and Comments

1. *State funding of private facilities.* Would the "under color of law" requirement be met if the mental health professional who is the object of a § 1983 action was employed by a private non-profit mental health center which receives 85% of its funding from state agencies and the rest from fees? See, *Rendell–Baker v. Kohn,* 457 U.S. 830, 102 S.Ct. 2764, 73 L.Ed.2d 418 (1982).

2. *The deprivation of federal rights requirement.* Section 1983 is intended to protect the patient from "the deprivation of any rights, privi-

leges, or immunities secured by the Constitution and laws" 42 U.S.C. § 1983. The statute covers only violations of rights guaranteed by the federal Constitution and federal laws and not those guaranteed by state law.

Two kinds of constitutional rights are protected by the Civil Rights Statutes: substantive rights and procedural rights. Substantive rights include those guaranteed by the Bill of Rights. Procedural rights are those protected by the due process clause of the Fourteenth Amendment. As might be expected, one of the most common procedurally grounded claims in the mental health treatment context involves irregularities in civil commitment. In fact, a violation may occur even when the psychiatric admission was ostensibly voluntary. For instance, in *Zinermon v. Burch,* ___ U.S. ___ (No. 87–1965, decided February 27, 1990), the Supreme Court held that a valid § 1983 claim was stated where the claimant charged that state officials knew or should have known that he was incompetent to give informed consent to his psychiatric admission. His admission under these circumstances, according to the Court, denied him his Constitutionally guaranteed procedural rights.

The imposition or the withholding of treatment may give grounds to an action under § 1983. In *Knecht v. Gillman,* 488 F.2d 1136 (8th Cir.1973), the plaintiff had been an inmate in a mental institution where the patients were given apomorphine, a drug that induces vomiting, when they violated hospital rules by, for example, swearing or lying. The court found that this use of apomorphine was not an accepted nor recognized form of treatment and that the use of this drug on an involuntary basis was cruel and inhuman punishment. The physician responsible for its administration was held liable in a civil rights action brought by the patient. In *Philipp v. Carey,* 517 F.Supp. 513 (N.D.N.Y.1981), the plaintiffs were mentally retarded voluntary residents of a state mental health facility, who complained that they were being given debilitating psychotropic drugs as a substitute for treatment and rehabilitation. The court found that they had a § 1983 cause of action for violation of Section 504 of the Rehabilitation Act, a federal law prohibiting the denial of benefits to handicapped persons by a facility receiving federal funding. 29 U.S.C. § 794.

A mentally ill patient may also attack the conditions of his confinement through a civil rights action. In *Jobson v. Henne,* 355 F.2d 129 (2d Cir.1966), the patient was assigned uncompensated work for up to sixteen hours a day. The work was not part of a therapy program, nor was it related to the patient's housekeeping needs. The court held that this stated a possible cause of action as a violation of the patient's Thirteenth Amendment right (freedom from involuntary servitude).

Other conditions of a patient's confinement may give rise to a civil rights action against a mental health professional. In *Gerrard v. Blackman,* 401 F.Supp. 1189 (N.D.Ill.1975), the court held that a psychiatrist who monitored an involuntary patient's calls to her attorney could be subject to a possible civil rights action. In *Jones v. Superintendent,* 370 F.Supp. 488 (W.D.Va.1974), the court refused to find a civil rights violation where the patient who was a vegetarian for religious reasons had been denied a special diet. The plaintiff was unable to show any physical injury, however, and the case suggests that an action might lie where there is such harm.

3. *Negligent deprivation of rights.* Whether negligent deprivations are actionable under § 1983 is not entirely clear. The U.S. Supreme Court has consistently rejected any state of mind requirement for section 1983. In *Daniels v. Williams,* 474 U.S. 327, 106 S.Ct. 662, 88 L.Ed.2d 662 (1986), however, the Court held that lack of due care by a state official could not "deprive" a person of life, liberty, or property under the fourteenth amendment. Thus, after *Daniels,* it is clear that a section 1983 action is not available where the plaintiff alleges only that he was negligently deprived of liberty or property without due process. The Court offered no guidance as to whether a person can be negligently deprived of a substantive right which has been incorporated into the Fourteenth Amendment. Additionally, *Daniels* leaves open the question of whether a state of mind short of intent, such as recklessness or gross negligence, is sufficient to violate the due process clause.

4. *Immunity under § 1983.* The need to give decision makers relative freedom to exercise discretionary judgment, has caused the Supreme Court to interpret § 1983 to provide officials sued under the Act with qualified immunity similar to that described in section II.A.d., Sovereign Immunity, supra. As a result, a plaintiff will not prevail in a § 1983 action unless the defendant's conduct violated "clearly established statutory or constitutional rights which a reasonable person would have known". *Harlow v. Fitzgerald,* 457 U.S. 800, 818, 102 S.Ct. 2727, 2738, 73 L.Ed.2d 396 (1982).

5. *Other civil rights statutes.* Although most psychiatric civil rights actions are brought under § 1983, two other sections should be noted. The first is 42 U.S.C. § 1985. This section is very similar to § 1983, but provides a remedy for a conspiracy to violate civil rights. The second is 18 U.S.C. § 242, which provides for criminal sanctions for a violation of civil rights by one acting under color of state law. The major difference between the civil and criminal statutes is intent. Criminal law generally is based on the assumption that the wrongdoer understands that he is doing something wrong and that he should be punished. Civil law, on the other hand, is simply a method of allocating losses. The intent requirement, therefore, in a criminal civil rights action is more stringent, and, indeed, the statute itself declares that the deprivation must be "willful." The U.S. Supreme Court has interpreted this to mean that the act must be done intentionally and with the specific intent to deprive the victim of a constitutional right. *Screws v. United States,* 325 U.S. 91, 65 S.Ct. 1031, 89 L.Ed. 1495 (1945). If, for example, the supervising psychiatrist of a mental hospital knew that a patient was sane and not dangerous, yet refused to authorize the patient's discharge, the psychiatrist could be held guilty of a criminal violation of the patient's rights.

Chapter Three

INFORMED CONSENT

I. INTRODUCTION

The fundamental principle that every person should have the right to determine what should be done with his body has deep-seated roots in our jurisprudence. In 1914 Justice Cardozo affirmed this basic right in *Schloendorff v. Society of New York Hospital*, 211 N.Y. 125, 129–130, 105 N.E. 92, 93 (1914), in the following terms:

> Every human being of adult years and sound mind has a right to determine what shall be done with his own body; and a surgeon who performs an operation without his patient's consent commits an assault, for which he is liable in damages.

For many years, however, the right of self-determination was honored more in the abstract than in reality. It is only relatively recently that the right has been given meaningful expression by courts and legislatures. The Supreme Court's 1973 disposition of the abortion cases provides the most dramatic evidence of this shift. Acknowledging the primacy of a woman's right to terminate an unwanted pregnancy, the Court rested its holding on the basic principle that every person has the right to determine what happens to his or her body.

This growing recognition of the individual's right to bodily self-determination can also be seen in another line of cases, those dealing with the prerogative of self-decision as to medical treatment. A limited right to self-determination had been a traditional part of our jurisprudence for many years. Courts were quite prepared, even before the turn of the century, to classify as a battery the rendering of medical treatment that involved a touching performed without the patient's approval or consent. The consent necessary to immunize the physician from liability was, however, very limited and required nothing more than the patient's general agreement to the proposed treatment. The patient had no recognized right to receive comprehensible information about the treatment's risks. Thus, a physician would escape liability if the patient agreed to treatment, even if the patient was totally unaware of the risks it involved.

Only since 1960 has the doctrine of consent emerged as something more than a mere technicality. In a series of cases decided in the early 1960's various state courts ruled that the patient could not give meaningful consent unless he had received adequate information about the risks of the therapy and any available alternative treatments. The courts found that consent based on inaccurate or incomplete information deprived the patient of the right to charter his own course as to treatment and use of his body.

The doctrine of informed consent in its present form comprises two separate elements. One involves the duty of *disclosure* of relevant information to the patient; the other pertains to the patient's *consent* to the proposed therapy. There is disagreement, however, on both the precise doctrinal source of this right as well as its actual scope and dimension. As the materials in this chapter make clear, in some jurisdictions informed consent is subsumed under the doctrine of assault and battery. In others, violations of this right are treated as a form of professional negligence. The implications of these different approaches are explored in the materials that follow.

It is important to note that the doctrine of informed consent has to date only been applied in medical cases. Even in the area of psychiatric malpractice, its application has been limited to physically intrusive treatment methods such as electro-convulsive or insulin shock therapy or the administration of psychotropic drugs. No reported cases have applied the doctrine to any psychotherapy, whether performed by a psychiatrist or a psychologist.

Two reasons may explain why the doctrine has been limited to the bio-medical field. One reason relates to the peculiarities of the law of damages. Recovery of monetary damages under some tort theories requires that the injured party has suffered some physical injury. Physical injury is, of course, a much more frequent result of surgery or drug therapy than of conventional psychotherapy.

Thus, in some states, a patient who has been deprived of the right to give informed consent to psychiatric or psychological treatment may have no compensable damages. In recent years, however, courts have demonstrated a marked tendency to expand compensation for non-physical injuries in tort law. A continuation of this trend may well result in exposing psychotherapists to increased risks of emotional distress liability under the informed consent doctrine.

There is, however, an additional but related problem in extending the doctrine beyond the medical field. A cause of action predicated on the lack of informed consent requires that the patient's injury be the direct and proximate cause of the treatment. This element of proof becomes increasingly difficult if an injury is not immediately identifiable as the direct consequence of the treatment. This point is illustrated by the following hypothetical fact situation. A patient feels that she is not advancing in her job as her intellectual potential might dictate due to excessive passivity and an inability to direct subordinates. On the therapist's recommendation, the patient undergoes assertiveness training. The training is successful to the extent that the patient has become much more assertive; however, her assertiveness and change of personality cause marital difficulties. Since her husband is unable to adjust to her new and more assertive personality, the patient now contends that she would not have consented to the therapy if she had been informed of its risks. In this situation the patient faces the significant difficulty of proving both that the psychotherapy in fact led to the personality change and that this fact was the proximate cause of the destruction of the marriage. While this burden of proof might not be altogether impossible to meet, it presents problems far more formidable than demonstrating that a particular physical injury was the direct and proximate cause of a surgical procedure. In spite of the various doctrinal and practical difficulties, it is likely that the concept

of informed consent will eventually be applied to non-medical treatment situations. The field of psychological research, which has in the
past been all too often characterized by a widespread disregard of any
notion of informed consent, would seem particularly vulnerable to this
form of legal regulation.

For those professionals whose activities are covered by the doctrine
of informed consent, the impact can be formidable. Under this doctrine
the possibility of civil liability no longer hinges on a departure from the
exercise of reasonable skill in providing treatment. Rather, professionals can face liability even when the treatment was flawless. Recovery
for the patient or research subject is predicated solely on the lack of
appropriate consent to treatment. The following materials provide an
overview of the doctrine's current development. Keep in mind, however, that the doctrine is still in its embryonic stage, and that major
issues remain to be resolved.

II. ORIGINS OF THE DOCTRINE OF
INFORMED CONSENT

A. AN EARLY CASE ESTABLISHING THE DUTY TO INFORM

MITCHELL v. ROBINSON

Supreme Court of Missouri, 1960.
334 S.W.2d 11.

BARRETT, COMMISSIONER.

William Mitchell has been awarded $15,000 damages against the
Doctors Robinson and their associates, particularly Dr. Jack DeMott,
for malpractice, and the essentially meritorious problem is whether
upon the record there is any evidence to support the jury's finding of
negligence.

Mitchell and Dr. DeMott were boyhood schoolmates in Independence, Kansas, attended Kansas University at the same time, and were
both living in Independence when Dr. DeMott began the practice of
medicine there. So when in 1951, at age 35, Mitchell was beset with
serious emotional problems he sought out Dr. DeMott who was then a
specialist in neurology and psychiatry and was then associated with
Doctor Robinson and the Neurological Hospital in Kansas City, Missouri. Mitchell had "a rather severe emotional illness," process schizophrenia, but he was not mentally incompetent; his illness was characterized by serious depression and rather severe anxiety, complicated by
alcoholism. It is not necessary at this point to detail his case history
and symptoms; it was the opinion of the doctors that he should have
"combined electro-shock and insulin subcoma therapy." The general
purpose of electroshock treatment is to build up the patient's "defenses
and controls and self-confidence" while insulin relieves "basic anxiety"

and "disturbance of the mood." The desired physical reaction and intended purpose of electroshock is to induce convulsive seizures of forty to fifty seconds duration. The desired physical reaction of insulin shock is the induction of unconsciousness, a "subcoma" state, but it is neither intended nor desired, as it is with electroshock, that the patient suffer a convulsion. One of the unpredictable results of insulin shock, however, is an unpreventable convulsion and one of the hazards of convulsions, whether from insulin or electroshock, is fractured vertebrae, fractured legs and various other injuries.

On October 25, 1951, Mitchell had his first electroshock treatment, the next day another, and, after two days' rest, his first insulin shock October 28 and the next day another, and on the 30th his third electroshock and on the 31st another insulin treatment. There were convulsions with the electroshock treatments but no untoward results; the insulin treatments came off with normal results and reactions except that on the 31st Mitchell suffered a convulsion and that particular treatment was successfully terminated by an intravenous injection of glucose. Insulin treatment, reduced to 25 units, was resumed November 2, but Mitchell went out for a walk and came in drunk and the treatments were "started over" again on November 4 with 25 units, increased to 40 units November 5 and on November 7, with his seventh insulin treatment of 40 units, he had "a hard generalized convulsion," a grand mal seizure, which resulted in a compression fracture of the fifth, sixth and seventh dorsal vertebrae. It is to recover damages for these specific injuries that Mitchell instituted this action.

These briefly noted facts are excerpted as background for certain basic distinctions in this and other malpractice cases and eventually to point up the problem precisely involved upon this appeal. The appellant doctors, relying on the general rules contend that their motions for a directed verdict should have been sustained because "There was no expert testimony to show that the insulin therapy administered to Mitchell failed to conform to the required standards of an ordinarily careful and prudent neurologist or psychiatrist in the community," indeed, the greater part of their brief is devoted to this subject. This phase of the appellants' argument has but little, if any, bearing upon the basic problem involved here; it may be that they could not anticipate just what position the plaintiff would take. But the plaintiff has made it perfectly clear that there is no claim of negligence in any of these general respects * * * [P]laintiff does not question the technique of administering the insulin, nor does he deny that it should have been administered. * * *

* * *

The defendants produced as a witness Dr. Pool, a radiologist connected with a veterans' hospital, Fort Roots Hospital, North Little Rock, Arkansas. While he was neither a neurologist nor a psychiatrist and disclaimed any special qualification in these fields he had made two case studies of the incidence of fractures from shock therapy as they occurred in his hospital. In one study of 46 insulin shock patients he testified that eighteen per cent of them sustained fractures, that in the course of combined electro and insulin shock treatment of 53 patients nineteen per cent sustained fractures, and in another group of 32 patients twenty-five per cent sustained fractures.

* * *

This finally brings us to the really meritorious question of whether in the circumstances of this case, the illness and treatment involved, the doctors were under a duty to inform the plaintiff that one of the hazards of insulin treatment is the fracture of bones not involved in either the illness or the treatment. That the hazard exists is beyond question; Dr. G. Wilse Robinson, Jr., said that fractured bones, serious paralysis of limbs, irreversible coma and even death were hazards incident to shock therapy and further that there are no completely reliable or successful precautions. In their amended answer the defendants "state that the fracture of bones is a danger and risk that is inherent in insulin shock therapy, and that compression fractures of the spine, and fractures of the limbs can and frequently do occur when said insulin shock therapy is properly administered." The plaintiff's principal claim here is that "There was evidence of a negligent failure to disclose to plaintiff the hazards of insulin treatment," and, of course, evidence that plaintiff would not have consented to the treatment had he known of the dangers. In his argument plaintiff states his position in this language: "He relies on defendants' negligent failure to warn him of the danger of injury from this therapy and on defendants' negligent assurance that there was no danger, and failure to use due care as submitted to the jury." The appellants, on the other hand, do not attempt to demonstrate or elaborate, they simply say that "Failure to inform Mitchell of the risks of the treatment, if there was such a failure, is not negligence." Thus, the serious hazards being admitted, the problem is whether in the circumstances of this record the doctors were under a duty to inform their patient of the hazards of the treatment, leaving to the patient the option of living with his illness or of taking the treatment and accepting its hazards.

* * *

* * * Mitchell testified that * * * Drs. Robinson and DeMott recommended the electroshock and insulin therapies, that he personally had no knowledge of the possibilities of fractures from insulin, that they explained the "process" to him "but there was nothing in his conversation to me that indicated any risk or disability as a result of the insulin treatment or any risk of disability at all." He categorically denied that either of the doctors advised him of the possibility of bone injuries or death from the treatments. He said that he asked Dr. DeMott if there was any danger and "His answer was that the treatments had only a temporary effect, a confusion that would last only a matter of an hour or so. He didn't say there would be any lasting effect at all"—in fact the doctor replied, "no danger."

* * *

Mitchell did not sign a written consent to the treatment; however, in his brief he repeatedly states that he needed the treatment and "Indeed, he consented to that," but, he says, he would not have consented had he been informed of the hazards. His then wife (they were divorced in 1952 and both have remarried) did sign a consent which contained this sentence: "This is to certify that I have been informed of the possible dangers of the shock treatment with curare and electro-shock, or with insulin in the case of William Mitchell and that I hereby give permission to the Neurological Hospital and staff to administer this treatment and request that this be done. We assume responsibility for any complications or accident resulting from the administration of these treatments." Mitchell testified that he did not authorize his wife to sign the consent and that he never heard of it until long after he had been discharged from the hospital and therefore had no notice from the consent of the hazards of the treatment. It is not necessary to say whether the consent Mitchell's wife signed was a valid assumption of the hazards of the treatment, the problem is whether it warned of the dangers * * *

* * *

While the fairly relevant cases may be indicative but inconclusive the authoritative literature is more specific and helpful to a positive and rather confident conclusion.

* * *

"* * * The proper solution is to recognize that *the doctor owes a duty to his patient to make reasonable disclosure of all significant facts,* i.e., the nature of the infirmity (so far as reasonably possible), the nature of the operation *and some of the more probable consequences and difficulties inherent in the proposed operation. It may be said that a doctor who fails to perform this duty is guilty of malpractice."* (Italics supplied.)

* * * There was no emergency here, it was not even claimed that Mitchell was critically or dangerously ill and that immediate spectacular treatment was imperative. He was "emotionally" ill and the treatment was "recommended," but it was not immediately necessary to save his life or even his sanity. The doctors said that he had "a rather severe emotional illness," he was "upset, agitated, anxious, depressed, crying." He had been drinking excessively, he was having marital difficulties, was not sleeping well, could not think things through, had unsuccessfully attempted to work for his father and later unsuccessfully attempted to work for his then father-in-law. As indicated, when Mitchell came to the doctors he was not mentally incompetent or in delirium, he had some understanding of his problems and the need for treatment.

In the particular circumstances of this record, considering the nature of Mitchell's illness and this rather new and radical procedure with its rather high incidence of serious and permanent injuries not connected with the illness, the doctors owed their patient in possession of his faculties the duty to inform him generally of the possible serious collateral hazards; and in the detailed circumstances there was a submissible fact issue of whether the doctors were negligent in failing to inform him of the dangers of shock therapy.

[The Court concluded that various errors in the instructions given the jury required reversal in spite of the fact that the plaintiff's pleadings and proof were sufficient to sustain a judgment.]

Questions and Comments

1. *Early case developments. Mitchell v. Robinson* is one of the earliest cases recognizing the therapist's duty to disclose collateral risk information. Shortly before the *Mitchell* decision was handed down, the Supreme Court of Kansas, in *Natanson v. Kline,* 186 Kan. 393, 350 P.2d 1093 (1960), *clarified,* 187 Kan. 186, 354 P.2d 670 (1960) (improper administration of radioactive cobalt therapy), expressly held that failure to disclose collateral risk data could constitute negligence. Though *Mitchell* and *Natanson* were decided within weeks of each other, most commentators agree that *Natanson* has been far more influential in shaping legal developments. Undoubtedly, one reason for this is that the *Natanson* opinion was better drafted, while the Mitchell court was somewhat "unclear about what it was up to." Capron, "Informed Consent In Catastrophic Disease Research and Treatment," 123 U.Pa.L.Rev. 340, 347 n. 20 (1974).

2. *Earlier doctrinal developments. Mitchell v. Robinson* and *Natanson v. Kline* are generally viewed as having ushered in the modern doctrine of informed consent. Prior to these cases, courts typically treated problems of consent as interlocked with the law of assault and battery, which insulated the physician from liability if the patient merely assented to the medical procedure. Adequate information was not a necessary component of a binding consent. The particular significance of the *Mitchell* and *Natanson* cases, and to some extent such earlier cases as *Salgo v. Leland Stanford Jr. University Board of Trustees,* 154 Cal.App.2d 560, 317 P.2d 170 (1957), is the court's recognition that a patient's consent cannot be meaningful or binding unless it is based upon sufficient information concerning the risks of the treatment. It is important to note that while a clear majority of states have accepted the *Mitchell–Natanson* approach, it has not been universally adopted. The trend, however, is clearly toward wider recognition of the therapist's duty to provide adequate information.

3. The insulin shock therapy which was the subject of plaintiff's action in *Mitchell v. Robinson* is no longer used. With increased reliance on electro-convulsive therapy, insulin induced shock was discontinued in the 1960's.

4. *Battery as a basis for recovery.* Numerous cases, some decided as early as the beginning of the century, used a theory of battery to impose liability on physicians who performed medical procedures without the patient's authorization. Typically, these cases involved one of two basic fact situations. In one the physician performed a medical or surgical procedure different than the one authorized by the patient. For instance, in *Hively v. Higgs,* 120 Or. 588, 253 P. 363 (1927), a surgeon who during an

operation on a patient's nose also removed the patient's tonsils was held liable for battery. Similarly, a dentist who had been authorized to extract two teeth, but removed eight while the patient was under sodium pentathol, was held liable in battery. *Moore v. Webb*, 345 S.W.2d 239 (Mo. App.1961).

The second situation leading to liability has involved the performance of a procedure consented to by the patient, but on a different part of the body than the patient had authorized. For instance, in *Mohr v. Williams*, 95 Minn. 261, 104 N.W. 12 (1905), the physician initially diagnosed the patient's right ear as requiring surgery (an ossiculectomy). The patient consented to undergo the recommended procedure, but during the operation the surgeon discovered a more serious defect in the left ear and performed an ossiculectomy on that instead. The court found that these facts established a basis for liability under a theory of battery. It is important to note, however, that in none of these early cases was liability predicated on the physician's failure to disclose information about collateral risks inherent in the treatment. Moreover, the physician could establish a complete defense with evidence that he had informed the patient of the planned procedure and that the patient had authorized the proposed treatment.

5. *Alternate theories.* The modern doctrine of informed consent has been applied under different doctrinal headings. Some courts have chosen to view the failure to inform as vitiating any technical consent which might have been given, thus rendering the physician liable for assault and battery. More commonly, however, courts have characterized violations of the duty to inform as giving rise to an action based on negligence. A few jurisdictions have permitted the plaintiff-patient to proceed on both a negligence and an assault and battery rationale. *See, e.g., Belcher v. Carter*, 13 Ohio App.2d 113, 234 N.E.2d 311 (1967).

Whether a jurisdiction appends informed consent to the doctrine of assault and battery rather than negligence is of more than theoretical interest and can have important practical implications for the litigants. At least four major consequences can follow the choice of one doctrine over the other. First, negligence actions generally are subject to a longer statute of limitations than those based on a theory of battery. A court's decision to subsume informed consent under battery may preclude a lawsuit that was still viable under the state's statute of limitations for negligence.

Second, the burden of proof imposed on the respective parties may vary with the theory chosen. For instance, when the action is based on battery, it is easier for the plaintiff to recover without introducing expert testimony to establish the prevailing medical practice as to the scope of disclosure. A full explanation of this point is provided in the notes following *Canterbury v. Spence*, 464 F.2d 772 (D.C.Cir.1972), which appears in the next section.

Third, the measure of damages may depend on which theory is utilized. Since battery is an intentional tort, the plaintiff may be able to recover punitive damages, particularly if he can show an element of malice. Also, under the battery theory the plaintiff may receive nominal damages even without a showing of actual injury. In negligence actions, on the other hand, damages are ordinarily awarded only in relation to the injuries actually suffered.

Fourth, under the terms of malpractice insurance policies, the defendant physician or therapist might not be covered if the action alleges battery, since intentional torts are specifically excluded in some policies.

6. *Question.* What type of information must be disclosed to the patient? Can disclosure be limited to the collateral risks of the proposed therapy or must the therapist also describe any alternative forms of therapy that may be available, as well as the collateral risks of each alternative? Consider these questions in the context of the cases which follow.

III. ELEMENTS OF THE DOCTRINE OF INFORMED CONSENT

A. THE DISCLOSURE REQUIREMENT

1. Standards Governing the Scope of Disclosure

As indicated in the preceding section, the doctrine of informed consent requires that the therapist disclose the collateral risks of the proposed treatment. However, a rule framed in these general terms leaves two issues unanswered. First, must there be disclosure of every risk, or is it sufficient if the physician informs the patient of only the more significant and probable adverse consequences? Second, is the adequacy of disclosure to be judged by what the medical profession regards as appropriate in the particular circumstances or by some other standard? The cases which follow represent two divergent approaches to the latter question.

AIKEN v. CLARY

Supreme Court of Missouri, 1965.
396 S.W.2d 668.

FINCH, JUDGE.

Plaintiff went to trial on Count III of a malpractice action wherein he alleged negligence of defendant in failing sufficiently to advise plaintiff of the hazards and risks involved in insulin shock therapy to enable plaintiff to give an informed consent for the treatment. Plaintiff alleged that as a result of such therapy administered by defendant he was caused to lapse into a coma and to suffer organic brain damage, resulting in total disability. He sought recovery of $150,000. The jury returned a verdict for defendant. After an unavailing motion for new trial, plaintiff appealed to this court.

* * * We proceed * * * to examine the evidence, which, insofar as pertinent to this assignment and viewed most favorably to plaintiff, was as follows:

After military service from 1941 to 1945 plaintiff entered employment of the Frisco Railroad, ultimately serving as an electrician in the diesel engine department. Early in 1961 plaintiff became irritable and "changed almost his entire personality." He was cross with the children, particularly a teen-age daughter, spent money on things for which he had never spent money before, and had trouble sleeping so that he lost a great amount of sleep and rest. His wife discussed with him the matter of seeing a doctor, but he maintained that his wife needed a doctor as much as he did, and that it was she who was "way out in left field." He agreed to see a doctor if she would, and they then consulted Dr. Lewis E. Jorel of Springfield, who previously had treated their daughter.

Following conferences by the doctor with both plaintiff and his wife, plaintiff entered St. John's Hospital at Springfield, Missouri, on June 3, 1961, for a complete physical examination.

[Following the administration of various tests and procedures, the plaintiff was found to have no physical disorder. Plaintiff was referred to Dr. Clary for a psychiatric examination. Dr. Clary diagnosed plaintiff as suffering from paranoid schizophrenia, and recommended both electric and insulin shock therapy. After consulting both his wife and his family physician, plaintiff gave his consent to ECT and insulin therapy.]

With respect to the information given by Dr. Clary to plaintiff in these conversations as to the nature of the treatment and the risks involved, plaintiff offered in evidence certain statements of the defendant given in an earlier deposition. That testimony was as follows:

"Q. When you talked to him previous to the moving down to psychiatry and signing the release, did you tell him what the possible effects of insulin shock therapy might be?

"A. I told him it would put him to sleep, I told him there was risks involved, I told him the same thing about electric shock therapy. I didn't belabor the point, I told him it was risky because this guy was real shook, but I told him it was risky, and he had no questions.

"Q. Did you tell him it might possibly result in his death?

"A. I implied it. In talking about the anesthetic, I said people take anesthetic, and there are hazards. Some people over-react to anesthetics, and insulin, I told him, it is like being put to sleep, there are risks involved. In terms of specifically telling him, 'This can kill you,' no, sir, I didn't.

"Q. Did you tell him it might possibly result in a delayed awakening, possible brain damage?

"A. No, I didn't tell him that."

Dr. Clary testified that he thought the plaintiff had the mental capacity at least to understand the ordinary affairs of life, understand what the treatment really was and what it might do to him. He again related what he had told plaintiff and stated that he tried to explain it to him on a level he would understand, and he thought plaintiff knew exactly what he was getting into. At the second conference between Dr. Clary and plaintiff, the latter agreed to take whatever treatment Dr. Clary recommended.

Accordingly, on June 9, 1961, a nurse in the psychiatric ward presented to plaintiff a form of "Consent to Shock Therapy." It read as follows: "I (We) hereby request and authorize Dr. Clary and whomever he may designate to assist him, to administer insulin and/or electroshock therapy to Mr. Aiken; and to continue to administer such therapy and such other supplemental treatment as he may deem advisable from time to time. The effect and nature of shock and/or insulin treatment have been fully explained to me (us), as well as the hazards involved. Notwithstanding the fact that there are risks to the patient inherent in this treatment, I (we) voluntarily accept the risks involved. No assurance has been made by anyone with respect to the results that may be obtained. I have been given a copy of the pamphlet 'Information to Relatives.'" The nurse testified that she did not explain anything about the dangers involved in the therapy when she presented the consent for signature. The plaintiff read the consent in her presence and she asked him if he had any questions, but he had none and he signed the consent.

Beginning on June 12, 1961, and continuing through June 22, 1961, plaintiff was given a series of shock treatments which involved insulin in increasing amounts of from 40 to 260 units. On June 22, 1961, plaintiff went into a deep coma. He suffered a delayed awakening from the insulin and did not respond to the procedures used for the purpose of bringing the patient out of the coma. A specialist in internal medicine was called in and plaintiff was transferred to the intensive care unit but the coma was prolonged and as a result plaintiff suffered brain damage.

Dr. Robert L. Lam, M.D., a specialist in neurology and psychiatry, testified for plaintiff that from an examination made by him at the Veterans Hospital in Little Rock, Arkansas, on January 16, 1964, his opinion was that plaintiff had severe organic brain damage, that he was totally incapacitated in terms of employment and that his condition was permanent as a result of the prolonged insulin coma. Plaintiff was still in the Veterans Hospital at the time of trial.

Dr. Lam was interrogated as to dangers in insulin shock therapy and he testified that the possible dangers or complications thereof are coma and death or prolonged coma resulting in various degrees of brain damage, or that there might be the production of epilepsy or localized paralysis, or there might be a vascular disturbance. In addition, he said that with convulsions that may occur one could have fractures of certain types, either of the vertebrae or the extremities. The doctor was not asked and did not undertake to testify as to the frequency of occurrence of such events, or any of them, and said that no doctor could predict which patient would be the one to have trouble, saying, "So that the only thing one can say is that, when one has a patient getting deep coma insulin, that there is a possibility that this could occur." Dr. Lam also testified that there was nothing improper in the administration of the insulin shock therapy and that the administration thereof was according to good medical practice. Dr. Lam was not asked about the adequacy of defendant's disclosures to plaintiff.

* * *

Defendant first asserts that plaintiff failed to make a submissible case because he failed to offer any expert medical evidence as to what a reasonably careful and prudent physician engaged in similar practice would do under the same or similar circumstances with respect to disclosure of risks involved in the proposed therapy. There is no dispute but that plaintiff did not offer any expert testimony on this matter of what a reasonably prudent practitioner would disclose. We must determine, therefore, whether plaintiff is required to offer such proof in order to make a submissible case.

The basic philosophy in malpractice cases is that the doctor is negligent by reason of the fact that he has failed to adhere to a standard of reasonable medical care, and that consequently the service rendered was substandard and negligent. In our judgment, this is true whether the alleged malpractice consists of improper care and treatment (the usual malpractice case) or whether it is based, as here, on an alleged failure to inform the patient sufficiently to enable him to make a judgment and give an informed consent if he concludes to accept the recommended treatment.

How, then, is a jury to determine whether a physician has been negligent in failing to inform his patient adequately to enable him to make an informed decision whether to consent to recommended treatment? What proof must a plaintiff offer? Obviously, in addition to evidence as to plaintiff's condition and the treatment proposed and administered, there must be testimony as to what risks are involved and what disclosures were made by the doctor. These necessarily are a part of plaintiff's case. Such evidence was offered by plaintiff in this case. The real issue here is whether plaintiff is required to go further and as a part of his case offer evidence as to a standard of medical conduct with reference to disclosures by the physician to his patient or whether this is a matter which the jury may decide without such expert testimony. There are cases from some states which hold that such expert testimony is necessary as a part of plaintiff's case and cases from other states holding that such evidence is not required.

* * *

We have reexamined this question and have concluded that the question of what disclosure of risks incident to proposed treatment should be made in a particular situation involves medical judgment and that expert testimony thereon should be required in malpractice cases involving that issue. The question to be determined by the jury is whether defendant doctor in that particular situation failed to adhere to a standard of reasonable care. These are not matters of common knowledge or within the experience of laymen. Expert medical evidence thereon is just as necessary as is such testimony on the correctness of the handling in cases involving surgery or treatment.

* * *

[Expert testimony as to the correctiveness of the level of disclosure required in a particular case would need to take into account such factors as] the state of the patient's health, the condition of his heart and nervous system, his mental state, and * * * among other things, whether the risks involved were mere remote possibilities or something which occurred with some sort of frequency or regularity. This determination involves medical judgment as to whether disclosure of possible risks may have such an adverse effect on the patient as to jeopardize success of the proposed therapy, no matter how expertly performed. (Defendant in this case testified that plaintiff was "real shook.") After a consideration of these and other proper factors, a reasonable medical practitioner, under some circumstances, would make full disclosure of all risks which had any reasonable likelihood of occurring, but in others the facts and circumstances would dictate a guarded or limited disclosure. In some cases the judgment would be less difficult than in others, but, in any event, it would be a medical judgment.

* * *

Accordingly, we hold that plaintiff, in order to sustain his burden of proof, is required to offer expert testimony to show what disclosures a reasonable medical practitioner, under the same or similar circumstances, would have made, or, stated another way, that the disclosures as made by the defendant do not meet the standard of what a reasonable medical practitioner would have disclosed under the same or similar circumstances. To whatever extent Mitchell v. Robinson is inconsistent with the views herein expressed, it is disapproved.

Once plaintiff has offered sufficient proof to make a submissible case, including the required expert testimony which we have discussed, then the ultimate determination of whether defendant did or did not fail to disclose to plaintiff in accordance with the standard of what a reasonable medical practitioner would have done is a jury question under proper instructions from the court.

* * *

In view of the fact that plaintiff made no offering of any expert testimony relative to the extent of disclosure a reasonable medical practitioner would have made under the same or similar circumstances, he failed to make a submissible case for the jury. However, we will not affirm this case on that basis for the reason that counsel for plaintiff asserted in the presentation of the case that in the case of Mitchell v. Robinson, supra, this court had stated that expert testimony is not necessary in cases involving extent of duty to warn, and that he relied thereon in offering no proof of that character. In the light of language used in the opinion of Mitchell v. Robinson, supra, it was reasonable for counsel to assume the lack of a requirement of such testimony in this case. Under those circumstances, we feel compelled to reverse and remand for a new trial in order to afford plaintiff an opportunity to offer expert testimony on the standard of disclosure required.

* * *

The judgment is reversed and the cause remanded for a new trial.

All of the Judges concur.

Questions and Comments

1. *Comment on* Aiken. Note that although the *Aiken* court sustained the defendant's legal argument, it reversed the judgment in defendant's favor and remanded the case for retrial. The court reached this unusual outcome on the basis that the plaintiff's lawyer had reasonably relied on the *Mitchell v. Robinson* opinion, which did not signal any requirement that a plaintiff must present expert testimony on the question of whether medical practitioners would make disclosures in similar circumstances. Normally when an attorney errs in this way, appellate courts are less forgiving than the *Aiken* court, and the client is precluded from a second opportunity to litigate the case.

2. Aiken *standard of disclosure.* Under *Aiken v. Clary* the scope of required disclosure is established by a determination of what a reasonable medical practitioner would disclose under the same or similar circumstances. This reasonableness standard is very flexible, for it allows the practitioner to take into account not only the remoteness of the possibility of adverse consequences but also whether "disclosure of possible risks may have such an adverse affect on the patient as to jeopardize success of the proposed therapy no matter how expertly performed." 396 S.W.2d 668, 674 (Mo.1965).

What specifically are the adverse effects that disclosure might engender? Does the *Aiken* court assume that psychological stress might result from knowledge of the risk and thereby impede recovery? Is there any evidence to support this assumption in the case of conventional medical treatment, including surgery? Is the risk of psychiatric complication following surgery more likely if the patient is also suffering from a psychiatric disorder? The scope of what is known as the "privilege of nondisclosure" is covered in greater detail in subsection 2, infra.

3. *Question.* Does *Aiken* in effect hold that if a particular risk is not normally disclosed by medical practitioners, the patient cannot therefore recover under an informed consent theory? If so, does this allow the medical profession to determine the actual scope of the doctrine of informed consent? Does this standard reflect an appropriate compromise between the patient's interests in receiving sufficient information upon which to base the decision to accept or reject treatment and the interest of the medical profession in being able to carry out its professional function without undue risk of liability?

4. *Hypothetical.* In the situation presented by the *Aiken* case (insulin coma therapy), would reasonable medical practice require the doctor to inform the patient of the risks of brain damage? What if the risk of brain damage is estimated to be only 0.1%?

Would the *Aiken* standard require disclosure of the risk of bone fracture, which is fairly rare when a muscle relaxant is administered?

What if a bone fracture occurs only once in every 8,000 cases in which a relaxant is used? *See generally* Krouner, *Shock Therapy and Psychiatric Malpractice: The Legal Accommodation to a Controversial Treatment,* 2 Forensic Sci. 397 (1973); see also Note, *Regulation of Electro-convulsive Therapy,* 75 Mich.L.Rev. 363, 367 (1976).

CANTERBURY v. SPENCE

United States Court of Appeals, District of Columbia Circuit, 1972.
464 F.2d 772.

SPOTTSWOOD W. ROBINSON, III, CIRCUIT JUDGE:

This appeal is from a judgment entered in the District Court on verdicts directed for the two appellees at the conclusion of plaintiff-appellant Canterbury's case in chief. His action sought damages for personal injuries allegedly sustained as a result of an operation negligently performed by appellee Spence, a negligent failure by Dr. Spence to disclose a risk of serious disability inherent in the operation, and negligent post-operative care by appellee Washington Hospital Center. On close examination of the record, we find evidence which required submission of these issues to the jury. We accordingly reverse the judgment as to each appellee and remand the case to the District Court for a new trial.

[In 1958, at the age of 19, appellant sought medical attention for severe pain between his shoulder blades. After tests revealed a "filling defect" in appellant's spine, Dr. Spence told the appellant that he required surgery to repair what Dr. Spence suspected was a ruptured disc. The surgery revealed a swollen spinal cord, dilated veins, and an absence of fat surrounding the spine. Dr. Spence attempted to relieve the pressure by surgically enlarging the outer wall of the spinal cord.

The day after surgery, the appellant fell off of his bed while voiding unassisted by hospital personnel. Several hours later he was virtually paralyzed from the waist down. Dr. Spence reopened the surgical wound "to allow the spinal cord greater room in which to pulsate". At the time of his 1968 trial, the appellant required crutches to walk, and still suffered from urine incontinence and paralysis of the bowels.

The damages claimed by appellant included pain and suffering, medical expenses, and loss of earnings.]

* * *

II

Appellant filed suit in the District Court on March 7, 1963, four years after the laminectomy and approximately two years after he attained his majority. The complaint stated several causes of action against each defendant. Against Dr. Spence it alleged, among other things, negligence in the performance of the laminectomy and failure to inform him beforehand of the risk involved. Against the hospital the complaint charged negligent post-operative care in permitting appellant to remain unattended after the laminectomy, in failing to provide a nurse or orderly to assist him at the time of his fall, and in failing to maintain a side rail on his bed. The answers denied the allegations of negligence.

* * *

Appellant introduced no evidence to show medical and hospital practices, if any, customarily pursued in regard to the critical aspects of the case, and only Dr. Spence, called as an adverse witness, testified on the issue of causality. Dr. Spence described the surgical procedures he utilized in the two operations and expressed his opinion that appellant's disabilities stemmed from his pre-operative condition as symptomized by the swollen, non-pulsating spinal cord. * * * Dr. Spence further testified that even without trauma paralysis can be anticipated "somewhere in the nature of one percent" of the laminectomies performed, a risk he termed "a very slight possibility." He felt that communication of that risk to the patient is not good medical practice because it might deter patients from undergoing needed surgery and might produce adverse psychological reactions which could preclude the success of the operation.

At the close of appellant's case in chief, each defendant moved for a directed verdict and the trial judge granted both motions. The basis of the ruling, he explained, was that appellant had failed to produce any medical evidence indicating negligence on Dr. Spence's part in diagnosing appellant's malady or in performing the laminectomy; that there was no proof that Dr. Spence's treatment was responsible for appellant's disabilities; and that notwithstanding some evidence to show negligent post-operative care, an absence of medical testimony to show causality precluded submission of the case against the hospital to the jury. The judge did not allude specifically to the alleged breach of duty by Dr. Spence to divulge the possible consequences of the laminectomy.

We reverse. The testimony of appellant and his mother that Dr. Spence did not reveal the risk of paralysis from the laminectomy made out a prima facie case of violation of the physician's duty to disclose which Dr. Spence's explanation did not negate as a matter of law. There was also testimony from which the jury could have found that the laminectomy was negligently performed by Dr. Spence, and that appellant's fall was the consequence of negligence on the part of the hospital. * * * These considerations entitled appellant to a new trial.

* * *

III

Suits charging failure by a physician adequately to disclose the risks and alternatives of proposed treatment are not innovations in American law. They date back a good half-century, and in the last decade they have multiplied rapidly. There is, nonetheless, disagreement among the courts and the commentators on many major questions, and there is no precedent of our own directly in point. For the tools enabling resolution of the issues on this appeal, we are forced to begin at first principles.

The root premise is the concept, fundamental in American jurisprudence, that "[e]very human being of adult years and sound mind has a right to determine what shall be done with his own body. * * *" True consent to what happens to one's self is the informed exercise of a choice, and that entails an opportunity to evaluate knowledgeably the options available and the risks attendant upon each. The average patient has little or no understanding of the medical arts, and ordinarily has only his physician to whom he can look for enlightenment with which to reach an intelligent decision. From these almost axiomatic considerations springs the need, and in turn the requirement, of a reasonable divulgence by physician to patient to make such a decision possible.

A physician is under a duty to treat his patient skillfully but proficiency in diagnosis and therapy is not the full measure of his responsibility. The cases demonstrate that the physician is under an obligation to communicate specific information to the patient when the exigencies of reasonable care call for it.

* * *

The context in which the duty of risk-disclosure arises is invariably the occasion for decision as to whether a particular treatment procedure is to be undertaken. To the physician, whose training enables a self-satisfying evaluation, the answer may seem clear, but it is the prerogative of the patient, not the physician, to determine for himself the direction in which his interests seem to lie. To enable the patient to chart his course understandably, some familiarity with the therapeutic alternatives and their hazards becomes essential.

* * *

We now find, as a part of the physician's overall obligation to the patient, a similar duty of reasonable disclosure of the choices with respect to proposed therapy and the dangers inherently and potentially involved.[31]

* * *

IV

Duty to disclose has gained recognition in a large number of American jurisdictions, but more largely on a different rationale. The

---

31. Some doubt has been expressed as to ability of physicians to suitably communicate their evaluations of risks and the advantages of optional treatment, and as to the lay patient's ability to understand what the physician tells him. We do not share these apprehensions. The discussion need not be a disquisition, and surely the physician is not compelled to give his patient a short medical education; the disclosure rule summons the physician only to a reasonable explanation. That means generally informing the patient in nontechnical terms as to what is at stake: the therapy alternatives open to him, the goals expectably to be achieved, and the risks that may ensue from particular treatment and no treatment. So informing the patient hardly taxes the physician, and it must be the exceptional patient who cannot comprehend such an explanation at least in a rough way.

majority of courts dealing with the problem have made the duty depend on whether it was the custom of physicians practicing in the community to make the particular disclosure to the patient. If so, the physician may be held liable for an unreasonable and injurious failure to divulge, but there can be no recovery unless the omission forsakes a practice prevalent in the profession. We agree that the physician's noncompliance with a professional custom to reveal, like any other departure from prevailing medical practice, may give rise to liability to the patient. We do not agree that the patient's cause of action is dependent upon the existence and nonperformance of a relevant professional tradition.

There are, in our view, formidable obstacles to acceptance of the notion that the physician's obligation to disclose is either germinated or limited by medical practice. To begin with, the reality of any discernible custom reflecting a professional concensus on communication of option and risk information to patients is open to serious doubt. We sense the danger that what in fact is no custom at all may be taken as an affirmative custom to maintain silence, and that physician-witnesses to the so-called custom may state merely their personal opinions as to what they or others would do under given conditions. We cannot gloss over the inconsistency between reliance on a general practice respecting divulgence and, on the other hand, realization that the myriad of variables among patients makes each case so different that its omission can rationally be justified only by the effect of its individual circumstances. Nor can we ignore the fact that to bind the disclosure obligation to medical usage is to arrogate the decision on revelation to the physician alone. Respect for the patient's right of self-determination on particular therapy demands a standard set by law for physicians rather than one which physicians may or may not impose upon themselves.

* * *

V

Once the circumstances give rise to a duty on the physician's part to inform his patient, the next inquiry is the scope of the disclosure the physician is legally obliged to make. The courts have frequently confronted this problem but no uniform standard defining the adequacy of the divulgence emerges from the decisions. Some have said "full" disclosure, a norm we are unwilling to adopt literally. It seems obviously prohibitive and unrealistic to expect physicians to discuss with their patients every risk of proposed treatment—no matter how small or remote—and generally unnecessary from the patient's viewpoint as well. Indeed, the cases speaking in terms of "full" disclosure appear to envision something less than total disclosure, leaving unanswered the question of just how much.

The larger number of courts, as might be expected, have applied tests framed with reference to prevailing fashion within the medical profession. Some have measured the disclosure by "good medical practice," others by what a reasonable practitioner would have bared under the circumstances, and still others by what medical custom in the community would demand. We have explored this rather considerable body of law but are unprepared to follow it. The duty to disclose, we have reasoned, arises from phenomena apart from medical custom and practice. The latter, we think, should no more establish the scope of the duty than its existence. Any definition of scope in terms purely of a professional standard is at odds with the patient's prerogative to decide on projected therapy himself. That prerogative, we have said, is at the very foundation of the duty to disclose, and both the patient's right to know and the physician's correlative obligation to tell him are diluted to the extent that its compass is dictated by the medical profession.

In our view, the patient's right of self-decision shapes the boundaries of the duty to reveal. That right can be effectively exercised only if the patient possesses enough information to enable an intelligent choice. The scope of the physician's communications to the patient, then, must be measured by the patient's need, and that need is the information material to the decision. Thus the test for determining whether a particular peril must be divulged is its materiality to the patient's decision: all risks potentially affecting the decision must be unmasked. And to safeguard the patient's interest in achieving his own determination on treatment, the law must itself set the standard for adequate disclosure.

* * *

In broad outline, we agree that "[a] risk is thus material when a reasonable person, in what the physician knows or should know to be the patient's position, would be likely to attach significance to the risk or cluster of risks in deciding whether or not to forego the proposed therapy."

The topics importantly demanding a communication of information are the inherent and potential hazards of the proposed treatment, the alternatives to that treatment, if any, and the results likely if the patient remains untreated. The factors contributing significance to the dangerousness of a medical technique are, of course, the incidence of injury and the degree of the harm threatened. A very small chance of death or serious disablement may well be significant; a potential disability which dramatically outweighs the potential benefit of the therapy or the detriments of the existing malady may summons discussion with the patient.

There is no bright line separating the significant from the insignificant; the answer in any case must abide a rule of reason. Some dangers—infection, for example—are inherent in any operation; there is no obligation to communicate those of which persons of average sophistication are aware. Even more clearly, the physician bears no responsibility for discussion of hazards the patient has already discovered, or those having no apparent materiality to patients' decision on therapy. The disclosure doctrine, like others marking lines between permissible and impermissible behavior in medical practice, is in essence a requirement of conduct prudent under the circumstances. Whenever nondisclosure of particular risk information is open to debate by reasonable-minded men, the issue is for the finder of the facts.

* * *

As in much malpractice litigation, recovery in nondisclosure lawsuits has hinged upon the patient's ability to prove through expert testimony that the physician's performance departed from medical custom. This is not surprising since, as we have pointed out, the majority of American jurisdictions have limited the patient's right to know to whatever boon can be found in medical practice.

* * *

The guiding consideration our decisions distill, however, is that medical facts are for medical experts and other facts are for any witnesses—expert or not—having sufficient knowledge and capacity to testify to them. It is evident that many of the issues typically involved in nondisclosure cases do not reside peculiarly within the medical domain. Lay witness testimony can competently establish a physician's failure to disclose particular risk information, the patient's lack of knowledge of the risk, and the adverse consequences following the treatment. Experts are unnecessary to a showing of the materiality of a risk to a patient's decision on treatment, or to the reasonably, expectable effect of risk disclosure on the decision. These conspicuous examples of permissible uses of nonexpert testimony illustrate the relative freedom of broad areas of the legal problem of risk nondisclosure from the demands for expert testimony that shackle plaintiffs' other types of medical malpractice litigation.

[The court next determined that the issues of whether the defendant Dr. Spence had performed the laminectomy negligently and whether the hospital was negligent in the aftercare should have been submitted to the jury.]

X

This brings us to the remaining question, common to all three causes of action: whether appellant's evidence was of such caliber as to require a submission to the jury. On the first, the evidence was clearly sufficient to raise an issue as to whether Dr. Spence's obligation to disclose information on risks was reasonably met or was excused by the surrounding circumstances. Appellant testified that Dr. Spence revealed to him nothing suggesting a hazard associated with the laminectomy. His mother testified that, in response to her specific inquiry, Dr. Spence informed her that the laminectomy was no more serious than any other operation. When, at trial, it developed from Dr. Spence's testimony that paralysis can be expected in one percent of laminectomies, it became the jury's responsibility to decide whether that peril was of sufficient magnitude to bring the disclosure duty into play.

[Reversed and remanded for new trial.]

Questions and Comments

1. *Adoption of the Aiken v. Clary standard.* Note that although the courts in *Aiken v. Clary* and *Canterbury v. Spence* anchored the duty of disclosure to the doctrine of negligence, the operational standard by which liability was to be determined was very different in each case. Most jurisdictions which have recognized the doctrine of informed consent (numbering 46 as of 1982) adhere to the *Aiken v. Clary* formulation of the appropriate standard. As of 1988, however, at least 14 jurisdictions had adopted the *Canterbury v. Spence* rule.

Jurisdictions which have rejected the professional standards rule have done so on the basis that under this standard disclosure "is totally subject to the whim of the physicians in the particular community" and vests the physician "with virtually unlimited discretion in establishing the proper scope of disclosure" and is "inconsistent with the patient's right to self-determination." *Largey v. Rothman,* 110 N.J. 204, 540 A.2d 504 (1988).

Jurisdictions which adhere to the professional standards rule give the following justifications: only physicians can determine the effect that a risk might have on a particular patient; the physician does not have enough time to give all the information patients may request; negligence normally evaluates the conduct of a reasonable actor, not the expectations of a reasonable victim; the physician should not be subjected to the hindsight of the patient and the second guessing of the jury. B. Furrow, S. Johnson, T. Jost, R. Schwartz, Health Law (1987).

2. *Meaning of "materiality".* *Canterbury* defines the breadth of required disclosure to include any risk which either singly or in combination with other risks would be deemed significant by the average patient in deciding whether to accept or forego the therapy. "Materiality" is the shorthand expression of this principle. Whether a particular risk or combination of risks was material in a given situation can be established by lay witnesses exclusively and, in all likelihood, will rest largely if not exclusively on the plaintiff's testimony that a particular risk would have been material to his decision. To what extent does this approach invite intentional or unintentional fabrication by the plaintiff? Does the *Canterbury* approach leave the possibility of therapist liability wide open and expose a professional to incalculable and unknown risks of liability? Does a standard that adopts a layman's definition of materiality give professionals adequate notice of what disclosure the law demands?

3. *Policy issues in the selection of standards.* Courts choosing among the various standards seek to find an appropriate balance between competing interests. There is, on the one hand, the interest of the patient to obtain all information necessary for a meaningful decision on the proposed therapy. In addition, the medical and other treating professions have an interest in carrying out their professional functions efficiently and with a minimum of open-ended risk of liability. The looser or more uncertain the

legal standard, the more difficult it becomes for professionals to adhere to a standard of conduct that will eliminate the risk of liability. And, finally, there is also a broader societal interest in maximizing access to needed professional services, which means, of course, that the cost of these services must be reasonable. As experience with malpractice shows, the greater the liability exposure of a profession, the higher the cost of malpractice insurance; higher premiums are in turn reflected in the fee structure and the costs of medical services. Does the majority rule outlined in *Aiken* or the minority rule of *Canterbury* better reconcile these competing interests?

4. *Disclosure of alternatives.* To what extent does either the majority or minority view require disclosure of additional alternative therapies? Could a therapist be held liable if he has disclosed all collateral risks of the proposed therapy but has failed to point out alternatives? Does either case speak to this point?

What if the undisclosed alternative involves even greater risk than the actual procedure? Consider *Logan v. Greenwich Hospital Association,* 191 Conn. 282, 465 A.2d 294 (1983). Plaintiff underwent a needle biopsy to obtain a specimen of kidney tissue. The procedure involved inserting a surgical needle into her back, under a local anesthetic, to extract the sample. Plaintiff's gall bladder was punctured during the biopsy, and abdominal surgery was required to remove it. At the time she gave her consent, the plaintiff was unaware of an alternate procedure, an open biopsy, which required an incision under general anesthetic. The defendants testified that the plaintiff was not informed about this alternative because the risk of complications was greater than with a needle biopsy. The trial court instructed the jury that there is a duty to warn of feasible alternatives but that "an alternative that is more hazardous is not a viable alternative." The jury returned a verdict for the defendants. On appeal, the Connecticut Supreme Court reversed. The court reasoned that the instruction was inconsistent with the view that patients must be provided with sufficient information to make an intelligent choice. Connecticut follows the *Canterbury v. Spence* standard. Would the result be different under the majority rule?

5. *Scope of duty to communicate.* What is the therapist's liability for non-disclosure of risk data not known by him? In the instance of established therapies, as distinguished from experimental therapies (which are considered separately in section IV, infra), the therapist has a duty to disclose only those risks known to him or that are generally known by a reasonably proficient practitioner. The *Canterbury* court defined this rule in the following terms:

> The category of risks which the physician should communicate is, of course, no broader than the complement [of risk] he could communicate. The duty to divulge may extend to any risk he actually knows, but he obviously cannot divulge any of which he may be unaware.

464 F.2d 772, 787 n. 84 (D.C.Cir.1972).

However, if the therapist is unaware of risks that are generally known by practitioners in the field, non-disclosure could give rise to a claim based on negligence. As noted by the court in *Canterbury:*

Nondisclosure of an unknown risk does not, strictly speaking, present a problem in terms of the duty to disclose although it very well might pose problems in terms of the physician's duties to have known of it and to have acted accordingly.

Id.

6. *Temporary aspects of materiality.* Is it possible that the materiality of the risk might change over period of time? For instance, the side effects of a particular medical drug may not be discovered until the drug has been in use for several years. When initially prescribed, the actual risks may have been unknown or perceived as less severe. To what extent does the *Canterbury* approach invite a court to gauge materiality by the state of knowledge prevailing at the time of trial rather than at the time of treatment? Would the *Aiken* requirement of expert testimony lessen this risk?

7. *Evidentiary problems.* The doctrine of informed consent under either the majority or minority approach poses particular problems for the adjudicatory process. In medical malpractice, resolution of the case requires the trier of fact to assess the *conduct* of the therapist. Liability will attach when the actions fall below normal professional standards. In an informed consent case, however, the therapist's performance is not an issue. In fact, liability can attach even if the defendant acted with optimum skill and proficiency. Resolution of the case depends entirely on whether disclosure of information was sufficient.

When the parties agree on what was communicated, all that must be adjudicated is whether this quantum of information was sufficient. Not infrequently, however, the extent of disclosure will be disputed by the parties. In this situation, the trier of fact must decide what the therapist in fact disclosed by weighing the credibility of the respective parties. Once the factual questions have been resolved, application of the governing legal standard will produce the verdict. This initial stage of fact determination imposes particular stresses on the adjudicatory system. Unless the disclosure has been reduced to writing, the only evidence available is the parties' conflicting testimony. Quite apart from the risk of intentional distortion, there is the possibility of inadvertent distortion, since a witness may be required to recollect the substance of verbal communication that took place several years earlier. In other areas of the law, where the communications between the parties form the cornerstone of the claim, the legal system has adopted special rules to guard against inaccurate recollection of facts. For instance, most contracts involving substantial claims cannot be enforced unless the terms have been reduced to writing.

Can therapists protect themselves against claims based on faulty patient recollection of what was disclosed? Is it feasible to make audio recordings of risk disclosure sessions? How long should the recordings be kept? Alternatively, is it feasible to reduce to writing a description of the risks of therapy and require the patient to read and sign such document? What problems is this procedure likely to produce? These issues are considered in greater detail in subsection C.2., infra.

8. *Informed consent to psychotherapy.* To date there have been no reported cases imposing liability on a psychotherapist on grounds of in-

formed consent where conventional verbal psychotherapy techniques were used. (But see, *Osheroff v. Chestnut Lodge*, discussed in Chapter Two, where the lack of informed consent was alleged but, as noted, the case was settled before it came to trial). This result is undoubtedly explained in large part by the evidentiary problems which would generally confront the patient-plaintiff in the proof of causation and damages. Putting aside these practical difficulties, are there not numerous situations in everyday practice which at least technically violate the rights of the patient to informed consent? To what extent would the doctrine of informed consent require disclosure in the following situations?

(a) There is a substantial body of expert opinion that long-term outpatient psychotherapy involves a significant risk of "negative effects." *See* Hadley and Strupp, *Contemporary Views of Negative Effects in Psychotherapy*, 33 Archives of General Psychiatry 1291 (1976). Is there any obligation on the part of the therapist to disclose the risks of the potentially negative effects prior to the commencement of a prolonged course of treatment?

(b) In some instances a patient who is close to decomposition may not tolerate intense psychoanalysis. In these cases the risk is that the analysis will in fact trigger decomposition. Must this risk be communicated when, in the analyst's view, there is any reasonable possibility that the analysis will result in decomposition?

(c) An established novelist has for some time suffered from intermittent bouts of anxiety and occasional episodes of depression. The novelist consults an analyst to explore the possibilities of treatment. At the initial interview the patient expresses some fear that successful treatment might detract from or at least reduce his creative abilities. In response to a direct question as to the risks of therapy the therapist answers: "To the extent that your creativity is the result of neurosis, there may be some loss, but your true creativity will be enhanced by the removal of neurotic blocks, inhibitions, and distortions." Would this reply constitute a sufficient disclosure of the risks inherent in therapy? *See* Jonas B. Robitscher, *The Powers of Psychiatry* (Boston: Houghton Mifflin, 1980).

9. *Exceptions to the duty to disclose.* In *Canterbury v. Spence*, the court recognized a medical privilege to withhold collateral risk data. The court's discussion of this point is reprinted in the following subsection.

2.   Exceptions to the Duty to Disclose
CANTERBURY v. SPENCE
United States Court of Appeals, District of Columbia Circuit, 1972.
464 F.2d 772.

(The main body of the opinion is set out in the preceding Section.)

VI

Two exceptions to the general rule of disclosure have been noted by the courts. Each is in the nature of a physician's privilege not to disclose, and the reasoning underlying them is appealing. Each, indeed, is but a recognition that, as important as is the patient's right to know, it is greatly outweighed by the magnitudinous circumstances giving rise to the privilege. The first comes into play when the patient is unconscious or otherwise incapable of consenting, and harm from a failure to treat is imminent and outweighs any harm threatened by the proposed treatment. When a genuine emergency of that sort arises, it is settled that the impracticality of conferring with the patient dispenses with need for it. Even in situations of that character the physician should, as current law requires, attempt to secure a relative's consent if possible. But if time is too short to accommodate discussion, obviously the physician should proceed with the treatment.

The second exception obtains when risk-disclosure poses such a threat of detriment to the patient as to become unfeasible or contraindicated from a medical point of view. It is recognized that patients occasionally become so ill or emotionally distraught on disclosure as to foreclose a rational decision, or complicate or hinder the treatment, or perhaps even pose psychological damage to the patient. Where that is so, the cases have generally held that the physician is armed with a privilege to keep the information from the patient, and we think it clear that portents of that type may justify the physician in action he deems medically warranted. The critical inquiry is whether the physician responded to a sound medical judgment that communication of the risk information would present a threat to the patient's well-being.

The physician's privilege to withhold information for therapeutic reasons must be carefully circumscribed, however, for otherwise it might devour the disclosure rule itself. The privilege does not accept the paternalistic notion that the physician may remain silent simply because divulgence might prompt the patient to forego therapy the physician feels the patient really needs. That attitude presumes instability or perversity for even the normal patient, and runs counter to the foundation principle that the patient should and ordinarily can make the choice for himself. Nor does the privilege contemplate operation save where the patient's reaction to risk information, as reasonably foreseen by the physician, is menacing. And even in a situation of that kind, disclosure to a close relative with a view to securing consent to the proposed treatment may be the only alternative open to the physician.

Questions and Comments

1. *Scope of the exception.* In its recognition of the exception to a therapist's duty to disclose, the court in *Canterbury v. Spence* adhered to the rule applicable in virtually all jurisdictions that have adopted the doctrine of informed consent. As the opinion clarifies, however, the exception is limited: it does not permit the therapist to remain silent "simply because the divulgence might prompt the patient to forego therapy the physician feels the patient really needs."

Presumably, non-disclosure is justified in three instances: first, where disclosure is likely to cause the patient to become so "ill or emotionally distraught" as to "foreclose a rational decision"; second, where the disclosure will "complicate or hinder the treatment"; and third, where the disclosure will result in "psychological damage to the patient." Unhappily, the *Canterbury* court, like other courts that have dealt with the exception, failed to provide much guidance as to the scope of the exception.

2. *Rules in other jurisdictions.* The California Supreme Court has articulated the medical disclosure exception in somewhat different terms. In *Cobbs v. Grant*, 8 Cal.3d 229, 104 Cal.Rptr. 505, 502 P.2d 1 (1972) the court observed:

A disclosure need not be made beyond that required within the medical community when a doctor can prove by a preponderance of the evidence he relied upon facts which would demonstrate to a reasonable man the disclosure would have so seriously upset the patient that the patient would not have been able to dispassionately weigh the risks of refusing to undergo the recommended treatment.

Id. at 516.

A minority of courts have also allowed the privilege of nondisclosure "where an explanation of every risk attendant upon a treatment procedure may well result in alarming a patient who is already apprehensive and who may, as a result, refuse to undertake surgery or treatment in which there is minimal risk * * *" *Woods v. Brumlop*, 71 N.M. 221, 228, 377 P.2d 520, 525 (1962). Can an exception explained in these terms be applied without devouring the disclosure rule itself?

3. *Interpreting the standard.* The standard set out in Note 1 raises at least two problems of interpretation. One is the degree of "psychological damage to the patient" which must be shown to justify non-disclosure. Would the risk of moderate to severe depression be a sufficient justification? Alternatively, would anticipation of a severe but transient anxiety reaction justify non-disclosure?

The second problem concerns the *source* or *cause* of the illness or emotional distress which "foreclose[s] a rational decision." Should the exception be construed to preclude only those situations where the disclosure itself caused the patient to become emotionally distraught, or is the exception intended to include those patients who, because of their mental illness, already have an irrational fear of the treatment? In other words, is it sufficient if, instead of being caused by disclosure, the irrationality is an underlying feature or symptom of the mental illness?

4. *Hypothetical.* The rule permitting non-disclosure of risks appears to have particular relevance when the patient is mentally ill. Assume the following situation: A hospitalized psychiatric patient, suffering from a number of phobias and delusions, believes that death will inevitably follow any prolonged period of impotency. In addition to the psychiatric disorder, the patient also suffers from high blood pressure. A commonly used drug for the treatment of high blood pressure is Inderal. One of the possible but unlikely side effects of this drug is impotency. Would the treating physi-

cian be justified in prescribing Inderal without disclosing to the patient the risk of impotency?

5. *Misrepresentation compared to nondisclosure.* Does the privilege to withhold information also allow a therapist to misrepresent the nature of the treatment or diagnosis to an emotionally disturbed patient in order to induce the patient to undergo needed therapy? In the somewhat unusual case of *Kraus v. Spielberg,* 37 Misc.2d 519, 236 N.Y.S.2d 143 (1962), the plaintiff, who had a tuberculosis phobia, consulted a physician because of acute stomach pains. To induce the patient to agree to chemotherapy treatment, the therapist led the plaintiff to believe that the tuberculous germs had spread to her stomach. In fact, however, the doctor had not verified the exact location of the tubercular condition. The plaintiff consented to the therapy and later suffered unpleasant side effects. Finding that the misrepresentation was necessary to induce the plaintiff to undergo needed treatment, the court held for the defendant-therapist. Is it likely that the case would be decided the same way today in jurisdictions recognizing the doctrine of informed consent?

6. *Waiver of right.* May a patient waive his right to be informed, and can the therapist rely on such waiver? This issue has not been conclusively resolved; however, the California Supreme Court has stated in *dictum:*

> "[A] medical doctor need not make disclosure of risks when the patient requests that he not be informed."

Cobbs v. Grant, 8 Cal.3d 229, 104 Cal.Rptr. 505, 516, 502 P.2d 1, 12 (1972).

BARCLAY v. CAMPBELL
Supreme Court of Texas, 1986.
704 S.W.2d 8.

McGEE, JUSTICE.

This is a medical malpractice case. Milton Barclay sued Dr. W. Lawrence Campbell, alleging that the doctor negligently prescribed certain drugs for Barclay and negligently failed to disclose to Barclay certain risks associated with the drugs. The trial court granted a partial directed verdict in favor of Dr. Campbell on informed consent * * *. The court of appeals affirmed the trial court judgment, holding that the trial court did not err in directing a verdict for Dr. Campbell on the issue of informed consent. 683 S.W.2d 498. We disagree. The issue of informed consent should have been submitted to the jury. Therefore, we reverse the judgment of the court of appeals and remand the cause to the trial court.

Barclay was referred to Dr. Campbell in January of 1978 by his employer's company physician. Dr. Campbell treated Barclay for mental illness and during the course of treatment prescribed certain neuroleptic drugs for Barclay. In a small percentage of cases, these drugs produce a condition known as tardive dyskinesia. This condition is marked by involuntary muscle movements. The evidence is undisputed that Dr. Campbell did not warn Barclay of the risks associated with the neuroleptic drugs, and Barclay now suffers from tardive dyskinesia.

This cause is governed by the Medical Liability and Insurance Improvement Act, TEX.REV.CIV.STAT.ANN. art. 4590i (Vernon Supp. 1985), enacted in 1977. * * * The Texas Medical Disclosure Panel was established by the Act to determine which risks related to medical care should be disclosed. Section 6.07(a) of the Act creates a rebuttable presumption of negligence when the physician has failed to disclose a risk found on the list. Section 6.07(b) provides that if the panel has made no determination concerning the disclosure of risks attendant to a particular medical procedure in question, the physician is under the "duty otherwise imposed by law." * * * In our case, the panel has not made a determination of risk disclosure associated with neuroleptic drug ingestion. Consequently, this cause falls under section 6.07(b) of the Act.

In *Peterson v. Shields*, 652 S.W.2d 929, 931 (Tex.1983), we held that the "duty otherwise imposed by law" meant the duty imposed by section 6.02 of the Act, that is, "to disclose the risks or hazards that could have influenced a reasonable person in making a decision to give or withhold consent." * * * Thus, the focus shifts from the "reasonable medical practitioner" standard to the "reasonable person" standard which asks what risks are material to making the decision to give or withhold consent to a particular medical procedure.

If no presumption has been established by the Act, the plaintiff must prove by expert testimony that the medical condition complained of is a risk inherent in the medical procedure performed. *Id.* The expert should also "testify to all other facts concerning the risk which show that knowledge of the risk could influence a reasonable person in making a decision to consent to the procedure." *Id.*

* * *

In our case, there was expert testimony introduced at trial that tardive dyskinesia is an inherent risk associated with neuroleptic drugs. Inherent means that the risk is one which exists in and is inseparable from the drug itself. Tardive dyskinesia arises from the use of the drug and not from any defect in the drug or negligent human intervention. Certain precautions must be taken in prescribing the drug due to the inherent risks associated with the medication.

* * * We hold that the expert testimony concerning the probabilities of contracting tardive dyskinesia is some evidence that the risk was material enough to influence a reasonable person in his decision to give or withhold consent to the procedure.

* * *

[T]he court of appeals held that the undisputed evidence established that Barclay did not have the reactions of a reasonable person. Relying on section 6.07(a)(2) of the Act, the court of appeals held that it was the legislature's intent to excuse a defendant who is negligent in failing to disclose a risk if it was not medically feasible to make the disclosure. The court of appeals concluded that even if the risk was material and, therefore, should have been disclosed, Dr. Campbell was excused from making the disclosure because it was not medically feasible. The testimony used to support this conclusion was that Barclay did not have the reactions of a reasonable person because he was suffering from schizophrenia. The consensus of the expert testimony was that had Barclay known of the risk of side effects like tardive dyskinesia, it probably would have caused him to refuse the treatment, no matter how minimal the risk and how great the counterveiling risk of refusing the medication.

While we appreciate the dilemma facing a psychiatrist in such a position, we hold that it was not the legislature's intent to take away an individual's right to make such decisions for himself just because his doctor does not believe his patient is reasonable. The court of appeals applied a subjective standard to determine if Barclay was entitled to be informed of the risk. The Act requires the application of an objective standard. The issue is not whether Barclay could have been influenced in making a decision whether to give or withhold consent to the procedure had he known of the risk. Rather, the issue is whether a "reasonable person" could have been influenced in making a decision whether to give or withhold consent to the procedure had he known of the risk. If a "reasonable person" could have been influenced, then Barclay was also entitled to be warned of the risk.

*   *   *

Barclay introduced the required expert testimony and, therefore, was entitled to issues on the question of informed consent. Barclay's mental illness does not foreclose his right to be informed of the risk if the jury finds the risk is material in the sense of one which could influence a reasonable person in making a decision to give or withhold consent to the procedure. We reverse the judgment of the court of appeals and remand the cause to the trial court for trial on the issue of informed consent.

B.   OTHER ELEMENTS NECESSARY TO ESTABLISH A CLAIM

1.   Causation

Mere non-disclosure of a risk is not sufficient to impose liability on the therapist. Liability results only if an *injury* occurs that would not have occurred *but for* the non-disclosure. Thus, a patient must prove that if the risk of injury had been disclosed, he would not have consented to the therapy that resulted in the injury. "Causation" is the shorthand legal term used to describe the relationship that must exist between the breach of duty (non-disclosure of a material fact) and the resulting injury.

*   *   *

CANTERBURY v. SPENCE

United States Court of Appeals, District of Columbia Circuit, 1972.
464 F.2d 772.

[The main body of the opinion is set forth at p. 180, supra].

A causal connection exists when, but only when, disclosure of significant risks incidental to treatment would have resulted in a decision against it. The patient obviously has no complaint if he would have submitted to the therapy notwithstanding awareness that the risk was one of its perils. On the other hand, the very purpose of the disclosure rule is to protect the patient against consequences which, if known, he would have avoided by foregoing the treatment. The more difficult question is whether the factual issue on causality calls for an objective or a subjective determination.

It has been assumed that the issue is to be resolved according to whether the factfinder believes the patient's testimony that he would not have agreed to the treatment if he had known of the danger which later ripened into injury. We think a technique which ties the factual conclusion on causation simply to the assessment of the patient's credibility is unsatisfactory.

* * *

[W]hen causality is explored at a post-injury trial with a professedly uninformed patient, the question whether he actually would have turned the treatment down if he had known the risks is purely hypothetical: "Viewed from the point at which he had to decide, would the patient have decided differently had he known something he did not know?" And the answer which the patient supplies hardly represents more than a guess, perhaps tinged by the circumstance that the uncommunicated hazard has in fact materialized.

In our view, this method of dealing with the issue on causation comes in second-best. It places the physician in jeopardy of the patient's hindsight and bitterness. It places the factfinder in the position of deciding whether a speculative answer to a hypothetical question is to be credited. It calls for a subjective determination solely on testimony of a patient-witness shadowed by the occurrence of the undisclosed risk.

Better it is, we believe, to resolve the causality issue on an objective basis: in terms of what a prudent person in the patient's position would have decided if suitably informed of all perils bearing significance. If adequate disclosure could reasonably be expected to have caused that person to decline the treatment because of the revelation of the kind of risk or danger that resulted in harm, causation is shown, but otherwise not. The patient's testimony is relevant on that score of course but it would not threaten to dominate the findings.

* * *

Questions and Comments

1. *Causation vs. materiality.* Causation must be distinguished from the element of materiality. Material risks, as noted previously, are those to which the patient is "likely to attach significance * * * in deciding whether or not to forego the proposed therapy." *Canterbury v. Spence,* 464 F.2d 772, 787 (D.C.Cir.1972). Not all material risks, of course, would prompt a patient to refuse therapy. In such a case, disclosure would be irrelevant to the patient's final decision. Waltz and Schoneman provide an example of this distinction: "(I)t would be reasonable to conclude that a patient who required brain surgery to survive would not have refused it even had he known of an undisclosed risk of speech impediment. At the same time the risk of a speech impediment could well be deemed to constitute nondisclosure of a material fact". Waltz and Schoneman, *Informed Consent to Therapy,* 64 Nw.U.L.Rev. 628, 648 (1970).

2. *Objective and subjective tests of causation.* The element of causation requires the fact-finder to determine whether the plaintiff would have foregone the therapy if he had been informed of the risk that actually materialized. In resolving this question, the fact-finder must decide how an individual would have acted under a hypothetical set of circumstances. Obviously, any decision of this type is at best an educated guess.

Basically two approaches can be used to determine causation. In one, the fact-finder focuses on the particular plaintiff and determines whether that individual would have foregone the therapy if the risk had been disclosed. This "subjective" approach focuses on the plaintiff's testimony. Thus, the plaintiff generally would prove causation by testifying that he would have foregone a particular therapy if he had been aware of the risk that eventually materialized. Of key importance here is the plaintiff's credibility as judged by the fact-finder. Only a minority of courts have adopted this approach. See *Scott v. Bradford,* 606 P.2d 554 (Okl.1979).

Alternatively, under the "objective" approach, as adopted by the court in *Canterbury v. Spence* the causation issue is posed not in terms of the particular plaintiff, but in terms of the effect that nondisclosure of a material risk would have on a reasonable person in plaintiff's position. While the plaintiff's testimony is still relevant, it is less influential; the issue is how a reasonable person in plaintiff's position—rather than the plaintiff himself—would have acted when faced with the disclosure risk. Undoubtedly, the outcome of informed consent cases is very much influenced by the court's choice of approach. Under the subjective approach causation is much less likely to be a barrier to recovery; consequently, the plaintiff has a greater chance of recovery than under the objective approach.

---

2. Damages

The previous subsection pointed out that a successful plaintiff must prove that a material risk of the therapy was not disclosed and that a reasonable person in the plaintiff's position would not have consented to the therapy had the risk been disclosed. What remains to be considered is the measure of damages applicable to this type of case. While few cases have addressed this question, it has generally been assumed that a successful plaintiff is entitled to damages to compensate for the loss or injury resulting from the risk that materialized. Thus, the measure of damages is generally the same as in a malpractice case. It has been argued that this rule is unduly harsh from the therapist's perspective and that the recovery should be reduced by an amount attributable to whatever injury or loss would have occurred if no therapy had been undertaken or if an alternative therapy had been adopted. Thus, under this view, if the plaintiff inevitably would have suffered physical deterioration if he had received no therapy whatsoever, that factor would reduce the amount of damages he can recover.

These general rules of damages may vary somewhat in the few jurisdictions that treat the doctrine of informed consent as a variant of an action in assault and battery. In those jurisdictions, because the basis of the claim is an "unauthorized touching," the therapist can be liable for monetary damages even if the plaintiff suffered no actual injury. Also, since battery is viewed as an intentional tort, the defendant can be assessed punitive or exemplary damages. However, most courts would not impose exemplary damages unless the physician was guilty of actual malice.

It is important to note that prevailing rules on damages significantly limit the impact of the doctrine of informed consent. Unless some *physical injury* results from the treatment, it is unlikely that a patient can recover anything more than nominal damages. Under the present state of the law, mental distress, fright, shock, humiliation, or similar violations of psychological integrity do not ordinarily constitute compensable injuries unless accompanied by physical impact. Thus, at least for the present, the doctrine of informed consent is limited to those professions that use treatment methods capable of inflicting physical harm. As a result, conventional psychotherapists, unless they also use treatment modalities such as drugs, which have the potential of inflicting physical harm, are relatively immune from liability. Undoubtedly, this explains in large part the relative absence of reported cases against non-medically trained psychotherapists for failure to secure the patient's informed consent. It also explains why behavioral science researchers, in spite of numerous reported violations of the requirements of informed consent, have escaped liability. However, the trend is clearly toward recognition of psychological harm as a sufficient basis for the recovery of monetary damages even when not associated with any physical injury. With these considerations in mind consider the following hypothetical fact situation:

A patient consults a psychotherapist to overcome his flying phobia, which in view of his occupational need to travel is proving to be an increasing handicap to his professional advancement. The therapist agrees to treat the patient, and over a period of the next three months

gives him a series of desensitization procedures coupled with hypnotherapy.

The patient is informed that he has made material progress and
the next step is to take a short flight. The patient is not alerted to the
possibility that he will feel great anxiety during the flight. In fact, the
therapist assures him that he is entirely ready to take the next step.
Pursuant to the therapist's recommendations, the patient secures a
ticket and boards an airline flight to the next city. Shortly after
takeoff, in spite of the patient's use of a tape-recorder designed to
facilitate self-hypnosis, the patient experiences a severe anxiety attack.
By the time the airplane lands 30 minutes later, the patient is in a
state of total collapse. He is taken by ambulance to the nearest
hospital and is placed under sedation. Upon release a week later, the
patient remains in a highly agitated and anxious state, which is
accompanied by insomnia. As a result of this condition he is absent
from work for the next three weeks. Upon his return to work, he
learns that during his absence he was considered but rejected for a
promotion, on the grounds that his records indicated that he had
health problems. Badly shaken by the experience and somewhat
angry at the therapist for having encouraged him to take the flight, he
consults an attorney to inquire whether he has any basis to sue the
therapist.

What is the attorney likely to advise? Would the result be different in
a jurisdiction which requires physical injury?

C. ISSUES PERTAINING TO PATIENT ACKNOWLEDGMENT AND UNDERSTANDING

1. Introduction

In its original form, legally sufficient consent required nothing
more than patient assent to the proposed treatment. Failure to obtain
consent subjected the therapist to liability for assault and battery. The
modern doctrine, on the other hand, requires that the consent be an
informed one.

The elements of informed consent are twofold. First, the therapist
must disclose information pertaining to the risks of the proposed
therapy. Second, as under the original doctrine, the patient must agree
to undergo the therapy. In law the agreement that the patient must
give to authorize the therapist to start the therapy is known as consent.

Two types of problems arise in connection with the element of
consent or agreement. One pertains to the evidentiary requirements
imposed by the legal system. In other words, what actions or expressions on the part of the patient will suffice to establish consent? A
second and more complex problem relates to the level of patient
understanding that must accompany the consent or agreement. More
specifically, does the legal system require that the patient understand
the nature and degree of risk that was disclosed? If so, can the
requisite level of understanding be presumed, or must the therapist

establish its existence? These interrelated issues are explained in the materials that follow.

Both legal opinions and the writings of legal commentators have advanced the view that "[t]o establish consent to a risk it must be shown that the patient was aware of the risk and assented to the encountering of it". Jon R. Waltz and Fred E. Inbau, *Medical Jurisprudence* (New York: Macmillan, 1971), p. 164. What these assertions leave unanswered, however, is whether the patient must have actual rather than imputed knowledge. Consider for a moment the legal efficacy of a consent given by a patient who has been fully informed of all risks and alternatives but who, unknown to the physician, fails to adequately understand the information he has received. Two different approaches can be followed in dealing with this problem.

One alternative focuses on the therapist's disclosure. If that disclosure is deemed adequate, in the sense that an ordinary patient would comprehend the information transmitted, awareness will be imputed without regard to the patient-plaintiff's *actual level of comprehension.* It is this approach that the *Canterbury v. Spence* court advocated. In a footnote, the court observed that "the physician discharges the duty when he makes a reasonable effort to convey sufficient information *although the patient, without fault of the physician, may not fully grasp it*". 464 F.2d 772, 780 n. 15 (D.C.Cir.1972) [emphasis added]. Thus, under this approach, the therapist has discharged his duty when he has made full disclosure in terms that would be comprehensible to the average patient.

Under the other approach, a patient's consent would not be effective unless he had *actual* knowledge and understanding of the therapist's disclosure. In the event of litigation, then, the fact-finder would be required to determine whether the *particular* patient-plaintiff had understood what the therapist had told him. One commentator has explained the rationale for this approach:

> Even when the information presented is adequate, therefore, the consenting process may be nothing more than a "ritual" if the patient-subject remains "uneducated and uncomprehending." To avoid this result, the physician could be held responsible for taking reasonable steps to ascertain whether the information presented has been understood, so that if it has not he may supplement it as needed or may convey the same information in a manner more comprehensible to the particular patient.

Capron, *Informed Consent in Catastrophic Disease Research and Treatment*, 123 U.Pa.L.Rev. 340, 414 (1974).

The weight of legal opinion has, however, rejected the "subjective" approach on a variety of grounds. As Waltz and Inbau have observed:

> One difficulty with this view is that the patient's testimony, undeniably admissible at trial, in fact controls the issue of consent. And the trial lawyer's healthy cynicism tells him that a claimant's testimony is sometimes susceptible to modification based upon hindsight. Another

difficulty is that it leaves no room for reasonable communication or interpretation mistakes by the physician; he assumes the risk of incorrectly concluding that the patient in fact understood and assented to the risks communicated. As the entire history of contract law attests, legal relationships based on communication cannot practicably be made to depend on the vagaries of the parties' subjective intent.

Jon Waltz and Fred Inbau, *Medical Jurisprudence* (New York: Macmillan Co., 1971), p. 165.

Comment

As a practical matter, the question whether the patient's awareness should be measured objectively or subjectively has only rarely arisen in modern informed consent cases. The reasons for this are twofold. First, modern cases have emphasized the element of disclosure. To the extent that the physician fails to inform the patient adequately, the question of awareness is typically never reached, since the case can be disposed of on that ground. Thus, the scope of patient awareness would only be an issue if the fact-finder determined that the therapist had given adequate disclosure, and the patient contended that he did not understand its content. Cases based on this type of contention are, however, very hard to win, which at least in part explains their absence. Moreover, a patient's case would be weakened by the dual contentions that there was insufficient disclosure and that he lacked awareness because he did not understand what was disclosed. While these are not necessarily inconsistent positions, the plaintiff's lawyer would be concerned that emphasis on the patient's lack of comprehension might buttress the defendant's contentions that there was full disclosure and that the patient, through no fault of the therapist, failed to understand what was said.

----

2. The Determination of Patient Assent: Evidentiary Problems

As has been noted, consent consists of the dual ingredients of awareness and assent. To establish consent to a risk it must be shown that the patient is made aware of the risk and knowingly assented to the treatment. Thus, in the event of litigation, the fact-finder must determine whether the patient's expressions in their totality (both verbal and nonverbal) support the conclusion that he assented to the treatment. The test is an objective one: intent is gauged by what is known as the reasonable person standard. Under this test the question is whether a reasonable therapist would have concluded from the patient's statements and behavior that the patient was aware of the risks that had been communicated and that he had manifested a willingness to undergo the therapy or procedure. Any other approach would, of course, subject the therapist to the unreasonable risk that a patient who manifests assent could subsequently deny it on the basis of unexpressed mental reservations.

When divorced from the question of knowledge, however, the element of assent is not likely to be an issue. The mere fact that the patient had some interaction with the therapist generally establishes assent to at least some form of treatment. But the issue is likely to be much broader. The crucial question for the fact-finder is usually not whether there was assent in the narrow sense, but whether the assent was coupled with sufficient knowledge and awareness. As might be expected, this factual determination poses problems of an evidentiary nature. Most commonly, an informed consent case will, if litigated, turn at least in part on the credibility of the parties to the action. The patient will contend that because of inadequate disclosure, he was not made aware of the risks of the treatment. The therapist, on the other hand, may have a substantially different recollection of what was disclosed. To lower the risk of erroneous recollection, a therapist would be wise to keep a written summary of the information communicated to the patient and a written record of a patient's consent.

Questions and Comments

1. *Empirical data on information recall.* What are the implications of various studies showing that within a relatively short period of time patients frequently lose recall of much of the medical data disclosed during the consent obtaining process? In one study which involved 200 cancer patients, it was found, for instance, that one day after receiving relevant information on the risks of chemotherapy, "[O]nly 60 per cent understood the purpose and the nature of the procedure, and only 55 per cent correctly listed even one major risk or complication." Cassileth, Zupkis, Sutton–Smith, and March, "Informed Consent—Why Are Its Goals Imperfectly Realized?" 302 New.Eng.J.Med. 896 (1980). *See also* Epstein and Lasagna, "Obtaining Informed Consent: Form or Substance?," 123 Arch Inter.Med. 682 (1969); Schultz, Pardee, Ensinck, "Are Research Subjects Really Informed?," 123 West.J.Med. 76 (1975).

Do studies such as the one described above call into question the overall utility of the informed consent doctrine? Do they at least point to the need for those providing treatment to maintain adequate records evidencing the disclosures made to the patient?

2. *Statutory requirements.* A number of states have enacted statutes that spell out the evidentiary requirements for informed consent to medical or surgical procedures. Typically, these statutes require that the attending physician provide the patient with a document that sets forth the procedures of treatment to be undertaken and the major risks. At the same time, they require that the patient sign a document acknowledging that the disclosure of information has been made and that all of his questions pertaining to the treatment have been answered. In turn, the fulfillment of these documentary requirements constitutes either *prima facie* or conclusive evidence that informed consent to treatment has been given. The Iowa statute illustrates this approach to proof of informed consent:

> A consent in writing to any medical or surgical procedure or course of procedures in patient care which meets the requirements of this

section shall create a presumption that informed consent was given. A consent in writing meets the requirements of this section if it:

1. Sets forth in general terms the nature and purpose of the procedure or procedures, together with the known risks, if any, of death, brain damage, quadriplegia, paraplegia, the loss or loss of function of any organ or limb, or disfiguring scars associated with such procedure or procedures, with the probability of each such risk if reasonably determinable.

2. Acknowledges that the disclosure of that information has been made and that all questions asked about the procedure or procedures have been answered in a satisfactory manner.

3. Is signed by the patient for whom the procedure is to be performed, or if the patient for any reason lacks legal capacity to consent, is signed by a person who has legal authority to consent on behalf of that patient in those circumstances.

Iowa Code Ann. § 147.137.

Note that the Iowa statute only requires disclosure of certain major risks that are itemized in Section 1 of the statute. Also, note that the statute does not require any information on alternative treatment.

In those states with statute regulating informed consent, the question of legislative preemption arises. A court in one of those states may have to determine whether the legislature has preempted the entire area or whether there is room for judicially developed remedies to supplement the statutory provisions.

3. *Effect of written form.* Is it possible for a patient who has signed a form that exhaustively lists the risks and hazards of the therapy to contend that although he signed the form he did not, in fact, understand its content? The answer to this question would presumably turn on whether under the law of the state controlling the disposition of the case, the signing of a statement is *conclusive* evidence of informed consent on the part of the patient. If it is only *prima facie* evidence, the patient's signature on a consent form would not preclude the contention that he was not, in fact, adequately informed. This suggests that for maximum protection the therapist should do more than obtain the patient's written consent on a form that recites the significant risks. In addition, the therapist should verbally explain the risks and alternatives and then enter a notation in the patient's file recounting the general nature of the conversation.

4. *Standardized forms.* Note that standardized consent forms that merely recite that the patient has been informed of "all risks" are likely to be of little legal protection. Valid consent requires disclosure of the specific risks and available alternative therapy.

Therefore, a summary consent form merely attesting that "all risks" have been communicated will not foreclose the admission of evidence that there was not, in fact, a sufficient disclosure. Not surprisingly, fairly detailed standardized consent forms are becoming more frequent. Illustrative of the standardized forms that have been developed is the one set out below for obtaining consent to electroshock therapy (ECT).

CONSENT TO ELECTRIC SHOCK THERAPY

A.M.

Date _____ Time _____ P.M.

1. I authorize Dr. _____, and assistants of his choice, to administer electric shock treatment, and relaxant drugs and other medication, to _____ and
(name of patient)
to continue such treatment at such intervals as he and his assistants may deem advisable.

2. I understand that this treatment consists of passing a controlled electric current between two electrodes applied to the patient's temples. In some instances, the patient may be given medication prior to treatment to reduce tension and produce muscular relaxation. I understand that the patient will not feel the electric current and will feel no pain. When the electric current is administered, the patient becomes unconscious and has strong convulsive muscular contractions which may last from 35 to 50 seconds. The patient gradually regains consciousness and his confusion clears within 15 to 60 minutes. The patient may experience headache and nausea.

3. I understand that the treatments may cause temporary confusion and memory impairment. I also understand that certain risks and complications are involved in the treatment. The most common risk is fracture and dislocation of the limbs and vertebrae. I acknowledge that these and other risks and complications of this procedure have been explained to me.

4. In addition to the foregoing, the strict care which will be required immediately following treatment and during convalescence has been fully explained to me.

5. The alternative methods of treatment have been explained and no guarantee or assurance has been given by anyone as to the results that may be obtained.

Signed _____

Witness _____

5. *Revocation of consent.* The right to consent implies the right to revoke any consent that has been given. Thus, a patient may withdraw his consent at any time before the treatment has been concluded. However, under the law of most states this principle does not apply to the consent given by a patient entering an institution through a voluntary admission procedure. Typically, laws governing admission to psychiatric facilities stipulate that a voluntary patient may be forcibly detained for a designated period even after he has withdrawn his voluntary admission consent. This problem is considered in greater detail in Chapter Eight.

_____

3. *Impediments to Valid Consent: Coercion and Duress*

Because the consent that the patient gives the therapist to authorize the treatment is an act having legal significance, it has attendant legal rights. There are, of course, numerous other instances in law where an individual's act establishes the responsibilities and rights of those who are a party to the transaction. Such is the case, for instance, in the law of contracts: an individual's acceptance of an offer creates a contract. In each instance some specific and intentional act has legal significance.

Because of the potentially far-reaching and important consequences that can attach, these legally significant acts will not be given effect unless they are voluntary. In fact, the law has traditionally refused to recognize or enforce any legally significant act that is the product of force or coercion. The reasons behind this principle are grounded in basic notions of fairness. Enforcement of involuntary acts would both recognize the legitimacy of force and violence and at the same time make the state a partner to the coercion.

While all are probably willing to accept a rule requiring consent to be voluntary, there may be less agreement as to exactly what conditions should render it involuntary. Unfortunately, the legal literature is not very informative on this question, at least in the context of consent to medical treatment. By what criteria then is the voluntariness of consent to be judged? To some extent the answer will depend on the particular model of behavior that one subscribes to. One can, for instance, adopt a free-will model, which perceives human behavior as the product of a free and autonomous will. Involuntary actions result when the free will is overwhelmed by some external force or pressure. An inquiry using this model will focus on an abstraction known as the "ordinary or reasonable man" and determine whether the pressures or forces exerted were of such magnitude as to override the free will of the model person. While this approach with its emphasis on free will may not accord with modern behaviorial science doctrines on the nature of man and the psychic apparatus, it is a workable one. Unlike other models presently available, it provides a frame of reference that judges and juries can use to decide specific cases in a manner generally acceptable to the public.

The issue, then, for the trier of fact is whether a particular set of circumstances was sufficiently coercive as to lead to the conclusion that, but for such pressure, consent would have been withheld. In making this decision, a judge or jury is likely to apply certain commonly held presumptions. We are all prepared, for instance, to assume that a decision reached at the point of a gun is likely to be involuntary. But other forms of duress or coercion aside from the threat of physical force may render the consent invalid. Even the promise of a benefit or the threat to withhold some privilege may constitute coercion under some circumstances. Certainly this would be the case if consent to participation in a biomedical research project were obtained from a prisoner serving an indeterminate sentence in exchange for a promise of early release. Consent here is likely to be viewed as coerced, not because the individual did not have an effective choice (as is the case when physical force is used or threatened), but rather because the "bargain" was basically unfair. The finding of unfairness here, of course, takes into account the particular vulnerability of the consenting individual. The perceived unfairness derives not so much from the inequality of the detriment in relation to the benefit, but rather from the particular vulnerability of the person giving the consent. What is called for in every case of this type is basically a moral judgment that takes into account the benefit in relation to the detriment and more important, the overall vulnerability of the consenting individual. This, of course, suggests that not every beneficial promise made to a prisoner that induces consent is necessarily coercive, thus rendering the consent invalid. An agreement by prisoners to donate blood in exchange for reasonable remuneration would not necessarily be viewed as unfair and therefore coercive. But even this conclusion is being challenged; some critics contend that the overall control that the institution or staff is likely to exercise over a prisoner or patient is sufficient to call into question the voluntary nature of consent to any medical procedure that is not of direct therapeutic benefit to the consenting person. However, this absolutist position has not found general acceptance; these cases are still decided on their own particular facts.

Whatever the actual dynamics of patient decision-making in an institution, the legal system assumes that treatment decisions made by a competent patient are voluntary unless shown, upon adequate proof, to be otherwise. As is further developed in Chapter Nine (Competency Determinations), *some* treatment decisions, particularly those pertaining to the treatment of psychiatric disorders, are not always subject to the informed consent requirement. In most jurisdictions, an institution, either by statute or judicial interpretation, is permitted to administer certain treatments, such as psychotropic medication, to involuntarily hospitalized patients without the patient's consent. In the treatment of nonpsychiatric disorders of institutionalized patients, the requirement of informed consent prevails, at least when the patient is legally competent and his consent is presumed voluntary unless shown to be otherwise.

This general presumption, however, does not necessarily apply when the treatment is administered in the experimental or research context. As we will see, the use of experimental treatment procedures on institutionalized patient-subjects, particularly if the procedures are physically intrusive, raise unique problems in determining the voluntariness of the patients' informed consent. Nor is this problem an insignificant one. While it is difficult to arrive at a numerical estimate, it is undoubtedly true that institutionalized persons have for many years been one of the prime sources of experimental subjects. In fact, the bulk of biomedical psychiatric research has by and large been carried out on institutionalized patients. It is, therefore, somewhat surprising that these practices have engendered relatively little litigation to date. In fact, only one decision, *Kaimowitz v. Department of Mental Health,* infra, has directly dealt with the issue of whether institutionalized persons have the capacity to give voluntary informed consent to intrusive experimental therapies. That decision, moreover, was only a trial court opinion; no appellate court has passed on the issues it sought to resolve. Nevertheless, the opinion is worth considering because it is the only decision that has come to grips with the extremely difficult questions underlying the application of any experimental procedures to institutionalized populations.

KAIMOWITZ v. DEPARTMENT OF MENTAL HEALTH FOR THE STATE OF MICHIGAN

Circuit Court for Wayne County, 1973.
Civil Action No. 73–19434–AW.

OPINION

This case came to this Court originally on a complaint for a Writ of Habeas Corpus brought by Plaintiff Kaimowitz on behalf of John Doe and the Medical Committee for Human Rights, alleging that John Doe was being illegally detained in the Lafayette Clinic for the purpose of experimental psychosurgery.

John Doe had been committed by the Kalamazoo County Circuit Court on January 11, 1955, to the Ionia State Hospital as a Criminal Sexual Psychopath, without a trial of criminal charges, under the terms of the then existing Criminal Sexual Psychopathic law. He had been charged with the murder and subsequent rape of a student nurse at the Kalamazoo State Hospital while he was confined there as a mental patient.

In 1972, Drs. Ernst Rodin and Jacques Gottlieb of the Lafayette Clinic, a facility of the Michigan Department of Mental Health, had filed a proposal "For the Study of Treatment of Uncontrollable Aggression."

This was funded by the Legislature of the State of Michigan for the fiscal year 1972. After more than 17 years at the Ionia State Hospital, John Doe was transferred to the Lafayette Clinic in November of 1972 as a suitable research subject for the Clinic's study of uncontrollable aggression.

Under the terms of the study, 24 criminal sexual psychopaths in the State's mental health system were to be subjects of experiment. The experiment was to compare the effects of surgery on the amygdaloid portion of the limbic system of the brain with the effect of the drug cyproterone acetate on the male hormone flow. The comparison was intended to show which, if either, could be used in controlling aggression of males in an institutional setting, and to afford lasting permanent relief from such aggression to the patient.

Substantial difficulties were encountered in locating a suitable patient population for the surgical procedures and a matched controlled group for the treatment by the anti-androgen drug. As a matter of fact, it was concluded that John Doe was the only known appropriate candidate available within the state mental health system for the surgical experiment.

The complete "Informed Consent" form signed by John Doe is as follows:

"Since conventional treatment efforts over a period of several years have not enabled me to control my outbursts of rage and anti-social behavior, I submit an application to be a subject in a research project which may offer me a form of effective therapy. This therapy is based upon the idea that episodes of anti-social rage and sexuality might be triggered by a disturbance in certain portions of my brain. I understand that in order to be certain that a significant brain disturbance exists, which might relate to my anti-social behavior, an initial operation will have to be performed. This procedure consists of placing fine wires into my brain, which will record the electrical activity from those structures which play a part in anger and sexuality. These electrical waves can then be studied to determine the presence of an abnormality.

"In addition electrical stimulation with weak currents passed through these wires will be done in order to find out if one or several points in the brain can trigger my episodes of violence or unlawful sexuality. In other words, this stimulation may cause me to want to commit an aggressive or sexual act, but every effort will be made to have a sufficient number of people present to control me. If the brain disturbance is limited to a small area, I understand that the investigators will destroy this part of my brain with an electrical current. If the abnormality comes from a larger part of my brain, I agree that it should be surgically removed, if the doctors determine that it can be done so, without risk of side effects. Should the electrical activity from the parts of my brain into which the wires have been placed reveal that there is no significant abnormality, the wires will simply be withdrawn.

"I realize that any operation on the brain carries a number of risks which may be slight but could be potentially serious. These risks include infection, bleeding, temporary or permanent weakness or paralysis of one or more of my legs or arms, difficulties with speech and thinking, as well as the ability to feel, touch, pain and temperature. Under extraordinary circumstances, it is also possible that I might not survive the operation.

"Fully aware of the risks detailed in the paragraphs above, I authorize the physicians of Lafayette Clinic and Providence Hospital to perform the procedures as outlined above.

October 27, 1972	/S/ Louis M. Smith
Date	Signature
Calvin Vanee	/S/ Emily T. Smith/Harry
	L. Smith
	Signature of responsible relative
	or guardian"

John Doe signed an "informed consent" form to become an experimental subject prior to his transfer from the Ionia State Hospital. He had obtained signatures from his parents giving consent for the experimental and innovative surgical procedures to be performed on his brain, and two separate three-man review committees were established by Dr. Rodin to review the scientific worthiness of the study and the validity of the consent obtained from Doe.

[Following a review of the research protocol both committees approved the proposal.]

Even though no experimental subjects were found to be available in the state mental health system other than John Doe, Dr. Rodin prepared to proceed with the experiment on Doe, and depth electrodes we e to be inserted into his brain on or about January 15, 1973.

Early in January, 1973, Plaintiff Kaimowitz, a legal services attorney, became aware of the work being contemplated on John Doe and made his concern known to the Detroit Free Press. Considerable newspaper publicity ensued and this action was filed shortly thereafter.

Upon the request of counsel, a Three–Judge Court was empanelled, * * * [and counsel was appointed to represent John Doe].

With the rush of publicity on the filing of the original suit, funds for the research project were stopped by * * * the Department of Mental Health, and the investigators, Drs. Gottlieb and Rodin, dropped their plans to pursue the research set out in the proposal. They reaffirmed at trial, however, their belief in the scientific, medical and ethical soundness of the proposal.

Three ultimate issues were framed for consideration by the Court. The first related to the constitutionality of the detention of Doe. The full statement of the second and third questions, to which this Opinion is addressed, are set forth in the text below.

[At an initial hearing on March 23, 1973 the Court determined that the detention of John Doe was unconstitutional and ordered his release. Following this development the state contended that consideration of the other issue—whether the proposed surgical procedures could be carried out on a subject in Doe's former status was now moot. In holding that the case had not been mooted and was appropriate for a declaratory judgment the court advanced the view that "even though the original experimental program was terminated, there was nothing that would prevent it from being instituted again in the near future" * * *]

The two issues framed for decision in this declaratory judgment action are as follows:

1. After failure of established therapies, may an adult or a legally appointed guardian, if the adult is involuntarily detained, at a facility within the jurisdiction of the State Department of Mental Health, give legally adequate consent to an innovative or experimental surgical procedure on the brain, if there is demonstrable physical abnormality of the brain, and the procedure is designed to ameliorate behavior, which is either personally tormenting to the patient, or so profoundly disruptive that the patient cannot safely live, or live with others?

2. If the answer to the above is yes, then is it legal in this State to undertake an innovative or experimental surgical procedure on the brain of an adult who is involuntarily detained at a facility within the jurisdiction of the State Department of Mental Health, if there is demonstrable physical abnormality of the brain, and the procedure is designed to ameliorate behavior, which is either personally tormenting to the patient, or so profoundly disruptive that the patient cannot safely live, or live with others?

Throughout this Opinion, the Court will use the term psychosurge·y to describe the proposed innovative or experimental surgical procedure defined in the questions for consideration by the Court.

At least two definitions of psychosurgery have been furnished the Court. Dr. Bertram S. Brown, Director of the National Institute of Mental Health, defined the term as follows in his prepared statement before the United States Senate Subcommittee on Health of the Committee on Labor and Public Welfare on February 23, 1973:

> "Psychosurgery can best be defined as a surgical removal or destruction of brain tissue or the cutting of brain tissue to disconnect one part of the brain from another, with the intent of altering the behavior, even though there may be no direct evidence of structural disease or damage to the brain."

Dr. Peter Breggin, a witness at the trial, defined psychosurgery as the destruction of normal brain tissue for the control of emotions or behavior or the destruction of abnormal brain tissue for the control of emotions or behavior, where the abnormal tissue has not been shown to be the cause of the emotions or behavior in question.

The psychosurgery involved in this litigation is a sub-class, narrower than that defined by Dr. Brown. The proposed psychosurgery we are concerned with encompasses only experimental psychosurgery where there are [no] demonstrable physical abnormalities in the brain. Therefore, temporal lobectomy, an established therapy for relief of clearly diagnosed epilepsy is not involved, nor are accepted neurological surgical procedures, for example, operations for Parkinsonism, or operations for the removal of tumors or the relief of stroke.

It is clear from the record in this case that the understanding of the limbic system of the brain and its function is very limited. Practically every witness and exhibit established how little is known of the relationship of the limbic system to human behavior, in the absence of some clearly defined clinical disease such as epilepsy.

The record in this case demonstrates that animal experimentation and non-intrusive human experimentation have not been exhausted in determining and studying brain function. Any experimentation on the human brain, especially when it involves an intrusive, irreversible procedure in a non life-threatening situation, should be undertaken with extreme caution, and then only when answers cannot be obtained from animal experimentation and from non-intrusive human experimentation.

Psychosurgery should never be undertaken upon involuntarily committed populations, when there is a high-risk low-benefits ratio as demonstrated in this case. This is because of the impossibility of obtaining truly informed consent from such populations. The reasons such informed consent cannot be obtained are set forth in detail subsequently in this Opinion.

* * *

The Court does not in any way desire to impede medical progress. We are much concerned with violence and the possible effect of brain disease on violence. Much research on the brain is necessary and must be carried on, but when it takes the form of psychosurgery, it cannot be undertaken on involuntarily detained populations. Other avenues of research must be utilized and developed.

As pointed out above, psychosurgery is clearly experimental, poses substantial danger to research subjects, and carries substantial unknown risks. There is no persuasive showing on this record that the type of psychosurgery we are concerned with would necessarily confer any substantial benefit on research subjects or significantly increase the body of scientific knowledge by providing answers to problems of deviant behavior.

The dangers of such surgery are undisputed. Though it may be urged, as did some of the witnesses in this case, that the incidents of morbidity and mortality are low from the procedures, all agree dangers are involved, and the benefits to the patients are uncertain.

Absent a clearly defined medical syndrome, nothing pinpoints the exact location in the brain of the cause of undesirable behavior so as to enable a surgeon to make a lesion, remove that portion of the brain, and thus affect undesirable behavior.

Psychosurgery flattens emotional responses, leads to lack of abstract reasoning ability, leads to a loss of capacity for new learning and causes general sedation and apathy. It can lead to impairment of memory, and in some instances unexpected responses to psychosurgery are observed. It has been found, for example, that heightened rage reaction can follow surgical intervention on the amygdala, just as placidity can.

It was unanimously agreed by all witnesses that psychosurgery does not, given the present state of the art, provide any assurance that a dangerously violent person can be restored to the community.

Simply stated, on this record there is no scientific basis for establishing that the removal or destruction of an area of the limbic brain would have any direct therapeutic effect in controlling aggressivity or improving tormenting personal behavior absent the showing of a well defined clinical syndrome such as epilepsy.

To advance scientific knowledge, it is true that doctors may desire to experiment on human beings, but the need for scientific inquiry must be reconciled with the inviolability which our society provides for a person's mind and body. Under a free government, one of a person's greatest rights is the right to inviolability of his person, and it is axiomatic that this right necessarily forbids the physician or surgeon from violating, without permission, the bodily integrity of his patient.

Generally, individuals are allowed free choice about whether to undergo experimental medical procedures. But the State has the po `er to modify this free choice concerning experimental medical procedures when it cannot be freely given, or when the result would be contrary to public policy. For example, it is obvious that a person may not consent to acts that will constitute murder, manslaughter, or mayhem upon himself. In short, there are times when the State for good reason should withhold a person's ability to consent to certain medical procedures.

It is elementary tort law that consent is the mechanism by which the patient grants the physician the power to act, and which protects the patient against unauthorized invasions of his person. This requirement protects one of society's most fundamental values, the inviolability of the individual. An operation performed upon a patient without his informed consent is the tort of battery, and a doctor and a hospital have no right to impose compulsory medical treatment against the patient's will. These elementary statements of tort law need no citation.

It is obvious that there must be close scrutiny of the adequacy of the consent when an experiment, as in this case, is dangerous, intrusive, irreversible, and of uncertain benefit to the patient and society.

Counsel for Drs. Rodin and Gottlieb argues that anyone who has ever been treated by a doctor for any relatively serious illness is likely to acknowledge that a competent doctor can get almost any patient to consent to almost anything. Counsel claims this is true because patients do not want to make decisions about complex medical matters and because there is the general problem of avoiding decision making in stress situations, characteristic of all human beings.

He further argues that a patient is always under duress when hospitalized and that in a hospital or institutional setting there is no such thing as a volunteer. Dr. Ingelfinger in Volume 287, page 466, of the New England Journal of Medicine (August 31, 1972) states:

"* * * The process of obtaining 'informed consent' with all its regulations and conditions, is no more than an elaborate ritual, a device that when the subject is uneducated and uncomprehending, confers no more than the semblance of propriety on human experimentation. The subject's only real protection, the public as well as the medical profession must recognize, depends on the conscience and compassion of the investigator and his peers."

Everything defendants' counsel argues militates against the obtaining of informed consent from involuntarily detained mental patients. If, as he agrees, truly informed consent cannot be given for regular surgical procedures by non-institutionalized persons, then certainly an adequate informed consent cannot be given by the involuntarily detained mental patient.

We do not agree that a truly informed consent cannot be given for a regular surgical procedure by a patient, institutionalized or not. The law has long recognized that such valid consent can be given. But we do hold that informed consent cannot be given by an involuntarily detained mental patient for experimental psychosurgery for the reasons set forth below.

Informed consent is a requirement of variable demands. Being certain that a patient has consented adequately to an operation, for example, is much more important when doctors are going to undertake an experimental, dangerous, and intrusive procedure than, for example, when they are going to remove an appendix. When a procedure is experimental, dangerous, and intrusive, special safeguards are necessary. The risk-benefit ratio must be carefully considered, and the question of consent thoroughly explored.

To be legally adequate, a subject's informed consent must be competent, knowing and voluntary.

In considering consent for experimentation, the ten principles known as the Nuremberg Code give guidance. They are found in the Judgment of the Court in *United States v. Karl Brandt.* There the Court said:

" * * * Certain basic principles must be observed in order to satisfy moral, ethical and legal concepts:

1. The Voluntary consent of the human subject is absolutely essential.

This means that the person involved should have legal capacity to give consent; should be so situated as to be able to exercise free power of choice, without the intervention of any element of force, fraud, deceit, duress, overreaching, or other ulterior form of constraint or coercion; and should have sufficient knowledge and comprehension to enable him to make an understanding and enlightened decision. This latter element requires that before the acceptance of an affirmative decision by the experimental subject there should be made known to him the nature, duration and purpose of the experiment; the methods and means by which it is to be conducted; all inconveniences and hazards reasonably to be expected; and the effects upon his health or person which may possibly come from his participation in the experiment.

The duty and responsibility for ascertaining the quality of the consent rests upon each individual who initiates, directs, or engages in the experiment. It is a personal duty and responsibility which may not be delegated to another with impunity.*

We must first look to the competency of the involuntarily detained mental patient to consent. Competency requires the ability of the subject to understand rationally the nature of the procedure, its risks, and other relevant information. The standard governing required disclosures by a doctor is what a reasonable patient needs to know in order to make an intelligent decision.

Although an involuntarily detained mental patient may have a sufficient I.Q. to intellectually comprehend his circumstances (in Dr. Rodin's experiment, a person was required to have at least an I.Q. of 80), the very nature of his incarceration diminishes the capacity to consent to psychosurgery. He is particularly vulnerable as a result of his mental condition, the deprivation stemming from involuntary confinement, and the effects of the phenomenon of "institutionalization."

The very moving testimony of John Doe in the instant case establishes this beyond any doubt. The fact of institutional confinement has special force in undermining the capacity of the mental patient to make a competent decision on this issue, even though he be intellectually competent to do so. In the routine of institutional life, most decisions are made for patients. For example, John Doe testified how extraordinary it was for him to be approached by Dr. Yudashkin about the possible submission to psychosurgery, and how unusual it was to be consulted by a physician about his preference.

Institutionalization tends to strip the individual of the support which permits him to maintain his sense of self-worth and the value of his own physical and mental integrity. An involuntarily confined mental patient clearly has diminished capacity for making a decision about irreversible experimental psychosurgery.

The second element of an informed consent is knowledge of the risk involved and the procedures to be undertaken. It was obvious from the record made in this case that the facts surrounding experimental brain surgery are profoundly uncertain, and the lack of knowledge on the subject makes a knowledgeable consent to psychosurgery literally impossible.

We turn now to the third element of an informed consent, that of voluntariness. It is obvious that the most important thing to a large number of involuntarily detained mental patients incarcerated for an unknown length of time, is freedom.

The Nuremberg standards require that the experimental subjects be so situated as to exercise free power of choice without the intervention of any element of force, fraud, deceit, duress, overreaching, or other *ulterior form of constraint or coercion.* It is impossible for an involuntarily detained mental patient to be free of ulterior forms of

* Trial of War Criminals before the Nuremberg Military Tribunals. Volumes 1 and 2, "The Medical Case," Washington, D.C.; U.S. Government Printing Office (1948) reprinted in 'Experimentation with Human Beings,' by Katz (Russel Sage Foundation (1972)) page 305.

restraint or coercion when his very release from the institution may depend upon his cooperating with the institutional authorities and giving consent to experimental surgery.

The privileges of an involuntarily detained patient and the rights he exercises in the institution are within the control of the institutional authorities. As was pointed out in the testimony of John Doe, such minor things as the right to have a lamp in his room, or the right to have ground privileges to go for a picnic with his family assumed major proportions. For 17 years he lived completely under the control of the hospital. Nearly every important aspect of his life was decided without any opportunity on his part to participate in the decision-making process.

* * *

Involuntarily confined mental patients live in an inherently coercive institutional environment. Indirect and subtle psychological coercion has profound effect upon the patient population. Involuntarily confined patients cannot reason as equals with the doctors and administrators over whether they should undergo psychosurgery. They are not able to voluntarily give informed consent because of the inherent inequality in their position.

It has been argued by defendants that because 13 criminal sexual psychopaths in the Ionia State Hospital wrote a letter indicating they did not want to be subjects of psychosurgery, that consent can be obtained and that the arguments about coercive pressure are not valid.

The Court does not feel that this necessarily follows. There is no showing of the circumstances under which the refusal of these thirteen patients was obtained, and there is no showing whatever that any effort was made to obtain the consent of these patients for such experimentation.

The fact that thirteen patients unilaterally wrote a letter saying they did not want to be subjects of psychosurgery is irrelevant to the question of whether they can consent to that which they are legally precluded from doing.

The law has always been meticulous in scrutinizing inequality in bargaining power and the possibility of undue influence in commercial fields and in the law of wills. It also has been most careful in excluding from criminal cases confessions where there was no clear showing of their completely voluntary nature after full understanding of the consequences. No lesser standard can apply to involuntarily detained mental patients.

The keystone to any intrusion upon the body of a person must be full, adequate and informed consent. The integrity of the individual must be protected from invasion into his body and personality not voluntarily agreed to. Consent is not an idle or symbolic act; it is a fundamental requirement for the protection of the individual's integrity.

We therefore conclude that involuntarily detained mental patients cannot give informed and adequate consent to experimental psychosurgical procedures on the brain.

[The petitioner challenged the proposed psychosurgery on the alternate ground that the procedure if carried out would violate his First Amendment rights. The Court held that in the absence of a compelling state interest, which the state had failed to demonstrate, an involuntarily detained mental patient may not be subjected to experimental psychosurgery without violating his First Amendment rights.]

For the reasons given, we conclude that the answer to question number one posed for decision is no.

In reaching this conclusion, we emphasize two things.

First, the conclusion is based upon the state of the knowledge as of the time of the writing of this Opinion. When the state of medical knowledge develops to the extent that the type of psychosurgical intervention proposed here becomes an accepted neurosurgical procedure and is no longer experimental, it is possible, with appropriate review mechanisms, that involuntarily detained mental patients could consent to such an operation.

Second, we specifically hold that an involuntarily detained mental patient today can give adequate consent to accepted neurosurgical procedures.

In view of the fact we have answered the first question in the negative, it is not necessary to proceed to a consideration of the second question, although we cannot refrain from noting that had the answer to the first question been yes, serious constitutional problems would have arisen with reference to the second question.

Questions and Comments

1. *Question.* If followed, does the *Kaimowitz* decision preclude any use of innovative psychosurgical procedures involving involuntary patients? Consider the three elements of effective consent focused on by the court: competency, voluntariness, and knowledge. The *Kaimowitz* court first declared that institutionalization vitiates the patient's *competence* to make important decisions by fostering dependence and eliminating the need to make autonomous choices. The court reasoned further that the inherent coercive atmosphere of the institution, in which the patient is dependent on the staff's goodwill for all privileges, renders *voluntary* decision-making impossible. Wouldn't the reasoning of the court effectively preclude an institutionalized patient from giving informed consent in *any* treatment context? Does the court properly balance the interests of a patient who may perceive the treatment as a means of possible recovery and release from the institution? How would this reasoning apply to a patient in need of a heart transplant?

The court also found that knowledge, the third element, could never be sufficient to support informed consent when experimental methods are involved. Wouldn't this conclusion also preclude *competent* persons from giving informed consent to experimental procedures?

A final, and even more incongruous, element of the court's reasoning is its suggestion that if greater knowledge of the dangers and risks involved in psychosurgery were available, then informed consent might be possible after all. Can this suggestion be reconciled with the court's findings that institutionalization eliminates both competence and voluntariness in patient decision-making?

2. *Comments on* Kaimowitz. Similar concerns were expressed in Note, Kaimowitz v. Department of Mental Health: *A Right to be Free from Experimental Psychosurgery?*, 54 B.U.L.Rev. 301 (1974) at 326:

> If *Kaimowitz* is followed, its determination of "public policy" would preclude a court from approving the consent of an involuntarily committed person to experimental psychosurgery even if consent had been found competent and voluntary by an acceptable review committee. Therefore, it is possible that experimental psychosurgery might someday be unavailable only to the small class of institutionalized persons who truly desire the operation. Ironically, then, the *Kaimowitz* per se rule may be creating a situation in which a "right" to be free from treatment could be used to deny the privilege to make personal medical decisions which the court was at pains to secure in John Doe's particular case.

See also, Annas, Glantz, Katz, *Informed Consent to Human Experimentation* (Cambridge, Mass., Ballinger Publishing Co., 1977) 147–151.

3. *Empirical evidence and the concept of inherent coercion.* The *Kaimowitz* opinion stands by itself as barring consent to organically intrusive experimental medical procedures. If construed broadly to bar consent to any non-therapeutic medical research, the *Kaimowitz* opinion cannot be reconciled with later cases such as *Bailey v. Lally,* 481 F.Supp. 203 (D.Md. 1979), which have rejected claims that institutionalization rendered invalid the consent given by prisoners to participate in a medical research program.

To what extent are the assumptions of the *Kaimowitz* court that institutionalized patients cannot give voluntary consent because the conditions of their confinement are inherently coercive supported by empirical data? While there is an absence of studies involving prisoners and non-psychiatric institutionalized persons, some data has been developed concerning severely disabled schizophrenic patients. According to Roth, Appelbaum, Lidz, Benson and Winslade, empirical evidence suggests that while this group of patients "may have difficulty in comprehension, they have the ability to and do say 'no' to many research procedures. Paranoid patients in particular, and in disproportionate numbers, refuse to participate in research. The study suggests that while there are problems involved in the recruitment of mentally disabled subjects for research, voluntariness is probably not the major issue. Other studies found that patients with schizophrenia, particularly paranoid schizophrenia, are less likely than other patients to volunteer for research participation." Roth, *et al., Informed Consent in Psychiatric Research*, 39 Rutgers Law Review, 425, 437–438 (1987).

4. *Critiques of* Kaimowitz. The result reached by the court in *Kaimowitz* has also been criticized on policy grounds. In this connection, consider the merits of the following commentary:

> The final point worth making about *Kaimowitz,* and the most important one from a practical standpoint, is that the main reasoning of the court quite ironically *goes against* a major thrust of liberal reform in the mental health-prison area in recent years. In trying to win for patients and/or prisoners the rights to do such things as vote, get married, manage their own money, consent (or refuse to consent) to *normal* medical procedures, etc., it has been necessary to insist again and again that one may not infer incompetence from the mere fact of institutionalization. A person might justifiably be committed to an institution and yet remain perfectly competent to manage—if not all— at least a very wide and complex range of his affairs; the mere fact of institutionalization, in other words, must not be allowed to demote an inmate from the status of an autonomous person and a bearer of rights. But now, in *Kaimowitz,* the court seems to be saying (by implication) that the above reform was all a mistake, that the mere fact of institutionalization *does* establish incompetence. The *Kaimowitz* decision was enthusiastically welcomed by liberals who seek to reduce the coercion experienced by inmates in total institutions. Ironically, the decision provides the basis for making the very coercion feared by liberals *easier* to justify!

Murphy, *Total Institutions and the Possibility of Consent to Organic Therapies,* 5 Human Rights 25, 37–38 (1975).

---

4. *Special Problems: Minors and the Mentally Disabled*

a. *Minors*

The previously discussed rule that medical treatment may be administered only with the patient's consent is generally deemed inapplicable in the case of minors. In order to protect children from their own inexperience, and to protect the interests of the parents who bear the financial responsibility for their children's support, the basic consent model for minors requires the substituted consent of the child's parents. Thus, children are for the most part legally incapable of consenting to their own medical treatment.

Although the substituted consent model is at least partially predicated on the interests of the parents, that interest must give way to the interests of the child in some cases. One purely practical exception to the parental consent rule permits treatment in cases of emergency when the parents are unavailable to consent to treatment necessary to save the child from death or irreparable injury. Because of the child's own legal incapacity to give consent, this exception is analogous to the emergency treatment of unconscious adults.

Two further exceptions to the rule requiring parental consent to treatment are premised on the realization that in certain situations the interests of parents and their children may not coincide. The first instills in the courts the power to order necessary medical treatment for a minor whose parents refuse to authorize needed treatment. These cases normally arise when the parents have religious convictions which forbid them to consent to certain types of medical treatment, such as surgery or blood transfusions. Where the child is in a life threatening situation or at risk of irreparable damage in the absence of treatment, courts will often override the wishes of the parents and provide the necessary substituted consent.

In addition to the "religious objection" cases, some state statutes provide for treatment in the absence of parental consent when the treatment is both necessary and relatively risk-free, and the parental consent requirement would have a "chilling effect" on the child's propensity to obtain treatment on his own. Such statutes allow the minor to provide the necessary consent to treatment involving venereal disease, pregnancy testing, contraception and drug dependency. A number of state statutes also authorize minors to receive mental health treatment without parental consent. An Illinois statute provides, for example, that: "Any minor fourteen years of age or older may request and receive counseling services or psychotherapy on an outpatient basis. The consent of the parent, guardian, or person in loco parentis shall not be necessary to authorize outpatient counseling or psychotherapy." Ill.—S.H.A. ch. 91½, ¶ 3–501(a).

Two other closely related exceptions to the parental consent requirement also permit minors to make their own treatment decisions. Under the emancipation doctrine, children who are in fact no longer subject to parental control, guidance, or financial support can give independent consent to treatment. Children can achieve emancipated status through acts of independence such as marriage or enlistment in the armed forces, through failure of the parents to meet their legal responsibilities, or through judicial decree. Similarly, a number of jurisdictions have adopted "mature minor" rules which give legal validity to consent to treatment given by older minors who demonstrate the intelligence and maturity of judgment necessary to satisfy the adult informed consent model. However, given the essentially subjective nature of these determinations, treating professionals are likely to seek parental consent and thereby avoid the threat of legal challenges.

Though the substituted consent model, with its exceptions applicable to minors, does afford some degree of guidance in the area of conventional therapeutic treatment, the application of these principles to research and experimentation remains clouded. Generally, both parents and the emancipated or mature minor may consent to experimentation when the objective is therapeutic. No legal guidelines have emerged, however, to deal with non-therapeutic research and experimentation.

Commentators have suggested that a workable rule must take into account both the risks involved and the potential benefit to be enjoyed by the child. Accordingly, experimentation and research that poses no significant risk should be able to proceed upon the consent of either parents or emancipated or mature minors. As the degree of risk increases, some question the utility of the parental consent model as an adequate safeguard of the interests of the child. See, Ellis, *The Rights of Children in Research and Treatment: A Conceptual Framework for Consent,* Proceedings, The Rights of Children as Research Subjects, University of Illinois at Urbana–Champaign, pp. 22–23, October 14–16, 1976. Because it is unlikely that potential risks to a research subject who is a minor will be tolerated on the basis of his or her imputed willingness to benefit children as a class, it may be impossible, absent direct benefit to the subject, to involve children in experimentation when they are unable to consent for themselves.

Comments

1. The United States Supreme Court relied on constitutional grounds to avoid the "chilling effect" of parental consent requirements in abortion cases. In holding that privacy rights were violated by a requirement that all minor women obtain parental consent before having an abortion, the Court in *Planned Parenthood of Central Missouri v. Danforth,* 428 U.S. 52, 74, 96 S.Ct. 2831, 2843, 49 L.Ed.2d 788 (1976) stated: "Constitutional rights do not mature and come into being magically only when one attains the state defined age of majority. Minors, as well as adults, are protected by the Constitution and have constitutional rights."

2. Although a rule requiring a direct benefit to any minor involved in experimentation may inhibit the study of many disorders unique to children, it is unlikely that the law will retreat from this position for some time. One of the leading advocates of this position has stated the case in no uncertain terms:

> No *adult* has the legal power to consent to experiments on an infant unless the treatment is for the benefit of the *infant.* * * * It is the lamentable use in experiments of such subjects as infant children, incompetents in mental institutions, unconsenting soldiers subject to military discipline—as has been done—that is indefensible; and no rational social order will or should tolerate it.

Burger, *Reflections on Law and Experimental Medicine,* 15 U.C.L.A.L.Rev. 436, 438 (1968).

———

b. Mentally Disabled

Recall that the doctrine of informed consent incorporates two elements: the communication of relevant information and assent predicated upon an adequate understanding of the communicated information. The application of this model in the mental health treatment context, however, raises particular problems. Psychiatric patients and those who are developmentally disabled are by definition more likely than the average population to suffer from impairments which may diminish or interfere with the requisite comprehension. In the instance of retardation, the barrier to understanding manifests itself at the cognitive level. In the case of mental illness, the impediment to informed consent is more likely to involve a distortion of the information provided or an impairment in the patient's ability to communicate his intentions. One commentator has provided the following description of the way that mental illness can interfere with the giving of informed consent:

> * * * how does one obtain consent from a severely ill catatonic schizophrenic who sits and stares at a blank wall all day, refusing to speak to anyone? Certainly if a patient is psychotic or hallucinating and cannot assimilate information about a proposed procedure, he does not have the capacity to reach a decision about the matter in question. Some mental patients are incapable of evaluating information in what most people would call a rational manner. A treatment decision might ordinarily be based on considerations of perceived personal objectives, or long-term versus short-term risks and benefits. But there are patients whose acceptance or rejection of a treatment is not made in relation to any "factual" information. To add to this dilemma, while a mental patient may refuse to give his consent to a procedure, his refusal may only be a manifestation of his illness, having little resemblance to his actual desires.

G. Annas, L. Glantz, and B. Katz, *Informed Consent to Human Experimentation: The Subject's Dilemma* (Cambridge, Mass.: Ballinger Publishing Co., 1977) at 152.

When it is clear that the patient's psychiatric condition precludes the giving of informed consent, non-emergency treatment cannot be administered without a judicial determination that the patient is legally incompetent and consent is provided by an appointed guardian. (The competency adjudication process and the mechanism for the giving of substituted consent are discussed in Chapter Nine.) Thus, unless the patient has already been adjudicated to be incompetent, any substantial doubt as to the patient's capacity to give consent would call for the initiation of competency proceedings by the physician or mental facility.

In some instances, however, the capacity of a particular patient to give informed consent will not be altogether clear. Assessments are frequently complicated by the fact that "competency is not necessarily a fixed state that can be assessed with equivalent results at any one of a number of times. Like the patient's mental status as a whole, a patient's competency may fluctuate as a function of the natural course of his or her illness, response to treatment, psychodynamic factors[,] * * * metabolic status, intercurrent illnesses, or the effects of medication." Appelbaum and Roth, *Clinical Issues on the Assessment of Competency*, 138 Am.J. of Psychiatry, 1462–1465 (1981). The physician's assessment may be further clouded by the lack of clear legal guidelines as to what constitutes capacity to consent (See infra, Chapter Seven, section II.A).

At the same time it would be impractical for those involved in treatment to seek an adjudication of incompetency whenever there is some element of doubt. Psychiatric commentators have noted that "[A]n immediate resort to the courts whenever the question of incompetency arises [would be] too time consuming and expensive." Appelbaum and Roth, at 1462. Furthermore, even an adjudication followed by a finding of competency would not necessarily establish the ability of the patient to give informed consent at some *later point in time*. Thus, those providing treatment theoretically may run some risk that a patient previously deemed legally competent would in subsequent litigation be found to have lacked capacity to give informed consent to treatment administered after the initial determination.

Exposure to liability is minimized, however, by the judicially announced rule that a "physician discharges the duty when he makes a reasonable effort to convey sufficient information although the patient, without fault of the physician, may not fully grasp it." *Canterbury v. Spence*, 464 F.2d 772, 780 n. 15 (D.C.Cir.1972). Thus if the clinical determination of capacity at the time of the giving of consent involves the exercise of due care, those providing treatment would be insulated from liability even if the assessment were subsequently deemed to have been erroneous.

Questions and Comments

1. In *Conservatorship of Waltz*, 180 Cal.App.3d 722, 227 Cal.Rptr. 436 (1986), the inpatient was found unable to give informed consent because of a psychotic fear reaction to even the discussion of the proposed ECT treatment. However, during rational periods, the patient expressed what would be considered a normal fear of ECT. The opposition to treatment manifested during a phase of competency governed. The court held that "even though he has a mental illness which causes him to be paranoid about ECT and many other things, this fact alone cannot be used to negate the presence of a rational fear of ECT which causes him to refuse treatment even during nonpsychotic moments."

The issue in *Waltz* concerned the patient's capacity to give informed consent. As elaborated in Chapter Nine, different regulatory approaches have been adopted to deal with this problem. In some states there are proceedings to determine the individual's overall competency. In the absence of competency, the power to give consent to medical treatment may be delegated to a guardian or conservator. Other states have adopted *limited* guardianship proceedings where the inquiry focuses on the individual's capacity in a particular sphere of activity. In some states, such as California, there are special provisions governing the giving of consent to intrusive psychiatric treatment modalities. Finally, New York uses nonjudicial Surrogate Decision Making Committees, composed of both professionals and interested lay people, to determine the patient's capacity to give informed consent and to determine the patient's best interests by considering the patient's values and preferences.

Different procedures also have been adopted by the states to control the administration of antipsychotic medication to prisoners. The procedures mandated by the state of Washington were sustained in *Washington v. Harper*, ___ U.S. ___, 110 S.Ct. 1028, 108 L.Ed.2d 178 (1990).

2. The capacity of psychiatric patients to understand and correctly interpret medical information has been the subject of numerous empirical studies. *See* Roth, *Competency to Consent to or Refuse Treatment*, in Psychiatry 1982: The American Psychiatric Annual Review, 350, L. Grinspoon, ed. (Washington, D.C.: American Psychiatric Press, 1982); Roth, Appelbaum, Lidz, Benson, Winslade, *Informed Consent in Psychiatric Research*, 39 Rutgers L.Rev. 425 (1987).

By and large, these studies indicate that psychotic patients frequently suffer severe impairment of competency to consent to medical treatment. For instance a 1978 study of hospitalized schizophrenic patients receiving antipsychotic medication included the following findings:

> "while the schizophrenic patients, as compared with medical patients, did not have defective understanding of the side effects and risks of medication, the schizophrenic patients were less knowledgeable about how their medication related to the nature of their problem. To the extent that schizophrenic patients fail to understand the nature of their problem, it may be anticipated that they will also fail to understand the risks and benefits of treatment or to weigh risks and benefits in deciding whether to accept treatment." *Id.* at 357.

Also, as reported by Roth, a study conducted in 1981 found "that even after having been carefully informed, most of the schizophrenic outpatients treated in a cognitive disorder clinic did not absorb or understand information about tardive dyskinesia." Id. On the other hand, a study of persons suffering from psychotic depression found that most patients in this category (more than 75 percent) "were able to understand the information the consent form gave about electro-convulsive treatment." Roth, 357–358. *See also*, Roth, Meisel, Lidz, *Tests of Competency to Consent to Treatment*, 134 Am.J. Psychiatry 279, 283 (1977); Roth and Appelbaum, *Obtaining Informed Consent for Research With Psychiatric Patients*, 6 Psychiatric Clinics of North America 551, 556–558 (1983); Benson, Roth, Appelbaum, Lidz, Winslade, *Information Disclosure, Subject Understanding, and Informed Consent in Psychiatric Research*, 12 Law and Human Behavior 455 (1988).

IV. RESEARCH AND INFORMED CONSENT

A. INTRODUCTION

Section III of this chapter considered the doctrine of informed consent in the context of treatment, including treatment modalities which are innovative or experimental. However, experimentation is not always limited to treatment intended to enhance the well-being of the subject. Specifically, in research situations, the activities in which the experimental subject is involved are primarily or wholly designed to develop or contribute to scientific or medical knowledge. Because the interests of the researcher and the subject are thus potentially in conflict, special regulations have been developed to protect the rights of experimental subjects.

The materials in this section will examine the legal regulation of both biomedical and behavioral research on human subjects. Since the risk to subjects is ordinarily greater in biomedical research, most current regulations were promulgated with that type of research in mind. Biomedical research may be defined as a scientific inquiry having a direct or immediate physical effect on the subject, which in turn produces some biological change. Biomedical research includes almost all medical research and psychiatric research aimed at the physiological origins of psychopathology.

Behavioral research is defined as a scientific inquiry into the factors determinative of human attitudes and behavior. In contrast to biomedical research, behavioral research generally involves no physical intrusion of the subject. Behavioral research may be divided into three categories, each distinguished by its effects on the subject's perception. One form consists of passive observation of the subject, with or without the subject's awareness. A second involves manipulation of the subject's environment without significant deception of the subject. A third also involves manipulation of the subject's environment, but coupled with overt deception of the subject.

B. PROFESSIONAL AND LEGAL REGULATION

The evolution of professional and legal standards to control research involving human subjects largely parallels the development of the doctrine of informed consent in the therapeutic treatment context. Thus, it was not until the early 1960's that courts, legislatures and professional organizations began to seriously search for methods to protect research subjects. Much of the impetus for this activity came from the disclosure of abuses in various research programs. For example, during the 1960's researchers at the Tuskegee Institute began a study of black males suffering from syphilis. The Tuskegee researchers intentionally deprived the subjects of treatment in order to study the degenerative effects of syphilis, a fact that, when revealed later, led to much criticism of the study and its researchers. In the social sciences, Stanley Milgram's obedience experiments, in which subjects were given the illusion that they were administering painful electric shocks to other persons, drew considerable criticism. Although these experiments are not typical of biomedical and behavioral research, fear of such overzealousness in the cause of science has been a primary motive for the regulation of human-subject research.

1. Self–Regulation

To a certain degree, researchers police their own activities through a process of self-questioning normally a part of any legitimate scientific inquiry. That scientists are encouraged to publish the results of their studies also affects the procedures utilized in research. Individual journals, for instance, can refuse to publish results of experiments that were not conducted in conformance with guidelines established by agencies such as the Department of Health and Human Services. Also, publication itself means that both the results and the research methods become available to the research community at large, which can then offer its own critique. The ethical codes and policy statements of professional organizations have also played a part in the process of self-regulation, particularly in the area of biomedical research. Internationally, the World Medical Association issued the Declaration of Helsinki in 1967 and a second document in 1975, known as Helsinki II. These policy statements espoused general principles, such as the necessity of fully informed consent, which have become the touchstone of both professional and legal regulation. In the United States, the American Medical Association's "Ethical Guidelines for Clinical Investigation" (1966) has had considerable influence on biomedical research methods, particularly in restricting the use of children and incompetent persons as subjects. Most of these guidelines, however, have only limited application to behavioral research. This gap has been partially filled by the Belmont Report, which was developed by the National Commission for the Protection of Human Subjects (an advisory group created by Congress to propose guidelines for federal regulations), and which presents the ethical principles applicable to all human-subject research. National Commission for the Protection of Human Subjects of Biomedical and Behavioral Research; *The Belmont Report: Ethical Principles and Guidelines for the Protection of Human Subjects of Research*, DHEW Pub. No. (OS) 78–0012 (1978).

2. Legal Regulation

Although a professional organization may impose sanctions on those members who violate organization guidelines, only the state can provide a remedy for subjects harmed by research or directly punish researchers and their sponsors. Legal regulation of human-subject research resulting from legislative and administrative agency action has had a significant impact on the conduct of human-subject research. However, these regulations have been designed as a means of preventing future injury to human subjects, not as means of remedying past injuries. Research subjects seeking compensation for injuries resulting from researcher misconduct must look to the law of torts, or the federal civil rights statutes for redress.

a. Statutory and Administrative Regulation

Congress and several state legislatures have shown their awareness of the public concern over the propriety of human-subject experimentation by enacting legislation. Congress created two regulatory mechanisms, both under the aegis of the Department of Health and Human Services (HHS) to insure the proper conduct of human-subject research. Both the Food and Drug Act of 1938 (21 U.S.C. § 355) and the National

Research Act of 1974 (42 U.S.C. 2891–2892) empower the Secretary of HHS to promulgate regulations affecting human-subject research. Several states, including New York and California, have also enacted legislation which in some respects parallels the federal regulation.

Two principal checks on biomedical and behavioral research are created by the HHS regulations. First, researchers must submit detailed protocols describing their proposed research to an Institutional Review Board (IRB) made up of representatives drawn from different academic disciplines. These IRBs must be established in each HHS-funded institution and oversee the conduct of all human-subject research; they are empowered to either prohibit or modify the research being proposed. 45 C.F.R. § 46.113. In reviewing proposals, the IRBs are under a mandate to insure that risks to human subjects are minimized. Moreover, each proposal must reasonably balance the risk to human subjects against the anticipated benefit of the research. 45 C.F.R. § 46.111(a)(1), (2). Where the proposed research involves pregnant women, fetuses, children, or prisoners, additional criteria must be met. The National Commission for the Protection of Human Subjects has proposed special regulations pertaining to the mentally infirm, but HHS has not adopted these proposed regulations. *See* 43 Fed.Reg. 11,328 (1978).

A second feature of the regulations is the requirement of informed consent of all subjects. Thus, as in the therapy situation, researchers must disclose all appropriate alternative procedures and all foreseeable risks. The HHS regulations also impose requirements in addition to those necessary where the intrusion is solely for therapeutic purposes. For instance, the researcher must also inform the subject that he or she may withdraw at any time. Additionally, the researcher must inform the subject of any compensation available should the subject suffer injury as a result of participation.

The Food and Drug Act of 1938 creates a second area of federal regulation of human-subject research. The act empowers the Secretary of HHS to approve the use of investigational drugs and medical devices. All researchers administering investigational drugs and devices must certify that the informed consent of either the subject or their proxies will be obtained. The regulations today require consent by the research subject or his legal representative except where four specific conditions are met, including the requirement of "a life threatening situation necessitating the use of the test article." 21 C.F.R. § 50.23.

A number of states, such as California and New York, have enacted legislation similar to the HHS regulations. *See* West's Ann.Cal.Penal Code §§ 2670–2678; N.Y.—McKinney's Pub.Health Law §§ 2440–2446. Like the HHS regulations, both New York and California require the subject's informed consent. Unlike HHS regulations, both the California and New York statutes cover all medical research conducted within the state, not just research in institutions receiving state funding. Neither the California nor the New York statutes explicitly cover behavioral research (unlike the HHS regulations, which cover all human-subject research but do explicitly exempt several categories of behavioral research including surveys, educational testing, and observation of public behavior. 45 C.F.R. § 46.101(b)).

As previously noted, neither federal nor most state regulations provides specific remedies for human subjects injured while participating in research. HHS merely denies funding to institutions with whom an offending researcher is affiliated, while California imposes criminal penalties on medical researchers who fail to obtain their subject's informed consent. West's Ann.Cal.Health & Safety Code § 21476. Some private remedy may nevertheless be available to an injured patient under state tort law or conceivably under one of the federal civil rights statutes. The scope of the Federal Civil Rights laws and their impact on the mental health treatment field is discussed in Chapter Two.

b. Private Remedies

Claims related to nontherapeutic research have rarely been the subject of litigation. Consequently, there is only a very limited body of case law defining the rights of research subjects under either the common law or the Constitution. Some attention, however, has been given to the validity of the informed consent of institutionalized persons. In *Kaimowitz v. Department of Mental Health for the State of Michigan,* which is set out in section III.C.3, supra, a Michigan trial court held that institutionalized patients could not give informed consent to highly intrusive experimental surgery. A similar issue was the subject of litigation in *Bailey v. Lally,* 481 F.Supp. 203 (D.Md.1979), which challenged the validity of the consent provided by persons participating in high-risk medical research involving exposure to infectious diseases. Documented informed consent was obtained, but the plaintiff prisoners claimed that subtle coercive factors in the prisoner's environment (*i.e.,* higher level of pay, better living conditions for subjects) vitiated their consent, thereby giving them a cause of action under federal civil right statutes. The district court held that the inducements offered to the prisoners did not amount to coercion negating their fully informed consent. In any event, the defendant researchers were found to have qualified immunity to suit under 42 U.S.C. § 1983.

Questions and Comments

1. *International standards.* An important contributing factor in the movement for reform not only in the U.S. but also in other countries was the disclosure of human rights abuses carried out under the guise of scientific experimentation by Nazi scientists during World War II. *See,* Ratnoff & Smith, *Human Laboratory Animals: Martyrs for Medicine,* 36 Ford.L.Rev. 673, 679 (1968). The World Medical Association has been at the forefront of efforts to develop international standards for the control of human experimentation. One result of these efforts is the first and second

Helsinki Declaration. *See, generally,* Jon R. Waltz and Fred E. Inbau, *Medical Jurisprudence,* pp. 381–383 (Macmillan Press, 1971).

The Tuskegee study and other abuses which stimulated the movement towards greater regulation are discussed in Nathan Hershey and Robert D. Miller, *Human Experimentation and the Law* (Germantown, Md.: Aspen System Corp., 1976) pp. 153–156.

2. *Legal challenges to government sponsored research on mind altering drugs.* A review of the suits brought in U.S. courts by persons alleged to have been harmed by covert U.S. government sponsored research on mind alt ring drugs are discussed in detail by Benson & Roth in *Law and Mental Health: International Perspectives,* Vol. 4, David N. Weisstub (Ed.) (Pergamon Press, 1988). The author concluded by noting that "By and large, the courts have not been sympathetic to lawsuits brought by persons who participated in these CIA experiments." Id. at 13.

3. *Commentaries on ethical and legal issues.* The ethical and legal issues which may be raised by experimentation with human subjects have been the subject of increasing attention by medical and legal scholars. *See, generally,* Paul A. Freund, ed., *Experimentations With Human Subjects,* (George Braziller, New York, 1970); Katz, Jay (with the assistance of Alexander Capron and Elenor Swift Glass), *Experimentation With Human Beings* (Russell Sage Foundation, New York, 1972); Symposium: *Medical Experimentation on Human Subjects,* 25 Case Wester.L.Rev. 431 (1975); National Academy of Sciences, *Experiments and Research With Humans: Values in Conflict* (Wash., D.C., 1975); George Annas, Leonard H. Glantz and Barbara F. Katz, *Informed Consent to Human Experimentation: The Subject's Dilemma* (Cambridge, Mass.: Ballinger Press, 1977).

4. *HHS regulations.* The HHS regulations under the National Research Act delegate to each institution's IRB the power to review all consent forms and procedures. But the regulations do not indicate to what degree IRB representatives should intervene in the consent process to insure that subjects are truly informed. Some commentators have argued that IRBs have concentrated too heavily on the review and revision of consent forms, suggesting that subjects might receive better protection if IRB representatives more frequently intervened in the consent process itself. *See,* Robertson, *Taking Consent Seriously: IRB Intervention in the Consent Process,* 4 IRB: A Review of Human Subject Research 10 (1982) (citing study by Gray (1975) in which 40% of subjects signing consent forms did not know they were involved in research).

5. *Definition of "risk of harm."* Under the HHS regulations, determinations of a subject's risks in proposed research have significant impact on whether the IRB will approve the proposed research. Accordingly, the definition of risk of harm will be pertinent to a court's determination of whether a researcher acted negligently. Neither state nor federal regulations, however, adequately define risk of harm. The HHS regulations define "minimal risk" as that risk of harm "not greater, considering probability and magnitude, than those ordinarily encountered in daily life * * *." 45 C.F.R. § 46.102. But such definitions say nothing about what kind of harm must be considered by IRBs. Risk of harm would certainly

include physical harm, but what kinds of psychological harm could be included?

Some individual IRBs have sought to eliminate this uncertainty by providing a definition of "risk of harm." For example, the University of Illinois's IRB provides researchers with lists of research examples. One list covers research involving minimal risk. A second list covers research involving greater than minimal risk (e.g., studies of the effects of prescribed tranquilizers on driving skills).

6. *Comment on* Bailey. In *Bailey v. Lally,* cited in the text above, the court found that researchers had not always informed prisoners that participation would not affect consideration for parole. However, the court concluded that this omission did not affect the validity of consent because researchers did not expressly promise parole board consideration of the subjects' participation.

Current regulations promulgated by the HHS would clearly prohibit the consent procedures followed in *Bailey.* Under special HHS regulations concerning prisoners, the researcher must inform each prisoner-subject that participation in research will have no effect on consideration of the prisoner-subject's parole. 45 C.F.R. § 46.305(a)(6). The *Bailey* case, however, illustrates the restrictive approach to the rights of human subjects which in the absence of specific regulation would apply.

C. SPECIAL PROBLEMS ASSOCIATED WITH BEHAVIORAL RESEARCH

In biomedical research the subject's knowledge about the research usually has little or no effect on research outcomes. In contrast, behavioral research frequently requires some deception of the subject as to the nature and purpose of the experiment. Consequently, strict imposition of the informed consent requirement would severely limit the behavioral research that could be conducted.

It has therefore been argued that some adjustment in the informed consent doctrine developed for biomedical research is called for in behavioral research. Moreover, it has been suggested that the need for strict informed consent standards is somewhat reduced by the nature of the risks posed by behavioral research, which rarely poses risk of physical harm. Some types of behavioral research, however, may expose the subject to risk of legally compensable psychological harm. Because the magnitude of these risks depends on the type of behavioral research conducted, it may be useful in evaluating current and proposed standards of informed consent to consider the legal implications associated with different types of behavioral research.

1. Passive Observation Studies

Passive observation of subjects in public places, without any modification of their environment, normally poses no risk of psychological harm. For example, in an experiment conducted by Bryan and Test (1967), the researchers measured the effect that the employment of black or white Santas as Salvation Army bell ringers had on frequency of donation. The mere act of giving or not giving constituted an experience of ordinary life which the researchers did not alter. Participants were completely unaware of ever having participated in the experiment.

In some instances, however, passive observation studies could subject the researcher to legal liability. For instance, in one controversial experiment by Humphreys (1970), the researcher stationed himself in public restrooms and posed as "lookout" for male homosexuals engaging in sex acts. By pretending to stand watch for intruders, the researcher was able to witness hundreds of sexual acts and sometimes follow up on these observations with interviews in which the purpose of the experiment was disclosed.

In this instance, even though the acts were committed in a public place, the nature of the activities plus the reasonable expectations of the parties would presumably give rise to protected privacy interests. Thus, by failing to inform the subjects of the true purpose of his presence, the researcher would in some jurisdictions become liable for invasion of privacy. See infra, Chapter Four. See also *Katz v. United States*, 389 U.S. 347, 88 S.Ct. 507, 19 L.Ed.2d 576 (1967); Fried, *Problems of Consent in Sex Research: Legal and Ethical Considerations in Ethical Issues in Sex Therapy and Research*, 31 (Masters, Johnson, Koldney, and Weems, ed. 1980).

An action for invasion of privacy occurs when the defendant publishes a matter concerning the private life of another which is highly offensive and is not of legitimate concern to the public. Restatement (Second) of Torts § 652D (1965). Thus, if an acquaintance of one of the subjects in the Humphreys's experiment had been able to identify the subject from the information presented in the published findings, the research might have constituted a form of invasion of privacy.

The HHS regulations promulgated under the National Research Act take into account the subject's right to privacy in research involving passive observation. The regulations generally exempt passive observation from coverage. Researchers lose the exemption, however, if (1) the researchers keep records which identify the subject, (2) publication of the records would expose the subject to legal liability or financial loss, and (3) the research concerns sensitive aspects of the subject's behavior. 45 C.F.R. § 46.101(b)(4).

2. *Surveys and Manipulation Studies Without Overt Deception*

A second type of behavioral research involves some manipulation of the subject's environment, but without any significant deception of the subject. One famous experiment by Meritz and Fowler (1944) involved the use of a "lost letter" technique to test the honesty of persons in various cities. Two different kinds of addressed envelopes were distributed, one containing a letter and the other containing a coin-shaped slug. The difference in the percentage of returns between the two kinds of letters was expected to indicate the honesty of the general population. The experiment would have been impossible to perform if informed consent had been required. The researchers, however, had no duty to inform because participation posed no risk to the subjects greater than that encountered in ordinary life.

Similarly, survey interviews normally create little risk of harm to the subject. But if the subject's responses concern sensitive or personal matters, the researcher has a legal duty to insure the anonymity of the subject. If the subject must be identified in the researcher's records, the researcher may need to take special precautions to insure that the subject's responses remain confidential. Again, HHS regulations exempt interviews and surveys, provided that the researcher maintain the subject's anonymity, the subject's responses do not place the subject at risk of legal liability, and the responses do not pertain to sensitive aspects of the subject's behavior. 45 C.F.R. § 46.101(b)(3).

3. Studies Involving Deception

A third type of behavioral research combines manipulation of the subject's environment with some form of deception. One study found that as much as 44% of recent research in social psychology involved deception of the subjects. Diener & Crandall, *Ethics in Social and Behavioral Research*, 74 (1978). Some social scientists have expressed concern that the use of deceit lessens public respect for the social sciences and may, because of participants' suspicions that researchers employ deception, become valueless as a research tool. Id. at 80.

Nevertheless, deceit is a necessity in some types of behavioral research. The research subject's knowledge of the manipulation would in many situations compromise the validity of the research outcome. Imposing traditional standards of informed consent on researchers would obviously preclude the conduct of research involving deception. Behavioral studies frequently entail manipulation of some external variables under controlled conditions. The HHS regulations recognize this problem by allowing an IRB to completely waive the informed consent requirement where the research poses no more than minimal risk to the subject. 45 C.F.R. § 46.117(c).

The nature and degree of risk of psychological harm varies with the type of deception employed by the researcher. Psychological harm might arise from the subject's misapprehension, intended by the researcher, of what appears to be an emergency situation. For example, in an experiment conducted by the United States Army, military recruits were placed in an aircraft and flown to an altitude of 5,000 feet. The researcher then instructed the pilot to turn off the plane's propellers. The subjects were allowed to overhear communications designed to convince them that the pilot would be forced to crash land the plane. The behavior of the subjects under these artificial stress conditions was monitored by researchers who were also aboard the aircraft.

The threat of psychological harm also might arise from a deception that causes subjects to misapprehend the nature of their own personalities. In a study by Bergin (1965) on dissonance theory, researchers falsely told male subjects that personality tests had revealed that the subjects had latent homosexual tendencies. Eventually, researchers "dehoaxed" the subjects, but not before many of the subjects suffered a blow to their self-esteem.

Either of these experiments could have exposed the researchers to liability for failure to obtain informed consent or for the tort of intentional infliction of emotional distress. To demonstrate intentional infliction of emotional distress, the plaintiff subject would have to show that the plaintiff's action amounted to conduct "so outrageous in character, and so extreme in degree, as to go beyond all possible bounds of decency." Restatement (Second) of Torts, § 46 comment d (1965). Some states have the added requirement that the emotional distress cause some physical manifestation of illness or injury. Thus, under current standards except in those states which do require a physical manifestation of the injury, the subjects in both the Army and Bergin studies could conceivably prevail in an action for intentional infliction of mental distress.

Questions and Comments

1. *Behavioral research and the requirement of informed consent.* It has been contended by some commentators that the low risk of injury from participation in behavioral research brings into question the necessity of applying the HHS regulations to behavioral research situations. See Pattullo, *Who Risks What in Social Research*, 2 IRB: A Review of Human Subject Research 1, 3 (1980). Cumbersome IRB procedures have undoubtedly discouraged some researchers from engaging in valuable scientific inquiry. See, Hunt, *Research Through Deception*, New York Times, Sept. 12, 1982, § 6 (Magazine) at 143. At the same time, the overwhelming consensus both within and outside the social sciences profession is that some regulation and institutional control of the actions of individual researchers is necessary.

2. *Debriefing.* Researchers employing deception have developed several safeguards to decrease the risks that subjects will become emotionally upset as a result of the deception. Most researchers as a matter of course debrief their subjects at the experiment's conclusion. In debriefing sessions, researchers meet with subjects and fully disclose the hoax. Disturbed subjects are comforted and reassured. To what extent does such debriefing protect against any psychological trauma which may have accompanied the experiment?

3. *Incompetent disclosure.* Behavioral and biomedical researchers have also developed several forms of "consent" that fall short of giving the subject all the information required to satisfy legal standards of informed consent. Some researchers have asked their subjects to consent to not

(R. & S.) Mental Health, 2d Ed. ACB—10

being informed of the real purposes of the experiment. Levine, *Consent to Incomplete Disclosure as an Alternative to Deception*, 4 IRB: A Review of Human Subject Research 10 (1982). Another technique consists of asking subjects to waive their right to disclosure without any forewarning to the subject that the research involves deception. Still another technique, heretofore used primarily in biomedical research, is to inform an incompetent subject's proxy of the experiment, but withhold the option of denying consent from the proxy. Within a specific period after the beginning of the experiment, however, the researcher must obtain the proxy's consent. The theory behind this technique, called "deferred consent," is that by delaying the consent decision, the subject's proxy will have more time to consider the matter and come to a "correct" decision. The HHS regulations under the National Research Act appear to authorize such techniques, but only if the research poses no more than minimal risk to the subject. 45 C.F.R. § 46.116(d). See, Fost & Robertson, *Deferring Consent with Incompetent Patients in an Intensive Care Unit*, 2 IRB: A Review of Human Subject Research 5 (1980). *Cf.*, Beauchamp, *The Ambiguities of "Deferred Consent,"* 2 IRB: A Review of Human Subject Research 6 (1980) (article critical of deferred consent technique).

Would any of these techniques provide a defendant researcher with a defense to an informed consent action filed on behalf of the incompetent subject?

Chapter Four

CONFIDENTIALITY, PRIVACY, AND PATIENT ACCESS TO RECORDS

Table of Sections

I. PROTECTION OF PRIVACY AND CONFIDENTIALITY

A. INTRODUCTION

1. *The Importance of Confidentiality in Psychotherapy*

Confidentiality is especially important in the unique setting of psychotherapy. The patient must reveal "his private personality, that which he keeps secret from the world," and "communicate all his thoughts, real and fantasy, to the therapist." Note, *Psychiatrists' Duty To The Public: Protection From Dangerous Patients*, 1976 U.Ill.L.F. 1103, 1112–1113. Typically, the attitudes expressed in therapy are grossly at variance with those of the patient's daily life. A minister, for example, may reveal hostile or aggressive impulses. Public disclosure of these communications could destroy the patient's reputation.

Confidentiality in psychotherapy is necessary not only to protect the patient from possible embarrassment, but also to accomplish treatment, which is the purpose of the relationship. A patient will not speak freely with a psychotherapist if public disclosure is likely, but effective treatment calls for true and complete communication by the patient of all his ideas and associations. To accomplish these complete revelations a patient must overcome inhibitions which "seek support from every possible source * * * including the possibility of disclosure." Goldstein & Katz, *Psychiatrist–Patient Privilege: The GAP Proposal and the Connecticut Statute*, 36 Conn.B.J. 175, 179 (1962). Thus, with remarkable uniformity, authoritative commentators assert that treatment through psychotherapy requires confidentiality to be successful.

Confidentiality fosters a related public interest: it induces the hesitant person in need of treatment to seek it. Receiving psychotherapy occasions social stigma; even in enlightened communities, patients in psychotherapy may be viewed with curiosity or suspicion. Furthermore, the stigma may exert an exaggerated effect upon persons who would benefit from therapy because they tend "to see themselves in the worst possible light." Confidentiality both as to the *fact* that a person is the patient of a psychiatrist, as well as to the *contents* of his communications, is thus important. By fostering treatment for those in need, confidentiality serves both the patient and society at large.

While the statement above relates particularly to psychotherapy, confidentiality is clearly important in the context of all psychiatric or psychological services. The results of personality and intelligence tests, for example, are no less sensitive than a patient's verbal confidences to a therapist. Of like sensitivity are disclosures by a student to a school counselor that he may have contracted a venereal disease or that he has been struggling with a drug or alcohol problem. This chapter begins a study of therapists' and counselors' obligations to maintain the confidentiality of patient and client information.

We say "begin" because the obligation of confidentiality raises a host of problems as it conflicts with such equally important societal values such as protecting the safety of the client as well as that of the community, meeting the obligations of fact finding in criminal and civil trials, and advancing scientific knowledge through research, debate, and teaching. It is these conflicts which must be balanced by courts and legislatures as they struggle to develop appropriate standards.

2. Professional/Ethical Foundations

The obligation of confidentiality is well recognized by the psychiatric profession. Psychiatrists, like other physicians, are ethically bound by the Hippocratic oath, which states in part, "Whatever, in connection with my professional practice, or not in connection with it, I see or hear, in the life of men, which ought not to be spoken of abroad, I will not divulge, as reckoning that all such should be kept secret."

The modern code of ethics promulgated by the American Medical Association reiterates this ancient injunction to maintain confidentiality. According to the code, breaches of confidentiality are permissible only when compelled by law or necessary to protect the welfare of the patient or community. In annotations to this code of ethics, the American Psychiatric Association has explained that confidentiality is essential to psychiatric treatment, not only because of the traditional ethical relationship between physician and patient, but also because of the special nature of psychiatric treatment.

Psychologists are similarly impressed with the practical and ethical importance of confidentiality in therapy. "Ethical Principles of Psychologists," the code of ethics of the American Psychological Association, provides that "[p]sychologists have a primary obligation to respect the confidentiality of information obtained from persons in the course of their work as psychologists." (Principle 5). Conditions which a psychologist must consider before divulging information in order to protect the client or society, to further the interests of the client, or to advance scientific knowledge also are set forth in the code. The conditions relate to such factors as the immediacy of danger, the scope and purpose of the disclosure, the client's awareness of the limits of confidentiality, and the client's consent to disclosure.

3. Legal Regulation

Various legal mechanisms exist to enforce the ethical obligation of confidentiality in psychiatric or psychological treatment. Perhaps the most obvious is enforcement of professional obligations set forth in licensing and certification statutes. Such statutes may include an express provision concerning the confidentiality of patient or client information. Statutory provisions mandating confidentiality frequently provide a corresponding testimonial "privilege," that is, a right on the part of the therapist to refuse to testify in court concerning his patients (see section II.D., infra). Violation of the statutory obligations of confidentiality may give rise to disciplinary proceedings and imposition of penalties as set forth in the statute. Penalties may range from a fine to license suspension or revocation.

In addition to, or in place of, explicit statutory provisions concerning confidentiality, a licensing or certification statute may incorporate a general obligation to adhere to the code of ethics promulgated by designated professional organizations. In the case of psychiatrists and psychologists, these codes include obligations to insure the confidentiality of patient or client information.

Even if the licensing statute does not expressly refer to the professional code of ethics, however, the mere fact that the profession is state-licensed or state-certified may *imply* an obligation on the part of practitioners to comply with professional ethical standards. Such an implied obligation was found, for example, in *Morra v. State Board of Examiners,* 212 Kan. 103, 510 P.2d 614 (1973). In that case, the court found an obligation to comply with professional ethical standards was implied by the state licensing statute.

Of course, the obligation of confidentiality would be meaningless if it did not extend to safeguarding patient and client records maintained by the therapist or by his employer. In some cases, the confidential patient records may be protected independently of the therapist's obligations, by a statute protecting institutional records generally. This is often the case in state hospitals for the mentally ill or retarded. In some states, similar statutes protect educational records maintained in public and private schools. Statutes of this sort usually provide that information contained in client records may not be disclosed, except for certain authorized purposes, without the client's knowledge or consent, or the knowledge and consent of his parent or guardian if the client is a minor or incompetent.

Perhaps the most effective and certainly the most common method to enforce a therapist's duty of confidentiality is the civil damage suit. A patient aggrieved by a therapist's wrongful disclosure of confidential information may sue the therapist under a number of legal theories.

A successful suit will result in an award of monetary damages for the disclosure itself; for any real injuries, such as damage to the patient's business or employment due to the disclosure; for non-economic losses, such as damage to the patient's reputation in the community; or for mental anguish caused by the disclosure. While monetary damages may not correct the injury, such awards, it is hoped, will assuage the patient's injured feelings, assure a legally sanctioned vent for righteous anger, and incidentally punish the malfeasant therapist and thereby deter abuse.

Although the nature of a patient's grievance may be readily understandable, the patient-plaintiff in a lawsuit must frame his complaint as an allegation of a wrong which is legally recognized. The torts which most commonly apply to improper disclosures of confidential information are defamation, invasion of privacy, and breach of duty arising from a confidential professional relationship. While these are distinct theories of wrong, very often a single act of wrongful disclosure will satisfy the elements of all three theories. In such cases the plaintiff will frequently elect to frame his complaint in terms of any one or all of these individual theories of liability.

The following materials examine briefly each of these separate doctrines. The first two—defamation and invasion of privacy—are not specific to the psychotherapist/patient relationship but apply to anyone who improperly communicates information concerning another. On the other hand, the tort of breach of the patient-therapist relationship is applicable only to those involved in rendering psychotherapeutic treatment.

Questions and Comments

1. *State law variations.* As noted above, some degree of confidentiality is desirable, if not essential, to the attainment of the goals of psychotherapy. At the same time, there is a general recognition that in some circumstances there are legitimate reasons for restricting the scope of confidentiality. One function of the legal system is to define an appropriate balance to be struck between these sometimes competing interests. It should, therefore, not be surprising that state legislatures have tended to resolve these competing claims in different ways with the result that significant differences exist in the degree of protection accorded under the laws of the various states.

Even within a particular state, the degree of protection accorded under state law, in a specific instance, may not always be immediately apparent. Confidentiality issues are frequently controlled by a series of overlapping and sometimes seemingly inconsistent laws. For instance, several states have enacted special psychotherapy confidentiality statutes which cover treatment rendered by mental health professionals. Typically, these laws make all patient disclosures and treatment records confidential with certain limited exceptions. The boundaries of the exceptions, however, frequently lack clear definition. Further, if the therapy was provided by a psychiatrist/physician, confidentiality issues will also be subject to the provisions of any medical records law the state may have adopted. Additionally, most states have enacted laws or adopted court rules specifically dealing with the testimonial privilege. These laws or rules may in turn conflict with the provisions contained in the medical records or psychotherapeutic treatment laws. In such instances, determining whether disclosure is either permitted or mandated requires that conflicts between the inconsistent legal provisions be resolved. In addition to statutory law, patient disclosures may be protected by common law principles such as the right to privacy. Here any determination of the patient's confidentiality rights must take into account the scope of these judicially formulated doctrines.

2. *Medical records legislation.* Several states also have enacted special legislation covering the confidentiality of *medical* records. Coverage under these laws tends to differ markedly from state to state. The different approaches have been summarized by Professor Winslade:

California, Rhode Island, and Montana have each enacted medical information statutes modeled after the AMA proposed legislation. The AMA Model Act requires the patient's written consent for any disclosure by a health care provider or third party recipient, or for redisclosure by recipients, unless the disclosure falls within one of eight exceptions. These exceptions include: (1) medical peer review committees; (2) medical and dental health care providers in an emergency; (3) "administration or operation of a provider" (which includes disclosure for accreditation, reimbursement, liability risk management, appraisal of defense, or prosecution, of legal actions); (4) program evaluations, management or financial audits, and scientific research; (5) third party payers for adjudicating claims; (6) employers, when necessary to administer employee benefits or worker compensation plans; (7) state insurance or other agencies to view claims or complaints by an insured; and, (8) public health or other disclosures as required by law.

Winslade, *Confidentiality of Medical Records,* 3 J. of Legal Medicine 497, 522 (1982).

3. *Special disclosure laws.* Numerous states have enacted special laws governing the disclosure of mental health treatment information. See, e.g., Mental Health and Development Disabilities Confidentiality Act §§ 1–17, Ill.–S.H.A. ch. 91½, ¶¶ 801–817, and see generally, Sloan and Hall, *Confidentiality of Psychotherapeutic Records,* 5 J. of Legal Medicine 435 (1984). In these states:

disclosure of mental health information is subject to greater restrictions than other health information. Special restrictions include the following: patients may consent to disclosure but a physician or therapist may be required to give additional consent; disclosures made without patient consent are permitted to courts but not to attorneys; less information may be released to insurers; a patient's presence in a facility may not be disclosed without consent; and, disclosures for research require Institutional Review Board approval and signing of confidentiality oaths. In more restrictive states, patient consent is required for virtually all disclosure if the patient is able to consent; furthermore, disclosure for such activities as audit, funding, licensure, statistical compilation, or research requires removal of patient identification. Examples of exceptions to consent requirements include child abuse reports, Secret Service reports, firearm ownership reports, and reports to specified law enforcement officials.

Winslade, *Confidentiality of Medical Records,* 3 J. of Legal Medicine 497, 524 (1982).

4. *Disclosure to third party recipients.* Insurers, employers, and government agencies are frequently the authorized recipients of medical records information. In a number of states such third party recipients of information are the subject of specific statutory regulation. However, as noted by one commentator:

[r]egulation of third party disclosures is particularly difficult under state law because the regulation often does not derive from a single area or set of statutes within state law. For example, in California, disclosure by insurers is governed by the Insurance Information and

Privacy Act, disclosure by employers is governed by the Confidentiality of Medical Information Act; and, disclosure by state and local government agencies is governed by the Information Practices Act of 1977 and by exclusions under the California Public Records Act. Each of these acts permits disclosure without consent under certain circumstances and excludes certain agencies or entities from coverage by the act. The result is a complex set of exceptions that few patients are likely to be sophisticated enough even to imagine, let alone understand.

Winslade, *Confidentiality of Medical Records,* 3 J. of Legal Medicine 497, 525 (1982).

5. *Federal legislation.* Aside from *state* law, treatment records may, in some limited instances, also be subject to federal regulation. For instance, a specific section of the U.S. Code governs the confidentiality of records of individuals who receive or have received treatment for drug dependency from programs that receive federal funds. See generally, 21 U.S.C. § 1175. See also, Sloan and Hall, *Confidentiality of Psychotherapeutic Records,* 5 J. of Legal Medicine 435, 448 (1984). Similar provisions apply to the confidentiality of records of persons who receive treatment for alcohol abuse under federally supported alcoholism treatment programs. 42 U.S.C. § 4582. Another federal law, the Family Education and Privacy Rights Act, also known as the Buckley Amendment, prohibits the disclosure of school counseling or treatment records "made or maintained by any physician, psychiatrist, psychologist, or any other recognized [treatment] professional." 20 U.S.C. § 1232g(a)(4)(B)(iv).

Occasionally, a breach of confidentiality may also violate the antifraud provisions of the federal securities law. In a recent case the SEC charged a psychiatrist with illegally using insider information gleaned in the course of treating a patient. The offending psychiatrist agreed to pay a civil penalty of $27,000 plus a sum equal to the illegal profit he had earned.

B. LEGAL REMEDIES FOR WRONGFUL DISCLOSURE

1. *General Remedies*

a. *Actions Based on Breach of Privacy*

A private remedy based on an infringement of privacy is today recognized in almost every jurisdiction *in either a limited or a more comprehensive form.* See Jon R. Waltz and Fred E. Inbau, *Medical Jurisprudence* (New York: MacMillan, 1971), Ch. 18. There are essentially four distinct types of privacy actions.

In one the privacy refers to a physical intrusion into a person's private affairs, such as wiretapping his telephone. In the second aspect of the doctrine the phrase refers to appropriation, *i.e.,* the use of another person's photograph or likeness for advertising without permission. A third form entails publication of incomplete or misleading information which places another person in a "false light" in the public eye. For instance, use of a person's photograph to illustrate a story about drug addicts, when that person is neither a drug addict nor has any relationship to the story, may violate his privacy rights. A fourth and final aspect of the right to privacy and the one that most concerns the therapist is the revelation of confidential information about the plaintiff. The action is founded on the premise that if information that the patient could reasonably expect to remain private is disclosed, a cause of action may arise based on that disclosure. This branch of privacy is most often referred to as the public disclosure of private facts and covers the disclosure of those matters that would be embarrassing to the average individual. The following case illustrates the application of this doctrine.

COMMONWEALTH v. WISEMAN

Supreme Judicial Court of Massachusetts, 1969.
356 Mass. 251, 249 N.E.2d 610.

CUTTER, JUSTICE.

This bill seeks, among other relief, to enjoin all showings of a film entitled "Titicut Follies," containing scenes at Massachusetts Correctional Institution at Bridgewater (Bridgewater), to which insane persons charged with crime and defective delinquents may be committed. The film was made between April 22, and June 29, 1966. Mr. Wiseman and Bridgewater Film Company, Inc. (BFC) appeal from an interlocutory decree, an order for a decree, and the final decree which enjoins showing the film "to any audience" and requires Mr. Wiseman and BFC to deliver up to the Attorney General for destruction specified films, negatives, and sound tapes. The plaintiffs appeal from the final decree because it did not order sums realized by various defendants from showing the film to be held for distribution as the court might direct.

The trial judge made a report of material facts. The evidence (2,556 pages of proceedings on eighteen trial days and sixty-four exhibits) is reported. The facts, except as otherwise indicated, are stated on the basis of the trial judge's findings and certain exhibits. The film has been shown to the Justices participating in this decision.

In 1965, Mr. Wiseman first requested permission from the Superintendent and from the Commissioner to make an educational documentary film concerning Bridgewater. His first request was denied. On January 28, 1966, permission was granted, subject to the receipt of a favorable opinion from the Attorney General (that the officials could grant permission) and to the conditions (a) that "the rights of the inmates and patients * * * [would be] fully protected," (b) that there would be used only "photographs of inmates and patients * * * legally competent to sign releases," (c) that a written release would be obtained "from each patient whose photograph is used in the film," and (d) that the film would not be released "without first having been * * * approved by the Commissioner and Superintendent." The existence of the final condition was the subject of conflicting evidence but there was oral testimony upon which the trial judge could reasonably conclude that it had been imposed.

* * *

In April, 1966, Mr. Wiseman and his film crew started work at Bridgewater. They were given free access to all departments except the treatment center for the sexually dangerous, whose director made "strong objections" in writing to any photography there without compliance with explicit written conditions. In three months, 80,000 feet of film were exposed. Pictures were made "of mentally incompetent patients * * * in the nude * * * [and] in the most personal and private situations."

In approaching the Commissioner and the Superintendent, Mr. Wiseman had indicated that he planned a documentary film about three people: an adult inmate, a youthful offender, and a correctional officer. It was to be an effort "to illustrate the various service performed—custodial, punitive, rehabilitative, and medical." The judge concluded (a) that the "plain import of [Mr.] Wiseman's representations was that his film was to be * * * non-commercial and non-sensational," whereas, in the judge's opinion, it was "crass * * * commercialism"; (b) that, in fact, the film "constitutes a most flagrant abuse [2] of the privilege * * * [Mr. Wiseman] was given"; and (c) that, instead of "a public service project," the film, as made, is "to be shown to the general public in movie houses."

* * *

In September, 1967, Mr. Wiseman made an agreement with Grove for distribution of the film for "showing to the general public * * * throughout the United States and Canada," with Mr. Wiseman to receive "50% of the theatrical gross receipts, and 75% from any television sale." Grove, for promotion of the film, was to have "complete control of the manner and means of distribution." The film was shown privately, and to the public for profit, in New York City in the autumn of 1967.

The trial judge ruled, inter alia, (a) that such "releases as may have been obtained [from inmates] are a nullity"; (b) "that the film is an unwarranted * * * intrusion * * * into the * * * right to privacy of each inmate" pictured, degrading "these persons in a manner clearly not warranted by any legitimate public concern"; (c) that the "right of the public to know" does not justify the unauthorized use of pictures showing identifiable persons "in such a manner as to * * * cause * * * humiliation"; (d) that "it is the responsibility of the State to protect" the inmates "against any such * * * exploitation"; and (e) that the Commonwealth is under "obligation * * * to protect the right of privacy of those * * * committed to its * * * custody."

2. Among the findings are the following: The film "is a hodge-podge of sequences * * * depicting mentally ill patients engaged in repetitive, incoherent, and obscene rantings * * *. The film is excessively preoccupied with nudity. * * * [N]aked inmates are shown desperately attempting to hide * * * their privates with their hands. * * * There is a scene of * * * [a priest] administering the last rites of the church to a dying patient [and] the preparation of corpse for burial. * * * A * * * patient, grossly deformed by * * * congenital brain damage, is paraded before the camera."

Reactions to the film set out in the record vary from the adversely critical conclusions of the trial judge to those expressed by witnesses who regarded it as fine journalistic reporting, as education, and as art.[5] The Attorney General (Mr. Richardson) testified that the film "was impressive in many ways * * * powerful in impact." He, however, expressed concern about the problem of obtaining valid releases, even from those "conceivably competent," since the releases would have been given before the inmates "could have any idea how they would be depicted." There was testimony from experts about the value of the film for instruction of medical and law students, and "exposture [sic] of conditions in a public institution."

* * *

1. [As an initial matter, the Court held that since the film constituted documentary evidence the appellate court could undertake its appraisal without regard to the findings of the trial court.]

2. The Commissioner and the Superintendent would have acted wisely if they had reduced any agreement to writing rather than to have risked the misunderstandings possible in oral discussions. They also might have avoided dispute if they had supervised the filming itself much more closely.

* * *

Early in the negotiations, Mr. Wiseman represented in writing that only pictures of inmates "legally competent to sign releases" would be used and that the "question of competency would * * * be determined by the Superintendent and his staff." In the 1966 request for the Attorney General's opinion, Mr. Wiseman was quoted as giving assurance that a written release would be obtained "from each * * * patient whose photograph is used." The latter assurance was quoted in the opinion (March 21, 1966) stating that the Superintendent had power to permit the film to be made. In the circumstances, the judge reasonably could conclude that these representations were a part of the arrangement.

The judge was also clearly justified in deciding on the basis of expert testimony, that some of sixty-two inmates identified as shown in the film were incompetent to understand a release and, on the basis of a stipulation, that releases were obtained only from eleven or twelve of the numerous inmates depicted. There was ample basis for concluding that Mr. Wiseman had not fulfilled important undertakings clearly designed to assure that the film would show only those consenting in

5. For example the Life review said, in part, "The Bridgewater atmosphere is one of aimless hopelessness. * * * A psychiatrist turns an interview with an inmate into a sadistic baiting, or, with malicious cheerfulness, forcefeeds a dying old man, while we wonder whether the ash from the doctor's carelessly dangling cigarette is really going to fall into the glop being funneled into the convulsively shuddering throat. A society's treatment of the least of its citizens * * * is perhaps the best measure of its civilization. The repulsive reality * * * forces us to contemplate our capacity for callousness. No one seeing this film can but believe that reform of the conditions it reports is urgent business. * * *

writing to their appearance in the film and competent to understand and to give such consent.

3. The film shows many inmates in situations which would be degrading to a person of normal mentality and sensitivity. Although to a casual observer most of the inmates portrayed make little or no specific individual impression, others are shown in close-up pictures. These inmates are sufficiently clearly exhibited (in some instances naked) to enable acquaintances to identify them. Many display distressing mental symptoms. There is a collective, indecent intrusion into the most private aspects of the lives of these unfortunate persons in the Commonwealth's custody.

We need not discuss to what extent in Massachusetts violation of privacy will give rise to tort liability *to individuals*. [Emphasis added]

We think, in any event, that Mr. Wiseman's massive, unrestrained invasion of the intimate lives of these State patients may be prevented by properly framed injunctive relief. The Commonwealth has standing and a duty to protect reasonably, and in a manner consistent with other public interests, the inmates from any invasions of their privacy substantially greater than those inevitably arising from the very fact of confinement.

There is a "general power of the Legislature, in its capacity as parens patriae, to make suitable provision for incompetent persons." A "comprehensive system for their care and custody" is contained in [Massachusetts statutory provisions]. The Legislature has exercised that power with specific reference to Bridgewater, among other institutions. These general provisions import all reasonable power, and the duty, to exercise proper controls over the persons confined and the conditions of their custody and to afford the inmates protection and kindness consistent with the terms and rehabilitative purposes of their commitments.

The Commissioner and Superintendent, under reasonable standards of custodial conduct, could hardly permit merely curious members of the public access to Bridgewater to view directly many activities of the type shown in the film. We think it equally inconsistent with their custodial duties to permit the general public (as opposed to members of groups with a legitimate, significant, interest) to view films showing inmates naked or exhibiting painful aspects of mental disease.

These considerations, taken with the failure of Mr. Wiseman to comply with the contractual condition that he obtain valid releases from all persons portrayed in the film, amply justify granting injunctive relief to the Commonwealth. The impracticability of affording relief to the inmates individually also supports granting this collective relief to the Commonwealth as parens patriae, in the interest of all the affected inmates. We give no weight to any direct interest of the Commonwealth itself in suppressing the film.

4. The defendants contend that no asserted interest of privacy may be protected from the publication of this film because the conditions at Bridgewater are matters of continuing public concern, as this court has recognized.

Indeed, it was concern over conditions at Bridgewater which led various public officials in 1965 and 1966 to consider a documentary film, in the hope that, if suitable, it might arouse public interest and lead to improvement.

Even an adequate presentation to the public of conditions at Bridgewater, however, would not necessitate the inclusion of some episodes shown in the film, nor would it justify the depiction of identifiable inmates, who had not given valid written consents and releases, naked or in other embarrassing situations. We agree with the trial judge that Mr. Wiseman's wide ranging photography amounted to "abuse of the privilege he was given to make a film" and a serious failure to comply with conditions reasonably imposed upon him. Mr. Wiseman could hardly have fairly believed that officials, solicitous about obtaining consent and releases from all inmates portrayed, could have been expected to approve this type of film for general distribution.

The record does not indicate to us that any inmate shown in the film, by reason of past conduct, had any special news interest as an individual. Each inmate's importance to the film was that he was an inmate of Bridgewater, that he suffered from some form of mental disease, and that he was undergoing in the Bridgewater facilities particular types of custody and treatment. Recognizable pictures of individuals, although perhaps resulting in more effective photography, were not essential. In the circumstances, there will be no unreasonable interference with any publication of matters of public concern if showing the film to the general public is prevented (a) to protect interests of the inmates in privacy, and (b) because Mr. Wiseman went unreasonably beyond the scope of the conditional permission to enter, and take pictures upon, State owned premises properly not generally open for public inspection and photography.

The case is distinguishable from decisions which have permitted publication of newsworthy events where the public interest in reasonable dissemination of news has been treated as more significant than the private interests in privacy. We need not now consider to what extent Mr. Wiseman could have been wholly excluded from making a film at Bridgewater. In this aspect of the case, we hold merely that he violated the permission given to him, reasonably interpreted, and did not comply with valid conditions that he obtain written releases.

* * *

5. That injunctive relief may be granted against showing the film to the general public on a commercial basis does not mean that all showings of the film must be prevented. As already indicated the film gives a striking picture of life at Bridgewater and of the problems affecting treatment at that or any similar institution. It is a film

which would be instructive to legislators, judges, lawyers, sociologists, social workers, doctors, psychiatrists, students in these or related fields, and organizations dealing with the social problems of custodial care and mental infirmity. The public interest in having such persons informed about Bridgewater, in our opinion, outweighs any countervailing interests of the inmates and of the Commonwealth (as parens patriae) in anonymity and privacy.

The effect upon inmates of showing the film to persons with a serious interest in rehabilitation, and with potential capacity to be helpful, is likely to be very different from the effect of its exhibition merely to satisfy general public curiosity. There is possibility that showings to specialized audiences may be of benefit to the public interest, to the inmates themselves, and to the conduct of an important State institution. Because of the character of such audiences, the likelihood of humiliation, even of identifiable inmates, is greatly reduced. In any event the likelihood of harm seems to us less than the probability of benefits.

* * * The decree is to be modified to permit (according to standards to be defined in the decree) the showing of the film to audiences of the specialized or professional character already mentioned.

*   *   *

[The Court held that individual inmates who had been filmed were not entitled to damages.]

Questions and Comments

1. *"Titicut Follies" revisited.* As indicated by the following news report, the film "Titicut Follies" continued to be the subject of judicial proceedings twenty years after the court rendered the above decision.

BOSTON, Sept. 29—A judge has said that a 22–year–old ban on the public showing of a film that depicts brutality in a state prison hospital for the mentally ill may be lifted if the faces of many of the inmates are blurred.

But the film maker, Frederick Wiseman, says that blurring faces is not technically feasible. Even if it were, he said, such an action would violate his right to free speech as a journalist and the public's right to know how state-supported institutions are run.

"The film would lose its meaning," said Mr. Wiseman, an award-winning director known for his unflinchingly realistic portrayal of the police, schools, hospitals and other institutions that bring people in contact with the state. "The whole point is that these are not faceless people. Their faces reflect the lives they've lived and how they've been treated."

Mr. Wiseman said today in an interview that he planned to appeal the latest ruling, handed down Sept. 22 by Judge Andrew G. Meyer of Suffolk Superior Court, to the Massachusetts Appeals Court.

New York Times, Sept. 30, 1989, p. 8 col. 6.

2. This action, which was brought by the state of Massachusetts, relied on the *parens patriae* power of the state to protect persons unable to care for themselves. The dimensions of this power will be explored in greater detail in Chapter Eight.

3. *Hypothetical.* Note that in *Wiseman* the defendant did not concede that the permission given by the authorities was conditioned on the obtaining of the consent of any inmates who would be included in the film. The trial court, however, accepted the state's version that the patients' consent was an express condition. Suppose the evidence had clearly indicated that no condition of consent had been imposed. Would the state have been able to enjoin the showing of the film under these facts? If so, on what theory?

4. *Capacity to consent.* Some inmates were so afflicted with mental illness as to lack capacity to consent to the filming. Could state authorities acting under the *parens patriae* power consent on behalf of these patients? If not, under what circumstances, if any, could they be filmed? Issues relating to this question are taken up in Chapter Nine.

5. *Privacy vs. public interest to know.* As noted in *Questions and Comments* 3 following Shaw v. Glickman, infra, numerous states authorize mental health professionals to disclose confidential communications during proceedings relating to involuntary hospitalizations. In the context of a commitment hearing, for instance, patients cannot assert the testimonial privilege to prevent their therapists from testifying. Yet, while there is no testimonial privilege, some states do recognize the patient's interest in maintaining the confidentiality of the hearing itself. Closely regulating access to the records of these hearings reduces unwarranted disclosure of private or potentially embarrassing information about the patient.

In some circumstances, however, outsiders or the general public will have a legitimate interest in the proper conduct of incompetency or involuntary commitment hearings. As the court noted in *Commonwealth v. Wiseman,* a public interest in the treatment of the mentally ill may sufficiently outweigh the patient's countervailing interest in privacy. To what extent should public concerns override privacy rights? Should disclosure be limited to cases where it is hoped that public attention will lead to improved conditions for patients, as in *Commonwealth v. Wiseman?*

Consider *In re New York News, Inc.,* 67 N.Y.2d 472, 503 N.Y.S.2d 714, 494 N.E.2d 1379 (1986). The New York Court of Appeals described the facts as follows:

> During the evening rush hour on October 22, 1985, at the Times Square subway station in Manhattan, appellant Mary Ventura, in what the police termed "an unprovoked assault", pushed a young woman into the path of an oncoming train, causing serious injury.
>
> * * *
>
> In the ensuing days, the newspapers reported that in July 1985 Ventura had been a psychiatric patient in Kings County Hospital, and that she had been released on September 27, 1985—only weeks before the assault—following a judicial proceeding under the Mental Hygiene Law. Her name and photograph, the details of the incident, her

hospitalization and her background were widely publicized. Ventura's mother and her neighbors made public statements about her hospitalization, her release and her past erratic, even violent behavior. Within two days of the incident, a spokesman for appellant Health and Hospitals Corporation (HHC) announced that the Judge who had presided at Ventura's retention hearing ordered release over the objection of psychiatrists, and the Judge and his law clerk responded that the psychiatric recommendation had been followed. Controversy immediately erupted over whether procedures for the release of mental patients, designed for the protection of both the patients and the public, were being properly applied—and if not where the fault lay.

After HHC's disclosure, New York News, Inc. petitioned for release of the retention hearing transcript, redacted to include only counsel's arguments, the psychiatrist's recommendation, and the court's determination. Although New York law limits disclosure to a party or to "someone properly interested," the paper argued that the press was "properly interested" because of the surrounding controversy. In holding that release was justified, the court noted that Ventura's assault and statements made by her mother and neighbors focused attention on her identity and condition; public apprehension concerning the proceeding which resulted in her release naturally resulted. The court concluded that blindly maintaining secrecy "even where a patient's identity is known * * * sacrifices a legitimate public interest in information regarding procedures for the release of mental patients." 494 N.E.2d at 1381.

Would the public have a similar interest in any "newsworthy" case? Contrast In re New York News with the cases in Section III of this chapter, "Patient Access to Records." If the press can now access a patient's sealed records, can a New York court ever assert a plausible argument for denying the patient access?

6. *Constitutional and legislative protection of privacy.* The *Wiseman* case is illustrative of the application of privacy as the basis for a right of action which may be asserted against private individuals. There is also a constitutionally based right to privacy, however, which can be invoked to limit only *governmental* intrusions. *Hawaii Psychiatric Society v. Ariyoshi,* 481 F.Supp. 1028 (D.Hawaii 1979) illustrates the application of this doctrine in the psychiatric sphere. In 1978, in an effort to curb Medicaid fraud, the legislature of the State of Hawaii adopted an administrative inspection scheme which required each health provider to maintain records fully describing the care being provided to Medicaid recipients and to make such records available to authorized state officials. A key provision in the statute authorized the issuance of administrative inspection warrants upon a showing of "probable cause." This provision in turn provided the statutory basis for the subsequent issuance of an administrative search warrant which authorized the inspection of a clinical psychologist's Medicaid records, including "therapeutic notes, patient history forms, medical records and reports, and diagnoses." Id. at 1034.

In *Ariyoshi* a psychologist, together with the Hawaii Psychiatric Society, challenged the constitutionality of the search warrant portion of the statute, both on its face and as applied to the plaintiff. The district court, in granting a preliminary injunction, concluded that it was highly probable that the statute violated constitutional prohibitions against invasion of privacy and unreasonable searches without the requisite compelling justification. Id.

7. *Protection in the age of computerization.* The existing rules designed to protect the privacy and confidentiality of patient's medical records were developed in an era when these records were maintained in the physician's office itself. Since that time, there have been significant changes in the way that medical data is recorded and stored. Several factors are responsible. The development of computerized data storage systems and data transmission networks that connect these systems make it possible to establish centralized medical record filing systems with virtually unlimited capacities. In addition, changes in the structure of the medical profession itself and in the way that medical care is financed have affected the locations and methods of the storage of patient's medical data.

The movement toward medical health care organizations and away from individual practice has been accompanied by increasing reliance on centralized computerized files. At the same time, health care is increasingly being financed through public and private insurance programs. In fact, it has been estimated that approximately 75% of all medical services are either totally or in part paid for by public or private insurance programs. Note, *Computers, the Disclosure of Medical Information, and the Fair Credit Reporting Act,* 3 Computer/Law Journal, 619 (1982); Dubro, *Your Medical Records. How Private Are They?* 3 Cal.Lawyer 33, 34 (April 1983). As a consequence of these changes, those involved in providing health care must share medical treatment information with those agencies which finance health care costs. The consent of the patient, which is usually required by insurance companies as a condition of reimbursement, authorizes this exchange of personal medical information.

Centralization of medical records has also been furthered by the formation of pooled record systems. By far the largest of these systems is that developed under the auspices of the Medical Information Board (MIB), which has collected data on over 11 million persons and is tied to a group of insurance companies that together write nearly 95% of the medical insurance policies issued in the United States. Note, *Computers, the Disclosure of Medical Information, and the Fair Credit Reporting Act,* 3 Computer/Law Journal 619 (1982). These files consist mainly of medical records supplied by the insurers themselves who obtain them directly from reporting physicians. Id. at 626. In the past such files even included data on sexual deviancy and social maladjustment, though this type of information was subsequently deleted by the MIB. Id.

Similar centralized data systems have been developed in the mental health field. The most comprehensive of these systems is the Multi–State Information System for Psychiatric Patient Records (MSIS), which collects data supplied by the institutions of at least seven states. Lawrence Tancredi, *Legal Issues in Psychiatric Care* (New York: Harper and Row, 1975), p. 55. It has been estimated that over 30% of the patients in state-operated mental hospitals in the U.S. are in facilities that in some way participate in this system. Jonas Robitscher, *The Powers of Psychiatry*

(Boston: Houghton Mifflin, 1980), p. 225. When insurance is provided by an employer, disclosure may also result from specific requests from the employer for information held by the insurance company. Note, *Computers, the Disclosure of Medical Information, and the Fair Credit Reporting Act*, 3 Computer/Law Journal 619, 626 (1982).

These changes, brought about by advanced data systems and a restructured medical profession, have led many to question the adequacy of traditional doctrines such as the law of privacy and defamation to provide sufficient safeguards to prevent abuses of these systems. A 1980 Senate bill attempted to address the problem of misuse of medical information at the federal level. The proposed Privacy of Medical Information Act would have required a record to be made of any agency or individual that gains access to a medical record bank. Strong lobbying by law enforcement and intelligence authorities, as well as by the medical profession itself, led to the defeat of the bill.

Limited efforts at controlling the release of medical information have also been undertaken on the state level. A number of states have enacted legislation promoting the confidentiality of psychiatric treatment records. Generally, these purport to prevent the disclosure of treatment information of those undergoing psychiatric therapy, excepting information sought for the purposes of research. Lawrence Tancredi, *Legal Issues in Psychiatric Care* (New York: Harper and Row, 1975), p. 56. At least one state, New York, has passed special legislation seeking to limit access to psychiatric records available for entry into computerized MSIS systems. Id. California has enacted legislation based on the National Association of Insurance Commissioners Model Bill. This act regulates some of the circumstances under which insurance companies disclose information to other agencies. The act also authorizes individual patients to inspect their insurance records and correct errors. Dubro, *Your Medical Records. How Private Are They?* 3 Cal.Lawyer 33, 36 (April 1983).

b. Defamation

Defamation is the tort of making a statement to a third person which tends to injure the reputation of another, that is, which tends to diminish the person's esteem and respect in the eyes of the community or to excite adverse or unpleasant opinions about him. When the statement is oral, the tort is called slander; when it is written, the tort is called libel. Sometimes courts require that the statement be made with malice or ill will toward the plaintiff. Even when the speaker made the statement without actual malice, however, he may be held liable for the injury to the plaintiff. In such cases the malice is said to be implied.

There are two defenses to any defamation action. One is truth; the second is privilege. The privilege in the law of defamation is not coextensive with the testimonial privilege to be discussed later. Privilege here means that certain statements which might otherwise be considered defamatory are immune from attack given the context in which they were spoken. For example, statements made by a therapist during the course of judicial or quasi-judicial proceedings are absolutely immune from legal challenge. This would apply to a therapist's testimony in commitment or malpractice trials.

It is also a general rule that defamatory statements, if made in good faith to discharge a legitimate duty with which the speaker is charged, or to advance a valid and important interest of the speaker, are privileged if the statements are made to anther person having a corresponding interest or responsibility. This interest need not necessarily be of a legal nature, but may arise from a moral or social imperative.

While a detailed analysis of the law of defamation is beyond the scope of these materials, it may be useful to consider a case which illustrates its application in the context of treatment.

HUGHLEY v. McDERMOTT
Court of Special Appeals of Maryland, 1987.
72 Md.App. 391, 530 A.2d 13.

KARWACKI, JUDGE.

David E. Hughley appeals from a summary judgment rendered against him by the Circuit Court of Prince George's County in the defamation action he filed against Michael T. McDermott, the appellee. We disagree with the hearing judge's conclusion that the pleadings, depositions, answers to interrogatories, admissions and affidavits filed in the proceeding showed that there was no genuine dispute between the parties as to any material fact and that the appellee was entitled to judgment as a matter of law. Consequently, under Rule 2–501, summary judgment was not appropriate, and we shall vacate that judgment and remand the case for trial.

We restate the questions presented by the parties as follows:

1. Did the appellee enjoy an absolute privilege in publishing the allegedly defamatory matter because of appellant's actual or implied consent to its publication?

2. Was the content of the publications actionable as defamation?

3. Did the appellee abuse the qualified privilege he enjoyed to publish the defamatory matter concerning the appellant?

* * *

The record before the hearing judge discloses the following "facts."

The appellant applied to the Maryland–National Capital Park and Planning Commission (MNCPPC) for the position of a Park Police Officer in October of 1981. He was accepted as a Park Police candidate on August 9, 1982. At that time he was advised that he would have to complete candidate training school, as well as a 12 month probationary period before final acceptance as a Park Police Officer. He worked as a police dispatcher through November of 1982 and then entered the Police Academy in Prince George's County. After completing his training at the Academy in April of 1983, he began field patrol training. When the appellant learned that he might be transferred to the horse mounted training unit, he wrote to Captain George Klotz, who was the commanding officer of that unit. He advised Captain Klotz that he had "no love of horses," and would be uncomfortable in mounted training. Captain Klotz met with the appellant, and the appellant explained his reservations about working with horses, relating his limited personal experiences with horses which included vivid childhood recollections of falling off a pony and of a disfiguring injury suffered by his uncle who was kicked in the face by a horse. Nevertheless, Captain Klotz informed the appellant that he was a "natural" for mounted training because he "was bowlegged and skinny," and convinced the appellant to "try" the mounted unit. He began training with the mounted unit on August 15, 1983.

The appellant's first contact with horses precipitated the onset of nausea which plagued the appellant whenever he rode a horse or was in a stall with one. His symptoms progressed from "mild stomach problems" to vomiting. At first the appellant was determined to overcome his fear which he felt produced the physical discomfort he experienced. At the conclusion of the first week of training the appellant informed Captain Klotz that he was "uncomfortable." On the morning of Monday, August 22, 1983, the appellant had stomach cramps and diarrhea, and called in sick. On the following Tuesday and Wednesday he participated in the program but advised his supervisors of his condition. The appellant was absent from work from August 25 until September 6 because he was experiencing leg, back and hip pain from riding horses. The appellant sought medical treatment from Dr. Gary Jones at his group health association for this problem.

When he returned to work on September 6, 1983, the appellant again spoke with Captain Klotz who insisted that the appellant complete mounted training, notwithstanding appellant's pleas that his illnesses were related to contact with horses. Later that day the appellant went to see Dr. Ann L.B. Williams, another physician at his group health association. On September 7, 1983, Dr. Williams, after consulting a psychiatrist, wrote a letter to MNCPPC on the appellant's behalf which recommended that the appellant be excused from mounted training because of his "extreme anxiety with associated physical symptoms" when around horses.

On September 12, 1983, appellant was summoned to appear before Lieutenant Robert Fox of the mounted unit. After they discussed the problems which appellant had experienced with horse mounted training, Lieutenant Fox told appellant that he would have to see the appellee. Two days later appellant received a telephone call from Lieutenant Fox advising him to report for an appointment with appellee that evening.

The appellee, a psychologist, had contracted with MNCPPC to act as its consultant and to provide counseling and referral services for its employees who needed help in resolving emotional problems which affected their work. The appellee met with the appellant for approximately 30 minutes on September 14, 1983.

At that meeting the appellant described his above mentioned unhappy childhood experiences with horses, and his observations as a Park Police candidate that several mounted officers had injured their knees as a result of horseback riding accidents. He chronicled his physical reactions to horseback riding and to being in a stall with a horse. He told the appellee that Captain Klotz insisted that he ride, and that other officers referred to the captain's methods of training as "Gestapo tactics." The appellee advised the appellant that he believed that the appellant had a real phobia of horses and that he would recommend his transfer from mounted training, but Colonel Leslie had told the appellee that if the appellant didn't ride, the appellant would be fired. The appellant informed the appellee about Dr. Williams' letter and that she had consulted a psychiatrist before rendering an opinion. The appellee suggested hypnosis to treat the appellant's phobia. The appellant refused this suggestion. The appellee insisted that he was going to recommend treatment. The appellant responded, "you are the psychiatrist, you can recommend anything you want to." The appellee responded, "I will do that, then. . . . They told me you had an authority problem but I don't think you have one, I don't think you are abnormal." Finally, the appellee agreed to provide a copy of his diagnosis to the appellant.

On September 29, 1983, the appellant was ordered to appear before Major Richard Belt of MNCPPC, Larry Brownlee of the Fraternal Order of Police, and the appellee. The appellee opened the meeting by stating that he had advised Major Belt that appellant's phobia of horses was real. Appellee next stated that he and appellant had agreed that appellant would submit to hypnosis to treat his phobia. At that point appellant interrupted and advised those present that he had not agreed to hypnosis. That contradiction precipitated an argument between appellant and appellee, and the meeting deteriorated. The appellee told the appellant to sign a "release" for his lawyers before leaving the meeting. The appellant complied. That document, preprinted with blanks which were completed in handwriting, is entitled "Consent for Release of Confidential Information." As completed and signed on September 29, 1983, it provided:

> I do hereby authorize Michael T. McDermott, Ph.D. to disclose to Major Belt the following information: Diagnosis and Recommendations for the purpose of suitability for mounted training.

In retaliation for the embarrassment which appellant's contradiction of appellee's report to his clients at the September 29, 1983 meeting had caused appellee, on October 4, 1983, the appellee wrote to Major Belt:

> At the request of Lt. Fox, I conducted an evaluation of POC David

Hughley on September 22, 1983.[1] As an outcome of this evaluation, a meeting was scheduled with you and Mr. Hughley on September 29, 1983. The purpose of these meetings was to determine if POC Hughley suffers a phobic reaction to horses which prevents him from receiving training in the Mounted Unit.

It is my opinion based on the session with Officer Hughley and conversation with other officers that no such phobic reaction exists and the symptoms of anxiety (stomach cramps) are presentations of false and grossly exaggerated symptoms. The symptoms appear to be produced to avoid working in the Mounted Unit and specifically to avoid working under the command of Captain Klotz. In a word, this is termed "malingering." Most notable in the process of arriving at this diagnosis was POC Hughley's lack of cooperation with the evaluation and prescribed treatment regimen.

I will supply you with a full detailed explanation of these findings in the near future. If I can be of further assistance in this matter, please feel free to call me.

As he had promised, the appellee supplemented that correspondence on October 22, 1983. On that date he related to Major Belt:

This report will elaborate on my letter of October 4, 1983 regarding POC Hughley in which I reported my findings that he was "malingering" in regard to work on the Mounted Unit.

* * *

[After detailing appellant's rejection of appellee's hypnotherapy recommendation, the appellee's report concluded:]

Based on his irascible mood, refusal to cooperate in any way to alleviate this situation at the Mounted Unit other than to be removed, the symptomatology occurring only when given an order, and his stated dislike of the Unit commander, I was forced to conclude that this was not a bona fide phobia but a manipulation to get out of a work assignment he did not like.

Beyond the issues in this incident, one must speculate on the viability of such an officer to be relied upon in the future to follow orders and deal with your organization in a forthright and honest manner. I would also question his ability to deal with authority in an orderly way and become a contributing member of the force. To date his actions have been a severe drain on all involved from supervisory personnel to fellow officers. The manipulations he demonstrated indicate there may be more pathological character issues involved here than just contempt for superiors. Other than with criminal elements, I have not seen an individual lie so boldly or so vehemently when to cooperate or to be truthful would only be in his best interest. In sum, one must wonder about his ability to be a police officer and carry out that task responsibly and honestly.

In summary I find that POC Hughley does not suffer from a phobia to horses which prevents his working in the Mounted Unit. I

---

1. Both the appellant and the appellee in their deposition testimony stated that the date of this interview was September 14, 1983.

did find that he was trying to avoid working in the Unit and specifically avoiding the command of Capt. Klotz. His exaggerated symptoms are false presentations aimed at reassignment.

If I can be more detailed or of further assistance in this matter, please call me.

The appellant was notified on October 18, 1983 of MNCPPC's intention to fire him, and he was officially terminated on December 2, 1983.

I.

Appellee contends that his publication of any defamatory matter in his letters of October 4 and 22, 1983, was absolutely privileged because the appellant consented to such publication. He posits that the record before the hearing judge indisputably showed that, (1) the appellant, at the time of his appointment with the appellee on September 14, 1983, was aware of the fact that the appellee would be reporting his diagnosis and recommendations with regard to the appellant's suspected phobia to the officials at MNCPPC, (2) the appellant implicitly consented to a lack of confidentiality in connection with that meeting by participating in the interview, and (3) the appellant expressly consented to the contents of appellee's reports to his employer by requesting a copy of the appellee's reports and by execution of the "Consent for Release of Confidential Information" on September 29, 1983. The hearing judge rejected the appellee's defense based upon absolute privilege as do we.

* * *

Appellant did not volunteer to see the appellee; he was ordered to that interview by one of his supervisors, Lieutenant Fox. Moreover, at the conclusion of the interview, appellant was advised by appellee that his phobia to horses was real and that the appellee would recommend to MNCPPC that appellant be transferred from the mounted unit. Finally, at the beginning of the meeting on September 29, 1983, appellee reported to those present that appellant's phobia was not feigned. Given these "facts," appellant could not reasonably be charged with knowledge either of the language of appellee's reports, or that appellee's reports would be defamatory when he consented to their publication.

II.

Appellee argues that the summary judgment of the court should be affirmed because his letters of October 4 and 22, 1983 contained only expressions of his opinions following his professional evaluation of the appellant. We are not persuaded.

Accepting, as we must, appellant's version of what occurred on September 14, 1983, the appellee diagnosed the appellant's condition as a genuine phobia to horses and advised him that he would recommend his transfer from the mounted unit. Appellee repeated his diagnosis at the commencement of the meeting on September 29, 1983. After appellant contradicted appellee's report at the meeting that appellant was willing to undergo hypnosis as a treatment for his phobia, they argued, and the meeting abruptly ended. Appellee in his letters which followed that disagreement knowingly falsified his earlier diagnosis. That knowing falsehood is the basis of the appellant's cause of action. * * * In the case *sub judice* the record before the hearing judge would support a finding by the trier of fact that the statements of the appellee, although couched as expressions of opinion, were calculated untruths which adversely affected the appellant's employment and were therefore defamatory.

* * *

III.

In granting the appellee's motion for summary judgment the hearing judge rested his decision on the ground that appellee enjoyed a qualified privilege for the defamatory statements he made in his letters of October 4 and 22, 1983 and that there was no evidence of an abuse of that privilege. We hold that he erred in his second conclusion.

The appellee, as a consultant retained by the appellant's employer to examine the appellant, enjoyed a qualified privilege to communicate defamatory information derived from that examination to the employer.

* * *

It is well settled, however, that the qualified privilege accorded to a defamatory communication published within the employer-employee relationship is defeasible where the publication is made with knowledge of its falsity or with reckless disregard for its truth. * * * Furthermore, where there is any evidence of such knowing falsity or reckless disregard for truth, the issue of whether the qualified privilege has been lost by its abuse must be resolved by the trier of fact and not as a matter of law by the court. * * * Since there was disputed evidence before the hearing judge in the instant case as to whether the appellee defamed the appellant in his letters of October 4 and 22, 1983, with knowledge that the information contained in those communications was false, the issue of appellee's forfeiture of his privilege by abuse was not one which could be resolved by summary judgment.

JUDGMENT VACATED; CASE REMANDED TO THE CIRCUIT COURT FOR FURTHER PROCEEDINGS CONSISTENT WITH THIS OPINION.

Questions

In *Hughley,* why was the psychologist's report defamatory? Was it because he had no clinical basis for changing his mind? What if during subsequent clinical sessions with the plaintiff, the psychologist changed his opinion regarding the basis of Hughley's reluctance to ride horses? What if the psychologist had simply been negligent in preparing his report?

2. *Remedies Arising From the Patient-Therapist Relationship*

DOE v. ROE

Supreme Court, New York County, 1977.
93 Misc.2d 201, 400 N.Y.S.2d 668.

MARTIN B. STECHER, JUSTICE:

This action for an injunction and for damages for breach of privacy is a matter of first impression in this State, and so far as I am able to ascertain, a matter of first impression in the United States. It arises out of the publication, verbatim, by a psychiatrist of a patient's disclosures during the course of a lengthy psychoanalysis. I have made and filed detailed findings of fact which are briefly summarized here.

Dr. Joan Roe is a physician who has practiced psychiatry for more than fifty years. Her husband, Peter Poe, has been a psychologist for some 25 years. The plaintiff and her late, former husband were each patients of Dr. Roe for many years. The defendants, eight years after the termination of treatment, published a book which reported verbatim and extensively the patients' thoughts, feelings, and emotions, their sexual and other fantasies and biographies, their most intimate personal relationships and the disintegration of their marriage. Interspersed among the footnotes are Roe's diagnoses of what purport to be the illnesses suffered by the patients and one of their children.

The defendants allege that the plaintiff consented to this publication. This defense is without substance. Consent was sought while the plaintiff was in therapy. It was never obtained in writing. In Dr. Roe's own words consent "was there one day and not there another day. That was the nature of the illness I was treating, unreliable." I need not deal with the value of an oral waiver of confidentiality given by a patient to a psychiatrist during the course of treatment. It is sufficient to conclude that not only did the defendants fail to obtain the plaintiff's consent to publication, they were well aware that they had none.

[The plaintiff contended that in the absence of a statutory provision expressly recognizing a cause of action against a therapist who wrongfully discloses confidential information, an action is impliedly authorized by various state laws including sections of the New York Civil Practice Law and Rules (Sec. 4504(a)) and provisions of the New York Licensing and Disciplinary Statutes (Ed.L. 6509 et seq.). Following a review of the text and history of these statutory provisions the court concluded that these sections standing by themselves did not authorize a private cause of action. The court next addressed the plaintiff's contention that other theories including the right to privacy and rights flowing from the contract between the therapist and patient grant a cause of action for wrongful disclosure.]

* * *

As hereafter indicated there are theories on which liability may be predicated other than violation of the CPLR [4504(a)], the licensing and disciplinary statutes [Ed.L. 6509 et seq.] and what I perceive as this State's public policy. In two of the very few cases which have come to grips with the issue of wrongful disclosure by physicians of patients' secrets [*Hammonds v. Aetna Casualty & Surety Company*, 243 F.Supp. 793 [N.D.Ohio, 1965]; and *Horne v. Patton*, 291 Ala. 701, 287 So.2d 824 [1973] the courts predicated their holdings on the numerous sources of obligation which arise out of the physician-patient relationship.

* * *

I too find that a physician, who enters into an agreement with a patient to provide medical attention, impliedly covenants to keep in confidence all disclosures made by the patient concerning the patient's physical or mental condition as well as all matters discovered by the physician in the course of examination or treatment. This is particularly and necessarily true of the psychiatric relationship, for in the dynamics of psychotherapy "(t)he patient is called upon to discuss in a candid and frank manner personal material of the most intimate and disturbing nature * * * He is expected to bring up all manner of socially unacceptable instincts and urges, immature wishes, perverse sexual thoughts—in short the unspeakable, the unthinkable, the repressed. To speak of such things to another human being requires an atmosphere of unusual trust, confidence and tolerance. * * *"

There can be little doubt that under the law of the State of New York and in a proper case, the contract of private parties to retain in confidence matter which should be kept in confidence will be enforced by injunction and compensated in damages.

The contract between the plaintiff and Dr. Roe is such a contract.

* * *

Every patient, and particularly every patient undergoing psychoanalysis, has such a right of privacy [emanating from the plaintiff's contract right to confidentiality and other state laws including the licensing and disciplinary statute and the New York civil practice law]. Under what circumstances can a person be expected to reveal sexual fantasies, infantile memories, passions of hate and love, one's most intimate relationship with one's spouse and others except upon the inferential agreement that such confessions will be forever entombed in the psychiatrist's memory, never to be revealed during the psychiatrist's lifetime or thereafter? The very needs of the profession itself require that confidentiality exist *and be enforced*. As pointed out in *Matter of Lifschutz*, 2 Cal.3d 415, 85 Cal.Rptr. 829, 467 P.2d 557 [1970] "a large segment of the psychiatric profession concurs in Dr. Lifschutz's strongly held belief that an absolute privilege of confidentiality is essential to the effective practice of psychotherapy" [*cf.* Annotation, 20 A.L.R.3d, 1109, 1112]. Despite the fact that in no New York case has such a wrong been remedied due, most likely, to the fact that so few physicians violate this fundamental obligation, it is time that the obligation not only be recognized but that the right of redress be recognized as well.

What label we affix to this wrong is unimportant [although the category of wrong could, under certain circumstances—such as determining the applicable statute of limitations—be significant]. It is generally accepted that "There is no necessity whatever that a tort must have a name. New and nameless torts are being recognized constantly". [Prosser, Torts (2d ed.), p. 3]. What is important is that there must be the infliction of intentional harm, resulting in damage, without legal excuses or justification.

* * *

The defendants contend that the physician's obligation of confidentiality is not absolute and must give way to the general public interest. The interest, as they see it in this case, is the scientific value of the publication.

It is not disputed that under our public policy the right of confidentiality is less than absolute. * * *

Despite the duty of confidentiality courts have recognized the duty of a psychiatrist to give warning where a patient clearly presents a danger to others to disclose the existence of a contagious disease, to report the use of "controlled substances" in certain situations and to report gunshot and other wounds.

In no case, however, has the curiosity or education of the medical profession superseded the duty of confidentiality. I do not reach the question of a psychiatrist's right to publish case histories where the identities are fully concealed for that is not our problem here, nor do I find it necessary to reach the issue of whether or not an important scientific discovery would take precedence over a patient's privilege of non-disclosure. I do not consider myself qualified to determine the contribution which this book may have made to the science or art of psychiatry. I do conclude, however, that if such contribution was the defendants' defense they have utterly failed in their proof that this volume represented a major contribution to scientific knowledge. The evidence is to the contrary and this defense must necessarily fail.

Nor is the argument available that by enjoining the further distribution of this book the court will be engaging in a "prior restraint" on publication.

* * *

There is no prior restraint in the case at bar. The book has been published and it does offend against the plaintiff's right of privacy, contractual and otherwise, not to have her innermost thoughts offered to all for the price of this book. There is no prior restraint and, therefore, no censorship within constitutional meaning.

* * *

The liability of Dr. Roe to respond in damages is clear, and Mr. Poe's liability is equally clear. True, he and the plaintiff were not involved in a physician-patient relationship and he certainly had no contractual relationship to her. But, the conclusion is unassailable that Poe, like anyone else with access to the book, knew that its source was the patient's production in psychoanalysis. He knew as well as, and perhaps better than Roe, of the absence of consent, of the failure to disguise. If anyone was the actor in seeing to it that the work was written, that it was manufactured, advertised and circulated, it was Poe. He is a co-author and a willing, indeed avid, co-violator of the patient's rights and is therefore equally liable.

The plaintiff seeks punitive damages and suggests that a proper measure of those damages, in addition to compensatory damage, is approximately $50,000, the sum plaintiff has thus far expended on and incurred for attorneys' fees.

* * *

In order to warrant an award of punitive damages, it must have been affirmatively demonstrated that the wrong committed was willful and malicious, that the act complained of was "morally culpable or * * * actuated by evil and reprehensible motives, not only to punish the defendant but to deter him, as well as others * * *"

Where the act complained of is willful, malicious and wanton, punitive damages are sometimes available to "express indignation at the defendants' wrong rather than a value set on plaintiff's loss." Certainly, the acts of the defendants here are such as to warrant an expression of indignation and punishment for the purpose of deterring similar acts by these defendants or others. The difficulty, however, is that the defendants' acts were not willful, malicious or wanton—they were merely stupid. I have no doubt that the defendants were of the opinion that they had sufficiently concealed the identity of the plaintiff and her family. I have no doubt that in addition to the commercial success they hoped to have, they believed that they were rendering a public service in publishing what they considered an in-depth description of the plaintiff's family. But there was no motive to harm. Under these circumstances, punitive damages are not available.

* * *

The plaintiff has suffered damage as a consequence of this publication. She suffered acute embarrassment on learning the extent to which friends, colleagues, employer, students and others, had read or read of the book. Her livelihood, as indicated in the findings, was threatened; but fortunately, the actual cash loss was only some $1,500. Medical attention, principally treatment with Dr. Lowenfeld, cost an additional $1,400. But beyond these sums the plaintiff suffered in health. She had insomnia and nightmares. She became reclusive as a consequence of the shame and humiliation induced by the book's publication and her well-being and emotional health were significantly impaired for three years. In my opinion the fair and reasonable value of the injury she sustained—to the extent it can be compensated in damages—is $20,000.

Damages, of course, do not provide an adequate remedy; for should the book circulate further, beyond the 220 copies already sold, the damage must accrue anew. The plaintiff is entitled to a judgment permanently enjoining the defendants, their heirs, successors and assigns from further violating the plaintiff's right to privacy whether by circulating this book or by otherwise disclosing any of the matters revealed by the plaintiff to Dr. Roe in the course of psychotherapy.

* * *

Questions and Comments

1. *Duty arises with treatment.* A duty of confidentiality does not arise unless a treatment relationship has been established between the patient and therapist. When it is clear from the outset that the physician or psychotherapist is examining or diagnosing a person at the request of a third party, no duty of confidentiality arises. Under these circumstances otherwise confidential matters may be included in the report that the therapist communicates to the third party.

2. *Waiver of confidentiality.* A patient may voluntarily waive the right of confidentiality. For instance, insurance companies frequently require an applicant to supply his medical background and, in that connection, request that the applicant authorize the insurance company to obtain information from any physician or other persons who may have provided health care in the past. Also, insurance carriers which provide coverage for psychological counseling often require reports of the services performed by the therapist as a condition for payment. In this situation, the patient may be asked to authorize certain disclosures to the insurance carrier. Disclosures even when authorized by the patient present some problems for the therapist. It is not always clear what information may be disclosed. Is it the fact of treatment or the diagnosis or may it include other information, such as the disability of the patient?

3. *Consent.* One of the defenses in *Doe v. Roe* was that the plaintiff had consented to the publication. The Court rejected the defense because "[i]t was sought while the patient was in therapy." Does this suggest that any consent to publication obtained in a course of treatment is not binding and cannot be relied on by the therapist? What considerations support this rule?

4. *Scope of permitted disclosure.* To what extent may a therapist disclose confidential information to other professionals without the patient's expressed consent? Similarly, what are the limits of disclosure for the purpose of research or the training of professionals? There is little developed case law on these points. However, as suggested by the court in *Wiseman* a professional appears to have somewhat greater latitude in being able to communicate information where the purpose involves the training of other professionals. The exact scope of this latitude has not been authoritatively resolved by decided cases. In any event, a treating professional can always obtain protection against subsequent claims by obtaining the patient's informed consent to having the information disclosed in the context of the publication of research findings or for training.

MacDONALD v. CLINGER

Supreme Court, Appellate Division, Fourth Department, 1982.
84 App.Div.2d 482, 446 N.Y.S.2d 801.

DENMAN, JUSTICE.

We here consider whether a psychiatrist must respond in damages to his former patient for disclosure of personal information learned during the course of treatment and, if he must, on what theory of recovery the action may be maintained. We hold that such wrongful disclosure is a breach of the fiduciary duty of confidentiality and gives rise to a cause of action sounding in tort.

The complaint alleges that during two extended courses of treatment with defendant, a psychiatrist, plaintiff revealed intimate details about himself which defendant later divulged to plaintiff's wife without justification and without consent. As a consequence of such disclosure, plaintiff alleges that his marriage deteriorated, that he lost his job, that he suffered financial difficulty and that he was caused such severe emotional distress that he required further psychiatric treatment. The complaint set forth three causes of action: breach of an implied contract; breach of confidence in violation of public policy; and breach of the right of privacy guaranteed by article 5 of the Civil Rights Law. Defendant moved to dismiss for failure to state a cause of action, asserting that there was in reality only one theory of recovery, that of breach of confidence, and that such action could not be maintained against him because his disclosure to plaintiff's wife was justified. The court dismissed the third cause of action but denied the motion with respect to the first two causes of action and this appeal ensued.

Research reveals few cases in American jurisprudence which treat the doctor-patient privilege in this context. That is undoubtedly due to the fact that the confidentiality of the relationship is a cardinal rule of the medical profession, faithfully adhered to in most instances, and thus has come to be justifiably relied upon by patients seeking advice and treatment. This physician-patient relationship is contractual in nature, whereby the physician, in agreeing to administer to the patient, impliedly covenants that the disclosures necessary to diagnosis and treatment of the patient's mental or physical condition will be kept in confidence.

Examination of cases which have addressed this problem makes it apparent that courts have immediately recognized a legally compensable injury in such wrongful disclosure based on a variety of grounds for recovery: public policy; right to privacy; breach of contract; breach of fiduciary duty. As the Supreme Court of Washington stated in *Smith v. Driscoll*, 94 Wash. 441, 442, 162 P. 572:

> Neither is it necessary to pursue at length the inquiry of whether a cause of action lies in favor of a patient against a physician for wrongfully divulging confidential communications. For the purposes

of what we shall say it will be assumed that, for so palpable a wrong, the law provides a remedy.

An excellent and carefully researched opinion exploring the legal ramifications of this confidentiality is *Doe v. Roe,* 93 Misc.2d 201, 400 N.Y.S.2d 668, a decision after a non-jury trial in which plaintiff sought injunctive relief and damages because of the verbatim publication by her former psychiatrist of extremely personal details of her life revealed during years of psychoanalysis. The court considered several proposed theories of recovery, including violation of public policy and breach of privacy rights. We agree with the court's observation that the several statutes and regulations requiring physicians to protect the confidentiality of information gained during treatment are clear evidence of the public policy of New York but that there is a more appropriate theory of recovery than one rooted in public policy.

Neither do we believe that an action for breach of the right of privacy may be maintained despite some current predictions to the contrary.

* * *

* * * I * * * find that a physician, who enters into an agreement with a patient to provide medical attention, impliedly covenants to keep in confidence all disclosures made by the patient concerning the patient's physical or mental condition as well as all matters discovered by the physician in the course of examination or treatment. This is particularly and necessarily true of the psychiatric relationship, for in the dynamics of psychotherapy "[t]he patient is called upon to discuss in a candid and frank manner personal material of the most intimate and disturbing nature * * * He is expected to bring up all manner of socially unacceptable instincts and urges, immature wishes, perverse sexual thoughts—in short, the unspeakable, the unthinkable, the repressed. To speak of such things to another human requires an atmosphere of unusual trust, confidence and tolerance. * * *"

* * *

It is obvious then that this relationship gives rise to an implied covenant which, when breached, is actionable. If plaintiff's recovery were limited to an action for breach of contract, however, he would generally be limited to economic loss flowing directly from the breach and would thus be precluded from recovering for mental distress, loss of his employment and the deterioration of his marriage. We believe that the relationship contemplates an additional duty springing from but extraneous to the contract and that the breach of such duty is actionable as a tort. Indeed, an action in tort for a breach of a duty of confidentiality and trust has long been acknowledged in the courts of this state.

* * * When such duty grows out of relations of trust and confidence, as that of the agent to his principal or the lawyer to his client, the ground of the duty is apparent, and the tort is, in general, easily separable from the mere breach of contract. * * *

* * *

Such duty, however, is not absolute, and its breach is actionable only if it is wrongful, that is to say, without justification or excuse. Although public policy favors the confidentiality described herein, there is a countervailing public interest to which it must yield in appropriate circumstances. Thus where a patient may be a danger to himself or others a physician is required to disclose to the extent necessary to protect a threatened interest.

* * *

Although the disclosure of medical information to a spouse may be justified under some circumstances, a more stringent standard should apply with respect to psychiatric information. One spouse often seeks counselling concerning personal problems that may affect the marital relationship. To permit disclosure to the other spouse in the absence of an overriding concern would deter the one in need from obtaining the help required. Disclosure of confidential information by a psychiatrist to a spouse will be justified whenever there is a danger to the patient, the spouse or another person; otherwise information should not be disclosed without authorization. Justification or excuse will depend upon a showing of circumstances and competing interests which support the need to disclose (cf. *Berry v. Moench,* 8 Utah 2d 191, 331 P.2d 814, *supra*). Because such showing is a matter of affirmative defense, defendant is not entitled to dismissal of the action.

The order should be modified to dismiss the cause of action for breach of contract and as modified should be affirmed.

Order modified on the law and as modified affirmed with costs to defendant.

SIMONS, J.P., concurs in a separate opinion.

SIMONS, JUSTICE Presiding (concurring).

Plaintiff seeks in this action to recover from defendant, his psychiatrist, for defendant's allegedly unjustified and damaging disclosure of confidential information about plaintiff's condition to plaintiff's wife. The members of the court are agreed that he may do so and that the action sounds in tort. We are divided about the nature of the cause of action, however, the majority believing it to be a "breach of fiduciary duty to confidentiality," while I believe the cause of action to be for malpractice. The difference is one of substance, for the majority hold plaintiff may recover if he submits evidence of the professional relationship, the disclosure of confidential information and damages. Once plaintiff does so, it is for the doctor to offer evidence of justification and for the jury to weigh it. Plaintiff's right to recover, as they see it, rests on proof of an unauthorized disclosure, the breach of an implied promise to hold confidential information received during treatment. In my view, plaintiff's right to recover must rest upon his proof that the disclosure was wrongful or unjustified.

When a physician undertakes treatment of a patient, he impliedly represents that he possesses, and the law places upon him the duty of possessing, the reasonable degree of learning and skill possessed by physicians in the community generally. Culpable fault exists if the physician fails to live up to this standard.

* * * Confidentiality, particularly in the case of a psychiatrist, is a significant and important aspect of medical treatment and a promise of non-disclosure may readily be implied from the physician-patient relationship. Thus, the relationship has elements of a contract, as plaintiff's first cause of action suggests, but commonly malpractice is a tort action predicated upon the physician's violation of his duty to supply the quality of care promised when he undertook to treat the patient. The physician's duty to honor this implied promise of confidentiality is merely another aspect of the treatment rendered and should be judged similarly.

The majority, by taking the cause of action out of the malpractice area, hold that all unauthorized disclosures, *prima facie,* violate reasonable medical care. The disclosure may be excused only if defendant proves that it was precipitated by danger to the patient, spouse or another. No other disclosure is permissible, apparently, even if mandated by statute. But further than that, the established rules of professional malpractice base liability upon an objective standard measured by the general quality of care of the professional community. The rule advanced by the majority permits the standard of care in unauthorized disclosure cases to be set by the jury. Thus, in every case of disclosure, the physician is exposed to the danger of a damage verdict resting upon the jury's subjective view of his explanation of his conduct even if it was in accordance with accepted medical practice. Thus, a jury disbelieving a physician's evaluation that a patient is assaultive or suicidal may hold the physician liable for the most limited but necessary disclosure relating to such common-place matters as advice to ensure that the patient takes prescribed medication or avoids stressful situations.

In short, to avoid a non-suit, a plaintiff should submit evidence of more than an unauthorized disclosure by the physician. There should be evidence that the physician has engaged in the unskilled practice of medicine. The relationship between the parties, after all, is medical, not fiduciary. The doctor is hired to treat the patient and his liability, if any, should be predicated upon his failure to do so properly.

* * *

Questions and Comments

1. *Disciplinary proceedings for breach of confidentiality.* Wrongful disclosure can lead to discipline by a regulatory authority. For instance, in *Mississippi State Board of Psychological Examiners v. Hosford,* 508 So.2d 1049 (Miss.1987), the psychologist had provided family counseling to a husband and wife. Later, during the couple's divorce proceeding, he

submitted an authorized affidavit to the court recommending the award of custody to the father. This recommendation was based in part on disclosures made by the wife during counseling. These facts were deemed sufficient to justify disciplinary action against the psychologist for his violation of the ethical principles of psychologists.

2. *Claim under contract theory.* Technically, a violation of a patient's right to confidentiality could be the basis for an action based on breach of a contract involving an implied covenant on the part of the therapist to maintain confidentiality. In fact this theory was the basis of a claim in *Allen v. Smith*, 368 S.E.2d 924 (W.Va.1988). While the court found a breach, it was unwilling to award damages for emotional distress alone.

3. *Defenses.* Regardless of the plaintiff-patient's choice of legal theory, the defendant-therapist may raise certain defenses whose merits will usually determine the outcome of the case. All of these defenses may best be understood as falling within four possible categories: absolute privilege, qualified privilege, patient consent, or absence of malice.

"Privilege" is a term frequently used in discussions about confidential information. Perhaps the best way to understand the term is to think of privilege as an exemption from liability which would otherwise attach to the actor's disclosure or withholding of information. A privilege may be either "absolute" or "qualified." An absolute privilege attaches whenever disclosure is compelled by law. Examples of compelled disclosure, which are treated in greater detail in section II of this chapter, includes reports of child abuse, drug dependency, or illnesses which pose a threat to the public safety, such as persons with venereal disease or other serious contagious diseases. Disclosure may also be compelled by courts or legislative and administrative agencies.

When disclosure of confidential information is not unequivocally mandated by law, a therapist's disclosures may nevertheless be immune under the doctrine of "qualified privilege," which allows disclosure only if certain conditions are met. The first condition is that the therapist's purpose in disclosing the confidential information must be to achieve some societal purpose of importance comparable to the patient's interest in preserving confidentiality. Such interests may include, for example, protection of the safety of another endangered by a violent patient or disclosures made in good faith in proceedings for the civil commitment of a patient. A second condition is that the disclosure be no greater than reasonably necessary to achieve the purpose sought. Third, the disclosure must be by a method which is appropriate under the circumstances to achieve the purpose sought. A therapist usually will not be liable, for example, for entrusting a confidential report to an office secretary for typing. He may incur liability, on the other hand, for submitting the report to the patient's employer, when such action is neither authorized nor necessary to achieve any legitimate purpose outweighing the patient's interest in confidentiality.

4. *The defense of consent.* If the patient or client has authorized disclosure, the therapist cannot be held liable for disclosures in compliance with the patient's authorization. The patient's consent thus constitutes a third possible defense in an action for wrongful disclosure. The issue of consent is not as simple as it may appear at first. First, it is not always

clear whether a patient has consented to disclosure. If disclosure of psychological reports to teachers and school officials is a routine practice at a psychological clinic, for example, can it be said that a patient who seeks counseling there has implicitly consented to such disclosures? See, *Iverson v. Frandsen,* 237 F.2d 898 (10th Cir.1956).

Second, even if the patient's express consent is obtained, the scope of consent is not always clear. A patient may consent to allow a therapist to disclose to the patient's prospective employer that he has received therapy. Does this consent authorize disclosure of the nature of the patient's problem? The nature or length of treatment? Specific facts about the patient relating to his suitability for employment?

II. LIMITATIONS ON THE DUTY OF CONFIDENTIALITY

A. INTRODUCTION

The preceding materials have explored doctrines which protect patients from unauthorized disclosures by professionals with whom they have entered into a patient-therapist relationship. The patient's rights of privacy, however, are not absolute, and in some circumstances a therapist may be under a legal duty to make disclosures to either agencies of the state or private citizens.

There are three situations where disclosure of information by the therapist may be *required.* One situation is created by compulsory reporting statutes which cover such matters as child abuse or narcotics addiction. The second category, which so far has been adopted by only a minority of states, is the obligation of a therapist to communicate to third parties the known dangerous propensities of the patient.

A third category of compelled disclosure is the duty to give testimony in a judicial proceeding. However, this duty is not applied universally, and in fact the legal system has carved out special exceptions for professionals, including physicians and psychotherapists. These exceptions fall within the ambit of what is known as the testimonial privilege, are fairly technical in nature, and do not apply with equal force in all jurisdictions. While any comprehensive treatment of the testimonial privilege is beyond the purview of these materials, subsection D below seeks to set forth the general legal framework governing the application of the privilege.

B. MANDATORY REPORTING REQUIREMENTS

Nearly all states have enacted laws which require physicians and mental health professionals to disclose to designated authorities certain types of patient information, even if the information would otherwise be confidential. Most states, for instance, require reporting to health authorities the fact that a patient is suffering from certain communicable diseases. *Hammonds v. Aetna Casualty & Surety Co.,* 243 F.Supp. 793 (N.D.Ohio 1965). Nearly all states also impose a duty on physicians or hospital administrators to report to police authorities any case where a patient appears for treatment of gunshot injuries. Jon R. Waltz and Fred E. Inbau, *Medical Jurisprudence* (New York: MacMillan, 1971), p. 364. Some states also require attending or consulting physicians to report the name of any person known to be a "habitual user of a narcotic drug." Id. at 365. Finally most states require any physician or mental health professional who has reasonable cause to suspect an incidence of child abuse to report such fact to a designated agency. Id. at 320–322. In some jurisdictions psychiatrists are covered by these provisions whereas other mental health professionals are not. There is an interplay between these reporting statutes and the testimonial privilege. It has been argued that mandatory reporting statutes lift the privilege of confidentiality granted by testimonial privilege statutes. The case set forth below addresses the question of whether the legislature, by requiring reporting, also intends to abrogate confidentiality rights.

DAYMUDE v. STATE

Court of Appeals of Indiana, First District, 1989.
540 N.E.2d 1263.

BAKER, JUDGE.

STATEMENT OF THE FACTS

The Greene County Division of the Indiana State Department of Public Welfare (Department) filed a petition in the Greene Circuit Court, Juvenile Docket, alleging that Daymude's 13–year–old daughter was a "child in need of services" as defined by IND.CODE 31–6–4–3. As provided by the CHINS statute, the Department, pursuant to court order, provided services to the child and her family. The daughter was admitted as an in-patient at Charter Hospital of Terre Haute (the hospital). In addition, the juvenile court ordered Daymude, the alleged victim, and her mother to undergo family counseling.

The hospital's clinical director referred the daughter's case to James Walker (Walker), a certified clinical mental health counselor working as an independent contractor for the hospital. Walker worked under the supervision of Dr. Mary Anne Johnson, the hospital's chief psychiatrist for the child and adolescent division. Walker developed and scheduled a treatment program in which the alleged victim and her family were to participate in a series of individual and group therapy sessions. During the course of a counseling session, Daymude disclosed information relating to alleged instances of sexual abuse.

On July 8, 1989, the State formally charged Daymude with child molesting and criminal deviate conduct in violation of IND.CODE 35–42–4–2 and 35–42–4–3, and with the offense of incest in violation of IND.CODE 35–26–1–3. Thereafter, the State sought to depose Walker regarding the content of communications between Walker and Daymude disclosed in the course of the family therapy. Daymude objected to the State's inquiry, insofar as it related to privileged and confidential communications between himself and Walker or any other member of the hospital's treatment team. The question was certified to the trial court and on January 31, 1989, the trial court overruled the defendant's objection and ordered Walker to answer such questions as were asked by the State pertaining to his communication with Daymude during the course of counseling. It is from this order that the instant interlocutory appeal is taken.

ISSUE

Whether the trial court erred in finding that Daymude's right to privileged communication with his health care provider was abrogated by IND.CODE 31–6–11–8 when that communication was undertaken subsequent to the State's involvement in allegations of child sexual abuse against Daymude, and when that communication was undertaken in the course of treatment and rehabilitation recommended by the State through its Department of Public Welfare.

DISCUSSION AND DECISION

Communications between a physician and a patient, of a confidential nature, are privileged and may not be disclosed by the physician without a waiver of that privilege by the patient. * * * This physician-patient privilege is codified in IND.CODE 34–1–14–5 which provides, in pertinent part:

The following persons shall not be competent witnesses:

. . .

4th. Physicians, as to matter communicated to them, as such, by patients, in the course of their professional business, or advice given in such cases, except as provided in IND.CODE 9–4–4.5–7.[1]

The privilege applies to those communications undertaken in the course of, and necessary to treatment.

However, in Indiana "*any individual* who has reason to believe that a child is a victim of child abuse or neglect shall make a report" as required by statute (emphasis added). IND.CODE 31–6–11–3. Thus, this language and the physician-patient privilege place conflicting duties upon a physician who learns of child abuse during the course of a physician-patient relationship. Consequently, the Indiana legislature adopted IND.CODE 31–6–11–8 which abrogates the physician-patient privilege when reporting child abuse. The abrogation statute states:

The privileged communication between a husband and wife, between a health care provider and that health care provider's patient, or between a school counselor and a student is not a ground for:

(1) excluding evidence in any judicial proceeding resulting from a report of a child who may be a victim of child abuse or neglect, or

---

1. IND.CODE 9–11–4–6, formerly 9–4–4.5–7, provides for the abrogation of the physician-patient privilege in certain cases involving chemical tests for purposes of Title 9, Criminal Investigations.

relating to the subject matter of such a report; or (2) failing to report as required by this chapter.

Id.

Daymude acknowledges that Walker, as a mental health professional had a duty under IND.CODE 31–6–11–3 to report suspected or known instances of child abuse or neglect even though such information is received in the course of confidential communications. *See* IND.CODE 31–6–11–3 (Duty to Report); IND.CODE 34–1–14–5 (Physician–Patient Privilege); IND.CODE 31–6–11–8 (Abrogation of Privilege). However, Daymude argues that the privilege is abrogated only in reporting child abuse, and that the abrogation does not extend to communications made during counseling ordered by the court as a result of CHINS proceedings.

Because of the special circumstances of this case, this appeal presents an issue of first impression for this court. However, we believe that the purpose of the reporting statutes and decisions from courts facing similar issues clearly support Daymude's contentions here.

The purpose of the Indiana reporting statute is:

[T]o encourage effective reporting of suspected or known incidents of child abuse or neglect, to provide in each county an effective child protection service to quickly investigate reports of child abuse or neglect, to provide protection for such a child from further abuse or neglect, and to provide rehabilitative services for such a child and his parent, guardian, or custodian.

IND.CODE 31–6–11–1. Thus, the reporting statute attempts to promote the reporting of child abuse cases, and thereafter, to provide a mechanism for the investigation of the abuse in order to protect the child and provide rehabilitative services for the child and parents, guardian, or custodian. The abrogation statute as set forth in IND.CODE 31–6–11–8 must be read in light of the purpose of the entire act.

Clearly, confidential communications between a health care provider and his patient are abrogated to the extent that the health care provider must report all suspected or known instances of child abuse. However, to extend the abrogation statute to information disclosed during Daymude's court ordered counseling goes beyond the purpose of the statute. The statute makes no mention of prosecuting alleged abusers, and instead only discusses means to facilitate the identification of the children who need the immediate attention of child welfare professionals.

* * *

In the present case, the reporting of child abuse is not an issue. The alleged abuse was reported long before Daymude made confidential statements to Walker. In fact the confidential communications arose only after the CHINS proceedings during which the court ordered Daymude to attend and participate in individual and family counseling sessions. Thus, because the alleged abuse already had been reported, the reporting statute's purpose had been served and the physician-patient privilege need not be abrogated further.

There is no question that the family therapy sessions are an integral and necessary part of the patient's diagnosis and treatment. If the physician-patient privilege is denied to those family members involved in CHINS counseling, then the alleged child abusers will be discouraged from openly and honestly communicating with their counselors. Without open and honest communications between the physician and the family members, the rehabilitative process will fail. Consequently, the child, whom the statute is designed to help and protect, is denied an opportunity for complete rehabilitation. As the *Andring* court stated:

> Once the abuse is discovered, however, the statute should not be construed, nor can the legislature have intended it to be construed, to permit total elimination of this important privilege. The central purpose of the child abuse reporting statute is the protection of children, not punishment of those who mistreat them.

Id.

* * *

In the present case, the physician-patient privilege arose as a direct result of therapy ordered by the court during a CHINS proceeding. The privileged communications were made long after the report of the child abuse. Since the abuse already had been reported, the purpose of the reporting statute had been fulfilled. To allow the abrogation of the privileged communication under these specific facts goes beyond the purpose of the statute. Thus, because of the specific facts of the present case, we hold that the physician-patient privilege is not abrogated with regard to confidential communications disclosed by a defendant while participating in counseling sessions ordered by a trial court pursuant to a report of child molesting.

For the above reasons, we reverse the trial court's ruling.

Judgment reversed.

RATLIFF, C.J., and ROBERTSON, J., concur.

Comments

Recent cases suggest that there are constitutional limits on the power of legislatures to impose medical reporting requirements. For instance, a majority of the justices of the Supreme Court have found broad state law requirements for notification of the parents of minors seeking an abortion to be constitutionally defective. *Bellotti v. Baird,* 443 U.S. 622, 99 S.Ct. 3035, 61 L.Ed.2d 797 (1979). But see, *H.L. v. Matheson,* 450 U.S. 398, 101 S.Ct. 1164, 67 L.Ed.2d 388 (1981).

In the psychiatric context a California appellate court has held that a state law provision that required institutions to notify a "responsible relative" of the patient prior to the administration of ECT or psychosurgery violated the patient's right to privacy. *Aden v. Younger,* 57 Cal.App.3d 662, 129 Cal.Rptr. 535 (1976).

C. DISCLOSURES OF THE DANGEROUS PROPENSITIES OF THE PATIENT

TARASOFF v. REGENTS OF THE UNIVERSITY OF CALIFORNIA

Supreme Court of California, 1976.
17 Cal.3d 425, 131 Cal.Rptr. 14, 551 P.2d 334.

(The opinion is set out at page 120, supra).

SHAW v. GLICKMAN

Court of Special Appeals of Maryland, 1980.
45 Md.App. 718, 415 A.2d 625.

[Plaintiff, Daniel Shaw, a dentist, had been undergoing group therapy treatment conducted by the defendant psychiatrist and his wife, a psychiatric nurse. Among the other patients in the group were Mr. and Mrs. Billian. Unknown to Mr. Billian, an amorous relationship developed between Mrs. Billian and Dr. Shaw. Upon learning of the extramarital affair, one of the therapists disclosed the information to Mr. Billian at a private therapy session. Some days later, Mr. Billian broke into Dr. Shaw's home. Finding his wife in bed with Dr. Shaw, Mr. Billian fired five shots at the doctor. Dr. Shaw filed an action to recover for his injuries, naming as defendants both Mr. Billian and the psychiatric team that had been conducting the group therapy sessions. The complaint charged that the defendant therapists had failed to warn him of Mr. Billian's "unstable and violent condition and the foreseeable and immediate danger that it presented to the plaintiff."]

GILBERT, CHIEF JUDGE:

* * *

Shaw points to *Tarasoff v. Regents of the University of California,* 17 Cal.3d 425, 131 Cal.Rptr. 14, 551 P.2d 334 (1976), as authority for the proposition that the psychotherapist-patient relationship imposes on the therapists a duty to control his patient and the concomitant duty to protect the patient's would-be victim.

* * *

The Court, in *Tarasoff,* noted that there was no question of a missed diagnosis or failure to predict the future conduct of the patient. What was involved was the fact that the patient did tell the therapist of the plan to kill Tatiana, and the therapist, while correctly predicting the event, negligently failed to warn the victim.

The court turned away the contention that "the therapist should be absolved of any responsibility for failing to act to protect the potential victim." Rather the court opined that "once a therapist . . . determine[s], or under applicable professional standards reasonably should have determined, that a patient poses a serious danger of violence to others, he bears a duty to exercise reasonable care to protect the foreseeable victim of that danger." The court concluded that each case must stand on its own facts, as measured against traditional negligence standards of reasonable care under the circumstances.

We neither accept nor reject the rationale of *Tarasoff* because, in our view, it is inapposite to the instant case.

Here there was no threat revealed to the "team" by Billian to kill or injure Dr. Shaw; there was apparently no confiding by Billian in the doctor or his staff, concerning any animosity or hatred toward Dr. Shaw. The record, at least, is devoid of the existence of any such feeling. Although Billian was known by Dr. Gallant to tote a gun, that fact does not give rise to the inference that Billian did so for the purpose of harming Dr. Shaw. The matter *sub judice* is unlike *Tarasoff* in that the intent to kill or injure was not disclosed.

Underlying Dr. Gallant's obligation to his patients was the Hippocratic oath. That oath, in pertinent part, states: "All that may come to my knowledge in the exercise of my profession or outside of my profession or in daily commerce with men, which ought not to be spread abroad, I will keep secret and will never reveal."

Of course, it may be argued that when as in *Tarasoff,* a patient informs a doctor of the patient's plan to kill another person, such information is not within the proscription of the Hippocratic oath, but rather "ought to be spread abroad" in order to prevent injury or loss of life. Clearly, had Billian confided in Dr. Gallant, or any of the team, that he, Billian, planned to shoot Dr. Shaw, Dr. Gallant would have faced a dilemma, *i.e.,* to breach Billian's confidence and tip off Shaw, or keep Billian's confidence and, figuratively speaking, throw Shaw to the wolves.

Even that dilemma is not without some legislative guidance. Md. Courts and Judicial Proceedings Code Ann. (1974) § 9–109(b) provides:

> "Unless otherwise provided, in all judicial, legislative, or administrative proceedings, a patient or his authorized representative has a privilege to refuse to disclose, and to prevent a witness from disclosing, communications relating to diagnosis or treatment of the patient's mental or emotional disorder."

* * *

The statute provides also for the exceptions to its tenets. None of the exceptions are germane to the issue before us, however. It seems to us that inasmuch as the statute confers a privilege of confidentiality on the communication between patient and psychiatrist-psychologist in judicial, legislative, or administrative proceedings, which privilege is that of the patient, no lesser privilege is existent when the matter is not judicial, legislative, or administrative. With the exception of those instances where the privilege of confidentiality is expressly prohibited, the lips of the psychiatrist or psychologist have been statutorily sealed shut subject solely to being unsealed by the patient or the patient's authorized representative.

We hold that under current Maryland law, it would have been a violation of the statute for Dr. Gallant or any member of his psychiatric team to disclose to Dr. Shaw any propensity on the part of Billian to invoke the old Solon law and shoot his wife's lover.

* * *

Because we believe no cause of action exists on the part of Dr. Shaw against the psychiatric team, under the circumstances of this case, we affirm the judgment of the Superior Court of Baltimore.

Judgment Affirmed.

Questions and Comments

1. *Some Questions.* What rationale led the *Shaw v. Glickman* court to reject the adoption of the *Tarasoff* doctrine? Could the court's decision be reversed by the legislature?

2. *Statutory exceptions to the privilege.* Since many states have enacted statutes protecting the confidentiality of psychotherapist-patient communications, other courts could similarly reject the *Tarasoff* doctrine in favor of the rationale of the *Shaw v. Glickman* court. Too few cases have been decided in other jurisdictions to indicate the direction in which the law is likely to develop.

3. *The duty to warn exception.* Note that the Maryland statute in *Shaw v. Glickman* provides certain exceptions to the privilege of confidentiality. The court found, however, that none of the statutory exceptions applied. Compare the approach adopted by the Vermont Supreme Court in *Peck v. Counseling Service of Addison County:*

> Defendant also argues that the therapist could not lawfully have warned the plaintiffs * * * because of the physician-patient privilege against disclosure of confidential information. 12 V.S.A. § 1612(a). * * * Defendant points out that the legislature has specified certain "public policy" exceptions to the physician-patient privilege, see, e.g., 33 V.S.A. §§ 683–684 (Supp.1984) (report of child abuse), 13 V.S.A. § 4012 (disclosure of gunshot wounds), 18 V.S.A. §§ 1152–1153 (report of abuse of the elderly), and that a therapist's duty to disclose the risk of harm posed by his or her patient to a foreseeable victim is not a recognized legislative exception. Given this, defendant argues that this Court is preempted from finding a duty-to-warn exception to the physician-patient privilege. The statutory exceptions to the physician-patient privilege indicate to this Court, however, that the privilege is not sacrosanct and can properly be waived in the interest of public policy under appropriate circumstances. A mental patient's threat of serious harm to an identified victim is an appropriate circumstance under which the physician-patient privilege may be waived.

499 A.2d at 426.

4. *Statutory exceptions.* Numerous states also authorize a physician or mental health professional to disclose any confidential information when

the patient's condition makes it necessary to set in motion commitment proceedings. For instance, in Illinois records and communications may be disclosed where it is "necessary to the provision of emergency medical care to a recipient" or in "commitment proceedings." Ill.—S.H.A. ch. 91½, ¶ 8–11 (Mental Health and Development Disability Confidentiality Act, 1979). In fact, failure of a therapist to initiate commitment where warranted could lead to civil liability for negligence. Thus, liability might attach where a therapist has failed to initiate civil commitment of a clearly suicidal patient.

. 5. *Disclosing limits of confidentiality to patients.* The normal rules pertaining to confidentiality are, of course, partially waived in those jurisdictions that adhere to *Tarasoff* since therapists have not only a duty but also a legal right to warn third persons of the dangerous propensities of their patients. In those jurisdictions where *Tarasoff* applies, should a therapist have an obligation to inform potential patients that confidentiality might be broken if the therapist later perceives the patient to be a threat to a third person? One commentator has suggested that failing to inform patients of the risk that their confidential communications will be disclosed could constitute a breach of the informed consent doctrine. See Note, *The Doctrine of Informed Consent Applied to Psychotherapy,* 72 Geo.L.J. 1637 (1984).

6. *Psychological harm as a basis for disclosure.* Should the threat of future *psychological* harm to third parties justify a psychologist's breach of a patient's confidentiality? In *Mississippi State Board of Psychological Examiners v. Hosford,* 508 So.2d 1049 (Miss.1987), the court held that the State Board of Psychological Examiners had the authority to limit the "clear danger" exception to the duty of confidentiality to "cases involving imminent danger to life and limb." In that case, the board had determined that the "clear danger" criteria did not include danger of emotional or psychological damage to a third party.

7. *Disclosure of past crimes.* May a therapist disclose information as to the patient's past commission of a crime? While such disclosure may constitute a breach of confidentiality, the violation cannot be asserted as a defense in a criminal proceeding. *State v. Beatty,* 770 S.W.2d 387 (Mo.App. 1989), (holding that a therapist's report that the patient had been involved in a robbery could not be raised as a defense in a criminal proceeding). The court in reality acknowledged that the patient might have a private cause of action against the therapist for a breach of confidentiality. What would be the extent of damages she could obtain? Should the term of imprisonment that resulted from the conviction be compensable?

D. JUDICIAL PROCEEDINGS AND THE TESTIMONIAL PRIV- ILEGE

1. Introduction

a. The Rationale for Compelled Disclosure

In many situations society, through an arm of government, needs information known only to a few. In these situations, according to an old maxim, the public has a right to every man's evidence. That is, each person has a duty to disclose information of vital importance to society. The duty to disclose arises when society's need to ascertain the truth outweighs the individual's interest in concealing the information. The public, through the coercive forces of government, may then compel disclosure. The usual contexts in which the need for information arises include civil and criminal trials and hearings and investigations by legislatures and administrative agencies. In each of these contexts, ascertaining the truth is essential to promote an important societal interest.

In a civil trial the dispute before the court may concern the interpretation of a contract, a disputed claim to property, or a claim for damages for an injury allegedly caused by another person's negligent conduct. The parties stand as adversaries competing to produce evidence helpful to their respective causes. The court, on behalf of society, seeks to achieve substantial justice between the parties. Ascertainment of the facts is essential in this task, but the basis of the court's decision must be limited to the evidence adduced at trial. Thus, not only do the individual parties have an interest in obtaining information, but the court, on behalf of society and in the interests of justice, seeks to assure each litigant's ability to obtain information necessary to his case.

The need for information is perhaps more dramatic in a criminal trial, where the guilt or innocence of an accused person is at stake. Society has a dual interest in ascertaining the facts in criminal cases. First, society seeks to assure that offenders are apprehended and punished. At trial, the state must prove beyond a reasonable doubt that the accused person is guilty as charged. Ascertaining the facts surrounding the crime is essential in this task. Second, and equally important, is the guarantee of a fair trial and a just verdict. In the interest of fairness, an accused person must have access to information necessary to his defense. Indeed, the federal Bill of Rights guarantees criminal defendants' right to compel witnesses' testimony, as do most state constitutions. The cause of justice is served by assuring the availability of information to both sides, so that the truth may emerge.

In addition to the familiar settings of trials, public need for information and an individual's corresponding duty to disclose may arise in the context of legislative hearings and investigations. Whether the area is securities regulation or care of the mentally ill, legislative decisions must rest in part on balancing diverse political interests. Equally important, the legislature needs access to factual information. Legislative fact-finding is accomplished through hearings and investigations during which the legislature may compel testimony. In investigating charges of widespread abuse in the care of the mentally ill, for example, the legislature may compel testimony from institution administrators, behavioral scientists, and professional organizations concerned with formulating standards of treatment.

The final setting in which a duty to disclose information is likely to arise is before an administrative agency. Administrative agencies may perform functions of each of the three branches of government. Pursuant to legislatively delegated authority, an agency may draft rules regulating an industry. The agency may be authorized to perform such executive functions as granting licenses and conducting investigations of alleged violations. Finally, an agency may serve as the primary tribunal for prosecuting alleged violations. See, Chapter One, Section II.C. In each capacity, fact-finding is essential. Like courts and legislatures, administrative agencies may have authority to compel testimony. More commonly, however, agencies must rely upon court orders to compel testimony from reluctant witnesses.

Whether the context is a trial, a hearing, or an investigation, the ascertainment of truth is paramount. The presiding governmental unit facilitates the endeavor by issuing subpoenae or by invoking a court's authority to issue subpoenae.

Aside from imposing a duty to disclose information, a subpoena affords a witness protection from certain adverse consequences which might otherwise flow from his appearance or disclosures. Witnesses are immune from civil liability for any statement made under oath. That is, a witness may not be sued for defamation, regardless of whether his testimony damages another person's reputation. This immunity from civil suit extends even to perjured testimony.

In some circumstances required information may be in written form. For example, in a suit for personal injuries, the records of a physician who treated the injured party may contain relevant information. Similarly, an accountant's records may contain information relevant to an investigation of a business merger which is suspected of violating antitrust laws. In such a case, the court or other tribunal may compel production of the documents in question by issuing a subpoena *duces tecum*, that is, a writ commanding production of the documents before the court.

b. Limitations on Disclosure: The Testimonial Privilege

Governmental authority to compel disclosure is not unlimited. It extends only as far as necessary to achieve the governmental purpose at hand. Thus, no witness may be compelled to testify concerning matters irrelevant to the case before the court or other tribunal.

Governmental authority is also limited when mandatory disclosure conflicts with rights or interests which are highly valued in a free society. To preserve important rights and interests, courts and other tribunals may recognize a "privilege" on the part of a witness to decline to answer certain questions. For example, no person may be compelled to make statements which might incriminate him. The privilege against self-incrimination is inherent in the American concept of liberty. Long recognized under the English common law, the privilege was incorporated in the Fifth Amendment to the federal Constitution and is made applicable to the states through the Fourteenth Amendment. Similarly, under the First Amendment guarantees of free speech and religion, no person may be compelled to state his political or religious beliefs under oath. Of course, a witness may waive the privilege and volunteer this information. The privilege merely protects against compulsory disclosure.

In addition to privileges which arise under the Constitution, legislatures may create testimonial privileges by statutes. In the absence of a statute or constitutional mandate, courts may recognize a privilege because of the importance of the interests thereby protected.

A testimonial privilege may protect certain *topics,* such as the witness' political or religious beliefs or information tending to incriminate the witness. Another form of privilege protects confidential communications in the context of certain relationships which society seeks to foster. When such a privilege is asserted, *neither* party to such a relationship may be compelled to disclose information exchanged in confidence. Relationships which traditionally have given rise to privileges of this sort include those between attorney and client, physician and patient, husband and wife, and priest and penitent. In recent years this privilege for confidential communications has been extended by statute or by courts in various states to such diverse professional groups as journalists, accountants, and psychotherapists.*

Traditionally, privilege for confidential communications is justified when four conditions are met. First, the relationship must be one which society seeks to foster. Second, the communications must originate in a confidence that they will not be disclosed. Third, the element of confidentiality must be essential to achieve the purpose of the relationship. Finally, injury to the relationship resulting from compelled disclosure must be greater than the benefit gained in correct disposal of litigation. Many courts, legislatures, and scholars have recognized that these conditions are clearly met in the psychotherapeutic relationship. Whether between a psychiatrist and a patient, or between a psychologist or other mental health professional and a client, the psychotherapeutic relationship is clearly one which society seeks to foster. Moreover, effective therapy is generally thought to require a patient's complete disclosure of his innermost thoughts and feelings. Fear of compulsory disclosure may inhibit a patient's ability to confide, and it may deter some persons from seeking psychotherapy. The assurance of confidentiality thus facilitates disclosures which are essential to effective treatment and induces hesitant persons to seek needed treatment.

* The reader may recall that the term "privilege" arises in many contexts. Generally, the term privilege refers to an exemption from liability for an action which would ordinarily give rise to liability. See, for example, the discussion of privilege as a defense to defamation in section I.B.1. of this chapter. In the present context, the action which would ordinarily give rise to liability is the withholding of subpoenaed testimony or information. Although the ordinary penalty for withholding subpoenaed information may be fine or imprisonment, the valid assertion of a recognized testimonial privilege exempts a witness from liability.

The availability and scope of testimonial privilege depend upon the profession of the psychotherapist and upon the law of the particular jurisdiction. Confidential communications between psychiatrist and patient are protected by physician-patient privilege statutes, which have been passed in about two-thirds of the states. In addition, statutes in a few states provide a comprehensive psychiatrist-patient privilege. In most states, statutes licensing psychologists provide a privilege for communications between psychologist and client. Finally, in a small number of states, statutes provide a privilege for other mental health professionals who provide psychotherapy, such as marriage counselors and social workers. Privilege statutes, however, are frequently ambiguous, and the availability and scope of the privilege in various contexts may be difficult to ascertain. The following materials illustrate some of the issues courts confront in applying the statutory provisions governing the privilege.

2. Conditions Giving Rise to the Privilege

a. The Course of Treatment Requirement

STATE v. COLE

Supreme Court of Iowa, 1980.
295 N.W.2d 29.

* * *

LARSON, JUSTICE.

This defendant appeals her conviction, in a jury-waived trial, of first-degree murder in violation of section 690.2, The Code 1977. She challenges the trial court's rulings in regard to psychiatric evidence secured by depositions and in-trial testimony * * * We affirm the trial court.

It is undisputed that on September 15, 1977, the defendant shot and killed Dr. Alan Tyler, her ex-husband, in his office at Wilden Clinic. Immediately after the shooting, she proceeded to the reception area and announced that she had "shot her husband." She then called the police and waited for them at the clinic. She was brought before a magistrate for an initial appearance where she was represented by Lawrence Scalise and Thomas Levis. At that time an order was signed by the magistrate to take the defendant to Iowa Lutheran Hospital "to undergo psychiatric and physical examination and evaluation." It is this order and the related evidence concerning the mental condition of the defendant which give rise to the most troublesome issues.

I. THE PSYCHIATRIC EVIDENCE

A. *Effect of the commitment order.* Pursuant to the court's order, the defendant was first examined by Dr. Michael Taylor, a psychiatrist who had been treating her on a private basis since before the shooting. He ceased his examination of her on September 30, 1977, at which time he was replaced by Dr. Vernon Varner. The defendant filed notice, * * * that she intended to rely upon the defense of diminished capacity. The State then sought to obtain psychiatric evidence through these doctors' depositions and in-trial testimony.

Upon application of the State, and over defendant's objections, pretrial depositions of Doctors Taylor and Varner were ordered by the court. Dr. Varner complied, and his deposition was taken. * * * Again over objection, the trial court permitted Dr. Taylor to testify at trial in the State's case in chief.

Defendant argues the trial court's rulings on the admissibility of the psychiatric evidence was erroneous because they violated her doctor-patient privilege, set out in section 622.10, The Code, as follows:

> No practicing attorney, counselor, physician, surgeon, or the stenographer or confidential clerk of any such person, who obtains such information by reason of his employment, minister of the gospel or priest of any denomination shall be allowed, in giving testimony, to disclose any confidential communication properly entrusted to him in his professional capacity, and necessary and proper to enable him to discharge the functions of his office according to the usual course of practice or discipline. Such prohibition shall not apply to cases where the person in whose favor the same is made waives the rights conferred. * * *

As the following authorities established, not every doctor-patient relationship provides a basis for exclusion of the doctor's testimony. In some cases the privilege never arises; in others it exists but is held to be waived by the patient. The privilege did not exist at common law, and its embodiment by statute has been criticized by at least one writer.

While our cases have evidenced no hostility to the rule itself, they have uniformly required three elements to be established: (1) the relationship of doctor-patient; (2) acquisition of the information or knowledge during this relationship; and (3) the necessity of the information to enable the doctor to treat the patient skillfully.

The order signed by the magistrate was as follows:

ORDER FOR PSYCHIATRIC EVALUATION AND REPORT

Now, on this 15th day of September, 1977, this matter having been brought to the attention of the court, and the court being fully advised of the charges against the defendant in the above captioned cause, and the present condition of the defendant; it is the considered opinion of this court that before further proceedings may be had an evaluation of the above-named defendant's physical and psychological state should be made by competent professionals in the fields of medicine and psychology in order that the court may be more fully advised and that the best interests of the parties and of justice may be realized.

* * *

The effect of [the Court's] order, and of the medical relationship which followed it, are determinative on the issue of whether or not the defendant could assert the doctor-patient privilege. In court-ordered evaluations, the third requirement of the privilege is lacking; the communication is not for the purpose of treatment but to determine the existence of a fact or condition for the benefit of the court. Therefore, "[t]he physician-patient privilege does not arise where on order of the court a defendant is examined to determine his mental or physical condition."

* * * The order clearly provided for evaluation and report to the court and made no provision for diagnosis or treatment.

The defendant, while acknowledging that the order appears to be for evaluation and report, argues it was really only intended to provide for her safekeeping in order to avoid a possible suicide. We do not believe the intentions of the parties can be properly used to countermand the unambiguous provisions of a court order.

* * *

Even if we were to consider the intentions of the parties, as appellant suggests, we do not believe the record supports her contention that "[t]he record unquestionably shows that Kathleen Cole was sent to Lutheran Hospital for the primary, if not the sole purpose, of obtaining diagnosis and treatment." Even under her own evidence, the commitment was for her protection; no one testified she was committed for treatment.

* * *

We find no reversible error; we therefore affirm the trial court.

Affirmed.

All Justices concur except HARRIS, J., who dissents, joined by REES and ALLBEE, JJ.

* * *

Questions and Comments

1. The *Cole* case affirms the basic rule that the privilege only attaches where the client's relationship to the psychologist or psychiatrist was in the course of treatment. Problems may arise in the application of this rule when the professional relationship involves both diagnosis undertaken as a result of a court order and treatment which is carried out at the initiative of the examining facility.

2. *Disclosure requirement.* Where the psychiatrist or psychologist examines a person on behalf of the court or an adverse party, is there any obligation on the part of the examiner to inform the person being examined as to the nature of the relationship and that any disclosures that are made will not be privileged? This question has only been addressed in the context of criminal cases where it has generally been held that, unless the person being examined is specifically informed that the purpose of the examination is not for treatment, any disclosures that may be made are not admissible in a subsequent criminal trial. See, *State v. Shaw,* 106 Ariz. 103, 471 P.2d 715 (1970) and *State v. Cole,* 295 N.W.2d 29, 34 (Iowa 1980).

3. *Scope of privilege.* In those jurisdictions where a privilege attaches to information or disclosures communicated in the course of psychotherapy,

the scope of such privilege may require judicial interpretation. An issue that has arisen is whether confidential information as used in statutes setting forth a privilege includes observations or any other information the therapist may have learned about the patient from sources other than the verbal communication of the patient himself. Illustratively, in *People v. Doe*, 103 Ill.App.3d 56, 58 Ill.Dec. 664, 430 N.E.2d 696 (1981), the psychiatric therapist was subpoenaed to appear before the grand jury and was presented with a drawing purporting to be a composite sketch of a person suspected of an ax murder. Claiming statutory privilege, the therapist refused to state whether she had seen anyone resembling the drawing even though there was independent evidence indicating that the person depicted by the composite drawing had been admitted to the psychiatric unit where the psychiatrist was working at the time. In finding the psychiatrist-patient privilege inapplicable, the court construed "communications" as used by the privilege statute to include only information obtained from conversations with the patient and not observations. Courts of other jurisdictions, however, have given a different interpretation to similar language. The American Psychiatric Association's proposed Model Law of Confidentiality of Health and Social Service Records specifically would extend the privilege to all "confidential information" which is defined to include "the fact that a person is or has been a patient/client." See, Sloan and Hall, *Confidentiality of Psychotherapeutic Records*, 5 J. of Legal Medicine 435, 463 (1984).

4. *Hospital admissions.* In some jurisdictions, the patient-psychotherapist privilege does not protect the existence of the fact of a hospital admission, the dates of hospitalization, or the purpose of the admission, so long as the purpose does not implicate a patient-psychotherapist communication. In *Commonwealth v. Clancy*, 402 Mass. 664, 524 N.E.2d 395 (1988), the court held that defense counsel was allowed this limited access to a witness' record without any showing of need, since this was not privileged information.

5. *Who is covered by privilege statutes?* It is sometimes difficult to determine whether a specific professional group, particularly in the mental health field, is covered by a particular privilege statute and, if so, the extent of the exemption. States have commonly enacted separate privilege statutes for various professional groups such as physicians, psychologists, marriage counselors, and social workers. Various problems are raised by the existence of multiple privilege statutes. For instance, in the absence of explicit legislative direction, should psychiatrists be entitled to the special privilege for psychologists which is normally broader and more comprehensive than the physician's privilege? In one jurisdiction the court held that the psychologist privilege did *not* cover psychiatrists. See *Ritt v. Ritt*, 98 N.J.Super. 590, 238 A.2d 196 (1967). In another state it was held that the psychologist privilege did cover psychiatrists, since the psychiatrist in question "worked with" the psychologist to whom the privilege applied. See *Day v. State*, 378 So.2d 1156 (Ala.Cr.App.1979), reversed sub nom. *Ex parte Day*, 378 So.2d 1159 (Ala.1979).

A number of states have enacted privilege statutes specifically covering social workers. However, the privilege is generally limited to social workers who are registered with the state. See *In re Westland,* 48 Ill.App.3d 172, 6 Ill.Dec. 331, 362 N.E.2d 1153, 1157 (1977).

Similar problems are encountered where the coverage of the privilege for psychologists and marriage counselors differ. For instance, in New Jersey the privilege for marriage counselors is virtually absolute, and confidential communications are not admissible in a divorce proceeding. However, under the Practicing Psychology Licensing Act the privilege would not necessarily bar the admission of confidential information in a divorce proceeding. In *Wichansky v. Wichansky,* 126 N.J.Super. 156, 313 A.2d 222 (1973), the court held that a psychologist who engages in marriage counseling is covered by the broader marriage counselor's privilege, even though he is not a licensed marriage counselor.

6. *Records covered.* When privilege protects confidential communications with a psychotherapist, the privilege extends as well to the patient records the psychotherapist maintains. Generally, such records are protected to the same extent as the communications they describe. When patient records are maintained at a hospital, school, or other public agency, however, the status of privilege is unclear. Similarly, when a patient is committed for treatment at a mental hospital, a variety of personnel may have access to his records. Courts, therefore, may regard the records as non-confidential and hence not privileged. On the other hand, other courts view nurses and ward staff as agents of the patient's psychiatrist and, accordingly, extend any applicable psychiatrist-patient or physician-patient privilege to hospital records.

Records at publicly funded hospitals pose additional problems. A few courts have found no confidential relationship between a resident-patient and psychiatrists employed at a state hospital, and hence no privilege for psychiatric records of state hospital patients. Additionally, courts sometimes treat state hospital records as public documents and therefore not privileged, or privileged under privilege statutes for government documents generally, and hence subject to waiver by the government, without consent of the patient. (See, for example, dissent in *Taylor v. United States,* 222 F.2d 398, 404 (D.C.Cir.1955) and New York cases cited therein.)

b. *Defining the Treatment Relationship*

STATE v. MILLER
Supreme Court of Oregon, 1985.
300 Or. 203, 709 P.2d 225.

CARSON, JUSTICE.

This case involves the scope of the psychotherapist-patient privilege in Oregon, under OEC 504.   *   *   *

FACTS

Defendant's case was tried to the court on stipulated facts. What follows is a summary of those facts.

Just before midnight on August 6, 1982, defendant telephoned his brother in California and told him that he had just "strangled a kid." Defendant's brother advised him to call a mental hospital or talk to someone who could help him with his problem. Minutes later, defendant telephoned Dammasch State Hospital and asked to speak to a doctor, giving a false name to the secretary-receptionist, Ms. Smith. When Ms. Smith asked him "what the problem [was]," he replied, "Murder. I just killed a man." Ms. Smith then said she would let him speak to a psychiatrist. She asked defendant for the telephone number from which he was calling; he told her the number, stating it was in a public telephone booth.

Ms. Smith telephoned the Clackamas County Sheriff's office, explained the situation, and gave them defendant's telephone number. Then Ms. Smith called Dr. Wendy Saville, the psychiatrist on duty that night at the hospital, and asked her to keep defendant on the line so that the Sheriff's office could "trace the call."

Dr. Saville talked to defendant for 10 or 15 minutes, asking him for background information, similar to what she usually obtained from a patient in a psychiatric interview. At trial, however, she testified that she was only talking to defendant so that the police could find him and that she only asked him about his background because it seemed the "safest" thing to talk about. When she questioned defendant about his name, he asked whether their conversation was confidential. Dr. Saville assured defendant that she would not disclose his confidences; only then did he give her his true name. During the conversation, defendant made a number of incriminating statements about his homosexual encounter with the victim, his fantasies and his role in the victim's death.

While defendant conversed with Dr. Saville, the Sheriff's office contacted the Portland Police Bureau, which located the telephone booth and sent a uniformed officer to investigate. When the officer arrived at the telephone booth and determined that defendant was the person talking to the state hospital, he physically removed defendant from the telephone booth, patted him down for weapons, found none, removed defendant's wallet and placed him in the locked rear passenger area of his patrol car.

The officer returned to the telephone booth to talk to Dr. Saville. She initially declined to give him any information about what defendant had told her because she believed it was a confidential communication protected by the psychotherapist-patient privilege. When the officer became "angry" and "pushed" her to tell him what happened, she told him that defendant told her he murdered someone.

The officer returned to the patrol car and questioned defendant. * * * During this questioning, defendant admitted that he had "hurt someone," that he "couldn't wake him up," and indicated that the person was in defendant's room in a residential hotel. Defendant then pulled his room keys out of his pocket and the officer took them.

The officer called for an ambulance, drove to the hotel one block away, entered the locked room using defendant's keys, and discovered the deceased victim's body. The officer returned to the car and for the first time advised defendant of his *Miranda* rights. Defendant did not respond to further police questioning.

Defendant's room was searched, and the victim's body and other evidence was removed. The next day, a search warrant was sought and issued, authorizing a search of defendant's room, from which other evidence was removed.

Defendant was charged with murder. He moved to suppress (1) his statements to Ms. Smith; (2) his statements to Dr. Saville; (3) his statements to the police officer; (4) evidence seized from his person; (5) evidence obtained during the warrantless entry and search of his room; and (6) all derivative evidence from the alleged illegalities. The trial court suppressed only his statements to the police officer, made during custodial interrogation without advice of *Miranda* rights and after he asserted his right to counsel. After a trial to the court, defendant was convicted of first degree manslaughter.

Defendant appealed to the Court of Appeals, which considered the case *in banc* and wrote four separate opinions. In the lead opinion, four members of the court relied upon the psychiatrist's statement that she was not diagnosing or treating defendant to conclude that no psychotherapist-patient relationship had been established and defendant could not claim the psychotherapist-patient privilege. The lead opinion also determined that even if defendant's communication to Dr. Saville was privileged, any error in admitting it was harmless because the statements were merely cumulative of the testimony of defendant's brother and the receptionist. * * *

Four judges dissented, three believing that defendant's statements to both the psychiatrist and the receptionist were privileged, and one judge determining that only defendant's statements to the psychiatrist were inadmissible. Two other judges specially concurred, agreeing with the dissenters that defendant's statements to the psychiatrist were privileged communications, but also agreeing with the lead opinion that the error in this case was harmless.

Defendant petitioned for review raising the same issues to this court. * * * For the reasons discussed below, we affirm the Court of Appeals.

DISCUSSION

I. *Psychotherapist–Patient Privilege*

The psychotherapist-patient privilege in Oregon is governed by OEC 504. The purpose of this privilege is to foster a relationship that is deemed important to society and one whose success is dependent upon full and free communication. Rule 504 combines the privileges for psychologists and psychiatrists, which were recognized separately under prior law, into a psychotherapist-patient privilege, which applies in both civil and criminal cases. Kirkpatrick, Oregon Evidence 160 (1982) (hereinafter cited as Kirkpatrick).

OEC 504(2) provides:

"A patient has a privilege to refuse to disclose and to prevent any other person from disclosing confidential communications made for the purposes of diagnosis or treatment of the patient's mental or emotional condition among the patient, the patient's psychotherapist or persons who are participating in the diagnosis or treatment under the direction of the psychotherapist, including members of the patient's family."

"Patient" is defined as "a person who consults or is examined or interviewed by a psychotherapist." OEC 504(1)(b).

"Psychotherapist" is defined as:

" * * * a person who is licensed, registered, certified or otherwise authorized under the laws of any state to engage in the diagnosis or treatment of a mental or emotional condition, or reasonably believed by the patient so to be, while so engaged." OEC 504(1)(c).

"Confidential communication" is defined as:

" * * * a communication not intended to be disclosed to third persons except: Persons present to further the interest of the patient in the consultation, examination or interview; persons reasonably necessary for the transmission of the communication; or persons who are participating in the diagnosis and treatment under the direction of the psychotherapist, including members of the patient's family." OEC 504(1)(a).

The need for the privilege is today widely recognized. * * * The parts of OEC 504 relevant herein were taken verbatim from proposed Federal Rule of Evidence 504. The need for the privilege is stated convincingly in the Advisory Committee's Note to Proposed FRE 504, as follows:

"Among physicians, the psychiatrist has a special need to maintain confidentiality. His capacity to help his patients is completely dependent upon their willingness and ability to talk freely. This makes it difficult if not impossible for him to function without being able to assure his patients of confidentiality and, indeed, privileged communication * * * [T]here is wide agreement that confidentiality is a *sine qua non* for successful psychiatric treatment. The relationship may well be likened to that of the priest-penitent or the lawyer-client. * * * A threat to secrecy blocks successful treatment." Report No. 45, Group for the Advancement of Psychiatry 92 (1960), *cited in* 56 FRD 183, 242 (1972).

The burden rests on the person seeking to assert the privilege to show that both that person and the nature of the testimony offered are within the ambit of the privilege.

A. STATEMENTS TO PSYCHIATRIST.

* * *

The communication must be "made for the purposes of diagnosis or treatment." OEC 504(2). The purpose of the communication may be inferred from the surrounding circumstances. A patient's reasonable belief that the communication is being made for the purposes of diagnosis or treatment will suffice. This point is more fully discussed *infra*.

The definition of a "psychotherapist" in OEC 504(1)(c) has two parts. The person must be both lawfully authorized to engage in diagnosis or treatment of the patient's mental or emotional condition (or reasonably believed by the patient so to be) and be "so engaged" when the communication which is intended to be kept confidential is made.

The trial court and four judges on the Court of Appeals seem to have concluded that defendant could not be a "patient" and invoke the privilege until a psychotherapist-patient relationship had been established that had been "agreed upon by both sides." They considered controlling the fact that defendant had not previously been a patient at the hospital, that the psychiatrist did not anticipate an ongoing psychotherapist-patient relationship to develop, and that she testified she was not actually diagnosing or treating defendant, but only keeping him on the telephone line until the police arrived.

* * *

Nothing in the legislative history of OEC 504 or proposed FRE 504 suggests that the phrase "while so engaged" should be limited to a contractual or employment relationship. It is likely that the requirement that a psychotherapist be "engaged" in diagnosis or treatment was intended to exclude communications to licensed mental health professionals engaged in non-clinical work, such as scientific research or teaching. The Legislative Commentary to OEC 504 states:

> "The definition of 'patient' in Rule 504 and 504–1 does not include a person submitting to examination *for scientific purposes*. This limitation agrees with the current Oregon requirement that a physician be consulted for treatment in order that the physician-patient privilege attach. * * *"

* * *

In light of the policy behind the rule and its similarity to the attorney-client privilege, we conclude that the psychotherapist-patient privilege protects communications made in an initial conference for the purpose of establishing a psychotherapist-patient relationship, even if such a relationship is never actually formed. The psychotherapist-patient privilege "necessarily includes communications made in the course of diagnostic interviews and examinations which might reasonably lead to psychotherapy." *Allred v. State*, 554 P.2d 411, 420 (Alaska 1976). This is required to encourage patients to discuss frankly and freely their mental or emotional problems so that the professional can accurately determine whether he or she is qualified to treat them. If information revealed during the initial conference indicates to either party that an ongoing professional relationship should not be formed, the confidences revealed in the initial consultation are protected nevertheless.

This is not to say, however, that a prospective patient who meets a person known to be a psychotherapist in a supermarket and immediately makes an unsolicited confession can claim the privilege solely because the patient intends the communication to be confidential and hopes to receive diagnosis or treatment. In order for statements made in an initial encounter to be covered by the privilege, the psychotherapist and patient must agree, or at least reasonably appear to agree, that they intend to establish a psychotherapist-patient relationship. There must be some indication from the psychotherapist that he or she is willing to embark upon such a relationship. An indication of this intent may be inferred from the circumstances. It might come from the setting alone. For example, if a prospective patient talks to a licensed psychotherapist in a professional practice setting, such as a mental health clinic or a private practice office, the patient could fairly infer that the psychotherapist has indicated a willingness to enter into a confidential relationship. The requisite willingness could also be shown by the psychotherapist's behavior, apart from the setting. If the prospective client in the above-stated supermarket example is assured by the psychotherapist that his statements will be kept confidential and is questioned about his problem, then the therapist has reasonably indicated a willingness to enter into a psychotherapist-patient relationship, and the privilege attaches when the first words are spoken.

Where a psychotherapist has given reasonable assurances to the patient that they are embarking upon a privileged relationship, an ulterior motive or purpose on the part of the psychotherapist will not prevent the patient from claiming the privilege. * * *

Thus, where a patient consults a psychotherapist for professional assistance for a mental or emotional problem and reasonably believes that the psychotherapist is willing to embark upon a professional relationship, the fact that the psychotherapist has a secret ulterior purpose for the interview or examination will not prevent the patient from claiming the privilege as to confidential communications. To hold otherwise would effectively transfer the privilege from the patient (who holds it under OEC 504(3)) to the psychotherapist. Such a shift is not supported by the language of the rule, its underlying policy, or caselaw.

Turning to the facts of this case, defendant herein specifically requested, and was assured of, confidentiality. Only then did he divulge his true name. This is a clear indication that defendant intended his conversation with the psychiatrist to be confidential.

At his brother's suggestion, defendant telephoned Dammasch State Hospital and asked to speak to a doctor. He was described as distraught and depressed. No one has disputed that he was seeking professional assistance for his emotional condition. He talked to a psychiatrist for 10 or 15 minutes, until the conversation was interrupted by the police officer removing him from the telephone booth. During this conversation the psychiatrist did not engage in "small talk" or idle chatter. She testified that she spoke to defendant and questioned him in much the same way she would have in a psychiatric interview. Based upon these facts, the only reasonable conclusion is that defendant reasonably believed that the communication was made "for the purposes of diagnosis or treatment."

We also conclude that, if Dr. Saville was a "psychotherapist" within the meaning of the rule, then defendant was a "patient" under OEC 504(1)(b), because he both "consulted" and was "interviewed by" her.

Dr. Saville was a licensed psychiatrist, authorized by statute "to engage in the diagnosis or treatment of a mental or emotional condition." The only dispute concerns whether she was "so engaged" while she was talking to defendant by telephone. She was the psychiatrist on duty at Dammasch State Hospital, a professional practice setting. She assured defendant of confidentiality and questioned him about his problem in the usual way that clinical interviews, as necessary precursors to diagnosis and treatment, are conducted. Although they had no prior psychotherapist-patient relationship and she testified that she did not anticipate forming one, it was not disputed that she led defendant reasonably to believe that she was willing to embark upon such a relationship. The fact that she had an ulterior purpose (keeping defendant on the telephone line until the police came) does not prevent him from claiming the privilege. We thus hold that defendant's statements to Dr. Saville were covered by the psychotherapist-patient privilege and should not have been admitted into evidence.

* * *

C. STATEMENTS TO SECRETARY–RECEPTIONIST.

The issue of when and to what extent communications made to agents and assistants of professional persons are protected by the evidentiary privileges is one with which many courts have wrestled.

OEC 504(1)(a) provides three separate categories of third persons to whom disclosures of confidential information are protected by the psychotherapist-patient privilege. The lead opinion in the Court of Appeals stated that the clause in OEC 504(1)(a) most applicable to the Dammasch State Hospital secretary-receptionist was the one which makes confidential those communications disclosed to "[p]ersons present to further the interest of the patient in the consultation, examination or interview." The opinion concluded that, because Ms. Smith was not physically present during defendant's consultation with the psychiatrist, the statements to Ms. Smith were not "confidential communications" within the meaning of OEC 504(1)(a).

We agree, however, with defendant and the dissent by Judge Richardson that the clause in OEC 504(1)(a) applicable to the secretary-receptionist is the one which renders confidential those communications to "persons reasonably necessary for the transmission of the communication." That clause contains no requirement that the person be present. * * *

* * *

The secretary-receptionist in the instant case testified that she had access to confidential patient information. One of her jobs on the graveyard shift was to collect information from persons entering the state hospital as patients. She also was responsible for screening incoming telephone calls to the psychiatrist on duty. She testified that all incoming calls to the state hospital come through her switchboard, making it impossible for anyone to talk to a psychotherapist without being put through by her. She was not merely a switchboard operator, however, because she testified that she was instructed to obtain the caller's name and determine if he or she was a former patient and the reason for the call, before connecting the caller with the psychiatrist.

When defendant called the state hospital, seeking professional services, he asked to speak to a doctor. Ms. Smith asked him what the problem was. A reasonable person in defendant's position could have believed he had to tell her his problem in order to get past her to talk to a doctor. In this circumstance, we believe that she was an assistant employed in the process of communication and thus was a person "reasonably necessary for the transmission of the communication," under OEC 504(1)(a). Defendant's statements to her are included within the scope of the psychotherapist-patient privilege. It was error to admit them at trial.

II. Harmless Error

The next inquiry is whether the error in admitting the testimony of the psychiatrist and secretary-receptionist was prejudicial. * * *

* * *

[A]fter review of the record, even absent the testimony of the secretary-receptionist and the psychiatrist, we are satisfied that there was substantial and convincing evidence of defendant's guilt, and we find there was very little, if any, likelihood that the evidential error affected the trial court's decision.

* * *

The decision of the Court of Appeals is affirmed.

Questions and Comments

1. *Rules of evidence.* Proposed Fed.R.Evid., Rule 504, discussed in *State v. Miller,* was eliminated from the Rules as finally adopted. As originally drafted, the Federal Rules of Evidence embodied specific testimonial privileges including the psychotherapist-patient privilege found in 504. See, Proposed Rules, 56 F.R.D. 183, 230–261 (1972). Congress, however, rejected the privilege rules approved by the Supreme Court and instead adopted Fed.R.Evid., Rule 501 which reads as follows:

> Except as otherwise required by the Constitution of the United States or provided by Act of Congress or in rules prescribed by the Supreme Court pursuant to statutory authority, the privilege of a witness, person, government, State, or political subdivision thereof shall be governed by the principles of the common law as they may be interpreted by the courts of the United States in the light of reason and

experience. However, in civil actions and proceedings, with respect to an element of a claim or defense as to which State law supplies the rule of decision, the privilege of a witness, person, government, State or political subdivision thereof shall be determined in accordance with State law.

As is indicated by the language of Rule 501, federal courts are to defer to state privilege rules in diversity cases; thus, the rule's applicability is primarily limited to federal criminal actions. In those situations where Rule 501 does control, courts are to look to federal common law in deciding whether to recognize a claimed privilege.

After Rule 501's adoption, the Courts of Appeals which considered the question refused to recognize a psychotherapist-patient privilege. See *United States v. Lindstrom,* 698 F.2d 1154 (11th Cir.1983); *United States v. Meagher,* 531 F.2d 752 (5th Cir.1976), cert. denied, 429 U.S. 853, 90 S.Ct. 146, 50 L.Ed.2d 128 (1976); *United States v. Witt,* 542 F.Supp. 696 (S.D.N.Y. 1982), affirmed, 697 F.2d 301 (2d Cir.1982). In 1983, however, the Court of Appeals for the Sixth Circuit held that the privilege should be recognized. *In re Zuniga,* 714 F.2d 632 (6th Cir.1983), cert. denied, 464 U.S. 983, 104 S.Ct. 426, 78 L.Ed.2d 361 (1983). The court concluded that the psychotherapist-patient privilege was "mandated by 'reason and experience.'" Id. at 639.

c. Scope of the Privilege: Communications Made in the Presence of Others

STATE v. ANDRING
Supreme Court of Minnesota, 1984.
342 N.W.2d 128.

WAHL, JUSTICE.

Defendant David Gerald Andring is charged with three counts of criminal sexual conduct in the second degree in violation of Minn.Stat. § 609.343 (1982). The two complaints setting out these counts allege that defendant had sexual contact with his 10–year–old stepdaughter and his 11–year–old niece. A hearing was held to consider a probable cause challenge to the complaints. Probable cause was found. Defendant was released on bond, pending trial, on condition that he have no contact with the alleged victims.

Defendant voluntarily entered the Crisis Intervention Unit at Bethesda Lutheran Medical Center (crisis unit) after the probable cause hearing but before trial. A social history of defendant was taken by a registered nurse; the admitting diagnosis was acute alcoholism and depression. During his stay, defendant received one-on-one counseling with staff physicians and other medical personnel. He also participated in a daily 2–hour group therapy session with other patients in the crisis unit, sessions which were supervised by physicians and registered nurses. Those present at the group therapy sessions were informed that such sessions were confidential and that only the staff would have access to information disclosed in the sessions. Defendant related his experience of sexual conduct with young girls (1) during one-on-one counseling sessions with registered nurses and a medical student, (2) during the taking of his social history with a registered nurse, and (3) during group therapy sessions.[1]

The state, in the course of its investigation of the case, learned of inculpatory disclosures made by defendant at the crisis unit. The state then moved for discovery and disclosure of defendant's medical records and statements made to crisis unit personnel. No request for disclosure from non-staff participants in the group therapy sessions was made. The trial court, after an extensive inquiry into the ramifications of the state's motion, denied the state's motion for discovery of statements made by defendant during the taking of his social history and during one-on-one therapy but granted the motion for discovery of defendant's disclosures made during group therapy sessions.

Considering the issue of confidentiality of group therapy disclosures as both important and doubtful, the trial court certified the following question to this court:

> Whether the scope of the physician-patient and/or registered nurse-patient privilege is to be extended to prevent disclosures of communications concerning Defendant's sexual conduct with minor children during group therapy sessions, a crime for which he has already been charged, where such group therapy sessions are an integral and necessary part of Defendant's diagnosis and treatment and consist of physicians and/or registered nurses and other patients, who participate in said group therapy sessions and are an aid to Defendant's diagnosis and treatment as well as their own, i.e., are such patients to be considered as agents of the physicians and/or registered nurses and/or do such patients come within the meaning of "being reasonably necessary for the accomplishment of the purpose of such a communication" so as to render the relationship confidential?

* * *

We now reach the question as to whether confidential group therapy sessions which are an integral and necessary part of a patient's diagnosis and treatment are to be included within the scope of the medical privilege. The troublesome aspect of this question lies in the fact that third parties, other patients and participants in the therapy, are present at the time the information is disclosed. Does their presence destroy the privilege?

McCormick, in discussing the issue of whether the presence of third parties renders a statement to a physician nonprivileged, argues that the court should analyze the problem in terms of whether the third persons are necessary and customary participants in the consultation or treatment and whether the communications were confidential for the purpose of aiding in diagnosis and treatment. McCormick's Handbook of the Law of Evidence, § 101 (E. Cleary 2d ed. 1972). Under this

---

1. The trial court found no reason to believe that any minor children other than defendant's stepdaughter and niece were involved in any of defendant's disclosures to the crisis unit's personnel.

approach, we conclude that the medical privilege must be construed to encompass statements made in group psychotherapy. The participants in group psychotherapy sessions are not casual third persons who are strangers to the psychiatrist/psychologist/nurse-patient relationship. Rather, every participant has such a relationship with the attending professional, and, in the group therapy setting, the participants actually become part of the diagnostic and therapeutic process for co-participants.

This point is more fully developed in Cross, *Privileged Communications Between Participants in Group Psychotherapy,* 1970 L. & Soc.Order 191, 196–98, 200–01 (1970):

> [T]he chief characteristic of group therapy that distinguishes it from individual analysis is that each patient becomes the therapeutic agent of the others * * *. Effective social interaction within the group is therefore a crucial prerequisite to group therapy. The type of interaction required can only be achieved, however, when group members respond to each other spontaneously, both in their speech and their actions * * *. No group participant would make himself vulnerable to community scorn and loss of spouse, job, or freedom by placing his most secret thoughts before the group, unless he could be assured of confidentiality. * * * [S]ociety should certainly foster a relationship that has an important prophylactic effect and thus shields both society and the patient from the consequences of antisocial behavior. * * * [A]lthough there may be occasional losses [of relevant important information] such sporadic occurrences are overshadowed by the potential destruction of the therapeutic relationship.

An interpretation which excluded group therapy from the scope of the psychotherapist-patient privilege would seriously limit the effectiveness of group psychotherapy as a therapeutic device. This would be particularly unfortunate because group therapy is a cost-effective method of psychotherapy in that it allows the therapist to treat a number of patients at the same time. It is also more effective with some patients, who, upon hearing other people reveal their innermost thoughts, are less reluctant to reveal their own. Many commentators agree that the psychotherapist-patient privilege should be extended to include group therapy. *See e.g.,* Smith, *Constitutional Privacy in Psychotherapy,* 49 Geo.Wash.L.Rev. 1, 51–52 (1980); Comment, *The Psychotherapist–Patient Privilege in Texas,* 18 Hous.L.Rev. 137, 161–62 (1980); 2 D. Louisell & C. Mueller, Federal Evidence § 216 (1978); Cross, *Privileged Communications Between Participants in Group Psychotherapy,* 1970 L. & Soc.Order 191. Because the confidentiality of communications made during group therapy is essential in maintaining its effectiveness as a therapeutic tool, we answer the certified question in the affirmative. We hold that the scope of the physician-patient/medical privilege extends to include confidential group psychotherapy sessions where such sessions are an integral and necessary part of a patient's diagnosis and treatment. We reverse the order of the trial court allowing disclosure of defendant's statements made during group therapy.

Certified question answered in the affirmative.

Reversed.

Questions and Comments

1. *Casual third party rule.* It is unclear to what extent multiple-person interactions are protected by the rules of privileged communication. If a "casual third party" is present during communications between patient and therapist, then such communications usually are not privileged. There is a presumption that the patient did not intend that the information remain confidential. Thus, persons in group therapy appear to be unprotected from other group members who may, without malice, reveal problems discussed during therapy to outsiders. (However, "the therapist may have aides present without destroying the confidential nature of the communication"). Schwitzgebel & Schwitzgebel, *Law and Psychological Practice* (New York: John Wiley & Sons, Inc., 1980).

2. *Marriage counselors.* Marriage counselors as well as psychotherapists in general are increasingly resorting to co-joint therapy of both the husband and wife. As a result, in some therapy sessions both spouses may be present. This practice presents a particular problem in terms of confidentiality, particularly where the parties may later be involved in litigation against each other such as in a divorce proceeding. To what extent, for instance, are decisions made during a therapy session in the presence of a spouse privileged? Under the traditional test no privilege would attach to prevent a spouse from testifying as to the communications made during a therapy session. At least one state (Colorado) has enacted legislation which

> prohibits the questioning of any persons who have participated in group therapy sessions "concerning any knowledge gained during the course of such therapy without the consent of the person or persons to whom the testimony sought relates."

Schwitzgebel at 209.

3. *Contracting around third party rules.* It has been suggested that disclosures by patient members of joint therapy groups could be controlled by having the members of the group enter into a contract prior to the commencement of the sessions binding each signatory to preserve the confidentiality of the sessions. See, Schwitzgebel at 209. It is not certain, however, that such contract could be enforced to prevent disclosure in a court proceeding. See also, Note, *Group Therapy and Privileged Communications,* 43 Ind.L.J. 93 (1967).

3. Waiver of the Privilege

A common element of psychotherapist-patient privilege is that its purpose is to protect the *patient's* interest in confidentiality. It is the patient, not the therapist, who is injured by compulsory public disclosure, for the patient is thereby deterred either from seeking needed treatment or from confiding fully during therapy. Privilege, therefore, belongs to the patient, not to the therapist, and a patient's assertion or waiver of privilege is binding upon the therapist. That is, if a patient asserts privilege, the therapist may not be compelled to testify, nor may he voluntarily testify concerning confidential communications. Similarly, if a patient waives privilege, the therapist may not invoke the privilege to refuse to testify.

A patient must assert or waive privilege when a party to litigation seeks to compel disclosure of confidential information. A litigant may compel testimony from the patient or from the psychotherapist by obtaining a subpoena issued by the court, and he may compel production of a psychotherapist's records by obtaining a subpoena *duces tecum*. The patient need not be a party to the litigation to assert the privilege.

A patient may waive privilege in two ways. First, he may simply fail to assert privilege when confidential information is sought by a party in litigation. That is, the patient may provide the information himself, or he may consent to its acquisition from the therapist. The therapist, however, is under an affirmative duty to assert the privilege for the patient if the patient is not present or is incapable of asserting privilege. Second, a patient may waive privilege by making his mental or emotional condition an element of a claim or defense. This form of waiver is often called the patient-litigant exception to privilege. In some jurisdictions a criminal defendant who raises an insanity defense, for example, may not invoke privilege to bar testimony concerning the results of a psychiatric interview to evaluate his sanity. See, e.g., *People v. Edney* at p. 302, *infra*. Similarly, a patient who initiates a malpractice suit against his therapist may not invoke the privilege to preclude testimony concerning the conduct of therapy. Finally, a patient makes his mental condition an element of a claim, and thereby waives privilege, when he seeks to recover damages for mental or emotional distress allegedly caused by another person's actions.

Generally, courts attempt to limit compulsory disclosures to those elements of the communications which are essential to the issues of a case. The practice reflects recognition of the sensitive nature of the information and accords with a general policy to protect witnesses and litigants from unnecessary harassment.

Privilege persists despite the termination of therapy, even after the patient's death. Although usually only a patient may waive privilege, in some circumstances a patient's personal representative, acting on behalf of the patient, may waive the privilege. Persons who may be granted this authority include the guardian of a mentally incompetent patient and the heirs or persons appointed to manage the estates of a deceased patient. Waiver of privilege after the death of a patient occurs most often in disputes concerning the patient's mental capacity at the time of making a will.

a. Circumstances Leading to Express or Implied Waiver of the Privilege

i. Civil Proceedings

IN RE LIFSCHUTZ

Supreme Court of California, 1970.
2 Cal.3d 415, 85 Cal.Rptr. 829, 467 P.2d 557.

TOBRINER, JUSTICE.

Dr. Joseph E. Lifschutz, a psychiatrist practicing in California, seeks a writ of habeas corpus to secure his release from the custody of the Sheriff of the County of San Mateo. Dr. Lifschutz was imprisoned after he was adjudged in contempt of court for refusing to obey an order of the San Mateo County Superior Court instructing him to answer questions and produce records relating to communications with a former patient. Dr. Lifschutz contends that this underlying court order was invalid as unconstitutionally infringing his personal constitutional right of privacy, his right effectively to practice his profession, and the constitutional privacy rights of his patients. He also attacks the order, or more specifically, the statutory provisions which authorize the compulsion of his testimony in these circumstances, as unconstitutionally denying him the equal protection of the laws since, under California law, clergymen could not be compelled to reveal certain confidential communications under these circumstances.

The instant proceeding arose out of a suit instituted by Joseph F. Housek against John Arabian on June 3, 1968, for damages resulting from an alleged assault. Housek's complaint alleged that the assault caused him "physical injuries, pain, suffering and severe mental and emotional distress." Defendant Abrabian [sic] deposed the plaintiff and during the course of that deposition Housek stated that he had received psychiatric treatment from Dr. Lifschutz over a six-month period approximately 10 years earlier. Nothing in the record indicates that the plaintiff revealed the nature or contents of any conversation with or treatment by Dr. Lifschutz.

Arabian then subpoenaed for deposition Dr. Lifschutz and all of his medical records relating to the treatment of Housek. Although Dr. Lifschutz appeared for the deposition, he refused to produce any of his medical records and refused to answer any questions relating to his treatment of patients; the psychiatrist declined even to disclose whether or not Housek had consulted him or had been his patient.

* * *

[Plaintiff] Housek has neither expressly claimed a psychotherapist-patient privilege, statutory or constitutional, nor expressly waived such a privilege.

In response to the psychiatrist's refusal to cooperate, defendant Arabian moved for an order of the superior court compelling the production of the subpenaed records and the answers to questions on deposition.

Relying on the patient-litigant exception of section 1016 of the Evidence Code, the superior court determined that because the plaintiff, in instituting the pending litigation, had tendered as an issue his mental and emotional condition, the statutory psychotherapist-patient (Evid.Code, § 1014) privilege did not apply. On December 20, 1968, the court therefore ordered Dr. Lifschutz to comply with the subpena and to answer questions posed during deposition. On January 15, 1969, defendant attempted to continue with the deposition of Dr. Lifschutz as ordered by the superior court, but petitioner remained resolute in his refusal to respond or produce records.

* * *

* * * Evidence Code, section 912, subdivision (a), provides that: " * * * the right of any person to claim a privilege provided by Section * * * 1014 (psychotherapist-patient privilege) * * * is waived with respect to a communication protected by such privilege if any holder of the privilege, without coercion, has disclosed a significant part of the communication or has consented to such disclosure made by anyone. Consent to disclosure is manifested by any statement or other conduct of the holder of the privilege indicating his consent to the disclosure, including his failure to claim the privilege in any proceeding in which he has the legal standing and opportunity to claim the privilege."

Since Housek, the holder of the privilege disclosed at a prior deposition that he has consulted Dr. Lifschutz for psychiatric treatment, he has waived whatever privilege he might have had to keep such information confidential. * * *

Defendant contended in the superior court, however, that *any* communication between the plaintiff and Dr. Lifschutz has lost its privileged status because the plaintiff has filed a personal injury action in which he claims recovery for "mental and emotional distress." Defendant relies on section 1016 of the Evidence Code, the patient-litigant exception to the psychotherapist-patient privilege, which provides that: "[t]here is no privilege under this article as to a communication relevant to an issue concerning the mental or emotional condition of the patient if such issue has been tendered by: (a) the patient * * *." To avoid the necessity for further contempt proceedings or delaying appellate review in the instant case, we have considered whether defendant has accurately identified the proper reach of the patient-litigant exception.

As we explain more fully below, the patient-litigant exception allows only a limited inquiry into the confidences of the psychotherapist-patient relationship, compelling disclosure of only those matters directly relevant to the nature of the specific "emotional or mental" condition which the patient has voluntarily disclosed and tendered in his pleadings or in answer to discovery inquiries. Furthermore, even when confidential information falls within this exception, trial courts, because of the intimate and potentially embarrassing nature of such communications, may utilize the protective measures at their disposal to avoid unwarranted intrusions into the confidences of the relationship.

In interpreting this exception we are necessarily mindful of the justifiable expectations of confidentiality that most individuals seeking psychotherapeutic treatment harbor. As has been aptly pointed out by Judge Edgerton in *Taylor v. United States* (1955) 95 U.S.App.D.C. 373, 222 F.2d 398, 401 (quoting from Guttmacher, M., et al., Psychiatry and the Law (1952) p. 272), " 'The psychiatric patient confides more utterly than anyone else in the world. He exposes to the therapist not only what his words directly express; he lays bare his entire self, his dreams, his fantasies, his sins, and his shame. Most patients who undergo psychotherapy know that this is what will be expected of them, and that they cannot get help except on that condition. * * * It would be too much to expect them to do so if they knew that all they say—and all that the psychiatrist learns from what they say—may be revealed to the whole world from a witness stand.' "

We believe that a patient's interest in keeping such confidential revelations from public purview, in retaining this substantial privacy, has deeper roots than the California statute and draws sustenance from our constitutional heritage.

                              *   *   *

Dr. Lifschutz presents a novel challenge, attempting to raise far-reaching questions of constitutional law. From the affidavits and correspondence included in the record we note that a large segment of the psychiatric profession concurs in Dr. Lifschutz's strongly held belief that an absolute privilege of confidentiality is essential to the effective practice of psychotherapy.

We recognize the growing importance of the psychiatric profession in our modern, ultracomplex society. The swiftness of change—economic, cultural, and moral—produces accelerated tensions in our society, and the potential for relief of such emotional disturbances offered by psychotherapy undoubtedly establishes it as a profession essential to the preservation of societal health and well-being. Furthermore, a growing consensus throughout the country, reflected in a trend of legislative enactments, acknowledges that an environment of confidentiality of treatment is vitally important to the successful operation of psychotherapy. California has embraced this view through the enactment of a broad, protective psychotherapist-patient privilege.

The nature of the actual interests involved in this case can only be properly evaluated against the California statutory background. Although petitioner, in pressing for judicial acceptance of a genuine and deeply held principle, seeks to cast the issue involved in this case in the broadest terms, we must properly address, in reality, a question of more modest dimensions. We do not face the alternatives of enshrouding the patient's communication to the psychotherapist in the black veil of absolute privilege or of exposing it to the white glare of absolute publicity. Our choice lies, rather, in the grey area.

Properly viewed, the broadest issue before our court is whether the Legislature, in attempting to accommodate the conceded need of confidentiality in the psychotherapeutic process with general societal needs of access to information for the ascertainment of truth in litigation, has unconstitutionally weighted its resolution in favor of disclosure by providing that a psychotherapist may be compelled to reveal relevant confidences of treatment when the patient tenders his mental or emotional condition in issue in litigation. For the reasons discussed below, we conclude that, under a properly limited interpretation, the litigant-patient exception to the psychotherapist-patient privilege, at issue in this case, does not unconstitutionally infringe the constitutional rights of privacy of either psychotherapists or psychotherapeutic patients. As we point out, however, because of the potential of invasion of patients' constitutional interests, trial courts should properly and carefully control compelled disclosures in this area in the light of accepted principles.

* * *

The primary contention of Dr. Lifschutz's attack on the judgment of contempt consists of the assertion of a constitutional right of a psychotherapist to absolute confidentiality in his communications with, and treatment of, patients. Although, as we understand it, the alleged right draws its substance primarily from the psychological needs and expectations of patients, Dr. Lifschutz claims that the Constitution grants him an absolute right to refuse to disclose such confidential communications, regardless of the wishes of a patient in a particular case.

[The court held that the privilege is that of the patient and that a psychotherapist has no constitutional right to assert the privilege in his own behalf.]

* * *

The second basis of petitioner's contention raises a more serious problem. Petitioner claims that if the state is authorized to compel disclosure of some psychotherapeutic communications, psychotherapy can no longer be practiced successfully. He asserts that the unique nature of psychotherapeutic treatment, involving a probing of the patient's subconscious thoughts and emotions, requires an environment of total confidentiality and absolute trust. Petitioner claims that unless a psychotherapist can truthfully assure his patient that all revelations will be held in strictest confidence and never disclosed, patients will be inhibited from participating fully in the psychotherapeutic process and proper treatment will be impossible. Petitioner concludes that the patient-litigation exception involved here conflicts with the preservation of an environment of absolute confidentiality and unconstitutionally constricts the field of medical practice.

Petitioner's argument, resting as it does on assertions of medical necessity, exemplifies the type of question to which the judiciary brings little expertise. Although petitioner has submitted affidavits of psychotherapists who concur in his assertion that total confidentiality is essential to the practice of their profession, we cannot blind ourselves to the fact that the practice of psychotherapy has grown, indeed flourished, in an environment of a non-absolute privilege. No state in the country recognizes as broad a privilege as petitioner claims is constitutionally compelled. Whether psychotherapy's development has progressed only because patients are ignorant of the existing legal environment can only be a matter for speculation; psychotherapists certainly have been aware of the limitations of their recognized privilege for some time.

Petitioner's broad assertion, moreover, overlooks the limited nature of the intrusion into psychotherapeutic privacy actually at issue in this case. As we explain more fully in part III infra, the patient-litigant exception of section 1016 of the Evidence Code compels disclosure of only those matters which the patient himself has chosen to reveal by tendering them in litigation. We do not know, of course, to what extent patients are deterred from seeking psychotherapeutic treatment by the knowledge that if, at some future date, they choose to place some aspect of their mental condition in issue in litigation, communications relevant to that issue may be revealed. We can only surmise that an understanding of the limits of section 1016, and the realization that the patient retains control over subsequent disclosure, may provide a measure of reassurance to the prospective patient.

* * *

In previous physician-patient privilege cases the exception [to the privilege of confidentiality] has been generally applied only to compel disclosure of medical treatment and communication concerning the very injury or impairment that was the subject matter of the litigation. There is certainly nothing to suggest that in the context of the more liberal psychotherapist-patient privilege this exception should be given a broader reading.

If the provision had as broad an effect as is suggested by petitioner, it might effectively deter many psychotherapeutic patients from instituting any general claim for mental suffering and damage out of fear of opening up all past communications to discovery. This result would clearly be an intolerable and overbroad intrusion into the patient's privacy, not sufficiently limited to the legitimate state interest embodied in the provision and would create opportunities for harassment and blackmail.

In light of these considerations, the "automatic" waiver of privilege contemplated by section 1016 must be construed not as a complete waiver of the privilege but only as a limited waiver concomitant with the purposes of the exception. Under section 1016 disclosure can be compelled only with respect to *those mental conditions* the patient-litigant has "disclose[d] * * * by bringing an action in which *they* are in issue" communications which are not directly relevant to those specific conditions do not fall within the terms of section 1016's exception and therefore remain privileged. Disclosure cannot be compelled with respect to other aspects of the patient-litigant's personality even though they may, in some sense, be "relevant" to the substantive issues of litigation. The patient thus is not obligated to sacrifice all privacy to seek redress for a specific mental or emotional injury; the scope of the inquiry permitted depends upon the nature of the injuries which the patient-litigant himself has brought before the court.

In some situations, the patient's pleadings may clearly demonstrate that his entire mental condition is being placed in issue and that records of past psychotherapy will clearly be relevant.

* * *

In other cases, however, the determination of the specific "mental condition" in issue may present more complex problems. The difficulties involved in analyzing the applicability of the exception in the instant case may be illustrative. The plaintiff's complaint, containing the typical allegations of "mental and emotional distress" arising out of a physical assault, does not specifically identify the nature of the "mental or emotional condition" at issue. In incorporating this allegation in his complaint, plaintiff obviously neither disclosed his entire medical history [of] treatment for mental or emotional conditions nor realistically waived his interest in maintaining the confidentiality of that treatment. The generality of the claim, however, does create the possibility that some feature of plaintiff's psychological history will be directly relevant to the determination of whether his emotional or mental distress can be properly attributed to the alleged assault. Although we doubt that the 10–year–old therapeutic treatment sought to be discovered from Dr. Lifschutz would be sufficiently relevant to a typical claim of "mental distress" to bring it within the exception of section 1016, we cannot determine from the present state of the record whether plaintiff's "mental and emotional" distress is merely the "normal" distress experienced as a result of physical assault or whether it includes unusual or particularly serious elements upon which prior history may be directly relevant.

Because only the patient, and not the party seeking disclosure, knows both the nature of the ailments for which recovery is sought and the general content of the psychotherapeutic communications, the burden rests upon the patient initially to submit some showing that a given confidential communication is not directly related to the issue he has tendered to the court. A patient may have to delimit his claimed "mental or emotional distress" or explain, in general terms, the object of the psychotherapy in order to illustrate that it is not reasonably probable that the psychotherapeutic communications sought are directly relevant to the mental condition that he has placed in issue. In determining whether communications sufficiently relate to the mental condition at issue to require disclosure, the court should heed the basic privacy interests involved in the privilege.

* * *

Inasmuch as plaintiff had already disclosed that he had consulted Dr. Lifschutz for psychotherapeutic treatment, petitioner could not properly have refused to answer at least that question concerning the communications; since neither plaintiff nor the psychotherapist has as yet made any claim that the subpenaed records are not directly relevant to the specific "mental and emotional" injuries for which plaintiff is claiming relief, Dr. Lifschutz had no right to refuse to produce the records. Thus the trial court's order requiring the production of records and the answering of questions was valid; the trial court properly adjudged Dr. Lifschutz in contempt of court for intentionally violating that valid court order.

The order to show cause is discharged and the petition for writ of habeas corpus is denied.

MOSK, Acting C.J., McCOMB, PETERS, BURKE, and SULLIVAN, JJ., and MOLINARI, J. pro tem., concur.

Questions and Comments

1. *Critique of the* Lifschutz *rule. Lifschutz* in effect requires the plaintiff-patient to "disclose at least part of the contents of protected communications to his lawyer and the trial judge as a condition to retaining its confidentiality of the communication." *Caesar v. Mountanos,* 542 F.2d 1064, 1075 (9th Cir.1976). This result has been criticized because it forces a plaintiff who wants to preserve confidentiality to elect either to make partial disclosure or possibly forego recovery for mental distress. Some, like Judge Hufstedler of the Ninth Circuit Court of Appeals, would avoid this problem by restricting compelled disclosures in a personal injury action to "the fact of treatment, the time and length of treatment, the cost of treatment, and the ultimate diagnosis unless the party seeking disclosure establishes in the trial court a compelling need for its production." *Caesar v. Mountanos,* 542 F.2d 1064, 1075 (9th Cir.1976), (Hufstedler, J., concurring and dissenting).

2. *Patient's waiver not absolute.* As noted in *In re Lifschutz,* the testimonial privilege belongs to the patient. Once the patient has waived the privilege, the psychiatrist or other mental health professional does not have standing to challenge that waiver. However, in some states, parties other than the patient have been given standing to challenge the waiver.

For instance, under New York law anyone having official custody of psychiatric records, such as "a treating hospital, physician or other institution" may request a protective order on the grounds that disclosure of all or part of the record "may be seriously detrimental to the interest of the patient, to uninvolved third parties, or to an important program of the custodian of the record." If granted, such protective order serves to immunize the records from disclosure "notwithstanding a valid waiver of the physician-patient privilege by the patient." See *Cynthia B. v. New Rochelle Hosp. Med. Ctr.,* 60 N.Y.2d 452, 470 N.Y.S.2d 122, 458 N.E.2d 363,

365 (1983). In the New Rochelle Hospital case the plaintiff/patient who was a litigant in a civil suit had waived the privilege. The facility sought a protective order of the psychiatric records on the grounds that "direct and unsupervised disclosure of psychiatric records may cause harm to the patient [plaintiff]." From an appeal of an order requiring disclosure, it was held that the lower court had not abused its discretion in directing unconditional release of the record.

ii. Criminal Proceedings

PEOPLE v. EDNEY
Court of Appeals of New York, 1976.
39 N.Y.2d 620, 385 N.Y.S.2d 23, 350 N.E.2d 400.

GABRIELLI, JUDGE.

Defendant was charged with kidnapping and the brutal killing of the eight-year-old daughter of his former girlfriend. He interposed the defense of insanity.

The jury found defendant guilty, as charged, of manslaughter, first degree and kidnapping in the first and second degrees. He was sentenced to a term of 25 years to life on the first degree kidnapping charge and to concurrent terms of up to 25 years on the other charges. The Appellate Division unanimously affirmed.

The critical and principal issue is whether the testimony of a psychiatrist, who had examined defendant prior to trial at the request of his attorney, was admissible over objections that the physician-patient and attorney-client privilege acted to bar its admission.

At trial, the prosecution showed that late in the afternoon on July 24, 1968, defendant grabbed Lisa Washington, the victim, off the street where she was playing with friends, and forcibly pushed her into a taxicab. At approximately 8:30 p.m., Lisa's aunt, with whom she was residing, received a call from defendant who stated that "If you don't get 'C' [the nickname of Lisa's mother] on the phone in the next couple of hours, I am going to rape and kill Lisa". A barmaid testified that defendant and a young girl were in the Nu–Way Lounge at about 9:30 p.m. and that she observed defendant leave the tavern with the girl, walk around a corner toward the back of the building, and return a short while later without her. Less than an hour later, police officers, responding to a call by a woman who had reported a disturbance in her backyard which adjoined the rear of the Nu–Way Lounge, found Lisa's lifeless body. She had been stabbed 11 times. The police questioned persons in the bar and learned of defendant's presence in the bar earlier in the evening with a little girl.

Defendant was located at his father's home early the next morning and taken into custody. As he was leaving with the officers, he was asked by his father whether he had "hurt that little child", to which he replied "I'm sorry, I'm sorry". Granules of dirt taken from defendant's trousers confirmed that defendant had been in the area behind the Nu–Way Lounge.

Following his arrest, and after receiving the standard preinterrogation admonitions defendant volunteered to a detective that he had been in the Nu–Way Lounge that evening, that he had been hearing voices which told him that God wanted Lisa, and that he might have killed Lisa but he was not sure. Taking the witness stand in his own defense, defendant testified that on the day in question, he had drunk large quantities of alcohol, had been smoking marijuana cigarettes, and that sometime after 9:00 p.m., he and Lisa had left the Nu–Way Lounge to go to his father's place; that he might have killed Lisa but he was not sure he had done so. He recalled walking to a cab across the street from the bar but could remember no more. He explained that he regained consciousness under a tree near his father's home and that he walked inside and blacked out; the next thing he was able to remember was someone pounding on him to wake up because the police were there.

A psychiatrist called by the defense testified that defendant suffered from paranoid schizophrenia of mild severity and that the condition was of long standing. It was his opinion that defendant was mentally ill to such an extent that he was unaware of the nature and quality of his act and did not know that his act was wrong.

In rebuttal, the prosecution called Dr. Daniel Schwartz, a psychiatrist, who originally examined defendant at the behest of defendant's attorney, who was not present during the examination. The defense unsuccessfully objected to his testifying on the ground that the attorney-client and physician-patient privileges barred his testimony. Dr. Schwartz described defendant as having an alcoholic psychosis which occasionally manifested itself through hallucinations and delusions; however, he found no evidence of an underlying disease or defect. It was his opinion that at the time of the murder defendant knew and appreciated the nature of his conduct and knew that such conduct was wrong.

Another rebuttal psychiatrist, who had independently examined the defendant for the prosecution, supported the conclusions of Dr. Schwartz that defendant knew and appreciated the nature of his conduct and that such conduct was wrong.

Two other psychiatrists, produced by the defense as surrebuttal witnesses, each testified that he was unable to form an opinion as to whether defendant knew or appreciated the nature of his acts, or whether such acts were wrong, although they did agree that defendant had some form of mental disease.

People v. Al–Kanani, 33 N.Y.2d 260, 351 N.Y.S.2d 969, 307 N.E.2d 43, is dispositive of the physician-patient privilege claim. There we held "that where insanity is asserted as a defense and * * * the defendant offers evidence tending to show his insanity in support of this plea, a complete waiver is effected, and the prosecution is then permitted to call psychiatric experts to testify regarding his sanity even though they may have treated the defendant. When the patient first fully discloses the evidence of his affliction, it is he who has given the public the full details of his case, thereby disclosing the secrets which the statute was designed to protect, thus creating a waiver removing it from the operation of the statute and once the privilege is thus waived, there is nothing left to protect against for once the revelation is made by the patient there is nothing further to disclose 'for when a secret is out it is out for all time and cannot be caught again like a bird, and put back in its cage. * * * The legislature did not intend to continue the privilege when there was no reason for its continuance and it would simply be an obstruction to public justice.' * * *."

Our holding in the case now before us comports with this rationale and is but a logical extension of our determination in *Al–Kanani*.

Equally unavailing to defendant is the claim that the attorney-client privilege bars admission of Dr. Schwartz' testimony. Essentially, defendant relies on decisions in other jurisdictions which have excluded such testimony apparently because a psychiatrist would inevitably be required to reveal a defendant's statements to him to justify his opinion and because a contrary rule would deter attorneys from freely seeking sound professional advice as to the soundness of an insanity plea. We do not find the reasoning of these cases compelling and, accordingly, do not follow them. Rather, we think the better rationale underlies the *Al–Kanani* rule that a plea of innocence by reason of insanity constitutes a complete and effective waiver by the defendant of any claim of privilege.

A defendant who seeks to introduce psychiatric testimony in support of his insanity plea may be required to disclose prior to trial the underlying basis of his alleged affliction to a prosecution psychiatrist. Hence, where, as here, a defendant reveals to the prosecution the very facts which would be secreted by the exercise of the privilege, reason does not compel the exclusion of expert testimony based on such facts, or cross-examination concerning the grounds for opinions based thereon. It follows that no harm accrues to the defense from seeking pretrial psychiatric advice where an insanity plea is actually entered, for in such circumstances, the underlying factual basis will be revealed to the prosecution psychiatrist. Conversely, were the defendant not to enter an insanity plea, no physician-patient waiver would occur and any information divulged to the psychiatrist would remain privileged. There is, therefore, no deterrent to seeking expert psychiatric advice for, in one instance, there will be disclosure to the prosecution in any event and, in the other, disclosure will never occur. In short, no reason appears why a criminal defendant who puts his sanity in issue should be permitted to thwart the introduction of testimony from a material witness who may be called at trial by invoking the attorney-client privilege anymore than he should be able to do so by invoking the physician-patient privilege.

This is not to say, however, that an attorney cannot consult a psychiatrist in order to obtain advice concerning the efficacy of an insanity plea or, for that matter, any trial strategy, without fear of later courtroom disclosure. The product of such a consultation is protected, of course, by the work product doctrine (see CPLR 3101). However, that doctrine affords protection only to facts and observations disclosed *by the attorney*. Thus, it is the information and observations of the attorney that are conveyed to the expert which may thus be subject to trial exclusion. The work product doctrine does not operate to insulate other disclosed information from public exposure.

It is significant that the underlying purpose of the attorney-client privilege would not be diminished by the admission of the testimony of Dr. Schwartz. The privilege is grounded in the salutary policy of encouraging "persons needing professional advice to disclose freely the facts in reference to which they seek advice, without fear that such facts will be made public to their disgrace or detriment by their attorney" * * * That policy is not harmed, however, by the admission of evidence which, in any event, in these circumstances would be available to the prosecution. Indeed, with respect to the testimony of Dr. Schwartz, it is readily apparent that the traditional and statutory requirements of an attorney-client relationship were simply not established (CPLR 4503, subd. [a]). We hold, therefore, that the privilege was inapplicable.

We find no merit in defendant's other contentions.

Accordingly, the order of the Appellate Division should be affirmed.

[The dissenting opinion of Judge Fuchsberg is omitted.]

STATE v. PRATT

Court of Appeals of Maryland, 1979.
284 Md. 516, 398 A.2d 421.

DIGGES, JUDGE.

The question presented by this criminal cause is one of first impression in this State, and yet, it involves "the oldest of the privileges for confidential communications"—that which exists between an attorney and his client. Stated succinctly, we are asked to decide whether this privilege was violated when, over objection, a psychiatrist, who was retained by defense counsel to examine his client in preparing an insanity defense, was permitted to testify at the instance of the prosecution. Because we conclude that this fundamental privilege was invaded, we will direct a new trial.

The factual background here is uncomplicated and may be briefly related. On the morning of October 23, 1976, respondent Margaret

Melton Pratt, after a sleepless night during which she contemplated the taking of her own life, shot and killed her still-slumbering husband, William S. Pratt, in their Montgomery County apartment. After the shooting, the wife packed an overnight bag and drove to a friend's farm near Front Royal, Virginia, to visit the gravesite of her dog; she stayed several hours and then proceeded to a nearby motel to spend the night. The next morning Mrs. Pratt returned to her home and, after a short stay there, began driving aimlessly around the Bethesda–Rockville area. Realizing she would eventually be apprehended, the respondent went to the Montgomery County police and informed them of her husband's death. The officers, after verifying Mrs. Pratt's story concerning what had taken place, arrested her for murder.

Upon being indicted by the grand jury for murder and related offenses, the respondent entered pleas of not guilty and interposed a defense of insanity at the time of the commission of the alleged crimes. Thereafter, the Circuit Court for Montgomery County, ordered that the Department of Health and Mental Hygiene conduct a mental examination of Mrs. Pratt to determine her "sanity or insanity at the present time and at the time of the commission of the crime, and * * * her competenc[y] to stand trial at the present time * * *." After an examination, the department, by its report dated December 30, 1976, informed the court that Mrs. Pratt was presently competent to stand trial and was sane at the time of the commission of the alleged offenses. Trial on the indictment began on April 18, 1977, and three days later the jury found Mrs. Pratt was sane at the time of the commission of the alleged crimes and guilty of both murder in the second degree and the use of a handgun in the commission of a felony.

Throughout the trial, Mrs. Pratt did not dispute that she had killed her husband but, instead, strenuously urged that she was insane at the time she fired the fatal shots. In support of her insanity plea, respondent presented two psychiatrists, Dr. Gerald Polin and Dr. Leon Yochelson, who testified that at the time of the act Mrs. Pratt was, in their opinion, suffering from a mental illness of such severity that she lacked substantial capacity to conform her conduct to the requirements of the law. In rebuttal, the State produced three psychiatrists, all of whom agreed that the respondent was suffering from some degree of mental disorder when the shooting took place. Nonetheless, two of these medical experts testified that, under Maryland law, Mrs. Pratt was legally responsible for her act. Of these two, one, Dr. Brian Crowley, had examined the accused at the request of her attorney after being retained by him to aid in preparing support for Mrs. Pratt's insanity plea. It is the evidence given by Dr. Crowley, who testified during the trial at the request of the State and over the objection of the defense, that precipitated the controversy now before us. On appeal to the Court of Special Appeals, that court concluded that the permitting of Dr. Crowley's testimony violated the attorney-client privilege and ordered a new trial. We agree.

In this State the attorney-client privilege, * * * is a rule of evidence that forever bars disclosure, without the consent of the client, of all communications that pass in confidence between the client and his attorney during the course of professional employment or as an incident of professional intercourse between them.

* * * While never given an explicit constitutional underpinning, the privilege is, nevertheless, closely tied to the federal, as well as this State's, constitutional guarantees of effective assistance of counsel and could, if limited too severely, make these basic guarantees virtually meaningless.

Initially we observe that, given the complexities of modern existence, few if any lawyers could, as a practical matter, represent the interest of their clients without a variety of nonlegal assistance. Recognizing this limitation, it is now almost universally accepted in this country that the scope of the attorney-client privilege, at least in criminal causes, embraces those agents whose services are required by the attorney in order that he may properly prepare his client's case. Consequently, in line with the views of the vast majority of the courts in our sister jurisdictions, we have no hesitancy in concluding that in criminal causes communications made by a defendant to an expert in order to equip that expert with the necessary information to provide the defendant's attorney with the tools to aid him in giving his client proper legal advice are within the scope of the attorney-client privilege.

This is uniquely so in cases concerning the question of a criminal defendant's sanity, because the need of an attorney to consult with a qualified medical expert is paramount. Such a medical expert not only provides testimony that usually is necessary at trial to support an insanity defense, but also "attunes the lay attorney to unfamiliar but central medical concepts and enables him, as an initial matter, to assess the soundness and advisability of offering the defense * * * and perhaps most importantly, * * * permits a lawyer inexpert in the science of psychiatry to probe intelligently the foundations of adverse testimony."

The State here does not dispute the inclusion of psychiatric communications within the scope of the attorney-client privilege; instead, it contends that when Mrs. Pratt interposed a defense of insanity, she waived the privilege with respect to all statements she may have made to any medical expert, whether in her employ or in that of the State. While there is little doubt that a client may waive this right to confidentiality, which may be done either expressly or impliedly, we have been made aware of only one decision in which a court, the New York Court of Appeals, has held that raising the defense of insanity, without more, is a relinquishment of the attorney-client privilege as to communications between the client and his alienist. In its opinion the court justified its conclusion that a defendant's insanity plea waived the attorney-client privilege on the following basis:

A defendant who seeks to introduce psychiatric testimony in support of his insanity plea may be required to disclose prior to trial the underlying basis of his alleged affliction to a prosecution psychiatrist. Hence, where, as here, a defendant reveals to the prosecution the very facts which would be secreted by the exercise of the privilege, reason does not compel the exclusion of expert testimony based on such facts, or cross-examination concerning the grounds for opinions based thereon. It follows that no harm accrues to the defense from seeking pretrial psychiatric advice where an insanity plea is actually entered, for in such circumstances, the underlying factual basis will be revealed to the prosecution psychiatrist. [*People v. Edney,* 39 N.Y.2d 620, 625, 385 N.Y.S.2d 23, 26, 350 N.E.2d 400, 403 (1976).]

While there appears to be some logic, at least in a technical sense, to New York's highest court's reasoning, nonetheless we find that the chilling effect such a result would have upon a client's willingness to confide in his attorney or any defense-employed consultants requires that we align ourselves with the overwhelming body of authority and reject that court's conclusion.

Moreover, a further drawback to the New York rule is the prejudice inherent in disclosing to the trier of fact that the source of this adverse testimony is an expert originally employed by the defendant. This factor will almost certainly carry added weight with the jury, which usually is the prosecution's principal purpose for producing the defense-employed psychiatrist as a witness. Note, *Protecting the Confidentiality of Pretrial Psychiatric Disclosures: A Survey of Standards,* 51 N.Y.U.L.Rev. 409, 411 (1976).

* * *

An additional consequence of the State's suggested waiver rule, if adopted by us, is that the defense, in essence, would be required to assist the prosecution in discharging its burden of proof. In Maryland, as in most other jurisdictions, the government not only bears the burden of showing that the defendant perpetrated the alleged criminal act, but, once the sanity of the accused has been placed in doubt by the defense, it is also saddled with the ultimate burden of proving, beyond a reasonable doubt, that the defendant was sane at the time he committed the act.

* * *

If, in its efforts to establish the mental responsibility of the accused following a plea of insanity, the State is permitted to utilize a psychiatrist hired by the defendant, both the defense attorney and his client will be inhibited from "consulting one or more experts, with possibly conflicting views, by the fear that in doing so [they] may be assisting the government in meeting its burden of proof on the [sanity] issue." Breaching the attorney-client privilege in this situation also would have the effect of inhibiting the free exercise of a defense attorney's informed judgment by confronting him with the likelihood that, in taking a step obviously crucial to his client's defense, he is creating a potential government witness who theretofore did not exist. The possible impact upon the federal and State constitutional rights of the defendant of a rule permitting such testimony further persuades us that we should be reluctant to hold there is a waiver, under the circumstances here, of the attorney-client privilege.

Accordingly, we affirm the judgment of the Court of Special Appeals, which comports with the ruling we make here.

Questions and Comments

A psychiatrist called upon to examine a criminal defendant on the issue of the defendant's sanity at the time of the offense may have performed the examination at the request of the defendant, the prosecutor, or the court. In the latter case the examiner is treated as an "independent" expert. Particularly complex Fifth and Sixth Amendment issues are raised when the prosecutor seeks to introduce evidence based on a psychiatric interview conducted by a court-appointed expert. The issues raised by such use are treated in the materials beginning in Chapter Six. What effect should a waiver made by the defendant in a criminal proceeding have in a subsequent civil suit? Compare *Novak v. Rathnam,* 106 Ill.2d 478, 88 Ill.Dec. 608, 478 N.E.2d 1334 (1985) with *Simpson v. Braider,* 104 F.R.D. 512 (D.D.C.1985). In *Novak,* the defendant, Rathnam, discharged Endicott from a mental health facility in Illinois. Endicott traveled to Florida where he shot and killed Novak's daughter. At his Florida murder trial Endicott called four psychiatrists, including Rathnam, in successfully asserting insanity as a defense. Thereafter, Novak filed a wrongful death action in Illinois alleging that Rathnam was negligent in approving Endicott's discharge. Rathnam refused to permit Novak to depose him, arguing that any information about his treatment of Endicott was privileged by state statute. The Illinois Supreme Court rejected Rathnam's claim that he could not testify unless Endicott waived the privilege. The court held that "[i]f there is a disclosure of confidential information by the individual for whose benefit the privilege exists, or if he permits such a disclosure, the privilege is waived and cannot be reasserted." 478 N.E.2d at 1337.

In contrast, the district court in *Simpson v. Braider* focused on the context of the defendant's disclosures in the criminal proceeding. "[T]hese revelations [about the defendant's history of mental health treatment] in the Superior Court criminal case, since they were made in defense of criminal charges, cannot be truly considered voluntary. There Justin Braider was an accused, a defendant, and these revelations were made only to protect his interests in that proceeding. These were not revelations undertaken on his own initiative, where he sought advantage such as where a person seeks to use information to obtain an advantage, but then invokes the privilege to preclude the adversary from challenging a claim." The district court concluded that no waiver should be implied from "circumstances indicating there was realistically no voluntary disclosure." 104 F.R.D. at 522–23.

Which is the better view? Does the passage from *People v. Al–Kanani,* quoted in *People v. Edney,* supra, implicitly reject the rationale articulated by the court in *Simpson v. Braider?*

4. Confrontation Clause Limitations on the Testimonial Privilege

PENNSYLVANIA v. RITCHIE

Supreme Court of the United States, 1987.
480 U.S. 39, 107 S.Ct. 989, 94 L.Ed.2d 40.

JUSTICE POWELL announced the judgment of the Court and delivered the opinion of the Court with respect to Parts I, II, III–B, III–C, and IV, and an opinion with respect to Part III–A in which THE CHIEF JUSTICE, JUSTICE WHITE, and JUSTICE O'CONNOR join.

The question presented in this case is whether and to what extent a State's interest in the confidentiality of its investigative files concerning child abuse must yield to a criminal defendant's Sixth and Fourteenth Amendment right to discover favorable evidence.

I

As part of its efforts to combat child abuse, the Commonwealth of Pennsylvania has established Children and Youth Services (CYS), a protective service agency charged with investigating cases of suspected mistreatment and neglect. In 1979, respondent George Ritchie was charged with rape, involuntary deviate sexual intercourse, incest, and corruption of a minor. The victim of the alleged attacks was his 13–year–old daughter, who claimed that she had been assaulted by Ritchie two or three times per week during the previous four years. The girl reported the incidents to the police, and the matter then was referred to the CYS.

During pretrial discovery, Ritchie served CYS with a subpoena, seeking access to the records concerning the daughter. Ritchie requested disclosure of the file related to the immediate charges, as well as certain records that he claimed were compiled in 1978, when CYS investigated a separate report by an unidentified source that Ritchie's children were being abused. CYS refused to comply with the subpoena, claiming that the records were privileged under Pennsylvania law. The relevant statute provides that all reports and other information obtained in the course of a CYS investigation must be kept confidential, subject to 11 specific exceptions.[2] One of those exceptions is that the Agency may disclose the reports to a "court of competent jurisdiction pursuant to a court order." Pa.Stat.Ann., Title 11, § 2215(a)(5) (Purdon Supp.1986).

---

2. The statute provides in part:

"(a) Except as provided in section 14 [Pa. Stat.Ann., Title 11, § 2214 (Purdon Supp. 1986)], reports made pursuant to this act including but not limited to report summaries of child abuse * * * and written reports * * * as well as any other information obtained, reports written or photographs or X-rays taken concerning alleged instances of child abuse in the possession of the department, a county children and

youth social service agency or a child protective service shall be confidential and shall only be made available to:

* * *

"(5) A court of competent jurisdiction pursuant to a court order." Pa.Stat.Ann., Title 11, § 2215(a) (Purdon Supp.1986).

At the time of trial the statute only provided five exceptions to the general rule of confidentiality, including the exception for court-ordered disclosure. * * *

Ritchie moved to have CYS sanctioned for failing to honor the subpoena, and the trial court held a hearing on the motion in chambers. Ritchie argued that he was entitled to the information because the file might contain the names of favorable witnesses, as well as other, unspecified exculpatory evidence. He also requested disclosure of a medical report that he believed was compiled during the 1978 CYS investigation. Although the trial judge acknowledged that he had not examined the entire CYS file, he accepted a CYS representative's assertion that there was no medical report in the record.[3] The judge then denied the motion and refused to order CYS to disclose the files.[4]

At trial, the main witness against Ritchie was his daughter. In an attempt to rebut her testimony, defense counsel cross-examined the girl at length, questioning her on all aspects of the alleged attacks, and her reasons for not reporting the incidents sooner. Except for routine evidentiary rulings, the trial judge placed no limitation on the scope of cross-examination. At the close of trial Ritchie was convicted by a jury on all counts, and the judge sentenced him to 3 to 10 years in prison.

On appeal to the Pennsylvania Superior Court, Ritchie claimed, *inter alia,* that the failure to disclose the contents of the CYS file violated the Confrontation Clause of the Sixth Amendment, as applied to the States through the Due Process Clause of the Fourteenth Amendment. The court agreed that there had been a constitutional violation, and accordingly vacated the conviction and remanded for further proceedings. * * *.

On appeal by the Commonwealth, the Supreme Court of Pennsylvania agreed that the conviction must be vacated and the case remanded to determine if a new trial is necessary. * * * [I]t concluded that Ritchie, through his lawyer, is entitled to review the entire file to search for any useful evidence. It stated: "When materials gathered become an arrow of inculpation, the person inculpated has a fundamental constitutional right to examine the provenance of the arrow and he who aims it." The Pennsylvania Court concluded that by denying access to the file, the trial court order had violated both the Confrontation Clause and the Compulsory Process Clause. The court was unpersuaded by the Commonwealth's argument that the trial judge already had examined the file and determined that it contained no relevant information. It ruled that the constitutional infirmity in this trial court's order was that Ritchie was unlawfully denied the opportunity to have the records reviewed by "the eyes and the perspective of an advocate," who may see relevance in places that a neutral judge would not.

In light of the substantial and conflicting interests held by the Commonwealth and Ritchie, we granted certiorari. 476 U.S. ___, 106

---

3. The trial judge stated that he did not read "50 pages or more of an extensive record." The judge had no knowledge of the case before the pretrial hearing.

4. There is no suggestion that the Commonwealth's prosecutor was given access to the file at any point in the proceedings, or that he was aware of its contents.

S.Ct. 2244, 90 L.Ed.2d 690 (1986). We now affirm in part, reverse in part, and remand for proceedings not inconsistent with this opinion.

II

[The plurality opinion rejects the defendant's contention that the Court lacked jurisdiction on the grounds that the decision below was not final.]

III

The Pennsylvania Supreme Court held that Ritchie, through his lawyer, has the right to examine the full contents of the CYS records. The court found that this right of access is required by both the Confrontation Clause and the Compulsory Process Clause. We discuss these constitutional provisions in turn.

A

The Confrontation Clause provides two types of protections for a criminal defendant: the right physically to face those who testify against him, and the right to conduct cross-examination. *Delaware v. Fensterer*, 474 U.S. ___, ___, 106 S.Ct 292, ___, 88 L.Ed.2d 15 (1985) (*per curiam*). Ritchie does not allege a violation of the former right. * * * Instead Ritchie claims that by denying him access to the information necessary to prepare his defense, the trial court interfered with his right of cross-examination.

Ritchie argues that he could not effectively question his daughter because, without the CYS material, he did not know which types of questions would best expose the weaknesses in her testimony. Had the files been disclosed, Ritchie argues that he might have been able to show that the daughter made statements to the CYS counselor that were inconsistent with her trial statements, or perhaps to reveal that the girl acted with an improper motive. * * *

The Pennsylvania Supreme Court accepted this argument, relying in part on our decision in *Davis v. Alaska*, [415 U.S. 308, 94 S.Ct. 1105, 39 L.Ed.2d 347 (1974)]. In *Davis* the trial judge prohibited defense counsel from questioning a witness about the latter's juvenile criminal record, because a state statute made this information presumptively confidential. We found that this restriction on cross-examination violated the Confrontation Clause, despite Alaska's legitimate interest in protecting the identity of juvenile offenders. The Pennsylvania Supreme Court apparently interpreted our decision in *Davis* to mean that a statutory privilege cannot be maintained when a defendant asserts a need, prior to trial, for the protected information that might be used at trial to impeach or otherwise undermine a witness' testimony.

If we were to accept this broad interpretation of *Davis,* the effect would be to transform the Confrontation Clause into a constitutionally-compelled rule of pretrial discovery. Nothing in the case law supports such a view. The opinions of this Court show that the right of confrontation is a *trial* right, designed to prevent improper restrictions on the types of questions that defense counsel may ask during cross-examination. The ability to question adverse witnesses, however, does not include the power to require the pretrial disclosure of any and all information that might be useful in contradicting unfavorable testimony.[9] Normally the right to confront one's accusers is satisfied if defense counsel receives wide latitude at trial to question witnesses. *Delaware v. Fensterer, supra,* 474 U.S., at ___, 106 S.Ct., at ___. In short, the Confrontation Clause only guarantees "an *opportunity* for effective cross-examination, not cross-examination that is effective in whatever way, and to whatever extent, the defense might wish." *Id.,* at ___, 106 S.Ct., at 295 (emphasis in original).

* * *

The lower court's reliance on *Davis v. Alaska* therefore is misplaced. There the state court had prohibited defense counsel from questioning the witness about his criminal record, even though that evidence might have affected the witness' credibility. The constitutional error in that case was *not* that Alaska made this information confidential; it was that the defendant was denied the right "to expose to the jury the facts from which jurors * * * could appropriately draw inferences relating to the reliability of the witness." 415 U.S., at 318, 94 S.Ct., at 1111. Similarly, in this case the Confrontation Clause was not violated by the withholding of the CYS file; it only would have been impermissible for the judge to have prevented Ritchie's lawyer from cross-examining the daughter. Because defense counsel was able to cross-examine all of the trial witnesses fully, we find that the Pennsylvania Supreme Court erred in holding that the failure to disclose the CYS file violated the Confrontation Clause.

B

The Pennsylvania Supreme Court also suggested that the failure to disclose the CYS file violated the Sixth Amendment's guarantee of compulsory process. Ritchie asserts that the trial court's ruling prevented him from learning the names of the "witnesses in his favor," as well as other evidence that might be contained in the file. Although the basis for the Pennsylvania Supreme Court's ruling on this point is unclear, it apparently concluded that the right of compulsory process includes the right to have the State's assistance in uncovering arguably useful information, without regard to the existence of a state-created restriction—here, the confidentiality of the files.

1

This Court has had little occasion to discuss the contours of the Compulsory Process Clause. * * *

9. This is not to suggest, of course, that there are no protections for pretrial discovery in criminal cases. See discussion in Part III(B), *infra.* We simply hold that with respect to this issue, the Confrontation Clause only protects a defendant's trial rights, and does not compel the pretrial production of information that might be useful in preparing for trial. * * *

* * * Instead, the Court traditionally has evaluated claims such as those raised by Ritchie under the broader protections of the Due Process Clause of the Fourteenth Amendment. Because the applicability of the Sixth Amendment to this type of case is unsettled, and because our Fourteenth Amendment precedents addressing the fundamental fairness of trials establish a clear framework for review, we adopt a due process analysis for purposes of this case. Although we conclude that compulsory process provides no *greater* protections in this area than those afforded by due process, we need not decide today whether and how the guarantees of the Compulsory Process Clause differ from those of the Fourteenth Amendment. It is enough to conclude that on these facts, Ritchie's claims more properly are considered by reference to due process.

2

It is well-settled that the Government has the obligation to turn over evidence in its possession that is both favorable to the accused and material to guilt or punishment. Although courts have used different terminologies to define "materiality," a majority of this Court has agreed, "[e]vidence is material only if there is a reasonable probability that, had the evidence been disclosed to the defense, the result of the proceeding would have been different. A 'reasonable probability' is a probability sufficient to undermine confidence in the outcome."

At this stage, of course, it is impossible to say whether any information in the CYS records may be relevant to Ritchie's claim of innocence, because neither the prosecution nor defense counsel has seen the information, and the trial judge acknowledged that he had not reviewed the full file. The Commonwealth, however, argues that no materiality inquiry is required, because a statute renders the contents of the file privileged. Requiring disclosure here, it is argued, would override the Commonwealth's compelling interest in confidentiality on the mere speculation that the file "might" have been useful to the defense.

Although we recognize that the public interest in protecting this type of sensitive information is strong, we do not agree that this interest necessarily prevents disclosure in all circumstances. This is not a case where a state statute grants CYS the absolute authority to shield its files from all eyes. Cf. 42 Pa.Cons.Stat. § 5945.1(b) (unqualified statutory privilege for communications between sexual assault counselors and victims).[14] Rather, the Pennsylvania law provides that the information shall be disclosed in certain circumstances, including when CYS is directed to do so by court order. Given that the Pennsylvania Legislature contemplated *some* use of CYS records in judicial proceedings, we cannot conclude that the statute prevents all disclosure in criminal prosecutions. In the absence of any apparent state policy to

---

14. We express no opinion on whether the result in this case would have been different if the statute had protected the CYS files from disclosure to *anyone,* including law-enforcement and judicial personnel.

the contrary, we therefore have no reason to believe that relevant information would not be disclosed when a court of competent jurisdiction determines that the information is "material" to the defense of the accused.

We therefore affirm the decision of the Pennsylvania Supreme Court to the extent it orders a remand for further proceedings. Ritchie is entitled to have the CYS file reviewed by the trial court to determine whether it contains information that probably would have changed the outcome of his trial. If it does, he must be given a new trial. If the records maintained by CYS contain no such information, or if the nondisclosure was harmless beyond a reasonable doubt, the lower court will be free to reinstate the prior conviction.

C

This ruling does not end our analysis, because the Pennsylvania Supreme Court did more than simply remand. It also held that defense counsel must be allowed to examine all of the confidential information, both relevant and irrelevant, and present arguments in favor of disclosure. The court apparently concluded that whenever a defendant alleges that protected evidence might be material, the appropriate method of assessing this claim is to grant full access to the disputed information, regardless of the State's interest in confidentiality. We cannot agree.

A defendant's right to discover exculpatory evidence does not include the unsupervised authority to search through the Commonwealth's files. Although the eye of an advocate may be helpful to a defendant in ferreting out information, this Court has never held—even in the absence of a statute restricting disclosure—that a defendant alone may make the determination as to the materiality of the information. Settled practice is to the contrary. In the typical case where a defendant makes only a general request for exculpatory material it is the State that decides which information must be disclosed. Unless defense counsel becomes aware that other exculpatory evidence was withheld and brings it to the court's attention, the prosecutor's decision on disclosure is final. Defense counsel has no constitutional right to conduct his own search of the State's files to argue relevance.

We find that Ritchie's interest (as well as that of the Commonwealth) in ensuring a fair trial can be protected fully by requiring that the CYS files be submitted only to the trial court for *in camera* review. Although this rule denies Ritchie the benefits of an "advocate's eye," we note that the trial court's discretion is not unbounded. If a defendant is aware of specific information contained in the file (*e.g.*, the medical report), he is free to request it directly from the court, and argue in favor of its materiality. Moreover, the duty to disclose is ongoing; information that may be deemed immaterial upon original examination may become important as the proceedings progress, and the court would be obligated to release information material to the fairness of the trial.

To allow full disclosure to defense counsel in this type of case would sacrifice unnecessarily the Commonwealth's compelling interest in protecting its child abuse information. If the CYS records were made available to defendants, even through counsel, it could have a seriously adverse effect on Pennsylvania's efforts to uncover and treat abuse. Child abuse is one of the most difficult crimes to detect and prosecute, in large part because there often are no witnesses except the victim. A child's feelings of vulnerability and guilt, and his or her unwillingness to come forward are particularly acute when the abuser is a parent. It therefore is essential that the child have a state-designated person to whom he may turn, and to do so with the assurance of confidentiality. Relatives and neighbors who suspect abuse also will be more willing to come forward if they know that their identities will be protected. Recognizing this, the Commonwealth—like all other States—has made a commendable effort to assure victims and witnesses that they may speak to the CYS counselors without fear of general disclosure. The Commonwealth's purpose would be frustrated if this confidential material had to be disclosed upon demand to a defendant charged with criminal child abuse, simply because a trial court may not recognize exculpatory evidence. Neither precedent nor common sense requires such a result.

IV

We agree that Ritchie is entitled to know whether the CYS file contains information that may have changed the outcome of his trial had it been disclosed. Thus we agree that a remand is necessary. We disagree with the decision of the Pennsylvania Supreme Court to the extent that it allows defense counsel access to the CYS file. An *in camera* review by the trial court will serve Ritchie's interest without destroying the Commonwealth's need to protect the confidentiality of those involved in child-abuse investigations. The decision of the Pennsylvania Supreme Court is affirmed in part, reversed in part, and remanded for further proceedings not inconsistent with this opinion.

It is so ordered.

JUSTICE BLACKMUN, concurring in part and concurring in the judgment.

I join Parts I, II, III–B, III–C, and IV of the Court's opinion. I write separately, however, because I do not accept the plurality's conclusion, as expressed in Part III–A of Justice Powell's opinion, that the Confrontation Clause protects only a defendant's trial rights and has no relevance to pretrial discovery. In this, I am in substantial agreement with much of what Justice Brennan says, *post,* in dissent. In my view, there might well be a confrontation violation if, as here, a defendant is denied pretrial access to information that would make possible effective cross-examination of a crucial prosecution witness.

*   *   *

Despite my disagreement with the plurality's reading of the Confrontation Clause, I am able to concur in the Court's judgment because, in my view, the procedure the Court has set out for the lower court to follow on remand is adequate to address any confrontation problem. Here I part company with Justice Brennan. Under the Court's prescribed procedure, the trial judge is directed to review the CYS file for "material" information. This information would certainly include such evidence as statements of the witness that might have been used to impeach her testimony by demonstrating any bias towards respondent or by revealing inconsistencies in her prior statements. * * *

JUSTICE BRENNAN, with whom JUSTICE MARSHALL joins, dissenting.

I join Justice Stevens' dissenting opinion regarding the lack of finality in this case. I write separately to challenge the Court's narrow reading of the Confrontation Clause as applicable only to events that occur at trial. That interpretation ignores the fact that the right of cross-examination also may be significantly infringed by events occurring outside the trial itself, such as the wholesale denial of access to material that would serve as the basis for a significant line of inquiry at trial. In this case, the trial court properly viewed Ritchie's vague speculations that the agency file might contain something useful as an insufficient basis for permitting general access to the file. However, in denying access to the prior statements of the victim the court deprived Ritchie of material crucial to any effort to impeach the victim at trial. I view this deprivation as a violation of the Confrontation Clause.

* * *

The right of a defendant to confront an accuser is intended fundamentally to provide an opportunity to subject *accusations* to critical scrutiny. Essential to testing a witness' account of events is the ability to compare that version with other versions the witness has earlier recounted. Denial of access to a witness' prior statements thus imposes a handicap that strikes at the heart of cross-examination.

* * *

The Court today adopts an interpretation of the Confrontation Clause unwarranted by previous case law and inconsistent with the underlying values of that constitutional provision. I therefore dissent.

JUSTICE STEVENS, with whom JUSTICE BRENNAN, JUSTICE MARSHALL, and JUSTICE SCALIA join, dissenting.

[Justice Stevens dissented on the grounds that the Court did not have jurisdiction to consider the case because in its present posture it lacked finality.]

Questions and Comments

1. *Absolute v. limited privilege.* As noted by Justice Powell in footnote 14 of *Ritchie,* the plurality opinion does not purport to decide whether the same result would have been reached in the case of an absolute privilege. The absolute privilege given by the plurality as an example, 42 Pa.Cons.Stat.Ann. § 5945.1, provides that a sexual assault counselor has "a

privilege not to be examined as a witness in any civil or criminal proceeding without the prior written consent of the victim being counseled by the counselor as to any confidential communication." Unlike the statute at issue in *Ritchie*, § 5945.1 creates no exceptions. The constitutionality of § 5945.1 has not yet been ruled on by any court.

In Massachusetts, however, where a very similar privilege has been enacted, the state's highest court has held that "in certain circumstances the absolute privilege ∗ ∗ ∗ must yield at trial to the constitutional right of a criminal defendant to have access to privileged communications." *Commonwealth v. Two Juveniles*, 397 Mass. 261, 266, 491 N.E.2d 234, 238 (1986). *See* Mass.Gen.Laws Ann. c. 233, § 20J. Adopting a standard similar to that articulated by the *Ritchie* plurality, the Massachusetts Supreme Judicial Court held that a defendant who demonstrates a legitimate need for otherwise privileged communications is entitled to have the trial court review the communications in camera and disclose to the defense those which are material. *Commonwealth v. Two Juveniles*, 397 Mass. at 268, 491 N.E.2d at 239.

2. In *Ritchie*, the court expressly noted that the Pennsylvania statutory privilege was only conditional rather than absolute. Whether *Ritchie* would require the same result when the state's statutory privilege is unconditional was an issue in *Commonwealth v. Kyle*, 367 Pa.Super. 484, 533 A.2d 120 (1987). In *Kyle*, the defendant was charged with rape, robbery, indecent assault, and deviate sexual intercourse. Subsequent to the attack, the victim received counseling from a licensed clinical psychologist. In an effort to review the substance of any statements made by the victim to the therapist and to prepare a defense strategy, the defendant made a pretrial request to inspect the psychologist's file or in the alternative, "to permit an in camera review of the file." The trial court determined that the records were privileged communications pursuant to the Pennsylvania law and consequently denied defendant's request. The victim was the principal witness for the prosecution. Following a three day trial, a conviction was obtained. The defendant subsequently appealed *inter alia* on the ground that the failure to disclose the contents of the psychologist's file denied him his rights guaranteed by the Confrontation Clause of the Sixth Amendment. In affirming the conviction, the court placed emphasis on the fact that *Ritchie* involved only a qualified statutory privilege. In distinguishing *Ritchie* the court observed:

> Although our disposition of this matter would be controlled by the due process analysis referred by the majority in *Ritchie*, it is at this point that we diverge from that case. Unlike the statutory conditional privilege at issue in *Ritchie*, the Pennsylvania law in this case grants an absolute privilege for communications between a licensed psychologist and a client. We are, therefore, presented with a situation where the interests of the accused in learning of favorable witnesses as well as obtaining arguably useful information directly conflicts with society's interest in maintaining confidentiality between a psychologist and a client. Although we are without clear guidelines as to the means of accommodating these interests, the *Ritchie* decision teaches that the rights of an accused are not without limitations. In *Ritchie*, the Court

noted that the public interest in protecting the CYS file was "strong." Because the statutory conditional privilege did not preclude all use of such information, however, the Court concluded that any material information in the file could be disclosed. *Ritchie*, ___ U.S. at ___, 107 S.Ct. at 1002. Based upon this reasoning, we conclude that a compelling public interest would justify the total non-disclosure of information.

Commonwealth v. Kyle, 367 Pa.Super. 484, 533 A.2d 120, 125 (1987).

III. PATIENT ACCESS TO RECORDS

GOTKIN v. MILLER

United States Court of Appeals, Second Circuit, 1975.
514 F.2d 125.

HAYS, CIRCUIT JUDGE:

Janet Gotkin, a former mental patient, and her husband Paul brought an action in the United States District Court for the Eastern District of New York under 42 U.S.C. § 1983 and 28 U.S.C. § 1343 (1970) seeking to have Mrs. Gotkin's records at Brooklyn State Hospital, Long Island Jewish–Hillside Medical Center, and Gracie Square Hospital made available to her. Judge Travia granted summary judgment in favor of the defendants. He held that the plaintiffs had failed to demonstrate that they had a constitutional right to inspect and copy Mrs. Gotkin's records. Gotkin v. Miller, 379 F.Supp. 859 (E.D.N.Y. 1974). We affirm.

I.

The facts are essentially undisputed. Between 1962 and 1970 Janet Gotkin was voluntarily hospitalized on several occasions mainly because of a series of suicide attempts. She has not received treatment since September, 1970. In April, 1973, the Gotkins contracted to write a book about Janet's experiences. In order to verify her recollections of various incidents, she wrote to three hospitals at which she had been a patient asking them to send her copies of her records. Brooklyn State Hospital and Long Island Jewish–Hillside Medical Center refused her request, and Gracie Square Hospital did not respond.

The Gotkins then filed suit against the directors of the three hospitals and the New York State Commissioner of Mental Hygiene, alleging that the policies of the hospitals against granting requests such as Mrs. Gotkin's violated the rights of former mental patients under the First, Fourth, Ninth, and Fourteenth Amendments of the United States Constitution. The complaint demanded declaratory and injunctive relief in favor of the Gotkins and all others similarly situated. The court granted the defendants' motion for summary judgment. It held that Paul Gotkin was not a proper plaintiff because he was not a former mental patient and had not requested access to his or his wife's records. 379 F.Supp. at 862. As to Janet Gotkin and other members of her purported class, the court held that former mental patients have no First Amendment right to receive information contained in their hospital records, 379 F.Supp. at 862–63; that the Fourth Amendment prohibition of unreasonable searches and seizures is inapplicable, id. 379 F.Supp. at 863; that plaintiffs enjoy no right of privacy entitling them to their records for purposes of publishing a book, id.; and that plaintiffs had not been deprived of "liberty" or "property" protected by the due process clause of the Fourteenth Amendment, id. 379 F.Supp. at 864–68.

II.

Appellants' main argument on this appeal is that the refusal by the hospitals to allow former mental patients to inspect their records deprives the patients of property without due process of law. We can find no basis for the proposition that mental patients have a constitutionally protected property interest in the direct and unrestricted access to their records which the appellants demand.

In Board of Regents of State Colleges v. Roth, 408 U.S. 564, (1972), the Supreme Court held that the Fourteenth Amendment is not an independent source of property rights. The due process clause protects only those property interests already acquired as a result of "existing rules or understandings that stem from an independent source such as state law—rules or understandings that secure certain benefits and that support claims of entitlement to those benefits." Id.

In an attempt to satisfy the *Roth* criteria, appellants argue that under New York case law, patients have a property interest in their hospital records. However, none of the cases cited by appellants indicates that patients have a right to unrestricted access to their records. The majority of the cited cases hold simply that under the discovery provisions of New York law, patients are entitled to a court order granting them access to their records for purposes of litigation.

* * *

New York statutory law also establishes that while patients may exercise a considerable degree of control over their records, they do not have the right to demand direct access to them. Under the Mental Hygiene Law records may not be released to third parties without the consent of the patient, except in certain enumerated situations. Section 17 of the Public Health Law provides for the release of medical records to a hospital or physician designated by the patient. These sections indicate the existence of substantial limitations on the right of access claimed by appellants. We therefore hold that the Fourteenth Amendment does not support appellants' claim that former mental patients have a constitutionally protected, unrestricted property right directly to inspect and copy their hospital records.

III.

Appellants also argue that the hospitals' policy violates the Fourteenth Amendment because it deprives former mental patients of liberty without due process of law. They claim that since the policy against unrestricted disclosure is in part based on the fear that such disclosure could have an adverse effect on the patient, the refusal by the hospitals to grant Mrs. Gotkin access to her records stigmatizes her as mentally ill, although she is now sane and competent.

We agree that the due process clause applies not only when one's physical liberty is threatened but also "[w]here a person's good name, reputation, honor, or integrity is at stake." Wisconsin v. Constantineau, 400 U.S. 433. However, the contention that Mrs. Gotkin is being stigmatized by the hospitals is without merit. No one has branded her as mentally ill or otherwise incompetent. Mrs. Gotkin has no valid claim of deprivation of liberty under the Fourteenth Amendment.

* * *

We agree with the district court that the defendants were entitled to summary judgment regardless of the outcome of these factual disputes. Plaintiffs in this action sought nothing short of unrestricted, direct access to Mrs. Gotkin's records. They failed to establish a constitutional basis for this claim, and it was therefore unnecessary for the district court to judge the wisdom of the hospitals' screening procedures or to decide if those procedures were properly administered.

Affirmed.

PALMER v. DURSO

Supreme Court, Special Term, Kings County, 1977.
90 Misc.2d 110, 393 N.Y.S.2d 898.

ARTHUR S. HIRSCH, JUSTICE.

On August 11, 1953 petitioner was certified by the Department of Mental Hygiene of the State of New York as a mentally incompetent person under Section 74 of the former Mental Hygiene Law and was confined in Brooklyn State Hospital for a period of six months. More than twenty-three years later, petitioner moved in this court last year to have the certification vacated and all records thereto expunged. His motion was denied and petitioner is proceeding *pro se* in appealing said motion to the Appellate Division.

The instant motion is for an order directing the release to petitioner of all sealed records relating to a Department of Mental Hygiene certification of petitioner on August 11, 1953 filed in the Office of the County Clerk of the County of Kings, which petitioner claims is necessary for the preparation of the appeal.

The relevant statute, Mental Hygiene Law 31.31 concerning sealed records of a hearing on an involuntary admission of a patient pursuant to medical certification provides:

(f) The papers in any proceeding under this article which are filed with the county clerk shall be sealed and shall be exhibited only to the parties to the proceeding or someone properly interested, upon order of the court.

As a party to the proceeding which resulted in the commitment, the petitioner is one of the designated persons listed in the statute who may have access to sealed records filed in the Office of the County Clerk, should the court decide petitioner's request for said records is legitimate and appropriate.

Respondent, County Clerk, in objecting to the release of the records argues that petitioner is merely seeking relief denied in his motion now being appealed. He contends that records of a patient in a mental hospital are of such confidential nature that public policy requires they not be revealed except on a strong showing of legitimate and proper call therefor. To buttress this contention, respondent cites a 1953 case (*Application of Hild,* Sup., 124 N.Y.S.2d 271.) The *Hild* court acknowledged that the purpose of the prevailing 1927 Mental Hygiene statute (comparable to the present statute) was to make records to a patient of a mental facility accessible, provided a commissioner or a judge of a court of record, after considering the facts of a given case, passed upon the propriety of the requested action. (Id. at 273[.]) The court, therefore, under appropriate circumstances could unseal records and make them available to former patients. The court in *Hild* denied the application only because petitioner had not shown that the records were germane to issues raised in a pending divorce action in a foreign state for which purpose they were to be used.

There is no question that the records in the instant case are competent, material and relevant to petitioner's appeal from an order denying his request to have those same records vacated and expunged. He is seeking in this motion to have access to the records unlike his initial motion in which he asked that they be destroyed. His ability to competently argue his appeal which he intends to do *pro se* may well hinge on his study of the very records that are the focal point of the proceeding.

In regard to respondent's reference to public policy, it is to be noted the Mental Hygiene Law which allows for concealment of mental institution records was enacted primarily to save patients from humiliation, embarrassment and disgrace (*Munzer v. Blaisdell,* 183 Misc. 773, 49 N.Y.S.2d 915). This rationale for keeping records sealed cannot seriously be applied to the instant situation as it is the petitioner who waived the privilege in order to prepare himself for the appeal. Public policy, especially in light of today's positive attitude towards openness and against bureaucratic concealment would demand that a litigant be facilitated in obtaining his records.

A second case is offered by respondent to support his objections (*Gotkin v. Miller* (D.C.1974) 379 F.Supp. 859, affd. 2 Cir., 514 F.2d 125). The United States District Court ruled that the withholding from plaintiff of records of certain mental hospitals was not a violation of plaintiff's constitutional rights. In *Gotkin,* the plaintiff had been a voluntary mental patient at mental hospitals for a series of threatened suicides. She wanted the record of her stay at these institutions to help her verify some data which she had included in a soon to be published book about her psychiatric experiences.

The court succinctly differentiated between plaintiff's need for the records as opposed to the needs of a litigant in a pending legal action (379 F.Supp. at 868). The petitioner in the instant action is of the latter group, having filed his notice of appeal in the Appellate Division of this state.

The use to which records will be put is a determinant factor in unsealing records of mental institutions. If an applicant needs to obtain information necessary to proceed with litigation, it is reasonable that he should be afforded the opportunity to review and to receive a copy of those records he needs including the order for his commitment, the papers upon which it was granted, as well as all records pertaining thereto. (*Lee v. State*, 183 Misc. 615, 49 N.Y.S.2d 836).

The court concludes petitioner has shown sufficient and legitimate need for records to be used in a pending litigation and further, that respondent has shown no public policy requiring a denial of petitioner's access to said records.

Accordingly, upon the foregoing papers, the petitioner's motion is granted. Petitioner may examine the sealed records of his commitment on file in the County Clerk's Office under such supervision as the County Clerk may deem proper.

Questions and Comments

1. *Legislation.* As the two preceding cases indicated, there was no common law right of a patient to information in his medical records. The patient was not perceived as having a property interest in the records nor as having an implied contractual right. In recent times various jurisdictions have passed specific legislation providing patients, and particularly those patients who have undergone psychotherapy, with a right of access to their records. A typical statute is that enacted by the State of Illinois in 1979, the Illinois Mental Health and Developmental Disabilities Confidentiality Act. This law provides that any recipient of mental health and developmental disabilities services "shall be entitled, upon request, to inspect and copy [his/her] record or any part thereof." Ill.—S.H.A. ch. 91½, ¶ 804. Moreover, the Illinois statute gives this right to any recipient who is 12 years of age or older.

It is, however, noteworthy that the Illinois statute like that of other states with similar legislation distinguishes between the "patient's record" and the therapist's "personal notes." The latter term is defined to include:

> (i) information disclosed to the therapist in confidence by other persons on condition that such information would never be disclosed to the recipient or other persons;

(ii) information disclosed to the therapist by the recipient which would be injurious to the recipient's relationships to other persons; and

(iii) the therapist's speculations, impressions, hunches, and reminders.

Thus, by restricting access to the patient's *official record,* these statutes make it possible for therapists to closely regulate and limit the amount of information that is actually available to the patient. Cf. California, which grants a patient access to his records unless in the view of the physician or administrative officer in question, release of such records to the patient would not "serve his best interests." West's Ann.Cal.Code § 5328.9.

2. *Policy questions.* What policy reasons support the recipient's access to the records of his mental health services? Are statutes which provide access merely protecting an abstract interest in the patient's right to know, or are there more practical reasons why the patient should have access to his records? Does the answer to this question depend in any sense on the scope of the therapist's authority to disclose information to third parties? In other words, to the extent that even the common law or statutory law of the state permits or at least does not prevent disclosure to third parties, the patient arguably may have a very substantial interest in screening his record so as to ensure that misinformation is not transmitted. However, if under the prevailing state law the therapist's powers to transmit to third parties are closely controlled, what is the patient's interest in gaining access to his records?

3. *Possible consequences.* Are there any possible negative consequences in a psychiatric patient gaining access to their records? Would a diagnosis which is merely tentative have the potential to become self-fulfilling if the patient learns of the tentative diagnosis? Is this problem greater or smaller in the case of children who are under treatment? Note, in this connection, that in some jurisdictions, such as Illinois, any recipient of services over the age of 12 has the right to inspect records maintained by a provider of services.

4. *Intended use of records.* At least one court has held that when a patient appeals an involuntary commitment order, due process requires that the patient be given access to the hearing record. See, *In re S.O.,* 342 Pa.Super. 215, 231, 492 A.2d 727, 735 (1985). Note that *Palmer v. Durso* distinguishes *Gotkin* by focusing on the use to which the different plaintiffs intended to put the records. In *Palmer,* the plaintiff was seeking to expunge a court order under which he had been committed 23 years earlier, while Mrs. Gotkin desired her hospital records to verify information for a book she was writing.

What is the possible impact of recent cases, which find that public interest in information on issues of public concern may at times justify disclosure, on the continued viability of the ruling in *Gotkin*? See, e.g., *In re New York News, Inc.,* 67 N.Y.2d 472, 503 N.Y.S.2d 714, 494 N.E.2d 1379 (1986) (p. 246, supra).

Part II

DEPRIVATIONS OF LIBERTY AND PROPERTY

INTRODUCTION

The government acts to deprive its citizens of liberty or property in a number of contexts. These interventions may be subdivided into three types. Under a *sanction* system, the goal of the government is punishment for past acts. The principal example of this type of intervention is the criminal justice process, which penalizes through incarceration or fines those who violate certain norms. Under a *control* system, the government deprives individuals of their liberty for the purpose of preventing future harm to others or themselves. The civil commitment process (at least that aspect which results in involuntary hospitalization of the "dangerous" mentally ill) might be seen as an exemplar of this model. Finally, under an *autonomy* system, the government acts to prevent "incompetent" choices and ensure that individuals capably exercise rights and privileges. One illustration of this type of intervention is the involuntary hospitalization of those found incompetent to stand trial for the purpose of restoring them to competency. Another is the coerced relinquishment of control over property or person which may occur pursuant to guardianship proceedings.

Part II of this book examines the impact of these types of state intervention on those considered to be mentally disabled. Under current law, mental disability assumes a significant role in the application of all three intervention modes. For instance, under the sanction model as applied in this country, the law has been unwilling to punish those who are considered "insane". With a few exceptions, application of the control model is predicated on a finding of mental disorder. Similarly, a finding of incompetency usually requires evidence of diagnosable mental disability.

Central to all three systems of intervention, therefore, is some concept of mental disorder. The first chapter of this part examines current thought on the nature of this phenomenon. The second chapter discusses an important subsidiary issue: our ability to identify who, if anyone, is "mentally disabled" and our ability to assess what the consequences of such disability are. With these preliminary issues

325

addressed, the next three chapters examine ways in which the sanction, control and autonomy systems affect the mentally disabled. The final chapter in Part II looks at legal issues connected with providing post-intervention treatment that concern all three models.

Chapter Five

THINKING ABOUT MENTAL DISORDER

Table of Sections

Virtually all of the laws we will be examining in this part of the book require a finding of "mental illness", "mental disorder," "mental disease or defect" or, to use the most archaic phrase, "lunacy or idiocy". Without some grasp of this problematic concept, these laws cannot be evaluated effectively. This chapter will try to address the following question: what might we mean when we use these phrases?

I. MODELS OF MENTAL DISORDER

There are several ways of thinking about mental condition. Lazare describes four such models, which can be distinguished along etiological lines.[a] The pure "medical" model posits that one's mental state results primarily from organic or chemical conditions within the body. The "psychologic" model suggests that one's personality is largely produced by patterns established during youth through interactions with one's family or family substitutes. The "behavioral" model treats behavior and any thoughts which may accompany it as the result of specific aversive or reinforcing events rather than some underlying pathology.

a. Lazare, "Hidden Conceptual Models in Clinical Psychiatry," 288 New England Journ.Med. 345 (1973).

The "social" model, similarly focusing on external determinants, fixes on relationships with social groups—family, peers, and institutions—as the primary influences on mental condition.

Each model contemplates the possibility of mental disorder and suggests ways of treating it. The medical model views mental disorder as the product of a diseased organ or an imbalance in chemicals; thus, the most effective treatment will usually involve medical modalities such as medication or surgery. The psychologic model sees mental problems as the product of childhood stresses; the treatment of choice here is psychotherapy designed to help the person "remember", clarify and deal with these early events. Behaviorists do not use disease language; instead they talk about maladaptive behavior, which they believe is a learned response to past events and is treated by conditioning the person against such behavior and reinforcing more acceptable behavior. The social model regards mental disorder as the result of social disorder, such as the death of a loved one, loss of a job, geographic displacement, or poor relationships, and suggests it is best treated by reorganizing the person's social system.

The law has preferred the medical model of mental disorder. To some extent, this preference is probably an accident of history; the medical tradition preceded the other three and thus was the first one encountered by the law. But there is also a philosophical reason for the law's attraction to the medical model: the correlation between the endogenous premise of that model and the law's individualized approach to justice. The other models, to a greater or lesser extent, focus on factors external to the individual as causes of behavior and thus potentially threaten the current foundations of the legal system. For example, imagine the impact abandonment of the medical model might have in a sanction system of intervention. Endorsement of the behavioral or social models of mental disorder could broaden enormously the scope of defenses based on lack of criminal responsibility, since these models suggest that exogenous factors, such as rewards for aggressive behavior or the impact of poverty and social class, cause mental abnormality.[b] Abandonment of the medical model would also have interesting implications for the control and autonomy systems of intervention. For instance, to the extent these systems allow coercive treatment in an effort to ameliorate mental disorder associated with dangerousness or incompetency, allegiance to the exogenous models of mental disorder might permit state intervention into the lives of persons other than the mentally disordered individual; according to the non-medical models, especially the social one, these other persons are contributors to the disorder.[c] This possibility is in obvious tension with our current conceptions of individual liberty.

b. See, e.g., Bazelon, "The Morality of the Criminal Law," 49 S.Cal.L.Rev. 385, 396 (1976) (arguing that social background, including poverty, should be considered in evaluating criminal responsibility).

c. D. Wexler, Mental Health Law 22 (1981).

A final introductory point is the relation of the various models to the different mental health professions. The medical model is most closely associated with psychiatrists, who must obtain a medical degree before beginning psychiatric residency. The psychologic model is also often connected with psychiatrists, but is most obviously aligned with psychoanalysts, most of whom rely on some version of the theories advanced by Sigmund Freud or his early disciples. Clinical psychologists, who are not medically trained but devote considerable study to research on human behavior, are usually identified with the behavioral model, first hypothesized by a psychologist, B.F. Skinner. And social workers receive training that is most likely to encourage adherence to the social model.

Of course, as Chapter One indicated, most mental health professionals develop an eclectic approach toward identification and treatment of mental problems. One is unlikely to find a clinician who is devoted entirely to one model over the other. Many clinical psychologists, for instance, reject behaviorism in its original form and take a very social approach to treatment. The important point for present purposes is that all of the models and most mental health professionals, regardless of guild, refer to and recognize the concept of mental abnormality. For instance, most mental health professionals are willing to apply the term "schizophrenia" to individuals who hallucinate, are out of touch with reality, and seem to speak in a disjointed, illogical fashion; most also would call a person who is diagnosed schizophrenic "mentally ill."

The remainder of this chapter explores the possible ways of looking at the concept of mental disorder. In thinking about these different approaches, the following vignettes may be helpful.

Case 1. John works at a 7-11; he is very quiet. One of his co-workers discovers that, each day after work, John spends several hours in the closet. When questioned about this, John says: "I've been doing it for three or four months, you know, it's where my mother used to put me." When asked what he does there, he explains: "I'm talking with Martians. They left me here to teach Earthlings about Mars. I'm also a rock star you know, but I'm getting smaller every day and pretty soon you won't be able to see me."

Case 2. Sam wants to set the world record for number of days on top of a flag pole. At the present time, he has been on a platform on top of a pole for 33 days. Although he is malnourished and dizzy from lack of food and sleep, he says he will not come down until he has stayed on the pole a total of 73 days, which will be a new record.

Case 3. Mary, a lawyer, says she feels hopeless and worthless. When asked why, she says she is single, has no good friends and no family, and thinks her work is meaningless. She is barely able to go to the office in the morning and in the evening she goes straight home, watches TV and falls asleep by 8 p.m. She cries frequently and sometimes wishes she were dead. She resists any attempts to "cheer her up" or get her involved socially.

Case 4. Cecelia goes to all-night worship service at her fundamentalist church. During the service she claims to hear voices talking to her, often speaks in tongues, and occasionally behaves in a wild way so that others have to restrain her. The monthly meetings are the only times she acts like this.

Case 5. Sarah is 21 and living with her parents. She says she has no idea what she wants to do with her life. She has been put on probation for shoplifting. She will hole up in her room with piles of junk food for days. When her mother or father tries to talk to her, Sarah often explodes with anger and usually retreats to her room. Recently, she has taken to sticking safety pins in her skin and letting them hang.

Case 6. Jimmy is a member of an ashram, a commune centered around Eastern religious beliefs. Since joining the ashram, Jimmy has been required to participate every day in a strenuous series of classes, meditation and prayer sessions, as well as street solicitations. He is constantly fatigued, has lost all sexual desire and sense of humor, and goes into trances quite frequently. He says he has found the true answer to "Life's Questions" and wants to continue at the ashram.

Case 7. As a child, Donald would torture small animals. He was always getting into fights with other children. By the time he was 25, he had been charged with several crimes, and convicted of burglary, two assaults and arson. When asked about these events, he merely states that they seemed like the thing to do at the time; he is only sorry that he got caught.

Case 8. Alyson, 55, lives in the country. She has drunk heavily for years. Recently she has become convinced that the cropdusters flying over her house are government airplanes bombarding her house with electronic particles. As evidence of this, she points to several places in her house where the foundations are weakened and notes the fact that her dog has mysteriously died. She also believes her house is being bugged by the government.

While reading the following materials, decide which, if any, of these individuals you would call "mentally ill" or "mentally disordered" and why.

II. MODERN CONCEPTIONS OF MENTAL DISORDER—DSM–III

Mental health professionals have studied and categorized human behavior for well over a century. The best known effort, in both clinical and legal circles, at attempting to classify mental and behavioral phenomena into categories is the American Psychiatric Association's

Diagnostic and Statistical Manual. The Manual is now in its third edition, and that edition was revised in 1987; thus the most recent nosological work of the APA bears the title DSM–III–R. The two third edition versions of the Manual are quite different from the first two editions. Unlike the earlier versions, DSM–III establishes concise criteria for each diagnosis, includes specific instructions with respect to differential diagnosis (which help clinicians distinguish between different diagnoses), suggests investigation of "psychosocial stressors" as well as "endogenous" factors, and was subjected to field tests to study the reliability of its categories.

The study of the Manual is important not only because it represents one of the most advanced attempts at understanding mental disorder but also because of its importance to the legal system. DSM–III states that "[t]he use of this manual for non-clinical purposes, such as determination of legal responsibility, competency or insanity, or justification for third-party payment, must be critically examined in each instance within the appropriate institutional context." Despite this admonition the legal profession has enthusiastically adopted the Manual's nomenclature for all sorts of legal purposes, and forensic clinicians, on the whole, have not objected. However one comes out on the worth of diagnostic information for legal purposes, a practicing attorney or forensic clinician is well-advised to be familiar with DSM–III and its successors.

A. THE STRUCTURE AND DEVELOPMENT OF DSM–III

Below are excerpts from the Manual explaining its organization and providing the criteria for several diagnoses that will figure prominently in the rest of this book.

DIAGNOSTIC AND STATISTICAL MANUAL OF MENTAL DISORDERS THIRD EDITION, REVISED

(Washington, D.C.: American Psychiatric Association, 1987).
pp. xxii–xxv.

* * *

Basic Features of DSM–III–R

Mental Disorder. Although this manual provides a classification of mental disorders, no definition adequately specifies precise boundaries for the concept "mental disorder" (this is also true for such concepts as physical disorder and mental and physical health). Nevertheless, it is useful to present a definition of mental disorder that has influenced the decision to include certain conditions in DSM–III and DSM–III–R as mental disorders and to exclude others.

In DSM–III–R each of the mental disorders is conceptualized as a clinically significant behavioral or psychological syndrome or pattern that occurs in a person and that is associated with present distress (a painful symptom) or disability (impairment in one or more important areas of functioning) or with a significantly increased risk of suffering death, pain, disability, or an important loss of freedom. In addition, this syndrome or pattern must not be merely an expectable response to a particular event, e.g., the death of a loved one. Whatever its original cause, it must currently be considered a manifestation of a behavioral, psychological, or biological dysfunction in the person. Neither deviant behavior, e.g., political, religious, or sexual, nor conflicts that are primarily between the individual and society are mental disorders unless the deviance or conflict is a symptom of a dysfunction in the person, as described above.

There is no assumption that each mental disorder is a discrete entity with sharp boundaries (discontinuity) between it and other mental disorders, or between it and no mental disorder. For example, there has been a continuing controversy concerning whether severe depressive disorder and mild depressive disorder differ from each other qualitatively (discontinuity between diagnostic entities) or quantitatively (a difference on a severity continuum). The inclusion of Major Depression and Dysthymia as separate categories in DSM-III-R is justified by the clinical usefulness of the distinction. This does not imply a resolution of the controversy concerning whether these conditions are in fact quantitatively or qualitatively different.

A common misconception is that a classification of mental disorders classifies people, when actually what are being classified are disorders that people have. For this reason, the text of DSM-III-R (as did the text of DSM-III) avoids the use of such expressions as "a schizophrenic" or "an alcoholic," and instead uses the more accurate, but admittedly more cumbersome, "a person with Schizophrenia" or "a person with Alcohol Dependence."

Another misconception is that all people described as having the same mental disorder are alike in all important ways. Although all the people described as having the same mental disorder have at least the defining features of the disorder, they may well differ in other important respects that may affect clinical management and outcome.

* * *

Descriptive Approach. For some of the mental disorders, the etiology or pathophysiologic processes are known. For example, in the Organic Mental Disorders, organic factors necessary for the development and maintenance of the disorders have been identified or are presumed. Another example is Adjustment Disorder, in which the disturbance, by definition, is a reaction to psychosocial stress.

For most of the DSM-III-R disorders, however, the etiology is unknown. Many theories have been advanced and buttressed by evidence—not always convincing—attempting to explain how these disorders come about. The approach taken in DSM-III-R is atheoretical with regard to etiology or pathophysiologic process, except with regard to disorders for which this is well established and therefore included in the definition of the disorder. Undoubtedly, over time, some of the disorders of unknown etiology will be found to have specific biological etiologies; others, to have specific psychological causes; and still others, to result mainly from an interplay of psychological, social, and biological factors.

The major justification for the generally atheoretical approach taken in DSM–III and DSM–III–R with regard to etiology is that the inclusion of etiologic theories would be an obstacle to use of the manual by clinicians of varying theoretical orientations, since it would not be possible to present all reasonable etiologic theories for each disorder. For example, Phobic Disorders are believed by many to represent a displacement of anxiety resulting from the breakdown of defense mechanisms that keep internal conflicts out of consciousness. Others explain phobias on the basis of learned avoidance responses to conditioned anxiety. Still others believe that certain phobias result from a dysregulation of basic biological systems mediating separation anxiety. In any case, clinicians and researchers can agree on the identification of mental disorders on the basis of their clinical manifestations without agreeing on how the disturbances come about.

DSM–III–R can be said to be "descriptive" in that the definitions of the disorders are generally limited to descriptions of the clinical features of the disorders. The characteristic features consist of easily identifiable behavioral signs or symptoms, such as disorientation, mood disturbance, or psychomotor agitation, which require a minimal amount of inference on the part of the observer. For some disorders, however, particularly the Personality Disorders, the criteria require much more inference on the part of the observer. An example of such a criterion in Borderline Personality Disorder is "marked and persistent identity disturbance manifested by uncertainty about at least two of the following: self-image, sexual orientation, long-term goals or career choice, type of friends desired, preferred values."

This descriptive approach is also used in the grouping of the mental disorders into diagnostic classes. All of the disorders without known etiology or pathophysiologic process are grouped into classes on the basis of shared clinical features. For this reason, in DSM–III and in DSM–III–R there is no diagnostic class of "neuroses," as there was in DSM–II.

*   *   *

Multiaxial Evaluation System. DSM–III–R has a multiaxial system for evaluation to ensure that certain information that may be of value in planning treatment and predicting outcome for each person is recorded on each of five axes. Axes I and II comprise the mental disorders; Axis III, physical disorders and conditions; and Axes IV and V, severity of psychosocial stressors and global assessment of functioning, respectively. In its entirety, the multiaxial system provides a biopsychosocial approach to assessment.

*   *   *

Comments

1. *Multi-axial approach.* The multi-axial approach to diagnosis, briefly described above, is new with the third edition of DSM. On Axis I, the evaluator indicates the person's "clinical syndrome". The major clinical syndrome categories are listed below:

Childhood disorders

Organic syndromes (e.g., senile dementia)

Psychoactive substance use disorders

Schizophrenia

Delusional (paranoid) disorders

Mood disorders (e.g., manic or depressive syndromes)

Anxiety disorders

Somato-form disorders (i.e., disorders which have physical symptoms but for which there are no demonstrable organic findings, e.g., hypochondriasis)

Dissociative disorders (e.g., multiple personality, psychogenic fugue)

Sexual disorders

Sleep disorders

Factitious (i.e., not genuine) disorders

Impulse control disorders not elsewhere classified (e.g., pyromania, pathological gambling)

Adjustment disorders (i.e. maladaptive reaction to a stressful event)

On Axis II are designated developmental disorders (e.g., mental retardation) and personality disorders (e.g., schizoid personality disorder, antisocial personality disorder). On Axis III, physical disorders and conditions are listed. On Axis IV, the clinician is to indicate the impact of psychosocial stressors on a scale from 1 (no acute events) to 6 (catastrophic stressors such as death of a child). Finally, to arrive at an overall picture, for Axis V the clinician is to "[c]onsider psychological, social and occupational functioning on a hypothetical continuum of mental health-illness," but to exclude from consideration "impairment in functioning due to physical (or environmental) limitations". Then the clinician must produce a rating on the Global Assessment Functioning (GAF) scale, with a score of 90 meaning absent or minimal symptoms and a score of 1 designating persistent danger of severely hurting self or others. Illustrations of diagnoses using the multi-axial approach are provided in DSM–III–R. One is replicated below (the numbers in Axes I and II are the diagnostic codes):

Axis I: 296.23 Major Depression, Single Episode, Severe without Psychotic Features

 303.90 Alcohol Dependence

Axis II: 301.60 Dependent Personality Disorder (Provisional, rule out Borderline Personality Disorder)

Axis III: Alcoholic cirrhosis of liver

Axis IV: Psychosocial stressors: anticipated retirement and change
           in residence, with loss of contact with friends. Severity:
           4—Moderate (predominately enduring circumstances)

Axis V: Current GAF: 44

          Highest GAF past year: 55

The Manual also provides "V Codes" for "conditions not attributable to a mental disorder that are a focus of attention or treatment."
These conditions include: academic problems; antisocial behavior; malingering; marital problems; noncompliance with medical treatment;
occupational problems; interpersonal problems; and uncomplicated
bereavement (due to death of a loved one). Again, the V Code is to be
used only if these conditions are not attributable to mental disorder.

2. *Development and testing of the manual.* The diagnostic system
described above is the result of a prolonged, multi-layered process. In 1974,
the American Psychiatric Association appointed a Task Force on Nomenclature and Statistics, headed by Robert L. Spitzer, to begin work revising
the second edition of the Diagnostic and Statistical Manual, which had
been in effect since 1968. From 1975 through 1979, successive Task Force
drafts of DSM–III were considered at the annual meeting of the American
Psychiatric Association as well as at a special meeting in 1976 which
focused entirely on DSM–III. Throughout that period, critiques were also
solicited from the rest of the psychiatric profession and groups of psychoanalysts, psychologists, and social workers as well. Finally, between 1977 and
1980, the diagnostic scheme was subjected to field trials to determine the
extent to which different clinicians arrive at the same diagnosis using the
DSM–III categories. In general, these tests revealed that interrater agreement for the major diagnostic categories (e.g., schizophrenia, manic-depressive psychosis) was quite high (between 69 and 85%). For other diagnostic
categories, the rate of agreement was lower (often below 50%).

DSM–III went into effect in 1980. In 1983, a Work Group was
appointed to begin revision of DSM–III. Twenty-six advisory committees
were formed to make recommendations in specific areas. According to the
introduction to DSM–III–R "[m]ost advisory committee decisions were the
result of a consensus that emerged among committee members. However,
several controversies, particularly in the areas of childhood, psychotic,
anxiety, and sleep disorders, could be resolved only by actually polling
committee members." DSM–III–R introduced about 200 changes in diagnostic guidelines and criteria (many of them minor) but was not subjected
to field trials.

3. *The future.* DSM–IV is expected sometime in the 1990's. Moreover, the approach adopted by the American Psychiatric Association has
been very influential at the international level. DSM–III was translated
into thirteen languages. DSM–III–R and its successors are likely to have a
major impact on the tenth revision of the International Classification of
Diseases, expected in 1992. Further assuring the Manual's longevity is its
use for insurance purposes and for legal purposes, both explored in subsequent materials.

B. SELECTED DIAGNOSES FROM DSM–III–R

DIAGNOSTIC & STATISTICAL MANUAL
3rd EDITION, REVISED.
(1987).

1. Developmental Disorders

Mental Retardation

A. Significantly subaverage general intellectual functioning: an IQ of 70 or below on an individually administered IQ test (for infants, a clinical judgment of significantly subaverage intellectual functioning, since available intelligence tests do not yield numerical IQ values).

B. Concurrent deficits or impairments in adaptive functioning, i.e., the person's effectiveness in meeting the standards expected for his or her age by his or her cultural group in areas such as social skills and responsibility, communication, daily living skills, personal independence, and self-sufficiency.

C. Onset before the age of 18.

Degrees of severity. There are four degrees of severity, reflecting the degree of intellectual impairment: Mild, Moderate, Severe, and Profound. IQ levels to be used as guides in distinguishing the four degrees of severity are:

Degree of severity	IQ
Mild	50–55 to approx. 70
Moderate	35–40 to 50–55
Severe	20–25 to 35–40
Profound	Below 20 or 25

2. Psychoses

Schizophrenia

A. Presence of characteristic psychotic symptoms in the active phase: either (1), (2), or (3) for at least one week (unless the symptoms are successfully treated):

(1) two of the following:

  (a) delusions

  (b) prominent hallucinations (throughout the day for several days or several times a week for several weeks, each hallucinatory experience not being limited to a few brief moments)

  (c) incoherence or marked loosening of associations

  (d) catatonic behavior

  (e) flat or grossly inappropriate affect

(2) bizarre delusions (i.e., involving a phenomenon that the person's culture would regard as totally implausible, e.g., thought broadcasting, being controlled by a dead person)

(3) prominent hallucinations [as defined in (1)(*b*) above] of a voice with content having no apparent relation to depression or elation, or a voice keeping up a running commentary on the person's behavior or thoughts, or two or more voices conversing with each other

B. During the course of the disturbance, functioning in such areas as work, social relations, and self-care is markedly below the highest level achieved before onset of the disturbance (or, when the onset is in childhood or adolescence, failure to achieve expected level of social development).

C. Schizoaffective Disorder and Mood Disorder with Psychotic Features have been ruled out, i.e., if a Major Depressive or Manic Syndrome has ever been present during an active phase of the disturbance, the total duration of all episodes of a mood syndrome has been brief relative to the total duration of the active and residual phases of the disturbance.

D. Continuous signs of the disturbance for at least six months. The six-month period must include an active phase (of at least one week, or less if symptoms have been successfully treated) during which there were psychotic symptoms characteristic of Schizophrenia (symptoms in A), with or without a prodromal or residual phase, as defined below.

Prodromal phase: A clear deterioration in functioning before the active phase of the disturbance that is not due to a disturbance in mood or to a Psychoactive Substance Use Disorder and that involves at least two of the symptoms listed below.

Residual phase: Following the active phase of the disturbance, persistence of at least two of the symptoms noted below, these not being due to a disturbance in mood or to a Psychoactive Substance Use Disorder.

Prodromal or Residual Symptoms:

(1) marked social isolation or withdrawal

(2) marked impairment in role functioning as wage-earner, student, or homemaker

(3) markedly peculiar behavior (e.g., collecting garbage, talking to self in public, hoarding food)

(4) marked impairment in personal hygiene and grooming

(5) blunted or inappropriate affect

(6) digressive, vague, overelaborate, or circumstantial speech, or poverty of speech, or poverty of content of speech

(7) odd beliefs or magical thinking, influencing behavior and inconsistent with cultural norms, e.g., superstitiousness,

belief in clairvoyance, telepathy, "sixth sense," "others can feel my feelings," overvalued ideas, ideas of reference

(8) unusual perceptual experiences, e.g., recurrent illusions, sensing the presence of a force or person not actually present

(9) marked lack of initiative, interests, or energy

Examples: Six months of prodromal symptoms with one week of symptoms from A; no prodromal symptoms with six months of symptoms from A; no prodromal symptoms with one week of symptoms from A and six months of residual symptoms.

E. It cannot be established that an organic factor initiated and maintained the disturbance.

F. If there is a history of Autistic Disorder, the additional diagnosis of Schizophrenia is made only if prominent delusions or hallucinations are also present.

Delusional Disorder

A. Nonbizarre delusion(s) (i.e., involving situations that occur in real life, such as being followed, poisoned, infected, loved at a distance, having a disease, being deceived by one's spouse or lover) of at least one month's duration.

B. Auditory or visual hallucinations, if present, are not prominent [as defined in Schizophrenia, A(1)(b)].

C. Apart from the delusion(s) or its ramifications, behavior is not obviously odd or bizarre.

D. If a Major Depressive or Manic Syndrome has been present during the delusional disturbance, the total duration of all episodes of the mood syndrome has been brief relative to the total duration of the delusional disturbance.

E. Has never met criterion A for Schizophrenia, and it cannot be established that an organic factor initiated and maintained the disturbance.

Specify type: The following types are based on the predominant delusional theme. If no single delusional theme predominates, specify as **Unspecified Type.**

Erotomanic Type

Delusional Disorder in which the predominant theme of the delusion(s) is that a person, usually of higher status, is in love with the subject.

Grandiose Type

Delusional Disorder in which the predominant theme of the delusion(s) is one of inflated worth, power, knowledge, identity, or special relationship to a deity or famous person.

Jealous Type

Delusional Disorder in which the predominant theme of the delusion(s) is that one's sexual partner is unfaithful.

Persecutory Type

Delusional Disorder in which the predominant theme of the delusion(s) is that one (or someone to whom one is close) is being malevolently treated in some way. People with this type of Delusional Disorder may repeatedly take their complaints of being mistreated to legal authorities.

Somatic Type

Delusional Disorder in which the predominant theme of the delusion(s) is that the person has some physical defect, disorder, or disease.

Unspecified Type

Delusional Disorder that does not fit any of the previous categories, e.g., persecutory and grandiose themes without a predominance of either; delusions of reference without malevolent content.

Brief Reactive Psychosis

A. Presence of at least one of the following symptoms indicating impaired reality testing (not culturally sanctioned):

   (1) incoherence or marked loosening of associations

   (2) delusions

   (3) hallucinations

   (4) catatonic or disorganized behavior

B. Emotional turmoil, i.e., rapid shifts from one intense affect to another, or overwhelming perplexity or confusion.

C. Appearance of the symptoms in A and B shortly after, and apparently in response to, one or more events that, singly or together, would be markedly stressful to almost anyone in similar circumstances in the person's culture.

D. Absence of the prodromal symptoms of Schizophrenia, and failure to meet the criteria for Schizotypal Personality Disorder before onset of the disturbance.

E. Duration of an episode of the disturbance of from a few hours to one month, with eventual full return to premorbid level of functioning. (When the diagnosis must be made without waiting for the expected recovery, it should be qualified as "provisional.")

F. Not due to a psychotic Mood Disorder (i.e., no full mood syndrome is present), and it cannot be established that an organic factor initiated and maintained the disturbance.

3. Mood Disorders

Manic Episode

Note: A "Manic Syndrome" is defined as including criteria A, B, and C below. A "Hypomanic Syndrome" is defined as including criteria A and B, but not C, i.e., no marked impairment.

A. A distinct period of abnormally and persistently elevated, expansive, or irritable mood.

B. During the period of mood disturbance, at least three of the following symptoms have persisted (four if the mood is only irritable) and have been present to a significant degree:

    (1) inflated self-esteem or grandiosity

    (2) decreased need for sleep, e.g., feels rested after only three hours of sleep

    (3) more talkative than usual or pressure to keep talking

    (4) flight of ideas or subjective experience that thoughts are racing

    (5) distractibility, i.e., attention too easily drawn to unimportant or irrelevant external stimuli

    (6) increase in goal-directed activity (either socially, at work or school, or sexually) or psychomotor agitation

    (7) excessive involvement in pleasurable activities which have a high potential for painful consequences, e.g., the person engages in unrestrained buying sprees, sexual indiscretions, or foolish business investments

C. Mood disturbance sufficiently severe to cause marked impairment in occupational functioning or in usual social activities or relationships with others, or to necessitate hospitalization to prevent harm to self or others.

D. At no time during the disturbance have there been delusions or hallucinations for as long as two weeks in the absence of prominent mood symptoms (i.e., before the mood symptoms developed or after they have remitted).

E. Not superimposed on Schizophrenia, Schizophreniform Disorder, Delusional Disorder, or Psychotic Disorder NOS.

F. It cannot be established that an organic factor initiated and maintained the disturbance. **Note:** Somatic antidepressant treatment (e.g., drugs, ECT) that apparently precipitates a mood disturbance should not be considered an etiologic organic factor.

Major Depressive Episode

Note: A "Major Depressive Syndrome" is defined as criterion A below.

A. At least five of the following symptoms have been present during the same two-week period and represent a change from previous functioning; at least one of the symptoms is either (1) depressed mood, or (2) loss of interest or pleasure. (Do not include symptoms that are clearly due to a physical condition, mood-incongruent delusions or hallucinations, incoherence, or marked loosening of associations.)

    (1) depressed mood (or can be irritable mood in children and adolescents) most of the day, nearly every day, as indicated either by subjective account or observation by others

    (2) markedly diminished interest or pleasure in all, or almost all, activities most of the day, nearly every day (as indicated either by subjective account or observation by others of apathy most of the time)

    (3) significant weight loss or weight gain when not dieting (e.g., more than 5% of body weight in a month), or decrease or increase in appetite nearly every day (in children, consider failure to make expected weight gains)

    (4) insomnia or hypersomnia nearly every day

    (5) psychomotor agitation or retardation nearly every day (observable by others, not merely subjective feelings of restlessness or being slowed down)

    (6) fatigue or loss of energy nearly every day

    (7) feelings of worthlessness or excessive or inappropriate guilt (which may be delusional) nearly every day (not merely self-reproach or guilt about being sick)

    (8) diminished ability to think or concentrate, or indecisiveness, nearly every day (either by subjective account or as observed by others)

    (9) recurrent thoughts of death (not just fear of dying), recurrent suicidal ideation without a specific plan, or a suicide attempt or a specific plan for committing suicide

B. (1) It cannot be established that an organic factor initiated and maintained the disturbance

    (2) The disturbance is not a normal reaction to the death of a loved one (Uncomplicated Bereavement)

    Note: Morbid preoccupation with worthlessness, suicidal ideation, marked functional impairment or psychomotor retardation, or prolonged duration suggest bereavement complicated by Major Depression.

C. At no time during the disturbance have there been delusions or hallucinations for as long as two weeks in the absence of prominent mood symptoms (i.e., before the mood symptoms developed or after they have remitted).

D. Not superimposed on Schizophrenia, Schizophreniform Disorder, Delusional Disorder, or Psychotic Disorder NOS.

Dysthymia

A. Depressed mood (or can be irritable mood in children and adolescents) for most of the day, more days than not, as indicated either by subjective account or observation by others, for at least two years (one year for children and adolescents)

B. Presence, while depressed, of at least two of the following:

(1) poor appetite or overeating

(2) insomnia or hypersomnia

(3) low energy or fatigue

(4) low self-esteem

(5) poor concentration or difficulty making decisions

(6) feelings of hopelessness

C. During a two-year period (one-year for children and adolescents) of the disturbance, never without the symptoms in A for more than two months at a time.

D. No evidence of an unequivocal Major Depressive Episode during the first two years (one year for children and adolescents) of the disturbance.

Note: There may have been a previous Major Depressive Episode, provided there was a full remission (no significant signs or symptoms for six months) before development of the Dysthymia. In addition, after these two years (one year in children or adolescents) of Dysthymia, there may be superimposed episodes of Major Depression, in which case both diagnoses are given.

E. Has never had a Manic Episode or an unequivocal Hypomanic Episode.

F. Not superimposed on a chronic psychotic disorder, such as Schizophrenia or Delusional Disorder.

G. It cannot be established that an organic factor initiated and maintained the disturbance, e.g., prolonged administration of an antihypertensive medication.

4. **Personality Disorders**

Paranoid Personality Disorder

A. A pervasive and unwarranted tendency, beginning by early adulthood and present in a variety of contexts, to interpret the actions of people as deliberately demeaning or threatening, as indicated by at least *four* of the following:

(1) expects, without sufficient basis, to be exploited or harmed by others

(2) questions, without justification, the loyalty or trustworthiness of friends or associates

(3) reads hidden demeaning or threatening meanings into benign remarks or events, e.g., suspects that a neighbor put out trash early to annoy him

(4) bears grudges or is unforgiving of insults or slights

(5) is reluctant to confide in others because of unwarranted fear that the information will be used against him or her

(6) is easily slighted and quick to react with anger or to counterattack

(7) questions, without justification, fidelity of spouse or sexual partner

B. Occurrence not exclusively during the course of Schizophrenia or a Delusional Disorder.

Schizoid Personality Disorder

A. A pervasive pattern of indifference to social relationships and a restricted range of emotional experience and expression, beginning by early adulthood and present in a variety of contexts, as indicated by at least *four* of the following:

(1) neither desires nor enjoys close relationships, including being part of a family

(2) almost always chooses solitary activities

(3) rarely, if ever, claims or appears to experience strong emotions, such as anger and joy

(4) indicates little if any desire to have sexual experiences with another person (age being taken into account)

(5) is indifferent to the praise and criticism of others

(6) has no close friends or confidants (or only one) other than first-degree relatives

(7) displays constricted affect, e.g., is aloof, cold, rarely reciprocates gestures or facial expressions, such as smiles or nods

B. Occurrence not exclusively during the course of Schizophrenia or a Delusional Disorder.

Schizotypal Personality Disorder

A. A pervasive pattern of deficits in interpersonal relatedness and peculiarities of ideation, appearance, and behavior, beginning by early adulthood and present in a variety of contexts, as indicated by at least *five* of the following:

(1) ideas of reference (excluding delusions of reference)

(2) excessive social anxiety, e.g., extreme discomfort in social situations involving unfamiliar people

(3) odd beliefs or magical thinking, influencing behavior and inconsistent with subcultural norms, e.g., superstitiousness, belief in clairvoyance, telepathy, or "sixth sense," "others can feel my feelings" (in children and adolescents, bizarre fantasies or preoccupations)

(4) unusual perceptual experiences, e.g., illusions, sensing the presence of a force or person not actually present (e.g., "I felt as if my dead mother were in the room with me")

(5) odd or eccentric behavior or appearance, e.g., unkempt, unusual mannerisms, talks to self

(6) no close friends or confidants (or only one) other than first-degree relatives

(7) odd speech (without loosening of associations or incoherence), e.g., speech that is impoverished, digressive, vague, or inappropriately abstract

(8) inappropriate or constricted affect, e.g., silly, aloof, rarely reciprocates gestures or facial expressions, such as smiles or nods

(9) suspiciousness or paranoid ideation

B. Occurrence not exclusively during the course of Schizophrenia or a Pervasive Developmental Disorder.

Antisocial Personality Disorder

A. Current age at least 18.

B. Evidence of Conduct Disorder with onset before age 15, as indicated by a history of *three* or more of the following:

(1) was often truant

(2) ran away from home overnight at least twice while living in parental or parental surrogate home (or once without returning)

(3) often initiated physical fights

(4) used a weapon in more than one fight

(5) forced someone into sexual activity with him or her

(6) was physically cruel to animals

(7) was physically cruel to other people

(8) deliberately destroyed others' property (other than by fire-setting)

(9) deliberately engaged in fire-setting

(10) often lied (other than to avoid physical or sexual abuse)

(11) has stolen without confrontation of a victim on more than one occasion (including forgery)

(12) has stolen with confrontation of a victim (e.g., mugging, purse-snatching, extortion, armed robbery)

C. A pattern of irresponsible and antisocial behavior since the age of 15, as indicated by at least *four* of the following:

(1) is unable to sustain consistent work behavior, as indicated by any of the following (including similar behavior in academic settings if the person is a student):

   (a) significant unemployment for six months or more within five years when expected to work and work was available

   (b) repeated absences from work unexplained by illness in self or family

   (c) abandonment of several jobs without realistic plans for others

(2) fails to conform to social norms with respect to lawful behavior, as indicated by repeatedly performing antisocial acts that are grounds for arrest (whether arrested or not), e.g., destroying property, harassing others, stealing, pursuing an illegal occupation

(3) is irritable and aggressive, as indicated by repeated physical fights or assaults (not required by one's job or to defend someone or oneself), including spouse- or child-beating

(4) repeatedly fails to honor financial obligations, as indicated by defaulting on debts or failing to provide child support or support for other dependents on a regular basis

(5) fails to plan ahead, or is impulsive, as indicated by one or both of the following:

   (a) traveling from place to place without a prearranged job or clear goal for the period of travel or clear idea about when the travel will terminate

   (b) lack of a fixed address for a month or more

(6) has no regard for the truth, as indicated by repeated lying, use of aliases, or "conning" others for personal profit or pleasure

(7) is reckless regarding his or her own or others' personal safety, as indicated by driving while intoxicated, or recurrent speeding

(8) if a parent or guardian, lacks ability to function as a responsible parent, as indicated by one or more of the following:

   (a) malnutrition of child

   (b) child's illness resulting from lack of minimal hygiene

   (c) failure to obtain medical care for a seriously ill child

(d) child's dependence on neighbors or nonresident relatives for food or shelter

(e) failure to arrange for a caretaker for young child when parent is away from home

(f) repeated squandering, on personal items, of money required for household necessities

(9) has never sustained a totally monogamous relationship for more than one year

(10) lacks remorse (feels justified in having hurt, mistreated, or stolen from another)

D. Occurrence of antisocial behavior not exclusively during the course of Schizophrenia or Manic Episodes.

Borderline Personality Disorder

A pervasive pattern of instability of mood, interpersonal relationships, and self-image, beginning by early adulthood and present in a variety of contexts, as indicated by at least *five* of the following:

(1) a pattern of unstable and intense interpersonal relationships characterized by alternating between extremes of overidealization and devaluation

(2) impulsiveness in at least two areas that are potentially self-damaging, e.g., spending, sex, substance use, shoplifting, reckless driving, binge eating (Do not include suicidal or self-multilating behavior covered in [5].)

(3) affective instability: marked shifts from baseline mood to depression, irritability, or anxiety, usually lasting a few hours and only rarely more than a few days

(4) inappropriate, intense anger or lack of control of anger, e.g., frequent displays of temper, constant anger, recurrent physical fights

(5) recurrent suicidal threats, gestures, or behavior, or self-mutilating behavior

(6) marked and persistent identity disturbance manifested by uncertainty about at least two of the following: self-image, sexual orientation, long-term goals or career choice, type of friends desired, preferred values

(7) chronic feelings of emptiness or boredom

(8) frantic efforts to avoid real or imagined abandonment (Do not include suicidal or self-mutilating behavior covered in [5].)

Histrionic Personality Disorder

A pervasive pattern of excessive emotionality and attention-seeking, beginning by early adulthood and present in a variety of contexts, as indicated by at least *four* of the following:

(1) constantly seeks or demands reassurance, approval, or praise

(2) is inappropriately sexually seductive in appearance or behavior

(3) is overly concerned with physical attractiveness

(4) expresses emotion with inappropriate exaggeration, e.g., embraces casual acquaintances with excessive ardor, uncontrollable sobbing on minor sentimental occasions, has temper tantrums

(5) is uncomfortable in situations in which he or she is not the center of attention

(6) displays rapidly shifting and shallow expression of emotions

(7) is self-centered, actions being directed toward obtaining immediate satisfaction; has no tolerance for the frustration of delayed gratification

(8) has a style of speech that is excessively impressionistic and lacking in detail, e.g., when asked to describe mother, can be no more specific than, "She was a beautiful person."

Narcissistic Personality Disorder

A pervasive pattern of grandiosity (in fantasy or behavior), lack of empathy, and hypersensitivity to the evaluation of others, beginning by early adulthood and present in a variety of contexts, as indicated by at least *five* of the following:

(1) reacts to criticism with feelings of rage, shame, or humiliation (even if not expressed)

(2) is interpersonally exploitative: takes advantage of others to achieve his or her own ends

(3) has a grandiose sense of self-importance, e.g., exaggerates achievements and talents, expects to be noticed as "special" without appropriate achievement

(4) believes that his or her problems are unique and can be understood only by other special people

(5) is preoccupied with fantasies of unlimited success, power, brilliance, beauty, or ideal love

(6) has a sense of entitlement: unreasonable expectation of especially favorable treatment, e.g., assumes that he or she does not have to wait in line when others must do so

(7) requires constant attention and admiration, e.g., keeps fishing for compliments

(8) lack of empathy: inability to recognize and experience how others feel, e.g., annoyance and surprise when a friend who is seriously ill cancels a date

(9) is preoccupied with feelings of envy

Dependent Personality Disorder

A pervasive pattern of dependent and submissive behavior, beginning by early adulthood and present in a variety of contexts, as indicated by at least *five* of the following:

(1) is unable to make everyday decisions without an excessive amount of advice or reassurance from others

(2) allows others to make most of his or her important decisions, e.g., where to live, what job to take

(3) agrees with people even when he or she believes they are wrong, because of fear of being rejected

(4) has difficulty initiating projects or doing things on his or her own

(5) volunteers to do things that are unpleasant or demeaning in order to get other people to like him or her

(6) feels uncomfortable or helpless when alone, or goes to great lengths to avoid being alone

(7) feels devastated or helpless when close relationships end

(8) is frequently preoccupied with fears of being abandoned

(9) is easily hurt by criticism or disapproval

Obsessive Compulsive Personality Disorder

A pervasive pattern of perfectionism and inflexibility, beginning by early adulthood and present in a variety of contexts, as indicated by at least *five* of the following:

(1) perfectionism that interferes with task completion, e.g., inability to complete a project because own overly strict standards are not met

(2) preoccupation with details, rules, lists, order, organization, or schedules to the extent that the major point of the activity is lost

(3) unreasonable insistence that others submit to exactly his or her way of doing things, or unreasonable reluctance to allow others to do things because of the conviction that they will not do them correctly

(4) excessive devotion to work and productivity to the exclusion of leisure activities and friendships (not accounted for by obvious economic necessity)

(5) indecisiveness: decision making is either avoided, postponed, or protracted, e.g., the person cannot get assignments done on

time because of ruminating about priorities (do not include if indecisiveness is due to excessive need for advice or reassurance from others)

(6) overconscientiousness, scrupulousness, and inflexibility about matters of morality, ethics, or values (not accounted for by cultural or religious identification)

(7) restricted expression of affection

(8) lack of generosity in giving time, money, or gifts when no personal gain is likely to result

(9) inability to discard worn-out or worthless objects even when they have no sentimental value

Passive Aggressive Personality Disorder

A pervasive pattern of passive resistance to demands for adequate social and occupational performance, beginning by early adulthood and present in a variety of contexts, as indicated by at least *five* of the following:

(1) procrastinates, i.e., puts off things that need to be done so that deadlines are not met

(2) becomes sulky, irritable, or argumentative when asked to do something he or she does not want to do

(3) seems to work deliberately slowly or to do a bad job on tasks that he or she really does not want to do

(4) protests, without justification, that others make unreasonable demands on him or her

(5) avoids obligations by claiming to have "forgotten"

(6) believes that he or she is doing a much better job than others think he or she is doing

(7) resents useful suggestions from others concerning how he or she could be more productive

(8) obstructs the efforts of others by failing to do his or her share of the work

(9) unreasonably criticizes or scorns people in positions of authority

Questions and Comments

1. *Additional information.* In addition to the diagnostic criteria, DSM–III–R provides information, when available, on associated features of each disorder, age at onset, course of the disorder, predisposing factors, prevalence, sex ratio, and familial pattern.

2. *Application of criteria.* Do any of the above diagnostic categories seem to apply to the eight cases described at the beginning of this chapter? Do any apply to you?

C. CRITICISMS OF DSM–III

DAVID GOLEMAN, "WHO'S MENTALLY ILL?"

11 Psychology Today 34–41.
(Jan. 1978).

* * *

Much of the controversy over *DSM–III* comes from its definition of the term "mental disorder." To qualify as a disorder, a patient's problem must, in its extreme form, cause him distress or disability. In some cases, the distress or disability may not be at all obvious. "Many schizophrenics and manics, particularly while acutely ill, deny subjective distress and object to being designated as ill," notes [Dr. Robert] Spitzer [Chair of the DSM–III Task Force].

"However, in the extreme form, these and similar conditions are regularly and intrinsically associated with disability and therefore are usefully categorized as disorders."

Under this definition, the manual recognizes habits like smoking as a treatable problem under certain circumstances. The definition of "tobacco-use disorder" proposed for *DSM–III* reads, in part: "This manual generally does not regard a condition or behavior as a mental or medical disorder if that condition has widespread social support for being regarded as 'normal'. . . . A heavy smoker who has no serious tobacco-caused or aggravated medical problems and who denies concern about smoking does not have tobacco-use disorder. . . . The use of tobacco is considered a mental disorder either when the use of the substance is directly associated with distress at the need to repeatedly use the substance; or, there is evidence of a serious tobacco-related medical disorder in an individual who is judged to be currently physiologically dependent upon tobacco."

If a smoker feels no distress when he can't have a cigarette, and if he has no physical symptoms, the diagnosis doesn't apply—although, as *DSM–III* notes, his habit makes him a likely candidate for developing the disorder. In a letter to the profession's trade paper *Psychiatric News,* Spitzer and a colleague, Dr. Jerome Jaffe, wrote that "tobacco-use disorder" is associated with "the three undesirable *D*'s that are the core criteria for the definition of mental disorder (distress, disability, or death). Because 'tobacco-use disorder' fits what we regard as a reasonable definition of medical and psychiatric disorder, it will be included in the proposed *DSM–III* classification, even if, unexplained, it invites derision."

Cigarette-smoking falls under "Drug–Use Disorders," a controversial category that also includes abuse of alcohol, marijuana, and more potent drugs. The manual acknowledges that the use of mood-altering drugs is common, but labels the strong desire to continue taking them a symptom of "drug-dependence disorder."

The problem of "caffeinism" comes under the heading of "Drug–Induced Organic Mental Disorders," a subsection that describes the specific effects on the brain of certain drugs. Some feel the standards set for diagnosing caffeinism are unrealistically low. One of the three criteria, for example, is recent consumption of the equivalent of two or three cups of coffee.

The publication of an early draft of *DSM–III*'s categories in *Psychiatric News* brought letters of protest—and ridicule. Richard Proctor, a psychiatrist in Winston–Salem, North Carolina, commented, tongue in cheek: "Since I use both tobacco and coffee, I hope that my hospital insurance and all of the other third-party carriers will cover the cost of hospitalization and treatment if I decide I would like to stop. . . . If, after prolonged hospitalization and treatment, I am still unable to abstain, I am more hopeful that I will be eligible for my disability benefits and my early Social Security benefits by reason of illness, since the use of tobacco and caffeine will be listed as official illnesses in *DSM–III*."

* * *

If the proposed new manual contains some seemingly trivial mental problems, it is because Spitzer's committee seeks to make it clearer, more comprehensive, and exact. For this reason, the committee has replaced a number of older, more traditional classifications with newer categories and a more thorough listing of symptoms. "The old manual," Spitzer explains, "would give you a description of a prototypical patient, but it would not tell you what clinical features had to be present before you could make the diagnosis. You had a rough feeling for what the patients were supposed to be like, but you didn't know what the borders of the condition were.

"Take schizophrenia. They'd mention delusions, hallucinations, thought disorder, impairment in social relations, flattening of affect [the patient's overall emotional tone or liveliness], and so on. But you never knew whether some or all of these had to be present before you made the diagnosis. They didn't specify because it's easier to be vague. That way you don't have to resolve differences of opinion. We take an activist view. We try to eliminate ambiguity and resolve differences." (The current manual devotes three pages to criteria for diagnosing different types of schizophrenia; the proposed revision, *DSM–III*, contains 17 pages of criteria.)

But many psychoanalysts disagree with the abandonment of the analyst's familiar categories in favor of strictly observable symptoms. One of them is John Schimel, who wrote an angry editorial in the April 1976 issue of the *Journal of the American Academy of Psychoanalysis*. "People are reduced to ciphers, symptoms," Schimel protested. "*Inferred* conditions [italics supplied for emphasis], such as neuroses, do not appear. Hysteria is reduced to Briquet's disorder, paralysis, paresis, aphonia, blindness, deafness, anesthesia. . . . I haven't seen one of these in years; I treat hysterics every day."

Schimel adds, "I do not find in *DSM–III* the kinds of neurotic patients I have worked with for thirty years, only disembodied fragments; I do not find the hysterics, the obsessionals, the anxiety-ridden, the socially or situationally afflicted. I believe the direction of *DSM–III* to be profoundly regressive, even antisocial . . . it does not fit the troubled human beings we see in our offices or hospital clinics; our patients are people, not target symptoms."

Attacks like Schimel's irk Spitzer, who feels they reflect a don't-confuse-me-with-facts attitude. "There are those who may be distressed not to find the category of neurosis, but that does not mean that the conditions that have traditionally been included in the neuroses have been eliminated," Spitzer says. "We have merely reclassified the conditions that were under the rubric of neuroses somewhat differently, and, we think, for good reasons. If neuroses have disappeared as a present classification, the neurotic subtypes remain. Depression, for example, is listed under 'Mood Disorders.' Obsessional neurosis is found under the category of 'Anxiety Disorders,' and so forth. The word 'hysterical,' with its confusing meaning, has been changed to 'histrionic'—all these concepts are understood better by reading the definitions than merely by looking at the names."

* * *

At the 1975 meeting of the American Psychiatric Association, members got their first look at a draft of *DSM–III*. Spitzer fielded an onslaught of objections with genial flexibility. A number of times he accepted the suggestions of critics on the spot, promising changes with comments such as, "That's a good idea. We hadn't thought of that." Spitzer's political style is one of accommodation. Rather than turn dissenters into enemies, he prefers to join them. [H]is consensus politics have resulted in a number of changes.

An alleged male bias in the early drafts of *DSM–III* riled feminists. They complained particularly about a category called "Gender–Identity Disorder of Childhood," which seemed to label certain tomboys as abnormal. The diagnosis applied to any girl who preferred to wear boys' clothes, play boys' games, hang out with boys instead of girls, fantasize about being a boy, or express the desire to become one. This description, says Ann Chappell, a San Francisco psychiatrist, can fit any normal tomboy who is alert to the greater freedom enjoyed by boys, who, for instance, are allowed to stay out later at night. It may be quite normal for a girl to want similar privileges, Chappell argues. "It certainly is destructive to call social awareness in sex role a mental disorder," she says. Chappell joined a group of like-minded psychiatrists serving on the APA's standing Committee on Women, which examined *DSM–III* for sexist bias. At the group's behest, the clause was rewritten to give tomboys a clean bill of mental health.

The heading called "Sexual Sadism" also drew strong objections from the Committee on Women. As defined at first, it included rapists and murderers who inflicted suffering on a nonconsenting partner for their own sexual excitement. The women's committee feared such a definition would allow an accused rapist to plead that he was suffering from mental illness and should go to a psychiatric hospital rather than a prison. To avoid this potential loophole, the manual task force rewrote the provision. It now specifies that the patient must have a compulsion to commit sadistic sexual violence, as demonstrated by repeated acts—a criterion most rapists could not meet.

One of Spitzer's most artful accommodations was over the new manual's treatment of homosexuality. Spitzer was one of those who objected to including homosexuality as a mental disorder in *DSM–III.* "Homosexuality" was dropped from later printings of *DSM–II* after the APA's vote in 1974. In the draft revision of the manual, it is replaced by "Homosexual–Conflict Disorder," which refers to someone who is distressed by an internal conflict over his homosexual arousal. In other words, if a homosexual feels no distress because of his sexual habits, then by the standards of *DSM–III,* he does not have a mental disorder.

Not everyone is happy with Spitzer's compromise on homosexuality. In a letter to *Psychiatric News,* Lewis Glickman, a Brooklyn psychiatrist, observed one of the ironies in the draft that has also been noted by others. Glickman expressed mock astonishment at the logic of a manual that would "include the smoker who wishes to give up smoking in the category of emotional illness, while eliminating the homosexual who wishes to continue his homosexuality."

The Vietnam Veterans' Working Group brought a new syndrome to the attention of the manual task force. New York psychiatrist Chaim Shatan, their coordinator, cited studies that found that 40 percent of American POWs from World War II and the Korean War had met violent deaths by suicide, homicide, or auto accidents. Shatan expressed fears that Vietnam vets, after a latency period of years with no evident problem, might suddenly begin to develop similar symptoms. "Survivors of combat, or other catastrophic manmade stress, experience far more enduring disorders than do survivors of natural disasters," Shatan said, during a panel session at last year's APA meeting. "We find that a symptom-free 'incubation period,' or delay of nine to 48 months or more, often precedes clinical symptoms and syndromes related to combat experience."

The manual task force enlarged its category of "Acute and Chronic Catastrophic Stress" to cover both natural disasters, such as floods, and "social" catastrophes, including combat. It also accepted a new subtype, "Post–Traumatic Stress Disorder," which would cover the delayed reactions Shatan fears would occur among Vietnam vets. The diagnosis helps establish the link between their current symptoms and their military experience, and thus makes it easier to justify veterans' benefits for treatment.

For both patients and therapists, a major impact of *DSM–III* will be financial. More and more therapy is paid for by third parties, whether through a health-insurance plan, Social Security, or another agency. Chaim Shatan notes that "the diagnostic act intervenes crucially in the lives of countless people—whether this result is intended or not."

Insurance companies vary in their policies toward the specific disorders they will compensate, but for any payment at all, a psychiatrist's diagnosis will most certainly have to be listed in *DSM–III*. This makes many psychotherapists uncomfortable. John Schimel described the overall problem this way:

"That which had been taken for granted, the need for treatment, now had to be defined and measured. It's not too difficult in defining pneumonia. It has not been too easy in many psychiatric conditions."

* * *

Questions and Comments

1. *Changes in DSM–III–R.* DSM–III–R reflected further changes in some of the diagnostic categories described in Goleman's article. For instance, "Caffeinism" is now "Caffeine Intoxication" and requires "recent consumption of caffeine, usually in excess of 250 mg., as well as at least five of the following signs: restlessness, nervousness, excitement, insomnia, flushed face, diuresis, gastrointestinal disturbance, muscle twitching, rambling flow of thought and speech, tachycardia or cardiac arrhythmia, periods of inexhaustibility, and psychomotor agitation. Tobacco use disorder is now lumped under the general category of "psychoactive substance dependence disorder," which requires at least three of the following: substance taken in larger amounts or over a longer period of time than the person intended; a persistent desire or one or more unsuccessful efforts to cut down or control substance use; a great deal of time spent in activities necessary to get the substance, take the substance (e.g., chain smoking), or recovering from its effects; frequent symptoms when expected to fulfill major role obligations at work, school, or home; important social, occupational, or recreational activities given up or reduced because of substance use; continued substance use despite knowledge of having a persistent or current social, psychological, or physical problem that is caused or exacerbated by the use of the substance; marked tolerance, meaning a need for markedly increased amounts of the substance in order to achieve the desired effect or markedly diminished effect with continued use of the same amount; characteristic withdrawal symptoms; substance often taken to relieve or avoid withdrawal symptoms.

2. *Reasons for overinclusiveness.* Assuming arguendo that the Manual is too expansive in its definition of mental disorder, why might this be the case? One reason was suggested by George Albee, past president of the American Psychological Association. In that organization's newsletter, the APA Monitor, Albee argued that DSM–III was an attempt by the American Psychiatric Association to preempt the territory of the other mental health professions by "turning every human problem in to a disease, in anticipation of the shower of health-plan gold that is over the horizon." Quoted in Goleman, supra at 34. Other reasons are suggested in the following materials.

III. MENTAL ILLNESS AS MYTH

Since the early 1960's, considerable controversy has been generated by the idea that mental illness is a "myth". This argument was originally advanced in this provocative form by Thomas Szasz, a psychiatrist who takes a psychoanalytic approach to treatment. The titles of Szasz' books indicate his general approach to the concept of mental illness: The Myth of Mental Illness (1961); The Manufacture of Madness (1970); Ideology and Insanity (1970); Ceremonial Chemistry: The Ritual Persecution of Drugs, Addicts, and Pushers (1974). The excerpts below represent summaries of ideas from his works and responses to them.

A. THE CLAIMS OF SZASZ AND "RADICAL PSYCHIATRY"

THOMAS SZASZ, IDEOLOGY AND INSANITY

(New York: Doubleday, 1970).
pp. 12–21.

THE MYTH OF MENTAL ILLNESS

My aim in this essay is to ask if there is such a thing as mental illness, and to argue that there is not. Of course, mental illness is not a thing or physical object; hence it can exist only in the same sort of way as do other theoretical concepts. Yet, to those who believe in them, familiar theories are likely to appear, sooner or later, as "objective truths" or "facts." During certain historical periods, explanatory concepts such as deities, witches, and instincts appeared not only as theories but as *self-evident causes* of a vast number of events. Today mental illness is widely regarded in a similar fashion, that is, as the cause of innumerable diverse happenings.

As an antidote to the complacent use of the notion of mental illness—as a self-evident phenomenon, theory, or cause—let us ask: What is meant when it is asserted that someone is mentally ill? In this essay I shall describe the main uses of the concept of mental illness, and I shall argue that this notion has outlived whatever cognitive usefulness it might have had and that it now functions as a myth.

[I]

The notion of mental illness derives its main support from such phenomena as syphilis of the brain or delirious conditions—intoxications, for instance—in which persons may manifest certain disorders of thinking and behavior. Correctly speaking, however, these are diseases of the brain, not of the mind. According to one school of thought, *all* so-called mental illness is of this type. The assumption is made that some neurological defect, perhaps a very subtle one, will ultimately be found to explain all the disorders of thinking and behavior. Many contemporary physicians, psychiatrists, and other scientists hold this view, which implies that people's troubles cannot be caused by conflicting personal needs, opinions, social aspirations, values, and so forth. These difficulties—which I think we may simply call *problems in living*—are thus attributed to physiochemical processes that in due time will be discovered (and no doubt corrected) by medical research.

Mental illnesses are thus regarded as basically similar to other diseases. The only difference, in this view, between mental and bodily disease is that the former, affecting the brain, manifests itself by means of mental symptoms; whereas the latter, affecting other organ systems—for example, the skin, liver, and so on—manifests itself by means of symptoms referable to those parts of the body.

In my opinion, this view is based on two fundamental errors. In the first place, a disease of the brain, analogous to a disease of the skin or bone, is a neurological defect, not a problem in living. For example, a *defect* in a person's visual field may be explained by correlating it with certain lesions in the nervous system. On the other hand, a person's *belief*—whether it be in Christianity, in Communism, or in the idea that his internal organs are rotting and that his body is already dead—cannot be explained by a defect or disease of the nervous system. Explanations of this sort of occurrence—assuming that one is interested in the belief itself and does not regard it simply as a symptom or expression of something else that is more interesting—must be sought along different lines.

The second error is epistemological. It consists of interpreting communications about ourselves and the world around us as symptoms of neurological functioning. This is an error not in observation or reasoning, but rather in the organization and expression of knowledge. In the present case, the error lies in making a dualism between mental and physical symptoms, a dualism that is a habit of speech and not the result of known observations. Let us see if this is so.

In medical practice, when we speak of physical disturbances we mean either signs (for example, fever) or symptoms (for example, pain). We speak of mental symptoms, on the other hand, when we refer to a patient's communications about himself, others, and the world about him. The patient might assert that he is Napoleon or that he is being persecuted by the Communists. These would be considered mental symptoms only if the observer believed that the patient was *not* Napoleon or that he was *not* being persecuted by the Communists. This makes it apparent that the statement "X is a mental symptom" involves rendering a judgment that entails a covert comparison between the patient's ideas, concepts, or beliefs and those of the observer and the society in which they live. The notion of mental symptom is therefore inextricably tied to the social, and particularly the ethical, context in which it is made, just as the notion of bodily symptom is tied to an anatomical and genetic context.

To sum up: For those who regard mental symptoms as signs of brain disease, the concept of mental illness is unnecessary and misleading. If they mean that people so labeled suffer from diseases of the brain, it would seem better, for the sake of clarity, to say that and not something else.

[II]

The term "mental illness" is also widely used to describe something quite different from a disease of the brain. Many people today take it for granted that living is an arduous affair. Its hardship for modern man derives, moreover, not so much from a struggle for biological survival as from the stresses and strains inherent in the social intercourse of complex human personalities. In this context, the notion of mental illness is used to identify or describe some feature of an individual's so-called personality. Mental illness—as a deformity of the personality, so to speak—is then regarded as the cause of human disharmony. It is implicit in this view that social intercourse between people is regarded as something inherently harmonious, its disturbance being due solely to the presence of "mental illness" in many people. Clearly, this is faulty reasoning, for it makes the abstraction "mental illness" into a cause of, even though this abstraction was originally created to serve only as a shorthand expression for, certain types of human behavior. It now becomes necessary to ask: What kinds of behavior are regarded as indicative of mental illness, and by whom?

The concept of illness, whether bodily or mental, implies deviation from some clearly defined norm. In the case of physical illness, the norm is the structural and functional integrity of the human body. Thus, although the desirability of physical health, as such, is an ethical value, what health is can be stated in anatomical and physiological terms. What is the norm, deviation from which is regarded as mental illness? This question cannot be easily answered. But whatever this norm may be, we can be certain of only one thing: namely, that it must be stated in terms of psychosocial, ethical, and legal concepts. For example, notions such as "excessive repression" and "acting out an unconscious impulse" illustrate the use of psychological concepts for judging so-called mental health and illness. The idea that chronic hostility, vengefulness, or divorce are indicative of mental illness is an illustration of the use of ethical norms (that is, the desirability of love, kindness, and a stable marriage relationship). Finally, the widespread psychiatric opinion that only a mentally ill person would commit homicide illustrates the use of a legal concept as a norm of mental health. In short, when one speaks of mental illness, the norm from which deviation is measured is a *psychosocial and ethical* standard. Yet, the remedy is sought in terms of *medical* measures that—it is hoped and assumed—are free from wide differences of ethical value. The definition of the disorder and the terms in which its remedy are sought are therefore at serious odds with one another. The practical significance of this covert conflict between the alleged nature of the defect and the actual remedy can hardly be exaggerated.

Having identified the norms used for measuring deviations in cases of mental illness, we shall now turn to the question, Who defines the norms and hence the deviation? Two basic answers may be offered: First, it may be the person himself—that is, the patient—who decides that he deviates from a norm; for example, an artist may believe that he suffers from a work inhibition; and he may implement this conclusion by seeking help *for himself* from a psychotherapist. Second, it may be someone other than the "patient" who decides that the latter is deviant—for example, relatives, physicians, legal authorities, society generally; a psychiatrist may then be hired by persons other than the "patient" to do something *to him* in order to correct the deviation.

* * *

Psychiatry is much more intimately related to problems of ethics than is medicine in general. I use the word "psychiatry" here to refer to the contemporary discipline concerned with problems in living, and not with diseases of the brain, which belong to neurology. Difficulties in human relations can be analyzed, interpreted, and given meaning only within specific social and ethical contexts. Accordingly, the psychiatrist's socio-ethical orientations will influence his ideas on what is wrong with the patient, on what deserves comment or interpretation, in what directions change might be desirable, and so forth. Even in medicine proper, these factors play a role, as illustrated by the divergent orientations that physicians, depending on their religious affiliations, have toward such things as birth control and therapeutic abortion. Can anyone really believe that a psychotherapist's ideas on religion, politics, and related issues play no role in his practical work? If, on the other hand, they do matter, what are we to infer from it? Does it not seem reasonable that perhaps we ought to have different psychiatric therapies—each recognized for the ethical positions that it embodies—for, say, Catholics and Jews, religious persons and atheists, democrats and Communists, white supermacists and Negroes, and so on?

[III]

[I]t seems to me that in our scientific theories of behavior we have failed to accept the simple fact that human relations are inherently fraught with difficulties, and to make them even relatively harmonious requires much patience and hard work. I submit that the idea of mental illness is now being put to work to obscure certain difficulties that at present may be inherent—not that they need to be unmodifiable—in the social intercourse of persons. If this is true, the concept functions as a disguise: instead of calling attention to conflicting human needs, aspirations, and values, the concept of mental illness provides an amoral and impersonal "thing"—an "illness"—as an explanation for problems in living. We may recall in this connection that not so long ago it was devils and witches that were held responsible for man's problems in living. The belief in mental illness, as something other than man's trouble in getting along with his fellow man, is the proper heir to the belief in demonology and witchcraft. Mental illness thus exists or is "real" in exactly the same sense in which witches existed or were "real."

* * *

I do not here propose to offer a new conception of "psychiatric illness" or a new form of "therapy." My aim is more modest and yet also more ambitious. It is to suggest that the phenomena now called mental illnesses be looked at afresh and more simply, that they be removed from the category of illnesses, and that they be regarded as the expressions of man's struggle with *the problem of how he should live.* This problem is obviously a vast one, its enormity reflecting not only man's inability to cope with his environment, but even more his increasing self-reflectiveness.

By problems in living, then, I refer to that explosive chain reaction that began with man's fall from divine grace by partaking of the fruit of the tree of knowledge. Man's awareness of himself and of the world about him seems to be a steadily expanding one, bringing in its wake an ever larger *burden of understanding.* This burden is to be expected and must not be misinterpreted. Our only rational means for easing it is more understanding, and appropriate action based on such understanding. The main alternative lies in acting as though the burden were not what in fact we perceive it to be, and taking refuge in an outmoded theological view of man. In such a view, man does not fashion his life and much of his world about him, but merely lives out his fate in a world created by superior beings. This may logically lead to pleading non-responsibility in the face of seemingly unfathomable problems and insurmountable difficulties. Yet, if man fails to take increasing responsibility for his actions, individually as well as collectively, it seems unlikely that some higher power or being would assume this task and carry this burden for him. Moreover, this seems hardly a propitious time in human history for obscuring the issue of man's responsibility for his actions by hiding it behind the skirt of an all-explaining conception of mental illness.

SZASZ, T., INTERVIEW

18 The New Physician 453–55.
(1969).

* * *

[Q:] [W]hy are people called mentally ill, if, as you say, they are not *really* ill?

SZASZ: Modern psychiatry may be said to have developed from the refinements of three interrelated phenomena: neurological diseases, malingering, and conversion hysteria. Neurological diseases are diseases of the nervous system, like neurosyphilis or multiple sclerosis. They present no conceptual problem. The problem for modern psychiatry really begins with persons who appear to have a neurological disease—seem to be paralyzed or blind—but who, when medically examined, display no abnormal neurological signs. In other words, they are physically normal and only mimic the picture of a neurological illness. Until the second half of the 19th century, persons of this kind were generally categorized as malingerers; that is, not sick. Modern psychiatrists, beginning with Charcot, and then much more actively, with Freud, claimed that these people were sick, suffering from an illness called "hysteria," and that they ought to be treated as patients. Two very important things were involved in this process of reclassification. One was the extension of the concept of illness from bodily disorder per se to what only looks like a bodily disorder but is actually a so-called mental disorder. The second was the recognition of the *sick role* as a sufficient criterion of illness (even in persons with healthy bodies), so that hypochondriacs, homosexuals, criminals, and people with all kinds of other deviant conduct could be, and were, classified as ill, mentally ill. With the development of modern psychiatry, the whole concept of illness has expanded; indeed it has become an almost infinitely elastic category capable of including anything psychiatrists want to place in it.

[Q:] Dr. Szasz, could you elaborate on the distinction between illness as a bodily disorder and the sick role, as a social performance?

SZASZ: Yes, I think this is a very important distinction. I believe that much confusion in psychiatry is due to a failure to distinguish between these two elementary concepts and the phenomena they designate.

Strictly speaking, an illness is a biological or physicochemical abnormality of the human body or its functioning. A person is sick if he has diabetes, a stroke, or cancer. Such diseases are physicochemical events, similar to natural events like solar eclipses or typhoons—except that they happen to the human body. It is important to emphasize that medical diseases are things that *happen* to human bodies, rather than things that people *do* with their bodies.

The sick role, on the other hand, is not a biological condition but a social status; it refers to a status of claiming illness by, for example, complaining of pain, fever, or weakness, and/or seeking medical attention. Like other social roles, such as father, husband, soldier, or college student, the sick role denotes a certain kind of relationship to other people in society.

* * *

[Q:] Now, how do you apply these concepts to mental illness? To schizophrenia, for example?

SZASZ: I view all behavior—"well" or "sick"—in the framework of symbolic action, or roles and games (in the serious, not frivolous, sense). This means that we can't talk about the problem as one of "mental illness" or "schizophrenia." Instead, we must identify it in behavioral terms, or, as I like to put it, in plain English. For example, let us assume that when we are talking about schizophrenia we mean a social situation where a person makes a patently false, self-aggrandizing claim. A poor, socially insignificant man may thus claim that he is

Jesus; or a poor, socially insignificant woman, that she is the Holy Virgin. If you look at this phenomenon simply, without any complicated psychiatric preconceptions or pretentions, you will notice that, whatever the *reason* for their action, such people make *false claims* about themselves. They impersonate; they pretend to be someone or something they are not. To me this is more like cheating in a game, or like fraudulent advertising—than it is like cancer or pneumonia. The simple fact, . . . is that in such cases we deal with conflicting claims, not with diseases.

* * *

In certain cases of interpersonal and social conflict, then, it sometimes happens that one party defines the other as "mentally sick" or "schizophrenic." This is one of the "solutions" our society provides for resolving such conflicts. In this sense, "schizophrenia" is an assigned or ascribed role—like convict or draftee. If we only looked at the "psychotic" as an individual cast in a role he does not want to be in—cast in it by his "loved ones," by his employer, by his psychiatrist, by society generally—we would at least be in a position to start to deal honestly with what we now call, quite misleadingly, the problem of "serious mental disease."

* * *

Questions and Comments

1. *Legal implications.* Much of Szasz' work attempts to develop the theme, alluded to at the end of the first excerpt, that the "myth of mental illness" is improperly used to "obscur[e] the issue of man's responsibility for his actions." Moore has summarized the legal implications of this position: "either the insanity defense should be abolished and those we call mentally ill punished like anyone else, or at the very least the phrase should play no part as a separate defense; the incompetency plea should either be abolished or highly limited; those we call mentally ill should be sued for breach of contract like anyone else, not excused from their contractual obligations because of supposed incapacity to contract; no one should be civilly committed for mental illness, for the mentally ill know their own good and have the capacity to act in accordance with such a conception no less than anyone else * * *; [and] anyone inside or outside a mental hospital should have the full civil rights of any citizen because he is just like any citizen." Moore, "Some Myths About 'Mental Illness' ", 18 Inquiry 233 (1975). In other words, if the legal system adopted Szasz' point of view, Part II of this book would be much shorter.

2. *The physical component of mental illness.* The primary thrust of Szasz' assault is aimed at the medical model of mental disorder. A major premise of his argument is that mental illness, unlike physical illness, has no bodily referent (which explains why mental retardation, which is commonly believed to be genetically transmitted, is exempted from the Szaszian attack). For much of what is labeled "mental illness", Szasz is right; there is not yet any proven biological correlate. But the medical model of illness does have some empirical support with respect to some behavioral phenomena. Even before Szasz began writing, for instance, it was clear

that manic behavior, hallucinations, and severe depression are responsive to certain types of medication, discussed in more detail later in this book. That these phenomena can be eliminated with chemicals suggests that they are physiologically rooted.

More recent research has sought to verify this theory, especially with respect to schizophrenia, which is the most widely used diagnosis and the paradigmatic "mental illness." For instance, there is evidence connecting schizophrenia with an excess level of dopamine in the body. Dopamine is a neurotransmitter, a substance which transmits information between nerve cells. Studies have shown that when amphetamines are given in high doses, a person's dopamine level rises at the same time symptoms which resemble schizophrenia occur. Additionally, when L-dopa, a drug which the body turns into dopamine, is given to persons with schizophrenia, it often makes them worse. Finally, drugs which are effective in treating schizophrenia clearly block dopamine action. Langer, Brown & Docherty, "Dopamine Receptor Supersensitivity and Schizophrenia: A Review," 7 Schizophrenia Bulletin 208 (1981). Studies of monozygotic twins (twins from the same zygote and thus with the same genetic material) also suggest that schizophrenia is genetically transmitted; for every twin pair from separate zygotes who are schizophrenic, five twin pairs from the same zygote are so designated. Gottesman, J.J. & Shields, J., Schizophrenia and Genetics (Academic Press: 1972). Finally, it has been claimed that the brains of those diagnosed as schizophrenic differ both in structure and function from other brains. Averback, "Structural Lesions of the Brain of Young Schizophrenics," 8 Canad. J. Neurol. Sciences 73 (1981); Stevens, "Neuropathology of Schizophrenia," 39 Arch. Gen. Psychiat. 1131 (1982).

Other researchers, however, discount these findings. Sarbin and Mancuso claim that the pharmacological studies are questionable because they do not reveal the extent to which anti-psychotic drugs might be antagonistic to *all* kinds of behavior, rather than just unwanted "schizophrenic" behavior.[d] After a review of the relevant research, they believed they could state "with high confidence" that the dopamine hypothesis "will fade into oblivion" just as other biological theories of schizophrenia have in the past. Sarbin and Mancuso also question the monozygotic twin studies, arguing that others' reaction to the usually poor physical status of such twins might explain the resulting similarity in behaviors. Finally, they note the inevitable difficulty of linking behavior correlated with brain structure, genetic make-up, excess dopamine or any other physiological trait to "schizophrenia," given the vagueness of the criteria for establishing the latter state. Sarbin & Mancuso, Schizophrenia: Medical Diagnosis or Moral Verdict? 144–150 (1980).

In his most recent book, Insanity: The Idea and Its Consequences (1987), Szasz repudiated research suggesting a biological correlate to mental disorders, calling it "either a monumental error, or a monumental fraud, or both." He claimed that the only profession which believes schizophrenia is a brain disease is psychiatry; none of the recent textbooks on pathology

d. For instance, many of these drugs produce "side effects" such as sedation, slowed movement and slurring of speech.

classify schizophrenia or any other psychiatric category as a disease, and internal medicine textbooks do so only because "the physician needs the psychiatrist to relieve him of the difficult patient", and thus "is often corrupted by him" to the extent that he is willing to "accept[ ] and legitimize[ ] the psychiatrist's classic claim that mental illness is like any other illness." (pp. 72–74).

3. *Other attacks on the mental illness concept.* Other theorists, although subscribing to the basic notion that mental illness is a meaningless term, reached this conclusion from perspectives differing from Szasz'.

R.D. Laing. R.D. Laing, who spent many years studying adolescents and others diagnosed as "schizophrenic," is well-known for his assertion that those who have been so diagnosed are not ill but are reacting in a sane and rational way to the intolerable emotional pressures placed on them by society and their families. R.D. Laing, The Politics of Experience (1967). He claimed that "*without exception* the experience and behavior that gets labelled schizophrenic is *a special strategy that a person invents in order to live in an unlivable situation.*" (id. at 114–15, emphasis in original). He also asserted: "What we call 'normal' is a product of repression, denial, splitting, projection, introjection and other forms of destructive action on experience ⁕ ⁕ ⁕ it is radically estranged from the structure of being." Laing & Esterson, Sanity, Madness, and the Family (1970).

Scheff and Labelling Theory. Building on Lemert's work, which suggested that conditions like radicalism, criminality, alcoholism and mental disorder tend to progress or worsen, Lemert, Social Pathology: A Systematic Approach to the Theory of Sociopathic Behavior (1951), Scheff argued that what psychiatrists call mental illness is largely a response to the shock of being labelled and treated as insane and the expectations that this labelling produces. Scheff, Being Mentally Ill: A Sociological Theory (1966). In other words, diagnosing someone mentally ill becomes a self-fulfilling prophecy. Sarbin argued further that labelling a person mentally ill is merely a means of designating "a special class of beings, to be feared or scorned, sometimes to be pitied, but nearly always to be degraded." Sarbin, "On the Futility of the Proposition that Some People be Labeled 'Mentally Ill' ", 31 J. Consult. Psychiat. 447 (1967). In partial support of these views, Goffman documented the pervasive effect of institutionalization on the lives of mental patients, who tend to view themselves as incompetent at leading a "normal life" outside the institution. Goffman, Asylums: Essays on the Social Situation of Mental Patients and Other Inmates (1961).

Other Sociological Perspectives. Krasner has suggested that the disease concept may be the creation of a "schizophrenia industry." Krasner, Foreword in Sarbin & Mancuso, supra. Krasner noted that " 'schizophrenia' as a disease metaphor has spawned thousands of jobs, not only for the psychiatric team (psychiatrist, clinical psychologist, and social worker), and other mental hospital employees, but also for the pharmaceutical, publishing, hospital supply, and related industries. The first task of any industry is to perpetuate itself and then to expand."

4. *Mental illness as a political construct.* As the above materials suggest, the writings of Szasz and others are permeated with the idea that

the concept of mental illness is used as a means of stigmatizing and controlling deviant or different behavior. Some research may support this view. For instance, beginning in the 1950's, several studies noted that the frequencies of different types of mental illness vary among socioeconomic classes, with the lower classes receiving "psychotic" diagnoses and being hospitalized proportionately more often than the upper classes. Hollingshead and Redlich, Social Class and Mental Illness: A Community Study (1958); Srole, Langner, Michael, et al, Mental Health in the Metropolis: The Midtown Manhattan Study (1962). Recent data from the National Institute of Mental Health indicate that non-whites are much more likely than whites to be hospitalized as mentally ill. Manderscheid & Barrett, eds., Mental Health, United States, 1987 (NIMH, 1988) (non-whites represent 31% of civil commitments and 37% of criminal commitments in state and county hospitals).

Research also suggests that women are much more likely to have "psychiatric careers" than men. Chesler, Women & Madness 312 (1972). The reason for this, according to Chesler, is that:

Men are generally allowed a greater range of 'acceptable' behaviors than are women. It can be argued that psychiatric hospitalization or labeling relates to what society considers 'unacceptable' behavior. Thus, since women are allowed fewer total behaviors *and are more strictly confined to their role-sphere than men are,* women, more than men, will commit more behaviors that are seen as 'ill' or 'unacceptable.'

Id. at 39 (note) (emphasis in original).

Finally, providing impetus for the mental illness-as-politics point of view are the accounts from the Soviet Union about the use of psychiatry to confine dissidents. See, e.g., Medvedev & Medvedev, A Question of Madness (translated by de Kadt) (1971). According to Roth, in that country, at least at one time, there was "a straightforward equation between being antisoviet and being mentally ill." Roth, Invited Address, "Uses of Psychiatry in the USSR and USA," October 7, 1988.

Some caveats to the research about American practices should be made. First, there could be explanations other than race or class for the differential in American hospitalization rates; for instance, those from upper classes are much more likely than others to be institutionalized in expensive, private institutions (which tend to be underrepresented in the studies reported). Are there any other possible explanations for the data reported above? Accepting the research at face value, does it necessarily support Szasz' thesis?

B. THE COUNTERATTACK ON AND ULTIMATE IMPACT OF SZASZIAN NOTIONS

MICHAEL MOORE, SOME MYTHS ABOUT MENTAL ILLNESS

18 Inquiry 233.
(1975).

* * *

[M]ental illness is not a myth. It is not some palpable falsehood propagated amongst the populace by power-mad psychiatrists, but a cruel and bitter reality that has been with the human race since antiquity. This is such an obvious truism that to have stated it twenty years ago would have been an embarrassment. Since the advent of radical psychiatry and its legal entourage, however, such truths need restatement. Even more, they need restatement in a form specifically addressed to the various senses in which mental illness has been thought to be a myth. Since on my reading of the radical psychiatrists there seem to be five distinguishable points they have in mind in thinking of mental illness as a myth, the discussion will proceed by considering them seriatim.

* * *

(A) THE MYTH AS A QUESTION OF ONTOLOGICAL STATUS: THERE IS NO SUCH THING AS MENTAL ILLNESS BECAUSE THERE IS NO REFERENT OF THE PHRASE

Mental illness is a myth because, stated popularly, 'there is neither such a thing as "insanity" nor such a thing as "mental disease". These terms do not identify entities having separate existence.'

Less popularly:

It is a term without ostensive referrent [sic] and lacking any, it cannot even be said to have outlived its usefulness, because there is no reason to think that it ever had any.

Szasz and his psychiatric and legal followers are suspicious of mental illness as an entity or thing; when looking into their ontology they see no such thing.

* * *

If the argument is that entity thinking is scientifically legitimate, but only about those entities referred to by terms capable of ostensive reference, such as 'Nixon', or 'St. Elizabeth's Hospital', the radical psychiatrists have a radically impoverished ontology—a nominalist ontology that would not admit the thinghood of abstract entities such as the number 2, squareness, shape, zoological species, or, more to the point perhaps, psychological states. Such a restricted ontology is characteristic neither of science nor of common understanding.

Indeed, in such a restrictive ontological system physical illnesses would not exist either. For the names of physical illnesses do not refer to concrete entities: 'Diseases are not things in the same sense as rocks, or trees, or rivers. Diseases . . . are not material.' Although diseases might be *caused* by the presence in the body of some such entity (as a cold may be caused by a virus), and although they might be associated with *symptoms* that are concrete entities (e.g. the fluid present in the sinuses), a physical illness is not (identical with) either its causes or its symptoms. The only thing one can fix as the referent of the names of various physical illnesses are states the ill are in, abstract entities incapable of being pointed at in some ostensive definition.

* * *

(B) The Myth as an Empirical Discovery: No One is in Fact Mentally Ill

Often mental illness is said to be a myth, not just in the sense that it doesn't exist, but also in the sense that no one is in fact mentally ill. The claim, in other words, denies not just that 'mental illness' is a name of some thing, but that 'mentally ill' is ever truly predicable of a person. The claim is that no one is really mentally ill.

This claim that mental illness is a myth is put forward as an empirical discovery: all of those people that have been thought to be mentally ill (i.e. irrational) are in fact just as rational as you and I. Szasz makes this claim when he argues that 'insane behavior no less than sane, is goal-directed and motivated . . .', and concludes from this that we should regard 'the behavior of the madman as perfectly rational from the point of view of the actor'. Braginsky, Braginsky, and Ring purport to have made the same 'discovery' regarding schizophrenics:

> the residents who remain in 'mental hospitals' are behaving in a perfectly rational manner to achieve a personally satisfying way of life—often the most satisfying of which they are capable . . . in a certain sense an individual *chooses* his career as a mental patient; it is not thrust upon him as a consequence of his somehow becoming 'mentally ill'. But in just what sense does the individual 'choose' his career? In our view, having and maintaining the status of a mental patient is the outcome of *purposive* behavior. Furthermore, given the life circumstances of most of the persons who become and remain residents of mental hospitals, their doing so evinces a realistic appraisal of their available alternatives; it is, in short, a *rational* choice.

* * *

The crunch for even this limited attempt at making out the behavior of the mentally ill as rational, comes in making more precise the nature of the beliefs and desires of mental patients in terms of which their actions are to be so adjudged. More specifically, the fudge occurs when [Szasz and others use] *unconscious* beliefs and desires to fill in where we all know that mental patients did not consciously guide their actions to achieve such goals in light of such beliefs.

* * *

[S]zasz can ignore the conscious/unconscious distinction only at the price of significance. What he fails to realize is that any behavior can be seen as rational (or as in accordance with rules of a game, or as furthering certain goals—Szasz's substitute criteria for consciousness), if one allows oneself the freedom to *invent* the beliefs and desires in terms of which the behavior is to be so viewed.

On occasion the empirical version of the myth claim is put forward without any extensive reliance on some supposed unconscious beliefs or desires of the mentally ill. R.D. Laing in particular explicitly disavows use of unconscious beliefs or desires in reaching his well known conclusion that *'without exception* the experience and behavior that gets labelled schizophrenic is *a special strategy that a person invents in order to live in an unlivable situation'.* Nonetheless such studies do not show schizophrenics to be as rational as everyone else, for the conscious beliefs such patients admittedly do have are themselves irrational beliefs; and actions that are predicated on irrational beliefs, and actors who hold them, are, in common understanding, irrational.

* * *

A convenient example is the case of 'Joan', a catatonic who was not one of Laing's patients but whose case Laing believed to afford 'striking confirmation' of his views regarding schizophrenia. Joan's own subsequent avowals were used by Laing in attributing to her catatonic withdrawal a rational basis. She recalled that when she was catatonic, she 'tried to be dead and grey and motionless'. She thought that her mother 'would like that': 'She could carry me around like a doll.' She also felt that she 'had to die to keep from dying. I know that sounds crazy but one time a boy hurt my feelings very much and I wanted to jump in front of a subway. Instead I went a little catatonic so I wouldn't feel anything'.

Laing finds in such statements the two typical motives for catatonic withdrawal. First, 'there is the primary guilt of having no right to life . . . and hence of being entitled at most only to a dead life'. Since Joan's parents had wanted a boy, and since 'she could not be anything other than what her parents wanted her to be', she sought to be 'nothing', i.e. a passive catatonic. Secondly, Joan's withdrawal was viewed by Laing as a defensive mechanism to avoid the loss of identity (Joan's metaphorical 'dying') with which she was threatened by any normal relationship with others:

> One no longer fears being crushed, engulfed, overwhelmed by realness and aliveness . . . since one is already dead [by the catatonic withdrawal]. Being dead, one cannot die, and one cannot kill. The anxieties attendant on the schizophrenic's phantastic omnipotence are undercut by living in a condition of phantastic impotence.

None of this would convince us that Joan or others like her were rational in effecting catatonic withdrawal (even if we were convinced that at least in her case the withdrawal was an *action* she performed for reasons at all). Her action (or non-action) is based on a series of beliefs that are irrational, including her belief in a disembodied self, a belief in her parents' complete determination of her worth, and a belief in her own omnipotence and impotence.

It is sometimes thought that the rationality of beliefs is not a matter that can be objectively judged and that calling them 'irrational' is simply a pejorative way of saying that they are false. The conclusion in the present context would be that people like Joan are thus as rational as the rest of us, only mistaken about certain facts. While the topic of rational belief is a difficult one, prima facie the most obvious way to differentiate beliefs that are irrational from those that are merely false is by looking at the influence relevant evidence would have on the holder of the belief. It is characteristic of irrational beliefs that their holder maintains them despite countervailing evidence, or despite inconsistencies with other beliefs he has. There is a 'fixed' or 'frozen' nature about such beliefs, in the sense that they are not corrigible by relevant evidence. Irrational beliefs are held with a strength (relative to other beliefs the actor has) disproportionate to the evidence known to the actor. Thus the man 'who believes very strongly that his brother is trying to poison him (in spite of appearances) and who believes, rather weakly by comparison, that Boston is north of New York, is likely to be flying in the face of the evidence and the claims that the evidence renders likely'—he is likely, in other words, to be irrational in his belief of his imminent poisoning.

The empirical version of the myth argument fails because it is, empirically, false. By our shared concept of what it is to be rational, the mentally ill are not as rational as the rest of the population. Only by muddling the concept of rationality have the radical psychiatrists appeared to call into question this obvious truth. Only by attributing unconscious beliefs and desires to the mentally ill for which there is no evidence, or only by referring to beliefs that are themselves irrational, can motives be found for the peculiar behavior symptomatic of mental illness. Neither of these moves satisfies what we usually mean by 'rational' as applied to actions and agents. One may, of course, like Humpty Dumpty, choose to make a word like 'rationality' mean what he pleases, but surely it is unhelpful when one does so to then present the manufactured match between the facts and the new criteria for the word as a discovery of new facts, previously overlooked because of the willful blindness of self-interested psychiatrists or whatever. To do so is to create one's own myths.

(C) THE MYTH AS A CATEGORY MISTAKE: MENTAL ILLNESS IS NOT
A PHYSICAL CAUSE

In *The Concept of Mind* Ryle made popular the notion of a category mistake.

* * *

By his examples, vocabulary, and explicit citation, Szasz makes it clear that he has read Ryle with approval. Thus he begins Part I of *Law, Liberty, and Psychiatry* by quoting Ryle on the nature of myths:

A myth is, of course, not a fairy story. It is the presentation of facts belonging in one category in the idioms belonging to another. To explode a myth is accordingly not to deny the facts but to re-allocate them.

'Mental illness' is a myth, then, in the same way that other mental terms are myths: it is as improper to place mental illness in the same category with real illnesses (read as physically caused illnesses) as it is to treat 'belief', 'desires', 'perception', etc. as the names of mechanical or paramechanical causes.

Szasz in fact makes a number of distinct uses of the doctrine of categorial differences in his attack on mental illness as a myth. [H]is primary use is to focus on 'mental' in the phrase 'mental illness' and to argue that mental illness is a myth because mind is a myth (and hence a sick mind is a myth).

* * *

What is a sick mind? Surely a large part of the appeal of the myth argument stems from the difficulty one has in answering this question. One may indeed be tempted by the radical psychiatrists' reply that only bodies can be sick and that minds are not the sorts of things that can be either healthy or ill. Yet a good deal of the attraction of this argument should be eliminated once it is realized that the difficulty we have in saying anything very intelligible about what a sick mind is, stems directly from the difficulty we have in saying anything very intelligible about what a mind is. For unless one is prepared to jettison our talk about minds *in toto*—as Szasz plainly is not—merely pointing out that 'mental illness' has no clearer reference than does 'mind' itself is hardly a sufficient basis for labeling it a myth.

* * *

The question, 'what is a sick mind?', can be left aside in favor of a more useful question: does 'mental illness' have as significant a descriptive/explanatory use as other mental expressions? If it doesn't, then 'myth' is as good a pejorative label as any; but if the phrase does have a significant use, then no amount of Rylean exorcism can suffice to eliminate it from our vocabulary.

* * *

While saying what 'illness' doesn't mean is considerably easier than saying what it does mean, being ill seems to involve something like being in a state of pain or discomfort, which, if not removed, may lead to premature death, and which for its duration incapacitates the patient from certain activities thought normal in our society. One might assume that such states are physically caused; but such assumptions are irrelevant to what we mean by 'illness'. There are presumably physical causes for our being in all kinds of states, such as being a thousand miles from Paris, or for being alert or angry, etc. *Whether* there are physical causes for such states, and if so, *whether* they are manifested by abnormal physical structures, is irrelevant to whether or not one is ill, alert, angry, or a thousand miles away from Paris. Merely discovering a physical deviation in no way tells us that the person whose body it is that deviates is ill. Rather, properly to predicate 'illness' of another we need to know such things as whether he is in pain, is incapacitated, or is dying.

The reason why this has been so well camouflaged by the radical psychiatrists is that the names of *particular* illnesses, such as 'polio', 'pneumonia', etc. do involve knowledge of physical causes . . . [W]hether one has polio or pneumonia is determined in part by knowledge of the virus involved. Yet whether one is ill (in general) is *not* determined by such causes; whether one is ill in general is determined by wholly different criteria, seemingly connected with pain, incapacitation, or hastened death.

Once one appreciates this, then the propriety of terming hysterics (mentally) ill is also evident. The activities for which one is incapacitated by a paralyzed arm do not differ a whit whether the paralysis is anatomical or hysterical; in neither case can one play baseball, tend father effectively, etc. The admittedly sincere reports of pain of an hysteric throat irritation are as good evidence that the hysteric feels pain as are such reports of one whose c-fibers are really jingling with physiological pain signals due to a physically caused throat irritation. More generally, those whose capacity to act rationally is diminished because their memory, perception, reasoning abilities, or other mental faculties are impaired, are incapacitated from a normal life in our society no less than is, e.g., the chronic alcoholic whose short-term memory banks have been physically damaged by his long-term drinking habits (Korsakoff's syndrome).

Being in a state properly called 'ill', then, does not depend on one's knowing, or even in the first instance on there being, any particular physiological condition. It depends on one's being in a state characterized, roughly, by pain, incapacitation, and the prospect of a hastened death. There is nothing mythical about such a state, whether it be due to a broken leg or a broken home.

* * *

(D) THE MYTH AS A DEDUCTION FROM EPISTEMOLOGICAL RELATIVITY: WE ARE EQUALLY MAD FROM THE EPISTEMOLOGICAL POINT OF VIEW OF THOSE WE LABEL MAD

'The quality of myth', Quine tells us, 'is relative . . . to the epistemological point of view'. Mental illness is a myth on the interpretation here discussed, because our current epistemology, in which we have concepts like 'mental illness', is itself a myth—judged of course from another epistemological point of view, not from our own. If one subscribes to the view that there is no judging between such basic points of view, then the argument of R.D. Laing and others—that from the point of view of those we label insane we are insane—has some sting. Attribute to those we label as mentally ill an epistemology; grant that, although it differs from ours, the relative merits cannot be judged; and our labeling of others as mentally ill is a myth because it presupposes what it cannot have, namely, a standard of judgment applicable to those judged as well as to those judging.

* * *

It seems to me that this position, and epistemological relativity in general, stems from a simple failure to take one's own epistemology seriously. Free as we might like to think we are in our most speculative moments to shop among competing epistemologies, ontologies, geometries, logics, like so many wares in the store window, we are in fact limited to small purchases at any one time—limited by the high prices of even small purchases. This is not, however, a tidy issue which needs resolution here.

(E) The Myth as an Evaluation Masquerading as an Explanation: the Abuse of the Normative Connotations of 'Mental Illness' by Orthodox Psychiatry

Sensitivity to the normative connotations of the concepts of 'mental health' and 'mental illness' is, I suspect, rather widespread. When one of the psychiatrists at the annual meeting of the American Psychiatric Association some years ago loudly diagnosed a women's libber who was disrupting the meeting, as a 'stupid, paranoid bitch', something other than a value-neutral explanation of her behavior was intended. The same suspicions are engendered when psychiatrists label homosexuals as mentally ill, or when 'mental health' is used as a synonym for whatever way of life is adjudged good. The radical psychiatrists build on these kinds of examples to argue that 'mental illness' and the predicate 'mentally ill' are used *only* to make evaluations of others' behavior, and that these terms are particularly effective as evaluations because they are paraded as value-neutral, scientific explanations: 'while allegedly describing conduct, psychiatrists often prescribe it.'

> The masquerading of promotive assertions in the guise of indicative sentences is of great practical significance in psychiatry. Statements concerning 'psychosis' or 'insanity' . . . almost always revolve around unclarified equations of these two linguistic forms. For example, the statement 'John Doe is psychotic' is ostensibly indicative and informative. Usually, however, it is promotive rather than informative . . .

It may seem curious to claim that 'mental illness' is used like 'bad' or 'wrong', or 'ugh'—that is, used to pass moral evaluations—when by our shared notions for moral responsibility we use the same phrase to *excuse* those who are mentally ill. To attribute a harmful action to the actor's mental illness, then, cannot always be exactly the same as attributing it, say, to his 'murderous personality'. What Szasz *sometimes* has in mind in saying that 'mental illness' is used prescriptively or promotively, is not that moral judgments are made with such use; rather, psychiatric usage of the phrase is often promotive, etc. in the quite different sense that the capability of being morally responsible is denied. 'Mental illness' for Szasz is evaluative often only in the sense that it denies the 'personhood' of those to whom it is applied:

> What better way is there . . . for degrading the culprit than to declare him incapable of knowing what he is doing . . . This is the general formula for the dehumanization and degradation of all those

persons whose conduct psychiatrists now deem to be 'caused' by mental illness.

Although needlessly stated in inflammatory terms (as if orthodox psychiatry were universally motivated by a desire to degrade the mentally ill), Szasz here suggests a very important feature of mental illness. 'Insanity' and 'mental illness' mean, and historically have meant, 'irrational'; to be insane, or to be mentally ill, is to fail to act rationally often enough to have the same assumption of rationality made about one as is made of most of humanity. And without that assumption being made, one cannot be fully regarded as a person, for our concept of what it is to be a person is centered on the notions of rationality introduced earlier. Unless we can perceive another being as acting for intelligible ends in light of rational beliefs, we cannot understand that being in the same fundamental way that we understand each other's actions in daily life. Such beings lack an essential attribute of our humanity. It is thus easy to appreciate that historically the insane have been likened to young children, the intoxicated, and wild beasts. For lacking rationality, the mentally ill are, as Bleuler said of his schizophrenic patients, stranger to us than the birds in our gardens.

Such statements are of course offensive to the ears of those concerned about the moral claims and legal rights of mental patients. Yet unless radical psychiatry and its lawyerly following can show, as I have argued earlier in this paper it has not, that those we label mentally ill are just as rational as everyone else, part of our fundamental explanatory scheme and part of our fundamental notion of personhood are not applicable to the mentally ill. This includes notions about their lack of responsibility and inability to choose and act upon their own conception of their good. If one believes (contra Szasz et al.) that there are in fact people who do not act rationally often enough for us to make the same assumption of rationality for them as we do for most of our fellows, then this 'evaluative' feature of the phrase 'mental illness' is accurate enough in its reflection of how the mentally ill fit into our fundamental conceptual scheme.

Szasz at other times seems to have in mind a second kind of normative use which we do on occasion make of 'mentally ill', in everyday expressions such as 'That was an insane thing to do' or 'That's crazy!'. In such usages we do seem to be expressing disapproval of the agent's ends and his actions, recommending that one ought not to do such things or seek such ends, etc. Thus Szasz is also right to note that at times 'mentally ill' or 'insane' can be used as terms of general disapproval:

> The difference between saying 'He is wrong' and 'He is mentally ill' is not factual but psychological.

Other examples with which we began this section were the diagnosis of the women's libber and the use of 'mental health' by some psychoanalysts, e.g. Erich Fromm, as if it were synonymous with 'good'.

To the extent that orthodox psychiatry uses these words in this way it is plainly abusing them. The phrase 'mental illness' and its companions are so abused not by being applied to those who are in fact irrational, but by being applied to persons whose actions are often rational but of whose ends prevailing psychiatric opinion does not approve. An action that is fully rational in each of the senses examined earlier cannot, without ignoring the meaning of the words, be said to be insane or due to mental illness, no matter how deviant may be the end pursued. The fact that homosexuals have a preference for a sexual relationship not shared by most of the populace is hardly a ground (as the APA with strong dissent implicitly recognized recently in its deletion of homosexuality as an illness) for labeling that preference irrational (ill). Homosexuals may (sometimes, often, or always) be mentally ill, if their capacity for rational action is significantly diminished below our expectations; such irrationality is hardly shown, however, by their unpopular sexual desires alone if those ends are pursued on the basis of rational and consistent beliefs, without conflict with other strong desires, and by relatively efficient means.

The mistake of radical psychiatry is to assume that mental illness is a myth just because the phrase can be so abused. The mistake is to assume that because words such as 'murder', 'greediness', 'mental illness', or even 'good' can be used to express attitudes, kindle emotions, pass evaluations and the like, they cannot also be used at the same time as a legitimate form of explanation and/or description, or at different times only as a description/explanation. Those moral philosophers who have raised another logical gulf between evaluative and descriptive statements, insufficiently stress the fact that words used in evaluations can also be used to express descriptions. Merely because a woman may call the doctor who through surgical error kills her husband a murderer, despite the fact that one of the main criteria for that term's proper use is not met (viz. *intentional* killing), is not sufficient to show that the term 'murderer' cannot have legitimate descriptive and explanatory uses.

* * *

Questions and Comments

1. *Definitions of mental illness.* In criticizing "radical psychiatry's" position that mental illness is a "myth", Moore develops his own definition of mental illness. What is it? How does it compare to the definition found in DSM–III–R? Another critic of radical psychiatry who tried to define "mental illness" is Kendell. In "The Concept of Disease and Its Implications for Psychiatry," 127 Brit.J.Psychiat. 305 (1975), Kendell rejected the idea that disease (whether mental or physical) can be defined in terms of suffering and incapacity or a complaint of some sort, since "[m]any people who we regard as ill neither complain nor suffer." Nor can disease be described with reference to need for treatment, since this "implies that no one can be ill until he has been recognized as such, and also gives doctors, and society, free rein to label all deviants as ill, thus opening the door to all

the inconsistences and abuses that Szasz has so vividly conjured up."
Instead, argued Kendell, disease should be defined in culturally neutral
terms, i.e., with reference to whether "the abnormality place[s] the individual at a 'biological disadvantage.'" According to Kendell, this notion
"[p]resumably . . . must embrace both increased mortality and reduced
fertility." Relying on empirical research with respect to the mortality and
fertility of various groups, he concluded that there is adequate evidence
that schizophrenia, manic-depressive illness, some sexual disorders (including homosexuality), and some forms of drug dependence "carry with them
an intrinsic biological disadvantage, and on these grounds are justifiably
regarded as illness."

Apply these various definitions to the eight cases at the beginning of
this chapter. Are they coherent? Helpful?

2. *The "radicals" and the Supreme Court.* It is clear that the United
States Supreme Court is unwilling to endorse the Szaszian position. The
Court has indicated on several occasions that the law may treat those
labelled mentally disordered differently from those who are not so labelled.
It has explicitly upheld commitment statutes,[e] and recognized the notion
that mental illness can form the predicate for an incompetency to stand
trial plea.[f] It has implicitly endorsed the insanity defense.[g] Moreover, in
City of Cleburne v. Cleburne Living Center, 473 U.S. 432, 105 S.Ct. 3249, 87
L.Ed.2d 313 (1985), it held that the mentally retarded (and, by implication,
the mentally ill) are not a suspect or quasi-suspect class for equal protection purposes. It gave four reasons for this holding:

> First, it is undeniable ＊ ＊ ＊ that those who are mentally retarded
> have a reduced ability to cope with and function in the everyday world.
> Nor are they all cut from the same pattern: as the testimony in this
> record indicates they range from those whose disability is not immedi-
> ately evident to those who must be constantly cared for. They are thus
> different, immutably so, in relevant respects, and the states' interest in
> dealing with and providing for them is plainly a legitimate one. How
> this large and diversified group is to be treated under the law is a
> difficult and often a technical matter, very much a task for legislators
> guided by qualified professionals and not by the perhaps ill-informed
> opinions of the judiciary. Heightened scrutiny inevitably involves
> substantive judgments about legislative decisions, and we doubt that
> the predicate for such judicial oversight is present where the classifica-
> tion deals with mental retardation.

> Second, the distinctive legislative response, both national and state, to
> the plight of those who are mentally retarded demonstrates not only
> that they have unique problems, but also that the lawmakers have
> been addressing their difficulties in a manner that belies a continuing
> antipathy or prejudice and a corresponding need for more intrusive

e. Addington v. Texas, 441 U.S. 418, 99
S.Ct. 1804, 60 L.Ed.2d 323 (1979); Jones v.
United States, 463 U.S. 354, 103 S.Ct. 3043,
77 L.Ed.2d 694 (1983).

f. Drope v. Missouri, 420 U.S. 162, 95
S.Ct. 896, 43 L.Ed.2d 103 (1975).

g. Leland v. Oregon, 343 U.S. 790, 72
S.Ct. 1002, 96 L.Ed. 1302 (1952); Ake v.
Oklahoma, 470 U.S. 68, 105 S.Ct. 1087, 84
L.Ed.2d 53 (1985).

oversight by the judiciary. [Here the Court described several federal and state legislative enactments barring discrimination against the mentally disordered and providing funding for them in several contexts].

* * *

Third, the legislative response, which could hardly have occurred and survived without public support, negates any claim that the mentally retarded are politically powerless in the sense that they have no ability to attract the attention of the lawmakers. Any minority can be said to be powerless to assert direct control over the legislature, but if that were a criterion for higher level scrutiny by the courts, much economic and social legislation would now be suspect.

Fourth, if the large and amorphous class of the mentally retarded were deemed quasi-suspect * * *, it would be difficult to find a principled way to distinguish a variety of other groups who have perhaps immutable disabilities setting them off from others, who cannot themselves mandate the desired legislative responses, and who can claim some degree of prejudice from at least part of the public at large. One need mention in this respect only the aging, the disabled, the mentally ill, and the infirm. We are reluctant to set out on that course and we decline to do so.

Cleburne is reprinted in full in Chapter Twelve. Its importance for present purposes is that it illustrates the Court's unwillingness to reject laws which treat the mentally disordered differently and thus suggests the Court's implicit acceptance of the idea that mental disorder exists.

3. *The impact of the radicals.* While no court has been willing to adopt the position that mental illness does not exist, the works of Szasz and other "radicals" heavily influenced the lawyers who brought the litigation, described in chapters Eight, Nine and Ten, which successfully sought changes in the civil commitment system and established various rights for the mentally disabled. Dietz, "Social Discrediting of Psychiatry: The Protasis of Legal Disfranchisement," 134 Am J.Psychiat. 1356, 1359 (1977). Similarly, many of the arguments made in the current debate over the continued validity of the insanity defense (described in Chapter Seven) revolve around Szasz' assertion that the defense diminishes the notion of human responsibility. Finally, Szasz' contention that many mental health professionals are engaged in moral evaluation rather than scientific investigation has helped trigger a major controversy about the usefulness of clinical opinion in the courts, the topic of the next chapter.

Chapter Six

MENTAL HEALTH PROFESSIONALS AND EXPERTISE

Table of Sections

I. INTRODUCTION

The law has adopted the position that mental disorder "exists". It also supposes that mental disorder is associated with legally relevant states such as insanity, dangerousness, or incompetence. The question then becomes how to identify who is mentally disordered and who, among this group, is insufficiently insane or sufficiently dangerous or incompetent to be deprived of his or her liberty or property. Traditionally, laypersons provided the evidence necessary to decide whether a person was insane, committable, or incompetent. But with the growth and acceptance of the mental health professions in the past century and a half, psychiatrists, and to a lesser extent psychologists and social workers, have all but taken over the evidence-production role and have even assumed the judicial role in some contexts. Such a development is not surprising, since these individuals were, and are, thought to know more about mental disorder and its effects than other groups.

Recently, however, the wisdom of this development has been questioned by several writers. Relying on an impressive array of research, these commentators have suggested that opinions reached by behavioral scientists lack sufficient reliability for legal purposes. Many conclude that the role of mental health professionals in their evidence-production role should be substantially circumscribed or even eliminated altogether.[a]

The first section of this chapter focuses on the debate about the appropriate scope of this role.[b] It looks at the core issue of when, if ever, testimony by mental health professionals should be prohibited or substantially limited. On the assumption that mental health professionals should be permitted to testify as experts in some or all of these contexts, the second section examines the types of professionals who should qualify as experts, the proper bases for expert opinions, and the form which those opinions should take.

II. ADMISSIBILITY OF CLINICAL OPINION TESTIMONY

To evaluate the admissibility issue, further knowledge of the topics the law requires mental health professionals to address is necessary. Also essential is some understanding of the law's framework for deciding when evidence is admissible.

Legally Relevant Behavior. To reiterate the introduction to this part of the book, one can think of government-sponsored deprivations of liberty under three rubrics: the sanction model, the control model, and the autonomy model. The differences between these models are developed in detail in following chapters. Here only enough will be said to make clear the types of issues that need to be addressed under each system when the mentally disabled are involved.

The sanction model, epitomized by the criminal justice system, is primarily concerned with gauging one's culpability. Only if a person is considered sufficiently culpable will he or she be sanctioned. Mental disorder is usually considered relevant under this model, because it is thought to diminish or eliminate one's culpability. An individual's responsibility for his or her acts is reduced, it is believed, to the extent mental disorder blunts perception and awareness or makes it difficult to control behavior.

A control system, exemplified by commitment, is not interested in culpability for past acts but in preventing future ones. Intervention is authorized if it is predicted that harm may occur. Mental disorder is

a. See, e.g., Faust & Ziskin, "The Expert Witness in Psychology and Psychiatry," 241 Science 31 (1988).

b. The extent to which clinicians should be allowed to function as legal decisionmakers is an issue left for later chapters.

considered relevant here because it may be related to a propensity toward harmful behavior directed at others or oneself. Its presence also allows the law to hypothesize that a person's dangerousness can be "treated", an hypothesis which, again, can only be proven by making a prediction (as to the person's responsiveness to treatment).

The autonomy model focuses on neither culpability for one's acts nor one's propensities but on one's ability to perform certain functions at the present time. Mental disorder is relevant here because it may make someone dysfunctional in legally relevant ways. It is thought to render a person unable to exercise his or her prerogatives in a capable manner.

In short, laws which contemplate depriving the mentally disordered of liberty pose four issues: (1) the mental disorder predicate; and whether mental disorder is connected with (2) one's responsibility for one's past actions (as with the insanity defense); or (3) one's future behavior (as with civil commitment); or (4) one's ability to function (as with competency to stand trial). Put functionally, the questions posed by the legal system focus on a person's: (1) normality; (2) responsibility; (3) propensity; and (4) competency.

Evidence Law: The Framework of Analysis. All four of these issues are difficult ones. Crucial to determining how they should be addressed is the law of evidence, since it regulates the types of information courts may consider. In this chapter, we will rely on the federal rules of evidence as the guiding source of evidence law, since they reflect the consensus view on the issues we are examining. A brief foray into these rules is necessary as an introduction.

All evidence, whether lay or expert, must clear what could be called "the relevance/prejudice hurdle". Under the federal rules of evidence, evidence is relevant if it has "any tendency to make the existence of any fact that is of consequence to the determination of the action more probable or less probable than it would be without the evidence." Fed.R.Evid., Rule 401. If evidence is found to be relevant, then it is generally admissible unless "its probative value is substantially outweighed by the danger of unfair prejudice, confusion of the issues, or misleading the jury, or by considerations of undue delay, waste of time, or needless presentation of cumulative evidence." Fed.R.Evid. 403. In short, the admissibility of testimony depends initially upon how one balances its probative value against its potential for misleading or confusing the factfinder.

When a witness wishes to go beyond a description of "facts" which he or she has observed or has knowledge of, and instead wants to offer an "opinion" about those facts, additional considerations come into play. Generally, only if the witness is qualified as an "expert" is opinion testimony permissible. Of course, any testimony is inferential to some extent. According to federal rule 701, even the lay witness may recite "opinions or inferences which are rationally based on the perception of the witness and helpful to a clear understanding of his testimony or the determination of a fact in issue". This rule recognizes that the difference between "facts" and "inferences" is difficult to discern at best, but that the lay witness generally must avoid conclusory language unless common everyday usage requires it to make the testimony understandable and helpful. On the other hand, the expert witness is not so limited. According to Rule 702, "[i]f scientific, technical, or other specialized knowledge will assist the trier of fact to understand the evidence or to determine a fact in issue, a witness qualified as an expert by knowledge, skill, experience, training, or education, may testify thereto in the form of an opinion or otherwise." Put another way, a witness with the appropriate qualifications may offer conclusory opinion testimony when it is based on specialized knowledge and will add to what the factfinder could discern for itself. Of course, the factual basis for the opinion can be and usually is brought out on direct or cross-examination.

Whereas lay witnesses providing evidence on normality, responsibility, propensity, or competency will normally be confined to giving descriptions of actions and speech that they observed and that are relevant to the issue at hand, mental health professionals are usually asked to offer an interpretation of such behavior. Thus, assuming appropriate education and training on the part of the proferred clinician witness (a topic discussed in section III of this chapter), determining the admissibility of his or her testimony must involve three related inquiries: (1) whether its probative value outweighs its potential prejudicial impact; (2) whether it is based on scientific, technical or other specialized knowledge; and (3) whether it will add to what the factfinder can determine for itself. In practice, these three issues can often be lumped together under the query: will the testimony assist the factfinder? But keeping them distinct may be helpful in the following discussion, which looks at the admissibility issue with respect to each of the topics identified above: normality, responsibility, propensity, and competency.

A. NORMALITY

Traditionally, the principal way mental health professionals have provided information about whether someone is mentally disordered (i.e., abnormal or "crazy") is by indicating whether the person has a diagnosis and what that diagnosis is. For example, in insanity cases, testimony as to whether the defendant was suffering from a "mental disease or defect" which rendered him insane at the time of the offense is usually framed in terms of diagnostic categories. The following excerpt from the trial of John Hinckley, who shot President Ronald Reagan and three others, captures the flavor of this type of testimony. The selections which follow argue that this type of testimony should be barred.

TESTIMONY IN THE HINCKLEY CASE

John Hinckley's attempted assassination of President Reagan took place on March 30, 1981 in the District of Columbia. His lawyers indicated that he would plead insanity; under the District of Columbia's test for insanity—the American Law Institute, or ALI test—the jury would thus have to decide whether, at the time of the offense, Hinckley was "substantially unable to appreciate the wrongfulness of his act or conform his behavior to the requirements of the law" as a result of "mental disease or defect." Over the seven month period between the assassination attempt and the trial, various mental health professionals for the defense and the prosecution interviewed Hinckley and collected information about his life in an effort to answer this question. The testimony of two of these clinicians on the preliminary issue of whether Hinckley had a "mental disease or defect" is set out below. William Carpenter was one of the defense's psychiatrists and Park Dietz was one of the prosecution's psychiatrists.

a). Direct Examination of William T. Carpenter, M.D.

Q. Doctor, yesterday, before we started the chronological development of your exhaustive interview process, I asked you whether you had an opinion as to whether Mr. Hinckley had suffered from a mental disease on March 30, 1981. Do you recall that question?

A. Yes.

Q. And your answer was?

A. Yes, that I had formed an opinion.

Q. Now, would you tell us how you diagnose the defendant's mental illness, mental disease?

A. Yes.

* * *

THE WITNESS: * * * I concluded then that on March 30th, and before, that he did have the following manifestations of mental illness, that he had blunted affect or restricted affect.

This process where he has an incapacity to have an ordinary emotional arousal that should be associated with events in life. Blunt affect is of critical importance because from the beginning of the descriptions of the major psychotic or major psychiatric illnesses the blunted affect has been one of the prime distinctions of the process of one of the psychotic illnesses, so that I concluded that he did have blunted affect and as a symptomatic expression of an illness process.

He also had what technically we would call an "autistic retreat from reality." The autistic refers to the process of pulling into your own inner mind and away from the outer realty * * *.

The third major symptom status that he had is the depression and the associated features, including the suicidal features that were present in Mr. Hinckley.

And the fourth—* * * [t]here was important illness derived manifestations of dysfunction and his ability to work and his ability to establish social bonds. And these were of a severe magnitude and help measure the impact of illness.

The diagnostic labels that I want to mention, as you say in psychiatry, in approaching diagnoses, there are two somewhat overlapping approaches and it may be important to mention both to you.

The American Psychiatric Association has recently accepted a revision in its diagnostic manual and this is called the Diagnostic and Statistical Manual. It is the third volume.

But it has the listing of the different categories of illness and the descriptions and criteria that go with these different categories and there are many different categories of illness.

This manual notices the fact that we cannot draw emphatically clear distinctions between different types of illnesses, that the manifestations of illnesses may overlap so we don't know exactly where to draw the dividing line.

We are better at drawing the dividing line as to whether illness is present or absent than precisely how to define each illness category. For that reason in this diagnostic manual that is used now in this psychiatrists are encouraged to make multiple diagnoses; that is, if a person meets criteria for a number of diagnoses.

So that Mr. Hinckley does meet either full or partial criteria for a large number of diagnoses listed in that manual. It is only useful to— for me to present in my diagnostic findings the way he fits into a couple of major categories.

The first category that I want to mention, it draws from a concept of schizophrenia, which is one of the major psychotic illnesses which was identified at the turn of the century and has usually lifetime implications in terms of the pattern of illness and the outcome of illness.

And conceptually linked to this are personality dysfunctions, that the term "schizotypal and schizoid personality" mean. To define these labels, "schizoid" refers to someone who is withdrawn from social contacts, aloof from them, a sense of the kind of tender feelings that are associated with tender feelings, usually implying a life-long pattern and may be used for a pattern of socialization and alienation.

The schizotypal personality is a very similar personality formation with the difference being that the person has either something eccentric or bizarre or their use of language gets—but some more severe symptoms than otherwise are similar.

And psychiatrists are directed if schizotypal features are there, to use that instead of the diagnosis of schizoid personality.

Mr. Hinckley did meet criteria for both schizotypal and schizoid. He also met criteria for schizophrenia. This is generally thought of as a more severe form of illness, but that has many of the same kinds of personality features, the development of illness is shown through the personality function that schizotypal and schizoid have.

And I would make, using the criteria of the Diagnostic and Statistical Manual, then from the American Psychiatric Association, a diagnosis of Mr. Hinckley of schizophrenia and would not use the label schizotypal and schizoid, because it is the same symptoms. If they are explained by schizophrenia, you would not resort to those.

Mr. Hinckley at this—to some extent on the point of view he had illness manifestation symptoms that meet the criteria for what is called a major affective disorder. For many years the two major severe psychiatric disorders were the schizophrenia and relating conditions and the manic depressive and related conditions.

Mr. Hinckley in his depression reached the criteria for major depressive disorder and, using DSM–III as a guide, one would make—I would make that diagnosis. The only reason to argue against making that diagnosis is if the presence of schizophrenia can potentially explain the disorder mood that he had, the depression that he had, one could account for the depressive components within the single diagnostic framework.

Those are the diagnoses that I would use in terms of DSM–III.

A more broadly used concept in the world for schizophrenia involves a concept which is called "process schizophrenia" and this term is the primary term that I have used in diagnosing Mr. Hinckley. This term is important because it implies a certain form of development of the illness, an illness that usually begins during adolescence or early adulthood. It has usually a slow development so that the first years in the illness will be the illness manifestation, begin with fairly subtle disorders and social functioning and in personality functioning, and it progresses to a more severe psychiatric disorder and psychotic disorder, and that is where the presence of the delusion and ideas of reference, this type of symptom comes in.

And in this concept people who have developed this disorder, in most instances they are persevering impairments in their health. It runs chronic on long-standing courses. So it is typically slow and gradual in development and once reaching the psychotic state, as the person continues to have continued dysfunction and a broad range of social and psychological measures.

Process schizophrenia, which is the diagnostic conclusion I have reached, is related both in concept and related in a genetic basis to the schizotypal and schizophrenic reference as well as overlapping with schizophrenia as defined in DSM–III so that the clinical diagnosis—that I concluded that the illness Mr. Hinckley had on and before March 30th is process schizophrenia.

[Excerpted from page 3295 through page 3304 of the trial transcript.]

* * *

b). *Cross–Examination*

Q. Now you testified Friday Mr. Hinckley had been suffering from what you called "process schizophrenia" from 1976, all the way back to 1976.

A. Well, expressing all the difficulties and pinpointing a beginning date for an illness, it began slowly and developed over time.

Q. But as best you can recall that is when he began to have—

A. I refer to '76 as when it began to reach the proportions that one could begin to consider schizophrenic illness present.

Q. In other words, you would have diagnosed him as process schizophrenic if you had seen him in 1976, from your testimony?

A. I don't know. That I would have if I had seen him. I don't know what I would have found out if I had seen him in 1976. Putting the development of the illness into a picture, you are always helped by subsequent developments. That is part of the very nature.

Q. All right.

A. And so when you find out that when symptoms have reached their greatest intensity in any illness, it helps you to interpret things that would be compatible with that illness as they developed earlier. It is like you went back to the earliest stages now that you know somebody had tuberculosis, if you had seen him when he had the first cough, you would have diagnosed it.

* * *

Q. Friday * * * [you testified that] * * * "his process schizophrenia did not become psychotic until 1976, right?" And you answered: "I think that would be the case." You still stick to that now?

A. Yes.

Q. And * * * your answer on the previous page to the same point, [was] "I don't think it was until about then," 1976, "that it developed to an intensity that it reached psychotic proportions." Right?

A. Right.

Q. Are you aware that Mr. Hinckley in the period of 1976 through 1980, was a student at Texas Tech University from time to time?

A. From time to time.

Q. Were you aware, then, as it comes to your attention, that during that period, '76 to '79, when he was there in certain courses he received As; did you learn that?

A. Yes.

Q. And he got some Bs.

A. Yes.

Q. And generally he kept a pretty good grade point average, right?

A. He had a lot of academic difficulty. He dropped a lot of courses because he was having difficulty with them. He had success in some courses.

Q. Well, Doctor, he got an A in writing, didn't he?

A. Yes.

Q. And he got this A in writing during this period you said he was suffering from process schizophrenia; right?

A. Yes.

Q. And you are aware, are you not, that in early 1977, he held a job at a place called Taylor's Supper Club in the Lakewood, Colorado area?

A. Yes, for about five months.

Q. Five months. And I take it you learned that he worked everyday at a busboy job there; right?

A. He didn't come to work quite everyday, but he did work fairly regularly during that period of time. Some absences.

Q. Right. And this is during a period of time when you say he suffered from process schizophrenia; right?

A. Yes.

Q. And you are also aware that in 1976, Mr. Hinckley traveled all by himself to California for several months; right?

A. Yes.

Q. And while he was there, he went trying to sell his songs; right?

A. Yes.

* * *

Q. And this is during a period of time when you say that Mr. Hinckley was a process schizophrenic; right?

A. Well, this is a time when I think it is beginning to develop its magnitude and it is this information from this very period of time that I would fit into that picture, yes.

Q. And then Mr. Hinckley got back from California all by himself in 1976; are you aware of that?

A. Oh, yes.

Q. I mean his parents didn't have to come out and bring him home in their car, did they?

A. Oh, certainly no.

Q. And this is during the time you said he was suffering from process schizophrenia; right?

A. Yes.

Q. You are aware in 1977, he spent a few weeks in California as well; right?

A. Yes.

Q. And again, he went out there by himself, did he not?

* * *

A. Yes.

Q. He didn't have any trouble getting out there. He didn't get lost in Arizona or run into the Grand Canyon, did he?

A. No.

Q. And while he was there he functioned pretty well, did he not?

A. Oh, no. He had impairments—you see, you may want to define "functioning" for me.

Q. He didn't get arrested by the police, he wasn't found walking around with no clothes on or anything of that sort while he was in California to 1977?

A. That's right and he never walked around without clothes.

[Excerpted from page 3517 through page 3524 of the trial transcript.]

c). *Prosecution Rebuttal Testimony (Park Elliott Dietz, M.D.)*

Q. All right. Now, let me ask you formally, if you determined whether at the time of the criminal conduct on March 30, 1981 the defendant Hinckley, as a result of mental disease or defect, lacked substantial capacity to conform his conduct to the requirements of the law?

A. I did make such a determination.

Q. What determination did you make?

A. That on March 30, 1981, as a result of mental disease or defect, Mr. Hinckley did not lack substantial capacity to conform his conduct to the requirements of the law.

* * *

Q. All right. Now, I take it you have some reasons for those conclusions?

A. Yes, I do.

Q. . . . [Y]ou have announced diagnosis of four mental disorders in Mr. Hinckley as of March 30, 1981. And you gave them certain labels, did you not?

A. Yes.

Q. Where did those labels come from?

A. Well, like other labels in medicine, these are derived from Greek and Latin words. These specific labels of mental disorder come from the official diagnostic system, the DSM–III.

Q. In each of the four instances that you mentioned were the diagnoses you announced from DSM–III?

A. Yes.

Q. All right. Now, in connection with DSM–III, can you tell us whether this book is designed for medical purposes or for legal purposes?

A. For medical purposes.

Q. And what do you mean by that?

A. I mean that this volume DSM–III is designed to allow physicians to make reliable diagnoses, to exchange information and know what they are talking about with one another, to be able to speak a common language. But that the diagnoses there do not automatically translate into anything legal and certain not into determination of criminal responsibility.

Q. And criminal responsibility to repeat has how many parts?

A. Depending on how one counts it, it would.

Q. As we have counted it, how many does it have?

A. Two.

Q. DSM–III deals with how many of those two parts?

A. One.

Q. Now, can you tell us, Doctor, with respect to the matter of mental disorders whether there is a range of mental disorders in DSM–III?

A. Yes, there is.

Q. Can you explain the range of mental disorders to the jury?

A. Well, DSM–III covers every conceivable sort of mental disorder from extremely serious to quite minor ones.

The types of disorders within the volume included such things as organic brain syndromes with psychosis, serious depressions with psychosis. Other serious disturbances of mood with psychosis.

It includes neuroses or what are now called anxiety disorders. It includes sorts of personality disorders that I've mentioned and will be talking more about. And it includes what we call situational stress disorders, when in a certain situation a person develops symptoms. For example, after a serious stressful incident.

It includes addictions of various kinds. It even includes tobacco dependence disorder. It ranges from minor to serious. From long-standing to brief. It includes a whole host of conditions.

Q. Can you compare that range in some way to the range that we all might be familiar with in functional medicine?

A. Well, for just about any system of the body there is a range of disorders that can occur. People may, for example, have the sniffles or a cold which is an infection of the respiratory system. They [(sic)] may have more serious infection of the respiratory system like pneumonia and can have life threatening disorders of the respiratory system like pneumonia in a very old person or lung cancer or serious injuries to the lungs.

Q. Does that same range exist in mental disorders?

A. A similar range does.

Q. A similar range. Now, you have already mentioned, actually, certain psychotic disorders, correct?

A. Yes.

Q. And can you briefly describe those in terms of the range of mental disorders?

A. Well, the psychotic disorders, I think, all would agree, are the most serious of the mental disorders. There are many different ways to look at seriousness. I think it is fair to say that the disorders associated with psychoses at least while an individual is psychotic are the most serious.

Q. Going down the range, if you will, can you tell us the next general category of disorders?

A. Well, again, it depends on how one classifies it but there is a group of nonpsychotic mental disorders and, generally speaking, the nonpsychotic disorders are considerably less serious than psychotic. Nonpsychotic disorders that are less serious, for example, include the anxiety disorders and the personality disorders. There are other examples.

Q. All right. You mentioned personality disorders. Where do they fit on this spectrum?

A. On the nonpsychotic, less serious side.

Q. And further down or further along are there any other set of disorders that you would care to comment on?

A. Farther down.

Q. Along the range, along the spectrum?

A. Well, the organic mental disorders one associates with psychoses are further up toward the serious end.

Q. All right.

A. Many of the anxiety disorders are toward the less serious end.

Q. In Mr. Hinckley's case, did you find and determine that he had a psychotic disorder?

A. No.

Q. Did you find and determine that Mr. Hinckley had any organic disorder?

A. No.

Q. Now, where in the range do the disorders that you found in Mr. Hinckley, that is to say, the dysthymic disorder, the narcissistic and the schizoid disorder and mixed personality disorders, fall?

A. These are all within them, the dysthymic is an affective disorder and this is on the less serious side.

* * *

Q. Before I go any further, you are aware of a category in DSM–III called Schizophrenia; is that right?

A. Yes.

Q. Is Schizoid Personality the same as Schizophrenia?

A. No, it is not.

Q. All right, and briefly at this point could you explain your answer?

A. Schizophrenia is a serious mental disorder in which a patient will at least sometimes and frequently for long times be psychotic.

Schizoid Personality Disorder is a personality disorder. It is not a functional psychotic disorder, as we refer to Schizophrenia.

An individual whose problem is Schizoid Personality Disorder does not become psychotic as a result of it, and does not develop some of the symptoms so characteristic of Schizophrenia such as delusions and hallucinations.

Q. Dr. Dietz, in DSM–III, are Schizoid Personality and Schizophrenia in the same categories or in different categories?

A. They are in different chapters altogether.

Q. Now could you tell us a little bit about the nature of the Schizoid Personality Disorder?

A. Yes, I can. As I have mentioned, this, this is the lonely personality disorder. As a consequence of that, people who have the features of Schizoid Personality Disorder tend to do loner sorts of things. Many of these people, for example, will engage in occupations that don't require much interaction with other people.

For example, cowboys frequently don't have to interact much with others and that's the kind of thing that can appeal to someone who is Schizoid.

Computer operators may not have to interact too much with other people. Even librarians, forest rangers. Now, this is not to say that there is any problem with people who engage in these occupations. It's to say that these are occupations that one can do without having to interact much with others. And people perform beautifully at those kinds of professions if, even if they have this disorder. It's a way to, to be able to function well without having to run into the problem that individuals with these disorders run into when they try to interact with others.

Q. Would people with this Schizoid Personality Disorder function in everyday life without any difficulty?

A. I wouldn't say without any difficulty, but I would say they certainly function in everyday life in many ways. The one way that they are not likely to function, and this is part of the definition, is that they don't have friends.

Q. Can they hold jobs?

A. Yes.

Q. Can they go to school?

A. Yes.

Q. Can they travel?

A. Yes.

Q. Now Schizoid Personality, does that mean a person is out of contact with reality or psychotic?

A. No, it does not.

Q. Could you explain to the jury what you saw in Mr. Hinckley on March 30th, 1981, to indicate that he suffered from a Schizoid Personality Disorder on that day?

A. Well, I think there are really only two features that are known to have been present on that date in Mr. Hinckley, and the first of those is what we describe as emotional coldness and aloofness. That is, being, being cruel and unemotional, not becoming involved emotionally with other people.

Q. Does that mean a person is out of contact with reality?

A. No, no, but it may mean that they have trouble making friends.

Q. All right. What are the other characteristics?

A. Well, another one that I think was observable that day was indifference to the feelings of others. There are, one of the things we use to diagnose many of these mental disorders is to, to say that if there is, there are certain things that must not be present, if it's present, then we can't make this diagnosis, and one of those in Mr. Hinckley's case that was not present on March 30, and which we have to make sure wasn't present was no eccentricities of speech, behavior or thought, and there was nothing eccentric about his speech, behavior or his thought that day, and there were many observers I have interviewed to determine that.

*   *   *

[Excerpted from page 6388 through page 6411 of the trial transcript.]

d). Cross-Examination

Q. Before we get into the substance of your testimony, I would like to extract an agreement I think we can reach, and that is that you share the view of other defense psychiatrists that Mr. Hinckley on March 30, 1981 was suffering from a mental disease? You do agree with that statement, do you not?

A. No, I do not.

Q. All right. Was it not your testimony on direct examination that Mr. Hinckley suffered a mental disease of dysthymic mental disorder?

A. No. I testified that Mr. Hinckley suffered in the past and indeed on March 30 from a mental disorder.

Q. Are you distinguishing between a mental disease and mental disorder?

A. Yes.

Q. I see.

Would you agree that on March 30, 1981 Mr. Hinckley had a mental illness in a broad sense?

A. I testified about a mental disorder, and I would have some difficulty agreeing with your statement that he suffered from a mental illness.

Q. All right, taking your term as a mental disorder, how do you distinguish that, sir, from a mental disease?

A. Well, a mental disorder is any of the diagnostic categories listed in DSM III, the guide book for mental disorders, and for the diagnosis of mental disorders. When one switches to the term mental disease or mental illness, one is suggesting that this is a sickness, that it has some kind of biological basis.

That is quite a difference.

Q. So it is your testimony that all of the descriptions of mental conditions in DSM III constitute mental disorders as compared or contrasted to mental diseases?

A. Yes, sir.

Q. Accepting your qualification, then, you will agree that on March 30, 1981 Mr. Hinckley suffered from a mental disorder?

A. Yes.

Q. And that the question before this Court and this jury would become as to the question of the severity of that disorder?

A. No, sir. The question before the jury is about his criminal responsibility.

* * *

[Excerpted from page 6388 through page 6411 of the trial transcript.]

* * *

Questions and Comments

1. *Use of DSM–III.* The witness' heavy reliance on the diagnostic categories found in the Third Edition of the American Psychiatric Association's Diagnostic and Statistical Manual (DSM–III) is typical. You may want to check the criteria for each diagnosis used by the experts by referring to Chapter Five. Consider also the following commentary on the Hinckley trial from Stone, past president of the APA:

> The discrepancies in the psychiatric testimony [at the Hinckley trial] would be much easier to understand if the defense and prosecution had agreed that there was a thought disorder but disagreed about its extent—for example, whether it was sufficient to be diagnosed psychosis, and whether it was sufficient to negate criminal responsibility. Such agreement would have placed Hinckley in the problem area of psychiatry's familiar nosological disputes. Thus, if both sides had agreed that he was a schizotypal personality or a paranoid personality and the defense said he had gone over into psychosis while the prosecution insisted he had not, every clinician would have understood the problem. How much thought disorder makes a psychosis? But here the prosecution specifically rejected the diagnoses of schizotypal personality and paranoid personality, the character disorders which suggest a thought disorder. This makes the discrepancies harder to understand and harder to explain to the cynics who believe psychiatrists can be hired to say anything.

A Suggested Diagnosis for John Hinckley

> Based on my own reading of the testimony of all the psychiatrists, I believe that before DSM–III, I would have diagnosed John Hinckley as a case of erotomania, and Freud's classic paper written in 1911 would have helped me to clarify Hinckley's psychopathology. Most clinicians have seen patients with delusions of love—a condition that is not that uncommon. There is even a French name for such delusions—Clerambault's syndrome. * * * But erotomania per se no longer appears in DSM–III, and one could debate whether it is or is not a psychosis. It is my own clinical and theoretical opinion that a delusion of love may protect the person against ego decompensation into florid psychosis, and this may have been the case with Hinckley. His pathological attachment to Jodie Foster [c] is in my view crucial not only to his diagnosis but also to his prognosis. It is interesting, however, that delusions of love seem to have disappeared from DSM–III. Such delusions do not make up a separate diagnosis and are not listed as a specific symptom in any of the diagnostic categories of the paranoid spectrum. Perhaps the Hinckley case may also lead us to reconsider this gap in DSM–III.[d]

c. Apparently, one reason Hinckley shot the president was to impress the actress Jodie Foster. His actions on the day of the offense were possibly meant to mimic the actions of a character who tried to shoot the president in the film Taxi Driver, in which Foster played a major role. [footnote by eds.]

d. The revised version of DSM–III (DSM–III–R) does include such a diagnosis.

Evaluating the Psychiatric Diagnoses

The defense psychiatrists themselves had trouble finding a place for Hinckley in DSM–III. Whether they were oriented psychoanalytically or biologically, their theoretical understanding of the underlying disorder caused them to fight the theoretical diagnostic categories of DSM–III. The defense's experts all had a more powerful commitment to their theory (biological, psychodynamic, or biopsychosocial) of Hinckley's psychiatric condition than they did to the diagnostic nomenclature in DSM–III. If they had been forbidden to use diagnoses (* * * some favor legislation that forbids diagnoses), they would have been released from a constraint against which they struggled. On the other hand, the prosecution witnesses seemed to have no theory about Hinckley's disorder and no real explanation of his actions except that he was a bad narcissistic person. Rather, they carefully and conscientiously applied DSM–III.

In evaluating these conclusions about the psychiatric testimony, several things should be kept in mind. First, the preparation and the quality of the psychiatric testimony in the Hinckley case was far superior to what one usually finds. Second, these experts appear to have genuinely and honestly come to their various conclusions. The Hinckley testimony is not an example of what happens when lawyers buy psychiatric experts for a price. The testimony may have been rehearsed, the experts may have been carefully sorted and selected by the lawyers, but these experts believed what they said. If Hinckley did not fall readily into any DSM–III category, if his disorder is in the gray area between psychosis and personality disorder, then we can see that there was room for honest disagreement. Third, * * * [i]f there was something flawed about the psychiatric testimony, it is in the sense one gets of the psychiatrists getting caught up in and succumbing to the adversarial process. There is a kind of overstatement in their testimony as though they had taken on the responsibility of convincing the jury and outwitting the opposition. Clinical working hypotheses became scientific truths. Clinical possibilities became certainties. And as these truths and certainties from one side meet contradictory truths and certainties from the other side, one has the feeling that psychiatry's credibility hangs in the balance.

A. Stone, Law, Psychiatry and Morality 92–93 (1984).

2. *The purpose of diagnosis in an insanity trial.* The witnesses obviously agree that Hinckley had *some* diagnosable mental disorder. But, given the wide array of behavior that can be called disordered and that is found in DSM–III, that finding alone is insufficient as a predicate for the insanity defense. The mental disorder must be a "serious" one. Why did Dietz insist on the term "mental disorder" as opposed to "mental disease"? Is the diagnostic testimony "relevant" to deciding whether Hinckley's mental disorder was serious? Does it "assist" the factfinder? Consider the following excerpt.

See "Delusional Disorders", p. 338 of this book. [footnote by eds.]

STEPHEN MORSE, CRAZY BEHAVIOR, MORALS &
SCIENCE: AN ANALYSIS OF MENTAL HEALTH LAW
51 S.Cal.L.Rev. 527, 604–613.
(1978).

* * *

The crucial question for the law is not, or at least should not be, whether the actor allegedly fits one of the mental health diagnostic categories, but whether the actor behaves crazily enough to warrant special legal treatment on moral and social grounds. The law must therefore decide on legal grounds and for legal purposes which cases fit this criterion of sufficient craziness. These decisions should not and cannot be totally dependent on scientific categories that may serve other purposes, and experts should not testify about whether an actor suffers from a mental disorder or even about whether the actor is normal. Conclusions about mental disorder or psychiatric normality are not particularly and precisely relevant to *legal* decisions about normality. Rather, for various reasons, experts should be limited to describing behavior to the factfinder that laypersons may not notice but that may be relevant to legal decisionmaking.

The first reason for limiting experts to descriptions of behavior is that their conclusions are based, in part, on mental health diagnostic categories that are generally overinclusive. These categories are much broader than the crazy behaviors that seem to compel special legal treatment. The various disorder categories delineated by both the present and proposed diagnostic manuals of the American Psychiatric Association may be ranged along a quantitative and qualitative continuum of craziness. Some categories seem to describe behavior that would be considered quite crazy, at least in its extreme forms, by anyone. Others describe behavior that would not be considered crazy and, at worst, would be considered normally quirky.

Thus, present definitions of mental disorder cover such a wide range of behavior that vast percentages of the population may be considered disordered, including most persons whom the legal system would not consider crazy or different enough to warrant special treatment. A large proportion of the diagnostic categories simply do not describe behavior that seems very crazy and the inexorable product of a deranged mind. If no conclusions about diagnosis, illness, disease, or abnormality are drawn by experts, the law will avoid the confusion engendered by the metaphysical complexities of the mental health debate about which behaviors ought to be labeled and considered illnesses. Further, whether behavior is considered disordered for clinical or research purposes should not be dispositive of legal decision-making where narrower moral and social definitions of craziness are appropriate.

The second reason for limiting experts to descriptions of behavior is that particular diagnoses do not *accurately* convey legally relevant information concerning the person's behavior. A diagnosis will not inform the law whether, how, or to what degree an actor behaves crazily. The major related reasons for this fact are that present psychiatric diagnoses are not highly reliable or descriptively precise.

In behavioral science, reliability is a complex construct, but for the purposes of legal decisionmaking about abnormality it can be defined as the accuracy of a diagnosis. The preeminent "measuring tool" used to make diagnoses is a human observer applying the present diagnostic categories to behavior. Unlike much physical disorder that often can be verified by various tests that measure pathology (whether or not the cause of the symptom, syndrome, or condition is known), there is no objective, empirical referent of *mental* disorder other than crazy behavior itself. Indeed, the only possible verification of the presence of mental disorder is by a consensus of those who have observed the actor's behavior. There is no postmortem pathological examination or other diagnostic procedure to verify conclusively whether or not a person suffered from a particular disorder or any disorder at all. Even if objectively verifiable referents other than behavior itself are present, an actor is not considered mentally disordered unless he behaves crazily.

In a sense, there is no such thing as an independently "correct" or "incorrect" mental health diagnosis; there are only agreed on and disagreed on diagnoses. The crucial issue, then, is the extent of agreement achieved by professional diagnosticians when they apply their categories of disorder to behavior itself. The best evidence of the reliability of present diagnostic categories indicates that if two professionals independently diagnose a person on the basis of the same or similar data, it is rare for them to agree on the diagnosis in more than half the cases. The large amount of disagreement is not narrowed appreciably by limiting the possible diagnoses to broad diagnostic categories. Thus, mental health diagnoses are not terribly reliable; people who do not have mental disorder or a specific disorder will be diagnosed as having it, and vice versa. Of course, in clear cases everyone will agree the actor is crazy, but such cases are few.

* * *

The major cause of diagnostic unreliability—criterion variance—further explains why particular diagnoses do not convey legally relevant information. Criterion variance is both a general cause of unreliability and a bar in specific cases to the ability of a diagnosis to convey precise information, even when observers agree on the diagnosis. The diagnostic categories of mental disorders are descriptions of allegedly recurring clusters of behaviors, that is, of recurring patterns of thoughts, feelings, and actions. It is hypothesized that each category describes a more or less distinguishable disorder. The present and proposed diagnostic categories, however, are vague and overlap; each includes a quite heterogeneous range of behavior. Some persons who receive the most severe diagnoses that seem to map legal craziness, such as "schizophrenia," may not be crazy enough to warrant special legal treatment. Vastly different behavior, ranging from only mildly to wildly crazy, may properly fit into the same and most serious diagnostic categories. Thus, even if two psychiatrists do agree on a diagnosis, it is impossible to know whether social and moral purposes will be served by special legal treatment unless the behavior itself is described to the factfinder.

*   *   *

*   *   * There is still a role, however, for expert assistance and expert testimony in deciding whether an actor is crazy.

Because experts interact with all types of crazy persons far more often than laypersons, they may be especially sensitive to or inquire about behavior that would go unnoticed by laypersons. Laypersons may not know to ask, for example, if a person hears voices, entertains crazy beliefs, or has trouble sleeping or staying awake. Because the expert is attuned to crazy behavior, he may help the factfinder attend to a fuller range of the actor's behavior. Nonetheless, the expert need not and should not report conclusions about mental disorder, abnormality, or even craziness; these are legal determinations for the judge or jury. It is far more precise and useful to the judge or jury if the expert simply describes his observations of behavior. For the legal question of normality, then, the relevant expertise of mental health professionals is not their ability to draw inferences from data or to form opinions. Rather, their special skill is observational—to perceive behaviors that nonexperts may fail to notice. The expert should describe, in as much precise but commonsense detail as possible, his observations of how the person thinks, feels, and acts. The test of relevance for the testimony of experts and laypersons alike should be whether their observations of the actor's behavior shed light on the question of whether the actor is crazy.

For example, experts should not testify that an actor is "hallucinatory and probably schizophrenic." Instead, the expert should testify that the actor told the expert that on some (specified) occasions, the actor heard or hears voices despite the fact that no one was or is talking to him and the voices told or tell him the following (specified) things. For another example, experts should not testify that an actor "suffers from loose associations when questioned on an ego-threatening topic and is therefore probably schizophrenic." Rather, the expert should testify that when the expert asked the actor certain (specified) questions about topics that seem to mean a lot to the actor, the actor responded in the following way (specified by examples). Of course, if laypersons such as family, friends, coworkers, or neighbors are aware of such behavior, they too can testify about it.

Using lay as well as expert testimony about the actor's behavior, the decisionmaker can then decide if the person is sufficiently crazy to be an appropriate candidate for the application of mental health laws. If the factfinder's response to the behavioral data it hears is "so what," then the actor probably does not meet the legal criterion of mental disorder; if the response is "that's crazy" or "he's crazy," then the criterion of mental abnormality may be met.

* * *

Questions and Comments

1. *The nature of Morse's argument about diagnoses.* Is Morse arguing that diagnostic testimony is irrelevant (i.e., has no tendency to make the fact at issue—craziness—more or less probable)? That it is relevant, but unduly misleading or confusing? Or that it is not based on specialized knowledge that adds to what the factfinder can determine for itself? Note that present practice usually requires witnesses to give the basis of their opinions. Federal Rule 705 states that "[t]he expert may testify in terms of opinion or inference and give his reasons therefore without prior disclosure of the underlying facts or data, unless the judge requires otherwise." But the Rule also states "[t]he expert may in any event be required to disclose the underlying facts or data on cross-examination." Thus, for example, in a part of the Hinckley trial testimony not included in the previous excerpt, the factual basis for the diagnoses given by the witnesses were brought out on direct and cross-examination. If diagnoses are accompanied by the descriptive data that Morse argues should be provided, are they helpful or merely superfluous? In Washington v. United States, 390 F.2d 444 (D.C. Cir.1967), Judge Bazelon, one of the country's most influential judges on mental health law matters, wrote that a trial judge should limit "use of medical labels [like] schizophrenia" and require experts to explain them, but should not bar them altogether, because "they sometimes provide a convenient and meaningful method of communication."

2. *The reliability of diagnoses.* Morse notes that, because diagnoses are constructs rather than "facts", there is no independent method of determining whether a diagnosis is correct or not correct (or "valid" or "invalid", to use behavioral science terminology). Rather validity can only be indirectly determined through an assessment of the extent to which different raters agree that a given diagnosis is correct (i.e., a "reliability" assessment). As Morse states, the reliability of most diagnoses is far from perfect. But field tests of the new diagnostic scheme introduced by DSM–III, conducted in two phases between 1977 and 1980, indicated that inter-rater agreement may be better than the one out of two ratio Morse, who relied on earlier data, reported in the above excerpt. The tests showed that for some major diagnostic categories the inter-rater agreement was quite high: organic disorders (79% in the first phase, 76% in the second phase); schizophrenia (81% in both phases), paranoid disorders (66% and 75%); mood disorders (69% and 83%); impulse disorders (28% and 80%); personality disorders (56% and 65%). This improved diagnostic reliability presumably resulted from the more precise diagnostic criteria found in DSM–III. In other words, the results of the field tests suggest that DSM–III has reduced the criterion variance of which Morse writes.

However, some have questioned the methodology of the DSM–III field tests, Kutchins & Kirk, "The Reliability of DSM–III: A Critical Review," 1986 Social Work Res. & Abstr. 3 (1986), and others have had difficulty replicating their results, at least in the emergency context. Lieberman & Baker, "The Reliability of Psychiatric Diagnosis in the Emergency Room," 36 Hosp. & Comm. Psychiat. 291 (1985) (41% agreement on schizophrenia, 50% agreement on mood disorders; 37% on organic disorder). Moreover, for sub-categories of the major diagnostic classifications (e.g., subtypes of schizophrenia, schizoid personality disorder), the agreement in the field trials was often much lower, in the 10 to 40% range. See also, Mellsop, et al. "The Reliability of Axis II of DSM–III," 139 Am J. Psychiat. 1360 (1982) (reliability of personality disorder diagnoses in everyday clinical setting ranged from 49% for antisocial personality to 1% for schizoid personality). See generally, Faust & Ziskin, "The Expert Witness in Psychology and Psychiatry," 241 Science 31 (1988).

3. *Other causes of unreliability.* Although, as Morse indicates, criterion variance is the major cause of diagnostic unreliability, there are other causes as well, which are worth noting not only because they may infect diagnostic assessments but also because they can influence assessments of responsibility, propensity, and competency as well.

ENNIS & LITWACK, PSYCHIATRY AND THE PRESUMPTION OF EXPERTISE: FLIPPING COINS IN THE COURTROOM
62 Cal.L.Rev. 693, 719–729.
(1974).

* * *

REASONS WHY PSYCHIATRIC JUDGMENTS ARE
UNRELIABLE AND INVALID

* * *

A. Orientation and Training

It has been suggested that psychiatrists are prone to diagnose mental illness and to perceive symptoms in ambiguous behavior because they are trained in medical school that it is safer to suspect illness and be wrong, than to reject illness and be wrong. In other words, "being a mental health professional may constitute a set to perceive mental illness. . . ."[90]

In addition, each school of psychiatry has a different view of what mental illness is, how it is caused, and how it should be treated. Substantial evidence suggests that psychiatric judgments are strongly influenced by these different schools of thought and training.

90. In one study two groups of graduate students in clinical psychology viewed a taped interview and were asked to evaluate the interviewee. One group represented the behaviorist and the other the psychoanalytic orientation. Behaviorists are trained to describe carefully the behavior an individual manifests but to refrain from making any judgments or inferences about that individual or his behavior; analysts are more willing to make such speculations. Half the clinicians were told the interviewee in the film was a "job applicant," and half were told he was a "patient." It was found that the behaviorists rated the subject approximately the same (on an adjustment rating scale) regardless of the "set;" the analysts, on the other hand, agreed with the behaviorists on adjustment of the "job applicant" but saw the "patient" as a much more disturbed person. . . .

Pasamanick, Dinitz, and Lefton, for example, inferred from their findings that:

> . . . despite their protestations that their point of view is always the individual patient, clinicians in fact may be so committed to a particular school of psychiatric thought that the patient's diagnosis and treatment is largely predetermined. Clinicians . . . may be selectively perceiving only those characteristics and attributes of their patients which are relevant to their own pre-conceived system of thought. As a consequence, they may be overlooking other patient characteristics which would be considered crucial by colleagues who are otherwise committed. . . .

B. Context

* * *

[T]he effect of "suggestion" or "set" was examined in a study in which an actor portrayed a healthy man while talking about himself in a diagnostic interview with a clinician. The interview was recorded and played to groups of a) graduate students in clinical psychology, b) psychiatrists, c) law students, and d) undergraduates. Before playing the tape, however, a prestige figure—a different person for each group—told the groups that the interview was interesting because the subject "looked neurotic but actually is quite psychotic." As a control four comparable groups heard the taped interview but were given no prestige suggestion for "psychosis." After hearing the tape, the groups were asked to assign the interviewee to one of 30 specified diagnostic categories. None of the control groups diagnosed the subject as psychotic, and the majority diagnosed him as healthy. By contrast, 60 percent of the psychiatrists, 30 percent of the undergraduates, 28 percent of the psychologists, 17 percent of the law students, and 11 percent of the graduate psychology students diagnosed psychosis. The authors conclude that prestige suggestion influences diagnosis, and that an initial diagnosis "may have a profound effect" upon a subsequent diagnosis by influencing "interpersonal perception, whether or not the [initial] diagnostic label refers to a disease which actually exists." In other words, clinicians often perceive what they expect to perceive and the impact of suggestion on clinical perception may be profound.

In a study of pseudo-patients, eight sane individuals feigning one symptom of schizophrenia were admitted to various mental hospitals with that diagnosis. Rosenhan found that even though immediately after admission the pseudo-patients ceased displaying that symptom and behaved normally,

> once a person is designated abnormal, all of his other behaviors and characteristics are colored by that label. Indeed, that label is so powerful that many of the pseudo-patient's normal behaviors were overlooked entirely or profoundly misinterpreted.

For example, when several of the pseudo-patients took notes of their experiences, that activity was noted in three of their records as "an aspect of their pathological behavior." The purpose of Rosenhan's study was to determine whether "the salient characteristics that lead to diagnoses reside in the patients themselves or in the environment and contexts in which observers find them." Although the pseudo-patients related absolutely normal life histories, Rosenhan found that "diagnoses were in no way affected by the relative health of the circumstances of a pseudo-patient's life. Rather, the reverse occurred: the perception of his circumstances was shaped entirely by the diagnosis."

C. Time

Since even "normal" people speak and behave differently from one day to the next, it is no less natural for an allegedly mentally ill individual to appear agitated one day and composed the next. Consequently, the timing of a prospective patient's examination may substantially influence the diagnosis he or she is given. In his 1967 review of studies, Zubin found that the consistency over time of specific diagnoses of nonorganic conditions is quite low, and that even the "broad diagnostic categories appear to display a low order of consistency [about 50 percent] over time." In a related study Edelman found that diagnostic impressions change by a fourth interview-therapy session about 25 percent of the time. He also noted that:

> The typical procedure for establishing a diagnosis is a single unstandardized interview, the results of which may be augmented by psychological testing. An implicit assumption of this procedure is that interviewee behavior has been adequately sampled in the allotted time span and that the interviewee is sufficiently motivated to reveal all pertinent information. Yet, there are numerous studies which indicate that interviewee behavior is mediated by complex process variables suggesting that such assumptions may not always be justified.

In other words, even if a patient's behavior is consistent over time, different aspects of that behavior may be observed at different times.

D. Class and Culture

There is considerable evidence that psychiatric judgments are strongly influenced by the socio-economic backgrounds of the clinician and patient. Philips and Draguns reviewed the literature from 1966 to 1969 and concluded:

> . . . The influence of the client's socio-economic class in facilitating the attribution of some, and impeding the application of other, nosological designations is particularly well documented . . . [T]he findings converge in suggesting social distance as the mediating variable. Across socio-economic or other subcultural lines, the middle class diagnostician is prone to assign categories of severe psycho-pathology. . . .

In a controlled experiment, Lee and Temerlin found that the diagnoses of psychiatric residents were highly influenced by the imagined socio-economic history of the patient (and by the perceived diagnoses of other, prestigious psychiatrists) independent of the clinical picture presented. A lower socio-economic history biased diagnosis toward greater illness and poorer prognosis. Similarly, according to studies conducted by Ordway, clinicians may be influenced to conclude that lower socio-economic class individuals are dangerous because such individuals are presumed to be impulsive and therefore more prone to violence.

* * *

E. Personal Bias

The factor which may most influence diagnosis is the clinician's own personality, value system, self-image, personal preferences, and attitudes. * * *

Grosz and Grossman present evidence suggesting that the clinicians' varying personal biases may account for the significant differences in their evaluation of ambiguous and emotionally charged case history data. They summarize their findings, as follows:

> . . . The more complex, ill-defined, ambiguous, unfamiliar and uninformative the data, the more strongly do the observer's set, focused attention, expectation, bias and other intra-observer conditions come into play and influence his perception, judgment, and decision. . . . The possibility exists that such judgments are less informative about the patient whom they are meant to describe than about the clinician who makes them. They may reveal the clinician's concepts of norms or his toleration of deviations compared to those of his peers, his clinical orientation and attitudes toward certain aspects of the patient's history, his clinical experience and interests, and perhaps even his own background and personality.

Their conclusions are borne out by others. For instance, Dickes, Simons, and Weisfogel demonstrate that the unconscious conflicts of clinicians often cause distortions in perception, and misapprehension of the patient's true condition. And in the context of sanity hearings Pugh found that the ultimate determinations are strongly influenced by the personal idiosyncracies of the examining psychiatrist.

Strupp found that therapists' perceptions of a patient presented in a film interview varied according to the therapist's experience and his attitude toward the patient. As an illustration of the latter factor, if for some reason the therapist disliked the patient the result was often a poor prognostic evaluation. Braginsky and Braginsky suggest a possible context in which a psychiatrist might develop a dislike for a patient. Their study showed that mental health professionals view patients who express radical political views as more disturbed than patients who voice the same psychiatric complaints, but whose political views are more conventional. They also discovered that voicing criticism of the mental health profession, whether from a radical or conservative perspective, may substantially increase a patient's psychopathology in the eyes of mental health professionals, while flattering the profession tends to decrease a patient's otherwise perceived symptomatology.

Numerous other studies confirm that the clinician's personal values and attitudes strongly influence diagnosis and judgment.

*   *   *

Questions and Comments

1. *Rosenhan Study: Labelling and normality.* Ennis and Litwak refer to the Rosenhan study, probably the most controversial of all the research addressing the problem of diagnostic reliability. In that study, as Ennis and Litwak report, eight "normal" individuals showed up at various mental hospitals with feigned symptoms (specifically, they all reported having an auditory hallucination). Otherwise they acted normally. All but one were diagnosed as schizophrenic and all were admitted to the hospital. Their behavior after admission was normal; they never again reported hearing unusual sounds or voices. Although all were eventually discharged (with a diagnosis of schizophrenia in remission), they spent an average of 19 days in the hospital, with the range from 7 to 52 days.

Some have argued that it would have been much more disturbing if the pseudopatients had *not* been admitted for further investigation, since auditory hallucinations are considered indicative of schizophrenia. Kety commented: "If I were to drink a quart of blood and, concealing what I had done, come to the emergency room of any hospital vomiting blood, the behavior of the staff would be quite predictable. If they labeled and treated me as having a bleeding ulcer, I doubt that I could argue convincingly that medical science does not know how to diagnose that condition." Kety, "From Rationalization to Reason," 131 Am.J.Psychiat. 957 (1974). Does Kety's response explain all of the phenomena observed by Rosenhan's pseudopatients? Spitzer has suggested that, to some extent at least, the study reflects staffing and resource problems rather than deficiencies in psychiatric judgement. Spitzer, "More on Pseudoscience in Science and the Case for Psychiatric Diagnosis," 33 Arch.Gen.Psychiat. 459 (1976).

2. *Implications of variance.* Ways of trying to minimize the effect of the distorting influences described by Ennis and Litwak and Rosenhan are for the most part self-evident, although not always successful. For example multiple interviews by independent interviewers might alleviate the effects of training, context, time and bias. See Bonnie & Slobogin, "The Role of Mental Health Professionals in the Criminal Process: The Case for Informed Speculation, 66 Va.L.Rev. 427, 496–522 (1981). Probably the best minimization technique, already alluded to, is to improve the criteria for decisionmaking. For instance, if diagnostic criteria are made more precise the possibility that observer bias would affect the ultimate diagnosis should be reduced. Thus, to the extent DSM–III has reduced criterion variance, the potential for other factors to cause variance should be reduced as well. The same relationship between precise criteria and the effects of biases, context and other factors exists in assessing responsibility, propensity and competency as well.

Nonetheless, it is probable that diagnostic and other criteria will always carry some ambiguity; greater precision is unlikely to remove entirely the effects of the influences described by Ennis and Litwak. Does this fact make all or most psychiatric judgments so suspect that they should be barred in legal proceedings? Does replacing diagnoses with "descriptive" information solve the problem? Or are "descriptions of facts" just as susceptible to the influences described above?

3. *The admissibility of other types of expert testimony.* Other types of expert testimony have significant validity and reliability problems as well. For instance, one study found that police crime labs misidentify paint samples 51 percent of the time, drug samples 18 percent of the time, blood samples 71 percent of the time, and firearms 28 percent of the time. Peterson, Fabricant, Field, Crime Laboratory Proficiency Testing Research Program: Final Report (1978). What are the probable reasons for these inaccuracy rates? Are they any more rectifiable than those which cause diagnostic unreliability?

The testimony of economists in antitrust cases is another interesting example of expertise in action. Battles of the experts in such cases are much more common than in insanity cases. As Younger noted:

> Unlike any other country, we submit many issues to the courts that don't turn on factual determinations at all. Should I.B.M. be broken up? Is it good for America to break up A.T. & T.? We pretend those are factual questions and call economists to testify, but they're simply a matter of opinion. And in virtually every case in this country in which experts end up on the witness stand there are vast possibilities for honest differences of opinion. In a case where opinions can reasonably differ on a question, each lawyer simply scouts around until he finds an expert who has an opinion that comports with his client's interest. Experts can testify in good faith and still be testifying to opposites.

Reported in Jenkins, "Expert's Day in Court," New York Times Magazine, Dec. 11, 1983, p. 98, col. 4. Despite the lack of precision in economic science, courts have allowed experts to offer opinions about market conditions, the opportunities for collusion, market behavior and whether industries conspired to form a cartel. See, e.g., In re Japanese Electronic Products, 723 F.2d 238, 280 (3d Cir.1983); reversed on other grounds, 475 U.S. 574, 106 S.Ct. 1348, 89 L.Ed.2d 538 (1986).

Similarly, despite the seeming subjectivity of the issues raised in obscenity trials under the prevailing test, see Roth v. United States, 354 U.S. 476, 77 S.Ct. 1304, 1 L.Ed.2d 1498 (1957), rehearing denied, 355 U.S. 852, 78 S.Ct. 8, 2 L.Ed.2d 60 (1957), witnesses have been permitted to offer opinions as to the dominant theme of an allegedly obscene work, the effect of that work on an "average man," and whether the work has any "redeeming social value." For instance, in Commonwealth v. Trainor, 374 Mass. 796, 374 N.E.2d 1216, 1220 (1978), the court stated "[w]here the question is whether portrayals of sexual conduct are 'obscene' under the statutory definition, it would be a rare case in which testimony from a qualified expert should be excluded on the ground that it would not be helpful to the trier of fact." Courts generally allow in such evidence and leave problems of uncertainty to the trier of fact. See generally, Stern, "Toward a Rationale for the Use of Expert Testimony in Obscenity Litigation," 20 Case Western Res.L.Rev. 523 (1969).

Do these examples from other legal arenas support retaining diagnostic and other psychiatric opinion testimony? A revamping of *all* expert testimony? Or are they different from psychiatric testimony in significant ways? Consider these questions again after reviewing the materials on responsibility assessments.

B. RESPONSIBILITY

The relationship between mental disorder and responsibility is most obviously raised by the insanity defense, but is also implicated by a number of criminal law doctrines. Generally, the criminal law assumes that the effect of mental disorder is either "cognitive" or "volitional". In the first instance, the focus is on one's awareness and perceptions about one's actions at the time of the offense; in the second, the emphasis is on one's ability to control one's behavior at the time of the offense. The following case deals with the mental health profession's expertise on the latter issue.

UNITED STATES v. LEWELLYN
United States Court of Appeals, Eighth Circuit, 1983.
723 F.2d 615.

FAGG, CIRCUIT JUDGE.

[Gary Lewellyn, a Des Moines stockbroker, was indicted on fifteen counts of embezzlement, making false statements, and mail fraud for converting over $17 million in money and securities from two Iowa banks. In response to the government's pretrial motion, the district court ruled that Lewellyn could not rely on a defense of insanity "by reason of pathological gambling" and excluded evidence related to that defense. Lewellyn was convicted on all counts. On appeal, he contended that the district court erred in precluding his insanity defense. The test for insanity was the ALI test, which recognizes a defense, *inter alia*, when "mental disease or defect" causes a person to lack "substantial capacity . . . to conform his conduct to the requirements of the law."]

We have recognized that in order to raise the issue of insanity a defendant must make a minimum showing. A defendant is presumed sane, but the introduction of evidence of insanity dispels the presumption and subjects the prosecution to the burden of proving sanity beyond a reasonable doubt. United States v. Dresser, 542 F.2d 737, 742 (8th Cir.1976), citing Davis v. United States, 160 U.S. 469, 486–88, 16 S.Ct. 353, 357–58, 40 L.Ed. 499 (1895). In *Dresser* we referred to this threshold showing as a "prima facie case of insanity." 542 F.2d at 742 n. 7.

[I]n the present case we need not decide whether pathological gambling may never be grounds for an insanity defense. In the particular circumstances of this case we are concerned with the connection between pathological gambling and collateral criminal activity. To make the required minimum showing of insanity Lewellyn had to show that at least some pathological gamblers lack substantial capacity to conform their conduct to the requirements of laws prohibiting criminal activities like embezzlement. We now turn to the record to determine whether Lewellyn made a showing which would have allowed him to rely on an insanity defense at trial.

DSM–III [i.e., Diagnostic and Statistical Manual of Mental Disorders (3d ed.1980)] contains the following description of pathological gambling:

> The essential features are a chronic and progressive failure to resist impulses to gamble and gambling behavior that compromises, disrupts, or damages personal, family, or vocational pursuits. The gambling preoccupation, urge, and activity increase during periods of stress. Problems that arise as a result of the gambling lead to an intensification of the gambling behavior. Characteristic problems include loss of work due to absences in order to gamble, defaulting on debts and other financial responsibilities, disrupted family relationships, borrowing money from illegal sources, forgery, fraud, embezzlement, and income tax evasion.
>
> Commonly these individuals have the attitude that money causes and is also the solution to all their problems. As the gambling increases, the individual is usually forced to lie in order to obtain money and to continue gambling, but hides the extent of the gambling. There is no serious attempt to budget or save money. When borrowing resources are strained, antisocial behavior in order to obtain money for more gambling is likely. Any criminal behavior—e.g., forgery, embezzlement, or fraud—is typically nonviolent. There is a conscious intent to return or repay the money.

Id. at 291. The diagnostic criteria for pathological gambling included in DSM–III are:

> A. The individual is chronically and progressively unable to resist impulses to gamble.
>
> B. Gambling compromises, disrupts, or damages family, personal, and vocational pursuits, as indicated by at least three of the following:
>
>> (1) arrest for forgery, fraud, embezzlement, or income tax evasion due to attempts to obtain money for gambling
>
> * * *
>
> C. The gambling is not due to Antisocial Personality Disorder.

Id. at 292–93.

The language of DSM–III does not establish that pathological gamblers may lack substantial capacity to refrain from engaging in embezzlement and similar criminal activities. Portions of DSM–III no doubt indicate that criminal activity is often associated with pathological gambling. DSM–III does not state, however, that pathological gamblers who engage in criminal conduct do so because they lack substantial capacity to conform their conduct to the requirements of law, nor does it state anything of equivalent meaning. It is not remarkable, though, that the language of DSM–III does not conform to the legal principles embodied in the ALI insanity rule.

> The purpose of DSM–III is to provide clear descriptions of diagnostic categories in order to enable clinicians and investigators to diagnose, communicate about, study, and treat various mental disorders. The use of this manual for nonclinical purposes, such as determination of legal responsibility, competency or insanity * * * must be critically examined in each instance within the appropriate institutional context.

Id. at 12. When we examine DSM–III carefully within the context of the criminal law we conclude that its language does not establish a relationship between pathological gambling and criminal activity sufficient to constitute insanity under the ALI standard. As a consequence, DSM–III does not alone supply the minimum showing Lewellyn was required to make before he could rely on an insanity defense.

Expert testimony adduced by Lewellyn, couched in terms more like those of the ALI insanity rule, does suggest the requisite connection between pathological gambling and criminal activity because it supports the proposition that some pathological gamblers lack substantial capacity to resist engaging in embezzlement and similar offenses. Dr. Julian Taber, a psychologist, testified that in some instances pathological gamblers are incapable of conforming their conduct to the requirements of law, and are unable to avoid behavior such as forgery, fraud, and embezzlement. Dr. Robert Custer, a psychiatrist, testified that in the late stage of pathological gambling individuals are unable to resist activities like embezzlement or fraud because they have to gamble and they have to obtain money in order to gamble.

Lewellyn is dependent on this scientific expert testimony to sustain his burden of making the required minimum showing that would permit him to rely on an insanity defense at trial. The expert testimony is essential because it supports a proposition not established in DSM–III: that some pathological gamblers lack substantial capacity to refrain from committing embezzlement and similar offenses. We note, however, that established principles control admissibility of scientific evidence. "[W]hile courts will go a long way in admitting expert testimony deduced from a well-recognized scientific principle or discovery, the thing from which the deduction is made must be sufficiently established to have gained general acceptance in the particular field in which it belongs." Frye v. United States, 293 F. 1013, 1014 (D.C.Cir. 1923). In deciding whether a scientific principle meets the Frye standard we have recognized reliability as "one of the most important factors" that should be considered. United States v. Alexander, 526 F.2d 161, 163 (8th Cir.1975). Because our analysis of the Frye rule would govern the admission at trial of expert testimony similar to that given at the pretrial hearing, this analysis is equally applicable in determining whether expert testimony adduced by Lewellyn is sufficient to constitute the required minimum showing of insanity.

Pathological gambling has received relatively little scientific attention. Dr. Custer testified that pathological gambling has only recently been recognized as a disease. Both Dr. Taber and Dr. Custer cited the inclusion of pathological gambling in DSM–III, published in 1980, as evidence that the condition is generally accepted as a mental disease by mental health professionals. Pathological gambling was not listed, however, in DSM–II, published in 1968.

From the testimony at the pretrial hearing it is apparent that few psychologists or psychiatrists have had much experience dealing with pathological gamblers. Dr. Taber estimated that there may be perhaps 20 psychologists with some in-depth experience working with pathological gamblers, but he said that to his knowledge he was the only psychologist devoted full-time to their treatment. Dr. Taber knew of no psychiatrist who would work full-time with pathological gamblers. Dr. Custer stated that probably not more than 20 or 25 doctors have had experience with pathological gambling.

There is accordingly little knowledge about pathological gambling within the community of mental health professionals. Dr. Taber testified that in talking with physicians, social workers, and psychologists, he had "found very prevalent ignorance or just lack of concern with the problem." Dr. Custer indicated that it is necessary to spend a significant amount of time working with pathological gamblers in order to understand the problem "because it is so new and there is so very little that has been known about it." Dr. Custer said he does not think many doctors know about pathological gambling, and that as a result they do not recognize it as a disease.

In order to make the necessary minimum showing of insanity Lewellyn was required to demonstrate that there is general acceptance in the fields of psychiatry and psychology of the principle that some pathological gamblers lack substantial capacity to conform their conduct to the requirements of laws prohibiting embezzlement and similar offenses. There is no evidence in the record, however, either in DSM–III or the expert testimony, that this principle is generally accepted in the mental health professions. Indeed, the record shows that the pathological gambling disorder itself has only recently been recognized in DSM–III, and that there is scant experience and limited knowledge concerning this problem. In our view, Lewellyn has failed to show that the opinions espoused by his expert witnesses possess the requisite indicia of scientific reliability.

Because we find that Lewellyn did not make the required minimum showing of insanity, we affirm the district court's exclusion of evidence pertaining to a defense of insanity by reason of pathological gambling.

Questions and Comments

1. *Pathological gambling and cognitive impairment.* The expert testimony that the defendant sought to introduce in *Lewellyn* was aimed at

showing volitional impairment at the time of the offense. Testimony about the effects of pathological gambling may also be presented to show cognitive impairment. For instance, Dr. Custer, one of the two mental health professionals involved in *Lewellyn,* testified as follows in *State v. Campanaro,* Union Country Indictment no. 632079 (Superior Court of New Jersey Criminal Division 1981):

Q. Doctor, is [the defendant] by virtue of the condition under which he labored at the time he drew the specific checks before you incapable of distinguishing right from wrong as regards that check?

A. Well, here's a man who was a law enforcement officer, who knows the law well, who knows about right and wrong but a man who is in a desperate strait. He is under a tremendous amount of stress at that point, does not consider right and wrong. I don't think that becomes part of his thinking process. His process then is to survive. He's losing his job, his family, his children, his reputation, everything is going down. So he functions this way, in an irrational way to which his judgment is that impaired.

*   *   *

Q. Is he capable of making a value judgment at that point?

A. No.

In this case, not only was the testimony admitted, but the defendant was acquitted by reason of insanity. Would the *Lewellyn* court have been more willing to admit this type of testimony?

2. *Presumptions and expert testimony.* The court in *Lewellyn* decided that the evidence presented by the defendant did not overcome the presumption of sanity and thus upheld its exclusion by the trial court. In most jurisdictions, the presumption of sanity functions only as a requirement that the defendant produce *some* evidence of insanity in order to get the issue to the jury; as one commentator summarized it, the usual approach is to hold that a "scintilla" of evidence satisfactorily rebuts the presumption. Goldstein, The Insanity Defense 113 (1967). However, the *Lewellyn* court, relying on precedent, stated that the presumption can be overcome only if a *prima facie* case of insanity is made out by the defendant, thus raising the threshold for admission. Put another way, in most jurisdictions, the defendant overcomes the presumption of sanity if relevant rebuttal evidence (i.e., evidence having any tendency to prove insanity) is presented. But here the court requires the defendant to "establish" insanity to the satisfaction of the court before the jury may hear the evidence.

3. *Diagnosis and responsibility.* Relying on the prima facie test for overcoming the presumption of sanity, the *Lewellyn* court found that the language in DSM–III about pathological gambling, by itself, was insufficient. Do you agree? If the court were to adopt the more typical "scintilla" or relevance rule in determining whether the presumption is met, would a diagnosis of pathological gambling be enough? Should a diagnosis, if believed, ever be sufficient by itself to overcome the presumption?

4. *The* Frye *Rule.* The defendant also relied on the testimony of Drs. Custer and Taber in support of his insanity defense. The court implies

that had this testimony been admissible, the defendant would have overcome the presumption of sanity and could have asserted an insanity
defense at trial. But it found the testimony inadmissible, relying on a
second evidentiary doctrine, announced in *Frye v. United States,* 293 Fed.
1013 (D.C.Cir.1923). As the court states, the "*Frye* rule" holds that "the
thing" from which scientific evidence is deduced "must be sufficiently
established to have gained general acceptance in the particular field in
which it belongs." Although it seems to add a barrier to admissibility
beyond those posed by the federal rules,[e] this rule has been widely applied
in determining the admissibility of many different types of scientific
evidence, including testimony based on neutron activation analysis, polygraph tests, and voice spectograph assessments. Its application to psychiatric and psychological testimony is much more recent.

Some have criticized the *Frye* rule on the ground that the "general
acceptance" standard is confusing and difficult to apply consistently. One
commentator has noted that, under the rule, "courts must decide *who* must
find the procedure acceptable, they must define exactly *what* must be
accepted, and they must determine what methods will be used to establish
general acceptance." Gianelli, "The Admissibility of Novel Scientific Evidence: Frye v. United States, A Half-Century Later," 80 Colum.L.Rev.
1197, 1208 (1980). Did the *Lewellyn* court properly address these issues?

A separate criticism of the *Frye* test has to do with its conceptual
underpinning. Many commentators reject the *Frye* rule as a means of
determining the admissibility of scientific testimony because they feel that
the traditional relevance/prejudice inquiry is a more sensitive tool for this
purpose. See, e.g., C. McCormick, Handbook of the Law of Evidence § 203,
at 491 (2d. ed. 1972); J. Richardson, Modern Scientific Evidence § 2.5
(1974). Implicit in the relevance inquiry is an accuracy assessment: evidence which is inaccurate has no tendency to make a proposition more or
less probable. But if it is not known whether evidence in a particular case
is inaccurate, as is often the case with scientific evidence, then exclusion
should only occur if the jury is likely to accept it unquestioningly. If, on
the other hand, problems with the evidence can be made clear to the jury,
it should be admitted and the jury allowed to make up its mind. In other
words, questions about the inaccuracy of expert testimony should go to the
weight of the evidence and not its admissibility. *Frye* held the opposite.

In response to this criticism, it could be argued that the *Frye* rule is
merely an application of the relevance/prejudice inquiry in the scientific
evidence context. That is, the courts which apply it have decided that
scientific evidence is, by its nature, so likely to persuade a jury that it must
be "screened" for accuracy before it is admitted. Does this reasoning apply
to psychiatric testimony?

5. *Reasonable Certainty.* In addition to presumption analysis and the
Frye rule, a third method of judicially "screening" psychiatric evidence
before it gets to the jury—also not explicitly endorsed by the federal rules—
is to decide whether it is based on "reasonable medical certainty" or

---

e. "It is not clear whether Rules 702
and 703 are intended to codify the *Frye* test
or whether they establish a less demanding
standard for scientific evidence." (S.
Saltzburg & K. Redden, Federal Rules of
Evidence Manual 452 (3d ed. 1982).

"reasonable psychological certainty." If an opinion cannot be offered with reasonable degree of certainty, then it is excluded. As with the *Frye* test, the ambiguity of the concept renders it difficult to apply. After analyzing the three possible bases for the "certainty rule"—preventing usurpation of the jury's role, assuring sufficiency of the evidence, and avoiding speculation—Martin concludes that "either the basis itself or its application through this admissibility rule is in all cases unsatisfactory." Martin, "The Uncertain Rule of Certainty: An Analysis and Proposal for a Federal Evidence Rule," 20 Wayne L.Rev. 781, 808 (1974). Martin points out that the differing backgrounds and orientations of legal and medical professionals make it unlikely that they mean the same thing when they speak of "reasonable medical certainty." Id. at 804–95. He also notes that most experts do not make specific quantitative determinations regarding their certainty in a particular opinion, often because it is impossible to do so. Id. at 806. He concludes that degree of certainty should not be a determinant of admissibility, and that gross speculation will be excluded on other grounds, e.g., because the evidence "cannot assist the trier, it is not relevant and wastes time, and it cannot be supported by facts." Id. at 808–09.

6. *Jury confusion.* A final consideration which has led some judges to exclude expert testimony is a fear that the jury will be confused by the testimony or attempts to rebut it. In a sense, this ground for exclusion is based on a premise opposite to that motivating the other screening rules, which act to prevent the jury from being too easily swayed, rather than befuddled, by expert testimony. The federal rules give the judge discretion to exclude testimony which creates a potential for jury confusion. Rule 403. But in United States v. Torniero, 735 F.2d 725 (2d Cir.1984), another pathological gambling case, the court found fault with the trial judge's ruling excluding expert testimony on this ground:

> This is not a case . . . where a specific piece of evidence or testimony of a particular expert would be eliminated. The effect of the preclusion here is to keep an entire line of argument from being presented to the jury. The unique character of the insanity defense militates against exclusion on the sole ground that the jury would be confused by the clashing opinions of experts. The insanity defense by its very nature is complex and perhaps even confusing at times. But, evidence submitted to a jury in many cases is frequently obfuscated. [E]ven in civil litigation, where non-perspicuous issues and abstruse evidence proliferate, we have never adopted a "complexity exception" to the right to jury trial.

7. *Novel defenses and substantive law.* The pathological gambling defense raised in *Lewellyn* is of recent vintage. To the extent they should be relied upon at all, use of the *Frye* rule and other screening devices is most easily justified in just such a situation, when novel and relatively untested scientific evidence is at issue. But in some cases involving novel defense arguments, reliance on these devices may serve another goal, one that is substantive rather than evidentiary. That is, they might be used to exclude evidence not because of its inaccuracy but because of its effect on accepted legal doctrine. Is it possible that the real concern of the *Lewellyn*

court was not that the testimony would be inaccurate or misleading, but that it might lead to an improper expansion of the insanity defense? See Bonnie, Compulsive Gambling and the Insanity Defense, 9 Newsletter of the Amer.Acad.Psychiat. & Law 6, 7 (1984).

In any event, the types of evidentiary issues raised in *Lewellyn* are seldom raised in more "routine" insanity cases. The next excerpt takes exception to this practice.

STEPHEN MORSE, CRAZY BEHAVIOR, MORALS & SCIENCE: AN ANALYSIS OF MENTAL HEALTH LAW

51 S.Cal.L.Rev. 527, 582–88, 618–19.
(1978).

[I]

. . . [T]he law is concerned with specific cases where an actor may be clearly crazy and where the craziness is clearly related to legally relevant behavior. . . . In terms of responsibility, . . . [i]ndividual cases of clear relationship may be separated into two types: *crazy urges* and *crazy reasons.* In each case, this section considers the particular factors that help one decide whether the actor could have behaved otherwise. Even assuming that the craziness was a causal variable, the critical question remains: Was the crazy urge uncontrollable or was the crazy reason and the legally relevant behavior based on it the inexorable result of a disturbed mind?

a. *Crazy urges:* The case of crazy urges refers to what is usually termed an "irresistible impulse." The actor may be perfectly rational cognitively, but he *feels* as if he must carry out a particular behavior and that he cannot prevent himself from doing so. He may be quite aware that the action he feels compelled to perform is weird, deviant, immoral, maladaptive, or the like. Still, he feels incapable of behaving otherwise. If the behavior felt to be compelled is weird, deviant, or immoral, we are inclined to believe that the urge is crazy, because no one would desire to behave in those ways when he comprehends how those behaviors were assessed. The prototypical case of a crazy urge is the sexual deviant, *e.g.,* a child molester, who knows that his actions are viewed as sick or evil (or both) by most persons, and yet who feels an overwhelming desire to molest children.

Is the child molester's behavior the irresistible effect of his crazy urge? To analyze this question we must first ask the threshold question of whether the actor's crazy urge is related to mental illness. This case is a clear example of the situation where craziness is diagnosed because the legally relevant behavior seems crazy itself and where no other significant evidence of mental disorder may exist. We assume that there must be some underlying abnormality because no rational person would choose to molest children unless he was "forced to" by circumstances beyond his control. [T]here is no evidence of underlying abnormality in such cases, but let us accept arguments that it is reasonable to call this person crazy because he experiences a perhaps inexplicable and crazy urge.

Is the urge irresistible? For at least two reasons, most persons would assume that the urge must be very strong. First, the molester reports that the urge is overwhelming. Second, it seems intuitively obvious that most persons would not "give in" to such an urge unless it was overpowering. Let us assume that, indeed, the urge is powerful and perhaps even tormenting to our molester. But could it have been resisted, albeit at the cost of frustration and discomfort? Do all persons who feel such urges give in to them, or are there some who resist?

Although there exists little systematic epidemiological study of such questions, it is clear from clinical practice that many persons report extremely strong "deviant" urges that are often a source of misery to them. Yet most persons do not engage in the urged behavior; indeed, many seek assistance from clergymen, doctors, counselors, and psychotherapists in order to defeat the urge. Holding that the urge is not overwhelming in such cases, but that it is overwhelming in the cases of those who give in, is tautological reasoning: the urge must be overwhelming because the person gave in. In terms more familiar to lawyers, we are faced with the difficulty of distinguishing between the irresistible impulse and the impulse not resisted.

There is no scientific measure of the strength of urges. Nor is there evidence of what percentage of people who experience various urges of various strengths act on those urges. Even if such measures and data were available, as they may be someday, the measured strength of the urge would not answer the question of whether the urge was irresistible. Such data may help us to identify how predisposing, in a statistical sense, the urge might be, but they would not answer the question of moral and legal responsibility. Where to draw the cutting point would clearly be a moral and legal determination. In the future, behavioral science may provide more precise information to help draw the line, but science alone cannot draw the line of legal responsibility.

At present, then, the determination of the irresistibility of crazy urges must rest on commonsense assessments of the craziness and strength of the urge. The data to be evaluated would be first, the report of the urged actor, and second, the craziness of the urged action. Whether certain urges are crazy is not a scientific question that needs expert answers. And whether the urge is sufficiently strong or crazy is a question that is answered by assessing the reported feelings of the actor and the sincerity of his report. There is simply no test for knowing when an urge is irresistible, and indeed, there is no reason to believe that there is any urge that is not, to some degree, resistible. Deciding whether an urge is irresistible is not a scientific decision.

b. *Crazy reasons:* It may also be believed that an actor had no free choice about whether to engage in certain behavior if the actor reports crazy reasons for his behavior. If an actor kills someone because he sincerely believes the victim was a hostile agent, we believe that the killing not only is related to the crazy belief as was seen above, but that it is the compelled result of the crazy belief. After all, no one would hold and act on such beliefs unless there were something uncontrollably wrong with him that caused him to have those beliefs.

Before we can determine whether an actor had control over his crazy reasons and consequent actions, we must first analyze the nature of a crazy reason. Following from our definition of craziness itself, we may define a crazy reason as one that is irrational and inexplicable. Of course, the degree of craziness of a reason varies along a lengthy continuum.

* * *

It may be very hard for a person to think straight; in some cases, crazy beliefs may powerfully compel the crazy person to act on them. But there is no certainty that an actor cannot control his crazy beliefs or, at least, control actions based on them. Indeed, even the craziest persons seem to behave quite normally or rationally a great deal of the time, especially if there is good reason to do so. On at least some occasions, including some instances when they are behaving crazily, crazy persons are clearly capable of playing by the usual rules. Nor do they always act on the basis of their crazy reasons. Moreover, the defects and disordered thinking that supposedly distinguish crazy persons from normal ones are very prevalent in the general population. * * * Even if it is found that the person typically seems out of touch with reality, reasons crazily, and gives mostly crazy reasons for his behavior, scientific evidence cannot demonstrate that such behavior is the result of mental disorder and that related legally relevant behavior is sufficiently unfree to ascribe nonresponsibility to the actor. At most it can be urged that a person who typically does not think "straight" is more or less predisposed to give crazy reasons and to act on them.

* * *

[II]

Whether an actor could have behaved otherwise and is legally and morally responsible for his legally relevant behavior cannot be determined scientifically. No diagnosis gives the answer to these questions, and there are no scientific tests to measure the strength of crazy urges or the strength of the actor's self-control. Nor are there tests to distinguish the person who *cannot* think straight or control himself from the person who *will not* think straight or control himself. Whether a person cannot or will not think straight or control himself is a moral and commonsense judgment that should be made by the legal decisionmaker.

Let us take an example to examine how experts might help or hinder legal decisions about responsibility. In a famous homicide case,[194] clinicians testified that the defendant killed the victim in order to avoid psychic disintegration and insanity. If this formulation is

194. People v. Gorshen, 51 Cal.2d 716, 336 P.2d 492 (1959).

correct, the defendant was faced with a very hard choice indeed—kill or psychically disintegrate—and the defendant would hardly seem as responsible as most criminal homicide defendants, or perhaps, responsible at all. Some clarifying questions, however, should be asked: (1) Are there hard data behind the theorizing that the killing was the inexorable or nearly inexorable result of threatened ego-disintegration?; and (2) What percentage of persons with such fears kill? The answer to question (1) is "no," and the answer to question (2) is that the data are unavailable although the actual percentage is probably quite low. Such fears are not a proven necessary or sufficient cause of homicidal behavior. In this case, as in all cases, the expert's assertion that the person could not have acted otherwise is really a moral guess and not a scientific fact. Justice would be better served if the expert drew no conclusions and simply described in ordinary language the cognitive and affective state of the defendant without intruding terms and theories of unproven accuracy and usefulness.[195]

* * *

RICHARD BONNIE & CHRISTOPHER SLOBOGIN, THE ROLE OF MENTAL HEALTH PROFESSIONALS IN THE CRIMINAL PROCESS: THE CASE FOR INFORMED SPECULATION

66 Va.L.Rev. 427, 461–64, 486–93.
(1980).

* * *

We concede that the central etiological theories and conceptual categories of the clinical behavioral disciplines have not been scientifically validated, and that few clinical opinions can be stated with a high degree of certainty. At best, opinions about psychological processes— beyond merely descriptive observations—are clinical probability judgments rooted in theoretical constructs that are more or less widely shared among mental health professionals.

According to the weight of authority, however, the fact that opinion testimony is uncertain does not by itself justify exclusion, as long as the evidence rises above mere conjecture or speculation. If it has any tendency to prove a fact, and is otherwise qualified as expert opinion, the evidence is admissible unless some overriding reason requires exclusion. The rationale for this position is that many observations, both scientific and lay, can be expressed only in terms of "probabilities" or "possibilities"; to deny the factfinder such evidence on this ground alone might deplete seriously the amount of information available.

---

195. Of course, an expert who tries to describe the person's past mental state faces grave difficulties. This probably cannot be done with substantial accuracy unless the expert had occasion to know or examine the actor at the past time in question. Thus, experts probably should never testify about an actor's mental state at a time when the expert had no direct knowledge of it. Still, descriptions of a present mental state may help a factfinder draw inferences about a past mental state provided that the time in question is not too remote and that there is some direct evidence of the actor's behavior at the past time.

Although Professor Morse acknowledges this general evidentiary principle, he asserts that "an exception should be made for mental health professionals, primarily because their expertise is limited on most issues and their unrestricted testimony tends to obscure the moral and social nature of the questions being asked." We do not think the case for an exception can be made. Particularly when the defendant determines whether expert testimony by mental health professionals will be introduced—typically the case in the reconstructive inquiries of the criminal law—the opinions of qualified witnesses within their sphere of specialized knowledge should be freely admitted.

A defendant's past psychological functioning cannot be reconstructed with scientific precision. The truth will remain very much in the shadows whether or not mental health professionals are permitted to offer their opinions. In formulating an evidentiary test, then, we should begin by comparing the knowledge of mental health professionals not with the knowledge of physicists about the laws of motion, but with that of laymen about psychological aberration and criminal behavior. We should ask whether the observations, intuitions, and hypotheses of clinicians offer a useful and acceptable supplement to those of Everyman.

Morse insists that inferences concerning the nature, extent, and consequences of mental dysfunction are within the range of lay experience and common sense. To some extent this is correct; the factfinder is competent to draw such inferences in the absence of expert testimony, and need not yield to such testimony even when undisputed.[118] Moreover, lay witnesses sometimes may express opinions on a defendant's mental condition. Nevertheless, we stress the incremental nature of the modern test: we must ask whether "specialized knowledge will assist the trier of fact," not whether the fact finder can manage when left to his own devices.

* * *

[In the responsibility assessment] setting the "factual" inquiry concerns the relationship, if any, between a defendant's aberrational psychological functioning and his behavior. We agree that categorizing the strength of that relationship, and evaluating it according to some externally derived moral gradient, is the responsibility of the judge or jury and not an appropriate subject for expert opinion. Professor Morse's exclusionary approach to expert testimony, however, also would preclude an expert from expressing any opinion regarding why a relationship may or may not exist between the defendant's psychological functioning and his criminal behavior. We think this would unnec-

118. It is generally accepted that an opinion of an expert, even if uncontradicted, need not be accepted by the jury as long as there is some evidence to support a contrary conclusion. This same concept has also been expressed as a requirement that a "jury may not arbitrarily disregard expert testimony. . . ." Of course, in ju-risdictions where the government bears the burden of proving the defendant's "sanity" beyond a reasonable doubt, a jury cannot find the defendant sane, even if they find the defendant's expert unbelievable, unless the government has presented some evidence from which sanity can be inferred.

essarily deprive the factfinder of helpful insights and would unfairly hamper the defendant's effort to present a case-in-exculpation or -mitigation.

Morse refers to the famous *Gorshen* case to illustrate his rationale. Gorshen shot his supervisor after a fight at work. A psychiatric witness testified that Gorshen was a chronic paranoid schizophrenic who for twenty years had experienced trances accompanied by auditory and visual hallucinations. He claimed to see and hear devils in disguise committing abnormal sexual acts, sometimes upon Gorshen himself. These experiences had intensified during the months before the crime.

On the day of the shooting, Gorshen had been drinking at work. His supervisor told him to go home, and a fight ensued. He then went home, obtained a pistol, returned, and shot the victim. According to the psychiatrist, Gorshen said, "All I was thinking about all of this time is to shoot O'Leary. I forgot about my family, I forgot about God's laws and human's laws and everything else. The only thing was to get that guy, get that guy, get that guy, like a hammer in the head."

The expert witness explained that during the period of the offense Gorshen was driven by an obsessive murderous rage aroused by the stress of the beating and by what he perceived as challenges to his manhood. Psychologically, this rage reflected a desperate attempt to ward off imminent and total disintegration of his personality:

> The strength of the obsession is proportioned not to the reality of danger but to the danger of the insanity. . . . [F]or this man to go insane means to be permanently in the world of these visions and under the influence of the devil. . . . [A]n individual in this state of crisis will do anything to avoid the threatened insanity. . . .

Professor Morse questions the highly speculative quality of this formulation, pointing out that no "hard data" support the hypothesis "that the killing was the inexorable or nearly inexorable result of threatened ego-disintegration," and that probably very few persons with such fears kill, although there are no data available. Of course, both of these points could have been made very effectively by skillful cross-examination. Skillful redirect examination in response might have brought out the psychodynamic concepts from which this formulation was derived, perhaps with descriptions from the clinical literature of the characteristics of violent behavior committed by individuals with comparable paranoid thought patterns.

Morse characterizes the *Gorshen* expert's testimony as "really a moral guess and not a scientific fact." Although explanatory clinical formulations by careful forensic specialists are hardly "scientific facts," they do represent something more than idiosyncratic "guesses." Such witnesses offer "informed speculation," essentially in the following form:

> I cannot assure you that this is what happened, and I cannot measure for you the impact that these intrapsychic variables had on the

defendant's behavior under the circumstances which existed at the time of the offense. Nonetheless, based on our operating theories of psychology, which we employ in our everyday clinical practice, and on my own study of the relevant literature concerning this type of psychological functioning and this type of criminal behavior, I think the following explanation(s) are possible (or probable).

These explanatory formulations can assist the factfinder, who must speculate in any event, by identifying "clinically reasonable" possibilities that otherwise may not occur to him. Appropriately instructed, the jury will know that these explanations are only possibilities and will not be misled.[192]

* * *

[Indeed] in the context of the reconstructive inquiries of the criminal law, the risk that a jury will give undue weight to such an expert opinion, notwithstanding any cautionary instructions, has been grossly exaggerated. If only the defense has offered psychiatric testimony, the natural skepticism of the jurors, and the corrective value of cross-examination, virtually eliminate the risk that the jury will abdicate its factfinding function to the experts. If each side has its own witness, expert "dominance" is not the problem, and the risk of confusion can be minimized by adequate preparation by counsel and by ordinary judicial supervision. In short, we see little disadvantage in admitting appropriately restricted opinion testimony by qualified mental health professionals.

Most important, the wholesale exclusion of such testimony would unduly restrict the defendant's opportunity to present relevant evidence in his defense, and would enhance the natural advantage enjoyed by the prosecution on reconstructive issues. In particular, a defendant's opportunity to carry his de facto burden of proving that he did not perceive, believe, expect, or intend what a normal person would have under the same circumstances—and that he therefore lacked the mens rea required for the offense—is undermined by rules which altogether exclude qualified opinion testimony or which allow such testimony only if the expert finds that the defendant's abnormal functioning was attributable to a mental disease or defect. Similarly, a defendant's opportunity to offer a plausible explanation for his behavior—and thereby to establish a meaningful case in exculpation or mitigation under the applicable responsibility doctrines—would be restricted severely and unjustifiably by rules that exclude explanatory formulations by qualified mental health professionals.

* * *

192. The *Gorshen* trial judge stated that "up till the time that [the defense expert] testified in this case, there was no explanation of why this crime was commit- ted. . . . [He is] the first person that has any reasonable explanation. Whether it's correct or not, I don't know."

Questions and Comments

1. *Levels of inference.* To make clearer the nature of the debate between Morse on the one hand and Bonnie & Slobogin on the other it might be helpful to conceptualize expert testimony as consisting of ascending levels of inference. For instance, in an insanity case, the progressive levels of inference might be as follows:

1. application of meaning (perception) to a behavioral image (e.g., "he was wringing his hands.")

2. perception of general mental state (e.g., "he appeared anxious.")

3. "formulation" of the perception of general mental state to fit into theoretical constructs or the research literature and/or to synthesize observations (e.g., "his anxiety during the interview was consistent with a general obsession with pleasing others.")

4. diagnosis (e.g., "his behavior on interview and reported history are consistent with a generalized anxiety disorder.")

5. relationship of formulation or diagnosis to legally relevant behavior (e.g., "at the time of the offense, his anxiety was so overwhelming that he failed to reflect upon the consequences of his behavior.")

6. elements of the ultimate legal issue (e.g., "although he was too anxious at the time of the offense to reflect upon the consequences of his behavior, he was aware of the wrongfulness of his acts.")

7. ultimate legal issue (e.g., "he was sane at the time of the offense.") [f]

At what level of testimony would Morse permit mental health professionals to testify? Bonnie & Slobogin? If you were a judge deciding the admissibility of clinical testimony on the responsibility issue in the *Gorshen* case, up to which level would you allow? If you instead relied on one of the screening rules discussed previously?

2. *The importance of context.* Bonnie & Slobogin refrain from taking a position on the admissibility of clinical opinion testimony outside the "reconstructive" setting assessing mental state at the time of the offense. What are the differences between this setting and other settings in which clinical opinion testimony might be offered? In particular, what are the differences between the reconstructive context and the predictive one, to be discussed below?

C. PROPENSITY

Predictions of behavior are required in many different legal settings. Most relevant to this book are the sentencing and commitment contexts, where predictions relevant to dangerousness and treatability are often called for. The following case addresses admissibility issues in the context where such predictions have their greatest impact: death penalty proceedings.

---

f. This example is adapted from G. Melton, J. Petrila, N. Poythress, C. Slobogin, Psychological Evaluations for the Courts 13–14 (Guilford Press, 1987).

BAREFOOT v. ESTELLE

Supreme Court of United States, 1983.
463 U.S. 880, 103 S.Ct. 3383, 77 L.Ed.2d 1090.

*   *   *

JUSTICE WHITE delivered the opinion of the Court.

*   *   *

On November 14, 1978, petitioner was convicted of the capital murder of a police officer in Bell County, Tex. A separate sentencing hearing before the same jury was then held to determine whether the death penalty should be imposed. Under Tex.Code Crim.Proc.Ann., Art. § 37.071 (Vernon 1981), two special questions were to be submitted to the jury: whether the conduct causing death was "committed deliberately and with reasonable expectation that the death of the deceased or another would result"; and whether "there is a probability that the defendant would commit criminal acts of violence that would constitute a continuing threat to society." The State introduced into evidence petitioner's prior convictions and his reputation for lawlessness. The State also called two psychiatrists, John Holbrook and James Grigson, who, in response to hypothetical questions, testified that petitioner would probably commit further acts of violence and represent a continuing threat to society. The jury answered both of the questions put to them in the affirmative, a result which required the imposition of the death penalty.

On appeal to the Texas Court of Criminal Appeals, petitioner urged, among other submissions, that the use of psychiatrists at the punishment hearing to make predictions about petitioner's future conduct was unconstitutional because psychiatrists, individually and as a class, are not competent to predict future dangerousness. Hence, their predictions are so likely to produce erroneous sentences that their use violated the Eighth and Fourteenth Amendments.

*   *   *

The suggestion that no psychiatrist's testimony may be presented with respect to a defendant's future dangerousness is somewhat like asking us to disinvent the wheel. In the first place, it is contrary to our cases. If the likelihood of a defendant's committing further crimes is a constitutionally acceptable criterion for imposing the death penalty, which it is, *Jurek v. Texas,* 428 U.S. 262, 96 S.Ct. 2950, 49 L.Ed.2d 929 (1976), and if it is not impossible for even a lay person sensibly to arrive at that conclusion, it makes little sense, if any, to submit that psychiatrists, out of the entire universe of persons who might have an opinion on the issue, would know so little about the subject that they should not be permitted to testify. In *Jurek,* seven Justices rejected the claim that it was impossible to predict future behavior and that dangerousness was therefore an invalid consideration in imposing the death penalty.

*   *   *

Although there was only lay testimony with respect to dangerousness in *Jurek,* there was no suggestion by the Court that the testimony of doctors would be inadmissible. To the contrary, the joint opinion announcing the judgment said that the jury should be presented with all of the relevant information.

* * *

Acceptance of petitioner's position that expert testimony about future dangerousness is far too unreliable to be admissible would immediately call into question those other contexts in which predictions of future behavior are constantly made. For example, in *O'Connor v. Donaldson,* 422 U.S. 563, 576, 95 S.Ct. 2486, 2494, 45 L.Ed. 2d 396 (1975), we held that a nondangerous mental hospital patient could not be held in confinement against his will. Later, speaking about the requirements for civil commitments, we said:

> "There may be factual issues in a commitment proceeding, but the factual aspects represent only the beginning of the inquiry. Whether the individual is mentally ill and dangerous to either himself or others and is in need of confined therapy turns on the *meaning* of the facts which must be interpreted by expert psychiatrists and psychologists." *Addington v. Texas,* 441 U.S. 418, 429, 99 S.Ct. 1804, 1811, 60 L.Ed.2d 323 (1979).

In the second place, the rules of evidence generally extant at the federal and state levels anticipate that relevant, unprivileged evidence should be admitted and its weight left to the factfinder, who would have the benefit of cross-examination and contrary evidence by the opposing party. Psychiatric testimony predicting dangerousness may be countered not only as erroneous in a particular case but also as generally so unreliable that it should be ignored. If the jury may make up its mind about future dangerousness unaided by psychiatric testimony, jurors should not be barred from hearing the views of the State's psychiatrists along with opposing views of the defendant's doctors.[5]

Third, petitioner's view mirrors the position expressed in the *amicus* brief of the American Psychiatric Association (APA).

* * *

[H]owever, [w]e are [not] convinced . . . that the view of the APA should be converted into a constitutional rule barring an entire category of expert testimony. We are not persuaded that such testimony is almost entirely unreliable and that the factfinder and the adversary system will not be competent to uncover, recognize, and take due account of its shortcomings.

The *amicus* does not suggest that there are not other views held by members of the Association or of the profession generally. Indeed, as

5. In this case, no evidence was offered by petitioner at trial to contradict the testimony of Doctors Holbrook and Grigson. Nor is there a contention that, despite petitioner's claim of indigence, the court refused to provide an expert for petitioner. In cases of indigency, Texas law provides for the payment of $500 for "expenses incurred for purposes of investigation and expert testimony." Tex.Code Crim.Proc. Ann., Art. 26.05, § 1(d) (Vernon Supp. 1982).

this case and others indicate, there are those doctors who are quite willing to testify at the sentencing hearing, who think, and will say, that they know what they are talking about, and who expressly disagree with the Association's point of view.[7] Furthermore, their qualifications as experts are regularly accepted by the courts. If they are so obviously wrong and should be discredited, there should be no insuperable problem in doing so by calling members of the Association who are of that view and who confidently assert that opinion in their *amicus* brief. Neither petitioner nor the Association suggests that psychiatrists are always wrong with respect to future dangerousness, only most of the time. Yet the submission is that this category of testimony should be excised entirely from all trials. We are unconvinced, however, at least as of now, that the adversary process cannot be trusted to sort out the reliable from the unreliable evidence and opinion about future dangerousness, particularly when the convicted felon has the opportunity to present his own side of the case.

* * *

JUSTICE BLACKMUN, with whom JUSTICE BRENNAN and JUSTICE MARSHALL join as to Parts I–IV, dissenting. . . . The Court holds that psychiatric testimony about a defendant's future dangerousness is admissible, despite the fact that such testimony is wrong two times out of three. The Court reaches this result—even in a capital case—because, it is said, the testimony is subject to cross-examination and impeachment. In the present state of psychiatric knowledge, this is too much for me. One may accept this in a routine lawsuit for money damages, but when a person's life is at stake—no matter how heinous his offense—a requirement of greater reliability should prevail. In a capital case, the specious testimony of a psychiatrist, colored in the eyes

---

7. At trial, Dr. Holbrook testified without contradiction that a psychiatrist could predict the future dangerousness of an individual, if given enough background information about the individual. Dr. Grigson obviously held a similar view. At the District Court hearing on the habeas petition, the State called two expert witnesses, Dr. George Parker, a psychologist, and Dr. Richard Koons, a psychiatrist. Both of these doctors agreed that accurate predictions of future dangerousness can be made if enough information is provided; furthermore, they both deemed it highly likely that an individual fitting the characteristics of the one in the Barefoot hypothetical would commit future acts of violence.

* * *

We are aware that many mental health professionals have questioned the usefulness of psychiatric predictions of future dangerousness in light of studies indicating that such predictions are often inaccurate.

. . . Dr. John Monahan, upon whom one of the State's experts relied as "the leading thinker on this issue," concluded that "the 'best' clinical research currently in existence indicates that *psychiatrists and psychologists are accurate in no more than one out of three predictions of violent behavior over a several-year period among institutionalized populations that had both committed violence in the past . . . and who were diagnosed as mentally ill.*" J. Monahan, The Clinical Prediction of Violent Behavior 47–49 (1981) (emphasis in original).

* * *

All of these professional doubts about the usefulness of psychiatric predictions can be called to the attention of the jury. Petitioner's entire argument, as well as that of Justice Blackmun's dissent, is founded on the premise that a jury will not be able to separate the wheat from the chaff. We do not share in this low evaluation of the adversary process.

of an impressionable jury by the inevitable untouchability of a medical specialist's words, equates with death itself.

I

At the sentencing hearing, the State established that Barefoot had two prior convictions for drug offenses and two prior convictions for unlawful possession of firearms. None of these convictions involved acts of violence. At the guilt stage of the trial, for the limited purpose of establishing that the crime was committed in order to evade police custody, the State had presented evidence that Barefoot had escaped from jail in New Mexico where he was being held on charges of statutory rape and unlawful restraint of a minor child with intent to commit sexual penetration against the child's will. The prosecution also called several character witnesses at the sentencing hearing, from towns in five States. Without mentioning particular examples of Barefoot's conduct, these witnesses testified that Barefoot's reputation for being a peaceable and lawabiding citizen was bad in their respective communities.

Last, the prosecution called Doctors Holbrook and Grigson, whose testimony extended over more than half the hearing. Neither had examined Barefoot or requested the opportunity to examine him. In the presence of the jury, and over defense counsel's objection, each was qualified as an expert psychiatrist witness. Doctor Holbrook detailed at length his training and experience as a psychiatrist, which included a position as chief of psychiatric services at the Texas Department of Corrections. He explained that he had previously performed many "criminal evaluations," and that he subsequently took the post at the Department of Corrections to observe the subjects of these evaluations so that he could "be certain those opinions that [he] had were accurate at the time of trial and pretrial." He then informed the jury that it was "within [his] *capacity as a doctor of psychiatry* to predict the future dangerousness of an individual within a *reasonable medical certainty*," (emphasis supplied), and that he could give "*an expert medical opinion* that would be *within reasonable psychiatric certainty* as to whether or not that individual would be dangerous to the degree that there would be a probability that that person would commit criminal acts of violence in the future that would constitute a continuing threat to society," (emphasis supplied).

Doctor Grigson also detailed his training and medical experience, which, he said, included examination of "between thirty and forty thousand individuals," including 8,000 charged with felonies, and at least 300 charged with murder. He testified that with enough information he would be able to "give *a medical opinion within reasonable psychiatric certainty* as to the psychological or psychiatric makeup of an individual," (emphasis supplied), and that this skill was "particular to the field of psychiatry and not to the average layman."

Each psychiatrist then was given an extended hypothetical question asking him to assume as true about Barefoot the four prior convictions for nonviolent offenses, the bad reputation for being law-abiding in various communities, the New Mexico escape, the events surrounding the murder for which he was on trial and, in Doctor Grigson's case, the New Mexico arrest. On the basis of the hypothetical question, Doctor Holbrook diagnosed Barefoot "within a reasonable psychiatr[ic] certainty," as a "criminal sociopath." He testified that he knew of no treatment that could change this condition, and that the condition would not change for the better but "may become accelerated" in the next few years. Finally, Doctor Holbrook testified that, "within reasonable psychiatric certainty," there was "a probability that the Thomas A. Barefoot in that hypothetical will commit criminal acts of violence in the future that would constitute a continuing threat to society," and that his opinion would not change if the "society" at issue was that within Texas prisons rather than society outside prison.

Doctor Grigson then testified that, on the basis of the hypothetical question, he could diagnose Barefoot "within reasonable psychiatric certainty" as an individual with "a fairly classical, typical, sociopathic personality disorder." He placed Barefoot in the "most severe category" of sociopaths (on a scale of one to ten, Barefoot was "above ten"), and stated that there was no known cure for the condition. Finally, Doctor Grigson testified that whether Barefoot was in society at large or in a prison society there was a *"one hundred percent and absolute"* chance that Barefoot would commit future acts of criminal violence that would constitute a continuing threat to society. (emphasis supplied).

On cross-examination, defense counsel questioned the psychiatrists about studies demonstrating that psychiatrists' predictions of future dangerousness are inherently unreliable. Doctor Holbrook indicated his familiarity with many of these studies but stated that he disagreed with their conclusions. Doctor Grigson stated that he was not familiar with most of these studies, and that their conclusions were accepted by only a "small minority group" of psychiatrists—"[i]t's not the American Psychiatric Association that believes that."

After an hour of deliberation, the jury answered "yes" to the two statutory questions, and Thomas Barefoot was sentenced to death.

II

* * *

The American Psychiatric Association (APA), participating in this case as *amicus curiae*, informs us that "[t]he unreliability of psychiatric predictions of long-term future dangerousness is by now an established fact within the profession." The APA's best estimate is that *two out of three* predictions of long-term future violence made by psychiatrists are wrong. The Court does not dispute this proposition, and indeed it could not do so; the evidence is overwhelming.

* * *

Neither the Court nor the State of Texas has cited a single reputable scientific source contradicting the unanimous conclusion of professionals in this field that psychiatric predictions of long-term future violence are wrong more often than they are right.[2]

The APA also concludes, as do researchers that have studied the issue, that psychiatrists simply have no expertise in predicting long-term future dangerousness. A layman with access to relevant statistics can do at least as well and possibly better; psychiatric training is not relevant to the factors that validly can be employed to make such predictions, and psychiatrists consistently err on the side of overpredicting violence. Thus, while Doctors Grigson and Holbrook were presented by the State and by self-proclamation as experts at predicting future dangerousness, the scientific literature makes crystal clear that they had no expertise whatever. Despite their claims that they were able to predict Barefoot's future behavior "within reasonable psychiatric certainty," or to a "one hundred percent and absolute" certainty, there was in fact no more than a one in three chance that they were correct.

* * *

III

A

Despite its recognition that the testimony at issue was probably wrong and certainly prejudicial, the Court holds this testimony admissible because the Court is "unconvinced . . . that the adversary process cannot be trusted to sort out the reliable from the unreliable evidence and opinion about future dangerousness." One can only wonder how juries are to separate valid from invalid expert opinions when the "experts" themselves are so obviously unable to do so. Indeed, the evidence suggests that juries are not effective at assessing the validity of scientific evidence. Giannelli, Scientific Evidence, 80 Colum.L.Rev., [1197], 1239–1240, and n. 319 (1980).

There can be no question that psychiatric predictions of future violence will have an undue effect on the ultimate verdict. Even judges tend to accept psychiatrists' recommendations about a defendant's

2. Among the many other studies reaching this conclusion are APA Task Force Report, Clinical Aspects of the Violent Individual 28 (1974) (90% error rate "[u]nfortunately . . . is the state of the art") (APA, Clinical Aspects); Steadman & Morrissey, The Statistical Prediction of Violent Behavior, 5 Law & Human Behavior 263, 271–273 (1981); Dix, Expert Prediction Testimony in Capital Sentencing: Evidentiary and Constitutional Considerations, 19 Am.Crim.L.Rev. 1, 16 (1981); Schwitzgebel, Prediction of Dangerousness and Its Implications for Treatment, in W. Curran, A. McGarry, & C. Petty, Modern Legal Medicine, Psychiatry, and Forensic Science 783, 784–786 (1980); Cocozza & Steadman, Prediction in Psychiatry: An Example of Misplaced Confidence in Experts, 25 Soc.Probs. 265, 272–273 (1978); Report of the (American Psychological Association's) Task Force on the Role of Psychology in the Criminal Justice System, 33 Am.Psychologist 1099, 1110 (1978); Steadman & Cocozza, Psychiatry, Dangerousness and the Repetitively Violent Offender, 69 J.Crim.L. & Criminology 226, 227, 230 (1978); Cocozza & Steadman, The Failure of Psychiatric Predictions of Dangerousness: Clear and Convincing Evidence, 29 Rutgers L.Rev. 1084, 1101 (1976); Diamond, The Psychiatric Prediction of Dangerousness, 123 U.Pa.L.Rev. 439, 451–452 (1974); Ennis & Litwack Psychiatry and the Presumption of Expertise: Flipping Coins in the Courtroom, 62 Calif.L. Rev. 693, 711–716 (1974). A relatively early study making this point is Rome, Identification of the Dangerous Offender, 42 F.R.D. 185 (1968).

dangerousness with little regard for cross-examination or other testimo- ny. Cocozza & Steadman, *supra* n. 2, 25 Soc.Probs., at 271 (in making involuntary commitment decisions, psychiatric predictions of future dangerousness accepted in 86.7% of cases). There is every reason to believe that inexperienced jurors will be still less capable of "separat[ing] the wheat from the chaff," despite the Court's blithe assumption to the contrary. The American Bar Association has warned repeatedly that sentencing juries are particularly incapable of dealing with information relating to "the likelihood that the defendant will commit other crimes," and similar predictive judgments. Relying on the ABA's conclusion, the joint opinion announcing the judgment in *Gregg v. Georgia,* 428 U.S., at 192, 96 S.Ct., at 2934, recognized that "[s]ince the members of a jury will have had little, if any, previous experience in sentencing, they are unlikely to be skilled in dealing with the information they are given." But the Court in this case, in its haste to praise the jury's ability to find the truth, apparently forgets this well-known and worrisome shortcoming.

As if to suggest that petitioner's position that unreliable expert testimony should be excluded is unheard of in the law, the Court relies on the proposition that the rules of evidence generally "anticipate that relevant, unprivileged evidence should be admitted and its weight left to the factfinder, who would have the benefit of cross-examination and contrary evidence by the opposing party." But the Court simply ignores hornbook law that, despite the availability of cross-examination and rebuttal witnesses, "opinion evidence is not admissible if the court believes that the state of the pertinent art or scientific knowledge does not permit a reasonable opinion to be asserted." Because it is feared that the jury will overestimate its probative value, polygraph evidence, for example, almost invariably is excluded from trials despite the fact that, at a conservative estimate, an experienced polygraph examiner can detect truth or deception correctly about 80 to 90 percent of the time. Ennis & Litwack, *supra* n. 2, at 736. In no area is purportedly "expert" testimony admitted for the jury's consideration where it cannot be demonstrated that it is correct more often than not. "It is inconceivable that a judgment could be considered an 'expert' judgment when it is less accurate than the flip of a coin." *Id.,* at 737. The risk that a jury will be incapable of separating "scientific" myth from reality is deemed unacceptably high.

B

The Constitution's mandate of reliability, with the stakes at life or death, precludes reliance on cross-examination and the opportunity to present rebuttal witnesses as an antidote for this distortion of the truth-finding process. Cross-examination is unlikely to reveal the fatuousness of psychiatric predictions because such predictions often rest, as was the case here, on psychiatric categories and intuitive clinical judgments not susceptible to cross-examination and rebuttal. Psychiatric categories have little or no demonstrated relationship to violence, and their use often obscures the unimpressive statistical or intuitive bases for prediction. The APA particularly condemns the use of the diagnosis employed by Doctors Grigson and Holbrook in this case, that of sociopathy:

> "In this area confusion reigns. The psychiatrist who is not careful can mislead the judge or jury into believing that a person has a major mental disease simply on the basis of a description of prior criminal behavior. Or a psychiatrist can mislead the court into believing that an individual is devoid of conscience on the basis of a description of criminal acts alone. . . . The profession of psychiatry has a responsibility to avoid inflicting this confusion upon the courts and to spare the defendant the harm that may result. . . . Given our uncertainty about the implications of the finding, the diagnosis of sociopathy . . . should not be used to justify or to support predictions of future conduct. There is no certainty in this area." Draft Report 30.

It is extremely unlikely that the adversary process will cut through the facade of superior knowledge. The Chief Justice long ago observed:

> "The very nature of the adversary system . . . complicates the use of scientific opinion evidence, particularly in the field of psychiatry. This system of partisan contention, of attack and counterattack, at its best is not ideally suited to developing an accurate portrait or profile of the human personality, especially in the area of abnormal behavior. Although under ideal conditions the adversary system can develop for a jury most of the necessary fact material for an adequate decision, such conditions are rarely achieved in the courtrooms in this country. These ideal conditions would include a highly skilled and experienced trial judge and highly skilled lawyers on both sides of the case, all of whom in addition to being well-trained in the law and in the techniques of advocacy would be sophisticated in matters of medicine, psychiatry, and psychology. It is far too rare that all three of the legal actors in the cast meet these standards." Burger, Psychiatrists, Lawyers, and the Courts, 28 Fed.Prob. 3, 6 (June 1964).

* * *

Nor is the presentation of psychiatric witnesses on behalf of the defense likely to remove the prejudicial taint of misleading testimony by prosecution psychiatrists. No reputable expert would be able to predict with confidence that the defendant will *not* be violent; at best, the witness will be able to give his opinion that all predictions of dangerousness are unreliable. Consequently, the jury will not be presented with the traditional battle of experts with opposing views on the ultimate question. Given a choice between an expert who says that he can predict with certainty that the defendant, whether confined in prison or free in society, will kill again, and an expert who says merely that no such prediction can be made, members of the jury charged by law with making the prediction surely will be tempted to opt for the expert who claims he can help them in performing their duty, and who predicts dire consequences if the defendant is not put to death.[13]

Moreover, even at best, the presentation of defense psychiatrists will convert the death sentence hearing into a battle of experts, with the Eighth Amendment's well-established requirement of individually focused sentencing a certain loser. The jury's attention inevitably will turn from an assessment of the propriety of sentencing to death the defendant before it to resolving a scientific dispute about the capabilities of psychiatrists to predict future violence. In such an atmosphere, there is every reason to believe that the jury may be distracted from its constitutional responsibility to consider "particularized mitigating factors," in passing on the defendant's future dangerousness.

*   *   *

IV

*   *   *

The Court . . . errs in suggesting that the exclusion of psychiatrists' predictions of future dangerousness would be contrary to the logic of *Jurek*. *Jurek* merely upheld Texas' substantive decision to condition the death sentence upon proof of a probability that the defendant will commit criminal acts of violence in the future. Whether the evidence offered by the prosecution to prove that probability is so unreliable as to violate a capital defendant's rights to due process is an entirely different matter, one raising only questions of fair procedure.

*   *   *

It makes sense to exclude psychiatric predictions of future violence while admitting lay testimony, because psychiatric predictions appear to come from trained mental health professionals, who purport to have special expertise. In view of the total scientific groundlessness of these predictions, psychiatric testimony is fatally misleading. Lay testimony, frankly based on statistical factors with demonstrated correlations to violent behavior, would not raise this substantial threat of unreliable and capricious sentencing decisions, inimical to the constitutional standards established in our cases; and such predictions are as accurate as any a psychiatrist could make.

*   *   *

---

13. "Although jurors may treat mitigating psychiatric evidence with skepticism, they may credit psychiatric evidence demonstrating aggravation. Especially when jurors' sensibilities are offended by a crime, they may seize upon evidence of dangerousness to justify an enhanced sentence." Dix, *supra* n. 2, at 43, n. 215. Thus, the danger of jury deference to expert opinions is particularly acute in death penalty cases. Expert testimony of this sort may permit juries to avoid the difficult and emotionally draining personal decisions concerning rational and just punishment. *Id.*, at 46. Doctor Grigson himself has noted both the superfluousness and the misleading effect of his testimony:

" 'I think you could do away with the psychiatrist in these cases. Just take any man off the street, show him what the guy's done, and most of these things are so clearcut he would say the same things I do. But I think the jurors feel a little better when a psychiatrist says it—somebody that's supposed to know more than they know.' " Bloom, Killers and Shrinks, Texas Monthly 64, 68 (July 1978) (quoting Doctor Grigson).

Questions and Comments

1. *Evidentiary analysis.* In arriving at their conclusions, both the majority and the dissent in *Barefoot* seem to structure their analysis primarily around the federal rules of evidence. The central arguments are over whether the jury will be able to "separate the wheat from the chaff" and whether psychiatrists can add anything to what the jury could figure out for itself. Dix, on the other hand, suggests applying the *Frye* rule in this context and concludes that, under this analysis, clinical prediction testimony should generally be excluded. Dix, "Expert Prediction Testimony in Capital Sentencing: Evidentiary and Constitutional Considerations," 19 Am Crim.L.Rev. 1, 19–21 (1981).

2. *Prediction testimony in other settings.* Many commentators have argued that clinical prediction testimony should be barred not just from capital sentencing proceedings but from other proceedings as well. See sources cited in note 2 of Blackmun's opinion in *Barefoot.* Even before *Barefoot,* however, the courts had been reticent about adopting such a position in capital cases, much less in other types of cases. See *People v. Murtishaw,* 29 Cal.3d 733, 767–75, 175 Cal.Rptr. 738, 758–63, 631 P.2d 446, 466–71 (1981). One court did prohibit clinical prediction testimony in civil commitment proceedings. *In re Wilson,* 33 Crim.L.Rep. (BNA) 2115 (D.C. Super.Ct. Apr. 14, 1983). But it stood alone and now, presumably, is nullified by *Barefoot.*

The majority in *Barefoot* states that a different holding "would immediately call into question those other contexts in which predictions of future behavior are constantly made." Does it make sense to say, as Justice Blackmun seems to be saying in his dissent, that clinical prediction testimony is too inaccurate for capital proceedings but is permissible in other proceedings, such as civil commitments? Within a particular setting (e.g., capital sentencing), does it make sense to bar clinical prediction testimony, but allow clinical testimony on normality and responsibility issues (which also are relevant at capital sentencing [g])?

3. *The accuracy of dangerousness assessments.* The Court quotes Monahan to the effect that, at best, clinical predictions of dangerousness are accurate no more than one out of three times. This conclusion is widely accepted. But it needs to be looked at more closely from at least three different perspectives.

(a) New Research. Much of the literature on predictive capacity focuses on the "false positive" rate, that is, the rate at which a positive finding of dangerousness is falsely or erroneously made. This terminology is used to emphasize the percentage of people who may be wrongfully sentenced to death or confined if decisions are based on dangerousness predictions. Putting Monahan's summary of the research in these terms, the "best" false positive rate obtained by clinical prediction studies has been around

---

g. For instance, the Model Penal Code's capital sentencing statute specifies as a mitigating circumstance the fact that, at the time of the murder, "the capacity of the defendant to appreciate the criminality [wrongfulness] of his conduct or to conform his conduct to the requirements of law was impaired as a result of mental disease or defect or intoxication." § 210.6(3)(g).

66%. Some studies have found false positive rates as high as 92%. See Wenk & Emrich, "Assaultive Youth: An Exploratory Study of the Assaultive Experience and Assaultive Potential of California Youth Authority Wards," 9 J. Res. Crime & Delinq. 171 (1972).

Recent research, relying on more sophisticated predictive models, has obtained better results. A Canadian study reported a false positive rate of 44%. Sepejak, Menzies, Webster & Jensen, "Clinical Predictions of Dangerousness: Two–Year Follow-up of 408 Pre–Trial Forensic Cases," 11 Bull. Am. Acad. Psychiat. & L. 171 (1983). Another study reported a 40% false positive rate. Klassen & O'Connor, "A Prospective Study of Predictors of Violence in Adult Male Mental Patients," 12 Law and Human Behavior 143 (1988). Whether such improved results can be replicated on a routine basis has not been shown.

(b) Methodological Problems. To some extent, the high false positive findings may be attributable to factors other than poor predictive capabilities. Most of the research relies on police or hospital records to determine whether a person predicted to be violent subsequently was so. But such records notoriously underreport the amount of violent acts committed, some suggest by a factor of ten. Meehl, The Insanity Defense, Minn. Psychol. 11, 15 (Summer, 1983). Thus, a number of the supposed "false positives" may simply be undiscovered "true positives" (i.e., individuals correctly predicted to be dangerous). As Monahan has suggested, it is possible that those who were arrested committed many of the unreported and unsolved crimes; if this is true, then the false positive rates may not be as grossly overstated as Meehl claims. Monahan, The Clinical Prediction of Violent Behavior 52–56 (NIMH 1981). But a recent study suggests that even taking this factor into account "more than one-quarter of the 'false positives' may not, in fact, be false positives if self reports are a valid measure of violence." Klassen & O'Connor, "Predicting Violence in Mental Patients: Cross–Validation of an Actuarial Scale," paper presented at the Annual Meeting of the American Public Health Association (1987).

A second methodological problem is that, with some of the studies, it is not clear that a prediction of dangerousness was even made. The most famous prediction research is the "Baxstrom study", which reported on the assaultive history of ex-prisoners after they were released or transferred to civil hospitals as a result of the Supreme Court's decision in *Baxstrom v. Herold,* 383 U.S. 107, 86 S.Ct. 760, 15 L.Ed.2d 620 (1966) (holding invalid New York's practice of transferring prisoners whose terms had expired to maximum security facilities for the "criminally insane"). In arriving at their 80% false positive rate, the researchers in this study assumed that the continued retention of the prisoners in the maximum security hospital (before the *Baxstrom* decision resulted in their release) was based on a specific determination of dangerousness. In fact no written evidence of such a determination existed; in other words, the continued detention of at least some of the *Baxstrom* patients may have been due to administrative inertia rather than clinical judgment. Allen, Book Review, 73 Mich.L.Rev. 1517, 1526 (1975).

A final methodological problem with the research literature on dangerousness results from the fact that, for obvious reasons, most of the studies cannot be based on "natural experiments" of the type involved in *Baxstrom*. That is, the *usual* response to a prediction of dangerousness, if one occurs, is to institutionalize, not release, the person thought to be violence-prone. Thus the clinical prediction that someone will be dangerous *in the community* is tested by reference to whether the person considered dangerous is assaultive *in the institution*. Because institutionalization and treatment may seriously curb the individual's assaultive behavior, the false positive rates reported in studies which use institutional violence as a criterion for violence may be significantly exaggerated. See Dix, "Clinical Evaluation of the "Dangerousness" of "Normal" Criminal Defendants," 66 Va.L.Rev. 523, 544 n. 82 (1980).

Because of these methodological problems, some have suggested that predictions of violence may meet the "clear and convincing" level of proof, at least when based on either a recent history of repeated violence, a more distant history of violence together with proof that the personality traits and attitudes that led to the past violence still exist, or unequivocal threats of serious intentions to commit violence. Litwack & Schlesinger, "Assessing and Predicting Violence: Research, Law, and Applications," in Weiner & Hess, eds., Handbook of Forensic Psychology 205, 224 (1987).

(c) Base Rates. Assuming psychiatric predictions of dangerousness are at best correct only one out of three times, Justice Blackmun claims that such predictions yield results that are less accurate than flipping a coin. The coin flipping analogy, first made by Ennis and Litwak in "Psychiatry and the Presumption of Expertise: Flipping Coins in the Courtroom," 62 Calif.L.Rev. 693 (1974), is seriously misleading to the extent it suggests that clinical predictions are no better than "chance." To discover why this is so, one must first determine the "base rate" for violent behavior among the population being evaluated for dangerousness. For instance, say that the base rate for violence in the general population is roughly one out of 300, meaning that only one person out of every 300 in the general population will commit a violent act in their lifetime. If a psychiatrist could predict accurately one-third of the time who was dangerous in the general population, his or her predictions would be much better than chance, specifically *100 times* better than a random selection from amongst the population. The populations involved in the research to which Monahan refers were usually institutionalized patients or criminals and tended to have a much higher base rate for violence than the general population, in the vicinity of one out of nine, rather than one out of 300. But a predictive accuracy ratio of one out of three for such a population would still be three times better than chance. This predictive ratio would be worse than chance only for a population with a base rate for violence higher than one out of three. Thus, the coin-flipping analogy would appear to be inapt. See Slobogin, "Dangerousness and Expertise," 133 Pa.L.Rev. 97, 110–14 (1984).

4. *Diagnosis and dangerousness.* Relevant both to predictive accuracy and to whether mental health professionals possess "specialized knowledge" about violence-proneness is the extent to which certain diagnoses can be viewed as indicative of dangerousness. The state's psychiatrists in

Barefoot diagnosed Barefoot as a "sociopath." The predecessor to this diagnosis was "psychopathy"; the analogous diagnosis in DSM–III–R is antisocial personality disorder (see 344–346). The general thrust of all three diagnoses is repeated antisocial behavior, accompanied by a lack of remorse or shame; no delusions are present. Forensic clinicians have often correlated this diagnosis with dangerousness. For instance, Dr. Grigson, who has testified for the state of Texas in scores of death penalty sentencing proceedings (and, as a result, has been dubbed 'Dr. Death' by the media [h]), usually couples his prediction that the defendant will be violent with a diagnosis of sociopathy.

There is some research supporting such a correlation. See, e.g., Vaillant, "Crime and Mental Illness in a Group of Psychopathic Personalities, 9 Med. Sci & L. 11 (1969) (psychopaths committed 23 times as many offenses as controls); Martin, Cloninger & Guze, "Female Criminality and the Prediction of Recidivism," 35 Arch. Gen. Psychiat. 207 (1978). Others have suggested that the diagnosis has no predictive power independent of that provided by the number and types of past antisocial acts committed by the individual labelled a sociopath. Gibbens, Pond, Stafford–Clark, "A Follow-up Study of Criminal Psychopaths," 105 J. Mental Sci. 108 (1969); Dix, supra, at 573. But more recent reports confirm that the psychopathy/sociopathy/antisocial diagnosis is highly correlated with violence proneness. Hare & McPherson, "Violent and Aggressive Behavior by Criminal Psychopaths," 7 Int'l J. Law & Psychiat. 35 (1984).

The evidence concerning the usefulness of other diagnoses in determining dangerousness is also mixed. As a group, mentally ill persons do not appear to be any more violent than non-mentally ill persons who have comparable histories of violent behavior. Monahan, supra, at 79–82. Even when the mentally ill are broken down into subcategories, little discrimination is possible. For instance, of seven recent studies comparing the violence proneness of those who are diagnosed paranoid schizophrenic and those with other diagnoses, four reported paranoid schizophrenics to have higher rates of violence, two reported them to have lower rates of violence, and one reported no differences. Krakowski, Volovka, & Brizer, "Violence and Psychopathology: A Longitudinal Study," 29 Comp. Psychiat. 131 (1986).

Finally, it should be noted that, diagnosis aside, theories about aggressive behavior exist which might have predictive value. For instance, Monahan has suggested that the literature concerning how people cope with stress may be relevant here. An evaluator could look at how an individual "appraises" situations (e.g., as provocative or accidental), what the person's typical expectations are in such situations (e.g., how one thinks one should act when a friend is assaulted), the type and intensity of the person's emotional reactions to stress (e.g., anger and hatred, or guilt, empathy, anxiety, and fear), and the manner in which the individual typically chooses to cope with stressful events (e.g., violence or withdrawal and avoidance). Monahan, supra at 109–112. To date, however, there is little research testing the predictive accuracy of such theories. See

h. See Time, June 1, 1981, at 64.

Novaco, Anger as a Clinical and Social Problem, in R. Blanchard and D. Blanchard (eds.), Advances in the Study of Aggression 1 (New York, 1986).

5. *Alternatives to clinical prediction testimony.* In his dissent in *Barefoot,* Justice Blackmun contends that "[l]ay testimony, frankly based on statistical factors with demonstrated correlations to violent behavior" could competently fill the gap created by prohibiting psychiatric testimony on dangerousness. This suggestion may have its own set of evidentiary problems, depending upon how it is implemented.

For instance, one factor which clearly has some predictive power with respect to future behavior is past behavior. Monahan, supra at 106. Perhaps, if this were the *only* type of propensity evidence allowed, no experts would be required. Where predictions are called for, evidence about relevant past behavior (e.g., past assaultive or self-harming acts, past treatment failures) could be provided by lay people (or mental health professionals acting as "fact" witnesses). But even within this relatively simple framework, fairness concerns might dictate that additional information be provided. Those individuals with histories of antisocial behavior— in other words, every person subjected to a sentencing proceeding and most persons subjected to commitment—might want to combat the inference of dangerousness thereby raised with statistical information showing the precise correlation between past and future behavior. (For example, the relevant statistics might show that of those individuals with one conviction for a crime against the person, only 1 out of 5 commit another such crime). If so, it may be that an expert (although not necessarily a mental health professional) would be needed to explain the methodology of the research and its results. See *State v. Davis,* 96 N.J. 611, 477 A.2d 308 (1984).

Moreover, there are many other factors besides past antisocial behavior which are "statistically correlated" with future behavior. For instance, research indicates that age, sex, race, IQ, socioeconomic and employment status, opiate and alcohol abuse, and marital status may be related to violence-proneness. Monahan, supra at 75–77. Both the state and the individual might want to introduce evidence about these factors, again probably requiring experts. An expert would also be needed to assist with or caution about combining statistical probabilities. For instance, the fact that an 18 year-old male has (let's assume) a 1 in 10 chance of committing an antisocial act, an opiate user a 2 out of 10 chance, and an exconvict a 2 out of 10 chance does not necessarily mean an 18 year-old drug user with one conviction has a 5 in 10 chance of committing another crime. Monahan, supra at 76.[i]

Other problems with statistical, or "demographic", prediction are explored in the excerpt below. Although the focus is on sentencing, many of the points are relevant to commitment as well.

---

i. Monahan and Walker suggest that at least some statistical information could be relayed via jury instructions. Monahan & Walker, "Social Frameworks: A New Use of Social Science in Law," 73 Va.L.Rev. 559, 592–98 (1987).

DANIEL GOODMAN, DEMOGRAPHIC EVIDENCE IN CAPITAL SENTENCING

39 Stanford L.Rev. 499, 508–27.
(1987).

* * *

OBJECTIONS TO THE USE OF DEMOGRAPHIC EVIDENCE

Demographic or actuarial evidence may be inappropriate for a variety of reasons. Some types of demographic evidence may be excludable on equal protection grounds. But the range of demographic evidence that is infirm on this basis is circumscribed by judicial interpretation limiting protection to suspect classes. A much wider range of demographic evidence may be inappropriate for policy reasons that are not overtly constitutional.

A.   Equal Protection Issues

The strongest basis for excluding demographic evidence would be that such evidence violates the equal protection clause of the fourteenth amendment—that the use of race-based or sex-based evidence, to use the clearest examples, is an impermissible discrimination against members of certain disadvantaged groups.

* * *

Nevertheless, there are difficulties with the constitutional attack. Not every rule that affects different racial groups differently violates the equal protection clause. With increasing clarity since the 1940s, the modern Court has refused to invalidate practices that are "de facto" discriminatory absent a showing of purposeful discrimination. The Court's 1976 decision in *Washington v. Davis* announced the Court's position regarding racially disproportionate impacts, holding constitutional a qualifying test for applicants to the Washington, D.C., police force that proportionately more blacks than whites failed. In finding the test racially neutral under the fourteenth amendment, the Court declared that its equal protection decisions "have not embraced the proposition that a law or other official act, without regard to whether it reflects a racially discriminatory purpose, is unconstitutional *solely* because it has a racially disproportionate impact." The requirement of *purposeful*, rather than simply "de facto," discrimination has been a constant theme in the Court's equal protection jurisprudence ever since.

* * *

However, [demographic] evidence . . . may be unconstitutional regardless of whether discriminatory intent lies behind its use, [if] it employ[s] an explicit racial categorization in determining the probable recidivism of members of various groups. Such overt racial classifications have been deemed "suspect" and subject to "the most rigid scrutiny" since the Court's decision in *Korematsu v. United States.* The Court subsequently has stated that strict scrutiny invalidates all racial categorizations not necessary to, or in an alternative phrasing, not narrowly tailored to, furthering a compelling state interest.

Thus, the strict scrutiny standard requires not only a "compelling" end but also a close "fit" between the objective and the means used to obtain it. In constitutional analysis, the requirement of narrowly tailored means, while less important in the area of economics and social welfare, becomes particularly acute in the area of criminal law. Although the predictive accuracy of demographic evidence is relevant to a determination of whether the means (allowing the use of the evidence) are "closely tailored" to the end, the question of whether these classifications are "necessary" to that end goes beyond the narrower inquiry of "fit." Even if such predictions are relatively accurate, they may not be "necessary" to jury deliberations. And if they are not necessary in the sense of being indispensable, the admission of the evidence becomes especially questionable in capital cases.

Moving from race to other types of categorizations, the equal protection scrutiny becomes less rigorous, the justification for concern less compelling. One notch below race are those categorizations termed "semi-suspect," which trigger heightened—but not strict—scrutiny. Heightened scrutiny has, over the years, been brought to bear to a greater or lesser degree on classifications based on gender, alienage, and illegitimacy. Of these, the Court has regarded gender-based classifications as the most appropriate area for intermediate-level scrutiny. The Court announced the standard of review for gender-based classifications in *Craig v. Boren:* "To withstand constitutional challenge, . . . classifications by gender must serve important governmental objectives and must be substantially related to achievement of those objectives."

Below the semi-suspect classes in the equal protection hierarchy are an infinite number of ways of dividing up the world. Some of these classifications involve characteristics that may aptly be called volitional; others involve classifications that are more properly termed nonvolitional. The definition of these two categories is necessarily inexact. Volitionality is more a spectrum than a rigid polarity. But it appears reasonably clear that there are some characteristics that are completely involuntary in the sense that they are unchosen by the individual, although it is considerably less clear, or less widely accepted, that there are characteristics that are completely voluntary or volitional. Our judgment of volitionality is partly a function of the degree to which we are willing to accept (or alternatively, to ignore) determinist arguments. But even for the "soft" determinist, some characteristics are more freely chosen than others.

Although classifications on the basis of nonvolitional or immutable traits (e.g., circumstances of birth) probably implicate equal protection concerns, classifications based on volitional characteristics (for example, past crimes) seem, under constitutional doctrine, to require no more than "rationality review." Even under rationality review, however, certain classifications may be so insupportable, or so unrelated to the ends sought, that the classification may be struck down.

A final concern in the equal protection area is the use of illegitimate surrogates, or "proxies," that closely track racial or other impermissible lines. These may be mere surrogates for race, or they may be factors that are "independent" in some sense, yet strongly predictive of future criminality. The problem, however, is that the latter category will also produce results that are similar to those arrived at using race. Given that race may indeed show a strong correlation with recidivism, and that disproportionate racial impacts do not automatically invalidate a classificatory scheme, disentangling permissible factors from impermissible factors may be extremely difficult. Indeed, whether a proxy or surrogate is legitimate is partly a statistical question but primarily a philosophical one, revolving around an inexact judgment about how closely a proxy may replicate the results produced using an illegitimate factor, and where the boundaries of equal protection are to be set. The crucial inquiry probably involves the motives of government officials, which may be impossible to ascertain. While proxies avoid the problem of the explicit use of race, they potentially avoid none of the invidious effects of racial classifications.

B. "Subconstitutional" Policy Issues

The equal protection attack on the use of demographic evidence is inherently limited. * * * [A] much wider range of demographic evidence may be infirm for a variety of policy reasons that are not of constitutional dimension.

1. Justice-by-the-numbers.

The use of social science statistics in judicial proceedings has always been a legitimate source of concern. Although certain types of statistical evidence are useful, probative, and objective, other types of calculation, offered as proof or as prediction, may threaten the equitable administration of justice. Statistical and probabilistic methods of proving guilt are fraught with pitfalls for the uninitiated, who may be unable to detect statistical sleight of hand or fail to realize that statistical generalizations are often inappropriate in individual cases. In many instances, such generalizations can offer only marginal assistance to a deliberating jury.

* * *

Predictive evidence based on recidivism rates is particularly susceptible to statistical ambiguity, such that some empirical conclusions drawn from this kind of evidence may be meaningless to a just and rational system of punishment. Recidivism rates can be determined for countless groups, and the focus need not be simply on physical characteristics but may include psychiatric profiles and a multitude of personal traits or life experiences. These categories range along a slippery continuum from the purely volitional to the purely nonvolitional. One author has suggested that where predictive techniques ignore the autonomy of the individual and rely instead on fixed factors over which the defendant has no control, they run counter to basic traditions of criminal law that stress free will and self-determination. The notion is a venerable one: that criminal guilt is predicated only upon actions over which the defendant exercised some control.

* * *

2. Status versus conduct.

The decisions of the Supreme Court and lower courts make it clear that individuals may be punished for conduct but not for "status." Thus, in 1962 the Supreme Court invalidated a California law making it a criminal offense for a person to "be addicted to the use of narcotics," holding that the state could not legitimately punish a person for a "status"—a mere condition not involving any action or "conduct."

* * *

It is a fundamental orthodoxy of our criminal justice system that the punishment should fit the crime and the individual, not the statistical history of the class of persons to which the defendant belongs. To allow a criminal defendant's sentence to be determined to any degree by his unchosen membership in a given race or class denies the very premise of self-determination upon which our criminal justice system is built. It raises the threat that defendants will be sentenced not on the basis of their personal merit or conduct, but on the basis of their "status."

3. Generalization versus individuation.

A procedure that allows judgments about an individual's blameworthiness to be based on statistical correlations to anonymous prior malefactors is deeply inconsistent with the general principles undergirding our system of law. There is no principle in our jurisprudence that supports the idea that a person might deserve more serious punishment because he is black, or less serious punishment because he is white. Judgments based on classifications that are less patently offensive may also threaten the notion that punishment is tied to individual blameworthiness. The requirement of individualized sentencing becomes particularly important where capital sentences are involved.

* * *

If this requirement is to be taken seriously, all admissible evidence must comport with it. Likewise, the ability to rebut a piece of evidence does not render it somehow more individualized. One observer has aptly noted that a "'battle of actuarial tables' is no substitute for personalized accounts."

4. Demographic versus psychiatric evidence.

The claim that demographic evidence violates the requirements of individualized sentencing inevitably raises the question of whether statistical evidence of this sort can be distinguished from psychiatric evidence, which the Supreme Court deemed admissible in *Barefoot v. Estelle*.

* * *

This note does not purport to judge the correctness of the Supreme Court's general conclusion in *Barefoot* that psychiatric evidence is sufficiently reliable to be admissible in court. Rather, given the judgment of the Court in that decision, it seeks an accommodation between, or a consistent rationale for, the rejection of demographic evidence and the continued admissibility of psychiatric evidence.

* * *

The key to the difference between these techniques . . . is the extent to which the defendant is able to rebut the inference that he will behave in the predicted manner. In clinical examination, an individual defendant can demonstrate his nonconformity to a statistical stereotype; in the courtroom, he cannot rebut the fact of his membership in a statistical class, but only, at best, the inference to be drawn from it. Actuarial evidence is not inherently or necessarily unfair, but in the judicial context it may disregard both the uniqueness and the autonomy of individuals. As an instrument of judicial decisionmaking, such evidence is in a very palpable way substantially less "relevant" to an individual's circumstances than is clinical psychiatric evidence. Unlike demographic studies, psychiatric evaluations are—at least in some sense—mediated through the individual. Clinical and statistical methods differ because "[a] clinical decisionmaker is not committed in advance of decision to the factors that will be considered and the rule for combining them. He is free to respond to individual differences whose relevance was not anticipated by any rule." Since the clinical approach recognizes the individuality of each defendant, it permits the psychiatrist or psychologist to alter in a particular case the general judgment of actuarial reckoning.

* * *

Demographic evidence, like purely statistical psychiatric evidence, presents a range of scores that indicates what behavior is typical for a member of a particular group. But it is impossible to say, simply on the basis of that evidence, where any particular *individual* will fall. The problem with demographic evidence in the courtroom setting is that it is of low probative value but highly susceptible to abuse. This problem of a *potentially misleading statistical probability curve* characterizes demographic evidence, as well as purely statistical psychiatric evidence.

The fact that all assessments are to some extent relational—that is, implicitly relative or based upon some unstated empirical assumptions—does not obviate the distinction between judicial methods that focus on the individual and those that are avowedly abstract or generic. And where those generic methods rely on statistics, their potential to mislead the jury outweighs their usefulness.

* * *

Questions and Comments

1. *Admissible statistical factors.* Actuarial devices are commonly used in some settings. For instance, the state of Michigan has developed such a device for use in making parole release decisions. It identifies as "very high" or "high" risk 40% of the prisoners who engage in post-release assaultive behavior (i.e., a 60% false positive rate), relying entirely on factors having to do with past antisocial conduct. However, in order to discriminate between prisoners who present a "low risk" and those who present a "very low" risk, the Michigan prediction table also allows consideration of marital status. In light of the arguments made by Goodman, should consideration of this factor be permissible if being unmarried resulted in greater confinement? Would it be permissible to include race as a factor on the table if it were shown that doing so would reduce the false positive rate for the very high and high risk categories to 10%? Employment opportunities? A diagnosis of antisocial personality?

2. *Comparing clinical and statistical evidence.* As the data on the Michigan prediction table indicate, actuarial devices developed to predict dangerousness generally have no more predictive accuracy than do mental health professionals. See Cocozza & Steadman, "Some Refinements in the Measurement and Prediction of Dangerous Behavior," 131 Am.J.Psychiat. 1012 (1974) (66% false positive rate for long-term predictions, using four variables); Convit, et al., "Predicting Assaultiveness in Psychiatric Inpatients: A Pilot Study," 39 Hosp.Comm.Psychiat. 429 (1988) (63% false positive rate using actuarial techniques).

However, the *probabilities* obtained by statistical information, as opposed to clinical assessment, are relatively accurate; for example, the probability of violent behavior associated with being a white male opiate user can be fairly reliably ascertained. Goodman asserts, nonetheless, that such statistical evidence lacks relevance because it is not "individualized", and is prejudicial because it is difficult to rebut and might mislead the factfinder; that is, in attempting to rebut statistical evidence that a white male opiate user with one conviction for violent crime has, say, a one in five chance of committing a violent act within the next five years, such a person might find it very difficult to convince the jury that other personal characteristics he possesses place him in the group of white male opiate users who will not commit another violent act within that time period.

How is clinical prediction testimony different? As the author admits, mental health professionals often rely on "unstated empirical assumptions" about relationships between certain traits (e.g., race, sex and opiate use) and certain behavior (e.g., violent behavior). If these assumptions are "unstated," how is it easier for the individual to rebut them?[j] Is the point that before arriving at a conclusion the clinician will observe all aspects of the individual and thus arrive at a fairer, less "stereotyped" assessment than would a jury hearing only demographic evidence and any rebuttal

---

j. Note that in *Barefoot,* Justice Blackmun concluded that psychiatric prediction testimony is difficult to rebut "because such predictions often rest . . . on psychiatric categories and intuitive clinical judgments . . .; their use often obscures the unimpressive statistical or intuitive bases for prediction."

information the individual cares to present? To what extent do you think this is the case, given what has been discussed about the reasons for variance in clinical assessments?

Would it be best to prohibit *both* clinical and statistical prediction evidence, permit both, or rely on only one type of evidence? If the latter, which one?

3. *Hypothetical questions.* In *Barefoot*, it will be remembered, both Dr. Grigson and Dr. Holbrook (the prosecution's witnesses) testified in answer to "hypothetical" questions. They did not interview Barefoot but rather were given information about his prior record and other aspects of his character and asked to formulate an opinion on that basis. Barefoot argued that use of hypotheticals is unconstitutional, both generally (because they allow testimony not based on personal examination), and in his particular case (because they allowed testimony that was based on controverted facts). The Court rejected these arguments, noting that hypothetical questions have long been in use and that, if the defendant was concerned about the accuracy of their assumptions in his particular case, he could have constructed his own questions using a different version of the facts. How is testimony based on a hypothetical question different from testimony based on statistical evidence? Should the same rule, whether it be admission or exclusion, be adopted for both?

4. *Substantive concerns.* Clearly, predicting future behavior is not easy, no matter which route is taken. Yet, as the majority in *Barefoot* noted, the Court has upheld the use of dangerousness as an aggravating factor in capital cases. Jurek v. Texas, 428 U.S. 262, 96 S.Ct. 2950, 49 L.Ed. 2d 929 (1976). Should *Jurek* be overturned? Should dangerousness be a criterion in *any* type of legal proceeding? Would it be consistent to jettison dangerousness as a justification for legal intervention, but not abnormality or incompetency? We will revisit these questions in subsequent chapters.

D. COMPETENCY

The "competency paradigm" permeates the law. One must be "competent" to stand trial, plead guilty or make a valid confession. If one is not "competent", a guardian may be appointed to manage one's affairs, treatment may be administered involuntarily, or one's will may be declared void. Mental health professionals are often called upon to help decide competency issues because it is usually assumed that mental disorder "causes" most, if not all, incompetency; indeed, many statutes require a finding that the incompetency results from mental disorder.

According to Grisso, legal competencies share a common structure consisting of several elements. First, the inquiry is always directed toward functional abilities, which refers to the "mental tasks" an individual can accomplish, and the specific knowledge, understanding or beliefs that may be necessary to perform them. For instance, with respect to competency to stand trial, an individual must be able to assist his or her attorney in preparing for and litigating the case, as well as have some capacity to understand the trial process and the charges. Second, legal competency constructs require causal inferences to explain an individual's functional abilities or deficits. For example, as noted above, many competency statutes require that the functional deficiency be "a result of" mental disorder or developmental disability. Third, each competency contemplates assessing the impact of a general environmental context to which a person must respond (such as criminal proceedings, police interrogations or hospitals). Fourth, legal competencies also require assessing *specific* interactive capacities in the person's particular situation. Thus, two defendants may be equally capable, in a general sense, of assisting their attorneys and understanding the charges, but if one is facing a much more complex charge than the other, he may be found incompetent while the other may be found competent. Finally, legal competency constructs require a judgment that "person-context incongruency is of a sufficient magnitude to warrant a finding of legal incompetency and its dispositional consequences." That is, a judgment must be made as to whether—in light of the person's functional deficiencies and their causes, and the way these will interact with the general environment and the particular demands of the person's situation—a specific disposition, such as hospitalization or deprivation of property, should occur. Grisso, Evaluating Competencies: Forensic Assessments and Instruments 14–28 (1986).

The evidentiary question is whether mental health professionals possess specialized knowledge that can assist the factfinder in answering any or all of the different types of questions raised by the competency issue. This subsection will focus on the mental health profession's expertise with respect to competency to stand trial, because of the relatively greater amount of legal and empirical material on the subject. Again, the commonly accepted legal test in this context consists of two prongs: (1) whether the person is able to assist the attorney in his or her defense; and (2) whether the person understands the nature of the charges and the trial process. In reading the sample competency to stand trial report below, taken from an actual case file,[k] consider the extent to which it helps answer these two questions in functional, causal, contextual, interactive and judgment/dispositional terms.

COMPETENCY REPORT

This [27 year old] patient was admitted on eight different occasions to the Broughton Hospital, Morgantown, North Carolina. His first hospitalization was on 28 March 1961 and he was discharged from the last, the eighth hospitalization, on 7 June 1969. His hospital records indicate that during the first few hospitalizations at Broughton it was felt that his main problem was a personality disorder, which was manifested primarily in anti-social behavior and excessive drinking.

k. This sample report is presented and analyzed in R. Roesch and S. Golding, "Competency to Stand Trial" 83–85 (1980).

During the last few hospitalizations at Broughton, however, it has become apparent that this patient is suffering of schizophrenia, he displayed bizarre behavior and ideations and obviously the patient was delusional.   The patient received a variety of different psychiatric treatments, his hospital course was rather unpredictable and also he has escaped a number of different occasions.

The personal past history indicates that he was born in 1942 in Shelby, North Carolina. This patient was reared mostly by his grand-parents and there is very little known about his birth and early development. It should be noted that his grandmother and two mater-nal uncles have been in Broughton Hospital as patients. Apparently he developed properly and at the usual age began school. He stopped his education at age 18 and was in the eleventh grade. It is stated that he has stopped his education on account of earning some money. Shortly after his school he entered the United States Air Force and remained in service for approximately six months. The reason for the separation was his emotional inability to adjust to service life. This patient is described while he was in high school as a fairly well adjusted individual who showed considerable interest in reading. From the age of 16 he began to drink, at times excessively. He has shown very little interest in the opposite sex and never married. Following his short service in the United States Air Force in 1960 this patient began to show disinterest in his environment and was reluctant to assume responsibilities. In 1961 he was hospitalized the first time in Brought-on. From here on until the present date this patient has been in and out of the hospital and obviously has shown evidence of a mental disturbance.

On admission the patient appeared to be alert but his affect[1] was rather fixed and at times inappropriate. He was well oriented in time, place and person.[m] He became somewhat confused and tense when he was asked about the circumstances under which he entered this Hospi-tal. He freely admitted to paranoid ideations and pedophilia. Obvi-ously the patient was very preoccupied and there was evidence of dissociation[n] of his thoughts. His hospital course was rather unevent-ful. On the ward the patient has presented no particular difficulties in his management. It is noted, that he is somewhat neglecting in his appearance and shows little interest in his environment. Generally speaking this patient appears to be tense and the psychomotor activity is somewhat increased.

During the consequent [sic] interviews the patient has expressed a great deal of his delusional system. It appears, that this patient firmly believes about his abilities to determine some individuals' future by looking in the sun. With an inappropriate affect the patient stated,

l. Emotional demeanor [eds.]

m. This is standard psychiatric jargon (oriented times three) suggesting a basic awareness of surroundings. [eds.]

n. Usually means distancing oneself from an idea, situation, or object. Not clear what it means here. [eds.]

that 'you wouldn't understand' just what those signs mean, neverthe-less he does and therefore he is a different individual from us.

He gave a rather coherent and detailed account of the incidence [sic] leading to his present charges. The patient stated, that he cannot resist to these impulses although he realizes the wrongness of such. During the interview the patient has become several times confused and irrelevant. He appears to be of above average intelligence and from that standpoint he is fully aware of his present legal situation.

The physical examination on admission revealed a well developed and nourished white male with a scar on the left knee, and otherwise the findings were essentially within normal limits. The laboratory findings were within normal, including a nonreactive VDRL.° The skull x-ray revealed a little irregularity at the outer side of the left antral sinus and this might possibly be the result of an old fracture. Otherwise the bony structure was normal and all other findings of the skull x-ray were normal. The chest x-ray was normal. The electroen-cephalogram was normal.

The psychological testing revealed a full-scale I.Q. of 98, which places this patient in the average intellectual functioning level.

Diagnosis: Schizophrenic Reaction, Chronic, Undifferentiated Type. APA Code: 295–90.

Recommendations: The examination and observations reveals that this patient is subject to a mental disturbance constituting insanity. This condition is manifested primarily in delusional thinking and inability to reason or to exercise proper judgment. This patient is fully aware of the wrongness of his alleged act, however, due to his mental disturbance he was unable to adhere to right and because of his disorganized thinking he is unable to assist in his own defense. He should continue hospitalization for a minimum necessary period of time as provided in G.S. 122–91 and 122–65 as being incompetent to stand trial at this time.

Questions and Comments

1. *The setting for competency determinations.* Adversarial hearings on competency to stand trial are rare. In many jurisdictions, the court making the competency determination usually relies entirely on a report or reports submitted by mental health professionals. Studies show that judges abide by the recommendations in such reports over 90% of the time. Petrila, "The Insanity Defense and Other Mental Health Dispositions in Missouri," 5 Int'l J.L.Psychiat. 81 (1982); R. Roesch & S. Golding, Compe-tency to Stand Trial 193 (1980) (35% of judges in North Carolina never disagree with hospital recommendations about competency; other 65% rarely or occasionally disagree). Should reports like the one above be admissible under these conditions? Are there sufficient facts about the defendant's mental state to aid the court in making a decision? How much

o. A test for syphilis. [eds.]

of the report is irrelevant and/or prejudicial? Is the report internally consistent?

2. *Diagnosis and competency.* Like the author of the report, many mental health professionals apparently equate psychosis (e.g., schizophrenia) with incompetency to stand trial. McGarry, "Competency for Trial and Due Process Via the State Hospital, 122 Am.J.Psychiat. 623 (1965) (100% correlation between psychosis and incompetency finding). But many courts have held that someone who is mentally ill might well be able to meet the relatively undemanding requirements of the competency standard; that is, they might be able to exhibit an understanding of the legal process and a capacity to recount relevant facts and the names of witnesses despite mental disability. See, e.g., *Swisher v. United States,* 237 F.Supp. 921 (W.D.Mo.1965). Based on what you can glean from the above report, do you agree? In any event, is the diagnostic information relevant to the competency issue?

3. *Competency protocols.* In an effort to assist the mental health professional in avoiding the pitfalls illustrated by the above report, a number of structured interview formats have been developed. The Competency Assessment Instrument (CAI), for instance, requires the evaluator to assess competency by looking at 13 different functions (e.g., "appraisal of available legal defenses", "capacity to testify relevantly"), and then producing a rating from 1 ("total incapacity") to 5 ("no incapacity"). Laboratory of Community Psychiatry, Competency to Stand Trial and Mental Illness 98–125 (1974). The Interdisciplinary Fitness Interview (IFI) requires the evaluator to rate on a scale of 0 through 2 (with 2 representing "substantial incapacity") the person's capacity with respect to five "legal items" (e.g., "capacity to appreciate the nature of the alleged crime, and to disclose pertinent facts, events and motives"; "quality of relationship with one's current attorney") and eleven "psycho-pathological items" (e.g., "delusional processes", "disturbances of memory/amnesia"); the evaluator must also rate on a 0–2 scale the weight given each particular dimension in the opinion formation process. Golding, Roesch, & Schreiber, "Assessment and Conceptualization of Competency to Stand Trial: Preliminary Data on the Interdisciplinary Fitness Interview," 8 Law & Hum.Behav. 321 (1984). Neither the CAI or the IFI equate a certain numerical score with a finding of competency; the numbers are merely meant to serve as a guide. In contrast, the Competency Screening Test (CST) consists of 22 sentence stems which the defendant is to complete (e.g., "When I go to court the lawyer will . . ."; When they say a man is innocent until proven guilty, I . . .") and the evaluator is to grade on a scale of 0–2 (with 2 being a "competent" answer). A score of 19 or below is supposed to indicate that the person requires further, more in-depth evaluation. A score of 20 or above means the person is competent. This device was developed specifically for use by laypeople as a device for screening out those who are clearly competent. Laboratory of Community Psychiatry, supra at 67. Are such devices a good way of improving competency evaluations and reports?

4. *Assistance to the factfinder.* Several studies have found that inter-rater agreement on competency to stand trial is quite high, usually over

90%. If mental health professionals are equating psychosis with incompetency, as recounted in note 2, this percentage may merely reflect the ability of clinicians to agree when someone is severely mentally ill. But even when clinicians understand and apply the specific competency criteria, reliability is very high, whether or not a structured interview format is used. Golding, Roesch, and Schreiber, supra 188–191 (97% agreement using IFI); Poythress & Stock, "Competency to Stand Trial: A Historical Review and Some New Data," 8 J.Psychiat.L. 131 (1980) (100% agreement between raters using unstructured interview). Thus, competency to stand trial determinations may be much more valid, or accurate, than normality, responsibility or propensity assessments.

Yet, it also appears that laypersons who have received a minimal amount of training can produce reliable conclusions on the competency issue, at least when using a structured interview format. Roesch & Golding, supra at 188–191 (90% agreement between trained laypersons and hospital evaluators using IFI). Moreover, Roesch & Golding state that "it appears that ward observations, psychological tests, and other data collected during hospitalization have little influence on the [competency to stand trial] determination." Roesch & Golding, supra at 190. What would be the Morsian argument in the competency to stand trial context? Who should be allowed to write competency reports and testify at competency hearings, and under what limitations?

III. IMPLEMENTATION ISSUES

Despite the arguments for eliminating or limiting expert testimony from mental health professionals, courts continue to permit such testimony on normality, responsibility, propensity and competency issues. This section addresses several topics related to how this testimony should be presented: which types of mental health professionals should be qualified to offer clinical opinions, when the state is required to provide the defendant/subject with such experts, when the state can obtain its own evaluation of the defendant/subject, what types of third party information experts may rely upon in forming their opinions, and the extent to which these opinions may embrace "ultimate" legal issues.

A. WHO IS AN EXPERT?

Federal Rule 702 defines an expert as one who is qualified to speak on a given issue "by knowledge, skill, experience, training or education." Arguably, any mental health professional—whether a psychiatrist, psychologist, social worker or psychiatric nurse—could possess specialized knowledge, skill, experience, training and education related to mental disorder and its consequences. But the courts have been cautious about opening the door to non-psychiatrists, as the following case illustrates.

JENKINS v. UNITED STATES

307 F.2d 637.

United States Court of Appeals, District of Columbia Circuit, 1962.

* * *

[W]e [will now] discuss . . . the [trial] court's instruction to the jury to disregard testimony of the three defense psychologists that appellant had a mental disease when he committed the crimes charged.

* * *

The first psychologist, Dr. Tirnauer, administered a battery of tests to appellant, studied his case history, and concluded he had been suffering from schizophrenia when he committed the crimes. In his opinion, the disease and the crimes were "related." The second psychologist, Dr. Margaret Ives, had reviewed Dr. Tirnauer's test results, had seen appellant at a staff conference, and had administered part of a Szondi profile test. She stated that appellant was suffering from schizophrenia and that his crimes were the product of the disease. The third psychologist, Dr. Levy, interpreted test results obtained by members of the District General staff in October 1959, and administered two additional tests shortly before trial. He testified that defendant had been suffering from schizophrenia on June 10, 1959, but could give no opinion concerning the relationship between the illness and the crimes. At the conclusion of the trial the court instructed the jury:

> "A psychologist is not competent to give a medical opinion as to a mental disease or defect. Therefore, you will not consider any evidence to the effect that the defendant was suffering from a mental disease or a mental defect on June 10, 1959, according to the testimony given by the psychologists."

The trial court apparently excluded these opinions because psychologists lack medical training. We agree with the weight of authority, however, that some psychologists are qualified to render expert testimony in the field of mental disorder.

* * *

The test . . . is whether the opinion offered will be likely to aid the trier in the search for truth. . . . Thus, non-medical witnesses who have had experience in electrical work may testify to the effects of electrical shock upon the human body. Optometrists, whose training includes instruction in the symptoms of certain eye diseases, may testify to the presence of a cataract discovered in the course of fitting glasses, and to the effect of a scar upon vision. A toxicologist has been permitted to testify to the effect of oxalic acid, a poison, upon the human eye. The kinds of witnesses whose opinions courts have received, *even though they lacked medical training and would not be permitted by law to treat the conditions they described,* are legion. The principle to be distilled from the cases is plain: if experience or training enables a proffered expert witness to form an opinion which would aid the jury, in the absence of some countervailing consideration, his testimony will be received.

* * *

[T]he Ph.D. in Clinical Psychology involves some—and often much—training and experience in the diagnosis and treatment of mental disorders. Typically, candidates are trained, *inter alia,* in general psychology, theory of personality and psychodynamics, psychopathology, diagnostic methods, therapeutic techniques, selected aspects of physiology and anatomy, and clinical methods. A one-year internship in a mental hospital is required for this degree. After graduation, many clinical psychologists administer and interpret diagnostic tests which elicit the patient's intellectual level, defenses, personality structure, attitudes, feelings, thought and perceptual processes. In many institutions and clinics their reports, which regularly include opinions concerning the presence or absence of mental disease or defect, are important aids to psychiatrists who customarily have the final responsibility for diagnosis. Some psychologists, moreover, regularly administer psychotherapy and related non-organic therapies in the treatment of certain types of mental disorders.

The determination of a psychologist's competence to render an expert opinion based on his findings as to the presence or absence of mental disease or defect must depend upon the nature and extent of his knowledge. It does not depend upon his claim to the title "psychologist." And that determination, after hearing, must be left in each case to the traditional discretion of the trial court subject to appellate review. Although there are no statutory criteria for licensing psychologists in the District of Columbia to assist trial courts, the American Psychological Association's list of approved graduate training programs provides some guidance. When completion of such training is followed by actual experience in the treatment and diagnosis of disease in association with psychiatrists or neurologists, the opinion of the psychologist may properly be received in evidence. We need not decide whether the three psychologists who testified for the defense at the trial under review were qualified to offer expert opinions since they may not be called to testify at the retrial. We hold only that the lack of a medical degree, and the lesser degree of responsibility for patient care which mental hospitals usually assign to psychologists, are not automatic disqualifications. Where relevant, these matters may be shown to affect the weight of their testimony, even though it be admitted in evidence. The critical factor in respect to admissibility is the actual experience of the witness and the probable probative value of his opinion. The trial judge should make a finding in respect to the individual qualifications of each challenged expert. Qualifications to express an opinion on a given topic are to be decided by the judge alone. The weight to be given any expert opinion admitted in evidence by the judge is exclusively for the jury. They should be so instructed.

* * *

BURGER, CIRCUIT JUDGE (concurring).

I concur in the remand because the court's basic holding that a psychologist is not barred as a matter of law from giving expert testimony about mental diseases makes it essential that we have a comprehensive record before us on the education and training of psychologists in general and clinical psychologists in particular.

* * *

At the outset certain factors should be kept in mind. The issue is not now and never was whether a psychologist's testimony is admissible in litigation where "sanity" is in issue. Such testimony has long been admissible in the form of psychological tests and the analysis and explanation of such tests by a psychologist. No one doubts that such matter is admissible. The real issue in dispute is whether the clinical psychologists in this case, by which we mean persons having degrees of Doctor of Philosophy in Psychology, and also additional training as clinical psychologists, are competent in a scientific sense and hence legally qualified

(1) to make a diagnosis of the existence and character of a mental disease, and

(2) whether there is a causal relationship between a disease and an unlawful act.

The issue can be stated also in terms of whether *medical* opinions and *medical* diagnoses can be made by and be the subject of expert testimony by a Doctor of Philosophy in Psychology with added clinical experience. For convenience I will hereafter refer to such a psychologist as a Clinical Psychologist.

While the issue is new to this court it is not new to medicine and psychiatry. In 1954 a Resolution was adopted by the American Medical Association, the Council of the American Psychiatric Association and the Executive Council of the American Psychoanalytical Association to the effect that psychologists and other related professional groups were autonomous and independent in matters where *medical* questions were *not* involved, but that where *diagnosis* and *treatment* of mental illness was involved the participation of psychologists "must be co-ordinated under medical responsibility." This Resolution, while not controlling on the courts is plainly entitled to great weight.

* * *

The cases cited by the majority concerning the optometrist, the toxicologist and other skilled specialists who are not medical doctors are not in any real sense relevant. Indeed they tend to divert us from the central issue. Of course an optometrist or the toxicologist is permitted to give *some* expert testimony within his competence just as a skilled shoemaker might be qualified to testify from long observation and experience as to the effect of wearing certain kinds of shoes, or a farrier to give expert testimony about the effect of certain types of shoeing on horses.

The heart of our problem is not whether a clinical psychologist is qualified to testify as an expert, for of course he is in some areas, but whether he is qualified to give expert testimony in the form of a diagnosis of a mental disease or illness, and to express an opinion on whether a stated mental disease "caused" the patient to commit a given unlawful act or "produced" that act. More rationally the question ought to be whether mental disease so substantially affected him that he was unable to control his conduct.

I agree with the majority that the scope of the training of the psychologist is of critical importance and that many factors other than academic degrees go to the admissibility and weight of the expert testimony. For example, if a general medical practitioner testified on the subject of mental disease, and gave a diagnosis of presence or absence of mental illness in opposition to a trained psychiatrist it would obviously be proper for the trial judge to tell the jury they could take into account the differences in training and experience in weighing the testimony of the one against the other. In the same way it would be proper, if a clinical psychologist is found qualified to testify as to the presence or absence of a mental disease and does so in opposition to a psychiatrist, to tell the jury they could take into account the difference in the education, training and experience of psychologists and psychiatrists and the absence of medical training in the former.

BASTIAN, CIRCUIT JUDGE, with whom WILBUR K. MILLER, CHIEF JUDGE, joins, dissenting.

* * *

In the first place, we think it must be concluded beyond doubt that the existence of a mental disease or defect is, first and foremost, a *medical* problem. The ascertainment of such a medical illness in a given individual with reference to kind, quality, degree and influence is, except in extreme cases, a highly unverifiable process, judged by any objective standard, even when undertaken by a *medical* doctor with years of special training in the detection of medical disturbances of the mind.

* * *

If the issue is so debatable among conceded professional medical experts, it is sheer folly, in our opinion, to attribute to a lay psychologist, who admittedly is not a doctor of medicine, such presumptive medical knowledge and diagnostic acuity as to entitle him to wear in a criminal courtroom the badge of an expert witness with respect to the existence of that elusive *medical* condition known as mental disease or defect.

* * *

We are not alone in our views on this precise issue. The American Psychiatric Association, an organization "comprised of those twelve thousand qualified Doctors of Medicine who specialize and practice as psychiatrists," in its amicus curiae brief, urges this court not to allow psychologists to qualify as experts to express opinions. We find in the brief this pertinent observation in regard to the proper medical ascertainment of mental disease or defect:

> "The diagnostic synthesis of *all data* collected is properly carried out only by an individual Doctor of Medicine with a broad training, experience, and familiarity with *all* of the areas indicated, and the diagnosis must reflect a comprehensive medical judgment in which the proper weight is given to all of the data available. Further, we know of no mental illness which does not have a biological as well as a psychological component. No facet of the data can be assumed to reflect the total diagnosis until viewed in the context of the total picture. A clinical psychologist, lacking *medical* training and the specialization required of the qualified psychiatrist, is not qualified to make this total *medical* diagnosis or to testify as a *medical* expert thereon." [Emphasis appears in amicus brief.]

The majority of the court ignores the above quoted wise counsel from the only undisputed experts now at work in the area of medical illness of the mind. In doing so, the court, we suggest, is bypassing all objective criteria in reaching the highly questionable and subjective conclusion that lay psychologists, whose opinions are predicated on the basis of test results, may qualify as experts on the medical question of the diagnosis of mental disease or defect, as well as experts concerning the causal relationship between a particular defendant's mental abnormality, as such may be "diagnosed" by these psychologists, and that defendant's criminal activity. In our opinion, the holding of the majority on this issue is wholly untenable. We would affirm the judgment and sentence of the District Court.

Questions and Comments

1. *Current state of the law.* Since *Jenkins* was decided in 1962, most states have provided by statute or case law that doctoral level clinical psychologists may offer opinions on insanity, as well as on other issues concerning the mentally disordered. See Gass, "The Psychologist as Expert Witness: Science in the Courtroom," 38 Md.L.Rev. 539, 544–554 (1979). But many states still refuse to allow psychologists as free a rein as psychiatrists. For instance, in insanity cases, some courts still limit psychologists to interpretations of psychological tests; testimony by psychologists about degree of cognitive or volitional impairment or causes of mental deficiencies is prohibited. *Commonwealth v. Williams,* 270 Pa. Super. 27, 410 A.2d 880 (1979); *People v. Manning,* 61 Ill.App.3d 558, 18 Ill. Dec. 763, 378 N.E.2d 227 (1978); *Spann v. Bees,* 32 Md.App. 313, 327 A.2d 801 (Spec.App.1974). Some courts still exclude psychologists from determinations of dangerousness in the criminal context. *State v. Williams,* 278 Md. 180, 361 A.2d 122 (1976). Many civil commitment provisions permit certification or testimony only by "physicians", Vernon's Ann.Tex. Const. art. 1, § 15a; N.Y.—McKinney's Mental Hygiene Law § 9.27, or, if they do allow psychologists to testify, require them to meet higher experiential standards than psychiatrists. West's Ann.Cal.Welf. & Inst.Code § 5251. A survey of guardianship statutes in the 50 states found 85 different provi-

sions which reserved the role of expert exclusively to physicians. Hafemeister & Sales, "Responsibilities of Psychologists Under Guardianship and Conservatorship Laws," 13 Prof.Psychol. 354 (1982). Moreover, in most states, masters level clinical psychologists, and masters and doctoral level social workers are barred entirely from testifying on most issues, see, e.g., *State v. Baucom*, 28 Or.App. 757, 561 P.2d 641 (1977), although some states do allow them to testify with respect to competency to stand trial. See Tenn.Code Ann. § 33–708; *People v. Parney*, 74 Mich.App. 173, 253 N.W.2d 698 (1977).

Finally, it has been noted that, even when psychologists are allowed to testify, judges and juries continue to view them (and therefore, presumably, social workers as well) as "second-class" experts. Perlin, "The Legal Status of the Psychologist in the Courtroom," 4 Men.Dis.L.Rptr. 194, 195–6 (1980). See also, Poythress, "Judicial Preference Regarding Expert Testimony," 10 Crim.Just. & Beh. 175 (1983).

2. *Justifications.* The limitations on and perceptions about expert qualifications of the various mental health professions can be interpreted as another illustration of the law's continued preference for the medical model of mental disorder. Such a preference clearly motivates the concurring and dissenting opinions in *Jenkins*. Are there other justifications for the law's current approach?

The psychiatric profession appears to continue to adhere to the position it took in 1954, described in *Jenkins*. In 1980, American Psychiatric Association President Donald Langsley acknowledged that psychologists, social workers, and others can and should be members of the "treatment team," but asserted that "it is [now] more appropriate than ever that the psychiatrist is the member of the team best equipped to perform triage, make differential diagnosis, [and to] plan and render treatment for a variety of psychological and somatic problems." Langsley, "Viewpoint, A Commentary by APA's President," Psychiatric News, Sept. 19, 1980, at 25, col. 1. If, as Langsley asserts, psychiatrists are superior at treatment and diagnosis then, presumably, they are superior at forensic tasks as well. In its opinions that have touched on the clinical testimony issue, the United States Supreme Court has lent considerable credence to this view—whether consciously or unconsciously is hard to say—by its tendency to speak only of psychiatrists, or to mention psychologists and other mental health professions only in passing. See, e.g., *Barefoot v. Estelle*, 463 U.S. 880, 103 S.Ct. 3383, 77 L.Ed.2d 1090 (1983) (speaking of the validity of "psychiatric" predictions of dangerousness); *Ake v. Oklahoma*, 470 U.S. 68, 105 S.Ct. 1087, 84 L.Ed.2d 53 (1985) (finding a constitutional right to "psychiatric assistance" in insanity and death penalty cases); Addington v. Texas, 441 U.S. 418, 99 S.Ct. 1804, 60 L.Ed.2d 323 (1979) (the "psychiatric diagnosis [necessary for civil commitment] is to a large extent based on medical 'impressions'").

Research indicates that non-psychiatrists may be just as competent as psychiatrists in addressing many forensic issues. Dix & Poythress, "Propriety of Medical Dominance of Forensic Mental Health Practice: The Empirical Evidence," 23 Ariz.L.Rev. 961, 971–984 (1981). Of particular interest, one study found that psychologists and social workers tend to do more thorough forensic evaluations and more comprehensive and more relevant forensic reports than their psychiatric colleagues. Petrella & Poythress, "The Quality of Forensic Examinations: An Interdiciplinary Study," 51 J. Consult. & Clinical Psychol. 76 (1983).

Morse has suggested that, under his scheme, described in section II of this chapter, "almost any person with extensive clinical experience with crazy persons should qualify as an expert." Morse, "Crazy Behavior, Morals and Science: An Analysis of Mental Health Law," 51 S.Cal.L.Rev. 527, 623–624 (1978). On the other hand, "[p]rofessionals without extensive, recent, and relevant mental health *clinical* experience, whatever their formal training, should not be qualified as experts" on these subjects. With respect to statistical evidence, "an expert from any field [e.g., sociology as well as psychiatry] who possesses data relevant to the specific . . . issue is competent to be qualified." Id. Do you agree?

3. *Knowledge of legal issues.* Clinical knowledge and training may not be enough to qualify a mental health professional as an expert witness. Many commentators have suggested that, unless the witness can demonstrate knowledge of the relevant legal test, he or she should remain unqualified regardless of clinical background. See, e.g., Pollack, "Forensic Psychiatry: A Specialty," 2 Bull.Am.Acad.Psychiat. & L. 1 (1974). For instance, as we saw in the previous section, failure on the part of clinicians to understand the legal test for competency to stand trial can lead to virtually useless reports or testimony. In an effort to remedy this situation, both disciplines have established forensic boards designed to provide certification of those members who have exhibited proficiency in forensic matters. See, "The American Board of Forensic Psychiatry, Inc., 1976," 4 Bull.Am.Acad.Psychiat. & L. 95 (1976). In a separate effort, several states have initiated, with some success, training programs for forensic clinicians in an attempt to eliminate excess psychiatric jargon, irrelevant detail and confusion about legal standards. Melton, Weithorn & Slobogin, Community Mental Health Centers and the Courts: An Evaluation of Community–Based Forensic Services 56–67 (1985).

B. THE RIGHT TO AN EXPERT EVALUATION

AKE v. OKLAHOMA

Supreme Court of the United States, 1985.
470 U.S. 68, 105 S.Ct. 1087, 84 L.Ed.2d 53.

JUSTICE MARSHALL delivered the opinion of the Court.

The issue in this case is whether the Constitution requires that an indigent defendant have access to the psychiatric examination and assistance necessary to prepare an effective defense based on his mental condition, when his sanity at the time of the offense is seriously in question.

I

Late in 1979, Glen Burton Ake was arrested and charged with murdering a couple and wounding their two children. He was arraigned in the District Court for Canadian County, Okla., in February

1980. His behavior at arraignment, and in other prearraignment incidents at the jail, was so bizarre that the trial judge *sua sponte* ordered him to be examined by a psychiatrist "for the purpose of advising with the Court as to his impressions of whether the Defendant may need an extended period of mental observation." The examining psychiatrist reported: "At times [Ake] appears to be frankly delusional. * * * He claims to be the 'sword of vengeance' of the Lord and that he will sit at the left hand of God in heaven." He diagnosed Ake as a probable paranoid schizophrenic and recommended a prolonged psychiatric evaluation to determine whether Ake was competent to stand trial.

In March, Ake was committed to a state hospital to be examined with respect to his "present sanity," i.e., his competency to stand trial. On April 10, less than six months after the incidents for which Ake was indicted, the chief forensic psychiatrist at the state hospital informed the court that Ake was not competent to stand trial. The court then held a competency hearing, at which a psychiatrist testified:

> "[Ake] is a psychotic * * * his psychiatric diagnosis was that of paranoid schizophrenia—chronic, with exacerbation, that is with current upset, and that in addition * * * he is dangerous. * * * [B]ecause of the severity of his mental illness and because of the intensities of his rage, his poor control, his delusions, he requires a maximum security facility within—I believe—the State Psychiatric Hospital system."

The court found Ake to be a "mentally ill person in need of care and treatment" and incompetent to stand trial, and ordered him committed to the state mental hospital.

Six weeks later, the chief forensic psychiatrist informed the court that Ake had become competent to stand trial. At the time, Ake was receiving 200 milligrams of Thorazine, an antipsychotic drug, three times daily, and the psychiatrist indicated that, if Ake continued to receive that dosage, his condition would remain stable. The State then resumed proceedings against Ake.

At a pretrial conference in June, Ake's attorney informed the court that his client would raise an insanity defense. To enable him to prepare and present such a defense adequately, the attorney stated, a psychiatrist would have to examine Ake with respect to his mental condition at the time of the offense. During Ake's 3–month stay at the state hospital, no inquiry had been made into his sanity at the time of the offense, and, as an indigent, Ake could not afford to pay for a psychiatrist. Counsel asked the court either to arrange to have a psychiatrist perform the examination, or to provide funds to allow the defense to arrange one. The trial judge rejected counsel's argument that the Federal Constitution requires that an indigent defendant receive the assistance of a psychiatrist when that assistance is necessary to the defense, and he denied the motion for a psychiatric evaluation at state expense on the basis of this Court's decision in *United*

States ex rel. Smith v. Baldi, 344 U.S. 561, 73 S.Ct. 391, 97 L.Ed. 549 (1953).

Ake was tried for two counts of murder in the first degree, a crime punishable by death in Oklahoma, and for two counts of shooting with intent to kill. At the guilt phase of trial, his sole defense was insanity. Although defense counsel called to the stand and questioned each of the psychiatrists who had examined Ake at the state hospital, none testified about his mental state at the time of the offense because none had examined him on that point. The prosecution, in turn, asked each of these psychiatrists whether he had performed or seen the results of any examination diagnosing Ake's mental state at the time of the offense, and each doctor replied that he had not. *As a result, there was no expert testimony for either side on Ake's sanity at the time of the offense.* The jurors were then instructed that Ake could be found not guilty by reason of insanity if he did not have the ability to distinguish right from wrong at the time of the alleged offense. They were further told that Ake was to be presumed sane at the time of the crime unless *he* presented evidence sufficient to raise a reasonable doubt about his sanity at that time. If he raised such a doubt in their minds, the jurors were informed, the burden of proof shifted to the State to prove sanity beyond a reasonable doubt. The jury rejected Ake's insanity defense and returned a verdict of guilty on all counts.

At the sentencing proceeding, the State asked for the death penalty. No new evidence was presented. The prosecutor relied significantly on the testimony of the state psychiatrists who had examined Ake, and who had testified at the guilt phase that Ake was dangerous to society, to establish the likelihood of his future dangerous behavior. Ake had no expert witness to rebut this testimony or to introduce on his behalf evidence in mitigation of his punishment. The jury sentenced Ake to death on each of the two murder counts, and to 500 years' imprisonment on each of the two counts of shooting with intent to kill.

On appeal to the Oklahoma Court of Criminal Appeals, Ake argued that, as an indigent defendant, he should have been provided the services of a court-appointed psychiatrist. The court rejected this argument, observing: "We have held numerous times that, the unique nature of capital cases notwithstanding, the State does not have the responsibility of providing such services to indigents charged with capital crimes." 663 P.2d 1, 6 (1983). Finding no error in Ake's other claims, the court affirmed the convictions and sentences. We granted certiorari. 465 U.S. 1099, 104 S.Ct. 1591, 80 L.Ed.2d 123 (1984).

We hold that when a defendant has made a preliminary showing that his sanity at the time of the offense is likely to be a significant factor at trial, the Constitution requires that a State provide access to a psychiatrist's assistance on this issue, if the defendant cannot otherwise afford one. Accordingly, we reverse.

* * *

III

This Court has long recognized that when a State brings its judicial power to bear on an indigent defendant in a criminal proceeding, it must take steps to assure that the defendant has a fair opportunity to present his defense. This elementary principle, grounded in significant part on the Fourteenth Amendment's due process guarantee of fundamental fairness, derives from the belief that justice cannot be equal where, simply as a result of his poverty, a defendant is denied the opportunity to participate meaningfully in a judicial proceeding in which his liberty is at stake. * * *

* * * We recognized long ago that mere access to the courthouse doors does not by itself assure a proper functioning of the adversary process, and that a criminal trial is fundamentally unfair if the State proceeds against an indigent defendant without making certain that he has access to the raw materials integral to the building of an effective defense. Thus, while the Court has not held that a State must purchase for the indigent defendant all the assistance that his wealthier counterpart might buy, see *Ross v. Moffitt,* 417 U.S. 600, 94 S.Ct. 2437, 41 L.Ed.2d 341 (1974), it has often reaffirmed that fundamental fairness entitles indigent defendants to "an adequate opportunity to present their claims fairly within the adversary system," *id.,* at 612, 94 S.Ct., at 2444. To implement this principle, we have focused on identifying the "basic tools of an adequate defense or appeal," *Britt v. North Carolina,* 404 U.S. 226, 227, 92 S.Ct. 431, 433, 30 L.Ed.2d 400 (1971), and we have required that such tools be provided to those defendants who cannot afford to pay for them.

To say that these basic tools must be provided is, of course, merely to begin our inquiry. In this case we must decide whether, and under what conditions, the participation of a psychiatrist is important enough to preparation of a defense to require the State to provide an indigent defendant with access to competent psychiatric assistance in preparing the defense. Three factors are relevant to this determination. The first is the private interest that will be affected by the action of the State. The second is the governmental interest that will be affected if the safeguard is to be provided. The third is the probable value of the additional or substitute procedural safeguards that are sought, and the risk of an erroneous deprivation of the affected interest if those safeguards are not provided. We turn, then, to apply this standard to the issue before us.

A

The private interest in the accuracy of a criminal proceeding that places an individual's life or liberty at risk is almost uniquely compelling. Indeed, the host of safeguards fashioned by this Court over the years to diminish the risk of erroneous conviction stands as a testament to that concern. The interest of the individual in the outcome of the

State's effort to overcome the presumption of innocence is obvious and weighs heavily in our analysis.

We consider, next, the interest of the State. Oklahoma asserts that to provide Ake with psychiatric assistance on the record before us would result in a staggering burden to the State. We are unpersuaded by this assertion. Many States, as well as the Federal Government, currently make psychiatric assistance available to indigent defendants, and they have not found the financial burden so great as to preclude this assistance. This is especially so when the obligation of the State is limited to provision of one competent psychiatrist, as it is in many States, and as we limit the right we recognize today. At the same time, it is difficult to identify any interest of the State, other than that in its economy, that weighs against recognition of this right. The State's interest in prevailing at trial—unlike that of a private litigant—is necessarily tempered by its interest in the fair and accurate adjudication of criminal cases. Thus, also unlike a private litigant, a State may not legitimately assert an interest in maintenance of a strategic advantage over the defense, if the result of that advantage is to cast a pall on the accuracy of the verdict obtained. We therefore conclude that the governmental interest in denying Ake the assistance of a psychiatrist is not substantial, in light of the compelling interest of both the State and the individual in accurate dispositions.

Last, we inquire into the probable value of the psychiatric assistance sought, and the risk of error in the proceeding if such assistance is not offered. We begin by considering the pivotal role that psychiatry has come to play in criminal proceedings. More than 40 States, as well as the Federal Government, have decided either through legislation or judicial decision that indigent defendants are entitled, under certain circumstances, to the assistance of a psychiatrist's expertise. For example, in subsection (e) of the Criminal Justice Act, 18 U.S.C. § 3006A, Congress has provided that indigent defendants shall receive the assistance of all experts "necessary for an adequate defense." Numerous state statutes guarantee reimbursement for expert services under a like standard. And in many States that have not assured access to psychiatrists through the legislative process, state courts have interpreted the State or Federal Constitution to require that psychiatric assistance be provided to indigent defendants when necessary for an adequate defense, or when insanity is at issue.

These statutes and court decisions reflect a reality that we recognize today, namely, that when the State has made the defendant's mental condition relevant to his criminal culpability and to the punishment he might suffer, the assistance of a psychiatrist may well be crucial to the defendant's ability to marshal his defense. In this role, psychiatrists gather facts, both through professional examination, interviews, and elsewhere, that they will share with the judge or jury; they analyze the information gathered and from it draw plausible conclusions about the defendant's mental condition, and about the effects of any disorder on behavior; and they offer opinions about how the defendant's mental condition might have affected his behavior at the time in question. They know the probative questions to ask of the opposing party's psychiatrists and how to interpret their answers. Unlike lay witnesses, who can merely describe symptoms they believe might be relevant to the defendant's mental state, psychiatrists can identify the "elusive and often deceptive" symptoms of insanity, *Solesbee v. Balkcom*, 339 U.S. 9, 12, 70 S.Ct. 457, 458, 94 L.Ed. 604 (1950), and tell the jury why their observations are relevant. Further, where permitted by evidentiary rules, psychiatrists can translate a medical diagnosis into language that will assist the trier of fact, and therefore offer evidence in a form that has meaning for the task at hand. Through this process of investigation, interpretation and testimony, psychiatrists ideally assist lay jurors, who generally have no training in psychiatric matters, to make a sensible and educated determination about the mental condition of the defendant at the time of the offense.

Psychiatry is not, however, an exact science, and psychiatrists disagree widely and frequently on what constitutes mental illness, on the appropriate diagnosis to be attached to given behavior and symptoms, on cure and treatment, and on likelihood of future dangerousness. Perhaps because there often is no single, accurate psychiatric conclusion on legal insanity in a given case, juries remain the primary factfinders on this issue, and they must resolve differences in opinion within the psychiatric profession on the basis of the evidence offered by each party. When jurors make this determination about issues that inevitably are complex and foreign, the testimony of psychiatrists can be crucial and "a virtual necessity if an insanity plea is to have any chance of success." By organizing a defendant's mental history, examination results and behavior, and other information, interpreting it in light of their expertise, and then laying out their investigative and analytic process to the jury, the psychiatrists for each party enable the jury to make its most accurate determination of the truth on the issue before them. It is for this reason that States rely on psychiatrists as examiners, consultants, and witnesses, and that private individuals do as well, when they can afford to do so. In so saying, we neither approve nor disapprove the widespread reliance on psychiatrists but instead recognize the unfairness of a contrary holding in light of the evolving practice.

The foregoing leads inexorably to the conclusion that, without the assistance of a psychiatrist to conduct a professional examination on issues relevant to the defense, to help determine whether the insanity defense is viable, to present testimony, and to assist in preparing the cross-examination of a State's psychiatric witnesses, the risk of an inaccurate resolution of sanity issues is extremely high. With such assistance, the defendant is fairly able to present at least enough information to the jury, in a meaningful manner, as to permit it to make a sensible determination.

A defendant's mental condition is not necessarily at issue in every criminal proceeding, however, and it is unlikely that psychiatric assistance of the kind we have described would be of probable value in cases where it is not. The risk of error from denial of such assistance, as well as its probable value, are most predictably at their height when the defendant's mental condition is seriously in question. When the defendant is able to make an *ex parte* threshold showing to the trial court that his sanity is likely to be a significant factor in his defense, the need for the assistance of a psychiatrist is readily apparent. It is in such cases that a defense may be devastated by the absence of a psychiatric examination and testimony; with such assistance, the defendant might have a reasonable chance of success. In such a circumstance, where the potential accuracy of the jury's determination is so dramatically enhanced, and where the interests of the individual and the State in an accurate proceeding are substantial, the State's interest in its fisc must yield. We therefore hold that when a defendant demonstrates to the trial judge that his sanity at the time of the offense is to be a significant factor at trial, the State must, at a minimum, assure the defendant access to a competent psychiatrist who will conduct an appropriate examination and assist in evaluation, preparation, and presentation of the defense. This is not to say, of course, that the indigent defendant has a constitutional right to choose a psychiatrist of his personal liking or to receive funds to hire his own. Our concern is that the indigent defendant have access to a competent psychiatrist for the purpose we have discussed, and as in the case of the provision of counsel we leave to the State the decision on how to implement this right.

B

Ake also was denied the means of presenting evidence to rebut the State's evidence of his future dangerousness. The foregoing discussion compels a similar conclusion in the context of a capital sentencing proceeding, when the State presents psychiatric evidence of the defendant's future dangerousness. We have repeatedly recognized the defendant's compelling interest in fair adjudication at the sentencing phase of a capital case. The State, too, has a profound interest in assuring that its ultimate sanction is not erroneously imposed, and we do not see why monetary considerations should be more persuasive in this context than at trial. The variable on which we must focus is, therefore, the probable value that the assistance of a psychiatrist will have in this area, and the risk attendant on its absence.

This Court has upheld the practice in many States of placing before the jury psychiatric testimony on the question of future dangerousness, see *Barefoot v. Estelle,* 463 U.S. 880, 896–905, 103 S.Ct. 3383, 3396–3400, 77 L.Ed.2d 1090 (1983), at least where the defendant has had access to an expert of his own, *id.,* n. 5. In so holding, the Court relied, in part, on the assumption that the factfinder would have before it both the views of the prosecutor's psychiatrists and the "opposing views of the defendant's doctors" and would therefore be competent to "uncover, recognize, and take due account of ∗ ∗ ∗ shortcomings" in predictions on this point. Without a psychiatrist's assistance, the defendant cannot offer a well-informed expert's opposing view, and thereby loses a significant opportunity to raise in the jurors' minds questions about the State's proof of an aggravating factor. In such a circumstance, where the consequence of error is so great, the relevance of responsive psychiatric testimony so evident, and the burden on the State so slim, due process requires access to a psychiatric examination on relevant issues, to the testimony of the psychiatrist, and to assistance in preparation at the sentencing phase.

The trial court in this case believed that our decision in United States ex rel. Smith v. Baldi, 344 U.S. 561, 73 S.Ct. 391, 97 L.Ed. 549 (1953), absolved it completely of the obligation to provide access to a psychiatrist. For two reasons, we disagree. First, neither *Smith,* nor McGarty v. O'Brien, 188 F.2d 151, 155 (CA1 1951), to which the majority cited in *Smith,* even suggested that the Constitution does not require any psychiatric examination or assistance whatsoever. Quite to the contrary, the record in *Smith* demonstrated that neutral psychiatrists in fact had examined the defendant as to his sanity and had testified on that subject at trial, and it was on that basis that the Court found no additional assistance was necessary. *Smith,* supra, at 568, 73 S.Ct. at 394; see also United States ex rel. Smith v. Baldi, 192 F.2d 540, 547 (CA3 1951). Similarly, in *McGarty,* the defendant had been examined by two psychiatrists who were not beholden to the prosecution. We therefore reject the State's contention that *Smith* supports the broad proposition that "[t]here is presently no constitutional right to have a psychiatric examination of a defendant's sanity at the time of the offense." At most it supports the proposition that there is no constitutional right to more psychiatric assistance than the defendant in *Smith* had received.

In any event, our disagreement with the State's reliance on *Smith* is more fundamental. That case was decided at a time when indigent defendants in state courts had no constitutional right to even the presence of counsel. Our recognition since then of elemental constitutional rights, each of which has enhanced the ability of an indigent defendant to attain a fair hearing, has signaled our increased commitment to assuring meaningful access to the judicial process.

IV

We turn now to apply these standards to the facts of this case. On the record before us, it is clear that Ake's mental state at the time of the offense was a substantial factor in his defense, and that the trial court was on notice of that fact when the request for a court-appointed psychiatrist was made. For one, Ake's sole defense was that of insanity. Second, Ake's behavior at arraignment, just four months after the offense, was so bizarre as to prompt the trial judge, *sua sponte,* to have him examined for competency. Third, a state psychiatrist shortly thereafter found Ake to be incompetent to stand trial, and suggested that he be committed. Fourth, when he was found to be competent six weeks later, it was only on the condition that he be sedated with large doses of Thorazine three times a day, during trial. Fifth, the psychiatrists who examined Ake for competency described to the trial court the severity of Ake's mental illness less than six months after the offense in question, and suggested that this mental illness might have begun many years earlier. Finally, Oklahoma recognizes a defense of insanity, under which the initial burden of producing evidence falls on the defendant. Taken together, these factors make clear that the question of Ake's sanity was likely to be a significant factor in his defense.

In addition, Ake's future dangerousness was a significant factor at the sentencing phase. The state psychiatrist who treated Ake at the state mental hospital testified at the guilt phase that, because of his mental illness, Ake posed a threat of continuing criminal violence. This testimony raised the issue of Ake's future dangerousness, which is an aggravating factor under Oklahoma's capital sentencing scheme, and on which the prosecutor relied at sentencing. We therefore conclude that Ake also was entitled to the assistance of a psychiatrist on this issue and that the denial of that assistance deprived him of due process.

Accordingly, we reverse and remand for a new trial.

It is so ordered.

CHIEF JUSTICE BURGER, concurring in the judgment.

This is a capital case in which the Court is asked to decide whether a State may refuse an indigent defendant "any opportunity whatsoever" to obtain psychiatric evidence for the preparation and presentation of a claim of insanity by way of defense when the defendant's legal sanity at the time of the offense was "seriously in issue."

The facts of the case and the question presented confine the actual holding of the Court. In capital cases the finality of the sentence imposed warrants protections that may or may not be required in other cases. Nothing in the Court's opinion reaches noncapital cases.

JUSTICE REHNQUIST, dissenting.

The Court holds that "when a defendant has made a preliminary showing that his sanity at the time of the offense is likely to be a significant factor at trial, the Constitution requires that a State provide access to a psychiatrist's assistance on this issue, if the defendant cannot otherwise afford one." I do not think that the facts of this case warrant the establishment of such a principle; and I think that even if the factual predicate of the Court's statement were established, the constitutional rule announced by the Court is far too broad. I would limit the rule to capital cases, and make clear that the entitlement is to an independent psychiatric evaluation, not to a defense consultant.

* * *

[E]ven if I were to agree with the Court that some right to a state-appointed psychiatrist should be recognized here, I would not grant the broad right to "access to a competent psychiatrist who will conduct an appropriate examination *and assist in evaluation, preparation, and presentation of the defense.*" A psychiatrist is not an attorney, whose job it is to advocate. His opinion is sought on a question that the State of Oklahoma treats as a question of *fact.* Since any "unfairness" in these cases would arise from the fact that the only competent witnesses on the question are being hired by the State, all the defendant should be entitled to is one competent opinion—whatever the witness' conclusion—from a psychiatrist who acts independently of the prosecutor's office. Although the independent psychiatrist should be available to answer defense counsel's questions prior to trial, and to testify if called, I see no reason why the defendant should be entitled to an opposing view, or to a "defense" advocate.

For the foregoing reasons, I would affirm the judgment of the Court of Criminal Appeals of Oklahoma.

Questions and Comments

1. *Implications of* Ake. As Justice Marshall points out, almost every state provides indigent defendants the opportunity to obtain, at state expense, an evaluation on sanity. Most states also provide evaluation services on sentencing issues in capital cases. Usually, these evaluations are performed by state hospital employees, although with increasing frequency they are conducted by community mental health professionals who receive payment from the courts for their services. If an indigent defendant receives evaluative assistance from a state employee, are the requirements of *Ake* met? Or can the defendant demand an expert who is not a regular employee of the state? In this regard, consider:

> If the indigent defendant could be guaranteed an 'impartial' evaluation by the state-employed clinician, then he should be satisfied with the opinion that results. But such a guarantee is not possible. Personal and professional predilections heavily influence clinical opinion. While it cannot be assumed that clinicians will find for the state merely because they are paid by it, as a practical matter, they are subject to institutional pressures that make it likely they will be 'prosecution-oriented',[265] at least in borderline cases. The bias inherent in their situation is suggested by the fact that, in most states, the indigent who requests an evaluation is sent to the same expert or experts who would be conducting the examination for the prosecution had the defendant been able to afford a private clinician. The state

---

265. A study involving interviews of former members of the federal prosecutor's office in the District of Columbia and [of] St. Elizabeth's Hospital, the District's forensic unit, found that the doctors frequently contacted the prosecutor's office, but rarely contacted the defense attorney. The study also noted that it was not un-common "for the hospital doctors to ask the prosecutor if he would oppose a certain diagnosis; if the prosecutor indicates opposition, the questioned diagnosis may never come to light." Chernoff & Schaffer, "Defending the Mentally Ill: Ethical Quicksand," 10 Am.Crim.L.Rev. 505, 510 (1972).

should not be allowed to force the defendant to accept such an evaluation on the ground that it is 'impartial' anymore than it should be
required to concede that the opinion of a private clinician offered by a
non-indigent defendant is scientifically objective.

Slobogin, "*Estelle v. Smith:* The Constitutional Contours of the Forensic
Evaluation," 31 Emory L.Journ. 71, 132–33 (1981).

Once a "competent psychiatrist" is selected, he or she is required,
under *Ake,* to "conduct an appropriate examination and assist in evaluation, preparation and presentation of the defense." Does this language
merely require, as Justice Rehnquist asserts, that the defendant be able to
ask questions of and elicit testimony from "a psychiatrist who acts independently of the prosecutor's office," or does it require something more? What
if the expert's conclusion is that the defendant is sane or dangerous—is this
expert able to "assist in evaluation, preparation and presentation of the
defense?" If not, does the due process clause entitle the defendant to
another expert? Does *Ake's* failure to overrule United States ex rel. Smith
v. Baldi, 344 U.S. 561, 73 S.Ct. 391, 97 L.Ed. 549 (1953), answer any of these
questions?

A number of states allow the defendant to seek an independent
evaluation if he or she is dissatisfied with the evaluator selected by the
court or with the results of the evaluation. S. Brakel, J. Parry and B.
Weiner, The Mentally Disabled and the Law 719 (1985). But in those
states which do not, *Ake* has brought no change. Lower court decisions
since *Ake* have condoned statutory procedures which permit a state-employed expert to report to the court or to the prosecution for transmittal to
the defense, as well as procedures which simply give the defense access to
the findings of the state's experts. See Note, "Expert Services and the
Indigent Criminal Defendant: The Constitutional Mandate of Ake v. Oklahoma, 84 Mich.L.Rev. 1326, 1348–49 nn. 150–52 (1986). Moreover, a
number of courts have held that in order to obtain an *Ake* evaluation the
defendant must make a "clear showing" that mental state is a "genuine" or
"real" issue, a showing which may be difficult without psychiatric assistance. Note, "The Indigent Defendant's Right to Psychiatric Assistance:
Ake v. Oklahoma, 17 N.Car.Cen.L.Journ. 208, 220–22 (1988).

2. *Sixth amendment analysis.* Note that *Ake* is based on the due
process clause. Some courts have held that the sixth amendment right to
effective assistance of counsel entitles the defendant to an "exploratory"
evaluation designed to assist the attorney in deciding what claims to make
and in preparing for the case. See, e.g., United States v. Edwards, 488 F.2d
1154, 1163 (5th Cir.1974) (stressing the "particularly critical interrelation
between expert psychiatric assistance and minimally effective representation of counsel"). See also Wood v. Zahradnick, 578 F.2d 980 (4th Cir.1978).
Does framing the right to expert assistance in sixth amendment terms offer
any advantages to the defendant? Perhaps worth noting is the Supreme
Court's decision in Wheat v. United States, 486 U.S. 153, 108 S.Ct. 1692,
100 L.Ed.2d 140 (1988), which stated that "a defendant may not insist on
representation by an attorney he cannot afford." If this is true for the
right to counsel, it is likely to be true for the right to expert assistance as
well.

3. *Expert assistance in other contexts.* Besides forming the basis for an insanity defense and for rebuttal of the state's case in capital sentencing, expert assistance may be useful in raising or rebutting a number of other claims in criminal cases. Discussed in the next chapter are various other "psychiatric" defenses (e.g., diminished capacity, automatism) which might result in acquittal, and various sentencing provisions which contemplate psychiatric testimony about past mental state and future dangerousness. As noted earlier in this chapter, competency to stand trial is also often viewed as a psychiatric issue. Most states provide expert assistance on the competency issue in the same fashion as they do for insanity claims, but few explicitly authorize such assistance for noncapital sentencing or responsibility issues other than insanity. See S. Brakel, J. Parry & B. Weiner, The Mentally Disabled and the Law 697–98, 719–29 (1985). Does anything in Justice Marshall's analysis in *Ake* foreclose a right to psychiatric assistance in these situations? Should it matter, as Marshall seems to suggest, whether a judge or a jury is the factfinder?

Expert assistance may also be necessary in noncriminal proceedings, such as civil commitment and guardianship hearings. Does *Ake* have implications for these types of proceedings or is it limited to criminal proceedings? The right to an independent expert in civil commitment is discussed further at pp. 729–730.

4. *State access to results.* As noted above, in many states the results of the indigent's evaluation are immediately made available to both the defense *and* the prosecution (as well as the court). Assuming this procedure does not compromise the expert's "independence", does state access nonetheless violate *Ake* to the extent it "chills" the exercise of the right to expert assistance by a defendant who is not sure how the evaluation will come out? Even if disclosing the results of the defense's exploratory evaluation to the prosecution does not violate *Ake*, does not state access run afoul of the attorney-client privilege and the associated right to effective assistance of counsel? An increasing number of states provide that the attorney-client privilege protects against disclosure of the results of the indigent's "exploratory" evaluation until the defendant decides to use them. See, e.g., West's Fla.S.A.R.Crim.Proc. 3.216(a).

A derivative issue arises when a *non*indigent defendant retains more than one expert, but decides to use only one or some of the experts at trial. May the prosecution call the unused expert or experts? The two leading cases on the issue, People v. Edney, 39 N.Y.2d 620, 385 N.Y.S.2d 23, 350 N.E.2d 400 (1976) and State v. Pratt, 284 Md. 516, 398 A.2d 421 (1979), are reprinted in Chapter Four; here they will only be summarized. *Edney* found that the state should have access to unused defense experts. Otherwise, the defendant would "be permitted to suppress any unfavorable psychiatric witness whom he had retained in the first instance, under the guise of the attorney-client privilege, while he endeavors to shop around for a friendly expert, and take unfriendly experts off the market." *Pratt,* on the other hand, rejected *Edney's* approach on the ground that it would discourage defense attorneys from seeking expert assistance and disturb the rapport between the defendant and the defense-retained expert. Are the concerns evinced by either court realistic? The American Bar Association Criminal Justice Mental Health Standards adopt *Pratt's* approach, but allow the prosecution access to unused defense experts if it can show a bad faith effort on the part of the defense to "gag" the available experts. Standard 7–3.3(b)(ii).

C. THE BASIS OF CLINICAL OPINION

Although mental health professionals increasingly rely on actuarial data, expert testimony still typically depends on the clinical evaluation process. For both criminal and civil cases, the primary source of information in this process is, of course, the interview of the person whose mental condition is at issue. The good evaluator also attempts to obtain as much third party information as possible to fill in gaps in the subject's story and for corroborative purposes. This section first discusses constitutional issues surrounding use of the defendant-subject as a source of clinical information; it then focuses on subconstitutional, evidentiary concerns which arise primarily in connection with use of third party information.

1. The Defendant as a Source: Constitutional Considerations

The fifth amendment states in part that "no person shall be compelled in any criminal case to be a witness against himself." The values said to underlie this right, summarized in Murphy v. Waterfront Commission, 378 U.S. 52, 55, 84 S.Ct. 1594, 1596, 12 L.Ed.2d 678 (1964), are manifold: the prevention of abuse by government officials, the protection of privacy, the fear that coerced statements will be unreliable, "our unwillingness to subject those suspected of crime to the cruel trilemma of self-accusation, perjury or contempt," the "preference for an accusatorial rather than an inquisitorial system of criminal justice", and "our sense of fair play which dictates 'a fair state-individual balance . . . by requiring the government in its contest with the individual to shoulder the entire load . . .'". The primary issue addressed here is whether the traditional attributes of the "accusatorial" system—which prevents the state from forcing the defendant to help it convict him or her—applies to state-requested psychiatric evaluations, or whether, instead, an "inquisitorial" approach—which relies more heavily on statements from the defendant—is permissible when the issue is the defendant's mental condition.

ESTELLE v. SMITH

Supreme Court of the United States, 1981.
451 U.S. 454, 101 S.Ct. 1866, 68 L.Ed.2d 359.

CHIEF JUSTICE BURGER, delivered the opinion of the Court.

We granted certiorari to consider whether the prosecution's use of psychiatric testimony at the sentencing phase of respondent's capital murder trial to establish his future dangerousness violated his constitutional rights.

I

A

On December 28, 1973, respondent Ernest Benjamin Smith was indicted for murder arising from his participation in the armed robbery of a grocery store during which a clerk was fatally shot, not by Smith, but by his accomplice. In accordance with Art. 1257(b)(2) of the Tex. Penal Code Ann. (Vernon 1974) concerning the punishment for murder with malice aforethought, the State of Texas announced its intention to seek the death penalty. Thereafter, a judge of the 195th Judicial District Court of Dallas County, Texas, informally ordered the State's attorney to arrange a psychiatric examination of Smith by Dr. James P. Grigson to determine Smith's competency to stand trial.[1]

Dr. Grigson, who interviewed Smith in jail for approximately 90 minutes, concluded that he was competent to stand trial. In a letter to the trial judge, Dr. Grigson reported his findings: "[I]t is my opinion that Ernest Benjamin Smith, Jr., is aware of the difference between right and wrong and is able to aid an attorney in his defense." This letter was filed with the court's papers in the case. Smith was then tried by a jury and convicted of murder.

In Texas, capital cases require bifurcated proceedings—a guilt phase and a penalty phase. If the defendant is found guilty, a separate proceeding before the same jury is held to fix the punishment. At the penalty phase, if the jury affirmatively answers three questions on which the State has the burden of proof beyond a reasonable doubt, the judge must impose the death sentence. See Tex.Code Crim.Proc.Ann., Arts. 37.071(c) and (e) (Vernon Supp.1980). One of the three critical issues to be resolved by the jury is "whether there is a probability that the defendant would commit criminal acts of violence that would constitute a continuing threat to society." Art. 37.071(b)(2). In other words, the jury must assess the defendant's future dangerousness.

At the commencement of Smith's sentencing hearing, the State rested "[s]ubject to the right to reopen." Defense counsel called three lay witnesses: Smith's stepmother, his aunt, and the man who owned the gun Smith carried during the robbery. Smith's relatives testified as to his good reputation and character. The owner of the pistol testified as to Smith's knowledge that it would not fire because of a mechanical defect. The State then called Dr. Grigson as a witness.

Defense counsel were aware from the trial court's file of the case that Dr. Grigson had submitted a psychiatric report in the form of a

---

1. This psychiatric evaluation was ordered even though defense counsel had not put into issue Smith's competency to stand trial or his sanity at the time of the offense. The trial judge later explained: "In all cases where the State has sought the death penalty, I have ordered a mental evaluation of the defendant to determine his competency to stand trial. I have done this for my benefit because I do not intend to be a participant in a case where the defendant receives the death penalty and his mental competency remains in doubt." See Tex.Code Crim.Proc.Ann., Art. 46.02 (Vernon 1979). No question as to the appropriateness of the trial judge's order for the examination has been raised by Smith.

letter advising the court that Smith was competent to stand trial. This report termed Smith "a severe sociopath," but it contained no more specific reference to his future dangerousness. Before trial, defense counsel had obtained an order requiring the State to disclose the witnesses it planned to use both at the guilt stage, and, if known, at the penalty stage. Subsequently, the trial court had granted a defense motion to bar the testimony during the State's case in chief of any witness whose name did not appear on that list. Dr. Grigson's name was not on the witness list, and defense counsel objected when he was called to the stand at the penalty phase.

In a hearing outside the presence of the jury, Dr. Grigson stated: (a) that he had not obtained permission from Smith's attorneys to examine him; (b) that he had discussed his conclusions and diagnosis with the State's attorney; and (c) that the prosecutor had requested him to testify and had told him, approximately five days before the sentencing hearing began, that his testimony probably would be needed within the week. The trial judge denied a defense motion to exclude Dr. Grigson's testimony on the ground that his name was not on the State's list of witnesses. Although no continuance was requested, the court then recessed for one hour following an acknowledgment by defense counsel that an hour was "all right."

After detailing his professional qualifications by way of foundation, Dr. Grigson testified before the jury on direct examination: (a) that Smith "is a very severe sociopath"; (b) that "he will continue his previous behavior"; (c) that his sociopathic condition will "only get worse"; (d) that he has no "regard for another human being's property or for their life, regardless of who it may be"; (e) that "[t]here is no treatment, no medicine ∗ ∗ ∗ that in any way at all modifies or changes this behavior"; (f) that he "is going to go ahead and commit other similar or same criminal acts if given the opportunity to do so"; and (g) that he "has no remorse or sorrow for what he has done." Dr. Grigson, whose testimony was based on information derived from his 90–minute "mental status examination" of Smith (*i.e.*, the examination ordered to determine Smith's competency to stand trial), was the State's only witness at the sentencing hearing.

The jury answered the three requisite questions in the affirmative, and, thus, under Texas law the death penalty for Smith was mandatory. The Texas Court of Criminal Appeals affirmed Smith's conviction and death sentence, *Smith v. State*, 540 S.W.2d 693 (Tex.Cr.App.1976), and we denied certiorari, 430 U.S. 922, 97 S.Ct. 1341, 51 L.Ed.2d 601 (1977).

B

After unsuccessfully seeking a writ of habeas corpus in the Texas state courts, Smith petitioned for such relief in the United States District Court for the Northern District of Texas pursuant to 28 U.S.C. § 2254. The District Court vacated Smith's death sentence because it found constitutional error in the admission of Dr. Grigson's testimony at the penalty phase. 445 F.Supp. 647 (1977). The court based its holding on the failure to advise Smith of his right to remain silent at the pretrial psychiatric examination and the failure to notify defense counsel in advance of the penalty phase that Dr. Grigson would testify. The court concluded that the death penalty had been imposed on Smith in violation of his Fifth and Fourteenth Amendment rights to due process and freedom from compelled self-incrimination, his Sixth Amendment right to the effective assistance of counsel, and his Eighth Amendment right to present complete evidence of mitigating circumstances.

The United States Court of Appeals for the Fifth Circuit affirmed. 602 F.2d 694 (1979). The court held that Smith's death sentence could not stand because the State's "surprise" use of Dr. Grigson as a witness, the consequences of which the court described as "devastating," denied Smith due process in that his attorneys were prevented from effectively challenging the psychiatric testimony. The court went on to hold that, under the Fifth and Sixth Amendments, "Texas may not use evidence based on a psychiatric examination of the defendant unless the defendant was warned, before the examination, that he had a right to remain silent; was allowed to terminate the examination when he wished; and was assisted by counsel in deciding whether to submit to the examination." Because Smith was not accorded these rights, his death sentence was set aside. While "leav[ing] to state authorities any questions that arise about the appropriate way to proceed when the state cannot legally execute a defendant whom it has sentenced to death," the court indicated that "the same testimony from Dr. Grigson, based on the same examination of Smith" could not be used against Smith at any future resentencing proceeding.

II

A

Of the several constitutional issues addressed by the District Court and the Court of Appeals, we turn first to whether the admission of Dr. Grigson's testimony at the penalty phase violated respondent's Fifth Amendment privilege against compelled self-incrimination because respondent was not advised before the pretrial psychiatric examination that he had a right to remain silent and that any statement he made could be used against him at a sentencing proceeding. Our initial inquiry must be whether the Fifth Amendment privilege is applicable in the circumstances of this case.

(1)

The State argues that respondent was not entitled to the protection of the Fifth Amendment because Dr. Grigson's testimony was used only to determine punishment after conviction, not to establish guilt. In the State's view, "incrimination is complete once guilt has been adjudicated," and, therefore, the Fifth Amendment privilege has no relevance to the penalty phase of a capital murder trial. We disagree.

The Fifth Amendment, made applicable to the states through the Fourteenth Amendment, commands that "[n]o person * * * shall be compelled in any criminal case to be a witness against himself." The essence of this basic constitutional principle is "the requirement that the State which proposes to convict *and punish* an individual produce the evidence against him by the independent labor of its officers, not by the simple, cruel expedient of forcing it from his own lips."

The Court has held that "the availability of the [Fifth Amendment] privilege does not turn upon the type of proceeding in which its protection is invoked, but upon the nature of the statement or admission and the exposure which it invites." *In re Gault,* 387 U.S. 1, 49, 87 S.Ct. 1428, 1455, 18 L.Ed.2d 527 (1967). In this case, the ultimate penalty of death was a potential consequence of what respondent told the examining psychiatrist. Just as the Fifth Amendment prevents a criminal defendant from being made " 'the deluded instrument of his own conviction,' " it protects him as well from being made the "deluded instrument" of his own execution.

We can discern no basis to distinguish between the guilt and penalty phases of respondent's capital murder trial so far as the protection of the Fifth Amendment privilege is concerned. Given the gravity of the decision to be made at the penalty phase, the State is not relieved of the obligation to observe fundamental constitutional guarantees. Any effort by the State to compel respondent to testify against his will at the sentencing hearing clearly would contravene the Fifth Amendment. Yet the State's attempt to establish respondent's future dangerousness by relying on the unwarned statements he made to Dr. Grigson similarly infringes Fifth Amendment values.

(2)

The State also urges that the Fifth Amendment privilege is inapposite here because respondent's communications to Dr. Grigson were nontestimonial in nature. The State seeks support from our cases holding that the Fifth Amendment is not violated where the evidence given by a defendant is neither related to some communicative act nor used for the testimonial content of what was said.

However, Dr. Grigson's diagnosis, as detailed in his testimony, was not based simply on his observation of respondent. Rather, Dr. Grigson drew his conclusions largely from respondent's account of the crime during their interview, and he placed particular emphasis on what he considered to be respondent's lack of remorse. Dr. Grigson's prognosis as to future dangerousness rested on statements respondent made, and remarks he omitted, in reciting the details of the crime. The Fifth Amendment privilege, therefore, is directly involved here because the State used as evidence against respondent the substance of his disclosures during the pretrial psychiatric examination.

The fact that respondent's statements were uttered in the context of a psychiatric examination does not automatically remove them from the reach of the Fifth Amendment. The state trial judge, *sua sponte,* ordered a psychiatric evaluation of respondent for the limited, neutral purpose of determining his competency to stand trial, but the results of that inquiry were used by the State for a much broader objective that was plainly adverse to respondent. Consequently, the interview with Dr. Grigson cannot be characterized as a routine competency examination restricted to ensuring that respondent understood the charges against him and was capable of assisting in his defense. Indeed, if the application of Dr. Grigson's findings had been confined to serving that function, no Fifth Amendment issue would have arisen.

Nor was the interview analogous to a sanity examination occasioned by a defendant's plea of not guilty by reason of insanity at the time of his offense. When a defendant asserts the insanity defense and introduces supporting psychiatric testimony, his silence may deprive the State of the only effective means it has of controverting his proof on an issue that he interjected into the case. Accordingly, several Courts of Appeals have held that, under such circumstances, a defendant can be required to submit to a sanity examination conducted by the prosecution's psychiatrist.[10]

Respondent, however, introduced no psychiatric evidence, nor had he indicated that he might do so. Instead, the State offered information obtained from the court-ordered competency examination as affirmative evidence to persuade the jury to return a sentence of death. Respondent's future dangerousness was a critical issue at the sentencing hearing, and one on which the State had the burden of proof beyond a reasonable doubt. See Tex.Code Crim.Proc.Ann., Arts. 37.071(b) and (c) (Vernon Supp.1980). To meet its burden, the State used respondent's own statements, unwittingly made without an awareness that he was assisting the State's efforts to obtain the death penalty. In these distinct circumstances, the Court of Appeals correctly concluded that the Fifth Amendment privilege was implicated.

(3)

In *Miranda v. Arizona,* 384 U.S. 436, 467, 86 S.Ct. 1602, 1624, 16 L.Ed.2d 694 (1966), the Court acknowledged that "the Fifth Amendment privilege is available outside of criminal court proceedings and serves to protect persons in all settings in which their freedom of action is curtailed in any significant way from being compelled to incriminate themselves." *Miranda* held that "the prosecution may not use statements, whether exculpatory or inculpatory, stemming from custodial interrogation of the defendant unless it demonstrates the use of procedural safeguards effective to secure the privilege against self-incrimination." Thus, absent other fully effective procedures, a person in custody must receive certain warnings before any official interrogation,

---

10. On the same theory, the Court of Appeals here carefully left open "the possibility that a defendant who wishes to use psychiatric evidence in his own behalf [on the issue of future dangerousness] can be precluded from using it unless he is [also] willing to be examined by a psychiatrist nominated by the state." 602 F.2d at 705.

including that he has a "right to remain silent" and that "anything said can and will be used against the individual in court." The purpose of these admonitions is to combat what the Court saw as "inherently compelling pressures" at work on the person and to provide him with an awareness of the Fifth Amendment privilege and the consequences of forgoing it, which is the prerequisite for "an intelligent decision as to its exercise."

The considerations calling for the accused to be warned prior to custodial interrogation apply with no less force to the pretrial psychiatric examination at issue here. Respondent was in custody at the Dallas County Jail when the examination was ordered and when it was conducted. That respondent was questioned by a psychiatrist designated by the trial court to conduct a neutral competency examination, rather than by a police officer, government informant, or prosecuting attorney, is immaterial. When Dr. Grigson went beyond simply reporting to the court on the issue of competence and testified for the prosecution at the penalty phase on the crucial issue of respondent's future dangerousness, his role changed and became essentially like that of an agent of the State recounting unwarned statements made in a postarrest custodial setting. During the psychiatric evaluation, respondent assuredly was "faced with a phase of the adversary system" and was "not in the presence of [a] perso[n] acting solely in his interest."

Yet he was given no indication that the compulsory examination would be used to gather evidence necessary to decide whether, if convicted, he should be sentenced to death. He was not informed that, accordingly, he had a constitutional right not to answer the questions put to him.

The Fifth Amendment privilege is "as broad as the mischief against which it seeks to guard," *Counselman v. Hitchcock*, 142 U.S. 547, 562, 12 S.Ct. 195, 198, 35 L.Ed. 1110 (1892), and the privilege is fulfilled only when a criminal defendant is guaranteed the right "to remain silent unless he chooses to speak in the unfettered exercise of his own will, and to suffer no penalty * * * for such silence." We agree with the Court of Appeals that respondent's Fifth Amendment rights were violated by the admission of Dr. Grigson's testimony at the penalty phase.

A criminal defendant, who neither initiates a psychiatric evaluation nor attempts to introduce any psychiatric evidence, may not be compelled to respond to a psychiatrist if his statements can be used against him at a capital sentencing proceeding. Because respondent did not voluntarily consent to the pretrial psychiatric examination after being informed of his right to remain silent and the possible use of his statements, the State could not rely on what he said to Dr. Grigson to establish his future dangerousness. If, upon being adequately warned, respondent had indicated that he would not answer Dr. Grigson's questions, the validly ordered competency examination nevertheless could have proceeded upon the condition that the results would be applied solely for that purpose. In such circumstances, the proper conduct and use of competency and sanity examinations are not frustrated, but the State must make its case on future dangerousness in some other way.

"Volunteered statements * * * are not barred by the Fifth Amendment," but under *Miranda v. Arizona, supra,* we must conclude that, when faced while in custody with a court-ordered psychiatric inquiry, respondent's statements to Dr. Grigson were not "given freely and voluntarily without any compelling influences" and, as such, could be used as the State did at the penalty phase only if respondent had been apprised of his rights and had knowingly decided to waive them. These safeguards of the Fifth Amendment privilege were not afforded respondent and, thus, his death sentence cannot stand.

B

When respondent was examined by Dr. Grigson, he already had been indicted and an attorney had been appointed to represent him. The Court of Appeals concluded that he had a Sixth Amendment right to the assistance of counsel before submitting to the pretrial psychiatric interview. We agree.

The Sixth Amendment, made applicable to the states through the Fourteenth Amendment, provides that "[i]n all criminal prosecutions, the accused shall enjoy the right * * * to have the assistance of counsel for his defense." The "vital" need for a lawyer's advice and aid during the pretrial phase was recognized by the Court nearly 50 years ago in *Powell v. Alabama,* 287 U.S. 45, 57, 71, 53 S.Ct. 55, 60, 65, 77 L.Ed. 158 (1932). Since then, we have held that the right to counsel granted by the Sixth Amendment means that a person is entitled to the help of a lawyer "at or after the time that adversary judicial proceedings have been initiated against him * * * whether by way of formal charge, preliminary hearing, indictment, information, or arraignment."

* * *

Here, respondent's Sixth Amendment right to counsel clearly had attached when Dr. Grigson examined him at the Dallas County Jail,[14] and their interview proved to be a "critical stage" of the aggregate proceedings against respondent. Defense counsel, however, were not

---

14. Because psychiatric examinations of the type at issue here are conducted after adversary proceedings have been instituted, we are not concerned in this case with the limited right to the appointment and presence of counsel recognized as a Fifth Amendment safeguard in *Miranda v. Arizona,* 384 U.S. 436, 471–473, 86 S.Ct. 1602, 1626–1627, 16 L.Ed.2d 694 (1966). See *Edwards v. Arizona,* 451 U.S. 477, 101 S.Ct. 1880, 68 L.Ed.2d 378. Rather, the issue before us is whether a defendant's Sixth Amendment right to the assistance of counsel is abridged when the defendant is not given prior opportunity to consult with counsel about his participation in the psychiatric examination.

Respondent does not assert, and the Court of Appeals did not find, any constitutional right to have counsel actually present during the examination. In fact, the Court of Appeals recognized that "an attorney present during the psychiatric interview could contribute little and might seriously disrupt the examination." 602 F.2d at 708. Cf. *Thornton v. Corcoran,* 132 U.S. App.D.C. 232, 242, 248, 407 F.2d 695, 705, 711 (1969) (opinion concurring in part and dissenting in part).

notified in advance that the psychiatric examination would encompass the issue of their client's future dangerousness, and respondent was denied the assistance of his attorneys in making the significant decision of whether to submit to the examination and to what end the psychiatrist's findings could be employed.

Because "[a] layman may not be aware of the precise scope, the nuances, and the boundaries of his Fifth Amendment privilege," the assertion of that right "often depends upon legal advice from someone who is trained and skilled in the subject matter." As the Court of Appeals observed, the decision to be made regarding the proposed psychiatric evaluation is "literally a life or death matter" and is "difficult * * * even for an attorney" because it requires "a knowledge of what other evidence is available, of the particular psychiatrist's biases and predilections, [and] of possible alternative strategies at the sentencing hearing." It follows logically from our precedents that a defendant should not be forced to resolve such an important issue without "the guiding hand of counsel."

Therefore, in addition to Fifth Amendment considerations, the death penalty was improperly imposed on respondent because the psychiatric examination on which Dr. Grigson testified at the penalty phase proceeded in violation of respondent's Sixth Amendment right to the assistance of counsel.

C

Our holding based on the Fifth and Sixth Amendments will not prevent the State in capital cases from proving the defendant's future dangerousness as required by statute. A defendant may request or consent to a psychiatric examination concerning future dangerousness in the hope of escaping the death penalty. In addition, a different situation arises where a defendant intends to introduce psychiatric evidence at the penalty phase. See n. 10, *supra.*

Moreover, under the Texas capital sentencing procedure, the inquiry necessary for the jury's resolution of the future dangerousness issue is in no sense confined to the province of psychiatric experts.
* * *

* * * While in no sense disapproving the use of psychiatric testimony bearing on the issue of future dangerousness, the inquiry mandated by Texas law does not require resort to medical experts.

III

Respondent's Fifth and Sixth Amendment rights were abridged by the State's introduction of Dr. Grigson's testimony at the penalty phase, and, as the Court of Appeals concluded, his death sentence must be vacated. Because respondent's underlying conviction has not been challenged and remains undisturbed, the State is free to conduct further proceedings not inconsistent with this opinion. Accordingly, the judgment of the Court of Appeals is

Affirmed.

[Concurring opinions by BRENNAN, MARSHALL, and STEWART, JJ., are omitted.]

JUSTICE REHNQUIST, concurring in the judgment.

I concur in the judgment because, under *Massiah v. United States,* 377 U.S. 201, 84 S.Ct. 1199, 12 L.Ed.2d 246 (1964), respondent's counsel should have been notified prior to Dr. Grigson's examination of respondent. As the Court notes * * *, respondent had been indicted and an attorney had been appointed to represent him. Counsel was entitled to be made aware of Dr. Grigson's activities involving his client and to advise and prepare his client accordingly. This is by no means to say that respondent had any right to have his counsel present at any examination. In this regard I join the Court's careful delimiting of the Sixth Amendment issue * * *.

Since this is enough to decide the case, I would not go on to consider the Fifth Amendment issues and cannot subscribe to the Court's resolution of them. I am not convinced that any Fifth Amendment rights were implicated by Dr. Grigson's examination of respondent. Although the psychiatrist examined respondent prior to trial, he only testified concerning the examination after respondent stood convicted. * * *

Even if there are Fifth Amendment rights involved in this case, respondent never invoked these rights when confronted with Dr. Grigson's questions. The Fifth Amendment privilege against compulsory self-incrimination is not self-executing. "Although *Miranda's* requirement of specific warnings creates a limited exception to the rule that the privilege must be claimed, the exception does not apply outside the context of the inherently coercive custodial interrogations for which it was designed." *Roberts v. United States,* 445 U.S. 552, 560, 100 S.Ct. 1358, 1364, 63 L.Ed.2d 622 (1980). The *Miranda* requirements were certainly not designed by this Court with psychiatric examinations in mind. Respondent was simply not in the inherently coercive situation considered in *Miranda.* He had already been indicted, and counsel had been appointed to represent him. No claim is raised that respondent's answers to Dr. Grigson's questions were "involuntary" in the normal sense of the word. Unlike the police officers in *Miranda,* Dr. Grigson was not questioning respondent in order to ascertain his guilt or innocence. Particularly since it is not necessary to decide this case, I would not extend the *Miranda* requirements to cover psychiatric examinations such as the one involved here.

Questions and Comments

1. *State access to the defendant; the necessity of warnings.* Estelle appears to hold that had Dr. Grigson given Smith warnings, to the effect

that he had the right to remain silent and that anything he said could be used against him at a subsequent capital sentencing proceeding, the prosecution could have relied on the results of the interview at that proceeding. Will the typical defendant being evaluated for competency or sanity understand such warnings? Or is the answer to this latter question irrelevant if, as *Estelle* now requires, the defendant's attorney is notified of the evaluation? [p]

More fundamentally, in the typical state-requested evaluation, will *Miranda*-type warnings be accurate? *Estelle* speaks only of when the defendant "neither initiates a psychiatric evaluation nor attempts to introduce any psychiatric evidence." What if, as is more likely to be the case, the defendant has already obtained or is about to obtain an evaluation (either privately or as authorized by *Ake*) and plans to introduce psychiatric testimony? May such a defendant constitutionally remain silent during a state-requested evaluation? Or may the state sanction non-cooperation? Put another way, does the accusatorial paradigm continue to apply or should it give way to the inquisitorial approach? The answers to these questions depend upon the precise issue about which the state is seeking information.

Sanity Evaluations. Assume that the state is seeking evaluation of the defendant's sanity. One of the first decisions to address the implications of the fifth amendment in this context, *Pope v. United States,* 372 F.2d 710 (8th Cir.1967), held that, once the defendant gives formal notice of an intent to raise an insanity defense, the state may compel an evaluation of the defendant; in other words, there is no right to remain silent during a state-requested evaluation once the defense is formally asserted. The court gave two reasons for this result. First, assertion of an insanity defense waives the fifth amendment privilege:

> [B]y raising the issue of insanity, by submitting to psychiatric and psychologic examination by his own examiners, and by presenting evidence as to mental incompetence from the lips of the defendant and these examiners, the defendant raised the issue for all purposes and . . . the government was appropriately granted leave to have the defendant examined by experts of its choice and to present their opinions in evidence.

Second, permitting the defendant to remain silent after asserting the defense would unfairly tip the "state-individual balance" in the defendant's favor:

> It would be a strange situation, indeed, if, first, the government is to be compelled to afford the defense ample psychiatric service and evidence at government expense and, second, if the government is to have the burden of proof, . . . and yet it is to be denied the opportunity to have

---

p. Perhaps relevant here is Colorado v. Connelly, 479 U.S. 157, 107 S.Ct. 515, 93 L.Ed.2d 473 (1986), in which the Court held that, so long as the defendant understands the warnings prior to interrogation by the police, the fact that mental illness may have "compelled" him or her to confess does not render the confession "involuntary" under either the due process clause or *Miranda*; the defendant's mental illness is relevant only to the extent state evidentiary law makes it so in assessing the reliability of the confession. See pp. 930–937 for further discussion of *Connelly*.

its own corresponding and verifying examination, a step which perhaps is the most trustworthy means of attempting to meet the burden.

Both the waiver and fairness rationales have been attacked. As to the waiver rationale, one court has pointed out: "It is difficult to understand how a waiver could be characterized as either voluntary or intentional if automatically triggered by a defendant's assertion of the defense of insanity." *Commonwealth v. Pomponi*, 447 Pa. 154, 160, 284 A.2d 708, 711 (1971). In response to the fairness argument, it has been argued that the prosecution does not require access to the defendant to meet its evidentiary burden but rather can rely on lay witnesses, cross-examination of the defendant's experts, and hypothetical questions addressed to its own experts. Meister, "*Miranda* on the Couch: An Approach to Problems of Self–Incrimination, Right to Counsel and *Miranda* Warnings in Pre–Trial Psychiatric Examinations of Criminal Defendants," 11 Colum.J.L. & Soc.Probs. 403, 425 (1975).

Nonetheless, most courts continue to agree with *Pope,* usually relying on the fairness rationale. The argument that the prosecution does not need its own evaluation of the defendant was forcefully rejected by Justice Scalia in an opinion he wrote while on the District of Columbia Circuit Court of Appeals:

> Appellant and *amici* would have us believe that the mere availability of cross-examination of the defendant's experts is sufficient to provide the necessary balance in the criminal process. That would perhaps be so if psychiatry were as exact a science as physics, so that, assuming the defense psychiatrist precisely described the data (consisting of his interview with the defendant), the error of his analysis could be demonstrated. It is, however, far from that. Ordinarily the only effective rebuttal of psychiatric opinion testimony is contradictory opinion testimony; and for that purpose . . . '[t]he basic tool of psychiatric study remains the personal interview, which requires rapport between the interviewer and the subject.'

> Our judgment that these practical considerations of fair but effective criminal process affect the interpretation and application of the Fifth Amendment privilege against self-incrimination is supported by the long line of Supreme Court precedent holding that the defendant in a criminal or even civil prosecution may not take the stand in his own behalf and then refuse to consent to cross-examination. The justification for this similarly 'coerced' testimony is precisely that which we apply to the present case. As said in *Brown* [*v. United States,* 356 U.S. 148, 78 S.Ct. 622, 2 L.Ed.2d 589 (1958)], a defendant cannot reasonably claim that the Fifth Amendment gives him not only this choice [whether to testify or not] but, if he elects to testify, an immunity from cross-examination on the matters he has himself put in dispute. It would make of the Fifth Amendment not only a humane safeguard against judicially coerced self-disclosure but a positive invitation to mutilate the truth a party offers to tell. . . . The interests of the other party and regard for the function of courts of justice to ascertain the truth become relevant, and prevail in the balance of considerations

determining the scope and limits of the privilege against self-incrimination.

United States v. Byers, 740 F.2d 1104 (D.C.Cir.1984).

Judge Bazelon, in a dissenting opinion in *Byers,* agreed that the fifth
amendment does not necessarily bar the state from obtaining its own post-
notice evaluation. But he argued that because the "state psychiatrist's aim
is diagnosis, not therapy" and "[h]is primary commitment is to his institution, not to his patient," the state-referred evaluation "poses a threat of
coercion similar to that in the interrogation deemed unconstitutional in
Miranda." Thus, he contended that the constitution requires that all such
interviews be taped. This step "would quiet our concern that psychiatrists
might manipulate or intimidate the defendant in an *in camera* interview"
and "help inform the court's judgment regarding the voluntariness and
reliability of the defendant's statement." Scalia responded that such a
requirement is not imposed even on police interrogators and that, in any
event, it stemmed from a concern over reliability, not compulsion; only the
latter is the proper focus of fifth amendment analysis. How should the
debate over the proper scope of the right to remain silent in the post-notice
context be resolved? What, if anything, does *Estelle* say about this issue?

The preceding discussion has focused on state evaluations after notice
of an insanity defense has been given. In many states, the prosecution
may obtain such an evaluation *before* the defendant has given formal notice
of an intent to raise an insanity defense. Should this practice be permitted? Why would the prosecution need such an evaluation? The American
Bar Association's Criminal Justice Mental Health Standards recommend
that, to guarantee the prosecution evaluation results that are "as fresh" as
those obtained by the defense, the state should be notified of a defense
evaluation within 48 hours and should be able to obtain its own evaluation
shortly thereafter. However, the results of this pre-notice evaluation are
to be disclosed to the prosecution only if and when the defense gives formal
notice of an intent to raise an insanity defense. Standard 7–3.4.

Capital Sentencing Evaluations. *Estelle* holds that the fifth amendment applies in the capital sentencing context. Does this mean that the
evaluation procedures applicable in the insanity context also apply to
capital sentencing evaluations? In other words, does *Estelle* hold that the
state is barred from compelling evaluation of the defendant on sentencing
issues such as dangerousness if the defendant does not intend to use clinical
testimony at sentencing? If the defendant *does* present clinical testimony
at the sentencing proceeding, but limits it to responsibility issues having to
do with culpability at the time of the offense, may the state compel an
evaluation of the defendant to determine propensity, i.e., dangerousness, or
is its examiner limited to addressing responsibility issues?

Other Contexts. In a footnote, the Court in *Estelle* cautioned that it
was not holding "that the same Fifth Amendment concerns are necessarily
presented by all types of interviews and examinations that might be
ordered or relied upon to inform a sentencing determination." 451 U.S. at
469 n. 13, 101 S.Ct. at 1876 n. 13. Thus, whether the defendant can refuse
to cooperate with a state-requested evaluation in the typical noncapital
sentencing context is unresolved. The Court *has* made clear, in *Allen v.*

Illinois, 478 U.S. 364, 106 S.Ct. 2988, 92 L.Ed.2d 296 (1986), that the fifth amendment does not apply to "special" sentencing evaluations and proceedings conducted pursuant to mentally disordered sex offender (MDSO) statutes, because the primary purpose of such statutes is "treatment", not punishment. For the same reason, the fifth amendment does not apply to competency to stand trial or civil commitment evaluations and proceedings. For present purposes,[q] the importance of *Allen* is that the state may compel an evaluation of the defendant in any of these contexts, at least when, as discussed below, the results of the evaluation are used only to adjudicate the issue for which the evaluation is sought.

2. *Sanctions.* In situations where there is no right to remain silent, but the defendant still refuses to cooperate,[r] a sanction is necessary. In insanity cases, the courts have imposed four different types of sanctions. They have: (1) prohibited the defendant from presenting any evidence of insanity; (2) allowed the defendant to make the insanity claim, but prohibited use of expert testimony to support it; (3) allowed the defendant to present clinical testimony but only that which is based on facts that were revealed to the state's expert as well (in those cases where there was partial, but not complete cooperation); and (4) allowed the defendant to present unrestricted clinical testimony but also allowed the prosecution to inform the factfinder about the defendant's refusal to cooperate with the state's expert. See Slobogin, *"Estelle v. Smith :* The Constitutional Contours of the Forensic Evaluation," 31 Emory L.J. 71, 103–104 (1981). Which option is fairest to both sides? Do any of these sanctions work when the defendant refuses to cooperate at an evaluation of competency to stand trial or on civil commitment issues? What would be an appropriate sanction in such situations?

3. *Use of evaluation results.* An issue separate from determining when the state may compel a defendant to undergo an evaluation is when, and for what purpose, the state may use the results of any evaluations that have taken place. Even when a compelled evaluation is permissible, prosecution use of its results may be limited or barred altogether. For instance, while the prosecution may compel the defendant to undergo a competency to stand trial evaluation, it may not, in most states, use the results of the evaluation for any purpose other than adjudication of competency. See, e.g., West's Fla.R.Crim.Proc. 3.211(e). Is such an approach required under *Estelle?* If not, should it be?

Most states have a similar rule with respect to the use of results from evaluations of mental state at the time of the offense. The federal rule is perhaps the most comprehensive:

q. *Allen* is reprinted at pp. 730–735, where its implications for civil commitment are discussed.

r. Defining "non-cooperation" is a difficult issue. As one court has stated:

The fact, amply demonstrated over the years, is that a failure of a defendant who pleads insanity . . . to cooperate most often reflects an even greater de-gree of insanity rather than less. He is not always controllable by his lawyer, and many a psychotic defendant, who may or may not be legally insane, refuses to be represented by a lawyer. In short, non-cooperation may be evidence of insanity.

Lee v. County Ct., 27 N.Y.2d 432, 448–492, 267 N.E.2d 452, 461–62, 318 N.Y.S.2d 705, 719 (1971).

> No statement made by the defendant in the course of any [psychiatric] examination . . ., whether the examination be with or without the consent of the defendant, no testimony by the expert based upon such statement, and no other fruits of the statement shall be admitted in evidence against the defendant in any criminal proceeding except on an issue respecting mental condition on which the defendant has introduced testimony.

Fed.R.Crim.Pro. 12.2. This rule prohibits three things: (1) prosecution use of evaluation results when the defendant has not asserted a clinically-based defense or claim; (2) when such a claim is asserted, prosecution use of evaluation results for purposes other than rebuttal of that claim (e.g., use of an evaluator solely to establish that the defendant committed the criminal act); (3) prosecution use of evidence derived from the results of the evaluation (e.g., introduction of a murder weapon discovered as a result of leads developed solely from the psychiatric evaluation). Is there a reason other than fear of compulsion or manipulation by the expert which underlies this extensive protection?

Even this degree of protection may not satisfy the dictates of the fifth amendment. For instance, if an insanity defense is raised, expert testimony is very likely to recount in detail the defendant's actions at the time of the offense. In cases where the defendant readily admits he or she committed the criminal act, such testimony presumably does not present a problem. But what if the defendant asserts not only an insanity defense, but also a "factual" defense (e.g., self-defense)? In jurisdictions where such dual pleading is permitted, the state's expert may disclose information, highly prejudicial to the factual defense, which was obtained during a compelled evaluation. Courts have resorted to two practices in such a situation. The first is an instruction to the jury cautioning that the expert testimony is to be considered only on the issue of insanity. The second is bifurcation of the trial, with the first stage addressing the factual defense, and the second addressing, if necessary, the insanity defense. The expert testimony would be deferred until the second stage, thus avoiding revelation of disclosures that were compelled from the defendant at a psychiatric evaluation during adjudication of the factual defense.

Should the rules with respect to using evaluation results change if the results come from a *defense*-requested evaluation? In Buchanan v. Kentucky, 483 U.S. 402, 107 S.Ct. 2906, 97 L.Ed.2d 336 (1987), the prosecution rebutted the defendant's psychiatric defense with the results of a post-offense evaluation that was conducted to determine whether the defendant required psychiatric hospitalization and was competent to stand trial; the evaluation had been jointly requested by the prosecution and the defense. The Supreme Court found no constitutional violation because, unlike in *Estelle*, the defendant had raised a psychiatric defense and the defendant had joined in the evaluation motion. Is *Buchanan* correctly decided? What are the possible consequences of the decision?

4. *The right to counsel.* According to *Estelle*, the sixth amendment's guarantee of a right to counsel "in all criminal prosecutions" requires that, after the initiation of formal proceedings against the defendant, any state-requested evaluation of the defendant must be preceded by notice to

counsel. Accord, Satterwhite v. Texas, 486 U.S. 249, 108 S.Ct. 1792, 100 L.Ed.2d 284 (1988). Presumably, this notice will permit counsel to explain the purpose of the evaluation to the defendant and to advise him or her whether to cooperate with the evaluator. However, the Supreme Court specifically avoided deciding whether there is a right to counsel's *presence* during the evaluation; if anything, it expressed some distaste for the idea. See n. 14.

Determining whether there should be a right to presence of counsel at state-requested evaluations is made difficult by the Court's somewhat muddled approach to the right to counsel generally. Under *United States v. Wade,* 388 U.S. 218, 87 S.Ct. 1926, 18 L.Ed.2d 1149 (1967), cited by *Estelle,* the right to counsel attached at any stage of the criminal prosecution which is deemed "critical"—that is, any stage where "the presence of counsel is necessary to preserve the defendant's basic right to a fair trial as affected by his right meaningfully to cross-examine the witnesses against him and to have effective assistance of counsel at the trial itself." In *Wade,* the Court found a right to counsel at post-indictment lineup identifications because (1) "the trial which might determine the accused's fate may well be not that in the courtroom but at the pretrial confrontation"; (2) "there is a serious difficulty in depicting what transpires at lineups", particularly if "the jury's choice is between the accused's unsupported version and that of the police officers present"; and (3) the "vagaries of eyewitness identification are well-known." If counsel is not present to observe, and thus enabled to reconstruct at trial, any irregularities in the identification process, these three factors create "a grave risk of erroneous conviction."

Wade's critical stage analysis was significantly modified, however, by United States v. Ash, 413 U.S. 300, 93 S.Ct. 2568, 37 L.Ed.2d 619 (1973), in which the Court found no right to counsel when the police show a witness photo displays for purposes of identification. Rejecting *Wade's* emphasis on whether the procedure in question might prejudice the defendant and whether counsel could alleviate the prejudice, the Court concluded that instead the key inquiry should be whether the procedure involves a "trial-like confrontation"—that is, whether it confronts the accused with the "intricacies of the law and the advocacy of the public prosecutor." *Wade's* approach, the Court stated, would give the right to counsel too broad a scope; as an example, the Court mentioned that critical stage analysis would improperly entitle the defendant to counsel at prosecutorial interviews of the victim and other witnesses.

Ash seemed to establish trial-like confrontation analysis as the test for the right to counsel. Yet, in *United States v. Henry,* 447 U.S. 264, 100 S.Ct. 2183, 65 L.Ed.2d 115 (1980), the Court held the right to counsel was violated when the government, after indictment, posted an informer in the defendant's prison cell, even though this ploy clearly did not involve a "trial-like confrontation".

Whether they apply the critical stage test or the trial-like confrontation test, most courts have held there is no right to have counsel present during state-requested clinical evaluations. Comment, "The Right to Counsel During Court–Ordered Psychiatric Examinations of Criminal Defendants," 26 Vill.L.Rev. 135 (1980). United States v. Byers, supra, is again illustrative. Then–Judge Scalia, relying on *Ash*, concluded for the majority that there is no right to counsel at a post-notice insanity evaluation. The defendant who has been advised of his or her rights by counsel prior to the evaluation "ha[s] no decisions in the nature of legal strategy or tactics to make" during the evaluation. Moreover, the "examining psychiatrist is not an adversary" or "expert in 'the intricacies of substantive and procedural criminal law.'" Scalia also registered practical objections to having counsel present during the evaluation:

> The 'procedural system' of the law, which is one justification for the presence of counsel and which, by the same token, the presence of counsel brings in its train, is evidently antithetical to psychiatric examination, a process informal and unstructured by design. Even if counsel were uncharacteristically to sit silent and interpose no procedural objections or suggestions, one can scarcely imagine a successful psychiatric examination in which the subject's eyes move back and forth between the doctor and his attorney. Nor would it help if the attorney were listening from outside the room, for the subject's attention would still wander where his eyes could not. And the attorney's presence in such a purely observational capacity, without ability to advise, suggest or object, would have no relationship to the Sixth Amendment's 'Assistance of Counsel.'

The latter observation also led Scalia to find, as he already had with respect to the fifth amendment, that the sixth amendment does not require taping of state-requested evaluations. He concluded: "It is enough, as far as the constitutional minima of the criminal process are concerned, that the defendant has the opportunity to contest the accuracy of witnesses' testimony by cross-examining them at trial, and introducing his own witnesses in rebuttal."

If *Wade* were applicable, how would you evaluate the result in *Byers*? Accepting *Ash* as the governing precedent, is Scalia's characterization of the psychiatrist as a non-adversary realistic? Is it consistent with *Estelle's* characterization of Dr. Grigson? Is it possible that the psychiatrist could be an "adversary" for fifth amendment purposes but not sixth amendment purposes? If so, does this mean there *is* a right to presence of counsel at *pre*-indictment state-requested evaluations (where the sixth amendment does not apply but *Miranda* clearly does), but not at *post*-indictment evaluations?

5. *Summary problems on evaluation issues.* How would you rule in the following scenarios and why? What are the counterarguments to your conclusions?

A. Assume Jones, charged with second degree murder, hires three mental health professionals to evaluate his sanity at the time of the offense. He then notifies the court and the prosecution that he intends to raise an insanity defense and that he intends to use the first two experts to support the defense. The prosecution wants to subpoena the third expert. Jones objects.

B. Same facts as A. The prosecution also wants to compel an evaluation of Jones. Jones objects.

C. The court grants the prosecution's motion in B. Jones's attorney requests to be present during the evaluation. The state objects.

D. At the state-requested evaluation, Jones will not talk about the day of the offense, claiming the state's expert is a CIA agent intent on "stealing my mind." The prosecution asks the court to sanction Jones.

E. Smith, who is indigent, is charged with capital murder. He has no documented history of mental disorder, but his attorney claims that Smith is suffering from severe depression and that the depression affects his ability to communicate at the present time and affected his behavior at the time of the offense. The attorney moves for a state-paid evaluation of Smith's competency to stand trial, his sanity, and issues related to capital sentencing, including whether he was under emotional stress at the time of the offense and his treatability. He specifically requests Dr. Black as the evaluator. Dr. Black is a private psychiatrist whose rates are very high. The state argues that Smith is not entitled to an evaluation of any sort and that, even if he is, an evaluation at the state hospital would be sufficient.

F. The court orders that Smith be evaluated at the state hospital on the competency, sanity and sentencing issues. Smith moves that the results of this evaluation be sent only to him. The state objects, arguing that it is entitled to the results as well.

G. The motion in F is granted. Smith indicates he will use expert testimony only at sentencing. The state moves for an evaluation on the competency issue. In support of its motion, the state points to the defense attorney's representations in E. Smith objects.

H. The court grants the state's motion in G. Smith is found competent to stand trial, tried and convicted of capital murder. At his capital sentencing proceeding he presents expert testimony to the effect that he was under extreme emotional distress at the time of the offense as a result of severe depression and that, with proper care, the prognosis for his condition is good. The state wants to introduce expert testimony, based on the results of the competency evaluation it obtained, that Smith is dangerous; dangerousness is an aggravating circumstance under the state's capital punishment statute. Smith objects, noting that no warnings were given him prior to the state's evaluation and that, in any event, he "opened the door" only on mitigation issues.

2. *Hearsay and Other Evidentiary Considerations*

Rarely will the testifying mental health professional have observed directly all of the behavioral or biological evidence upon which he or she relies. For instance, in evaluating a criminal accused who has asserted an insanity defense, the mental health professional will not only interview the defendant, but interview, or obtain statements made by, family, friends and witnesses of the alleged offense. Various types of records—medical, psychological, criminal, educational, and occupational—will be acquired. Clinical reports from other mental health professionals (e.g., psychological test results, social histories) are also usually obtained.

Unless the individuals who possess or created this information are produced at trial, the evidence is "hearsay"—that is, statements from declarants who are not in court. Hearsay is generally considered inadmissible because the declarant cannot be subjected to cross-examination. Federal Rule of Evidence, Rule 802. Of course, there are several exceptions to this rule. For instance, pre-trial statements by the person who is the subject of legal proceedings are admissible, even if the person does not take the witness stand and undergo cross-examination, under the party admissions exception.[s] Documentary information may also be admissible under the so-called "business records" exception to the hearsay rule, if the custodian of the record or "other qualified witness" can attest to the fact that the document was kept as a regular practice of the business or profession.[t] But much of the third party information which mental health professionals rely upon is hearsay for which there is not a traditionally accepted exception. The following case addresses this problem.

UNITED STATES v. SIMS

United States Court of Appeals, Ninth Circuit, 1975.
514 F.2d 147.

* * *

The substance of this appeal . . . involves the opinion expressed by a psychiatrist who testified for [the Government]. His opening testimony revealed that he based his opinion regarding appellant's mental state on his own examination of appellant, other psychiatric reports, and information derived from conversations with Government attorneys and IRS agents. The Government psychiatrist concluded that there was no evidence to support the contention that appellant lacked the capacity to appreciate the wrongfulness of his acts or to conform his conduct to the law. He added that appellant's "excessive amount of religiosity" was not "delusional thinking."

During cross-examination, appellant's counsel questioned the psychiatrist concerning the basis for his opinion, specifically in regard to appellant's pre–1971 conduct, which counsel contended to be free from aberration. "[I]s it a fact . . . that at least from the facts we know, that Mr. Sims had been practicing as a tax preparer, according to information you have, for at least ten years before he had any difficulty

---

s. Under the federal rules, if the party admission is offered *against* the party, then it is not hearsay to begin with. Rule 801(d)(2).

t. Rule 803(6) creates an exception to the hearsay rule for records of regularly conducted activity, i.e.: "[a] memorandum, report, record, or data compilation, in any form, of acts, events, conditions, opinions, or diagnoses, made at or near the time by, or from information transmitted by, a person with knowledge, if kept in the course of a regularly conducted business activity, and if it was the regular practice of that business activity to make the memorandum, report, record, or data compilation, all as shown by the testimony of the custodian or other qualified witness, unless the source of information or the method or circumstances of preparation indicate lack of trustworthiness. The term "business" as used in this paragraph includes business, institution, association, profession, occupation, and calling of every kind, whether or not conducted for profit."

with the law[?]" asked appellant's counsel. The psychiatrist then revealed that he had learned from IRS agents that appellant had been investigated for "alleged irregularities" prior to 1971. He added that this information was taken into account in reaching his opinion on appellant's sanity. The information came solely from out-of-court sources.[1]

The court thereupon *sua sponte* admonished the jury to consider the hearsay evidence only ". . . with reference to the basis for the doctor's opinion . . ." and not ". . . in any way in a determination as to whether the defendant did or did not commit the offenses that are charged. . . ."

Appellant moved that the Government psychiatrist's entire testimony be stricken because it was based on hearsay evidence unavailable to appellant prior to trial. The motion was denied, as was appellant's motion for a mistrial, thus forming the basis of this appeal.

* * *

The traditional rule is that an expert opinion is inadmissible if it is based upon information obtained out of court from third parties. The rationale behind this rule is that the trier of fact should not be presented with evidence grounded on otherwise inadmissible hearsay statements not subject to cross-examination and other forms of verification.

However, recent decisions, especially in the Federal courts, indicate there is a strong emerging trend in favor of admissibility. The new rule has been endorsed as the better reasoned and preferable approach in McCormick, Evidence § 15 (1972). *See also* 3 Wigmore, Evidence § 688 (1970).

The rationale in favor of the admissibility of expert testimony based on hearsay is that the expert is fully capable of judging for himself what is, or is not, a reliable basis for his opinion. This relates directly to one of the functions of the expert witness, namely to lend his special expertise to the issue before him. In so doing, various experts customarily rely on evidence not independently admissible in the courtroom. [T]he opinion ". . . is regarded as evidence in its own right and not as hearsay in disguise." In a sense, the expert synthesizes the primary source material—be it hearsay or not—into properly admissible evidence in opinion form. The trier of fact is then capable of judging the credibility of the witness as it would that of anyone else giving expert testimony. This rule respects the functions and abilities

1. The hardcore of the testimony here under challenge is as follows:

*   *   *   *   *

"Q Did some investigating agent tell you that Mr. Sims may have been in some difficulty before 1971 with the law?

*   *   *   *   *

"A Yes.

*   *   *   *   *

"Q This was in the private interview with these agents—

"A Yes.

"Q —that you had, and these private interviews and this private information is one of the reasons you reached this opinion?

"A It was taken into account in reaching an opinion, yes."

of both the expert witness and the trier of fact, while assuring that the requirement of witness confrontation is fulfilled.

Fully consistent with this view, though not yet controlling, is Rule 703 of the Federal Rules of Evidence for the United States Courts and Magistrates, effective July 1, 1975, which reads:

"The facts or data in the particular case upon which an expert bases an opinion or inference may be those perceived by or made known to him at or before the hearing. If of a type reasonably relied upon by experts in the particular field in forming opinions or inferences upon the subject, the facts or data need not be admissible in evidence." 65 F.R.D. 139, 152.

The rule merely codifies the law recently stated in the above-cited authorities.

It seems logical that an expert, such as a psychiatrist in formulating an opinion in a case such as this, should be permitted to interview the agents who made the investigation leading up to the indictment and secure from them relevant facts developed during the investigation. Because of his professional background, knowledge, and experience, we should, in circumstances such as these, leave to the expert the assessment of the reliability of the statements on which he bases his expert opinion. He should not be precluded, in forming an opinion, from interviewing those who for one reason or another have had occasion to investigate and study the defendant's background. Years of experience teach the expert to separate the wheat from the chaff and to use only those sources and kinds of information which are of a type reasonably relied upon by similar experts in arriving at sound opinions on the subject.

We do not open the gates to a wholesale use of all types of hearsay in formulating expert opinions. We only approve the use of that type of information upon which experts may reasonably rely. This follows the spirit of the Federal Rules of Evidence, *supra*. Upon admission of such evidence, it then, of course, becomes necessary for the court to instruct the jury that the hearsay evidence is to be considered solely as a basis for the expert opinion and not as substantive evidence. This the district court here did *sua sponte*.

CONCLUSION

After thorough consideration of all relevant factors, we conclude that no error was committed in admitting the expert's opinion. Finding no error, we affirm the district court's conviction of appellant.

Affirmed.

Questions and Comments

1. *Rule 703.* As the *Sims* court notes, Rule 703 significantly modifies the traditional rule. The Advisory Committee's Note on the new rule justified this change with the following words:

[The] rule is designed . . . to bring the judicial practice into line with the practice of the experts themselves when not in court. Thus a physician in his own practice bases his diagnosis on information from numerous sources and of considerable variety, including statements by patients and relatives, reports and opinions from nurses, technicians and other doctors, hospital records, and X rays. Most of them are admissible in evidence, but only with the expenditure of substantial time in producing and examining various authenticating witnesses. The physician makes life-and-death decisions in reliance upon them. His validation, expertly performed and subject to cross-examination, ought to suffice for judicial purposes.

56 F.R.D. 183, 283.

Are the Committee's rationale and the *Sims* court's reasoning persuasive when the expert testimony at issue is from mental health professionals? See Note, "Hearsay Bases of Psychiatric Opinion Testimony: A Critique of Federal Rule of Evidence 703," 51 S.Cal.L.Rev. 129 (1977). What if, for instance, the hearsay is an account of the defendant's early childhood from the defendant's parents? A description of apparently illegal conduct committed by the defendant, related to the clinician by the victim (or, as in *Sims*, by an IRS agent)? A diagnosis given the defendant ten years ago by a psychiatrist?

2. *Other bases for testimony.* Information which forms the basis of a clinical opinion may be inadmissible for reasons other than the hearsay rule. For instance, mental health professionals sometimes administer sodium amytal (a disinhibiting drug) or use hypnosis during their interview process. Although such techniques are not viewed as "truth determinants" by experienced clinicians, they may provide valuable information that the subject has "repressed" or "suppressed." Packer, "The Use of Hypnotic Techniques in the Evaluation of Criminal Defendants," 305, 319–20 (1981). The statements of a person who is under the influence of hypnosis or amytal are usually barred, not on hearsay grounds (because the statements are usually party admissions), but because of the unreliability of the technique used. See, e.g., *State v. Pierce*, 263 S.C. 23, 207 S.E.2d 414 (1974); *State v. Chase*, 206 Kan. 352, 480 P.2d 62 (1971). The courts that reach this result generally rely on some version of the *Frye* rule, discussed in sections IIB and C of this chapter.

Evidence may also be excluded for constitutional reasons. For instance, soon after the attempted assassination of President Reagan, John Hinckley's hotel room in Washington, D.C. was searched and a diary, containing a wealth of information relevant to his mental state, was discovered. The trial court held that since the police did not have a warrant or probable cause at the time of the search, the diary was inadmissible.

3. *Explaining the opinion.* Suppose a clinician offers an opinion based in whole or in part on hearsay, the results of an amytal or hypnosis interview, or illegally seized evidence. Suppose further that the court finds that the evidence is not independently admissible, but that it is of the type reasonably relied upon by mental health professionals. Should the court allow the opinion but exclude the evidence? See Greenfield v. Common-

wealth, 214 Va. 710, 204 S.E.2d 414 (1974). Or should it, like the court in *Sims*, allow both the opinion and the statements, with an instruction telling the jury that the problems with the latter should be considered only in evaluating the strength of the opinion? See Spector & Foster, "Admissibility of Hypnotic Statements: Is the Law of Evidence Susceptible?" 38 Ohio St.L.J. 568, 597–601 (1977). Under the first approach, how is the clinician to explain the opinion? Under the second, can the jury be trusted to follow the instruction?

4. *Judicial monitoring of evaluation process.* A final issue which could arise under Rule 703 is whether a clinical opinion is admissible when the facts undergirding it, although "reasonably relied upon", are so minimal that most clinicians would consider them an insufficient basis for an opinion. For instance, one study of the civil commitment process in a midwestern city found that clinicians often perform only cursory evaluations and seem to assume the person is ill. Scheff, "The Societal Reaction to Deviance: Ascriptive Elements in the Psychiatric Screening of Mental Patients in a Midwestern State," 11 Social Probs. 401 (1964). As another example, the evaluation procedures of Dr. Grigson, the psychiatrist who testified in *Estelle v. Smith* and *Barefoot v. Estelle*, appear to fall far short of the ideal. In *Estelle,* he conducted a 90–minute interview on the basis of which he purported to be able to deliver opinions about not only the subject's dangerousness but also his competency to stand trial and sanity. *Estelle v. Smith,* 451 U.S. 454, 457, 459–60, 101 S.Ct. 1866, 1870, 1871, 68 L.Ed.2d 359 (1981). In *Barefoot,* he based his opinion about the defendant's dangerousness on a brief hypothetical question. Yet, according to Monahan, a comprehensive evaluation of dangerousness would include a personal interview, as well as data collection designed to investigate the person's history, future environment, reactions to stress, and base rate for violence based on actuarial factors. Monahan, The Clinical Prediction of Violent Behavior 101–23 (NIMH, 1981).

The mental health professions have yet formally to establish even minimum standards for forensic evaluations. Until they do, the courts are unlikely to hold that any particular evaluation procedure provides an unreasonably small amount of data upon which to base an opinion. Cf. Monahan & Walker, "Social Science Research in Law: A New Paradigm," 43 Am.Psychol. 564 (1988) (arguing that the methodology of social science research should be evaluated by judges, relying on information provided by social scientists, and that their decisions about the adequacy of methodology should have the force of precedent).

5. *Differing contexts.* It should be noted that in some settings the hearsay rule and other exclusionary evidence rules may not apply with the same force as they do in criminal cases. For instance, some courts have held that hearsay is admissible in civil commitment proceedings. This position might have an impact on Rule 703 analysis (see Chapter Eight).

D. THE ULTIMATE ISSUE ISSUE

One final limitation on expert testimony may exist, even if one assumes that clinical opinion testimony is generally admissible, and even if it is offered by a qualified mental health professional who has relied solely on permissible sources of information. Traditionally, a witness, whether expert or lay, was barred from addressing the "ultimate" legal issue (e.g., in this context, sanity, competency, or committability). Usually, the reason given for this rule was that such an opinion usurped the function of the factfinder. As originally promulgated, Federal Rule 704 specifically did away with the ultimate issue limitation on testimony. It stated: "Testimony in the form of an opinion or inference otherwise admissible is not objectionable because it embraces an ultimate issue to be decided by the trier of fact." The Advisory Committee justified this change for two reasons. First, it contended that the rule was impossible to enforce, because witnesses would merely paraphrase their testimony in an effort to avoid the ultimate issue language. Second, it noted that the old rule tended to deprive the factfinder of helpful testimony. "Thus . . . in cases of medical causation, witnesses were sometimes required to couch their opinions in cautious phrases of 'might or could,' rather than 'did,' though the result was to deprive many opinions of the positiveness to which they were entitled, accompanied by the hazard of a ruling of insufficiency to support a verdict." The Committee also pointed out that opinion testimony must still be helpful to the trier of fact under Rules 701 and 702, which should "afford ample assurances against the admission of opinions which would merely tell the jury what result to reach . . . [or which are] phrased in terms of inadequately explored legal criteria." 56 F.R.D. 183, 284.

However, in 1984, largely in response to the outcome of John Hinckley's trial, Congress added paragraph (b) to Rule 704. It reads: "No expert witness testifying with respect to the mental state or condition of a defendant in a criminal case may state an opinion or inference as to whether the defendant did or did not have the mental state or condition constituting an element of the crime charged or of a defense thereto. Such ultimate issues are matters for the trier of fact alone." The purpose of this amendment to Rule 704, according to the Report of the House Committee on the Judiciary, "is to eliminate the confusing spectacle of competing expert witnesses testifying to directly contradictory conclusions as to the ultimate legal issue to be found by the trier of fact." H.R.Report 98–1030, 98th cong., 2d Sess., p. 230.

In reading the following case, think about whether it makes sense for Congress to have singled out clinical testimony in this way.

UNITED STATES v. EDWARDS

United States Court of Appeals, Eleventh Circuit, 1987.
819 F.2d 262.

*   *   *

VANCE, CIRCUIT JUDGE:

Roland Edwards was charged with unarmed bank robbery under 18 U.S.C. § 2113(a). He pleaded not guilty by reason of insanity. After a two day trial, a jury returned a verdict of guilty. Edwards appeals, claiming that the district court allowed improper psychiatric testimony. He argues that the district court erred in permitting a government witness to give opinion testimony in violation of Fed.R.Evid. 704(b). We affirm.

*   *   *

At trial Edwards did not contest his role in the bank robbery, but argued that he was insane at the time that he committed the offense. Edwards' ex-wife and an old friend testified that they believed Edwards to be incapable of criminal activity. The crux of the defense case, however, was the testimony of Doctor Adolfo Vilasuso, a board-certified psychiatrist. Doctor Vilasuso examined Edwards approximately six times during October, 1985 and continued seeing Edwards once or twice a week up to the date of trial in February, 1986. Doctor Vilasuso noted that Edwards had endured a difficult past and stated that he thought Edwards was "off the wall." Doctor Vilasuso testified that he had a "very, very strong suspicion" that Edwards suffered from "manic-depressive" illness during April, 1984. The government countered with the rebuttal testimony of Doctor Albert Jaslow, another psychiatrist. Doctor Jaslow concluded from Edwards' description of events that Edwards was not in "an active manic state" at the time of the robbery because Edwards' actions were reasonably well controlled and goal directed.

The testimony at issue concerns Doctor Jaslow's analysis of Edwards' frustration with his financial problems at the time of the robbery:

Q [by Prosecutor]:
     What sort of things were going on that would have depressed him?

A [by Doctor Jaslow]:
     His inability to come to grips with his financial problems; inability to handle the relationship with the I.R.S., who were after him and who were not permitting him to, according to him, of course, to settle down sufficiently so he could gain enough monies to take care of the financial problems and so on. These were bothering him tremendously, of course.

Q: Were these feelings understandable, in your opinion?

Defense Counsel: Objection. It's improper. That's not a proper question for a doctor.

The Court: Overruled.

A: Under the circumstances of the responsibilities, the problems that he had, it was quite understandable. He would be disturbed; it was quite understandable he would be upset. It's quite understandable he would be frantically trying to find ways to modify his situation so he could get on with his life.

Edwards contends that the trial court erred in allowing this testimony because it contained a psychiatrist's opinion concerning his sanity, the ultimate issue at trial. We disagree. "In resolving the complex issue of criminal responsibility, it is of critical importance that the defendant's entire relevant symptomatology be brought before the jury and explained." It has long been the position of our court that this is the only way a jury may become sufficiently informed so as to make a determination of a defendant's legal sanity. This was also the attitude of Congress when it passed Rule 704(b):

> Psychiatrists, of course, must be permitted to testify fully about the defendant's diagnosis, mental state and motivation (in clinical and commonsense terms) at the time of the alleged act so as to permit the jury or judge to reach the ultimate conclusion about which they and only they are expert.

Congress did not enact Rule 704(b) so as to limit the flow of diagnostic and clinical information. Every actual fact concerning the defendant's mental condition is still as admissible after the enactment of Rule 704(b) as it was before. Rather, the Rule "changes the style of question and answer that can be used to establish both the offense and the defense thereto." The prohibition is directed at a narrowly and precisely defined evil:

> When, however, "ultimate issue" questions are formulated by the law and put to the expert witness who must then say "yea" or "nay," then the expert witness is required to make a leap in logic. He no longer addresses himself to medical concepts but instead must infer or intuit what is in fact unspeakable, namely, the probable relationship between medical concepts and legal or moral constructs such as free will. These impermissible leaps in logic made by expert witnesses confuse the jury.

S.Rep. No. 225, 98th Cong., 1st Sess. 231 (quoting APA Statement on the Insanity Defense, Dec. 1982, at 18), *reprinted in* 1984 U.S.Code Cong. & Admin.News 3182, 3412–18. Accordingly, Rule 704(b) forbids only "conclusions as to the ultimate legal issue to be found by the trier of fact." *Id.* at 3412. See, e.g., *United States v. Hillsberg,* 812 F.2d 328, 331 (7th Cir.1987) (expert cannot state opinion as to whether defendant had the capacity to conform his conduct to the law); *United States v. Buchbinder,* 796 F.2d 910, 917 (7th Cir.1986) (expert could not testify as to whether defendant had the requisite mental state to defraud, but could testify as to the extent of defendant's depression over son's death).

The ultimate legal issue at Edwards' trial was whether Edwards "lack[ed] substantial capacity either to appreciate the wrongfulness of his conduct or to conform his conduct to the requirements of law." In fact, the challenged statements offer no conclusions at all about Edwards. Doctor Jaslow was simply observing that people who are not insane can nevertheless become frantic over a financial crisis.

The prosecution placed Doctor Jaslow on the stand to dispute Doctor Vilasuso's diagnosis. Using a common sense generalization, Doctor Jaslow explained why the defendant's behavior—his frantic efforts to pay bills, his manifestations of energy, his lack of sleep, and his feelings of depression—did not necessarily indicate an active manic state. We think that the doctor played exactly the kind of role which Congress contemplated for the expert witness:

> [I]t is clear that the psychiatrist's first obligation and expertise in the courtroom is to "do psychiatry," i.e., to present medical information and opinion about the defendant's mental state and motivation and to explain in detail the reason for his medical-psychiatric conclusions.

S.Rep. No. 225, supra, at 3413. We conclude that the district court committed no error in permitting this testimony.

AFFIRMED.

Questions and Comments

1. *Justification for the ultimate issue ban.* The *Edwards* court quotes the American Psychiatric Association to the effect that testimony on the ultimate issue involves the expert in a "leap of logic" from medical concepts to legal or moral ones. If Dr. Jaslow had testified that Edwards could appreciate the wrongfulness of the robbery or control his behavior at that time, would his testimony have intruded more into moral considerations than his actual testimony? How does one draw the line between "medical" or "clinical" concepts on the one hand, and moral concepts on the other? Does the language of Rule 704(b) help? Is Rule 704(b) necessary, given the existence of Rule 702 (requiring expert testimony to be based on specialized knowledge, skill, education, etc.)?

2. *The ABA position.* Ultimate legal language can usually be subdivided into two types. "Ultimate" conclusions directly address the dispositive legal issue, e.g., whether a person is or is not "incompetent", "insane", "committable" and so on. In contrast, a penultimate conclusion does not reach this level of generalization but only speaks to the relevant legal test: for example, testimony that, under the American Law Institute test for insanity, a person accused of crime does or does not "as a result of mental disease or defect, lack substantial capacity to understand the wrongfulness of his act or to conform his behavior to the requirements of the law." Rule 704(b) is apparently meant to bar both types of testimony in federal court. The American Bar Association, on the other hand, distinguishes between the two. While barring testimony on the ultimate issue, the ABA would permit penultimate testimony, at least in insanity cases, because the language of the legal test (e.g., concerning a person's ability to "appreciate" the wrongfulness of his or her acts) expresses a concept which has clinical content. However, the ABA would forbid use of such language if statutory provisions or appellate decisions have given it particular legal content. American Bar Association, Criminal Justice Mental Health Standards, commentary to standard 7–6.6, pp. 336–338 (Little, Brown: 1987). Is the ABA claiming that penultimate testimony does not involve a moral issue, or that it combines clinical and moral issues? Whatever the answer to this question, why does further definition of the penultimate language through statute or appellate decision change the situation?

3. *Ultimate language and the adversary process.* As noted, the reason given by Congress for adopting Rule 704(b) is the desire "to eliminate the confusing spectacle of competing expert witnesses testifying to directly contradictory conclusions as to the ultimate legal issue to be found by the trier of fact." Aren't contradictory conclusions the inevitable result of the adversary process? On the other hand, if a proceeding is *not* effectively adversarial (as is often true with competency and commitment determinations, for instance), should the expert be allowed to give *any* opinion (legal or otherwise)? See Slobogin, "The 'Ultimate Issue' Issue," 7 Behav.Sciences & Law 259 (1989).

It has been suggested that judges rely more heavily on the authority granted them under the federal rules and many state rules to appoint a "neutral" expert who would testify for the court rather than either of the parties. Golding, "Mental Health Professionals and the Courts: The Ethics of Expertise," Int'l J.L. & Psychiat. (in press). Federal rule 706 provides:

> [T]he court may on its own motion or on the motion of any party enter an order to show cause why expert witnesses should not be appointed, and may request the parties to submit nominations. The court may appoint any expert witnesses agreed upon by the parties, and may appoint expert witnesses of its own selection. . . . A witness so appointed shall advise the parties of the witness' findings, if any; the witness' deposition may be taken by any party; and the witness may be called to testify by the court or any party. The witness shall be subject to cross-examination by each party, including a party calling the witness.

Will witnesses "appointed by the court" rather than retained by the parties be less likely to act in an "adversarial" manner? If so, would this be a good thing?

4. *Education of the legal profession.* To some extent, poor communication in court is the fault of mental health professionals who are ignorant of, or unwilling to call attention to, the limits of their expertise. But ultimately the blame has to fall on the legal system. Research indicates that many judges and lawyers *prefer* conclusory testimony. Melton, Weithorn & Slobogin, Community Mental Centers & the Courts: An Evaluation of Community–Based Forensic Services 94–5, 99 (1985). Lawyers often are unfamiliar with the law, not to mention basic behavioral science concepts. Rosenberg & McGarry, "Competency for Trial: The Making of an Expert," 128 Am.J.Psychiat. 82 (1972) (only 10 of 28 criminal attorneys knew competency to stand trial standard). And even when they have some understanding of both, they may make little effort to use the tools of their trade in exposing spurious testimony. Poythress, "Psychiatric Expertise in Civil Commitment: Training Attorneys to Cope with Expert Testimony," 2 Law. & Hum.Behav. 1 (1978) (lawyers taught the inadequacies of clinical testimony persisted in avoiding careful cross-examination in commitment proceedings because of paternalistic attitudes). As Bonnie stated:

> The bench and bar are ultimately responsible for improving the administration of justice. If judges and juries are confused or misled by expert testimony, this usually means there has been poor lawyering. If experts give conclusory testimony, encompassing so-called ultimate

issues—and fail to explain the bases for their opinions—the fault lies with the bench and bar, not with the experts. If forensic evaluators do not have access to the same information and reach different opinions for this reason, the fault lies with the legal system, not with the experts.

Bonnie, "Morality, Equality, and Expertise: Renegotiating the Relationship Between Psychiatry and the Criminal Law," 12 Bull.Am.Acad.Psychiat. & L. 5, 5–6 (1984).

Chapter Seven

MENTAL DISABILITY AND CRIMINAL LAW

I. INTRODUCTION

The role of mental disability in determining whether those charged with crime should be punished and, if so, to what extent, is potentially quite broad. To understand why this is so, one must first analyze the purposes of criminal punishment. Most criminal law scholars would agree that criminal punishment has five possible purposes: retribution, general deterrence, specific deterrence, incapacitation, and rehabilitation. Under retributive theory, punishment is imposed when a person makes a choice which deserves blame because it offends certain shared moral sensibilities; in such a situation, the person owes society a debt which must be paid. Deterrence theory, on the other hand, views punishment as a means of dissuading persons from committing acts which harm society, whether or not they are "blameworthy". General deterrence refers to the impact of punishment on others, while specific deterrence refers to its impact on the particular offender. Punishment is justified on incapacitative grounds when necessary to prevent an individual from committing crime again. Similarly, punishment is justified on rehabilitation grounds if treatment would prevent a person from engaging in further criminal behavior.

Upon close examination, it should become clear that, in deciding *what* to punish, the focus is on retribution and general deterrence. Only in determining *how much* we want to punish do specific deterrence, incapacitation, and rehabilitation assume great significance. Put another way, the first two purposes logically are the primary considerations in defining the type of behavior that should be subject to criminal sanction, while the latter three are most usefully considered at sentencing in determining the type and scope of sanction once an individual has been identified as an offender. For instance, every jurisdiction makes knowingly killing another without justification or excuse a crime. In describing why, it makes sense to say that this type of conduct deserves punishment (i.e., requires societal vengeance), or that punishing it will serve as a disincentive to others who are contemplating such an act. In contrast, it makes little sense to say that such conduct is criminal because everyone who engages in it is in need of further (specific) deterrence, incapacitation, treatment, or some combination thereof. In fact, there are probably many individuals who commit unjustified and unexcused homicide who are not particularly dangerous or treatable. Only at sentencing, once a person has been found guilty of conduct which is considered blameworthy or in need of deterrence, can considerations of specific deterrence, incapacitation and rehabilitation be meaningfully considered in shaping the precise punishment to be meted out to each individual.

There may be a second, more complicated reason for considering only retributive and general deterrent goals in defining the elements of criminal liability. Our criminal justice system is founded on the assumption that we are autonomous beings who can justly be punished; although science may suggest that some or all behavior is "determined" by biological or environmental forces, thus rendering us nonresponsible, the law assumes we have "free will." For purposes of criminal punishment, it has further been assumed that this will is not manifested until the person acts. Thoughts alone are not enough to establish criminal liability. Packer justified this position in part by noting that historically "we have not been sufficiently stirred by the danger presented or sufficiently confident of our ability to discern propensities in the absence of conduct to use the instruments of the criminal law [to punish thoughts alone]." But even if we were, the assumption of free will should stand, according to Packer: "the capacity of the individual human being to live his life in reasonable freedom from socially imposed external constraints (the only kind with which the law is concerned) would be fatally impaired unless the law provided a locus poenitentiae, a point of no return beyond which external constraints may be imposed but before which the individual is free—not free of whatever compulsions determinists tell us he labors under but free of the very specific social compulsions of the law." Packer, The Limits of the Criminal Sanction 73–75 (1968).

The moral assumptions that persons have free will and can thus be punished, but only once their will has been manifested through behavior, are relatively easily implemented under either retributive or deterrence theory. In Anglo–American jurisprudence, for instance, retributivists hold that a person is not blameworthy unless he or she has acted on a wrong choice, since until that point no harm has occurred; similarly, according to deterrence theory, punishment is meant to prevent harm, which is absent unless there is conduct. On the other hand, deciding whether specific deterrence, incapacitation, and rehabilitation is necessary for a particular individual does not require that any particular act be committed; instead this determination relies on a prediction of behavior—in essence, whether this person will commit crime if he or she is not confined and treated. While past behavior may be useful in making this prediction, it need not be of any particular type or seriousness; moreover, in theory at least, it is not necessary at all.[a] To base a finding of guilt solely on such a prediction, rather than on a demonstration of a specific act the person has committed, could seriously undermine the moral assumption that we control our behavior. However, once a person is convicted for a (blameworthy, deterrence-worthy) act, allowing predictions to govern the type and duration of punishment is not as repugnant to this principle. Thus, again, while the three individual prevention goals should probably not be relied upon in defining the scope of criminal liability, they are usefully considered at sentencing.

This brief summary of the purposes of criminal punishment and their importance to the two stages of the criminal justice system, although highly simplified, helps put in perspective the role of mental disability in the criminal law. At the guilt adjudication stage, mental disability is theoretically relevant whenever it renders a person's decision to act less blameworthy or more difficult to deter. For instance, the oldest criminal law doctrine focusing specifically on the mentally disabled—the insanity defense—is often justified on the ground that the insane are so irrational in their behavior, or so unable to control themselves, that they do not deserve to be punished, and are unlikely to understand or pay attention to criminal sanctions. As Goldstein has stated: "It would be widely regarded as incalculably cruel and unjust to incarcerate men who are not personally responsible in order to serve social functions. The notion of 'desert' or culpability is too deeply rooted." Further, "[u]nder the deterrent theory, . . . the insanity defense describes the man who is sufficiently different from the rest of us that he cannot be used as an effective example and who, in quite

a. See pp. 429–431.

personal terms, cannot be expected to approach events mindful of the warnings sent to him by the criminal code." Goldstein, The Insanity Defense 13–14 (1967). For the same reasons, when a person's "actions" are "involuntary" (as when an epileptic seizure results in death of another), criminal punishment may be inappropriate, a notion recognized by the "automatism" defense. Indeed, anyone whose mental state at the time of the offense is "abnormal" might be able to argue that his or her culpability and deterrability was diminished at that time.

The impact of mental disability at sentencing is potentially even greater, because here specific deterrence, incapacitative and rehabilitative concerns, as well as retributive and general deterrence considerations, may enter in. Evidence of mental condition could be very useful in finetuning the punishment imposed, either as a "mitigating factor" (e.g., to show diminished responsibility or to suggest amenability to treatment outside the prison setting), or as an "aggravating factor" (e.g., as proof of dangerousness).

Over the past century, the criminal law has, with some significant exceptions, moved toward full realization of the possibilities outlined above. Here these developments will only be outlined, in order to place them in historical perspective. More detailed discussion occurs in the body of this chapter.

Particularly significant has been the increasing relevance of mental disability in determining criminal liability. The tendency toward expansion of the insanity defense is well known. Even more significant are developments with respect to the mental state element (mens rea) of criminal offenses. The common law usually required proof only of "objective", or inferred, intent rather than "subjective", or actual, intent. Thus, the prosecution could often secure conviction if it showed that the accused committed the criminal act under circumstances in which a "reasonable person" would intend such an act; the accused's actual intent was irrelevant. Probably the single most important trend in the substantive criminal law during this century has been the continuing erosion of this position. The highly influential Model Penal Code, officially promulgated in 1962 by the American Law Institute, expresses a strong preference for criminal liability based solely on proof of criminal intent or awareness of the risk of harm. Following logically from this proposition, the Code permits evidence of mental abnormality to be introduced not only the insanity issue, but also on the issue of whether the accused could form the intent associated with the alleged crime whenever that intent is subjective—sometimes called the "diminished capacity" defense. Additionally, the Model Penal Code's definitions of defensive doctrines such as mistake of fact, duress, self-defense and provocation—doctrines which were traditionally defined in "objective" terms (e.g., would a "reasonable" person be provoked to kill under given circumstances)—permit the defendant to submit evidence about his or her own feelings, desires, urges, and thoughts at the time of the offense. Theoretically, evidence of mental abnormality is relevant under any of these defenses.

The types of evidence an offender can present at sentencing—traditionally limited to pleas for mercy—have also expanded considerably over the past century. In many states, offenders may now submit virtually any mitigating information they can muster, including evidence of mental abnormality. Indeed, in death penalty cases, the Supreme Court has held that offenders have a constitutional right to offer such evidence. At the same time, the state is often permitted to introduce evidence of dangerousness or untreatability at sentencing.

While mental abnormality has thus become increasingly relevant in the determination of whether and what type of punishment should be imposed, there are also signs that courts and legislatures are reconsidering the wisdom of this development. For instance, in the 1980's several jurisdictions, many of them responding to the outcome of John Hinckley's trial on charges of attempting to assassinate President Reagan, significantly reduced the scope of the insanity defense. In a separate effort to curb the impact of the insanity defense, many states have adopted the "guilty but mentally ill" verdict as an intermediate option between insanity and a straight finding of guilt. Moreover, several states have rejected or severely limited the Model Penal Code's recommendation that mental abnormality be considered on the issue of intent, and many courts have demonstrated antipathy toward broadening other defenses.

Similar developments have occurred in the non-capital sentencing setting. Beginning in the 1970's, several states have moved toward "determinate sentencing", or sentencing schemes which provide decisionmakers with relatively little leeway in setting punishment. In an effort to remove discretion from decisionmakers, the thrust of these reforms has been to base sentence lengths primarily on backward-looking culpability assessments rather than on forward-looking assessments of dangerousness, treatability and so on.

To some extent, these differing views on the role of mental disability in the criminal justice system are a function of varying perceptions about the limits of clinical expertise, a topic discussed in the previous chapter. But at bottom they stem from assumptions about the fundamental purposes of the criminal sanction. The primary aim of this chapter is to examine these assumptions in an effort to provoke thought on the extent to which mental disability ought to be relevant to the doctrines of the substantive criminal law. The first section examines doctrines relevant to mental state at the time of the offense, including the defenses of insanity, "diminished capacity," and "automatism", and the guilty but mentally ill verdict. The second section looks at sentencing. In particular, it will focus on capital sentencing—the area in which sentencing law is most highly developed—and those special sentencing situations in which mental disability plays a significant role.

II. CRIMINAL RESPONSIBILITY

As explained above, the primary justifications for exculpatory and mitigating criminal law doctrines based on mental abnormality flow from retributive and deterrence theory. The criminal law assumes "free will", the capacity to make and act upon choices. But the law is also willing to assume that mental disability reduces this capacity, thus making the person less blameworthy and less able to obey the law's mandates. The assumption that the mentally disabled are incapable of being minimally rational or are less deterrable than others has been called more of an "intuitive hunch" than an empirically verified fact. See Morse, "Treating Crazy People Less Specially," 90 West.Va.L.Rev. 353, 370 (1988). Moreover, as Hart has pointed out, the deterrence rationale for defenses based on mental disability may be logically flawed because, even if some persons are undeterrable as a result of mental disorder, permitting such defenses may *encourage* others to commit crime in the hope that they can escape conviction through feigning mental disability. Hart, Punishment and Responsibility 18–20 (1968). Despite these possible problems, the central question remains the extent to which retributive or deterrence theory requires or suggests that inroads be made on the free will paradigm.

The possible impact of specific deterrence, incapacitation, and rehabilitation concerns should also be mentioned, however. For reasons given earlier, in deciding upon the proper scope of defenses based on mental disability one should generally not engage in the predictive inquiry required by the individual prevention goals of punishment. Nonetheless, these goals probably do influence legislatures and courts in deciding how to frame defenses based on mental disability. For instance, as Goldstein has noted, one view of the insanity defense "sees the defense almost entirely as a path to treatment in a mental hospital. . . . The tacit assumption is that a paternal state can put [the acquittee] right by psychotherapy or by judicious social planning, if only the 'helping' professions are provided with the resources to do the job." Goldstein, The Insanity Defense 14 (1967). As another example, consider from the incapacitative perspective the impact of narrowing the insanity defense. In most states, those adjudged insane are confined in a mental hospital for as long as they are considered mentally disordered and dangerous. If the insanity defense was abolished or its scope reduced significantly, individuals considered to be violent who previously might have been found insane and hospitalized indefinitely would be convicted and released from secure confinement at the end of their sentence, perhaps much earlier than they would have been had they been committed as insane. By changing the substantive law, the government would be deprived of a flexible dispositional device. As these examples illustrate, the extent to which policymakers want to implement rehabilitative and incapacitative goals might influence their efforts to define defenses based on mental disability.

These considerations should be kept in mind throughout the following materials.

A. THE INSANITY DEFENSE [b]

1. A Brief History

This section discusses the various formulations of the insanity defense that have been advanced through the years. A later section discusses whether the defense should be abolished, after examining its alternatives. As should become clear, the various tests set out below are the result of many variables, including changes in medical knowledge, the criminal justice system, and attitudes of society toward the mentally disabled.

Early Development. The idea of a defense to criminal responsibility based on mental disability goes back as far as the ancient Greek and Hebrew civilizations. English case law, which heavily influenced early American courts, has long recognized the concept. At least as early as 1300, records show that English kings were pardoning murderers because their crimes were committed "while suffering from madness." Over the next several centuries, many different formulations of the defense emerged. Sir Edward Coke, a famous legal scholar of the late 16th and early 17th century, felt that "idiots" and "madmen" who "wholly loseth their memory and understanding" should be found insane. Sir Matthew Hale, Chief Justice of the King's Bench in the 17th century, concluded in his private papers that the "best measure" for determining insanity was whether the accused had "as great understanding as ordinarily a child of fourteen hath." In 1723 Justice Tracy held that in order to be found insane "a man must be totally deprived of his understanding and memory so as not to know what he is doing, no more than an infant, brute or a wild beast." At about the same time, other English courts were excusing those who lacked the capacity to distinguish "good from evil" or "right from wrong."

The M'Naghten Test. It was this latter approach that, in slightly modified form, became the so-called "M'Naghten test" of insanity. In response to controversy surrounding the insanity acquittal of Daniel M'Naghten on a charge of murdering the private secretary of Prime Minister Robert Peel, the House of Lords announced the following rule:

> To establish a defense on the ground of insanity, it must be clearly proved that, at the time of the committing of the act, the party accused was laboring under such a defect of reason, from disease of the mind, as not to know the nature and quality of the act he was doing; or, if he did know it, that he did not know he was doing what was wrong.

This formulation, announced in 1843, became the accepted rule in both England and the United States.

b. This and the following descriptions in the text about criminal responsibility doctrines are adapted from Melton, Petrila, Poythress & Slobogin, *Psychological Evalu-* *ation for the Courts: A Handbook for Mental Health Professionals and Lawyers* Chap. 6 (1987).

Criticism of the test was immediate, especially from the medical community. Indeed, five years before the House of Lords' pronouncement, Sir Isaac Ray, a noted American physician, had argued that the "insane mind" is often "perfectly rational, and displays the exercise of a sound and well-balanced mind." Thus, according to Ray, a defense based on mental illness that focuses merely on cognitive impairment is incomplete; the defendant's ability to control his or her acts must also be considered. Although directed at the law as it existed in 1838, Ray's comments applied with equal force to the M'Naghten test, which varied only slightly from its predecessors.

A second criticism of the rule was its rigidity. Even if one accepts the premise that cognitive dysfunction is the only appropriate focus of the insanity defense, the M'Naghten rule, it was claimed, did not fairly pose the question; a literal interpretation of the M'Naghten test would seldom, if ever, lead to exculpation. In the words of one psychiatrist, "[if the test language were taken seriously,] it would excuse only those totally deteriorated, drooling hopeless psychotics of long-standing, and congenital idiots."

The Irresistible Impulse Test. In the United States, the legal response to the first criticism came in the form of a supplementary test for insanity, which eventually came to be called the "irresistible impulse" rule. One of the first courts to adopt the rule described it as follows:

> [The defendant is not] legally responsible if the two following conditions concur: (1) If, by reason of the duress of . . . mental disease he had so far lost the power to choose between the right and wrong, and to avoid doing the act in question, as that his free agency was at the time destroyed; (2) and if, at the same time, the alleged crime was so connected with such mental disease, in the relation of cause and effect, as to have been the product of it solely.

Parsons v. State, 81 Ala. 577, 596, 2 So. 854 (1886). The adoption of the test was usually justified on the ground that those offenders who could not control their behavior at the time of the offense were not deterrable by criminal sanctions; therefore, no legitimate moral or policy purpose was served by convicting them.

The "irresistible impulse" test met resistance from several fronts. Many in the legal community believed that impulsivity could easily be feigned, and feared that the test would lead to numerous invalid insanity acquittals. From the medical side came the criticism that a separate "control" test furthered the mistaken impression that the human psyche is compartmentalized into cognitive and volitional components. And, like M'Naghten, the test was seen as too rigid, excusing only those who were totally unable to prevent their unlawful behavior.

The Durham Rule. In 1954, partly in response to the latter two contentions and the criticisms of M'Naghten, the federal District of Columbia Court of Appeals adopted the "product test" for insanity—a rule originally devised by Sir Isaac Ray and adopted by the New

Hampshire Supreme Court in 1870, but one that had received little notice since that time. As set forth in *Durham v. United States*, 214 F.2d 862 (D.C.Cir.1954), the test stated simply that "an accused is not criminally responsible if his unlawful act was the product of mental disease or defect." Judge Bazelon, the author of the *Durham* opinion, hoped the rule would encourage mental health professionals to explain all aspects of a defendant's personality and functioning by removing legal strictures on such professionals' testimony.

In time, however, this lack of guidance became a problem in itself. The product test asked essentially two questions: (1) Did mental disease or defect exist at the time of the offense? (2) Was the offense the product of this disease or defect? The *Durham* court failed to define either "mental disease" or "product." Trial courts had particular difficulty dealing with the meaning of the former term, since it was no longer modified by functional criteria, as it had been in earlier tests. The problem surfaced dramatically in 1957 when staff members at St. Elizabeth Hospital, which provides the District of Columbia courts with most of their experts on the insanity issue, suddenly voted to incorporate the personality disorders, including the so-called "sociopathic personality," within the definition of "mental disease" for purposes of the insanity defense. Since many criminal offenders have some type of personality disorder, this weekend change in hospital policy had a major impact in the courts.

In *McDonald v. United States*, 312 F.2d 847 (D.C.Cir.1962), the District of Columbia Court of Appeals finally conceded that trial courts required some guidelines in implementing the product test, and declared that henceforth "the jury should be told that a mental disease or defect includes any abnormal condition of the mind which substantially affects mental or emotional processes and substantially impairs behavior controls." With the judicial gloss added by *MacDonald*, the difference between the product test and a test combining M'Naghten and the "irresistible impulse" rule was reduced substantially. Even so, definitional problems persisted, and *Durham* was finally overruled in 1972. New Hampshire remains the only state to follow the test.

The American Law Institute Test. In place of the product test, the District of Columbia Court of Appeals adopted still another version of the insanity test, which was first proposed a year after the *Durham* decision. This test, drafted by the American Law Institute (ALI), was an attempt to deal with most of the problems associated with previous tests by avoiding the "all-or-nothing" language of the M'Naghten and "irresistible impulse" formulations, while retaining some specific guidelines for the jury. The rule reads as follows: "A person is not responsible for criminal conduct if at the time of such conduct as a result of mental disease or defect he lacks substantial capacity either to appreciate the criminality [wrongfulness] of his conduct or to conform his conduct to the requirements of the law." This language combines the notions underlying both the M'Naghten and irresistible impulse formulations, but makes it clear that a defendant's cognitive or volitional impairment at the time of the offense need only be "substantial," rather than total, in order to merit an insanity defense.

The ALI's proposal also included a second paragraph, which, according to its drafters, was designed specifically "to exclude from the concept of 'mental disease or defect' the case of so called 'psychopathic personality.'" It states: "As used in this Article, the terms mental disease or defect do not include an abnormality manifested only by repeated criminal or otherwise anti-social conduct." Interestingly, this proposal was published two years before the St. Elizabeth's incident.

The ALI test proved to be a popular one: Over the next two decades, a majority of the country's jurisdictions adopted the first paragraph, and many of these also adopted the second.

Rejection of Medical Model. Nonetheless, the ALI test came under attack as well. One criticism was that the ALI test, as well as all of the tests that preceded it, relied too heavily on the so-called "medical model." Judge Bazelon, the author of the failed *Durham* test, was the most prominent proponent of this point of view. In a concurring opinion in *United States v. Brawner*, 471 F.2d 969 (D.C.Cir.1972), the decision which overturned *Durham*, he argued that a person should be found insane "if at the time of his unlawful conduct his mental or emotional processes or behavior controls were impaired to such an extent that he cannot justly be held responsible for his act." This test does away with the "mental disease or defect" requirement, as well as any specific requirement of functional impairment. It gives the factfinder virtually limitless discretion to decide the types of "impairment" which excuse one for one's behavior. No state has adopted the test.[c]

Several other proposed formulations also eschew the mental disease or defect predicate, but more explicitly require the jury to focus on the accused's mental state. For instance, Moore argued that the inquiry should focus on whether the accused is "so irrational as to be nonresponsible." According to Moore,

> One is a moral agent only if one is a rational agent. Only if we can see another being as one who acts to achieve some rational end in light of some rational beliefs will we understand him in the same fundamental way that we understand ourselves and our fellow persons in everyday life. We regard as moral agents only those beings we can understand in this way.

In determining whether the accused is rational, Moore explained, one should look at the intelligibility, consistency and coherency of the desires and beliefs that motivate the offense. Moore, Law & Psychiatry: Rethinking the Relationship 244–45, 207 (1985). In a similar vein, Fingarette and Hasse asserted that a "lack of capacity for rational conduct" is the core of insanity. Fingarette and Hasse, Mental Disabil-

---

c. Rhode Island excuses those who cannot justly be held responsible as a result of mental disease or defect. *State v. Johnson*, 121 R.I. 254, 399 A.2d 469, 476 (1979).

ities and Criminal Responsibility 218 (1979).[d] Although using different language, Morse tried to capture the same idea with his proposal: "A defendant is not guilty by reason of insanity if at the time of the offense the defendant was extremely crazy and the craziness affected the criminal behavior." According to Morse, "this test tracks the moral issues with greater honesty and precision, is more workable, and will not lead to the acquittal of more defendants than present tests or reformed versions of present tests." Morse, "Excusing the Crazy: The Insanity Defense Reconsidered," 58 S.Cal.L.Rev. 780 (1985). No jurisdiction has adopted any of these tests.

Elimination of Volitional Prong. A more popular (and the most recent) trend in insanity jurisprudence has been to attack the volitional prong of the defense. Soon after the insanity acquittal of John Hinckley, both the American Bar Association and the American Psychiatric Association recommended the elimination of the so-called "control" inquiry, although they continued to support the "appreciation" prong of the ALI's test, thereby indicating an unwillingness to return to the original M'Naghten formulation. The ABA's test reads as follows: "[A] person is not responsible for criminal conduct if, at the time of such conduct, and as a result of mental disease or defect, that person was unable to appreciate the wrongfulness of such conduct." American Bar Association, Criminal Justice Mental Health Standards, Standard 7–6.1 (1987). Echoing past criticism, both the ABA and the APA reasoned that if mistakes do occur in the administration of the insanity defense, they are most likely to result from utilizing a volitional test. The commentary to the ABA's standard stated: "Clinicians can be more precise and arrive at more reliable conclusions about awareness, perceptions, and understanding of an event than about the 'causes' of a person's behavior, especially when the determinants of behavior are felt to be unconscious."

In 1984, the United States Congress adopted an insanity test for the federal courts which essentially tracked the ABA proposal. The legislation, found in Title 18 of the United States Code, states:

§ 20. Insanity Defense.

(a) Affirmative Defense.—It is an affirmative defense to a prosecution under any federal statute that, at the time of the commission of acts constituting the offense, the defendant, as a result of severe mental disease or defect, was unable to appreciate the nature and quality or

---

d. Sendor also views irrationality as the proper test, but explains its importance somewhat differently:

[R]ationality is not important standing alone, but rather as a condition for engaging in conduct that others can interpret. When a mentally ill person injures legally protected interests through

irrational conduct, we excuse the individual because we do not interpret his conduct as expressing disrespect for those interests.

Sendor, "Crime as Communication: An Interpretive Theory of the Insanity Defense and the Mental Elements of Crime," 74 Geo.L.J. 1371, 1415 (1986).

the wrongfulness of his acts.   Mental disease or defect does not otherwise constitute a defense.

 Several states have followed this lead.

Questions and Comments

1. *Effect of the language.* In terms of outcome, does it matter which of the various formulations described above are incorporated into jury instructions? Using a mock case based on the facts of *Durham*, Professor Simon asked ten juries to decide the case under the *M'Naghten* standard and ten juries to decide the case under the *Durham* standard. She found a very small, although statistically significant, chance that jurors were more likely to find the defendant insane under the latter test. Simon, The Jury and the Defense of Insanity 215 (1967). A more recent study used five mock cases and six different instructions: the "wild beast" test, M'Naghten, M'Naghten plus irresistible impulse, *Durham*, the ALI test and the test developed by Fingarette and Hasse. It found no overall significant differences among the six instructions. Finkel, Shaw, Bercaw & Koch, "Insanity Defenses: From the Jurors's Perspective," 9 L & Psychol.Rev. 77 (1985). Goldstein came to a similar conclusion after an extensive survey of the cases. Goldstein, The Insanity Defense 213–14 (1967).

On the other hand, a review of studies looking at the effect of changes in the insanity standard in five states concluded that, despite methodological flaws, the research suggests that differences in acquittal rates can result when the M'Naghten test is replaced by the ALI test. Kielitz, "Researching and Reforming the Insanity Defense," in Brooks & Winick, Current Issues in Mental Disability Law 47, 57–61 (1987). Moreover, as the American Bar Association has pointed out:

> the impact of particular language on decisions made *before* a jury retires to deliberate also must be considered—the decisions of experts whether or not to testify and, if so, the formulation of their testimony; the strategic decisions by defense counsel relating to the insanity defense, direct and cross-examination, and summation; and trial court rulings on the legal sufficiency of the evidence to raise a jury question.

ABA, Criminal Justice Mental Health Standards, Commentary to Standard 7–6.1 at 343 (1989). The ABA concluded that the difference in outcome in jurisdictions with a test which included a volitional prong and those that did not might be significant. Finally, even if the language makes no appreciable difference in terms of specific case resolutions, it may have an important effect symbolically and on the public's perception of the criminal justice system.

2. *Burden and standard of proof.* Another aspect of jury instructions in insanity cases concerns the burden and standard of proof that apply when the defense is asserted. By far the majority of the states require the defendant to prove insanity by the preponderance of the evidence standard. About one-third of the states place the burden of disproving insanity on the prosecution beyond a reasonable doubt. Until 1984, federal jurisdictions followed this practice. After the Hinckley case, however, in the same legislation that changed the federal insanity test, the burden was switched

dramatically, to require that the *defendant* show insanity by *clear and convincing evidence.* 18 U.S.C. § 20(b). Arizona has also adopted this approach. Ariz.Rev.Stat. § 13–502.

The American Bar Association would vary the burden depending upon the test being used. It would require the prosecution to disprove insanity beyond a reasonable doubt under its cognitive-only test. When the test includes the volitional prong, however, the ABA would place the burden on the defendant to prove insanity by a preponderance of the evidence, on the theory, summarized above, that application of the volitional test is more prone to mistakes. American Bar Association, Criminal Justice Mental Health Standards, Standard 7–6.9 (1987).

Apparently, none of these approaches is unconstitutional. In *Leland v. Oregon,* 343 U.S. 790, 72 S.Ct. 1002, 96 L.Ed. 1302 (1952) the Supreme Court held that a state rule requiring the defendant to prove insanity beyond a reasonable doubt did not deny a state defendant his federal constitutional right to due process of law. Almost two decades later, the Court held that the prosecution must prove beyond a reasonable doubt "every fact necessary to constitute proof of the crime with which [the defendant] is charged." In re Winship, 397 U.S. 358, 90 S.Ct. 1068, 25 L.Ed.2d 368 (1970). *Winship* suggested that *Leland* was no longer good law. But in 1976 the Court dismissed, for want of a substantial federal question, an appeal of a conviction under an instruction placing the burden of proving insanity on the defendant by a preponderance of the evidence. *Rivera v. Delaware,* 429 U.S. 877, 97 S.Ct. 226, 50 L.Ed.2d 160 (1976). In dissenting to the dismissal, Justice Brennan wrote:

> In *Mullaney [v. Wilbur,* 421 U.S. 684, 95 S.Ct. 1881, 44 L.Ed.2d 508 (1975)], we considered a Maine rule that placed upon a criminal defendant charged with murder the burden of proving by a preponderance of the evidence that he had acted in the heat of passion on sudden impulse in order to reduce the homicide to manslaughter. We concluded that this rule did not comport with the due process requirement, as defined in *In re Winship* . . . that the prosecution must prove beyond a reasonable doubt every fact necessary to constitute the crime charged. . . . Like the state rule invalidated in *Mullaney,* which implied malice unless the accused negated it, the plea of insanity, whether or not the State chooses to characterize it as an affirmative defense, relates to the accused's state of mind, an essential element of the crime. . . .

429 U.S. at 878–80, 97 S.Ct. at 226–27 (Brennan, dissenting). As Brennan suggests, it seems clear that, at least in some cases, evidence of insanity might be relevant to whether the defendant had the required mental state for the crime charged (such as intent or knowledge). Dix has suggested an argument in support of the Court's position in *Rivera,* however. He notes that because the insanity defense almost always relies on relatively untrustworthy or perplexing expert testimony, telling juries "that they must acquit if this evidence raises a reasonable doubt . . . may [create] an unacceptably high risk of unjustified acquittals due to what are actually 'unreasonable' doubts generated simply by confusion." Dix, Criminal Responsibility and Mental Impairment in American Criminal Law, in 1 Law

and Mental Health: International Perspectives 1, 24 (1984). Does this argument necessarily justify placing the burden on the defendant?

It may be that the choice of a particular burden or standard of proof is primarily of symbolic value. The data that exist suggest little or no relationship between a particular burden of proof and outcome. One informal study sampled the acquittal rates of five states, three of which used the ALI test and two of which used M'Naghten. Only one of the five placed the burden on the defendant. That state, which used the ALI test, had the second highest acquittal rate overall and the *highest* acquittal rate of the three states that used the ALI test. Melton, et al., supra note b, at 125, n. 109.

3. *Consequences of an insanity acquittal.* A third issue that might be addressed in instructions to the jury is the impact of an insanity acquittal. As noted earlier, most states confine insanity acquittees in mental institutions for as long as they remain mentally ill and dangerous.[e] The precise duration of post-acquittal confinement is therefore unknown at the time of trial and could be either much shorter or much longer than the sentence that would have been imposed had the person been found guilty. In most states, the jury is not informed of these facts, just as, in the typical criminal trial, they are kept in the dark about possible sentences, on the theory that dispositional information may improperly influence its decision. About a third of the states, however, authorize an instruction about the consequences of an insanity acquittal. The American Bar Association, which also adopts this position, supported its view as follows:

> [D]espite instructions cautioning them to consider only the evidence they have heard, jurors who are not informed about dispositional consequences will speculate about the practical results of a nonresponsibility verdict and, in ignorance of reality, will convict persons who are not criminally responsible in order to protect society. Jurors surely know, without being told, what happens to most convicted offenders, as well as defendants who are acquitted outright; the proposed instruction provides the same level of knowledge with respect to the fate of persons acquitted by reason of insanity.

Empirical evidence as to jurors' understanding of dispositional consequences is spotty. Simon found that the overwhelming majority of jurors are aware, without being instructed, that dangerous persons are not released upon acquittal by reason of insanity, R. Simon, The Jury and the Defense of Insanity 38 (1967), but she later admitted that her methodology may have produced inaccurate results. Schwartz, "Should Juries Be Informed of the Consequences of the Insanity Verdict?", 8 J. Psychiat. & L. 167, 173–74 (1980). Morris found that, overall, jurors have inconsistent perceptions about disposition. Morris, "Whither Thou Goest?: An Inquiry into Jurors' Perceptions of the Consequences of a Successful Insanity Defense," 14 San Diego L.Rev. 1058 (1977). If you were a defense attorney, would you want dispositional instructions? A prosecutor? Would you also

---

e. The criteria and procedures for commitment of insanity acquittees are discussed in detail at pp. 756–770.

want instructions on the average duration of hospitalization for insanity acquittees?

4. *The reality of the insanity defense.* The public's position regarding the defense of insanity seems to be heavily influenced by the perception that the defense is frequently raised and widely abused. For instance, a survey taken in Wyoming revealed that the "average" resident in that state believed the defense was raised in 43% of all criminal cases in Wyoming between 1970 and 1972 and that it was successful 38% of the time. In fact, however, only 102 defendants—fewer than half of 1% of those arrested in Wyoming during the period relevant to the survey— raised the plea, and only one person out of these 102 was acquitted. Pasewark, Seidenzahl & Pantle, "Opinions About the Insanity Plea," 8 J.Forensic Psychiat. 8 (1981). Nationwide, the insanity defense appears to be raised in less than 1% of all criminal cases and appears to be successful about 25% of the time. Steadman, Pantle & Pasewark, "Factors Associated with a Successful Insanity Defense," 140 Am.J.Psychiat. 401 (1983). It should also be noted that in many states a sizeable proportion (over 70%) of acquittals by reason of insanity result from plea-bargaining or quasi-plea-bargaining with the prosecution; in these cases the prosecution agrees that the defendant should be acquitted, and there is no opportunity to "fool" a judge or jury. Rogers, Bloom & Manson, "Insanity Defenses: Contested or Conceded?" 141 Am.J.Psychiat. 885 (1984).

The public also seems to believe that those who successfully assert the insanity defense are released from custody quickly, thus endangering the public. In fact, although as noted above confinement time varies widely, the *average* duration of confinement for persons acquitted by reason of insanity roughly correlates with the time they would have spent in prison had they been convicted of the crime charged. Moreover, current evidence suggests that, as a group, acquittees who are released are no more dangerous than felons who are released on parole or after serving their time. See, e.g., Pantle, Pasewark & Steadman, "Comparing Institutionalization Periods and Subsequent Arrests of Insanity Acquittees and Convicted Felons," 8 J.Psychiat. & L. 305 (1980).

2. Cognitive Impairment

THE HEADS CASE

Shortly after midnight on August 22, 1977, Charles Heads shot and killed the husband of his wife's sister in Shreveport, La. Heads, a resident of Houston, had traveled to Shreveport in search of his wife, who had departed from Houston with their three children four days before in an effort to leave him. During those four days, Heads had taken a leave of absence from work and made repeated local and long distance phone calls to locate his family. He also visited his wife's parents home, again in an effort to find his wife and children. Finally he called his wife's sister. The sister's denial of knowledge about his wife's whereabouts arose his suspicion and he drove to her home, although it was nearing midnight. No one answered his repeated knocks on the doors and windows. Heads then kicked in a door leading from the carport, entered and found his sister-in-law's husband at the end of the bedroom hall, armed with a pistol.

Though the evidence is not clear as to the precise moment when the shooting began, both the victim's wife and Heads' wife testified that Heads began firing his pistol shortly after breaking into the house. The sister-in-law's husband informed the defendant that he, too, was armed and did not want to be forced to shoot him. But Heads continued firing his pistol down the bedroom hallway until he had emptied the pistol of bullets. He then ran to his car, retrieved a rifle from the trunk, and returned, firing several blasts, one of which struck the victim in the eye, killing him.

At his first trial, despite a plea of insanity, Heads was convicted of first degree murder. See *State v. Heads,* 385 So.3d 230 (La.1980). According to Heads' attorney, "the insanity defense at this first trial never got off the ground because neither of the psychiatrists who had examined the defendant had found evidence of any recognized mental disorder." Although Heads had had a difficult tour in Vietnam and "many suspected a Vietnam connection" to the killing, "no one could articulate it. The defendant himself denied any connection in his testimony under oath." Jack, "The Vietnam Connection: Charles Heads' Verdict," 9 Crim.Def. 7, 8 (1982).

Heads' conviction was overturned on unrelated grounds and his case was set for retrial. Between the two trials, the American Psychiatric Association issued the third edition of its Diagnostic and Statistical Manual, in which it recognized the so-called Post–Traumatic Stress Disorder (PTSD), with the following criteria:

    A. Existence of a recognizable stressor that would evoke significant symptoms of distress in almost everyone [such as rape or assault, military combat, earthquakes, torture and car accidents].

    B. Reexperiencing of the trauma as evidenced by at least one of the following:

        (1) recurrent and intrusive recollections of event;

        (2) recurrent dreams of the event;

        (3) sudden acting or feeling as if the traumatic were reoccuring, because of an association with an environmental or ideational stimulus;

    C. Numbing of responsiveness to or reduced involvement with the external world, beginning some time after the trauma, as shown by at least one of the following:

        (1) markedly diminished interest in one or more significant activities;

        (2) feeling of detachment or estrangement from others;

        (3) constricted affect [emotion];

D. At least two of the following symptoms that were not present before the trauma:

(1) hyperalterness or exaggerated startle response;

(2) sleep disturbance;

(3) guilt about surviving when others have not, or about behavior required for survival;

(4) memory impairment or trouble concentrating;

(5) avoidance of activities that arouse recollection of the traumatic event;

(6) intensification of symptoms by exposure to events that symbolize or resemble the traumatic event.

The Manual notes that, "[i]n rare instances there are dissociative states, lasting from a few seconds to several hours, or even days, during which components of the event are relived, and the person behaves as though experiencing the event at that moment." Under "Associated Features", the Manual states: "Increased irritability may be associated with sporadic and unpredictable explosions of aggressive behavior, upon even minimal or no provocation."

At Heads' second trial, Heads again asserted an insanity defense, this time relying on a PTSD diagnosis. Under Louisiana law: "If the circumstances indicate that because of a mental disease or defect the offender was incapable of distinguishing between right and wrong with reference to the conduct in question, the offender shall be exempt from criminal responsibility." At trial, Heads presented three experts who testified that he had been incapable of distinguishing right from wrong at the time of the killing because of post-traumatic stress. Reliance on the PTSD allowed the defense not only to construct a plausible theory of insanity but to introduce evidence normally not admissible: a film comparing Vietnam and World War II, extensive testimony by Vietnam veterans describing the war, and considerable testimony about Heads' childhood.

There follows a facsimile of the closing arguments for the defense and the prosecution at Heads' second trial, based in part on a description of the trial by Heads' attorney Jack, see Jack, supra, and in part on other cases in which a PTSD defense has been raised. See, e.g., *Louisiana v. Sharp*, 418 So.2d 1344 (La.1982).

DEFENSE ARGUMENT

The evidence shows that, while he was in Vietnam, Charles Heads experienced incredible trauma. Usually he was able to deal with the stress created by his horrible sojourn there. But when the anxiety created by Vietnam combined with the stress of his family leaving him, as happened on the night of the killing, Charles was not himself. On that night, he was literally unaware of what he was doing.

Charles has not had an easy life. He grew up in a section of Houston which once called itself "The Murder Capitol of the World."

When he was nine years old, his mother was killed by his father, who was sentenced to life imprisonment for this and another murder. Yet Charles managed to finish elementary and high school.

Eight months after graduation, he enlisted in the Marines, where he volunteered for the First Reconnaissance Battalion. As a Reconner, he was part of an "elite within an elite"; his mission was to collect intelligence about enemy activities deep in hostile country, staying out on lightly armed patrols for several days to a week in an attempt to locate the VietCong. By his 20th birthday, Charles had his first confirmed kill. Six more followed, including a woman and an old man. The duties of a Reconner, according to the experts, were "extraordinarily stressful." As Dr. John Yost testified, it was not just the stress of combat, but the stress of waiting for something horrible to happen. No place was secure or safe. Everybody who was not an American was the enemy.

After nine months, Charles' days as a Reconner came to an abrupt end when his sixteen man patrol was ambushed one misty morning by an estimated battalion-sized VC regular unit. Charles was the point man and was hit first, twice in the gut. Eventually, those surviving the patrol were saved by an airstrike and airlifted out. Charles was considered too badly wounded to continue his tour in Vietnam. He can remember very little about his nine months in Vietnam or the ambush, although he did remember being shot in the gut.

Dr. Williams, a psychologist and a Marine Corps company commander in Vietnam, testified here at trial that this memory deficit and Charles' difficulty in talking about his Vietnam experience reflected the "psychological defense mechanism of denial." He stated that Charles had probably "used" this defense mechanism in overcoming the catastrophes of his childhood and it stood him in good stead when he returned to the United States. He became a postal employee, as did his wife. Together, they earned over $30,000 a year and, to outward appearances, Charles seemed to have put Vietnam behind him.

However, as his wife testified, Charles experienced many restless, sleepness nights. He also had many nightmares, in which he relived painful memories about the war. It was one of these nightmares, a particularly severe one, which frightened his wife so much that she took the children and went to Shreveport. Dr. John Wilson testified that Charles was on the "extreme edge of vulnerability in terms of his capacity to cope with stress." Indeed, on one occasion two years before the killing and five years after he left Vietnam, when his wife briefly left him, he vaulted onto the roof of his house with a rifle, assumed the assault position, and fired harmlessly for a few minutes into the tops of the trees in the neighborhood. This was significant evidence that Charles was a victim of the post-traumatic stress syndrome, the diagnosis given Charles by all three of our experts. Yet there were no vet centers or outreach centers, no rap groups to help him out.

When his wife left with the children shortly before the killing, Charles lost his only support system. When he went unanswered at his sister-in-law's house he felt rejected and bereft. According to the doctors, it was at this point that the post-traumatic stress triggered his violent action. As it turned out, it was shortly after midnight, the ground and foliage were wet with two inches of rain that had fallen that day, the humidity was 100% and ground fog was beginning to form. According to Charles, his attention momentarily centered on the treeline in the small field across the street. This field, according to seven other Vietnam vets who had seen it or a videotape of it, symbolized or resembled Vietnam. To Charles, "It was just like Vietnam, in a way—that last patrol when we were ambushed, the way the mist hung in the trees." Charles said he was "hit" with a "boom", and he turned back toward the house. He says he was "on automatic." From this moment until he killed, his behavior was, according to the testimony of the vets, like that of a trained Marine Reconner surviving by cleaning out a hooch. When asked whether Charles was aware of the wrongness of the killing, Dr. Williams, a vet himself, replied: "Are you kidding? They gave us ice cream for that."

When the police arrived minutes later, they found Charles wandering in a daze inside the house in the midst of frantically scurrying children, his arms hanging at his side, in one hand the barrel of his own weapon, in the other the barrel of the weapon he had secured from his brother-in-law's body. They led him quietly away. The battle was over. Ladies and gentlemen of the jury, do not let this battle be for naught. Charles was not himself on the night of the killing. He thought he was in Vietnam. He did not know that what he was doing was wrong; he thought he was fighting for his country.

PROSECUTION ARGUMENT

Ladies and gentlemen of the jury, there is no doubt that Vietnam was a stressful environment. But Vietnam is not on trial here; Mr. Charles Heads is. He did not kill because he thought he was in Vietnam. He killed because he was upset his wife had left him and because she was unwilling to take him back or respond to his entreaties. In an overreaction to the sight of a gun, he intentionally and deliberately killed a man. If Vietnam is relevant at all here, it is relevant only because it made Mr. Heads better able and more willing to use violence to achieve his ends.

The defense experts testified that Mr. Heads is suffering from something called post-traumatic stress syndrome. Even assuming there is such a thing, and that Mr. Heads meets the criteria, the defense does not explain why most veterans who experienced the same stresses do not act violently. The defense presented witnesses from the same Reconner patrol who have never committed any violent acts since leaving Vietnam. Having bad dreams is one thing; acting them out is another.

But this whole Vietnam fantasy idea—that Mr. Heads thought he was in Vietnam on the night of the killing, and that he thought his relative was an ambushing VietCong—is preposterous in any event. The prosecution's expert provided a much more plausible explanation. Mr. Heads was not crazy on the night of the murder; he was just angry. The prosecution expert testified that the defendant has an "explosive personality disorder." Mr. Heads has stored up a lot of anger, starting with his father's murder of his mother. Every once in awhile, when a similar rejection occurs, this anger comes out, like the time his wife left him and he went up on the roof to let off a few rounds. This explosiveness, in fact, was one of the reasons his wife left him the final time, as she admitted.

These tantrums might have been pretty intense. But they were not signs of insanity. And they also were infrequent. Most of the time, Mr. Heads' behavior was entirely normal, even right before the murder. During the four days prior to the killing he made several calls, visited his wife's parents' home, and made personal visits to mutual friends and acquaintances. None of these people reported anything out of the ordinary. He rode his bicycle, listened to music, and studied his Vietnam photo album. This was the kind of normal behavior that he exhibited throughout the entire seven years after he left Vietnam.

So why did he act so violently on the night of the murder? By his own admission, he remembers thinking the day before the murder that he wished he were back in the service where, as he stated, "we were one big family, where you were close, where you could count on each other, where people didn't lie to you." To Mr. Heads, his wife was not acting like family, could not be counted on, and had lied to him. He was angry at her, so angry he made sure he had guns with him when he went to her sister's. When she rejected him by not answering his knocks, he exploded. Again, this is not the reaction of a diseased man. It is the reaction of a man who has a lot of pent-up anger and who acts aggressively on those occasions when he can no longer hold it in. Not only did he know it was wrong to kill on the night of the murder, he probably did not feel particularly bad about it, given his experience with killing in Vietnam. It is a sad thing, but combat makes some people less sensitive to the taking of life.

The state is asking that you convict Mr. Heads of first degree murder. The evidence shows that he intentionally brought weapons with him to the house in which he thought his wife was located, intentionally brought a pistol with him when he first entered the house and then, although he had not been fired upon himself, intentionally ran back to his car to get another weapon. He then intentionally shot to kill. He acted with deliberation and without adequate provocation.[f]

f. Heads was acquitted by reason of insanity at his second trial.

Questions and Comments

1. *Mental disease or defect and the cognitive prong.* Every insanity test currently in use requires a threshold finding of mental disease or defect. Historically, mental disease referred to mental illness and mental defect referred to mental retardation. But further definition was usually imprecise. What role does this concept play in fixing the exculpatory scope of the insanity defense? How should it be defined?

One possible approach is to equate the law's definition of mental disease or defect with the psychiatric definition of mental disorder. In the *Heads* case, for instance, it appears that the "recognition" of the PTSD by the American Psychiatric Association had a significant impact on the legal outcome. Would the aims of the legal system be met by a simple correlation between the law's definition of mental disease or defect and the disorders found in DSM–III, assuming that the law recognized only those disorders which have received "general acceptance" in the behavioral science community and can be reliably diagnosed?[g]

Gerard has argued that DSM–III should provide only the starting point for the law's analysis. Noting that psychiatry, and in particular the Freudian revolution, vastly expanded the behaviors that are labelled "ill", he posits three additional criteria that a disorder must meet before it qualifies as a "mental disease or defect" for purposes of the insanity defense. First, the disorder must meet the "traditional" definition of disease, which Gerard says is a phenomenon that is "based upon a clear description that (a) identifies the signs and symptoms, their mode of onset and chronology, (b) distinguishes the disease from others, and (c) predicts the untreated outcome with reasonable certainty on the basis of careful follow-up studies." Second, the disorder must *"characteristically"* interfere with "a person's ability to make normal choices about legally relevant behavior." Third, it must result from "physical malfunction." If not scientifically provable, this last criterion may be inferred only when the person's "behavior is irrational in the sense of being contrary to the person's own self-interest in the short range, when viewed objectively . . . and . . . compulsive in the sense of being impervious to influence by the person's environment." Applying these criteria, he concludes that, at present, only four DSM–III disorders justify invoking the insanity defense: moderate or worse mental retardation; schizophrenia; the affective disorders (mania and depression); and brain syndromes that were not induced by the voluntary ingestion of some substance, like drugs or alcohol. Gerard, "The Usefulness of the Medical Model to the Legal System," in Brooks & Winick, Current Issues in Mental Disability Law 135, 154–168 (1987) (emphasis in original).

On the other hand, LaFave and Scott, after surveying application of the various insanity tests by the courts, concluded that "any mental

g. The "general acceptance" or *Frye* test of admissibility is discussed at pp. 403–408. Many courts have permitted testimony based on evidence of post-traumatic stress syndrome, despite the recency of its development, on the ground that it is a generally accepted diagnosis. See Erlander, "Post–Traumatic Stress Disorder: Vietnam Veterans and the Law," 1 Behavioral Sciences and the Law 25 (1983).

abnormality, be it psychosis, neurosis, organic brain disorder, or congenital intellectual deficiency . . . will suffice *if* it has caused the consequences described in the second part of the test." LaFave & Scott, Criminal Law 312 (1986) (emphasis in original). In other words, the mental disease or defect predicate is relatively unimportant; what is important is whether the individual was so cognitively or volitionally impaired at the time of the offense that exculpation is necessary. In a similar vein, the ALI test leaves mental disease or defect undefined except to exclude "abnormality manifested only by repeated or otherwise anti-social conduct." This approach allows an insanity defense based on any diagnosis found in DSM–III (other than perhaps anti-social personality) that the courts are willing to recognize as sufficiently trustworthy. Presumably, it also allows a defense based on conditions not found in the Manual, as was true of the post-traumatic stress disorder prior to DSM–III. (See also, Zamora v. Florida, 361 So.2d 776 (Fla.App.1978), in which the defendant argued he was insane, ultimately unsuccessfully, based on "involuntary subliminal television intoxication" which produced a lessened appreciation of the wrongfulness of killing).

Others have adopted an intermediate position, which requires that the mental disease or defect be serious. The new federal statute, for example, provides that the mental condition must be "severe." According to the House Committee, this word was added "to emphasize that nonpsychotic behavior disorders or neuroses such as an 'inadequate personality,' 'immature personality,' or a pattern of 'antisocial tendencies' do not constitute the defense." H.R.Rep. No. 98–1030, 98th Cong., 2nd Sess. 229 (1984). The American Psychiatric Association would permit an insanity defense based only on "those severely abnormal mental conditions that grossly and demonstrably impair a person's perception or understanding of reality and that are not attributable primarily to the voluntary ingestion of alcohol or other psychoactive substances." APA, Statement on the Insanity Defense 12 (1983).

In defining mental disease or defect, the analysis may differ depending upon whether one is applying a cognitive as opposed to a volitional test. Focusing solely on the cognitive prong of the insanity defense for present purposes, which of the various formulations described above do you prefer? Would Heads have a "mental disease or defect" under your formulation? Note that one study has found that 20 to 30 percent of all Vietnam veterans "would be formally diagnosable" as experiencing a Post–Traumatic Stress Disorder. Egendorf, "The Postwar Healing of Vietnam Veterans: Recent Research," 33 Hosp. & Comm. Psychiat. 901 (1981). Another study found that, in 1979, 25% of the inmates in state prisons were veterans. Reported in 9 Crim.Def. 18 (1982).

2. *Know v. Appreciate.* Whatever the definition of mental disease or defect, it must cause, under the typical formulations of the cognitive prong, either a failure to "know" (under M'Naghten) or a "substantial inability to appreciate" (under ALI) the wrongness of the act. Although the M'Naghten test seems more rigid, Professor Goldstein's study of evidence presented and instructions given in jurisdictions which use that test indicates that the language is construed liberally, when it is defined at all. Goldstein, The Insanity Defense 49–53 (1967).

With respect to the difference between the "knowledge" and "appreciation" formulations, consider some of the facts developed in United States v.
Hinckley, in which John Hinckley was charged with attempting to assassinate the president of the United States in 1981. Before the attempt,
Hinckley had never been charged with a criminal offense. But he seemed
very interested in violent action. He read several books on famous assassi-
nations. He joined the Nazi Party and then was expelled in November,
1979, apparently because the party was alarmed over his open advocacy of
violence. He subsequently tried to organize on his own a group called The
American Front, which was designed to alert white Protestants to the
threat posed by minority groups.

According to evidence derived from Hinckley's diaries, his letters to his
parents and interviews with Hinckley, the key aspects of his mental state
at the time of the offense revolved around his obsession with the actress
Jodie Foster. This preoccupation began in 1976, when Hinckley first
viewed the film Taxi Driver. The film's main character, Travis Bickle,
rescues Iris, a child-prostitute played by Foster, from her pimp. Hinckley
identified strongly with Bickle, who, like Hinckley, was a loner and
alienated from society. Over the next several years, he bought an army
jacket and boots like Bickle's, acquired the same number of weapons that
Bickle had possessed, and tried to develop a relationship with Foster. He
left cards at her door, spoke with her over the telephone twice and tried to
reach her on several other occasions. Rejected by these advances, he did
what Bickle had done when rebuffed by women; he began to stalk the
president of the United States, at that time Jimmy Carter. On two
occasions he was near enough to Carter to attempt an assassination, but he
made no move.

After Ronald Reagan became president, Hinckley continued to think
about some action against the chief executive as a way of improving his
relationship with Foster. He copied a skyjacking note contained in a
biography of a skyjacker, intending to use it to force President Reagan to
resign and to have Jodie Foster brought to him. A postcard written to
Foster in mid-February of 1981 contained a message promising Foster that
one day she and Hinckley would occupy the White House together. Shortly before this, on New Year's Eve, 1980, he recorded a monologue. He
noted that, as usual, he was alone and afraid. He proclaimed Jodie Foster
to be the only thing that mattered in his life and made allusions to a death
pact between himself and Foster and to his own suicide. Poetry written
during the same period explored similar themes: mental deterioration,
suicide, alienation, and an assassination that receives world-wide publicity.

On March 30, the day of the assassination attempt, he was in Washington, D.C. From the newspaper, he read of President Reagan's itinerary for
the day. It was at this point that he decided to kill President Reagan. He
showered, took some Valium to calm his nerves, and loaded his .22 caliber
revolver with six Devastator bullets, ammunition which explodes on impact
with the skin. Travis Bickle had achieved a similar effect in Taxi Driver
by carving crosses on the tops of bullets. At about 12:45 he sat down to
write a letter to Jodie Foster. He described how he had repeatedly tried to
gain her attention and affection, but that time was running out. In order

to win her respect and love, he was willing to give up his freedom or possibly even his life in the perpetration of what he called a "historic deed." Shortly after finishing the letter, he concealed his weapon in the pocket of his raincoat and took a cab to the Washington Hilton, where Reagan was scheduled to speak. As Reagan came out of the hotel, Hinckley drew his revolver and fired six rounds, wounding four men, including the President.

One of the defense experts testified that on the day of the assassination Hinckley was preoccupied with two things: "the termination of his own existence" and accomplishing a "union with Jodie Foster through death, after life . . . .". The President and the other victims "were bit players who were there in a way to help him to accomplish the two major roles [which] . . . weighed far heavier in his emotional appreciation." The prosecution's expert emphasized the degree of planning involved in carrying out the attempt, the concealment of the weapon, Hinckley's admission that he knew the Secret Service might try to kill an assassin, and his decision to shoot when "[t]he Secret Service and the others in the presidential entourage looked the other way." On these facts, might one reasonably arrive at different conclusions about Hinckley's insanity, depending upon whether the test focused on "knowledge" of wrongfulness rather than on "substantial inability to appreciate" wrongfulness?[h]

Under a flexible definition of appreciation, even hardened criminals might have an insanity defense, given their lack of remorse for their criminal activity. This possibility perhaps explains the second paragraph of the ALI test excluding those whose mental illness is evidenced solely by repeated antisocial acts. The California Supreme Court offered further elaboration for the exception:

> [T]he assertion of the insanity defense by recidivists with no apparent sign of mental illness except their penchant for criminal behavior would burden the legal system, bring the insanity defense into disrepute, and imperil the ability of persons with definite mental illness to assert that defense. . . . To classify persons with 'antisocial personality' as insane would put in the mental institutions persons for whom there is currently no suitable treatment, and who would be a constant danger to the staff and other inmates. Mental hospitals are not designed for this kind of person; prisons are.

People v. Fields, 35 Cal.3d 329, 371–72, 197 Cal.Rptr. 803, 830–81, 673 P.2d 680, 707–08 (1983). Consider, in response, this excerpt from *United States v. Currens,* 290 F.2d 751, 774 n. 32 (3d Cir.1961):

> Our study has . . . revealed two very persuasive reasons why this court should not hold that evidence of psychopathy is insufficient, as a matter of law, to put sanity or mental illness in issue. First, it is clear that as the majority of experts use the term, a psychopath is very distinguishable from one who merely demonstrates recurrent criminal behavior . . . [From our survey], it can be seen that in many cases the

adjective 'psychopathic' will be applied by experts to persons who are very ill indeed.

Our second reason for not holding that psychopaths are 'sane' as a matter of law is based on the vagaries of the term itself. In each individual case all the pertinent symptoms of the accused should be put before the court and jury and the accused's criminal responsibility should be developed from the totality of his symptoms. . . . The criminal law is not concerned with . . . classifications but with the fundamental issue of criminal responsibility.

Are *Fields* and *Currens* necessarily inconsistent?

The Louisiana insanity law under which Heads was tried seems closer to the M'Naghten "knowledge" test than to the ALI "appreciation" language. If one accepts the defense theory of the case, is it plausible that Heads not only did not "appreciate" but did not "know" that his act was wrong? If one accepts the *prosecution's* theory of the case, does Heads have a plausible argument under either approach?

3. *Criminality v. Wrongfulness.* The final aspect of the cognitive tests has to do with whether "wrongness" is objectively or subjectively defined. The original M'Naghten decision permitted an insanity defense only if the accused did not know the act was *legally* wrong. Moreover, in cases where the delusion was "partial"—meaning, apparently, that it affects only the accused's thinking about the offense and not other aspects of his life—then he would not have an insanity defense even if he thought his act was legal, unless the delusion, if true, would justify the act. As the House of Lords stated:

> For example, if, under the influence of his delusion, he supposes another man to be in the act of attempting to take away his life, and he kills that man, as he supposes, in self-defense, he would be exempt from punishment. If his delusion was that the deceased had inflicted a serious injury to his character and fortune, and he killed him in revenge for such supposed injury, he would be liable to punishment.

Subsequently, several American courts rejected this view, at least in part. For instance, in *People v. Schmidt,* 216 N.Y. 324, 110 N.E. 945 (1915), Judge Cardozo stated that if a person has "an insane delusion that God has appeared to [him] and ordained the commission of a crime, we think it cannot be said of the offender that he knows the act to be wrong." This language would appear to permit an insanity acquittal of a person who, though knowing his act was legally wrong, felt "morally justified" in committing it because of mental illness. However, Judge Cardozo also expressed caution about this rule:

> The anarchist is not at liberty to break the law because he reasons that all government is wrong. The devotee of a religious cult that enjoins polygamy or human sacrifice as a duty is not thereby relieved from responsibility before the law.

The drafters of the ALI test did not attempt to resolve this issue. Instead they provided two options, the "legal wrong" approach encapsulated by the word "criminality" and the "moral wrong" approach represented by the word "wrongfulness." The states are divided evenly on the question. Washington takes a hybrid approach. It generally follows the criminality rule. According to the Washington Supreme Court, "[i]f wrong meant moral wrong judged by the individual's own conscience, this would seriously undermine the criminal law, for it would allow one who violated the law to be excused from criminal responsibility solely because, in his own conscience, his act was not morally wrong." *State v. Crenshaw*, 98 Wash.2d 789, 659 P.2d 488 (1983). However, *Crenshaw* also created a "deific decree" exception to the general rule that "wrong" means legal wrong, thus allowing a defense in a case like the one described by Cardozo in *Schmidt*. The court then upheld the homicide conviction of a person who claimed he was a member of the Moscovites—apparently a religious group which believes there is a "duty to assassinate an unfaithful spouse". The defendant had killed his wife because he "knew", despite the absence of objective evidence, that she had been unfaithful. There was also evidence that the defendant had been hospitalized on several occasions with a diagnosis of paranoia.

Assuming the other criteria for insanity are met, does Heads have an insanity defense under the criminality approach? The wrongfulness approach?

4. *Alternative formulations.* Most mentally ill people who commit violent acts have some idea that their act is against the law. Only rarely, as in the oft-used but probably unrealistic example of the man who strangles his wife thinking she is a lemon, will they have no idea they are committing a crime. Is the legal wrong approach thus too restrictive? Does the "deific decree" exception, or use of the "appreciation" language, broaden the rule sufficiently? If neither of these solutions are acceptable and the moral wrong approach must be adopted, how does one restrict that approach to avoid acquittal of anyone who has a strongly held belief that he or she is "in the right"? Does the mental disease or defect predicate handle this problem?

Several scholars reject knowledge of wrongness as the proper test for insanity. As noted in the introduction to this section some have suggested that insanity should be equated with "irrationality" or "craziness." Do these tests better capture the moral scope of the insanity defense?

3. *Volitional Impairment*

United States v. Pollard [i]

Marmion Pollard, in April, 1956, had been for several years a member of the Detroit Police Department. He was an apparently well-adjusted, highly intelligent black officer on the force, of an active nature, pleasing personality, and happy disposition. His rating as a member of the Police Department was excellent, and his intelligence quotient, as appeared from the examination of the Department, was

i. The "majority" opinion in this book's version of *Pollard* is taken from the district court opinion in the *Pollard* case, 171 F.Supp 474 (E.D.Mich.1959), and the dissenting opinion is taken from the circuit court of appeals decision reversing the district court, 282 F.2d 450 (6th Cir.1960), mandate clarified, 285 F.2d 81 (6th Cir. 1960).

very high. He was married and had four children. He was a good
husband and father and had never been in any trouble. He left a
Detroit high school, where he was a good student, when he was in the
twelfth grade, to enlist in the Navy, earning, after his full service there,
an honorable discharge.

In April, 1956, while he was on police duty, his wife and small
daughter were brutally murdered in their home by a drunken neighbor.
After the murder, Pollard's three other children, all sons, continued to
live with him and his mother-in-law, who cared for the children and the
home. Gradually, Pollard became the victim of chronic depression or
melancholia, appearing generally to be overcome with fatigue, bursting
into tears and crying and sobbing for considerable periods, and repeatedly threatening to commit suicide with his police gun. His brother-in-
law on one occasion prevented him from deliberately running onto a
thru-way, where he probably would have been killed by swift-moving
cars. On another occasion, his brother-in-law found him lying on the
floor in his home, sobbing; his body was so limp he could hardly be
lifted to the bed. After many of these incidents, Pollard seemed to
recover and would become suddenly cheerful with no memory of what
had happened.

His fellow officers in the Police Department noticed various
changes about him after the death of his wife. They weren't abrupt
changes. Sometimes a week would pass and he would seem all right;
but then he would do something out of the ordinary. In the course of
his duties as a policeman, on one day he would insist upon enforcing
the law and issue loitering tickets for violation of ordinances, and the
next day, he would express an opinion that he did not see anything
wrong with such conduct. When asked a question by his fellow
policemen, while driving with them in a scout car, he would sometimes
be silent for about ten minutes, and then answer the question as though
he had just been asked. Sometimes when he came to work with a
fellow officer, they might talk to each other normally. Other times he
would sit for two hours at a time and say nothing. This was a change
from his prior general demeanor, when he had always been very lively
and talkative. Once when he drove the scout car, he constantly beat on
the steering wheel with his fist for approximately half an hour. When,
on this occasion, he was asked if anything was wrong, he acted as
though he didn't know he was doing it, and would continue. It should
also be noted, however, that a police lieutenant of the Detroit Police
Department testified that the defendant's police work, during the
period with which we are now concerned, as evidenced by his efficiency
rating and his written duty reports, was, if anything, more effective
than his service prior to the death of his wife.

A little more than two years after the murder of his wife and
daughter, Pollard remarried, on May 22, 1958. On the day before his
remarriage, Pollard attempted to hold up a branch of the Detroit Bank
& Trust Company about eleven o'clock in the morning. With a gun, he

threatened the teller, ordering her to fill up a paper bag with money. The teller did so and handed the bag to Pollard, who ordered a bank official to accompany him to the exit. As they approached the door, the official suddenly threw his arms around Pollard, who then dropped the bag of money and ran out of the building.

About 4:00 P.M., on the same day, he entered the Chene–Medbury Branch of the Bank of the Commonwealth and walked to a railing behind which a bank employee was sitting. He pointed his gun at the man and told him to sit quietly. The employee, however, did not obey this order but instead raised an alarm, whereupon the defendant ran from the bank and again escaped.

The defendant later admitted to agents of the Federal Bureau of Investigation that after his abortive attempts to rob the two banks, he decided to rob a third bank and actually proceeded on the same day to an unnamed bank he had selected but decided not to make the attempt when he discovered that the bank was "too wide open"—had too much window area so that the possibility of apprehension was enhanced.

On June 3, at about 3:00 P.M., the defendant entered the Woodrow Wilson–Davison Branch of the Bank of the Commonwealth and went directly to an enclosure behind which a male and female employee were sitting at desks facing each other. Defendant held his gun under a jacket which he carried over his right arm. He ordered the woman employee to come out from behind the railing. In doing so, she grasped the edge of her desk. Defendant, in the belief that she may have pushed an alarm button, decided to leave but ordered the woman to accompany him out of the bank. When they reached the street, he told her to walk ahead of him, but not to attract attention. Defendant noticed a police car approaching the bank and waited until it passed him, then ran across an empty lot to his car and again escaped.

On June 11, 1958, he attempted to hold up a grocery market. He was thwarted in the attempt when the proprietor screamed and, becoming frightened, the defendant fled. In so doing, he abandoned his automobile in back of the market where he had parked it during the holdup attempt. Routinely, this car was placed under surveillance and later when the defendant, dressed in his Detroit Police Officer's uniform, attempted to get in it, he was arrested by detectives of the Detroit Police Force.

After his apprehension, the defendant confessed to eleven other robberies, or attempted robberies.

The three psychiatrists who submitted the written reports, all qualified and respected members of their profession, testified that in their opinion the defendant, at the time he committed the criminal acts, knew the difference between right and wrong and knew that the acts he committed were wrong but was suffering from a "traumatic neurosis" or "dissociative reaction", characterized by moods of depression and severe feelings of guilt, induced by the traumatic effect of the death of his wife and child and his belief that he was responsible for their deaths because by his absence from home he left them exposed to the actions of the crazed, drunken neighbor. They further stated that he had an unconscious desire to be punished by society to expiate these guilt feelings and that the governing power of his mind was so destroyed or impaired that he was unable to resist the commission of the criminal acts. In their opinion, however, the defendant was not then, nor is he now, psychotic or committable to a mental institution.

Counsel for defendant contends that since all the medical testimony was to the effect that the defendant was suffering from an irresistible impulse at the time of the commission of the offenses, this Court must accept this uncontroverted expert testimony and find him not guilty by reason of insanity.

* * *

Psychiatry and law approach the problem of human behavior from different philosophical perspectives. Psychiatry purports to be scientific and takes a deterministic position with regard to behavior. "Its view of human nature is expressed in terms of drives and dispositions which, like mechanical forces, operate in accordance with universal laws of causation." Hall, "Psychiatry and Criminal Responsibility", 65 Yale Law Journal 761, 764. For psychiatry, what we do is determined by what we are, and there is little or no room for moral or ethical judgments. In a sense, all criminal behavior, whether it be the acts of the rapist, the forger, the embezzler, the sender of licentious literature through the mails or tax evasion by a reputable businessman, is evidence of mental disease. But the uncritical adoption of this point of view would completely do away with the concept of criminal responsibility. Dangell, Criminal Law, Sec. 128; White, Insanity and the Criminal Law, at page 26; Weihofen, "Crime, Law and Psychiatry", 4 Kansas Law Review 377, 386. Criminal law is "a practical, rational, normative science which, although it draws upon theoretical science, also is concerned to pass judgment on human conduct. Its view of human nature asserts the reality of free choice and rejects the thesis that the conduct of normal adults is a mere expression of imperious psychological necessity. Given the additional purpose to evaluate conduct, some degree of autonomy is a necessary postulate." Hall, supra at page 764.

The psychiatrists, as hereinbefore related, testified that the defendant suffered from severe feelings of depression and guilt; and that in their opinion he had an irresistible impulse to commit criminal acts, an unconscious desire to be apprehended and punished; and that he geared his behavior to the accomplishment of this end. However, his entire pattern of conduct during the period of his criminal activities militates against this conclusion. His conscious desire not to be apprehended and punished was demonstrably greater than his unconscious desire to the contrary. After his apprehension, despite searching interrogation for over five hours by Detroit Police Officers and by agents of the Federal Bureau of Investigation, he denied any participation in criminal conduct of any kind. It was only after he was positively identified by bank personnel that he finally admitted that he did attempt to perpetrate the bank robberies. The trial judge asked one of the psychiatrists to explain this apparent inconsistency. In answer, he stated that although the defendant had an unconscious desire to be apprehended and punished, when the possibility of apprehension became direct and immediate, the more dominating desire for self-preservation asserted itself. This explanation may have merit if applied to individual acts. However, the validity of a theory that attempts to explain the behavior of a person must be determined in light of that person's entire behavioral pattern and not with reference to isolated acts which are extracted from the pattern. The defendant's pattern of behavior of May 21, 1958, discloses that the desire for self-preservation was not fleeting and momentary but continuing, consistent and dominant. What, then, becomes of the theory of irresistible impulse? Looking to the events of that day, we are asked to believe, first, that the defendant, acting pursuant to an irresistible impulse, selected a bank site to rob, entered the bank to accomplish that end, purposely failed in the attempt and when the end he sought, apprehension, was in view, escaped because of the dominance, at the moment of ultimate accomplishment, of the stronger drive for self-preservation. We must then believe that when the defendant knew he was apparently free from detection, his compulsive state reasserted itself and that he again went through the steps of planning, abortive attempt and escape. And if we acquiesce in this theory, what other psychiatric theory explains his subsequent conduct—his plan to rob a third unnamed bank and the rejection of that plan because of his subjective belief that the possibility of apprehension would be too great? If the theory remains the same, then it appears that in the latter case, the fear of apprehension and punishment tipped "the scales enough to make resistible an impulse otherwise irresistible." It is a logical inference that, in reality, the other robbery attempts were made as the result of impulses that the defendant did not choose voluntarily to resist because, to him, the possibility of success outweighed the likelihood of detection which is in essence a motivation for all criminal conduct. The impulse being resistible, the defendant is accountable for his criminal conduct.

Psychiatrists admit that the line between irresistible impulse and acts which are the result of impulses not resisted is not easy to trace. To the extent that the line may be traced, the distinguishing motivation of the action, whether the act is performed to satisfy an intrinsic need or is the result of extrinsic provocation, is a determining factor. Admittedly, motivations may be mixed. However, all the facts have clearly established that defendant's criminal activity was planned to satisfy an extrinsic need by a reasoned but anti-social method. The defendant had financial problems of varying degrees of intensity throughout his life. He had financial difficulties during his first marriage. He was now embarking upon a second marriage. He was about to undertake the responsibility of supporting not only a wife and himself, but also four children, three of them the product of his first marriage. In statements given to agents of the Federal Bureau of Investigation admitting his criminal activity, he stated: "Inasmuch as I was about to marry my second wife, I decided that I would not lead the same type of financially insecure life that I led with my first wife. I needed about $5,000 in order to buy a home. My only purpose in deciding to rob a bank was to obtain $5,000 and if I obtained the money, I did not intend to continue robbing." Defendant's entire pattern of conduct was consistent with this expressed motivation.

Life does not always proceed on an even keel. Periods of depression, feelings of guilt and inadequacy are experienced by many of us. Defendant was a devoted husband and loving father. His feelings of despondency and depression induced by the brutal killing of his wife and infant daughter were not unnatural. How else the defendant should have reacted to his tragic loss we are not told. His conduct throughout this crucial period did not cause any concern among his colleagues. All stated unequivocally that in their opinion he was sane. Significant also is the fact that his present wife married him on May 22, 1958, after a year of courtship. It is a permissible inference that defendant's conduct relative to his mental condition, as related by her, did not suggest to her that the defendant was insane.

We are satisfied beyond a reasonable doubt that the defendant committed the acts for which he is now charged and that when he committed them he was legally sane.

DISSENT

If the mere preponderance of evidence created a reasonable doubt as to whether appellant acted under an irresistible impulse, the government did not prove his guilt. When there has been created, by the evidence, a reasonable doubt as to whether an accused person acted under an irresistible impulse, the burden is upon the prosecution to establish, beyond a reasonable doubt, that he did not act under an irresistible impulse.

In the instant case, the psychiatric witnesses had unanimously agreed that Pollard suffered from severe feelings of depression and guilt; that, in their opinion, he had an irresistible impulse to commit criminal acts; an unconscious desire to be apprehended and punished; and that he geared his behavior to the accomplishment of this end. The court, however, states that his entire pattern of conduct during the period of his criminal activities militated against this conclusion, and that his conscious desire not to be apprehended and punished was demonstrably greater than his unconscious desire to the contrary. Without drawing any conclusions from the foregoing as to whether appellant's conscious or unconscious desires were the stronger, it can be said that acts that appear rational are not to be taken by the factfinder as evidence of sanity, where all of the other evidence in the case is proof of a defendant's mental unsoundness.

It should also be mentioned that in the Report of the Neuropsychiatric Staff Conference of the Medical Center for Federal Prisoners, it was pointed out that the attempted robberies by Pollard were bizarre and ineffectively planned and executed; that when he tried to leave one bank, he ordered a bank official to follow behind him instead of ahead of him, which resulted in his being caught from behind and barely escaping after a struggle, during which he dropped the paper bag of money he had collected; that on the various occasions of his attempted robberies, he would suddenly enter a bank that he had never seen before, without prior knowledge of the arrangement of the premises, or of the personnel. Taken in consideration with all of the other factors, such conduct, on the part of a highly intelligent police officer with a knowledge of how crimes are committed, has about it nothing of sanity.

It is emphasized by the government that Pollard was motivated to attempt the bank robberies because of his need for financial security. The claimed motivation seems pointless. Pollard, during his first marriage, had been receiving the regular salary of a policeman with promotions, of approximately $450 a month. His first wife, at that time, was receiving about $300 a month as a clerk with the Michigan Unemployment Compensation Commission. Their joint income was almost twice what a regular policeman's salary would be. His second wife, at the time of her marriage to him, had money of her own— enough to pay her own bills, and take care of her daughter with the money which was paid for support by her former husband. She had previously held a position for six years with the Michigan Bell Telephone Company. She considered herself to be relatively comfortable financially. Between the time of Pollard's arrest on June 11, 1958, and his trial, she had, herself, paid off about $700 in bills that he had owed. Pollard's financial condition could not be considered a reasonable motivation for his attempted bank robberies. As far as income went, he was much better off than most other policemen and if such a financial condition could be considered a reasonable motivation for Pollard's attempted robberies, every other policeman in the department would have had twice the motivation to commit such crimes as Pollard had.

Certain distinctions have been drawn by courts in applying the rule of irresistible impulse. While anger, greed, and passion are said, in ordinary parlance, to result in acts because of desires that have become irresistible, this is not, in law, the "irresistible impulse" that results from a mental defect or mental disease. Further, it is held that "emotional insanity," which is an unbridled passion lasting just long enough to enable the act complained of to be done, and then subsiding, does not relieve the accused of accountability, even in those jurisdictions where the doctrine of irresistible impulse, arising out of a mental defect, is recognized. Moreover, to like effect, in *Bell v. State,* 120 Ark. 530, 180 S.W. 186, 196 (1915), the court although sustaining the doctrine of irresistible impulse as a defense to crime, distinguished between such impulse and "emotional" insanity, as follows: "But it must be remembered that one who is otherwise sane will not be excused from a crime he has committed while his reason is temporarily dethroned not by disease, but by anger, jealousy, or other passion."

From all of the evidence of the lay and expert witnesses, however, it cannot be affirmatively concluded that Pollard was sane. Obviously, as a result of the murder of his wife and child while he was absent from his home, he was suffering from some grave disorder, and that disorder was, in the opinion of all the psychiatric and medical experts, a disassociative reaction resulting in Pollard's commission of the acts charged because of an irresistible impulse.

Questions and Comments

1. *Volition, causation and compulsion.* The "majority" opinion cites several commentators to the effect that the "deterministic" premise of psychiatry, if given full sway, could "do away with the concept of criminal responsibility". This concern is most often voiced when discussing application of the volitional tests for insanity, because these tests directly pose the question of whether a person could control his or her behavior. If mental health professionals answer this question honestly, the argument goes, they will always say that an individual's acts are caused by various endogenous or exogenous factors over which the individual had little or no control.

In *Pollard,* for instance, the psychiatric testimony suggested that Pollard was not aware of his true reasons for acting, and thus, in some sense, he was not "in control of" his actions. Another common type of case in which "lack-of-control" defenses are raised involves defendants diagnosed as having "impulse disorders" such as kleptomania, pyromania, or pedophilia. Other examples are legion. For example, in *People v. Yukl,* 83 Misc.2d 364, 372 N.Y.S.2d 313 (1975), the defendant raised an insanity defense relying on evidence that individuals with an extra Y (or male) chromosome are particularly aggressive, and thus less able to control their behavior. See Note, "The XYY Chromosomal Abnormality: Use and Misuse in the Legal Process," 9 Harv.J.Legis. 469 (1972). Several cases have involved claims that the type of posttraumatic stress syndrome raised in *Heads* not only made it difficult for the defendant to distinguish right from wrong, but also "compelled" the defendant to act violently. See, e.g., *Louisiana v. Sharp,* 418 So.2d 1344 (1982) (defendant had "uncontrollable 'rage reaction'" as a result of PTSD). Unusual plasma androgen levels are said to "overinfluence" sexual offenders. Rada, "Plasma Androgens and the Sex Offender," 8 Bull.Am.Acad.Psychiat. & L. 456 (1980). It has also been asserted that women, just prior to or during early menstruation, may be prone to uncontrollable impulses resulting in violence. See Note, "Premenstrual Syndrome: A Criminal Defense," 59 Notre Dame L.Rev. 253 (1983).

Other defenses have been predicated on pressures that appear to be as much "external" as "internal". In *United States v. Alexander and Murdock,* 471 F.2d 923 (D.C.Cir.1972), for instance, the evidence showed that Murdock grew up in the Watts section of Los Angeles in a large family with little love or attention and no father. He became "greatly preoccupied with the unfair treatment of negroes in this country and believe[d] that racial war is inevitable." Early one morning, Murdock and his companions became involved in an argument with a group of Marines, all of whom were white. Murdock admitted that, during the altercation, which took place in a hamburger shop, he drew his fully loaded gun and emptied it. He killed two of the Marines, even though he had not seen any weapons. As they drove from the scene, he took his companion's gun and continued firing into the restaurant. In explanation, he said that just before he began firing he had heard someone say "Get out, you black bastards". He also claimed he saw Marines advancing toward him, although the surviving Marines denied this allegation. His attorney argued that Murdock was unable to control his conduct because of a "deepseated emotional disorder that was rooted in his 'rotten social background.'" Id. at 957–59.

How should the criminal law respond to these types of claims? In "Responsibility and the Unconscious," 53 So.Cal.L.Rev. 1563 (1980), Moore draws a distinction between "causation" on the one hand and "compulsion" on the other:

> Everyone is undoubtedly caused to act as they do by a myriad of environmental, physiological, or psychological factors. Yet to say that any actions are caused, for example, by an unhappy childhood, a chemical imbalance, or a belief that it is raining, is not to say the actions are compelled. One must point to something other than causation to make out the excuse of compulsion. . . .

Moore then uses the *Pollard* case to illustrate his point.

> Suppose Pollard did unconsciously feel guilty at the death of his first wife and child. He may have felt guilty because he had not been there; alternatively, he may have felt guilty because he had unconsciously wished to kill them himself. In either case, could such unconscious guilt *compel* Pollard to do an act for which he would be punished?

In answering this question, Moore compares Pollard to the kleptomaniac (a person who appears to experience a strong urge to steal). The kleptomaniac, according to Moore, feels compelled to steal and knows he is yielding to the compulsion, "yet he does not know the object of his passionate desire. . . . A few thefts readily tell him it is not the stolen objects themselves." Pollard on the other hand, "had a perfectly intelligible, conscious motive for acting. In such circumstances one is often more reluctant to accept as a factual matter that some unconscious emotion really explains his behavior."

Even accepting Moore's distinction between causation and compulsion, one may have difficulty differentiating between the two in an individual case. Do you agree with Moore that Pollard was probably not "compelled" by his unconscious guilt to commit the robberies and attempted robberies? As another example, assume that research shows that men with an extra Y chromosome are significantly more likely to commit violent acts than men with normal chromosomal structure. Should the decision as to whether an "XYY" defendant has an insanity defense depend upon whether he had "a perfectly intelligible, conscious motive for acting" (which will normally be the case)? Finally, using Moore's compulsion-causation distinction, how do you evaluate Murdock's claim?

2. *Reform efforts.* The previous note identified two concerns associated with the volitional prong. The first is that it could swallow up the criminal law by providing an excuse for everyone, particularly as the behavioral sciences become more sophisticated. The second is that, even if the volitional prong can theoretically be limited, as Moore has tried to do, difficulties associated with determining who is properly excused under the test could lead to mistake or abuse. Of the reforms advanced to address these problems, three stand out.

Elimination of Volitional Prong. The first, of course, is abolition of the volitional prong, a step the U.S. Congress took in the Insanity Defense Reform Act of 1984. Is this solution justifiable, assuming that there are people who knowingly commit crime but apparently "can't help themselves?" Consider the following comment by Bonnie, an opponent of the volitional tests:

> It might be argued, of course, that the risk of mistake should be tolerated if the volitional prong of the defense is morally necessary. The question may be put this way: Are there clinically identifiable cases involving defendants whose behavior controls were so pathologically impaired that they ought to be acquitted although their ability to appreciate the wrongfulness of their actions was unimpaired? I do not think so. The most clinically compelling cases of volitional impairment involve the so-called impulse disorders—pyromania, kleptomania, and the like. These disorders involve severely abnormal compulsions that ought to be taken into account in sentencing, but the exculpation of pyromaniacs would be out of touch with commonly shared moral intuitions.

Bonnie, "The Moral Basis of the Insanity Defense," 69 A.B.A.J. 194, 197 (1983). Do you agree that the conviction of pyromaniacs for arson and kleptomaniacs for theft is in "touch with commonly shared moral intuitions"?[j] Under Bonnie's approach, would Pollard be convicted and the psychiatric testimony relegated to a sentencing hearing? Or is the expert testimony in this case possibly relevant to cognitive impairment as well?

Related to this latter question, as well as the movement toward elimination of the volitional prong, consider the effect of adopting an "irrationality" test for insanity. Would volitional impairment be irrelevant under this test? If Pollard's real reason for committing the robberies was to assuage his guilt by getting caught, was he rational? How would a kleptomaniac fare under such a test? An "XYY" defendant? Consider this excerpt from Fingarette, The Meaning of Insanity, 160–172 (1972), an advocate of the rationality test:

> We may find it congenial to speak idiomatically of the insane person as one who is driven, or seized, or overwhelmed, or possessed by fear,

---

j. One study in Maryland concluded that manic patients are often severely impaired in their capacity to control behavior, while their cognitive impairment is less striking. As a result, the authors asserted, elimination of the volitional prong could lead to conviction of "a class of psychotic patients whose illness is clearest in symptomatology, most likely biologic in origin, most eminently treatable and potentially most disruptive in penal detention." Governor's Task Force to Review the Defense of Insanity, State of Maryland (reported in R. Simon & D. Aaronson, The Insanity Defense 167 (1988)).

anxiety, emotions or delusions. Yet there is one literal truth we must never lose sight of: it is the person himself who initiates and carries out the deed, it is his desire, his mood, his passion, his belief which is at issue, and it is he who acts to satisfy this desire, or to express this mood, emotion, or belief of his. Even if his motive is unconscious, it is his motive, and it is he who acts out of this motive.

From this premise, Fingarette argues that "[t]here is a crucial difference between saying a person lacks capacity to conform to law (that is, cannot conform to law) and saying that he does not control his conduct in the way a normal person does." Virtually all nonresponsible insane persons can control their conduct in the latter sense. What distinguishes them from responsible sane people "is the way in which [they come] to adopt one or another course of action"—the fact that they do so irrationally.

Tightening the Definition of Mental Disease. An alternative solution to the dangers of mistake or abuse associated with the volitional prong is to narrow the definition of mental disease or defect for purposes of the insanity defense. The traditional unstructured approach is illustrated by the "dissent" in *Pollard,* which cited several authorities for the proposition that the irresistible impulse must result from a persistent disease, rather than a "temporary", "normal" reaction. Along these lines is *United States v. Lyons,* 731 F.2d 243 (5th Cir.1984), which held that drug addiction is not a mental disease or defect for purposes of the insanity defense unless it causes "actual drug-induced or drug-aggravated psychosis, or physical damage to the brain or nervous system". Other attempts to narrow the mental disease or defect predicate have been described in the previous discussion of the cognitive prong. The most restrictive definitions are found in the federal statute, which limits the insanity defense to "severe" diseases, and in the recommendation of the American Psychiatric Association, which would only permit an insanity defense based on proof of "conditions that grossly and demonstrably impair a person's perception or understanding of reality." Neither the federal statute nor the APA recognize a volitional impairment defense. But if their approach to the mental disease or defect predicate were applied in the volitional context, would persons with impulse disorders (e.g., the kleptomaniac) and personality disorders (e.g., Murdock) have a defense under a control test? Would Pollard? Would the volitional prong have any significance independently of the cognitive prong?

Tightening the Definition of Volitional Impairment. A final reform, more widely espoused when the volitional prong was first adopted than presently, is to require that the impulsive act be truly "irresistible." This concept has been colloquially captured by the "policeman at the elbow" rubric: would the accused have committed the act had a policeman been present at the time? Even kleptomaniacs try to elude detection, and thus would probably not have a defense under a tightened volitional prong. However, determining whether the impulse was irresistible or merely not resisted will still be difficult for some cases. For instance, Hinckley committed his assassination attempt in the midst of several policemen and Secret Service agents. But was his attempt "irresistible"?

3. *Research on the volitional prong.* Recent empirical evidence suggests that the concern over mistake or abuse which underlies the foregoing proposals may be unwarranted. Relying on results obtained by trained mental health professionals using a structured interview format, one study found that, while neither determination is likely to lead to highly reliable results, interrater agreement on the volitional and cognitive prongs was virtually identical. Rogers, "Empiricism v. Emotionalism," 42 Am.Psychol. 840, 841–42 (1987). Using the same interview format, a second study found that reliance on the volitional prong resulted in 23.5% fewer insanity recommendations from mental health professionals than did use of the cognitive prong. Rogers & Clark, "Diogenes Revisited: Another Search for the Ultimate NGRI Standard," Paper presented at American Academy of Psychiatry and Law meeting, Albuquerque (October, 1985). Assume that research eventually substantiates that psychiatric assessment of volitional impairment is at least as reliable as assessment of cognitive impairment, as well as less likely to result in acquittal. How would these findings affect your attitude toward eliminating the volitional prong or, if that prong is retained, narrowing the definition of mental disease or defect or increasing the level of control required?

4. *The Supreme Court and the volitional prong.* While the Supreme Court has yet to rule squarely on the constitutional status of the insanity defense, it has handed down several decisions that might relate to the necessity of the volitional prong. In *Leland v. Oregon,* 343 U.S. 790, 72 S.Ct. 1002, 96 L.Ed. 1302 (1952), rehearing denied, 344 U.S. 848, 73 S.Ct. 4, 97 L.Ed. 659 (1952), it held that, given the state of knowledge at that time, due process did not mandate use of an insanity test any broader than the traditional M'Naghten formulation. However, in *Robinson v. California,* 370 U.S. 660, 82 S.Ct. 1417, 8 L.Ed.2d 758 (1962) and *Powell v. Texas,* 392 U.S. 514, 88 S.Ct. 2145, 20 L.Ed.2d 1254 (1968), the Court suggested that some aspects of volition must be considered in gauging criminal liability. *Robinson* held that the Eighth Amendment's prohibition against cruel and unusual punishment bars punishing someone merely for being addicted to heroin. In *Powell* five justices interpreted this holding as a ban on convicting a person for an "irresistible urge," at least under certain circumstances. While the majority in *Powell* decided that an alcoholic could constitutionally by convicted for being drunk *in public,* Justice White wrote a concurring opinion in which he stated that, after *Robinson,* "the chronic alcoholic with an irresistible urge to consume alcohol should not be punishable [merely] for drinking or for being drunk", a statement with which the four dissenters agreed. Does this language, if it reflects the position of a majority of the Court, require states to provide an "irresistible impulse" insanity defense?

B. THE AUTOMATISM DEFENSE

NOTE ON AUTOMATISM

Except for strict liability offenses, which are not relevant to the topic of this chapter, every crime is comprised of at least two elements: (1) the physical conduct associated with the crime (known as the "actus reus"); and (2) the mental state, or level of intent, associated with the crime (known as the "mens rea"). To convict an individual of a particular crime, the state must prove beyond a reasonable doubt that the defendant committed the actus reus with the requisite mens rea for that crime.

The automatism defense developed out of the law's attempt to define the actus reus concept. The actus reus contemplates a voluntary physical act. For instance, if A pushes B's arm into C, B cannot be convicted of assault even though B's arm committed the actual touching, because B's act was not voluntary. It could also be said that B did not intend to commit the assault, and thus did not have the mens rea for the crime. But a distinction is usually made between an act over which there is no conscious control and a conscious action with unintended consequences. The assault above is an example of the first type of act and has traditionally been analyzed under the voluntariness requirement of the actus reus. An example of the latter situation would be if B, in tapping C, meant only to frighten him but instead killed him; B's act would be voluntary, but he would not have the mens rea for murder.

The automatism (or "unconsciousness") defense recognizes that some criminal acts may be committed "involuntarily," even though no third party (like A in the example above) is involved. The classic example of the "automaton" is the person who commits an offense while sleep-walking; courts have held that such an individual does not have conscious control of his or her physical actions and therefore acts involuntarily. See, e.g., *Fain v. Commonwealth*, 78 Ky. 183 (1879). Other situations in which the defense might be implicated arise when a crime occurs during a state of unconsciousness induced by concussion following a head injury; by shock created by bullet wounds; or by metabolic disorders such as anoxia, hypoglycemia, or the involuntary ingestion of alcohol or drugs. Events caused by epilepsy are probably best placed in this category as well.

Several courts have limited the automatism defense by holding that a person claiming to have been affected by one of the above-named conditions at the time of the offense cannot prevail with the defense if the disability has been experienced on previous occasions and steps reasonably could have been taken to prevent the criminal occurrence. Thus, if a man knows he is subject to epileptic seizures, loses control of a car because of a seizure, and kills someone in the process, he may not be able to take advantage of the defense. See, e.g., *People v. Decina*, 2 N.Y.2d 133, 157 N.Y.S.2d 558, 138 N.E.2d 799 (1956).

Conceptually, the automatism defense differs from the insanity defense in three ways. First, insane persons, unlike "automatons," are generally conscious of their acts but either do not understand the true nature of the acts or cannot stop themselves from performing them. Second, while there is some dispute over whether sanity is an element that must be proven for each offense, the prosecution clearly bears the burden of establishing the actus reus and thus bears the burden of negating an automatism claim beyond a reasonable doubt. Finally, to prevail, a person alleging insanity must be found to have a mental disease or defect; there is no such requirement when automatism is involved.

Questions and Comments

1. *Application.* As indicated above, the automatism defense contemplates a loss of conscious control over one's bodily movements. Does either Heads or Pollard have a viable automatism claim? In *People v. Lisnow*, 88 Cal.App.3d Supp. 21, 26–27, 151 Cal.Rptr. 621, 623 (1978), the court held that a Vietnam veteran who struck a maitre d' in a restaurant for "no apparent reason" and then went into the parking lot and engaged in other "acts of violence" while in a "dreamlike" state was entitled to an instruction on the automatism defense. See also, Apostle, "The Unconsciousness Defense as Applied to Post Traumatic Stress Disorder in a Vietnam Veteran," 8 Bull.Am.Acad.Psychiat. & L. 426 (1980). In a jurisdiction where the volitional prong of the insanity test is eliminated, would the automatism defense take up the slack? Why or why not?

2. *Incapacitation concerns.* Most commentators agree that an epileptic seizure is best characterized as an involuntary act rather than an "irresistible impulse," because the seizure is not triggered by the individual's conscious, or even unconscious, processes. Yet courts in Britain, where the law of automatism is well developed, have rejected automatism defenses based on epilepsy and instead have permitted only claims of insanity, on the explicit ground that to do otherwise would result in immediate release of dangerous individuals. See, e.g., *Bratty v. Attorney–General for Northern Ireland*, 3 All E.R. 535 (1961). Why might commitment statutes for insanity acquittees not apply to those acquitted on an automatism defense? Is there any way to avoid distorting the insanity doctrine while at the same time protecting the public in the latter type of case?

C. EXPERT TESTIMONY ON MENS REA (THE DIMINISHED CAPACITY DOCTRINE)

NOTE ON MENS REA

The principal device the law uses to grade culpability is mental state. A person who deliberately plans a crime is more culpable than one who accidentally commits one. Under the common law, courts developed literally scores of "mens rea" terms to describe various levels of culpability. Unfortunately, these terms—"willful and wanton," "with a depraved heart," and so on—were more colorful than descriptive. Over the years, two generic categories were created to help categorize these diverse mental states, although they were only partially successful in doing so. "Specific intent" was meant to designate the mens rea for those crimes that require a further intention beyond that identified with the physical act connected with the offense (e.g., "premeditated" murder, "aggravated" assault, assault "with intent to rape"). "General intent" crimes, on the other hand, were those that merely required proof that the defendant was conscious or should have been conscious of his or her physical actions at the time of the offense (e.g., manslaughter, assault, rape).

Because neither the original mens rea terms nor the concepts of specific and general intent were necessarily self-defining, modern statutory codes have attempted to be more precise on issues relating to mental state. Most influential in this regard has been the ALI's Model Penal Code formulation, which attempts to simplify the mens rea inquiry by specifying a total of four levels of mens rea. In descending order of culpability, they are (1) "purpose," requiring proof that the offender intended the relevant conduct or result; (2) "knowledge," requiring proof that the offender was aware of the conduct or result; (3) "recklessness," requiring proof that the offender consciously disregarded "a substantial and unjustifiable risk" that he or she was engaging in the conduct or causing a result; and (4) "negligence," requiring proof that the offender should have been aware of "a substantial and unjustifiable risk" that he or she was engaging in the conduct or causing a result. The first two mental states clearly focus on subjective mental state, "negligence" is commonly said to be objectively defined, and "recklessness" falls somewhere in between. Although the common-law terms are so amorphous that equating them with Model Penal Code mental states is a somewhat risky venture, it is probably fair to say that "specific intent" most closely coincides with "purpose" and "knowledge," while "general intent" can be analogized to "recklessness" and "negligence."

As will become clear below, distinguishing between subjective mental states (purpose, knowledge, and specific intent) and objectively defined mental states (negligence, general intent) is important in understanding the courts' approach to clinical input on mens rea. It is also important to recognize that the mens rea inquiry described above is quite distinct from the insanity inquiry. While it may be true that persons who meet the M'Naghten test may also be incapable of forming the requisite intent for an offense, it is theoretically and practically possible for insane persons to have the appropriate mens rea. Their *reasons* for committing acts may be so "crazy" that no jury would be willing to hold them criminally responsible, even though their knowledge of what they were doing was relatively unimpaired. To use the *M'Naghten* case as an example, Daniel M'Naghten probably met the mens rea requirements for the crime charged (i.e., knowingly shooting at another with the purpose of killing him), but he was nonetheless found insane.

Out of this distinction has developed the so-called "diminished capacity" concept. In its broadest sense, the diminished capacity doctrine permits the accused to introduce clinical testimony focusing directly on the mens rea for the crime charged, without having to assert an insanity defense.[k] If the testimony negates the mens rea, the

k. As the American Bar Association has pointed out, the phrase "diminished capacity" can be misleading since it implies a "quasi-insanity defense" that the defendant is acquitted only of that charge and may still be prosecuted on lesser charges. Thus, a person charged with first degree murder might be able to escape conviction on that charge if clinical testimony shows that he or she did not kill purposely or knowingly (or with specific intent). However, conviction may still occur on a lesser charge requiring a lesser intent (e.g. manslaughter or assault). The following materials evaluate the ramifications of this idea.

JOHNSON v. STATE

Court of Appeals of Maryland, 1982.
292 Md. 405, 439 A.2d 542.

* * *

DIGGES, JUDGE.

Lawrence Johnson was convicted, after removal of this criminal cause from Baltimore County, by a jury in the Circuit Court for Calvert County of first degree murder (both premeditated and in the commission of a felony), first degree rape, kidnapping, and use of a handgun during the commission of a felony or a crime of violence. The same jury subsequently sentenced Johnson to death for the murder.

* * *

The sordid chronicle of this crime spree was related by the appellant, Lawrence Johnson, at trial. It began on the early morning of February 23, 1980, when he was suddenly awakened by a friend, Amos Batts, while perched on the couch at the home of his cousin, Dwayne Mayers. At the urging of Batts, Johnson followed his friend outside to a car being operated by the cousin. It soon became apparent to Johnson that Mayers and Batts had stolen the vehicle during the night and had abducted its owner, Betty Toulson, in the process. Although Johnson had earlier declined to participate when the other two decided to obtain some money through crime, the defendant this time joined them in the car with the victim. After a brief discussion, Mayers started the vehicle and drove around while the three men smoked "parsley flakes sprayed with some kind of embalming fluid." The victim remained silent throughout this journey "with her head down." Later, after driving to a remote area of Baltimore County, Mayers stopped the car and asked whether his companions "wanted to have sex" with their prisoner. Mayers and the appellant eventually raped the woman on the back seat of her car. The trio then drove the victim to another location nearby where Mayers stripped Ms. Toulson of her

defendant must prove, when in fact the underlying notion is merely a recognition that clinical testimony may be just as relevant to the mens rea inquiry as evidence of mistake or intoxication. See commentary to ABA Criminal Justice Mental Health Standard 7–6.2. This book will nonetheless use the phrase "diminished capacity doctrine" because, as subsequent materials make clear, most jurisdictions have developed special rules with respect to clinical mens rea testimony that go far beyond the simple relevance notion that usually applies to other mens rea testimony. At the same time, in recognition of the fact that the prosecution bears the burden of proving beyond a reasonable doubt that the defendant had the requisite mens rea, this book avoids calling the diminished capacity notion a "defense."

coat and pocketbook. After discussing the problem presented by the victim's knowledge of their identities, Mayers returned to the automobile, removed a pistol from under the seat, and presented it to appellant with instructions to kill the woman. Johnson led her into the woods and complied with the directive. Ms. Toulson's snow-covered body was recovered five days later; she had received fatal shots in the head and chest.

* * *

Johnson . . . asserts that the trial court erred in not admitting certain psychological evidence at trial where he sought to use this information, not to establish his legal insanity, but rather, to demonstrate that he lacked a sufficient mental capacity to form the requisite intent to commit murder in the first degree. As an aid to an understanding of this issue we set out its factual predicate.

At trial, the defense called Dr. Ernest Kamm, a clinical psychologist at the Clifton T. Perkins Hospital Center. Dr. Kamm had conducted a psychological examination of Johnson as part of the court ordered evaluation performed by the Perkins staff and had prepared a report of his findings. Counsel for Johnson proffered that he wished to use Dr. Kamm's entire report and testimony "to go to the mitigation of First Degree Murder and any specific [intent] crimes," rather than to raise the issue of defendant's sanity. The court allowed the psychologist to read to the jury only parts of his report relating to intelligence tests he had administered to Johnson and his conclusion, based on those tests, that the defendant "functions at the borderline intellectual level (I.Q. 72) . . ."[6] Appellant urges that the entire report is relevant to his

---

6. We reproduce here in full Dr. Kamm's psychological report with emphasis indicating the portions read to the jury:

TESTS ADMINISTERED:

WAIS

Bender–Gestalt

Holtsman Inkblot Technique

Color Pyramid Test

TEST BEHAVIOR:

The patient is a 19–year old youth of medium height and build who presented a neat and clean appearance. He was extremely sullen and hostile, and his co-operation for interview and test was poor. In view of this test results have to be considered tentative.

TEST RESULTS:

On the WAIS he earned a Verbal I.Q. of 78, a Performance I.Q. of 68, and a Full Scale I.Q. of 72 which places him within the borderline range of intelligence. His potential, as gauged by his abstract reasoning, is at least within the low average range. Intellectual efficiency is decreased by a combination of edu-

cational deprivation and negativism. There are some signs which point in the direction of bizarre thinking and a tenuous hold on reality. E.G. on Card 22 of the Holtzman he saw "the devil," and on Card 27 he saw "God over water." But these should be interpreted with caution, as they may also be attempts to embarrass and express contempt for the examiner by giving nonsensical answers.

The personality picture is that of an extremely deprived individual who does not expect any affection and emotional support from either parental figure. He perceives the mother figure as domineering, but distant and devoid of warmth and understanding and the father figure as hostile and threatening. Yet he has conjured up the image of an idealized, all wise and all loving father surrogate with whom he will compare any male elder. Since such a person is bound to fall short of his ideal he is apt to equate this person with the real father figure whom he sees in negative terms and reject him. As a result he not only has trouble with authority figures, but perceives the

defense of "diminished capacity"—that is, he did not have sufficient mental capacity to form the requisite specific intent to commit some of the crimes with which he is charged. Consequently, the argument goes, it was error to keep that information from the jury when it determines the guilt issue. In order to decide whether this ruling on the evidence was erroneous, however, we must first examine whether the criminal defense known as "diminished capacity," or as it is sometimes called, "diminished responsibility," is recognized in this State. Only if such a doctrine exists in our jurisprudence is defendant arguably entitled to produce evidence in support of it. Because we here determine, however, that this State does not recognize diminished capacity as a legal doctrine operating to negate specific criminal intent, it was not error to exclude evidence in support of it.

* * *

The states are less than unanimous in their resolution of the question whether application of diminished capacity to criminal trials on the issue of guilt represents a legally sound resolution of the pressing problem of how the criminal law should treat evidence of mental abnormality that does not establish the actor's legal insanity. It is generally recognized, however, that adoption of the concept of diminished capacity as a separate defense involves "a fundamental change in the common law theory of [criminal] responsibility," *Fisher v. United States,* 328 U.S. 463, 476, 66 S.Ct. 1318, 1325, 90 L.Ed. 1382 (1946). This is true because the introduction of expert psychiatric testimony concerning the defendant's mental aberrations when the basic sanity of the accused is not at issue conflicts with the governing principle of the criminal law that all legally sane individuals are equally capable of forming and possessing the same types and degrees of intent. Consequently, an individual determined to be "sane" within the traditional constructs of the criminal law is held accountable for his action, regardless of his particular disabilities, weaknesses, poverty, religious beliefs, social deprivation or educational background. The most that is proper to do with such information is to weigh it during sentencing.

[The court then traced the development of insanity defense law in Maryland from the common law adoption of the M'Naghten test to the legislature's enactment, in 1970, of an insanity test almost identical to the ALI test].

* * *

We here reaffirm our position that "the concepts of both diminished capacity and insanity involve a moral choice by the community to withhold a finding of responsibility and its consequence of punish-

world about him as a cold inhospitable place where he does not have a chance.

CONCLUSION:

The patient functions at the borderline intellectual level (I.Q. 72), but his potential is at least within the low average *range. He can be described as a severely deprived individual with a hostile and negative orientation and an* [sic.] *severe authority problem.* Contact with reality is difficult to evaluate on account of his poor productivity resulting from extreme negativism.

ment," and on this basis are indistinguishable.[10]   Accordingly, because the legislature, reflecting community morals, has, by its definition of criminal insanity already determined which states of mental disorder ought to relieve one from criminal responsibility, this court is without authority to impose our views in this regard even if they differed.

* * *

What has just been iterated does not mean, however, that evidence of a defendant's mental abnormality which does not establish his insanity has been totally precluded from the consideration of those operating the machinery of our criminal justice system. Such evidence typically constitutes part of the range of data upon which the trial judge, following establishment of guilt, focuses attention when sentencing the individual accused. Such use of this information squares with the practice prevailing in our jurisprudence of permitting the judge wide latitude in making individualized sentencing decisions after consideration of information both in aggravation and mitigation of penalty.

* * *

ELDRIDGE, JUDGE, dissenting:

* * *

The defendant Johnson, *inter alia,* was charged with murder in the first degree under Maryland Code (1957, 1976 Repl.Vol.), Art. 27, § 407. In order to constitute first degree murder under § 407, the homicide must be a "wilful, deliberate and premeditated killing." Consequently, the State had the burden of proving the existence of these three elements. The mental condition of the defendant is obviously relevant

---

10. Given the primary assumption in the criminal law concerning a defendant's criminal culpability regardless of his lesser abilities, whatever they may be, and "recognizing the unique position of the concept of insanity in the framework of criminal responsibility," *Bethea v. United States,* 365 A.2d 64, 86 (D.C.App.1976), we cannot agree with those courts which easily declare that evidence of a legally sane defendant's mental impairment is always probative on the factual question of whether a particular accused entertained the requisite mental state. There is a fundamental difference between evidence demonstrating that the defendant did not *as a fact* possess the requisite mental state, here premeditation and deliberation, as opposed to evidence establishing that the defendant was *generally less capable* than a normal person of forming a requisite *mens rea.* Certainly, we recognize the basic proposition that the state must prove every element of a crime beyond a reasonable doubt including specific intent if necessary, and that an accused is entitled to rebut the state's case. The doctrine of diminished capacity, in our view, however, does not operate to demonstrate that, as a fact, a defendant did not entertain a requisite mental state; rather,

the principle is used to establish a legally sane but mentally impaired defendant's diminished culpability for a particular criminal act.

Moreover, facile comparison of the doctrine of diminished capacity with the rule allowing certain evidence of a defendant's intoxication on the issue of *mens rea* does not withstand scrutiny. The degree of intoxication necessary to negate *mens rea* is great and is comparable with that degree of mental incapacity that will render a defendant legally insane. As noted in *State v. Gover,* 267 Md. 602, 608, 298 A.2d 378, 382 (1973):

> If the trier of fact determines that at the time the alleged criminal act occurred, the accused had become so inebriated that he possessed no reason or understanding, then he has reached that stage of intoxication that renders him incapable of forming the requisite *mens rea* which is a necessary element of all specific intent crimes.

Lesser degrees of incapacity, whether produced by intoxication or organic mental impairment, will not relieve a defendant of full responsibility for his acts.

to willfulness, deliberation and premeditation. Evidence designed to show that a particular defendant was incapable of having the requisite mental state is nothing more or less than evidence designed to show that he did not commit the crime with which he was charged.

As Justice Powell stated for the Supreme Court in *Chambers v. Mississippi,* 410 U.S. 284, 302, 93 S.Ct. 1038, 1049, 35 L.Ed.2d 297 (1973), "[f]ew rights are more fundamental than that of an accused to present witnesses in his own defense." By holding that one accused of first degree murder is no longer entitled to present relevant testimony of his mental condition for the purpose of negating the elements of first degree murder, the majority today imposes an unjustified limitation upon the right of a criminal defendant to present evidence in his own behalf.

* * *

COLE and DAVIDSON, JJ., have authorized me to state that they concur with the views expressed herein.

Questions and Comments

1. *Legal status of diminished capacity doctrine.* Approximately half the states disagree with the result in *Johnson* and permit clinical testimony relevant to mens rea, at least under certain circumstances. Some courts have held, as suggested by the *Johnson* dissent, that this position is constitutionally mandated. In *Commonwealth v. Walzack,* 468 Pa. 210, 360 A.2d 914, 920 (1976), for instance, the Pennsylvania Supreme Court held that, under the Pennsylvania constitution, due process requires the admission of psychiatric testimony that is relevant to the mens rea issue. The court stated: "It is inconsistent with fundamental principles of American jurisprudence to preclude an accused from offering relevant and competent evidence to dispute the charge against him." See also, *Hendershott v. People,* 653 P.2d 385, 394 (Colo.1982).

The drafters of the Model Penal Code came to the same conclusion on policy grounds. Section 4.02(1) of the Code provides: "Evidence that the defendant suffered from a mental disease or defect is admissible whenever it is relevant to prove that the defendant did not have a state of mind that is an element of the crime." In support of this provision, the drafters stated: "If states of mind such as deliberation or premeditation are accorded legal significance, psychiatric evidence should be admissible when relevant to prove or disprove their existence to the same extent as any other evidence." Model Penal Code, Comments to § 4.02, 193 (Tent.Draft No. 4, 1955). More recently, the American Bar Association, finding that "logical relevance" so requires, has recommended an identical rule. American Bar Association Criminal Justice Mental Health Standard 7–6.2 (1987).

2. *Diminished capacity v. diminished responsibility.* To be distinguished from the diminished capacity idea, which focuses on the defendant's mens rea, is what is sometimes called the "partial" or "diminished responsibility" defense, which permits the factfinder to consider mitigating evidence of cognitive or volitional impairment that neither constitutes insanity nor negates mens rea. In Great Britain, for instance, a sane

defendant for whom the actus reus and mens rea of murder have been proven may nonetheless be convicted only of manslaughter if the defense shows that at the time of the killing the defendant "was suffering from such abnormality of mind . . . as substantially impaired his mental responsibility for acts and omissions in . . . the killing." English Homicide Act, 5 & 6 Eliz. II, ch. 11, § 2. To date, no American court has recognized the diminished responsibility defense. If it were recognized and made applicable to all crimes (rather than just homicide, as in Great Britain), how would one gauge its mitigating impact? Morse has suggested that, if such a defense were permitted, it should lead to a sentence one-half the length normally received for the crime. Morse, "Diminished Capacity: A Moral and Legal Conundrum," 2 Int'l J.Psychiat. 271 (1979).

One criticism of the diminished capacity doctrine is that, while it is theoretically distinguishable from diminished responsibility, in practice it will open the door wide to undifferentiated psychiatric testimony similar to that contemplated by the latter doctrine. For instance, the majority in *Johnson* asserted in footnote 10 that the diminished capacity doctrine "does not operate to demonstrate that, as a fact, a defendant did not entertain a requisite mental state; rather, the principle is used to establish a legally sane but mentally impaired defendant's diminished culpability for a particular criminal act." In perhaps the leading case supporting this position, *Bethea v. United States*, 365 A.2d 64 (D.C.App.1976), the District of Columbia Court of Appeals stated:

> The concept of mens rea involves what is ultimately the fiction of determining the actual thoughts or mental processes of the accused. It is obvious that a certain resolution of this issue is beyond the ken of scientist and laymen alike. Only by inference can the existence of intent—or the differentiation between its forms, such as general or specific—be determined. The law presumes that all individuals are capable of the mental processes which bear the jurisprudential label 'mens rea'; that is, the law presumes sanity . . . The concept of insanity is simply a device the law employs to define the outer limits of that segment of the general population to whom these presumptions concerning the capacity for criminal intent shall not be applied. The line between the sane and the insane for the purposes of criminal adjudication is not drawn because for one group the actual existence of the necessary mental state (or lack thereof) can be determined with any greater certainty, but rather because those whom the law declares insane are demonstrably so aberrational in their psychiatric characteristics that they are incapable of possessing the specified state of mind. Within the range of individuals who are not 'insane', the law does not recognize the readily demonstrable fact that as between individual criminal defendants the nature and development of their mental capabilities may vary greatly. . . . By contradicting the presumptions inherent in the doctrine of mens rea, the theory of diminished capacity inevitably opens the door to variable or sliding scales of criminal responsibility. We should not lightly undertake such a revolutionary change in our criminal justice system.

Id. at 88–89.

Consider the expert evidence in *Johnson*. Is it relevant to diminished capacity or only to diminished responsibility? Put another way, if the *Johnson* court had been willing to allow clinical testimony on mens rea, could it properly have excluded the defendant's expert testimony in any event, or would such exclusion have been improper?

3. *Diminished capacity and volitional impairment.* As one way of distinguishing diminished capacity from diminished responsibility, it is often said that the latter might involve either cognitive or volitional impairment, whereas the diminished capacity doctrine contemplates only evidence of cognitive dysfunction relevant to the capacity to form intent. In this regard, consider *Commonwealth v. Terry*, 513 Pa. 381, 521 A.2d 398 (1987). There Terry, a prison inmate, killed a prison guard with a baseball bat he had hidden in his trousers. The incident occurred when Terry was returning to the cellblock from the prison yard and the guard gave him a slight shove. According to Terry, this contact reminded him of a prior altercation with this particular guard; when the guard was momentarily distracted, Terry retrieved the bat and clubbed him. At trial, a state trooper testified that shortly after the incident the defendant had told him that he had been looking for someone to kill because it would enhance his standing among the prisoners; he chose the guard because of the prior conflict.

In his defense, Terry argued that he should be convicted only of second degree murder, not premeditated, first degree murder. A psychologist at the defendant's trial testified that the defendant suffered from a "dyssocial personality with paranoid hysterical and explosive features and organic brain syndrome with epileptic seizures." The expert also noted that at one point in the past the defendant had believed guards were injecting poison into his ankles and crippling him; the expert attributed this belief to psychosis. According to the psychologist, on the day of the offense:

> the resentment and rage that he felt . . . brought him to the point where he did make a decision and that decision was that he would protect himself and not let himself be beaten again. So that he decided to protect himself, and if somebody hurt him, he would hurt them. However, what I believe happened at that moment, then, within that context, is that when the [guard] grabbed him, he went into a rage; it was immediate, it was reactive, it was based on an emotional response. He didn't stop and deliberate and think and form the intent. He reacted.

Id. at 405. The Pennsylvania Supreme Court, upholding Terry's conviction and death sentence, found this testimony irrelevant to the diminished capacity issue, because it "directly advances impulsive rage as negating premeditation." According to past caselaw, "only 'mental disorders affecting cognitive functions necessary to form specific intent' are admissible." Id. at 404. Do you agree with the court that the expert's testimony was irrelevant to the mens rea issue? Is it accurate to say that diminished capacity testimony should only concern cognitive impairment?

4. *The California experiment.* One possible way of avoiding the problems associated with differentiating and defining diminished capacity and diminished responsibility is to redefine the mens rea required for

conviction. In a series of decisions beginning in 1964, the California Supreme Court did just that in connection with the law of homicide. In *People v. Wolff,* 61 Cal.2d 795, 40 Cal.Rptr. 271, 394 P.2d 959 (1964), the court held that premeditation (for first degree murder) requires not only that the defendant sanely intend or plan the killing but that "[he] maturely and meaningfully reflect upon the gravity of his contemplated act." Subsequently, the court held that, for second degree murder, the prosecution must show not only that the defendant intended to kill but that he had "[a]n awareness of the obligation to act within the general body of laws regulating society . . .". *People v. Conley,* 64 Cal.2d 310, 49 Cal.Rptr. 815, 411 P.2d 911 (1966). Finally, in *People v. Poddar,* 10 Cal.3d 750, 111 Cal. Rptr. 910, 518 P.2d 342 (1974), the court held that the mens rea for murder also required that the defendant be able "to act in accordance with . . . the law." The effect of these decisions redefining the mens rea for murder was to permit psychiatric testimony about cognitive and volitional impairment similar to that contemplated by the diminished responsibility doctrine. For a fuller treatment of these cases, see Arenella, "The Diminished Capacity and Diminished Responsibility Defenses: Two Children of a Doomed Marriage," 77 Colum.L.Rev. 827, 836–849 (1977).

In 1981, the California legislature enacted a statute which nullified these judicial developments. West's Ann.Cal.Penal Code §§ 188, 189, 21. The legislature also enacted, however, a provision permitting evidence of mental disease or defect if it is offered to show the absence of specific intent. West's Ann.Cal.Penal Code § 28.

5. *Limitations on clinical mens rea testimony.* Although many states permit clinical testimony that is relevant to mens rea (as opposed to diminished responsibility), they have done so cautiously. Most have placed limitations on such testimony beyond those constraints that are imposed by the rules of evidence on all expert opinion evidence.[1] The principal limitations are of three types.

The Mental Disease or Defect Limitation. The first limitation is a requirement, imposed explicitly in several states and implicitly in any state which adopts the Model Penal Code language, that the diminished capacity be associated with a "mental disease or defect" similar to that required for the insanity defense. See, e.g., *State v. Humanik,* 199 N.J.Super. 283, 489 A.2d 691 (A.D.1985). Is such a requirement justifiable? Are the reasons for the mental disease or defect predicate in the insanity context applicable when the issue is whether the defendant had the requisite mental state at the time of the offense?

In *United States v. Bright,* 517 F.2d 584 (2d Cir.1975), the defendant was charged with three counts of violating a statute which penalizes anyone who knowingly possesses stolen mail. It was undisputed that Bright had had in her possession nine welfare checks that had been stolen from the mail and that she had cashed at least three of them. Her defense was that she had not known they were stolen. She had been given the checks by one Fred Scott, an acquaintance of her boyfriend Leslie; Scott gave Bright the checks to cash for him on the pretense that he had no bank

---

1. See Chapter Six for a thorough treatment of these limitations.

account of his own. She testified that, although the checks were clearly made out to someone other than Scott, she had believed everything Scott had told her about the checks and had not suspected their source. In addition to her own testimony, she proffered the testimony of a psychiatrist, Dr. Weiss, who stated in part:

> [T]hough I do not consider Mrs. Bright to have been suffering mental illness, I believe that her dependent, childlike character structure unconsciously 'needed' to believe that these men would never involve her in illegal activities and that Leslie could do no wrong. I believe that at the time of the alleged crime, because of this unconscious 'need', she did not think that the checks had been stolen. . . . I do not believe that she knew that the checks that she allegedly possessed were stolen as a result of her need to deny the possibility that the men involved would in any way take advantage of her. This passive-dependent personality disorder rendered her incapable of understanding this.

Although the court appeared to be unwilling to foreclose a diminished capacity argument under all circumstances, it upheld the exclusion of the expert testimony, primarily because no mental disease analogous to that required for the insanity defense was found to be present:

> Couched in simpler language [the psychiatrist] was prepared to testify that [Bright] was a gullible person but a person unaffected either by psychosis or neurosis. . . .

> The mind and motivation of an accused who is not on the other side of the line [drawn by the insanity defense] is, by the judgment of experience, left to the jury to probe. The complexity of the fears and long-suppressed traumatic experiences of a lifetime is in the personality of all of us. All humankind is heir to defects of personality.

> To transmute the effect of instability, of undue reliance on another, of unrequited love, of sudden anger, of the host of attitudes and syndromes that are a part of daily living, into opinion evidence to the jury for exculpation or condemnation is to go beyond the boundaries of current knowledge. The shallower the conception the deeper runs the danger that the jury may be misled. . . .

> In short, [Bright] asks us to go beyond the boundaries of conventional psychiatric opinion testimony. We think the testimony offered was not sufficiently grounded in scientific support to make us reach or, indeed, cross the present frontier of admissibility. On the instant appeal we need decide no more than that [the trial judge] did not abuse her discretion in rejecting the opinion evidence.

Is it true, as suggested by the *Bright* court, that clinical testimony is less reliable if it is not based on a finding of significant mental disorder? Is such testimony any more suspect than the testimony offered in *Heads* or *Pollard?* If it is, why not let the rules of evidence governing the admission of expert testimony take care of the problem rather than resorting to a mental disease limitation? Perhaps the rules of evidence are insufficient protection against testimony on the "outer boundaries?" Or is there another concern—similar to that evinced by the *Johnson* court—underlying the court's position?

Because the psychiatric testimony was excluded, the sole basis for Bright's assertion—that she did not know the checks were stolen because she was abnormally willing to believe those upon whom she depended emotionally—was her own testimony. Consider the following comment about the *Bright* case.

> [E]xclusion [of the psychiatric testimony] compromises [Bright's] ability to persuade the factfinder not to draw inferences about her beliefs on the basis of what a normal person would have believed under the circumstances. Because [Bright] carries a de-facto burden of proof on this issue, the exclusion of expert testimony in effect holds her to the standards of a normally suspicious person, selectively redefining the offense to apply objective standards to her and subjective standards to everyone else.

Bonnie & Slobogin, "The Role of Mental Health Professionals in the Criminal Process: The Case for Informed Speculation," 66 Va.L.Rev. 427, 480–81 (1980). Is this concern, assuming it exists, sufficiently significant to outweigh the concerns identified by the *Bright* court?

The Capacity Limitation. A second reason given by the *Bright* court for excluding the psychiatric testimony in that case centered on the form in which the testimony was offered. The court noted that the psychiatrist went beyond stating that Bright "did not have the capacity to form a specific intent to commit the crime" and instead directly asserted that Bright did not believe the checks were stolen. The court suggested that diminished capacity testimony should address *only* the capacity of the defendant to harbor the required mental state, not whether the defendant actually had that mental state. Several other courts have explicitly required that psychiatric testimony on mens rea be couched in terms of the defendant's "capacity." See, e.g., *Simpson v. State,* 269 Ind. 495, 381 N.E.2d 1229 (1978); *State v. Craig,* 82 Wash.2d 777, 514 P.2d 151 (1973). What is the purpose of this limitation?

Most formulations of the diminished capacity doctrine do not limit clinical testimony in this way. See Model Penal Code § 4.01(1). At least one state explicitly *forbids* capacity testimony, and provides that "[e]vidence of mental disease, mental defect, or mental disorder is admissible solely on the issue of whether or not the accused actually formed a required specific intent, premeditated, deliberated, or harbored malice aforethought, when a specific intent crime is charged." West's Ann.Cal. Penal Code § 28(a). What is the purpose of this prohibition?

Consider *Waine v. State,* 37 Md.App. 222, 377 A.2d 509 (1977). There the defendant was charged with two counts of first degree murder. In his defense, he called a psychiatrist who testified off the record that the defendant was a passive person and that, in his opinion, violence on the part of the defendant would be very unlikely. The psychiatrist also stated, again off the record, that there "is no way in the world I can say he didn't commit these [homicides] but I can say according to his lifestyle, this would be totally out of character." After hearing the proffer of the psychiatrist, the trial court allowed the psychiatrist to testify as to the "psychiatric makeup" of the defendant—to the effect that he was a "passivist"—but did not allow him to testify as to "whether or not this person might possibly be able to commit an act of violence . . ., or did in fact commit, possibly or not possibly, an act of violence . . . at the time these people were killed." The Maryland Court of Special Appeals upheld this ruling. Apparently, it was willing to allow this and like testimony, short of the "ultimate conclusion" as to whether the defendant committed the murders, because of a perceived analogy to evidentiary rules permitting criminal defendants to present "character evidence".[m] Note that *Waine* was decided by a Maryland intermediate appellate court five years before the Maryland Supreme Court's decision in *Johnson.* Should *Waine* be decided the same way today? See *Kanaras v. State,* 54 Md.App. 568, 460 A.2d 61, 73 (1983) (upholding *Waine*).

Crime Limitation. Finally, most states restrict the admissibility of clinical evidence to certain types of crimes. This third limitation is itself of two types. One approach permits clinical testimony only in cases where defendants are charged with some type of intentional homicide. For instance, although the Pennsylvania Supreme Court has held that competent evidence of diminished capacity cannot constitutionally be prohibited, *Walzack,* supra, it has nonetheless limited such evidence to murder cases. *Commonwealth v. Garcia,* 505 Pa. 304, 479 A.2d 473, 477 (1984). A second approach admits clinical testimony on mens rea for any crime involving specific intent, but does not admit such evidence for crimes involving general intent. In "Model Penal Code" jurisdictions, an analogous result is achieved by permitting expert evidence for any element requiring purpose or knowledge, but barring such evidence when the mens rea is recklessness or negligence. See *State v. Thompson,* 695 S.W.2d 154, 159 (Mo.App.1985) and cases cited therein.

The murder-only rule plainly violates the premise of the diminished capacity doctrine, since mental abnormality can lead to the absence of mens rea for other crimes as well. Expanding the doctrine's applicability to all specific intent crimes does not necessarily solve this problem. If the mens rea for general intent crimes (or recklessness and negligence) were truly "objectively" defined, then diminished capacity evidence would indeed be irrelevant in such cases. But such is not always the case.

Looking first at the Model Penal Code approach to mens rea, it is clear that even negligence contemplates some degree of investigation into the defendant's actual mental state. Section 2.02(2)d of the Model Penal Code states:

> A person acts negligently with respect to a material element of an offense when he should be aware of a substantial and unjustifiable risk that the material element exists or will result from his conduct. The risk must be of such a nature and degree that the actor's failure to

---

m. Cf. Fed.R.Evid., Rule 404(a)(1) ("Evidence of a person's character or a trait of character is not admissible for the purpose of proving action in conformity therewith on a particular occasion, except [when it is] evidence of a pertinent trait of character offered by an accused, or by the prosecution to rebut the same."); Fed.R.Evid., Rule 405(a) ("In all cases in which evidence of character or a trait of character of a person is admissible, proof may be made by testimony as to reputation or by testimony in the form of an opinion. . . .")

perceive it, *considering the nature and purpose of his conduct and the circumstances known to him,* involves a gross deviation from the standard of care that a reasonable person would observe *in the actor's situation.*

(Emphasis supplied). Under § 213.4 of the Code, the crime of sexual assault is defined as, *inter alia,* "sexual contact with another . . . [when] (6) the other person is less than 16 years old and the actor is at least four years older than the other person." It is a defense to this crime if the victim was between 10 and 16 and the actor had a non-negligent belief that the victim was older than 16. See §§ 213.6; 1.13(16). Suppose a defendant wants to submit expert testimony that, due to mental illness or mental retardation, he thought a person with whom he admittedly had sexual contact was over 16 (even though a "normal" person should have known otherwise). Under the above definition of negligence, could not one make a plausible argument that such testimony should be admissible on diminished capacity grounds?

The same sort of problem occurs under the common law in distinguishing specific and general intent crimes, primarily because the courts are so idiosyncratic in defining these terms. In *State v. McVey,* 376 N.W.2d 585 (Iowa 1985), for instance, the defendant was charged under a statute which makes it theft for a person to "[exercise] control over stolen property, knowing such property to have been stolen, or having reasonable cause to believe that such property has been stolen, unless the person's purpose is to promptly restore it to the owner or to deliver it to an appropriate public officer." West's Ann.Iowa Code 714.1(4). According to prior case law, the Iowa Supreme Court noted, "the mens rea of this offense requires proof that the accused actually believe the property is stolen." But case law had also established that the offense did not require proof of "specific intent". Rather "[t]he offense is a general intent crime because it is complete without intent to do a further act or achieve a further consequence." Id. at 586. The court then upheld the trial court's exclusion of psychiatric evidence proffered to show that the defendant did not know that an automobile in which he was apprehended was stolen. The court noted that, although Iowa courts had long recognized that a diminished capacity defense "is available to any crime in which specific intent is an element," expanding it to general intent crimes would be unsound:

> In practical terms a court's refusal to recognize the relevancy of evidence of mental impairment short of legal insanity results from the court's understanding of the legislative intention concerning the blameworthiness of the defendant's conduct. To the extent evidence of mental impairment that does not meet the legal insanity standard permits an accused to avoid responsibility for otherwise culpable conduct, the policy inherent in the insanity defense is undermined.

If the defendant's evidence proves that he did not know the car was stolen, is he blameworthy? Is this case any different from *Bright?*

The usual justification given for limiting diminished capacity evidence to certain types of mens rea is not the one advanced by the Iowa Supreme Court but rather stems from a utilitarian rationale: if no such limitation were imposed, some mentally ill defendants (including those who ordinarily would have pleaded insanity and thus been committed) would be able to use clinical evidence to elude confinement completely. The public is protected in states limiting clinical testimony on mens rea to murder cases because a defendant who escapes a murder conviction through using diminished capacity evidence can still be convicted of manslaughter. Similarly, in those states which have adopted the specific intent limitation, the defendant who successfully argues diminished capacity can still usually be convicted of a lesser included offense requiring only general intent.

In *People v. Wetmore*, 22 Cal.3d 318, 149 Cal.Rptr. 265, 583 P.2d 1308 (1978), the defendant was charged with burglary after being discovered in another person's apartment wearing that person's clothes and cooking his food. The defendant credibly showed that as a result of mental illness he had come to believe that he owned the apartment. He had lived in the apartment for three days prior to his arrest and been shocked and embarrassed when the police arrived and informed him that the apartment was not his. In overturning his conviction for burglary (for which there was no lesser included offense), the California Supreme Court stated:

> We reject the suggestion that we sustain the trial court by holding that a defense of diminished capacity cannot be raised whenever, owing to the lack of a lesser included offense, it might result in the defendant's acquittal. A defendant who, because of diminished capacity, does not entertain the specific intent required for a particular crime is entitled to be acquitted of that crime. If he cannot be convicted of a lesser offense and cannot safely be released, the state's remedy is to institute civil commitment proceedings, not to convict him of a specific-intent crime which he did not commit.

In California, the relevant civil commitment statute permits confinement of any person who "as a result of mental disorder [is] a danger to others, or to himself, or gravely disabled." Confinement under the first two criteria may last only 90 days unless the person "has threatened, attempted, or actually inflicted physical harm to another during his period of post-certification treatment." Is the court's solution sufficiently protective of the public? Would it be wise to amend the civil commitment statute to permit longer confinement of those acquitted on diminished capacity grounds? Or should we condone conviction of *some* offense, even one for which the defendant did not have the required mental state, as a compromise between retributive and utilitarian notions?

D. OTHER DEFENSES

NOTE ON SELF–DEFENSE, PROVOCATION AND DURESS

In adjudicating guilt, evidence of mental abnormality is most likely to be considered relevant to insanity, automatism or diminished capacity. Increasingly, however, psychiatric and psychological testimony has been proffered in support of other claims. This development is a direct outgrowth of the criminal law's movement toward a subjective definition of culpability. To illustrate this development and its ramifications, this section looks briefly at three criminal law doctrines: self-defense, provocation, and duress.

The traditional approach to self-defense is summarized by LaFave and Scott as follows: "One who is not the aggressor in an encounter is justified in using a reasonable amount of force against his adversary when he reasonably believes that he is in immediate danger of unlawful bodily harm from his adversary and that the use of such force is necessary to avoid this danger." LaFave & Scott, Criminal Law, at 454 (1986). In a majority of jurisdictions a person may use deadly force to repel an attack which is reasonably believed to be deadly even if he or she could safely retreat from the attack; however, in a "strong minority" of jurisdictions, one must retreat before using deadly force, if the retreat can be accomplished safely. Even in the minority jurisdictions, one need not retreat if the attack takes place in the defendant's house, on the theory that one is entitled to stand firm in one's home. Id. at 46–61. A valid self-defense claim leads to acquittal on any charge.

The provocation "defense", on the other hand, is available only in homicide cases and, rather than acquittal, leads to reduction of the charge from murder to voluntary manslaughter. In most jurisdictions, this reduction occurs when the defendant can show that (1) the killing was in reaction to provocation that, while insufficient to justify the killing, would cause the "reasonable" person to lose control; (2) this provocation in fact provoked the defendant; (3) a "reasonable" person so provoked would not have cooled off in the interval of time between the provocation and the delivery of the final blow; and (4) the defendant did not in fact cool off. LaFave & Scott, supra, § 7.10(a). The provocation defense has sometimes been characterized as imperfect self-defense because it recognizes that some types of provocation, although they do not justify the use of deadly force in return, might make a "reasonable" person impulsively kill someone, and thus should be given mitigating (but not exculpatory) effect. The common law identified a number of situations in which such provocation might occur, e.g., serious battery not rising to deadly force, serious assault (i.e., attempted battery), mutual combat not involving deadly force, and discovery of adultery by the offended spouse.

Finally, the defense of duress is recognized when a person's unlawful threat causes the defendant reasonably to believe that the only way to avoid imminent death or serious bodily injury to him or herself or to another is to engage in conduct which violates the criminal law, and the defendant acts on that belief. LaFave & Scott, supra, at 432–33. Duress is not normally a defense, however, to intentional homicide, since the rationale for the defense is generally thought to be that acquittal should be permitted only when the defendant, faced with a choice of evils, chooses to do the lesser evil.

It should be clear even from this brief description that, under the common law, "reasonableness" language dominates the definition of these defenses. Use of such language presumably renders mental abnormality irrelevant, since a person who is mentally disordered at the time of the offense never acts "reasonably". The reasonable person is the "normal" person as defined by the judge or members of the jury. Thus, for instance, with respect to provocation, in most jurisdictions "the defendant's special mental qualities . . . are not to be considered." LaFave & Scott, supra, at 659.

Modern developments in these three areas demonstrate an increasing willingness to consider the personal characteristics of the accused in deciding whether a defense is available. The Model Penal Code is representative. The Code permits "the use of force upon or toward another person . . . when the actor believes that such force is immediately necessary for the purpose of protecting himself against the use of unlawful force by such person on the present occasion." Model Penal Code § 3.04. This formulation makes the actor's beliefs relevant to a self-defense claim regardless of how "unreasonable" they are. The provision of the Code which is analogous to the common law provocation doctrine is somewhat more objectively defined but still incorporates subjective elements. It states that a homicide which would otherwise be murder is manslaughter if it "is committed under the influence of extreme mental or emotional disturbance for which there is reasonable explanation or excuse[,] . . . the reasonableness of such explanation or excuse [to] be determined from the viewpoint of a person in the actor's situation under the circumstances as he believes them to be." Model Penal Code § 210.3. Similarly, with respect to duress, the Code provides for an affirmative defense when a person commits a crime "because he was coerced to do so by the use of, or a threat to use, unlawful force against his person or the person of another, which a person of reasonable firmness in his situation would have been unable to resist." Model Penal Code § 2.09(1). The defense is not available when the "actor recklessly placed himself in a situation in which it was probable that he would be subjected to duress." Id. § 2.09(2).

JAHNKE v. STATE

Supreme Court of Wyoming, 1984.
682 P.2d 991.

THOMAS, JUSTICE.

The essential questions presented in this case arise out of a notion that a victim of abuse has some special justification for patricide.

*   *   *

The appellant's father, Richard Chester Jahnke, died on November 16, 1982, as a result of gunshot wounds. Those gunshot wounds were inflicted by the appellant, and that fact has never been an issue in this case.

*   *   *

The material facts relating to the death of the appellant's father can be briefly stated. On the night of his death the father took the mother out to dinner, apparently to celebrate the anniversary of their meeting. Earlier the appellant had been involved in a violent altercation with his father, and he had been warned not to be at the home when the father and mother returned. During the absence of his parents the appellant made elaborate preparation for the final confrontation with his father. He changed into dark clothing and prepared a number of weapons which he positioned at various places throughout the family home that he selected to serve as "backup" positions in case he was not successful in his first effort to kill his father. These weapons included two shotguns, three rifles, a .38 caliber pistol and a Marine knife. In addition, he armed his sister, Deborah, with a .30 caliber M–1 carbine which he taught her how to operate so that she could protect herself in the event that he failed in his efforts. The appellant removed the family pets from the garage to the basement to protect them from injury in a potential exchange of gunfire between him and his father, and he closed the garage door. He then waited inside the darkened garage in a position where he could not be seen but which permitted him to view the lighted driveway on the other side of the garage door. Shortly before 6:30 p.m. the parents returned, and the appellant's father got out of the vehicle and came to the garage door. The appellant was armed with a 12–gauge shotgun loaded with slugs, and when he could see the head and shoulders of his father through the spacing of the slats of the shade covering the windows of the garage door, he blew his R.O.T.C. command-sergeant-major's whistle for courage, and he opened fire. All six cartridges in the shotgun were expended, and four of them in one way or another struck the father.

* * *

After the shooting, and while the mother still was screaming in the driveway, the appellant and his sister exited the family home through a window in the mother's bedroom, which was at the far end of the house from the garage. The appellant and his sister then went separate ways, and the appellant was arrested at the home of his girl friend. Prior to the arrival of authorities the appellant told his girl friend's father that he had shot his dad for revenge. Subsequently, after being advised of his constitutional rights, the appellant made a statement in which he explained he had shot his father "for past things."

[Jahnke was convicted of voluntary manslaughter and sentenced to 5 to 15 years. On appeal he argued that the trial court erroneously excluded expert testimony describing him as a victim of the "battered person syndrome" who was in constant fear of serious bodily harm from his father but at the same time unable to leave the site of the battering.]

It is clear that self-defense is circumscribed by circumstances involving a confrontation, usually encompassing some overt act or acts by the deceased, which would induce a reasonable person to fear that his life was in danger or that at least he was threatened with great bodily harm.

* * *

Although many people, and the public media, seem to be prepared to espouse the notion that a victim of abuse is entitled to kill the abuser that special justification defense is antithetical to the mores of modern civilized society. It is difficult enough to justify capital punishment as an appropriate response of society to criminal acts even after the circumstances have been carefully evaluated by a number of people. To permit capital punishment to be imposed upon the subjective conclusion of the individual that prior acts and conduct of the deceased justified the killing would amount to a leap into the abyss of anarchy.

*   *   *

This record contained no evidence that the appellant was under either actual or threatened assault by his father at the time of the shooting. Reliance upon the justification of self-defense requires a showing of an actual or threatened imminent attack by the deceased.

Absent [such] a showing, the reasonableness of appellant's conduct at the time was not an issue in the case, and the trial court, at the time it made its ruling, properly excluded the hearsay testimony sought to be elicited from the forensic psychiatrist.

*   *   *

ROSE, JUSTICE, dissenting, with whom CARDINE, JUSTICE, joins

*   *   *

This case concerns itself with what happens—or can happen—and did happen when a cruel, ill-tempered, insensitive man roams, gun in hand, through his years of family life as a battering bully—a bully who, since his two children were babies, beat both of them and his wife regularly and unmercifully. Particularly, this appeal has to do with a 16–year–old boy who could stand his father's abuse no longer—who could not find solace or friendship in the public services which had been established for the purpose of providing aid, comfort and advice to abused family members—and who had no place to go or friends to help either him or his sister for whose protection he felt responsible and so— in fear and fright, and with fragmented emotion, Richard Jahnke shot and killed his father one night in November of 1982.

*   *   *

The Reasonableness of Self–Defense

*   *   *

In contemplating the overall problem which brings on my dissent, it is initially necessary to be aware of at least these following facts:

Richard Jahnke, a sensitive boy who had never been in any sort of trouble in his life, had been beaten regularly and unmercifully by his father since he was two years old. On the night of the homicide he had received a severe beating, and when his father and mother left the house to go to dinner that night, his father said:

"I'm disgusted with the shit you turned out to be. I don't want you to be here when I get back."

The father also said:

"I don't care what I have to do, I'm going to get rid of you. I don't know how but I'm going to get rid of you, you bastard."

The boy felt he had to protect his sister who was hysterical when the mother and father left for dinner. He did not believe that there was any place or anyone where or to whom they could go for safety. The mother testified that the elder Jahnke always carried a gun, and Richard believed he had one with him that night. Mrs. Jahnke said that when the father said to Richard, "I'm going to get rid of you"—

> "He was trying to frighten him and maybe do something else besides just throwing him out of the house."

When Richard was in the garage after having stationed his father's guns around the house for "backup," he reflected upon past confrontations with his father and he was afraid the father would kill him when he returned and found what Richard had done with the guns. Even as he contemplated these things, the father drove the car into the driveway. Richard said he wanted to go and hug him and tell him he loved him, but he remembered when he had done this before, he had received a beating for his efforts. He knew from past experience that when his father "stomped" after him that he was in for a beating. He testified about how his father approached the garage door that night:

> "A. Yes. I remember he was stomping. When he stomped down the hall when he was really mad and really prepared to beat someone up, beat on one of us. I remember being a little kid, just sitting in my room. My dad stomping after me to hit me, that I could never stop him. This time I stopped him."

*   *   *

[In] the *ordinary* self-defense situation where there are no psychiatric implications and where the jury is permitted to know what the accused knew about the violent character of his victim, there need be no expert testimony touching upon the reasonableness of the defendant's behavior. In normal circumstances, these are things that jurors can fathom for themselves. However, when the beatings of 14 years have—or may have—caused the accused to harbor types of fear, anxiety and apprehension with which the nonbrutalized juror is unfamiliar and which result in the taking of unusual defensive measures which, in the ordinary circumstances, might be thought about as premature, excessive or lacking in escape efforts by those who are uninformed about the fear and anxiety that permeate the world of the brutalized—then expert testimony is necessary to explain the battered-person syndrome and the way these people respond to what they understand to be the imminence of danger and to explain their propensity to employ deadly force in their self-defensive conduct. Given this information, the jury is then qualified to decide the reasonableness of a self-defense defendant's acts at the time and place in question.

The Proffered Testimony of the Forensic Psychiatrist

Dr. McDonald, a forensic psychiatrist, was offered by the defendant for the purpose of testifying about the behavior of battered children— that Richard was a battered child—all as an aid to the triers of fact with respect to their obligation to decide whether or not this defendant—as a battered person—behaved reasonably on the night of November 16, 1982, but the court would not permit the jury to hear the testimony.

The defendant suggests that his offer of proof represented that Dr. McDonald would testify that:

1. The doctor had diagnosed Richard Jahnke as a battered child, based on interviews with him and upon other information.

2. Battered children behave differently from other children, and perceive things differently from other children.

3. Because he was a battered child, Jahnke reasonably believed himself to be in immediate danger on the night he shot his father, and perceived himself as acting in self-defense.

* * *

The doctor described an extensive background of Richard receiving physical abuse from his father. His earliest memory was of his father beating him, his mother and his sister. Between the ages of four and 12, there was seldom a day without some sort of punishment by his father. The punishment became less frequent between 12 and 15—more like every other day, but there were more beatings when his father used his fists on him. He was beaten with his father's fists every couple of weeks between 15 and 16. He would be beaten for such things as not cleaning the basement the right way—for walking along with his mouth open—for spending too much time polishing his ROTC uniform. At one juncture, the doctor testified that the children were forced to eat with plastic spoons and forks because their father did not like the noise they made while eating with ordinary utensils. Dr. McDonald testified that Richard related that he would be beaten for things like defending his sister. If Richard would react to verbal abuse by changing facial expression, the father would physically abuse him. When Richard and his mother had an argument, she would call him a "bastard" and report him to his father who would beat him.

On May 2, 1982, after a severe beating by his father, he ran out of the house in his bare feet, then put his sneakers on and ran five miles to his ROTC instructor's home. He sat outside the instructor's house, afraid to go in, and was finally discovered there by the instructor. The doctor explained that children who are victims of abuse are often reluctant to report their problems to others. In Richard's case, he believed for many years that child beatings were the normal behavior for a father. He was humiliated by the abuse and even had trouble reporting it to the ROTC instructor with whom he had a close relationship. On this occasion, however, the instructor and Richard went to the sheriff to report the abuse. The family was then interviewed together, and Richard chose to return home rather than go to a foster home, principally because he saw himself as the protector of his mother and sister.

Richard believed the May visit to the sheriff's office was useless even though his father did not beat him for a week or more. When he returned from reporting his beating to the sheriff, he put a chair against his door every night so his father could not get in. A week and a half after the sheriff's incident, the father exclaimed, "That bastard reported me to the Sheriff," and would say things like

> "I'll give him something that he can really complain about, that is if he can talk,"

the implication being that he would be in a condition that would prevent him from talking about anything.

* * *

[T]he doctor took other factors into account to reach his evaluation conclusion. For example, the beatings and verbal abuse had an adverse effect on Richard's psychological development. He testified that the boy does not have the ability to handle stress that other young people of his age have and any ability he does have in this regard has come about as a developed defensive mechanism against the brutality of his father. That was the problem on November 16, 1982—that is, when his mother turned on him, blaming him for all the trouble with her marriage and in the home generally, and when she kept calling him a bastard and throwing things at him it was too much for him to stand. He felt victimized when his mother reported him to his father that night because she reported things that he had never said about her. This series of events and its repercussions, together with his father's beating him that night and the father's threat that he should leave home, was more than Richard Jahnke could handle. In addition, according to Dr. McDonald, he was afraid of another beating when his father and mother returned from dinner. Therefore, taking all of these things into account, he was under unusual and, for him, unbearable pressure on the evening of November 16, 1982.

* * *

The Insanity Misconception

Both the State and the trial court believed the defendant was urging an insanity or diminished-capacity defense and thus were of the opinion that the proffered testimony was irrelevant.

The theory of Richard Jahnke's defense was misunderstood by the prosecuting attorney, the trial court and now, I submit, this court.

* * *

In these proceedings, the mental state of Richard Jahnke was not offered as a defense as would be the case with an insanity plea. Neither his mental capacity nor his intent to commit the crime was in issue. Rather, the specific defense is self-defense, which requires a showing that Jahnke reasonably believed it was necessary to use deadly force to prevent imminent death or great bodily harm to himself. In this situation, the expert testimony is offered, when the battered defendant pleads self-defense, as an aid to the jury in interpreting the surrounding circumstances as they affected the reasonableness of his belief. The expert testimony offered was secondary to the defense asserted. Given the opportunity, the defendant would not seek to show through the expert testimony that the mental and physical mistreatment which he suffered affected his mental state so that he *could not be responsible* for his actions; rather, the testimony was offered to show that, because he suffered from 14 years of brutalizing, *it was reasonable* for him to have remained in the home—to have prepared to respond to the beating that he had been promised would surely come and to have believed at that time and place that he was in imminent danger.

* * *

It is because a jury would not understand and would not be expected to understand why Richard Jahnke would remain in that environment and believe that he was in imminent danger that the expert testimony is critical to aid and assist them in evaluating these conditions, circumstances and behavior patterns.

* * *

Questions and Comments

1. *Analyzing* Jahnke. Assuming that it otherwise met the criteria for expert testimony,[n] should the psychiatric opinion and associated factual evidence in *Jahnke* have been admitted under the traditional definition of self-defense? Provocation? Under the Model Penal Code's definitions of self-defense and provocation? Is the expert's testimony relevant to mens rea or insanity issues? Or is it irrelevant to criminal liability? Note that one week after the court's decision, the governor commuted Jahnke's sentence to three years.

If, instead of killing his father, the defendant had stolen something in order to prove that he was "tough" rather than "sensitive" and thus avoid further beatings, should he have a duress defense to a charge of theft?

2. *The battered spouse syndrome.* The issues raised in *Jahnke* were presaged in a number of cases involving women charged with killing their husbands after suffering through years of abuse. According to Dr. Lenore Walker, who is often credited with recognizing the "battered wife syndrome", some women who are subjected to abuse by their husbands develop what has come to be called "learned helplessness". Because of low self-esteem, passivity, an inability to express terror and anger, and inculcation of traditional societal attitudes toward females, these women believe that the batterer is all-powerful, that they are to blame for the battering, and that no one can help them. Emotionally and financially dependent upon the battering husband, and perhaps fearful of being stigmatized as failures, they develop "coping" responses rather than "escape" responses as a method of surviving the relationship. In other words, rather than leaving the batterer, they remain with him and put up with the beatings. The battering cycle usually proceeds through three stages. The first phase— the "tension-building" stage—involves minor battering incidents and verbal

n. In a part of the opinion not reprinted, the majority suggested that the "battered-child syndrome" was not a "generally accepted diagnosis". See discussion of the general acceptance doctrine at pp. 403–408.

abuse, during which the woman tries to placate the man and be as passive as possible to stave off further violence. Phase two is the "acute battering incident", usually precipitated by some event in the man's life outside the relationship, but sometimes triggered by the woman when she can no longer tolerate or control her reaction to the man's phase one actions. Phase three is characterized by contrition and reconciliation on the part of the man; he often promises to seek professional help, stop drinking and refrain from further violence. Sometimes, however, the normal cycle is disrupted during phase one or two. The woman either precipitates an incident or fights back and the husband is killed or badly hurt. See L. Walker, The Battered Woman (1979).

Evidence of the syndrome is introduced to support a number of legal theories, including insanity and diminished capacity, but it is most often offered to support a self-defense claim. The courts are split as to whether evidence of the syndrome is relevant to such a claim. See Cross, "The Expert as Educator: A Proposed Approach to the Use of Battered Women Syndrome Expert Testimony," 35 Vand.L.Rev. 753 (1982). In *State v. Kelly,* 97 N.J. 178, 478 A.2d 364 (1984), the court permitted evidence about the syndrome in a homicide case:

> At the heart of the claim of self-defense was defendant's story that she had been repeatedly subjected to "beatings" over the course of her marriage. While defendant's testimony was somewhat lacking in detail, a juror could infer from the use of the word "beatings," as well as the detail given concerning some of these events (the choking, the biting, the use of fists), that these physical assaults posed a risk of serious injury or death. When that regular pattern of serious physical abuse is combined with defendant's claim that the decedent sometimes threatened to kill her, defendant's statement that on this occasion she thought she might be killed when she saw Mr. Kelly running toward her could be found to reflect a reasonable fear; that is, it could so be found if the jury believed Gladys Kelly's story of the prior beatings, if it believed her story of the prior threats, and, of course, if it believed her story of the events of that particular day.

> The crucial issue of fact on which this expert's testimony would bear is why, given such allegedly severe and constant beatings, combined with threats to kill, defendant had not long ago left decedent. Whether raised by the prosecutor as a factual issue or not, our own common knowledge tells us that most of us, including the ordinary juror, would ask himself or herself just such a question. And our knowledge is bolstered by the experts' knowledge, for the experts point out that one of the common myths, apparently believed by most people, is that battered wives are free to leave. To some, this misconception is followed by the observation that the battered wife is masochistic, proven by her refusal to leave despite the severe beatings; to others, however, the fact that the battered wife stays on unquestionably suggests that the "beatings" could not have been too bad for if they had been, she certainly would have left. The expert could clear up these myths, by explaining that one of the common characteristics of a battered wife is her inability to leave despite such constant beatings;

her "learned helplessness"; her lack of anywhere to go; her feeling that if she tried to leave, she would be subjected to even more merciless treatment; her belief in the omnipotence of her battering husband; and sometimes her hope that her husband will change his ways.

* * *

It would not be proper for the expert to express the opinion that defendant's belief on that day was reasonable, not because this is the ultimate issue, but because the area of expert knowledge relates, in this regard, to the reasons for defendant's failure to leave her husband. Either the jury accepts or rejects that explanation and, based on that, credits defendant's stories about the beatings she suffered. No expert is needed, however, once the jury has made up its mind on those issues, to tell the jury the logical conclusion, namely, that a person who has in fact been severely and continuously beaten might very well reasonably fear that the imminent beating she was about to suffer could be either life-threatening or pose a risk of serious injury. What the expert could state was that defendant had the battered-woman's syndrome, and could explain that syndrome in detail, relating its characteristics to defendant, but only to enable the jury better to determine the honesty and reasonableness of defendant's belief. Depending on its content, the expert's testimony might also enable the jury to find that the battered wife, because of the prior beatings, numerous beatings, as often as once a week, for seven years, from the day they were married to the day he died, is particularly able to predict accurately the likely extent of violence in any attack on her. That conclusion could significantly affect the jury's evaluation of the reasonableness of defendant's fear for her life.

3. *The outer boundaries of culpability.* In contrast to the court in *Kelly*, the majority in *Jahnke* asserts that allowing self-defense in such abuse cases would be "antithetical to the mores of modern civilized society." Consider, in support of this position, the following excerpt from Justice Holmes' The Common Law (1881), arguing that the deterrent purpose of the criminal law must take precedence over the retributive goal.

[T]here can be no case in which the law-maker makes certain conduct criminal without his thereby showing a wish and purpose to prevent that conduct. Prevention would accordingly seem to be the chief and only universal purpose of punishment. The law threatens certain pains if you do certain things, intending thereby to give you a new motive for not doing them. If you persist in doing them, it has to inflict the pains in order that its threats may continue to be believed.

If this is a true account of the law as it stands, the law does undoubtedly treat the individual as a means to an end, and uses him as a tool to increase the general welfare at his own expense. It has been suggested above, that this course is perfectly proper; but even if it is wrong, our criminal law follows it, and the theory of our criminal law must be shaped accordingly . . .

If the foregoing arguments are sound, it is already manifest that liability to punishment cannot be finally and absolutely determined by considering the actual personal unworthiness of the criminal alone.

That consideration will govern only so far as the public welfare permits or demands. And if we take into account the general result which the criminal law is intended to bring about, we shall see that the actual state of mind accompanying a criminal act plays a different part from what is commonly supposed.

For the most part, the purpose of the criminal law is only to induce external conformity to rule. All law is directed to conditions of things manifest to the senses. And whether it brings those conditions to pass immediately by the use of force, as when it protects a house from a mob of soldiers, or appropriates private property to public use, or hangs a man in pursuance of a judicial sentence, or whether it brings them about mediately through men's fears, its object is equally an external result. In directing itself against robbery or murder, for instance, its purpose is to put a stop to the actual physical taking and keeping of other men's goods, or the actual poisoning, shooting, stabbing, and otherwise putting to death of other men. If those things are not done, the law forbidding them is equally satisfied, whatever the motive.

Considering this purely external purpose of the law together with the fact that it is ready to sacrifice the individual so far as necessary in order to accomplish that purpose, we can see more readily than before that the actual degree of personal guilt involved in any particular transgression cannot be the only element, if it is an element at all, in the liability incurred . . .

It is not intended to deny that criminal liability . . . is founded on blameworthiness. Such a denial would shock the moral sense of any civilized community; or, to put it another way, a law which punished conduct which would not be blameworthy in the average member of the community would be too severe for that community to bear. It is only intended to point out that, when we are dealing with that part of the law which aims more directly than any other at establishing standards of conduct, we should expect there more than elsewhere to find that the tests of liability are external, and independent of the degree of evil in the particular person's motives or intentions. The conclusion follows directly from the nature of the standards to which conformity is required. These are not only external, as was shown above, but they are of general application. They do not merely require that every man should get as near as he can to the best conduct possible for him. They require him at his own peril to come up to a certain height. They take no account of incapacities, unless the weakness is so marked as to fall into well-known exceptions, such as infancy or madness. They assume that every man is as able as every other to behave as they command. If they fall on any one class harder than on another, it is on the weakest. For it is precisely to those who are most likely to err by temperament, ignorance, or folly, that the threats of the law are the most dangerous.

The reconciliation of the doctrine that liability is founded on blameworthiness with the existence of liability where the party is not to blame . . . is founded in the conception of the average man, the man of ordinary intelligence and reasonable prudence. Liability is said to arise out of such conduct as would be blameworthy in him. But he is an ideal being, represented by the jury when they are appealed to, and his conduct is an external or objective standard when applied to any given individual. That individual may be morally without stain, because he has less than ordinary intelligence or prudence. But he is required to have those qualities at his peril. If he has them, he will not, as a general rule, incur liability without blameworthiness.

E. ABOLITION OF THE INSANITY DEFENSE

This topic has been reserved until now because proposals to abolish the insanity defense cannot properly be evaluated until one has some grasp of the framework of the criminal law. For instance, one could reasonably conclude that eliminating the insanity defense would change little if the automatism, diminished capacity, self-defense, and duress doctrines were given their full potential scope.

NOTE ON THE MENS REA ALTERNATIVE

The most prominent proposal to abolish the insanity defense has been termed the "mens rea" alternative. Although most jurisdictions retain the insanity defense, at least four states (Montana, Utah, Idaho, and Colorado) have adopted this alternative, which replaces the defense with a provision allowing acquittal if the accused, as a result of mental disability, lacked the mens rea for the crime charged. In Montana, for instance, the defendant is to be acquitted if the jury finds that "due to a mental disease or defect he could not have had a particular state of mind that is an essential element of the offense charged." Other evidence of cognitive or volitional impairment due to mental disability is admissible only at sentencing; if the sentencing court finds that the offender "was suffering from a mental disease or defect which rendered him unable to appreciate the criminality of his conduct or to conform his conduct to the requirements of law," it may "sentence him to be committed to the custody of the director of the department of institutions to be placed in an appropriate institution for custody, care, and treatment for a definite time not to exceed the maximum term of imprisonment that could be imposed." Mont.Code Ann. 46–14–201(2), 46–14–311, 46–14–312. The provisions relating to the disposition of those who are acquitted by reason of mental disease or defect are similar to typical commitment statutes for insanity acquittees. Id.

The American Medical Association, in a report released shortly after the Hinckley verdict, supported this approach. See "Insanity Defense in Criminal Trials and Limitations of Psychiatric Testimony: Report of the Board of Trustees," 251 J.Am.Medical Ass. 2967 (1984). The Association's report stated in part:

> The essential goal of an exculpatory test for insanity is to identify the point at which a defendant's mental condition has become so impaired that society may confidently conclude that he has lost his free will. Psychiatric concepts of mental illness are ill-suited to this task. . . .
> Because free will is an article of faith, rather than a concept that can

be explained in medical terms, it is impossible for psychiatrists to determine whether a mental impairment has affected the defendant's capacity for voluntary choice, or caused him to commit the particular act in question.

* * *

Even under a truncated test of insanity limited to cognitive impairments, the inscrutable cause-and-effect relationship between mental illness and free will remains the central question. . . . Meaningful reform can be achieved only if the focus of the inquiry is shifted away from the elusive notion of free will, and its relationship to mental disease, and back to the relatively objective standards of *mens rea* where it fell traditionally.

The AMA also asserted that several practical problems associated with the insanity defense would be solved by its approach.

Most significantly, perhaps, abandonment of the moral pretense of the insanity defense in favor of a *mens rea* concept may lead to a more realistic appreciation of the relationship between mental impairment and criminal behavior. Some observers of the criminal justice system maintain that this relationship extends far beyond its manifestations in the case of those few offenders acquitted on claims of insanity; recognition of a special defense applicable to these few detracts from the legitimate treatment needs of the many. *Mens rea* proposals seek to correct this myopic focus of the insanity defense by emphasizing considerations of mercy and appropriate treatment for all mentally disordered offenders.

Additionally, according to the AMA, the mens rea approach would make expert testimony on volitional impairment irrelevant, and "diminish the scope and importance of psychiatric testimony relating to cognitive impairment in the vast majority of cases." Thus, for example, "psychiatric testimony would not be permitted to establish that a defendant's conscious premeditation or deliberation was the consequence of a mental disorder or that his intent to kill was motivated by unconscious aberrational influences."

Questions and Comments

1. *Constitutional status of the insanity defense.* In *State v. Korell*, 213 Mont. 316, 690 P.2d 992 (1984), the Montana Supreme Court upheld the constitutionality of the statute described above. Abolishing the insanity defense, the court concluded, does not violate the federal constitution so long as mental impairment is taken into account at sentencing. No modern court has explicitly held that the constitution mandates an insanity defense.[o] In 1910, the Washington Supreme Court declared unconstitutional a scheme which reserved the insanity issue until the sentencing stage. It stated that preventing the accused from offering evidence tending to prove that "he was insane at the time to the extent that he could not comprehend the nature and quality of the act—in other words, if he had no

o. See p. 527 for a discussion of Supreme Court cases bearing on this issue.

will to control the physical act of his physical body—. . . . is in our opinion as much a violation of his constitutional right to trial by jury as to take from him the right to offer evidence before the jury tending to show that he did not physically commit the act or physically set in motion a train of events resulting in the act." State v. Strasburg, 60 Wash. 106, 110 P. 1020 (1910). See also, State v. Lange, 168 La. 958, 123 So. 639 (1929); Sinclair v. State, 161 Miss. 142, 132 So. 581 (1931).

Even if there are no constitutional problems with eliminating the insanity defense, the mens rea alternative may run afoul of the due process clause if it is meant to bar the automatism defense as well. Like mens rea, the actus reus is a fundamental element of each offense. Thus, analogous to those cases finding that the admission of diminished capacity evidence is constitutionally mandated, the due process clause might prohibit exclusion of evidence relevant to the "involuntariness" of the accused's act.

2. *Evaluating the theory behind the mens rea alternative.* Constitutional concerns aside, does limiting evidence concerning mental disease or defect to the mens rea issue capture the universe of mental disabled people who should have their disability accorded exculpatory effect? The American Bar Association rejected the mens rea alternative, noting that it would permit conviction of any defendants who "knew what they were doing at the time of an offense and possessed the intent to commit it." According to the ABA:

> The issue of criminal blameworthiness merits deeper inquiry because it implies a certain *quality* of knowledge and intent transcending a minimal awareness and purposefulness. Otherwise, for example, a defendant who knowingly and intentionally killed his son under the psychotic delusion that he was the biblical Abraham, and his son the biblical Isaac, could be held criminally responsible.

In response, consider this argument from Morris, a vigorous advocate of the mens rea approach:

> It too often is overlooked that one group's exculpation from criminal responsibility confirms the inculpation of other groups. Why not permit the defense of dwelling in a Negro ghetto? Such a defense would not be morally indefensible. Adverse social and subcultural background is statistically more criminogenic than is psychosis; like insanity, it also severely circumscribes the freedom of choice which a non-deterministic criminal law . . . attributes to accused persons. True, a defense of social adversity would politically be intolerable; but that does not vitiate the analogy for my purposes. [Some might argue] that insanity destroys, undermines, diminishes man's capacity to reject what is wrong and to adhere to what is right. So does the ghetto— more so. But surely, [it will be replied,] I would not have us punish the sick. Indeed I would, if [one insists] on punishing the grossly deprived. To the extent that criminal sanctions serve punitive purposes, I fail to see the difference between these two defenses. To the extent that they serve rehabilitative, treatment, and curative purposes I fail to see the need for the difference.
>
> . . . . It seems clear that there are different degrees of moral turpitude in criminal conduct and that the mental health or illness of an actor is

relevant to an assessment of that degree—as are many other factors in a crime's social setting and historical antecedents. This does not mean, however, that we are obliged to quantify these pressures for purposes of a moral assessment . . . leading to conclusions as to criminal responsibility.

Morris, "Psychiatry and the Dangerous Criminal," 41 S.Cal.L.Rev. 514, 520–21 (1968). Is Morris' equation of poverty and mental illness for purposes of determining criminal responsibility persuasive? See Morse, "Excusing the Crazy: The Insanity Defense Reconsidered," 58 S.Cal.L.Rev. 779, 788–90, 793–95 (1985). If it is, why isn't it an argument for *expanding* the insanity defense rather than for its abolition?

3. *Evaluating the practical impact of the mens rea alternative.* Is the AMA correct in asserting that the mens rea alternative will reduce psychiatric testimony and acquittals based on mental disability? Dershowitz has argued that it will not:

> The clash of experts testifying about the defendant's state of mind will continue, as it has for more than a century. The battlefield may shift from the issue of right versus wrong to the equally troublesome issue of intent, but the jurors will hear testimony not substantially different— or more informative—from what they hear today.
>
> In the last analysis, it is the jury that decides whether an accused is to be convicted or acquitted. No matter how the law reads, it is a deeply entrenched human feeling that those who are grossly disturbed— whether they are called 'madmen,' 'lunatics,' 'insane,' or 'mentally ill'—should not be punished like ordinary criminals. This feeling, which is as old as recorded history, is unlikely to be rooted out by new legislation.

Dershowitz, "Abolishing the Insanity Defense," 9 Crim.L.Bull. 434, 438–39 (1973). Current empirical evidence on the impact of the mens rea alternative is inconclusive. In a study of the impact of Montana's legislative changes in 1979 abolishing the insanity defense and limiting the mental disability defense to mens rea, researchers looked at various factors for the three years prior to and the three years after the reform. They found that the proportion of defendants who claimed a defense based on mental disease or defect was virtually unchanged between the pre and post periods. However, of those who claimed a psychiatric defense, 22.7% were successful and 49.3% were found guilty in the pre-reform period, while 2.3% were successful and 60.9% were found guilty in the post-reform period. At the same time, the number of psychiatric cases which were dismissed rose from 17.3% to 29.9% between the two periods, suggesting to the researchers that, after the reform, many of those who would have been found not guilty by reason of insanity were found incompetent to stand trial instead. They also found that, after the reform, a smaller percentage of those who raised a defense were imprisoned (35.4 to 29.1) or hospitalized (30.0 to 16.3) and a greater percentage were put on probation, conditional release or released altogether (25.7 to 46.5). Callahan, et al., "The Impact of Montana's Insanity Defense Abolition," paper published by Policy Research Associates, Inc. (July, 1988).

4. *Bifurcation.* An alternative which is functionally similar to the mens rea approach is to "bifurcate" the trial, adjudicating the issue of "factual guilt" at the first stage and leaving the insanity issue to the second stage. Bifurcation was first proposed as a method of (1) alleviating jury confusion by avoiding complex psychiatric testimony about insanity until after the defendant had been found "guilty" of the crime; (2) eliminating the risk of the jury returning a verdict of insanity out of sympathy for a mentally ill, but guilty, defendant; and (3) conserving judicial resources where the defendant was acquitted at the first stage.[p] The difference between the bifurcation and mens rea approaches is that in the former the insanity issue is still litigated at trial (albeit at the second stage), while in the latter any psychiatric information not relevant to mens rea is considered only at sentencing.

As originally conceived, bifurcation was different from the mens rea alternative in an additional way: psychiatric testimony was to be excluded entirely from the first stage. But, as discussed previously, most courts found this scheme unconstitutional on the ground that such evidence could not be excluded if it was relevant to mens rea. See, e.g., *Sanchez v. State,* 567 P.2d 270 (Wyo.1977); but see, *Steele v. State,* 97 Wis.2d 72, 294 N.W.2d 2 (1980). According to the American Bar Association, once this position is accepted, "mandatory bifurcation loses its allure" because "relevant evidence of mental abnormality must be allowed at the first stage as well as the second, which uselessly duplicates evidence and nullifies many of the supposed advantages of bifurcation." ABA Criminal Justice Mental Health Standards, commentary to Standard 7–6.7, p. 341 (1987). Can the same type of claim be leveled at the mens rea approach?

5. *Abolition of insanity and mens rea defenses.* A final approach has been most forcefully presented by Lady Wooton in her book Crime and the Criminal Law (1963). She too suggests a bifurcated approach to determining the appropriate punishment, but with a significant difference. The first stage would consider only whether the defendant committed an antisocial act. *No* consideration of mental state, psychiatric or otherwise, would take place at this stage. At the second stage, the appropriate disposition of the defendant would be decided, based on expert opinion if deemed necessary or desirable. Lady Wooton defended her proposal as follows:

> The law, of course, always requires clear-cut distinctions. The responsible and sane stand on one side of the line, the irresponsible or insane on the other: every single defendant must be appropriately classified. Yet natura non facit saltum: in reality we are all strung out along a continuum which reaches from the most responsible to the most hopelessly weak-willed and weak-minded; and in many cases the degree of our responsibility almost certainly varies from time to time in accordance with our circumstances or physiological condition. In

p. Bifurcation was also supported by a fourth reason—protecting the fifth amendment right of a defendant who wanted to assert both a not guilty plea and a plea of not guilty by reason of insanity, without having to present possibly damaging psychiatric testimony during the adjudication of the first plea. Bifurcation allows adjudication of the factual defense at the first stage while adjudication of the second plea, if necessary, is reserved for the second stage. See pp. 471–476.

short, the "vital distinction between illness and evil" is anything but clear-cut. Indeed the worst feature of all the formulae that have been tried—McNaghten, Durham, British Homicide Act, or what have you— is their insistence on a hard and fast and totally unrealistic line between the sheep and the goats. Anyone who has followed trials in which this issue has been raised will be well aware of the sophisticated forensic subtleties for which it offers opportunity. Is careful planning of a crime consistent with diminished responsibility? Is it possible that a man should be fully responsible when he seizes a stick in the entrance to a house, but only partially so when he uses it to beat an old gentleman in bed upstairs? In these and the many similar examples which can be culled from trials in which the defendant's mens rea is in issue, all contact with reality seems to have been lost.

Clearly the only way to avoid getting entangled in these niceties and absurdities is to demote the concept of blame from its dominant position in the criminal process. If we could emancipate ourselves from the deep-rooted tradition that the basic function of the criminal law is to identify and punish wickedness, all this farcical hairsplitting about the limits of mental abnormality could be done away with. Questions of the accused's mental condition could be ignored in the actual trial, the purpose of which would be to establish responsibility in a purely physical sense for the actus reus without reference to the presence, or absence, of malicious intent. Mens rea would thus no longer be written into the definition of every crime. Only after the accused's physical responsibility for a forbidden action had been proved would it be permissible to inquire into his mental condition, in order to determine how best he could be dealt with. In other words an offender's state of mind would be regarded as relevant, not to the measure of his guilt, or to the crime of which he should be convicted, but to the choice of the treatment most appropriate to his case.

* * *

Hitherto, of course, strict liability has generally been restricted to such statutory offenses as are generally regarded as of minor importance. In such cases disregard of mens rea is defended on the dual ground, first, that the number of these offenses is so enormous that life is simply not long enough to inquire in every case into the accused's motivation or mental state (imagine what would happen, for example, in a busy city court which disposes of some 300 parking offenses in a morning if proof of mens rea were required in every case!); and, second, that in any case these offenses are not "truly criminal" and do not involve any serious "moral turpitude."

Yet could not an equally compelling argument be made the other way round; i.e., in favor of eliminating the requirement of mens rea from particularly grave offenses such as homicide or rape? Crimes such as these are just as damaging to their victims whether they are the result of calculated wickedness or of insane delusions. Is it not, therefore, proper that anyone who is suspected of having committed such an actus reus should be liable to answer for it in a criminal court, whatever the state of his mind—so long, that is, as he is not too ill to be able to instruct counsel or to understand court proceedings?

* * *

Obviously, if the essential purpose of a criminal court is to punish the blameworthy as they deserve, the compassionworthy must be rescued from its clutches. But, were this obsession with the punitive once dispelled, the courts could be free to deal with every lawbreaker in whatever way, consonant with the moral standards of the community, seemed best calculated to discourage future lawbreaking. Their eyes would be on the future, not on the past. Nor need they be bound by rigid diagnostic categories.

* * *

It follows logically that, once the practice of classifying offenders into the wicked and the weak-minded is abandoned, the similar distinction between prisons and hospitals becomes equally inappropriate. Already hybrid institutions, such as Grendon Underwood in Britain and similar establishments in the United States, are beginning to make their appearance; and suggestions that the courts should simply pass "custodial" sentences without specifying under what conditions, penal or medical, this sentence is to be served are much in the air, and much to be commended. Obviously, in the case of sentences of any considerable duration, the court is in no position to forecast what kind of regime will be best suited to an offender several years ahead. Hence the need for a variety of institutions and for easy transfer from one to another without inhibiting labels, at the discretion of those who are in continuous touch with persons under detention. Nor must this be read as merely a plea for the "soft" treatment of offenders. If the weaker vessels need the protection of a kindly environment, there are others for whom a more demanding regime is certainly indicated; and the response of a single individual to different types of treatment is not necessarily constant throughout his history.

Wooton, "Book Review of A. Goldstein, The Insanity Defense," 77 Yale L.J. 1019, 1028–1032 (1968).

Is Wooton's proposal coherent? Can it be seen as the logical extension of Holmes' arguments excerpted at pp. 553–555, or does it stray too far from Holmes' premise? Under her proposal, what happens to the person who wants to plead self-defense or duress? To what extent does her proposal undercut what was described in the introduction to this chapter as the central assumption of our criminal justice system—that we have "free will"? Consider the following from Hermann, The Insanity Defense, 91–93 (1983):

An influential critique of the concept of responsibility has come from behaviorists who maintain that the determination of responsibility, in a moral or traditional legal sense, with elements of culpability and blameworthiness, is meaningless and reflects a fallacious understanding of human behavior. At the same time, it is argued that there should be a reformulation of the utilitarian objectives of the criminal law into one that can be stated succinctly as crime-preventive. Such a view [has been] urged quite eloquently by Lady Wooton . . .

* * *

Even assuming the soundness of the determinism of the behaviorist view, there is a fundamental mistake in supposing that law is unrealistic in retaining the concepts of responsibility and punishment. This mistake stems from the assumption that ethics and law have the same point of view with regard to responsibility as does science. Unlike science, the ethical and legal systems are moral enterprises. The ascription of responsibility promotes ethical and legal values. Thus, even if it were true that a person cannot control the determinants of his conduct, and therefore is not free and responsible in some ultimate libertarian sense, the interest of law and ethics in minimizing socially harmful conduct is promoted by fostering feelings of responsibility in society. This need not be regarded as some "noble lie" but, rather, should be viewed in terms of an "as if" constituting an example of a pragmatic sense of truth. Ethical prohibitions and criminal law sanctions can themselves act as a determinant of choices, thereby assuring that actors will avoid condemnation and sanction. The influence of attribution of responsibility has been suggested by one commentator who observed: "[T]he individual who perceives himself as free and responsible behaves very differently than the individual who believes that he lacks choice and responsibility. In general, the direction of this difference is toward a higher level of awareness, initiative, achievement, independence and complexity for those who perceive themselves as freely choosing to behave in certain ways and as responsible for the behavior." Moreover, the criminal sanction with its corollary of blameworthiness strengthens the resolve of persons to obey the law.

Another significant legal purpose is served by treating persons as responsible and blameworthy when they violate the law. By requiring guilt before criminal sanctions can be applied, the law-abiding person is protected from governmental interference. As one commentator succinctly stated: "The rule of law now guards the innocent, but its protective wall would not survive the dissolution of criminal responsibility." Elimination of the principle of responsibility would result in every attitude, disposition, or accidental movement seen by the state as undesirable, becoming a potential source of coercive intervention in the life of any and every citizen no matter how well intentioned he might be.

6. *Tort liability.* By way of comparison to the foregoing materials, note that traditionally an "insane" person could not escape tort liability by reason of mental disability, at least in a negligence action. See Prosser, Torts 1030. As described by the court in *Jolley v. Powell,* 299 So.2d 647 (Fla.2d D.C.A.1974):

[L]iability without subjective fault, under some circumstances, is one price men pay for membership in society. The sane and the insane, the awkward and the coordinated are equally liable for their acts or omissions. In such cases, we do not decide fault, rather we determine upon whom our society imposes the burden of redress for a given injury. As Holmes implied in his 'awkward man' parable, a principle at least co-equal with that of the fault principle in the law of torts is that the innocent victim should have redress.

* * *

We therefore reiterate, when the predicate for a wrongful death action is unintentional tort the standard against which such tort is measured is the objective, "reasonable man standard" and the subjective state of mind of the tortfeasor is irrelevant.

A small number of courts reject this view. As stated in *Fitzgerald v. Lawhorn,* 29 Conn.Supp. 511, 294 A.2d 338 (Com.Pl.1972):

If a child too young cannot be held liable in negligence, then an insane person would not be held liable; it is unjust to hold one responsible for a wrong that he is incapable of avoiding; a man who is so devoid of intelligence or reason as to be unable to apprehend danger and do something to avoid it cannot be held negligent. . . .

As the above implies, mental disability is usually considered a defense in intentional tort and punitive damage actions.

How is Lady Wooton's approach to criminal liability different from the traditional approach to civil liability?

F. THE "GUILTY BUT MENTALLY ILL" PLEA

A final reform aims not at abolishing the insanity defense, but at reducing the number of insanity pleas and acquittals by offering an alternative to the insanity verdict. Since 1976, at least 12 states have passed statutes authorizing the factfinder to return a verdict of "guilty but mentally ill" (GBMI). Although there are many different versions of the GBMI concept, most proposals work basically as follows: A defendant who pleads not guilty by reason of insanity may be found not guilty, guilty, insane, or, in the alternative, guilty but mentally ill at the time of the offense. If the jury makes the last mentioned finding, the defendant may be sentenced to any term appropriate for the offense, with the opportunity for treatment in a mental hospital during that period. Thus, jurors in insanity cases are given three sets of instructions with respect to the ultimate verdict they may reach: One explains under what circumstances a defendant may be found guilty of the crime charged; one describes the state's test for insanity; and one informs the jury when a defendant who is guilty beyond a reasonable doubt but not insane may be found GBMI. See, e.g., Mich.Comp.Laws Ann. § 768.36; Ill.—S.H.A. ch. 38, ¶ 115–2(b); Ky.Rev.Stat. 504.120. The definition of mental illness found in the last of these instructions varies from state to state, but usually borrows heavily from the definition of mental illness in the state's civil commitment statute. In Michigan, for instance, the definition is taken directly from the mental health code and states that mental illness is "[a] substantial disorder of thought or mood which significantly impairs judgment, behavior, capacity to recognize reality, or ability to cope with the ordinary demands of life." Mich.Comp.Laws Ann. § 330.1400a.

As the following case illustrates, a person who is found guilty but mentally ill is subject to the same dispositions as a person found guilty of the crime charged.

PEOPLE v. CREWS

Supreme Court of Illinois, 1988.
122 Ill.2d 266, 119 Ill.Dec. 308, 522 N.E.2d 1167.

* * *

JUSTICE MILLER delivered the opinion of the court:

The defendant, William Crews, pleaded guilty but mentally ill to one count each of murder and attempted murder in the circuit court of Randolph County. The trial judge sentenced the defendant to death for the murder conviction and imposed a 30–year prison term for the conviction for attempted murder. The defendant's execution was stayed pending direct review by this court.

The defendant's convictions stem from his attack on two correctional officers at Menard Correctional Center on November 30, 1984. The defendant was an inmate of Menard at the time of the offenses and was serving a 20–to–60–year term for an earlier murder conviction. The attack occurred on the gallery outside the defendant's cell. The defendant stabbed correctional officer Cecil Harbison to death with a shank and wounded another guard, Lamont Gilbert. The defendant then fled from the gallery, and he was captured moments later on the ground floor of the cellhouse.

The defendant initially pleaded not guilty to the charges here, but he later asked to change his plea to guilty but mentally ill (GBMI). As required by statute (see Ill.Rev.Stat.1983, ch. 38, pars. 113–4(d), 115–2(b)), the trial judge ordered the defendant to undergo a psychological examination, and a hearing was held in August 1985 on the defendant's mental condition. At the hearing, defense counsel presented the testimony of three psychiatrists—Drs. Pichardo, Vallabhaneni, and Parwatikar—who had treated the defendant at Menard Correctional Center or Menard Psychiatric Center. Dr. Pichardo first saw the defendant in February 1980 and last saw him in the middle of September 1984, a little more than two months before the defendant's attack on the two guards. Dr. Pichardo believed that the defendant was suffering from a mental illness during that period, but he could not say whether the defendant had a judgment-impairing, substantial disorder of thought, mood, or behavior. According to Dr. Pichardo, the defendant had attempted to commit suicide in April 1980.

Dr. Vallabhaneni saw the defendant several days after his attack on the guards and believed that at the time of the offenses the defendant was suffering from a mental illness and that his judgment was impaired, but he did not have a specific diagnosis for the defendant's condition.

Dr. Parwatikar believed that at the time of the offenses the defendant was mentally ill, in that he had a substantial disorder of mood, thought, or behavior. Dr. Parwatikar saw the defendant on December 2, 1984, two days after the offenses here, and his diagnosis then was of an intermittent explosive disorder.

The State disputed the defendant's contention that he was mentally ill at the time of the offenses. Dr. Daniel Cuneo, a clinical psychologist, testified in the State's behalf at the hearing. Dr. Cuneo had interviewed the defendant on two occasions—in March 1985 and in August 1985—and, based on those examinations, as well as on his review of the defendant's records, Dr. Cuneo concluded that the defendant was malingering and that he had an antisocial personality disorder. Dr. Cuneo believed that the defendant was only feigning mental illness.

The State also introduced into evidence statements the defendant made to authorities concerning the offenses here. In an initial statement given on the night of his attack on the two guards, the defendant said simply that he had gone berserk, and he did not provide a motive for his acts. In a statement given the next day, however, the defendant explained that he attacked the officers because he resented an order Harbison had given him shortly before that. The State also presented testimony from two inmates who spoke with the defendant in the period following his attack on the two guards. They testified that the defendant told them that he was trying to convince psychiatrists that he was crazy. Also, one of the inmates recalled that on the day of the occurrence here the defendant mentioned the name of a friend who had been killed earlier that year and made a comment suggesting that the friend's death should be avenged. Finally, the State presented evidence of the defendant's extensive history of disciplinary violations since 1974, when he began serving the prison sentence for his earlier murder conviction. These disciplinary tickets included 16 violations of rules, 10 assaults, 5 instances of damaging property, 19 instances of disobeying orders, and 11 instances of possession of contraband or dangerous weapons.

The trial judge accepted the defendant's GBMI plea, finding that there was a factual basis that the defendant was mentally ill when he committed the offenses here. The State then requested a death penalty hearing, and the defendant waived his right to a jury for that purpose. The defendant, who was born in 1952 and therefore 18 or older at the time of the offenses, was eligible for the death penalty because the murder victim was a correctional officer.

[Under the Illinois death penalty statute, the sentencing authority is to consider both aggravating and mitigating circumstances in deciding between life imprisonment and death. The prosecution must prove the existence of one aggravating circumstance (such as a significant history of criminal conduct); if it does so, the death penalty may be imposed unless the defense can convince the factfinder that mitigating factors outweigh the aggravating factor or factors. One of the mitigating factors listed in the Illinois statute is proof that the defendant "was under the influence of extreme mental or emotional disturbance" at the time of the offense.]

Dr. Cuneo testified in the State's behalf at the sentencing hearing, and he repeated his earlier diagnosis that the defendant had an antisocial personality disorder. Dr. Cuneo did not believe that the defendant was functioning under an extreme mental or emotional disturbance at the time of the offenses. Dr. Cuneo also said that he was familiar with capital sentencing in Illinois and that he did not know of any case in which a defendant received the death sentence after being found guilty but mentally ill.

* * *

The defendant did not present any testimony at the sentencing hearing. Included in a presentence investigation report, however, was a report dated August 5, 1985, by a psychiatrist, Dr. Moisy Shopper, who had examined the defendant and reviewed his prison file. Dr. Shopper described the defendant's suicide attempt in April 1980 and noted parallels between that event and the defendant's later attack on the two guards. Also, Dr. Shopper described the defendant's condition at the time of the offense as "an acute paranoid psychotic state with marked depressive features."

The trial judge sentenced the defendant to death for the murder conviction. The trial judge did not believe that imposition of the death penalty was precluded by the defendant's GBMI plea. The trial judge found that the defendant had a significant history of criminal conduct, and he did not believe that the defendant was acting under the influence of an extreme mental or emotional disturbance sufficient to preclude imposition of the death penalty.

* * *

The defendant . . . argues that the legislature did not intend the death penalty to be available as a possible punishment for GBMI offenders.

* * *

In support of this argument, the defendant relies on section 5–2–6 of the Unified Code of Corrections (Ill.Rev.Stat.1983, ch. 38, par. 1005–2–6). Section 5–2–6 bears the heading "Sentencing and Treatment of Defendant Found Guilty but Mentally Ill," and the defendant contends that certain provisions in the statute signify the legislature's intent to preclude the death penalty as a possible punishment for GBMI offenders.

* * *

Although we agree with the defendant that section 5–2–6 of the Unified Code of Corrections is applicable to GBMI offenders, we do not believe that the statute may be understood as precluding the imposition of the death penalty. To the contrary, the plain language of the statute indicates otherwise. Section 5–2–6(a) provides, "The court may impose any sentence upon the defendant which could be imposed pursuant to law upon a defendant who had been convicted of the same offense without a finding of mental illness." Clearly, that language leaves available for GBMI offenders the full range of sentences—including the death penalty—that may be imposed on persons who are guilty of offenses and who are not mentally ill. This is entirely consistent with the legislature's definition of the term "mental illness" as a condition distinct from insanity. Section 6–2(c) of the Criminal Code of 1961 provides, "A person who, at the time of the commission of a criminal offense, was not insane but was suffering from a mental illness, is not relieved of criminal responsibility for his conduct and may be found guilty but mentally ill." (Ill.Rev.Stat.1983, ch. 38, par. 6–2(c).) Section 6–2(d) of the Criminal Code of 1961 provides, "For purposes of this Section, 'mental illness' or 'mentally ill' means a substantial disorder of thought, mood, or behavior which afflicted a person at the time of the commission of the offense and which impaired that person's judgment, but not to the extent that he is unable to appreciate the wrongfulness of his behavior or is unable to conform his conduct to the requirements of law." (Ill.Rev.Stat.1983, ch. 38, par. 6–2(d).) A GBMI offender is no less guilty than one who is guilty and not mentally ill; unlike insanity, a GBMI finding or plea does not relieve an offender of criminal responsibility for his conduct. By its plain terms, section 5–2–6(a) authorizes imposition on a GBMI offender of any sentence that could be imposed on one convicted of the same offense without the additional finding of mental illness; the death penalty therefore is available as a sentence for GBMI offenders who have been convicted of murder (see Ill.Rev.Stat.1983, ch. 38, par. 1005–5–3(c)(1)).

* * *

Opposing that interpretation of section 5–2–6 of the Unified Code of Corrections, the defendant argues that sentencing a GBMI offender to death would be inconsistent with the treatment alternatives prescribed for GBMI offenders in section 5–2–6 of the Unified Code of Corrections. The provisions concerning treatment do not pertain to defendants sentenced to death, however. Rather, they apply to persons sentenced to terms of imprisonment (see Ill.Rev.Stat.1983, ch. 38, pars. 1005–2–6(b), (c), (d)) and to those placed on probation or sentenced to a term of periodic imprisonment or a period of conditional discharge (see Ill.Rev. Stat.1983, ch. 38, par. 1005–2–6(e)). The statute thus does not mandate what is referred to in the dissent as the "meaningless" requirement of treatment for one awaiting execution. Having rejected the defendant's interpretation of section 5–2–6, we conclude that the statute does not preclude imposition of the death penalty on GBMI offenders.

* * *

The defendant also contends that the trial judge's stated reasons for imposing the death penalty in this case were inconsistent with his earlier finding of a factual basis for the defendant's GBMI plea. * * * The defendant contends that the trial judge's decision to accept the GBMI plea cannot be reconciled with his later statement, made at the sentencing hearing, that the defendant "may not have been under an extreme mental or emotional disturbance."

The defendant's argument assumes that mental illness, as that term is applied to GBMI offenders, is more serious than the mitigating circumstance of extreme mental or emotional disturbance, as that term is used in the death penalty statute. * * * We have already concluded that the legislature authorized imposition of the death penalty on GBMI offenders, and, consistent with that holding, we do not believe that a finding of mental illness necessarily establishes the mitigating circumstance of extreme mental or emotional disturbance. It is important to note here that the distinction between mental illness and the statutory mitigating circumstance of extreme mental or emotional disturbance does not mean that a GBMI plea or finding is irrelevant in a capital case. Because mitigating circumstances are not limited to those specifically enumerated in section 9–1(c) of the Criminal Code of 1961 (Ill.Rev.Stat.1983, ch. 38, par. 9–1(c)), evidence of a defendant's mental illness is admissible at a capital sentencing hearing regardless of the relationship between the GBMI provisions and the statutory mitigating circumstance of extreme mental or emotional disturbance. The trial judge's decision here to sentence the defendant to death was not contrary to the findings he made in accepting the defendant's GBMI plea. In accordance with the provisions of section 9–1(h) of the Criminal Code of 1961 (Ill.Rev.Stat.1983, ch. 38, par. 9–1(h)), the trial judge balanced the conflicting evidence and found that any mental or emotional disturbance of the defendant was not sufficient to preclude imposition of the death penalty.

* * *

JUSTICE SIMON, dissenting.

* * *

A sentence of death is completely inconsistent with the goals of the GBMI statutory provisions—providing treatment for the mentally ill as well as punishing them for the crimes they committed. During a reading of the GBMI bill on the Senate floor, the bill's co-sponsor, Senator Adeline J. Geo–Karis, emphasized this goal of treatment, stating that a "guilty but mentally ill defendant, for example, can be . . . sentenced exactly as a healthy defendant charged with the same crime, except that his sentence, either to probation, periodic imprisonment, or to the penitentiary, must include psychiatric and psychological treatment or counseling." The bill as enacted includes this requirement of treatment for the offender's mental illness. The statute also requires the Department of Corrections to make periodic inquiry and examination "concerning the nature, extent, continuance, and treatment of the defendant's mental illness" for those GBMI offenders who are imprisoned. The Department of Corrections is also to provide psychological, psychiatric and other counseling and treatment to the defendant and may transfer the inmate to the Department of Mental Health if necessary. This treatment requirement, however, would be meaningless for someone who is going to be put to death. "In view of the statutory treatment rights that underlie a GBMI verdict, to order death as a GBMI's treatment would not only be contrary to the legislature's objectives, but also would be morally reprehensible." Note, "Disposition of the Mentally Ill Offender in Illinois—'Guilty But Mentally Ill,'" 31 DePaul L.Rev. 869, 889–90 (1982).

* * *

[T]he majority [also] concludes that a finding of mental illness does not necessarily establish the mitigating circumstance of mental or emotional disturbance. On the contrary, a finding of mental illness is a recognition of the likelihood of a more serious disorder than the mental state of an extreme emotional disturbance.

Under Illinois law, a finding of mental illness is a recognition that the defendant's judgment at the time of the offense was seriously impaired, a mental state exceeded only by insanity, a complete defense. The legislature has provided for a special verdict form for GBMI defendants. Thus mental illness is unique among mitigating factors because it is the only one that can be incorporated into the judgment at trial. Finally, in order for a GBMI plea to be accepted, the defendant must be examined by a clinical psychologist or psychiatrist, the judge must examine the psychiatric or psychological report or reports and conduct a hearing on the issue of the defendant's mental health.

A finding of extreme mental or emotional disturbance requires none of the above procedures, indicating that the standard for this mitigating factor is much less stringent than that for mental illness. The failure to require a psychological or psychiatric examination to establish an extreme mental or emotional disturbance indicates that it can be established without a finding of mental illness, thus making it a much broader, less serious condition than mental illness. This is evidenced by cases where an extreme mental or emotional disturbance has been found without a finding that the defendant was mentally ill at the time of the offense. Moreover, a finding of extreme mental or emotional disturbance does not necessitate treatment for the offender, and there is no special verdict form for this type of disturbance.

The conclusion of the trial court and the majority that a finding of mental illness does not necessarily establish the mitigating factor of extreme mental or emotional disturbance is therefore clearly in error. By failing to recognize that mental illness is a more serious condition than extreme mental or emotional disturbance, the sentencing court did not give proper weight to the defendant's illness as a mitigating factor, and, a new sentencing hearing is required.

* * *

Questions and Comments

1. *The GBMI verdict as a finding of diminished responsibility.* The court states that a person who is found guilty but mentally ill "is no less guilty than one who is guilty and not mentally ill." Clearly, as the court points out, the Illinois legislature did not want the verdict to be a finding of diminished responsibility that would reduce the degree of crime for which the defendant is convicted. But a GBMI verdict could still function as a

determination of diminished responsibility that is implemented at *sentencing;* under this interpretation, the defendant found guilty but mentally ill would be convicted of the crime charged but would be entitled to greater mitigation at sentencing than someone found merely guilty of the same charge.   Such an approach might seem particularly appealing in the capital sentencing context.[q] Does the majority in *Crews* hold that the evidence of mental illness associated with the GBMI verdict is irrelevant to the extreme mental or emotional distress issue, relevant but not dispositive, or dispositive on that issue but not dispositive of the ultimate decision with respect to the death penalty?   Of these three positions and the dissent's position that the verdict precludes imposition of the death penalty, which is the correct reading of legislative intent?

If one agrees with the majority's position, is there any point in having a distinct verdict indicating that the defendant is guilty of the offense and was also mentally ill (but not insane) during its commission? Or is it accurate to say, as Slovenko has asserted, that one might as well have a verdict called "guilty but flat feet"? Slovenko, "The Insanity Defense in the Wake of the Hinckley Trial," 14 Rutgers L.J. 373, 393 (1983).

2. *The GBMI verdict and treatment.*   Some have contended that, whatever the impact of the GBMI verdict in assessing the degree of culpability or punishment, it does afford better *conditions* of punishment. Mickenberg has contended that "although . . . GBMI does not reduce the degree of crime for which defendants are responsible, it does provide necessary and acceptable mitigation in the form of psychiatric assistance for the convicts while they serve their sentences." Mickenberg, "A Pleasant Surprise: The Guilty But Mentally Ill Verdict Has Both Succeeded in Its Own Right and Successfully Preserved the Traditional Role of the Insanity Defense," 55 Cinn.L.Rev. 943, 990 (1987). Isn't the holding in *Crews* inconsistent with this position?

Arguably, if the point of the GBMI scheme is to facilitate treatment for mentally ill offenders, it is both inefficient and unnecessary. A finding by a judge or jury that an offender was mentally ill *at the time of the offense* is not likely to be very useful in determining the offender's treatment needs (a fact which is recognized by provisions in most GBMI legislation—like Illinois'—requiring a post-conviction treatment assessment by mental health professionals). Moreover, every state already provides that mentally ill prisoners be treated. In Illinois, for instance, well before passage of the state's guilty but mentally ill statute, the legislature required the Department of Corrections to ascertain whether *any* person committed to it needed psychiatric treatment, and authorized transfer of prisoners requiring such treatment to special facilities within the Department or to mental hospitals. Ill.—S.H.A. ch. 28, ¶ 1003–8–5. Research indicates that although GBMI legislation has focused attention on the paucity of treatment resources available to prisoners generally, it has not meant that those who are found guilty but mentally ill are more likely to receive treatment than those who are simply convicted and sentenced and are subsequently found to need treatment. Smith & Hall, "Evaluating Michigan's Guilty But

q. The role of mental abnormality in in greater detail in the next section, where
capital sentencing proceedings is discussed the *Crews* case will be revisited.

Mentally Ill Verdict: An Empirical Study," 16 Mich.J.Law Ref. 77, 104–106 (1982). Nor are most courts, whatever the original intent of the GBMI legislation, willing to redress this situation by according those found guilty but mentally ill special treatment status. See, e.g., *People v. Marshall*, 114 Ill.App.3d 217, 70 Ill.Dec. 91, 102, 448 N.E.2d 969, 980 (1983); *People v. Sharif*, 87 Mich.App. 196, 200–01, 274 N.W.2d 17, 19–20 (1978). Is this stance wrong? If not, how does the verdict provide "mitigation", as that word is used by Mickenberg, that would not ordinarily be available without the verdict?

3. *The GBMI verdict as a device for easing the factfinder's burden.* Questions about its conceptual underpinnings aside, might the GBMI verdict be sanctioned on the ground that it makes the difficult choice about criminal responsibility easier? In her study of jury reaction to the insanity defense, Simon found:

> Many of the jurors felt constrained by the verdict limitations placed upon them by the court. They would like to have a way of easing the choice between acquitting the defendant on grounds of insanity and finding him guilty. The former designation goes further than they want to go in distinguishing the defendant from the ordinary criminal, and the latter allows for no distinction. In many instances, the jury would have liked to declare the defendant guilty, but insane. That kind of verdict would permit the jurors to condemn the defendant's behavior . . . [and fulfill] their desire to commit the defendant to an institution that both punished and treated.

R. Simon, The Jury and the Defense of Insanity 178 (1967).

Presumably, if the verdict were functioning in the way described by Simon, it would occasion a reduction in insanity acquittals. Certainly this was the hope of many who advocated adoption of the GBMI scheme. Yet a study of Michigan's GBMI reform found that the acquittal rate remained the same after passage of the statute. Smith & Hall, supra, at 100–102. In a mammoth multi-state study, the National Center for State Courts provided data from other states that suggested the same conclusion, although there is some indication that the verdict reduced the acquittal rate marginally in one or two states. See Slobogin, "The Guilty But Mentally Ill Verdict: An Idea Whose Time Should Not Have Come," 53 Geo.Wash.L. Rev. 494, 507–08 (1985).

To what extent does any reduction in the insanity acquittal rate caused by the verdict result from "improper" conviction of the insane, rather than prevention of "inappropriate" insanity acquittals? Although such things are obviously difficult to measure, it appears that most persons found guilty but mentally ill are more likely to have characteristics normally associated with guilt, rather than with insanity. Smith & Hall, supra, at 95–100; Criss & Racine, "Impact of Change in Legal Standard for Those Adjudicated Not Guilty By Reason of Insanity," 8 Bull.Am.Acad.Psychiat. & L. 261 (1980). But see, *People v. Murphy*, 416 Mich. 453, 331 N.W.2d 152 (1982), in which the Michigan Supreme Court struck down a verdict of guilty but mentally ill and directed an insanity acquittal, noting that even the prosecution's expert agreed that the defendant was out of touch with reality and unable to control his behavior or appreciate the wrongfulness of his acts at the time of the offense. See also, *Michigan v. Fultz,* 111 Mich. App. 587, 314 N.W.2d 702 (1981).

III. SENTENCING

Once convicted, an offender is subjected to the sentencing process. Evidence of mental disorder could have a significantly greater impact here than at trial, for at least two reasons. First, many of the concerns that underlie proposals to restrict the role of mental disability in adjudicating guilt—i.e., the diminishment of the free will paradigm implied by broad psychiatric defenses, the threat to public safety if acquittal occurs, the spectre of confusing battles of the experts—are likely to lessen appreciably once the accused is convicted and decision-making takes place in the relatively informal sentencing atmosphere. Indeed, as previous material has suggested, one frequently suggested alternative to considering mental abnormality at trial is to shift most or all psychiatric inquiries to the sentencing stage. A second reason mental disorder is likely to play a greater role at sentencing was noted in the introduction to this chapter: once the question shifts from identifying who is to be punished to determining what kind of punishment should be imposed, attention may focus not just on retributive and general deterrence objectives but also on concerns connected with individual prevention, such as dangerousness and rehabilitative potential. Addressing these issues opens up the inquiry beyond the backward-looking culpability assessments required at trial by necessitating predictions about mentally disordered individuals.

This section will look at the role evidence of mental disability plays in two different sentencing contexts: capital sentencing and special track sentencing, in particular sentencing of those identified as "mentally disordered sex offenders". These two settings raise most starkly the tensions created by consideration of mental disability at the sentencing phase.

A. CAPITAL SENTENCING
NOTE ON SUPREME COURT CASES

Because "death is different," the constitutionality of the death penalty and the procedures for imposing it have been subjected to intense judicial scrutiny, primarily under the Eighth Amendment's ban on cruel and unusual punishment and the Fourteenth Amendment's due process clause. As a result, sentencing criteria in death penalty cases are far more developed than in other cases; most pertinent to our purposes, death penalty litigation has provided the most explicit consideration of the relationship between mental disability and criminal punishment. There follows a brief summary of the Supreme Court's pronouncements concerning the death penalty and the state statutes which attempt to implement those decisions, focusing in particular on material which bears on this relationship.

In 1972, the Supreme Court decided *Furman v. Georgia,* 408 U.S. 238, 92 S.Ct. 2726, 33 L.Ed.2d 346 (1972), which overturned the death sentences in four cases, by a vote of 5–4. In addition to a brief per curiam opinion announcing the court's decision, each of the nine justices wrote an opinion. Although there was no clear majority rationale, *Furman* was widely understood, under either an Eighth Amendment or due process rationale, to prohibit death penalty statutes that left the sentencing decision to the unguided discretion of the jury. For instance, in voting to overturn the death sentences, Justice Douglas spoke of the discriminatory impact of the death penalty on poor, black defendants. Justice Stewart asserted that the death penalty was "wantonly and freakishly imposed" and that death sentences were "cruel and unusual in the same way that being struck by lightning is cruel and unusual." Justice White believed that there was "no meaningful basis for distinguishing the few cases in which [the death penalty] is imposed from the many cases in which it is not." In addition to these three justices, two justices, Brennan and Marshall, concluded that the death penalty is unconstitutional under all circumstances.

Thirty-five states rewrote their statutes in response to *Furman.* Roughly half of these states removed jury discretion by making the death penalty mandatory in certain situations. The other half left the jury considerable decisionmaking power but attempted to set clearer guidelines as to how to exercise it, usually by instructing the jury to weigh specified aggravating and mitigating circumstances. In five cases decided together in 1976, the Court found the former type of statute unconstitutional, but upheld the second type of statute.

One of the statutes that withstood constitutional scrutiny was Georgia's. See *Gregg v. Georgia,* 428 U.S. 153, 96 S.Ct. 2909, 49 L.Ed.2d 859 (1976). A later decision of the Court, *Zant v. Stephens,* 462 U.S. 862, 103 S.Ct. 2733, 77 L.Ed.2d 235 (1983), summarized why the statute was upheld:

> [Our] approval of Georgia's capital sentencing procedure in [*Gregg*] rested primarily on two features of the scheme: that the jury was required to find at least one valid statutory aggravating circumstance and to identify it in writing, and that the state supreme court reviewed the record of every death penalty proceeding to determine whether the sentence was arbitrary or disproportionate. These elements, the opinion concluded, adequately protected against the wanton and freakish imposition of the death penalty. This conclusion rested . . . on the fundamental requirement that . . . an aggravating circumstance must genuinely narrow the class of persons eligible for the death penalty and must reasonably justify the imposition of a more severe sentence on the defendant compared to others found guilty of murder.

North Carolina's mandatory statute, on the other hand, was found unconstitutional. See *Woodson v. North Carolina,* 428 U.S. 280, 96 S.Ct. 2978, 49 L.Ed.2d 944 (1976). Although the Court gave several reasons for this holding, the following language has assumed the most significance in later cases:

A third constitutional shortcoming of the North Carolina statute is its failure to allow the particularized consideration of relevant aspects of the character and record of each convicted defendant before the imposition upon him of a sentence of death. . . . A process that accords no significance to relevant facets of the character and record of the individual offender or the circumstances of the particular offense excludes from consideration in fixing the ultimate punishment of death the possibility of compassionate or mitigating factors stemming from the diverse frailties of humankind. . . .

. . . Consideration of both offender and the offense in order to arrive at a just and appropriate sentence has been viewed as a progressive and humanizing development. While the prevailing practice of individualizing sentencing determinations generally reflects simply enlightened policy rather than a constitutional imperative, we believe that in capital cases the fundamental respect for humanity underlying the eighth amendment requires consideration of the character and record of the individual offender and the circumstances of the particular offense as a constitutionally indispensable part of the process of inflicting the penalty of death.

This conclusion rests squarely on the predicate that the penalty of death is qualitatively different from a sentence of imprisonment, however long. Death, in its finality, differs more from life imprisonment than a 100–year prison term differs from one of only a year or two. Because of that qualitative difference, there is a corresponding difference in the need for reliability in the determination that death is the appropriate punishment in a specific case.

The central message of the 1976 cases appeared to be that while the jury may not be given unlimited discretion, neither may it be prevented from considering information relevant to the offender's characteristics. In two subsequent cases, the Supreme Court reinforced the latter notion. In *Lockett v. Ohio*, 438 U.S. 586, 98 S.Ct. 2954, 57 L.Ed. 2d 973 (1978), seven members of the Court struck down a death penalty statute which required the judge to impose the death penalty unless the defendant proved one of three mitigating circumstances—that the victim had induced or facilitated the offense; that the defendant was "under duress, coercion or strong provocation"; or that the offense was "primarily the product of psychosis or mental deficiency." In an opinion joined by four justices,[r] the Court stated that this statute improperly prevented individualization of the sentencing decision: "The eighth and 14th amendments require that the sentencer, in all but the rarest kind of capital case, not be precluded from considering, *as a mitigating factor,* any aspect of a defendant's character or record

r. Two other members of the Court, Justices Blackmun and White, concurred in the result because the defendant, who had waited in the "getaway car" during the commission of the robbery murder, may not have been sufficiently involved in the crime. Justice Marshall also joined the result, adhering to his opinion in *Furman* that the death penalty is unconstitutional under all circumstances. Justice Brennan, who had indicated in several opinions that he shared this view, did not participate. Only Justice Rehnquist dissented.

and any of the circumstances of the offense that the defendant proffers as a basis for a sentence less than death." (emphasis in original). In *Eddings v. Oklahoma*, 455 U.S. 104, 102 S.Ct. 869, 71 L.Ed.2d 1 (1982), the Court reversed, 5–4, the death sentence of a 16 year-old because the sentencing judge had failed to consider evidence of the defendant's "turbulent family history, of beatings by a harsh father and of severe emotional disturbance." Again, the Court made clear that relevant mitigating evidence should not be excluded, although the factfinder has discretion to give it little or no weight.

As a result of these developments, modern death penalty schemes provide that before a person convicted of capital murder[s] can be sentenced to death the factfinder must find at least one aggravating circumstance and find further that any mitigating circumstances that exist do not make imposition of the death penalty inappropriate. As the Court stated in *Zant,* to be sufficiently "aggravating" to justify the death penalty, a circumstance "must genuinely narrow the class of persons eligible for the death penalty and must reasonably justify the imposition of a more severe sentence on the defendant compared to others found guilty of murder." Typical aggravating factors found in state statutes (many of them copied from the Model Penal Code's death penalty provisions) include murder which is committed: (1) against certain types of persons (e.g., a police officer, a correctional officer, or a judge); (2) while the person is under sentence of imprisonment; (3) for "pecuniary gain"; (4) in the course of certain felonies, such as rape, robbery, arson and kidnapping; (5) for the purpose of avoiding arrest; and (6) in a particularly heinous, cruel or vile manner. Other aggravating circumstances focus on the person rather than the capital murder itself, e.g., murder committed by (7) someone who has been convicted of prior violent felonies; and (8) someone considered likely to commit violent acts in the future (the "dangerousness" criterion). In most states, the listed factors are exclusive. In some, so long as a statutory predicate for the death penalty has been established, consideration of non-statutory aggravating factors is permissible.

In addition to listing aggravating circumstances, which is apparently required under the Court's cases, most state statutes also list mitigating factors that must be considered by the jury. Again borrowing from the Model Penal Code, most states recognize mitigation for any person who (1) was a juvenile at the time of the murder; (2) was only a "minor" participant in the murder; or (3) has no significant prior criminal history. A good number of state statutes also copy verbatim or with slight variation three other mitigation provisions found in the Model Penal Code: (4) "the defendant acted under duress or under the domination of another person;" (5) "the murder was committed while the defendant was under the influence of extreme mental or emotional

---

s. The Court's cases appear to hold that the death penalty may be imposed only on defendants who "intended that a killing take place or that lethal force be used." *Enmund v. Florida*, 458 U.S. 782, 102 S.Ct. 3368, 73 L.Ed.2d 1140 (1982); see also, *Coker v. Georgia*, 433 U.S. 584, 97 S.Ct. 2861, 53 L.Ed.2d 982 (1977).

disturbance;" and (6) "at the time of the murder, the capacity of the defendant to appreciate the criminality [wrongfulness] of his conduct or to conform his conduct to the requirements of the law was impaired as a result of mental disease or defect." [t] Model Penal Code § 210.6(4)(b), (f), (g). A few states also include as mitigating factors: (7) that the defendant believed the murder to be morally justified or committed under extenuating circumstances; and (8) that the defendant is not dangerous. Note that, after *Lockett,* statutory mitigating factors are not to be considered exclusive. They are meant to focus the factfinder's attention on those circumstances most likely to have mitigating impact.

A final question is how aggravating and mitigating circumstances are to be balanced against one another. Under the Model Penal Code's provisions, the factfinder may consider a death sentence only if it finds that "there are no mitigating circumstances sufficiently substantial to call for leniency." Model Penal Code § 210.6(2). Connecticut makes the death penalty even harder to obtain, by prohibiting its imposition if *any* statutory mitigating criterion is found. On the other hand, most state statutes are similar to Alabama's law, which provides that "the trial court shall determine whether the aggravating circumstances it finds to exist outweigh the mitigating circumstances it finds to exist." Ala.Code 1975, § 13A–5–47(e).

Questions and Comments

1. *Mental disability and aggravating circumstances.* The dangerousness criterion, found in a handful of state statutes,[u] is the aggravating circumstance most likely to occasion expert testimony on the impact of mental disorder. Indeed, in Barefoot v. Estelle, reprinted at pp. 418–426, the Supreme Court specifically upheld the admissibility of psychiatric testimony on "future dangerousness". The predicate for *Barefoot* was *Jurek v. Texas,* 428 U.S. 262, 96 S.Ct. 2950, 49 L.Ed.2d 929 (1976), one of the five 1976 death penalty cases. There, the Supreme Court upheld a Texas statute which included as an aggravating factor proof that "there is a probability that the defendant would commit criminal acts of violence that would constitute a continuing threat to society." To the petitioner's argument that it is impossible to predict future behavior and that the statutory language is so vague as to be meaningless, the Court responded:

It is, of course, not easy to predict future behavior. The fact that such a determination is difficult, however, does not mean that it cannot be made. Indeed, prediction of future criminal conduct is an essential element in many of the decisions rendered throughout our criminal

---

t. In *Penry v. Lynaugh,* ___ U.S. ___, 109 S.Ct. 2934, 106 L.Ed.2d 256 (1989), the Supreme Court held that sentencing a mentally retarded person to death is not cruel and unusual punishment under the Eighth Amendment, "so long as [the] sentencer[ ] can consider and give effect to mitigating evidence of mental retardation in imposing sentence." Thus, when a mentally retarded defendant is involved, con-sideration of something akin to the "lack of capacity" mitigant is clearly constitutionally required.

u. At least six states explicitly make dangerousness an aggravating circumstance (Idaho, Oklahoma, South Carolina, Texas, Virginia, and Washington) and two others recognize nondangerousness as a mitigating circumstance.

justice system. The decision whether to admit a defendant to bail, for instance, must often turn on a judge's prediction of the defendant's future conduct. And any sentencing authority must predict a convicted person's probable future conduct when it engages in the process of determining what punishment to impose. For those sentenced to prison, these same predictions must be made by parole authorities. The task that a Texas jury must perform in answering the statutory question in issue is thus basically no different from the task performed countless times each day throughout the American system of criminal justice. What is essential is that the jury have before it all possible relevant information about the individual defendant whose fate it must determine. Texas law clearly assures that all such evidence will be adduced.

Although only three justices joined this language, the other opinions in *Jurek* made it clear that, as *Barefoot* later put it, "seven Justices rejected the claim that it was impossible to predict future behavior and that dangerousness was therefore an invalid consideration in imposing the death penalty."

Strong evidence exists that a prediction, whether by mental health professionals or laypersons, that someone will cause harm to others is more often wrong than right.[v] Should "proof" of dangerousness be sufficient, by itself, to impose the death sentence on a person convicted of capital murder? Does it "genuinely narrow the class of persons eligible for the death penalty" as reliably as do other aggravating circumstances?

2. *Mental disability and mitigating circumstances.* Of the mitigating circumstances typically listed in state death penalty statutes, four focus on the defendant's mental state at the time of the offense. Using the Model Penal Code language, they are: (a) whether the defendant was "under duress or under the domination of another person;" (b) whether the defendant was suffering from "extreme mental or emotional disturbance"; (c) whether "the capacity of the defendant to appreciate the criminality [wrongfulness] of his conduct or to conform his conduct to the requirements of law was impaired as a result of mental disease or defect or intoxication"; and (d) whether "the murder was committed under circumstances which the defendant believed to provide a moral justification or extenuation for his conduct." All of these mitigating criteria have obvious analogues to defenses which are usually available at trial. The first is similar to the duress defense,[w] the second to the provocation defense, the third to the insanity defense, and the fourth to the self-defense doctrine. How does the language used to define the mitigating factors differ from the usual formulations of the defenses? Some state statutes use even broader language. For instance, with respect to the second mental state factor, some states omit the word "extreme." With respect to the third factor, some states omit the words "mental disease or defect."

Permissible Limitations. The essential preliminary question in determining the proper mitigating circumstances is whether there should be *any*

v. See pp. 418–438.

w. Note that although the "duress" factor appears to be identical to the duress defense, it provides meaningful mitigation because the duress defense is usually unavailable in homicide cases.

limitation on the type of mental state evidence which can be presented in mitigation at a death penalty proceeding. Arguably, given the gravity of the penalty, the usual concerns about wide-open consideration of a defendant's psychology should be suspended. In *Lockett,* the Court stated that restricting mitigating claims is impermissible because it "creates the risk that the death penalty will be imposed in spite of factors which may call for a less severe penalty." However, in a footnote, it also cautioned that "nothing in this opinion limits the traditional authority of a court to exclude, as irrelevant, evidence not bearing on the defendant's character, prior record, or the circumstances of his offense." Does this footnote limit mental state evidence in any way?

Consider *North Carolina v. Boyd,* 311 N.C. 408, 319 S.E.2d 189 (1984), cert. denied, 471 U.S. 1030, 105 S.Ct. 2052, 85 L.Ed.2d 324 (1985). In that case, Boyd was convicted of murdering a former girlfriend who had recently left him. At his sentencing hearing, he presented the following evidence: (1) his father had been an alcoholic who had abandoned his family when Boyd was young; (2) his grandfather—whom he had come to view as a father—had then died; (3) he had a history of losing jobs and repeated imprisonment; and (4) his life since adolescence had been characterized by drug and alcohol abuse. He also proffered testimony by a sociologist to the effect that his crime and life history conformed to a common pattern that distinguishes those who kill intimates from those who kill others. In particular, according to the sociologist, those who, like Boyd, suffer repeated deep personal losses often develop strong feelings of self-destructiveness which may cause them to kill a loved one as a way of destroying part of themselves. Thus, the sociologist testified, the defendant's crime could be seen "primarily as a depression-caused self-destructive act, closely related to the impulse of suicide, resulting from a life history of an inordinate number of losses beginning with the abandonment by the defendant's father and the death of his grandfather and culminating with the threatened loss of [the victim]." The expert also testified that Boyd told him during an interview that he so feared the end of his relationship with the girlfriend that he had contemplated suicide shortly before the murder. The defense attorney explained that the testimony was designed to "link together all of the defendant's mitigating evidence into a unified whole which explained the apparent contradiction of killing the person the defendant loved the most." The trial court excluded the sociologist's testimony. In a somewhat ambiguous opinion, the North Carolina Supreme Court upheld this ruling, either on the ground that the testimony was irrelevant or that it was relevant but was of so little weight that its exclusion was not a proper ground for vacating the death sentence. The United States Supreme Court denied certiorari, over a vigorous dissent by Justice Marshall, which Justice Brennan joined. Should the expert testimony have been admitted? Should it make a difference that the North Carolina statute did not include as an aggravating factor the dangerousness criterion?

Consider also the United States Supreme Court's opinion in *Skipper v. South Carolina,* 476 U.S. 1, 106 S.Ct. 1669, 90 L.Ed.2d 1 (1986), involving a statute which listed dangerousness as an aggravating circumstance. In that case, the prosecutor, in attempting to prove dangerousness, made references during both cross-examination and closing argument to Skipper's allegedly violent behavior in prison. Nonetheless, the South Carolina Supreme Court upheld the trial court's exclusion of three defense witnesses—two prison guards and a "regular visitor" to the prison—who would have testified that Skipper had "made a good adjustment" during his time spent in jail. A unanimous Court held that this exclusion violated the constitution. Six members of the Court found, under *Lockett* and *Eddings,* that "evidence that the defendant would not pose a danger if spared (but incarcerated) must be considered potentially mitigating [and] may not be excluded from the sentencer's consideration." However, Justice Powell, joined by Chief Justice Burger and Justice Rehnquist, disagreed with this broad ruling, and concurred only in the result. Powell concluded that had the state not argued that Skipper was dangerous, the lower court's ruling excluding evidence of nondangerousness should have been upheld despite *Lockett* and *Eddings.*

> I see no reason why a State could not, consistent with [eighth amendment principles], exclude evidence of a defendant's good behavior in jail following his arrest, as long as the evidence is not offered to rebut testimony or argument such as that tendered by the prosecution here. Such evidence has no bearing at all on the "circumstances of the offense," since it concerns the defendant's behavior after the crime has been committed. Nor does it say anything necessarily relevant about a defendant's "character or record," as that phrase was used in *Lockett* and *Eddings.*

> Those decisions clearly focus on evidence that lessens the defendant's culpability for the crime for which he was convicted. . . . The type of evidence [they] required to be admitted . . . pertained to conduct and circumstances *prior* to the crime, and to the nature and extent of the defendant's participation in the crime. In this case, for the first time, the Court classifies as "mitigating" conduct that occurred *after* the crime and after the accused has been charged. Almost by definition, such conduct neither excuses the defendant's crime nor reduces his responsibility for its commission. It cannot, therefore, properly be considered "mitigating evidence" that the sentencer must consider under the Constitution.

Powell also argued that even if a person's ability to adjust to prison life were within the scope of permissible mitigating evidence, a state could reasonably exclude evidence of conduct in prison while awaiting trial or sentencing. Because a prisoner awaiting sentence "has every incentive to behave flawlessly in prison if good behavior might cause the sentencing authority to spare his life", a court might determine that such evidence has little or no probative value as to his conduct after sentence is imposed.

Should the holding in *Skipper* be limited in the manner suggested by Powell? If so, would it mean that psychiatric testimony to the effect that a defendant is not dangerous or is "treatable" should be excluded unless the prosecution raises the dangerousness issue? What if the relevant state statute recognizes nondangerousness as a mitigating factor?

Applying the Statutory Factors. A separate question is whether particular evidence, assuming it is admissible, meets the relevant statutory mitigating criteria. Because these criteria are not exclusive, one might conclude that the answer to this question doesn't matter; even if a court or jury determines that the defendant's evidence does not meet a particular criterion, the defendant can still argue it has mitigating value. But in a state like Connecticut, where proof of any statutory mitigating factor precludes the death penalty, the definition of a particular factor can assume extreme importance. Even in those states where the aggravating and mitigating circumstances are balanced against one another, the definition may be significant, since proof of statutory mitigating factors are likely to carry more weight than proof of nonstatutory factors.

Many courts have demonstrated a reluctance to define the statutory factors broadly. For instance, in *Illinois v. Crews,* reprinted at pp. 564–569, the Illinois Supreme Court refused to equate a guilty but mentally ill ruling with extreme mental or emotional distress; more significantly, it was unwilling to overturn the trial judge's ruling in the case that the defendant's evidence of mental illness, which was not insignificant, met this or any other statutory factor. Was it right? Assuming so, should it have ruled differently had the Illinois statutory language, as is true with other statutes, not included the word "extreme"?

Consider also two other cases discussed in the previous materials, *Johnson v. State,* reprinted at pp. 531–535, and *Jahnke v. Wyoming,* reprinted at pp. 545–551. Johnson was convicted of capital murder. Does the evidence of mental disability presented in that case prove a statutory mitigating circumstance? The death penalty was not sought in Jahnke's case, although it was within the prosecutor's authority to do so. Had Jahnke been convicted of capital murder, would he have been able to prove any of the typical statutory mitigating circumstances associated with mental disability?

3. *Mental disability as both an aggravating and a mitigating circumstance.* In many cases evidence of mental disability is relevant both to aggravating and mitigating circumstances. In *Miller v. State,* 373 So.2d 882 (Fla.1979), the facts adduced at trial were as follows. Miller was released from county jail on the morning of the murder, where he had been incarcerated for possession of a concealed weapon (a fishing knife). He wandered around Ft. Myers and bought a fishing knife similar to the one which had been taken from him by the police. An employee in the store where the weapon was purchased stated that Miller was "wild looking" and was mumbling angrily to himself. This employee called the police and followed Miller to two nearby bars. Finally the employee saw Miller leaving in a taxi cab with a woman driver and contacted the taxi company to inform it of the apparent danger. The woman taxi driver was found murdered a short while later, having been stabbed nine times. Miller had apparently raped her when she was dead or dying. When Miller was arrested at the bus station that evening, his pants were still covered with blood. Blood-soaked money, some of which had been taken from the taxi driver, was found in his pockets.

After Miller was charged with this crime, he was found incompetent to stand trial and was committed to a state mental hospital. Two and a half years later, after being heavily medicated, he was found to be competent to stand trial and convicted of capital murder. At the sentencing hearing psychiatric testimony suggested that Miller was suffering from paranoid schizophrenia and hallucinations. He had been committed to mental hospitals on several previous occasions, and had a long history of drug abuse. Testimony also indicated that Miller had a severe hatred of his mother, and had planned to kill her after his release from the Lee County Jail, just prior to this murder. Apparently this hatred arose in part from the fact that his mother, who had been married four times, had refused any contact with her son for several years. On several previous occasions, Miller suffered hallucinations in which he saw his mother in other persons, in a "yellow haze." On at least one previous occasion, he had senselessly assaulted another woman during such hallucinations. Miller testified that at the time of the capital murder, he saw his mother's face on the 56 year-old woman taxi driver, in a "yellow haze," and proceeded to stab her to death.

The jury recommended a death sentence. In Florida, as in most states, the trial judge must decide if this penalty is appropriate. The relevant portions of the Florida Supreme Court's description of the judge's deliberations and its analysis of the judge's conclusions follows:

> The trial court found that the evidence introduced at the sentencing hearing proved beyond a reasonable doubt three statutory aggravating circumstances: (1) the defendant was previously convicted of a felony involving the threat of violence to another person; (2) the murder was committed while the defendant was engaged in the commission of or attempt to commit robbery, and was thus committed for pecuniary gain; and (3) the murder was especially heinous, atrocious, and cruel.

> In addition, the trial court found several mitigating circumstances to exist: (1) the murder was committed while the defendant was under the influence of extreme mental disturbance; (2) the defendant acted under mental duress; (3) due to mental sickness, the defendant's capacity and ability to conform his conduct to the requirements of law were substantially impaired. In addition, the trial court specifically found from the evidence presented at the sentencing hearing that the defendant was suffering from mental illness at the time the murder was committed.

Based upon these factual findings, the trial judge explained the reasoning which led him to conclude that the death penalty was appropriate:

> [I]n weighing the aggravating and mitigating factors, I have to conclude that the aggravating factors are such that the reality of Florida law wherein life imprisonment is not, in fact, life imprisonment; and, in fact, the defendant would be subject to be released into society—In other words, it doesn't mean life imprisonment and there is a substantial chance he could be released into society. And the testimony overwhelmingly establishes that the mental sickness or illness that he suffers from is such that he will never recover from it, it will only be repressed by the use of drugs.

> Thus, in light of that fact, in light of the aggravating factors here, I have to conclude the only certain punishment and the only assurance society can receive that this man never again commits

to another human being what he did to that lady, is that the ultimate sentence of death is imposed.

If the law in Florida were such that life imprisonment meant the ability to live in a prison environment for the entire, remainder of one's life, I would have the conclusion that there would be sufficient mitigating factors to offset the aggravating factors, and allow him to live in prison.

But since that is not the case, the reality is that life imprisonment does not mean that, I conclude in this case that the aggravating factors heavily outweigh the mitigating factors.

The heinousness of the crime, the way in which it was committed speaks for itself. Now I, as the Judge, must therefore impose the sentence of death and do so.

It is clear from the trial judge's sentencing order that he considered as an aggravating factor the defendant's allegedly incurable and dangerous mental illness. The use of this nonstatutory aggravating factor as a controlling circumstance tipping the balance in favor of the death penalty was improper. The aggravating circumstances specified in the statute are exclusive, and no others may be used for that purpose. This court [has] stated: "We must guard against any unauthorized aggravating factor going into the equation which might tip the scales of the weighing process in favor of death."

Strict application of the sentencing statute is necessary because the sentencing authority's discretion must be "guided and channeled" by requiring an examination of specific factors that argue in favor of or against imposition of the death penalty, thus eliminating total arbitrariness and capriciousness in its imposition. The trial judge's use of the defendant's mental illness, and his resulting propensity to commit violent acts, as an aggravating factor favoring the imposition of the death penalty appears contrary to the legislative intent as set forth in the statute. The legislature has not authorized consideration of the probability of recurring violent acts by the defendant if he is released on parole in the distant future. To the contrary, a large number of the statutory mitigating factors reflect a legislative determination to mitigate the death penalty in favor of a life sentence for those persons whose responsibility for their violent actions has been substantially diminished as a result of a mental illness, uncontrolled emotional state of mind, or drug abuse.

If dangerousness *had* been an aggravating circumstance under the Florida death penalty scheme (or if Florida were one of the states in which non-statutory aggravating factors may be considered once at least one statutory factor is proven), would the trial judge's ruling have been appropriate? Consider another Florida case, *Huckaby v. State,* 343 So.2d 29 (Fla. 1977). There the Florida Supreme Court held that, although there was insufficient proof of insanity, the evidence showed Huckaby's mental illness motivated his murder of members of his family. The court reversed the trial court's imposition of the death penalty and held that the mitigating circumstances outweighed the aggravating circumstances. It explained:

> Our decision here is based on the causal relationship between the mitigating and aggravating circumstances. The heinous and atrocious manner in which this crime was perpetrated, and the harm to which the members of Huckaby's family were exposed, were the direct consequence of his mental illness, so far as the record reveals.

Note that one of the aggravating factors found by the trial judge in *Miller* was the heinousness of the crime. In light of *Huckaby,* is this finding permissible? How do you think the Florida Supreme Court would answer the question at the beginning of this paragraph?

More generally, in cases such as *Miller* and *Huckaby,* how should one balance the desire to accord mitigating impact to mental disability on the one hand and, on the other, the two goals of incapacitating the very dangerous (who may be mentally ill) and punishing severely those who commit particularly heinous crimes (perhaps because of mental illness)? Should the conclusion as to when the mitigating impact of mental disability "trumps" its aggravating aspects differ depending upon whether the aggravating aspect is dangerousness or vileness of the crime?

B. NON–CAPITAL SENTENCING

1. History: Retribution v. Incapacitation/Rehabilitation

The history of sentencing outside the capital punishment setting reflects the tension between two different models: the retribution/deterrence model and the incapacitation/rehabilitation model. Under the first model, the type and duration of punishment is determined by assessing the offender's blameworthiness (as indicated by the offense committed and perhaps other criminal behavior as well) and the message punishment will send to others. Under the second model, the type and duration of punishment is dependent upon the offender's perceived dangerousness and the extent to which those criminal propensities can be reduced through treatment. Because information about blameworthiness of the offender and the deterrent value of particular punishments is usually known at the time of sentencing, the first model is more likely to result in determinate sentences, or at least sentences with a relatively narrow range. Conversely, the second model is more likely to produce indeterminate sentences with no specific termination point because, at the time of sentencing, it is not known how long a person will have to be incapacitated and treated before he or she is considered nondangerous. It is sometimes suggested that under the first model the effort is to fit the punishment to the crime, while under the second, punishment is designed to fit the criminal. This statement is somewhat misleading, because the blameworthiness assessment called for by the first model may consider individual traits (such as mental state at the time of the offense), while the dangerousness assessment mandated by the second model may in practice focus on the type of crime committed by the offender more than any other single factor. But it is fair to say that, as a general matter, the second model places more emphasis on individualization of punishment than does the first.

In the United States, the retribution/deterrence model dominated sentencing practices until the mid–19th century. Sentences tended to be uniform for each type of crime; an offender's rehabilitative potential was usually ignored. After the Civil War, concurrent with optimism that the causes of crime could be identified and treated, movement toward the incapacitation/rehabilitation approach gained momentum. By 1922, 37 states had enacted indeterminate sentencing statutes, and 7 others had parole systems functionally similar to the indeterminate sentence. The remaining states set maximum sentences for each crime, but allowed the judge and parole board to determine when within that time limit release would occur. In 1948, the United States Supreme Court seemed to approve of this trend when it described as the "prevalent modern philosophy of penology" the idea that "the punishment should fit the offender and not merely the crime. . . . Retribution is no longer the dominant objective of the criminal law. Reformation and rehabilitation of offenders have become important goals of criminal jurisprudence." Williams v. New York, 337 U.S. 241 (1948).

However, in the mid–1970's a countertrend emerged, often labelled the "just deserts" movement. Advocates of this approach believed that "those whose criminal actions are equally reprehensible deserve like amounts of punishment." VonHirsch & Hanrahan, "Determinate Penalty Systems in America: An Overview," 27 Crime & Delinq. 289, 294 (1981). Today, several states and, since 1986, the federal government, require imposition of "fixed" or "presumptive" sentences, or permit sentences only within a very narrow range, unless a showing is made that the offender should be treated differently. Under most of these schemes, variance from the legislated sentence is permissible only on culpability grounds; concerns about dangerousness or rehabilitation are not supposed to influence the sentencing authority. For instance, under the federal Sentencing Reform Act of 1984 the court is generally limited to imposing a sentence with a small range, the maximum of which may not exceed the minimum by more than the greater of 25% or six months. 28 U.S.C. § 994(a). Parole is abolished, 18 U.S.C. § 3624(a)(b), and rehabilitation rejected as a purpose of punishment. 28 U.S.C. § 994(k).

These vacillations in sentencing policy reflect several different influences. The just deserts variant of the retribution/deterrence model is founded on the belief that culpability is the touchstone of punishment: while incapacitation and rehabilitation goals may be achieved through punishment indirectly, they should not determine its scope; indeed, even the deterrence objective is deemphasized. The movement also seems to be a product of disenchantment with prison rehabilitation efforts, a belief that neither dangerousness nor treatability predictions are very accurate, and a desire to reduce sentencing disparity and indeterminancy, which are believed to be inequitable and have harmful psychological effects on inmates. See generally, VonHirsch, Doing Justice (1976).

The incapacitation/rehabilitation model still has many adherents, however. For instance, Dr. Halleck argues that because it refuses to consider dangerousness as a punishment variable, the retribution/ deterrence model of sentencing is less protective of society; at the same time, because it incarcerates nondangerous, treatable individuals for long periods of time, it is unnecessarily harsh, ignores different people's susceptibility to punishment, and dehumanizes justice and society. Halleck, The Mentally Disordered Offender 191–93, 198–99 (1987). He asserts that "indeterminate programs have usually released offenders earlier than determinate programs, and they have almost always provided greater numbers of offenders with greater opportunities for freedom." Id. at 199. Compared to the retribution/deterrence model, the incapacitation/rehabilitation approach "is less discriminatory, imposes less pain on offenders as a group, and is especially merciful toward selected offenders who can be released when they are judged to be nondangerous to society." Id. at 202. See also Clear, Hewitt, & Regoli, "Discretion and the Determinate Sentence: Its Distribution, Control, and Effect on Time Served," 24 Crime & Delinq. 428 (1978) (concluding that Indiana's determinate statute has been a failure because it continues to allow prosecutorial and judicial discretion and permits "untenably heavy penalties").

The two models differ significantly in their treatment of evidence concerning psychological makeup. Theoretically, under the incapacitation/rehabilitation approach to sentencing, all aspects of an individual's personality are relevant, including every shade of mental disability. Sentencing under this model

> is premised on the assumption that a sentencing judge, armed with an intimate knowledge of the offender's character and background and aided by scientific and clinical evaluations, can determine an appropriate sentence and treatment program that will rehabilitate the offender. Under this model, the sentencing judge seeks to define the offender's exact personality and social situations, and then prescribes an 'individualized' sentence and treatment program.

Dershowitz, "The Role of Psychiatry in the Sentencing Process," 1 Int'l J.L.Psychiat. 63, 66 (1978). In those states which follow this approach or variations on it, sentencing criteria are rarely specified because the information that may be considered by the judge is so wide-ranging.

Under the retributive/deterrence model, on the other hand, only those aspects of mental disability relevant to blameworthiness may be considered and, in most state statutes which reflect the influence of this model, these features are specifically identified as aggravating and mitigating factors. For instance, under the Minnesota sentencing scheme, the judge must normally impose a sentence based on the crime committed and the offender's previous criminal history unless specified aggravating or mitigating circumstances are shown. Included in the statute as mitigating factors are the following:

(1) the offender played a minor or passive role in the crime or participated under circumstances of coercion or duress.

(2) the offender, because of physical or mental impairment, lacked substantial capacity for judgment when the offense was committed.

(3) other substantial grounds exist which tend to excuse or mitigate the offender's culpability, although not amounting to a defense.

See "Research Project: Minnesota Sentencing Guidelines," 5 Hamline L.Rev. 293, 412–15 (1982). In some states, proof of an aggravating or mitigating factor can result in a substantial variance from the presumptive sentence. For instance, in Arizona the judge may increase the sentence by up to 25% if an aggravating factor is shown and reduce the sentence by up to 50% if a mitigating circumstance is proven. Arizona R.S. §§ 13–502, 13–7–1, 13–7–2.

To the extent the retribution/deterrence model of sentencing is concerned with mental disability, this book's materials on capital sentencing discuss many of the pertinent issues; [x] little further discussion is warranted. The legal issues connected with the incapacitation/ rehabilitation model are worth delving into in more detail. Examples of statutes which adopt this approach are numerous. At the federal level, for instance, they range from the Narcotic Addict Rehabilitation Act, 18 U.S.C. §§ 4251 et seq., which permits the addict with charges pending to elect treatment for a specified period of time, to the Youth Correction Act, 18 U.S.C. §§ 5005 et seq., which, before its repeal in 1986, granted the courts authority to sentence persons between 21 and 26 to indeterminate confinement not to exceed four years for "corrective and preventive guidance and training designed to protect the public by correcting the antisocial tendencies of youth offenders." Id. § 5006(f). Probably the purest expression of the incapacitation/rehabilitation model, however, is found in statutes providing for the indeterminate confinement of those found to be "mentally disordered sex offenders." We now turn to an examination of these statutes.

2. Mentally Disordered Sex Offender Statutes [y]

In the early part of the twentieth century, a number of states passed legislation aimed at diverting into special indeterminate treatment programs a category of offenders who came to be known as "defective delinquents". Many of these states had already adopted an indeterminate sentencing system. Thus, apparently, the impetus for

---

x. Although they usually do not include predictive criteria such as dangerousness and treatability, determinate sentencing statutes are otherwise similar to capital sentencing statutes in structure; thus, many of the same legal issues may arise (e.g., when is a particular mitigating factor proven, how does the court "count" mental disability which is both mitigating and aggravating).

y. Most of this introduction is taken from Dix, "Special Dispositional Alternatives for Abnormal Offenders," in Monahan & Steadman, Mentally Disordered Offenders: Perspectives from Law and Social Science 133, 134–145 (1983).

these initial special sentencing programs was to remove from the regular prison system particularly disruptive and hard to treat offenders. Although some states still have such statutes, they have rarely been enthusiastically implemented.[z]

Much more popular were statutes aimed at diverting those charged with sex offenses, the first of which was passed by Michigan in 1937. At one time, over 25 states had such statutes, which come to be called mentally disordered sex offender (MDSO) statutes. S. Brakel & R. Rock, The Mentally Disabled and the Law 341 (1971). Apparently programs singling out sex offenders succeeded where the defective delinquent statutes did not because sex offenders were believed to be particularly likely to recidivate if not treated and at the same time particularly amenable to treatment. Additionally, sex offenders, especially pedophiles, tend to be mistreated by other prisoners and were often segregated from the rest of the prison population in any event.

MDSO statutes vary considerably both substantively and procedurally. A MDSO "commitment proceeding" usually can only be triggered by conviction of a sex offense. However, several states permitted such a proceeding upon indictment for a sex offense, and at least one state— Illinois—authorizes initiation of MDSO proceedings after an individual is charged with *any* offense. Commitment as a MDSO usually requires a showing that the person is predisposed to commit sexual offenses as a result of "mental disease or defect". A few statutes also require a separate showing of repeated sexual misconduct (in Illinois, because the proceeding is initiated by indictment, the subject must have "demonstrated propensities towards acts of sexual assault or acts of sexual molestation of children"); a few other states require a showing of treatability. Under most of the original statutes, commitment as a MDSO resulted in indeterminate confinement, with release dependent upon initiation of discharge proceedings by the superintendent of the treating facility and approval by the committing court. More recently, many statutes limit the time of confinement to the maximum term that could have been imposed for the crime committed by the offender, although in some of these states commitment may be renewed if a new commitment proceeding is held at which more stringent criteria are met.

For the same reasons determinate sentencing is gaining popularity, MDSO statutes are disappearing. At present, perhaps only fifteen states have such laws. American Bar Association, Criminal Justice Mental Health Standards 7–424 n. 20. Nonetheless, they are worth looking at because they are a good illustration of the incapacitation/rehabilitation model of sentencing. Moreover, the pendulum is likely to swing back toward this model if rehabilitative techniques are improved.

---

z. An exception was the Maryland Defective Delinquent Act, Art. 31B (1964), which was frequently used to confine defective delinquents indeterminately until 1978, when the duration of confinement was limited to the maximum sentence that would have been received. See Kohlmeyer, "The First Year of Operation Under the New Patuxent Laws," 7 Bull.Amer.Acad. Psychiat. & L. 95 (1979). The Act was repealed in 1989.

STATE v. LITTLE
Supreme Court of Nebraska, 1978.
199 Neb. 772, 261 N.W.2d 847.

C. THOMAS WHITE, JUSTICE.

The defendant, a 58–year–old male, was charged with indecent exposure and fondling the sexual organs of a minor boy under the age of 16 years. Following pleas of guilty to each count by the defendant, and at defendant's request, proceedings were initiated under sections 29–2901 to 29–2910, R.R.S.1943, the Nebraska Sexual Sociopath Act. The trial court, pursuant to that statute, suspended further proceedings and ordered an examination of the defendant. The court found the defendant to be an untreatable sexual sociopath and committed him to the Nebraska Penal and Correctional Complex.

The medical and criminal history of the defendant-appellant was introduced at the trial. The defendant had twice been convicted and committed in other states for sexual offenses involving minor children. It is not necessary to detail the factual situation of this case except to state that the evidence that the defendant is a sexual sociopath is overwhelming.

The defendant does not allege error in the proceedings or in the determination that he is a sexual sociopath. His complaint is focused on the place of confinement and the uncertain duration of the confinement under the sexual sociopath statutes. The defendant's challenge to the constitutionality of the statutes rests on two alternative bases: (1) The indefinite term of commitment to the Nebraska penal complex was an enhancement of defendant's sentence which violates the defendant's right to equal protection of the law; and (2) an order of commitment to the Nebraska penal complex of a person who is determined to be a sexual sociopath for an indefinite period is in violation of the Constitution's clause against cruel and unusual punishment since it is punishment for a status or because it is disproportionate to the nature of the offense.

* * *

The defendant's equal protection argument is two-pronged. First, he claims he is denied equal protection because his sentence is enhanced under the sexual sociopath statute rather than the habitual offender statute. A person convicted of a third felony may have his punishment enhanced under the terms of sections 29–2221 and 29–2222, R.R.S.1943, as a habitual criminal. The theory is that defendant's past crimes operate to aggravate his guilt to justify heavier penalties. The defendant concedes the constitutionality of the habitual offender statutes. The defendant points out that while the habitual offender may have his penalty enhanced to a stated number of years, the sexual sociopath found to be untreatable may have the statutory penalty further increased, in effect, to a life sentence without possibility of parole. Thus, the defendant says since this condition is indistinguishable from the other, the differing treatment is violative of equal protection.

The placement of the sexual sociopath in a distinct category is a permissible classification. In *State ex rel. Pearson v. Probate Court*, 205 Minn. 545, 287 N.W. 297, an alleged sexual psychopath, committed under Minnesota law, unsuccessfully challenged the sex offender law on an equal protection basis. The Minnesota Supreme Court held that the Equal Protection Clause did not prohibit a state from classifying the sex offender in a special category, and providing special procedures for dealing with a person in this group where the behavior of the members showed that they were actually dangerous and incapable of controlling their sexual impulses. On appeal, the United States Supreme Court affirmed the decision of the Minnesota Court. *Minnesota ex rel. Pearson v. Probate Court*, 309 U.S. 270, 60 S.Ct. 523, 84 L.Ed. 744.

Equal protection does not require that all persons be dealt with identically, but it does require that the distinction made have some relevance to the purpose for which the classification is made. The question becomes whether the distinction of differing treatment made by the Legislature is reasonable in that it is relevant to the purpose of the initial classification. We hold that classification of sexual sociopaths apart from habitual criminals and the differing disposition it generates is a reasonable one. The classifications of habitual criminals and sexual sociopaths encompass groups of individuals with distinct characteristics. Habitual criminal laws provide that the repetition of criminal conduct aggravates the guilt and justifies greater punishment. The sexual sociopath statutes, sections 29–2901 to 29–2910, R.R.S.1943, proceed on the premise that the sexual sociopath is neither normal nor legally insane and on the idea that the commission of sex crimes is evidence of a mental disorder which should be treated if found treatable. The statutes provide that the offender, the sexual sociopath, shall be treated and held at the facility for treatment. If found to be untreatable and dangerous, the sexual sociopath is held at the Nebraska Penal and Correctional Complex separate from other prisoners. The purposes of the habitual offender law and the sexual sociopath law are alike in that both are for the protection of society. On the one hand, the protection is from a dangerous criminal offender and on the other, from a person who is found to be dangerous to society by reason of his sexual proclivities. However, differing purposes are emphasized for the purposes of the incarceration. For the habitual offender, the purpose is punishment only; and for the sexual sociopath, the purpose is treatment, if possible, and only incidentally punitive.

The defendant's second equal protection argument relates to the [fact that most] incurably mentally ill, dangerous persons [are confined] to the regional center [a] [while incurable sex sociopaths are confined] to

a. The "regional center" is a state hospital designed to treat those convicted under the Sexual Sociopath Act, as well as others who have sex-related problems. [eds.]

the Nebraska Penal and Correctional Complex. We conclude again that these are distinct classifications marked by a distinguishing characteristic which is determinative. [T]he Legislature could have reasonably determined that the public health and safety required that those previously convicted on a sex offense and deemed untreatable may be appropriately held in the Nebraska Penal and Correctional Complex rather than in the regional center due to the fact of the prior conviction of the crime.

Defendant's next assignment of error relates to the length of the possible duration of the confinement as constituting cruel and unusual punishment. In support of the contention, defendant first argues that the punishment of an untreatable sexual sociopath is punishment for a status and thereby violates *Robinson v. California*, 370 U.S. 660, 82 S.Ct. 1417, 8 L.Ed.2d 758. In *Robinson*, the defendant had been arrested after a police officer had observed needle marks on his arm. The defendant was convicted under a statute that made it an offense to use or be addicted to narcotics despite the fact that it was never proven the defendant had used drugs while in the jurisdiction. According to the Supreme Court, the effect of the statute was to allow a conviction for the mere status of addiction rather than from the actual use of drugs. It was suggested that punishment for the status of being addicted to drugs is just as repugnant to traditional ideas of fairness and justice as punishment for a physical illness such as leprosy or venereal disease or a mental illness. The court held that a status offense was one where there is no actus reus present and the imposition of any punishment for such an offense violates the cruel and unusual punishment prohibition of the Eighth Amendment.

We do not find *Robinson v. California, supra,* controlling on the issue of the constitutionality of confinement under Nebraska's Sexual Sociopath Act. As we have pointed out, section 29–2902, R.R.S.1943, provides that a proceeding under the act may only be instituted following a criminal conviction. The conviction is the actus reus that was absent in *Robinson v. California, supra,* and distinguishes it from that case.

*   *   *

Defendant's major argument that the confinement of untreatable sexual sociopaths dictated by statute constitutes cruel and unusual punishment rests on the premise that the sentence is disproportionate to the nature of the offense. Defendant states correctly, that the indeterminate confinement may well be a life sentence. After the initial determination by the court of untreatability under section 29–2903(3), R.R.S.1943, the sexual sociopath is confined to the Nebraska Penal and Correctional Complex indefinitely without treatment.

[T]he statute does provide a procedure whereby a sexual sociopath may seek his release. Section 29–2906(2), R.R.S.1943, provides that: "A motion for a hearing to determine whether the defendant is a sexual sociopath may be made by or on behalf of the defendant at one-year intervals after initial commitment." A hearing may be held if the District Court determines that there is probable cause to believe that the defendant is no longer a sexual sociopath. The defendant is eligible for release only after a psychiatric evaluation shows that he is fit for discharge. He is still subject to sentence under the original criminal charge.

We cannot ignore the reality that, even with this procedure for discharge, the indefinite term of confinement may easily become a life sentence. Once the designation of untreatability is made, the statute places the sexual sociopath in legal limbo. The defendant is sent to a segregated portion of the penal complex with no evidence that he is given other than custodial care. By the terms of the statute, he is given no treatment. He is expected to bear the burden of proving he has somehow recovered in the vacuum situation in which the statute places him.

A proceeding for investigation and for commitment of an alleged sexual sociopath is civil in nature. The nature and duration of civil commitment must bear some reasonable relation to the purpose for which an individual is committed. *Jackson v. Indiana*, 406 U.S. 715, 92 S.Ct. 1845, 32 L.Ed.2d 435. We stated earlier that the purpose that differentiates the Sexual Sociopath Act from a criminal statute is the element of treatment. Despite the labeling of the initial commitment as civil, the statutes' provisions for possible life confinement, without any provisions for treatability or review of treatability, make the statutes penal in nature.

                              *   *   *

In *People v. Feagley*, 535 P.2d 373 (1975), the statute provided for annual review of the case of each mentally disordered sex offender to determine whether he might have become "amenable" to treatment in a hospital facility. The court held that this was not enough—confinement without treatment for any length of time constitutes cruel and unusual punishment. The court based the holding on the finding that without ongoing treatment, the confinement of the untreatable sexual sociopath is punishment for a status under *Robinson v. California, supra*, ...

We do not embrace the California court's status rationale since, as we held earlier, we do not believe the Nebraska statute constitutes punishment merely for status. However, we agree with the California court that treatment is a necessary part of a statutory scheme involving sexual sociopaths. The Nebraska statute has no provision for even review of treatability once the initial determination of untreatability is made. As defendant points out, under the terms of the Sexual Sociopath Act: "For appellant and other untreatable sexual sociopaths, even the milieu of hope and opportunity of a treatment facility is foreclosed." Thus, without more, the untreatable sexual sociopath faces a probable life sentence. As such, the statute is penal in nature and the sentence under it is so disproportionate to the offense committed in this case as to constitute cruel and unusual punishment.

Section 29–2903(3), R.R.S.1943, says the Nebraska Penal and Correctional Complex shall "detain, house, and care" for the sexual sociopath when he is in the penal complex. The "care" of such an individual must include, at the very least, some effort to make the possibility of treatment open to him. Thus, we hold that an annual evaluation by qualified professional personnel must be made of each sexual sociopath housed in the penal complex and an annual review of treatability be made by the District Court from which such individual was originally committed.

AFFIRMED.

Questions and Comments

1. *Habitual offender laws and the Supreme Court.* In *State ex rel. Pearson v. Probate Court,* 309 U.S. 270, 60 S.Ct. 523, 84 L.Ed. 744 (1940), cited in *Little,* the Supreme Court rejected an equal protection claim similar to the first claim made in *Little.* In justifying this decision, the Court stated:

> [T]he legislature is free to recognize degrees of harm, and it may confine its restrictions to those classes of cases where the need is deemed to be clearest. If the law 'presumably hits the evil where it is most felt, it is not to be overthrown because there are other instances to which it might have been applied.'

309 U.S. at 275, 60 S.Ct. at 526. The Supreme Court has also held that confinement for *life* under the type of habitual offender statute mentioned in *Little* (the "three-time loser" statute) is not a violation of the eighth amendment, at least so long as there is the possibility of parole. Solem v. Helm, 463 U.S. 277, 103 S.Ct. 3001, 77 L.Ed.2d 637 (1983).

2. *The Import of* Little. Although the court in *Little* seemed sympathetic to the defendant's eighth amendment claim, note that it affirmed the constitutionality of Nebraska's Sexual Sociopath Act, as well as the defendant's placement under it. Moreover, the court did not require that those committed under the Act receive treatment, but merely mandated that the state conduct an annual evaluation of treatability. Can this holding be squared with equal protection principles? Eighth amendment principles? (Consider the reasoning in *People v. Feagley,* cited in *Little*). Should it matter under either analysis whether commitment occurs after conviction as opposed to while charges are pending, as permitted under some MDSO statutes? The court also cites *Jackson v. Indiana,* which is a due process case holding that the nature and duration of confinement must bear some relation to its purpose. Would a due process argument have been more profitable for the defendant?

More generally, should dangerousness and/or treatability ever form the sole bases for determining the length of sentence? Or should retributive and deterrent objectives determine the sentence range within which a sentence may be imposed based on incapacitive, rehabilitative and other goals?

3. *Research on MDSO statutes.* Perhaps relevant to the constitutional issues is research on the duration and success of confinement under

MDSO programs. The two available studies indicate that, on average, prisoners convicted of sex crimes are confined much longer than MDSOs who are released. One California study found that while the 122 persons convicted of sex crimes and released from California prisons in 1973 had served a mean of 54 months, the 180 MDSOs released from the state hospital as nondangerous in that year had served an average of 17.7 months, and the 80 MDSOs believed to be dangerous but who were nonetheless released or transferred to prison in that year had served a mean of 21.5 months. Sturgeon & Taylor, "Report of a Five–Year Follow–Up Study of Mentally Disordered Sex Offenders Released from Atascadero State Hospital in 1973," 6 Law & Hum.Beh. 31 (1982). The second study found that MDSOs spent, on average, four to six months less time institutionalized than did persons sent to prison for a sex crime. Ransley, "Repeal of the Wisconsin Sex Crimes Act," 1980 Wisc.L.Rev. 941. Of course, both of these studies focused on MDSOs who were released; they do not take into account MDSOs who had not been released and may never be.

Sturgeon & Taylor also found that, after release, the reconviction rates for sex crimes for MDSOs considered dangerous and for prisoners previously convicted of sex crimes were almost identical (24% v. 25%) and were twice the reconviction rate for MDSOs considered nondangerous (12%). However they also state that "none of these data prove that any particular treatment is effective in helping to rehabilitate sex offenders" and that "[t]he initial discriminating process which channels offenders either to prison or to the hospital may account for more of the outcome differences between these two groups than differences in treatment." Id. at 62.

4. *MDSO commitment procedures.* Most courts consider MDSO statutes as hybrids, part criminal and part civil. Although it eventually expresses reservations about its claim, initially the *Little* court referred to the Nebraska MDSO process as "civil in nature", apparently because of its emphasis on treatment. Many courts agree with this characterization of MDSO statutes; indeed, in *Allen v. Illinois,* 478 U.S. 364, 106 S.Ct. 2988, 92 L.Ed.2d 296 (1986), the U.S. Supreme Court, relying on this rationale, found that the privilege against self-incrimination does not apply at such proceedings.[b] In justifying this decision, it stated in part:

> Petitioner [a "sexually dangerous person" confined in a psychiatric center in the state's maximum security prison complex] has not demonstrated, and the record does not suggest, that "sexually dangerous persons" in Illinois are confined under conditions incompatible with the State's asserted interest in treatment. Had petitioner shown, for example, that the confinement of such persons imposes on them a regimen which is essentially identical to that imposed upon felons with no need for psychiatric care, this might well be a different case. But the record here tells us little or nothing about the regimen at the psychiatric center, and it certainly does not show that there are no relevant differences between confinement there and confinement in the other parts of the maximum-security complex. Indeed, counsel for the state assures us that under Illinois law sexually dangerous persons must not be treated like ordinary prisoners. We therefore cannot say

b. *Allen* is reprinted at pp. 730–735.

that the conditions of petitioner's confinement themselves amount to "punishment" and thus render "criminal" the proceedings which led to confinement.

478 U.S. at 373–74, 106 S.Ct. at 2994. The treatment premise of MDSO statutes may lead the Court to hold that other rights associated with the criminal trial do not apply to the MDSO process. Cf. *Addington v. Texas*, 441 U.S. 418, 99 S.Ct. 1804, 60 L.Ed.2d 323 (1979) (holding that clear and convincing standard of proof, rather than the criminal reasonable doubt standard, applies in civil commitment proceedings).

On the other hand, in *Specht v. Patterson*, 386 U.S. 605, 87 S.Ct. 1209, 18 L.Ed.2d 326 (1967), the Supreme Court held that persons subject to MDSO proceedings are entitled to certain procedural rights beyond those constitutionally required in non-capital sentencing proceedings (which the Court has indicated may be quite informal[c]). Because a MDSO statute requires a finding of dangerousness due to mental disorder it raises a distinct issue involving "the making of a new charge leading to criminal punishment." Id. at 610, 87 S.Ct. at 1212. Thus, at the least, according to *Specht*, the person subjected to a MDSO proceeding is entitled to "be present with counsel, have the opportunity to be heard, be confronted with witnesses against him, have the right to cross-examine, and to offer evidence of his own." Id. Given the holding in *Little*, how much procedure should be due offenders subject to the Nebraska statute?

5. *MDSO commitment standards.* Presumably the definition of "mental disease or defect" found in most MDSO statutes is meant to be different from the definition of that phrase under the insanity test. In fact, Sturgeon & Taylor found that 49% of those admitted as mentally disordered sex offenders were diagnosed merely as having some variant of "sexual deviation." Thirty-six percent suffered from "personality disorders" and only 11 of the 260 MDSOs received any psychotic diagnosis. Sturgeon & Taylor, supra at 43. The Group for the Advancement of Psychiatry has asserted that "[s]ex psychopathy is a . . . meaningless grouping from a diagnostic and treatment standpoint." GAP, Psychiatry and Sex Psychopath Legislation: The 30s to the 80s, 936 (1977).

As to the "danger" that the person subjected to MDSO proceedings must pose before commitment is possible, most courts have interpreted the vague statutory language extremely broadly. For instance, in *State v. Hungerford*, 84 Wis.2d 236, 267 N.W.2d 258 (1978), the Wisconsin Supreme Court held that a prediction of physical harm is not required, and that "moral" harm alone might be sufficient. In rare contrast is *Millard v. Harris*, 406 F.2d 964 (D.C.Cir.1968), in which Judge Bazelon interpreted the following language: "The term 'sexual psychopath' means a person, not insane, who by a course of repeated misconduct in sexual matters has evidenced such lack of power to control his sexual impulses as to be dangerous to other persons because he is likely to attack or otherwise inflict injury, loss, pain, or other evil on the objects of his desire." 22 D.C. Code § 3503(1) (1967). The appellant had been charged with exhibitionism and the trial court had found that he was likely to engage again in public

c. See *Williams v. New York*, 337 U.S. 241, 69 S.Ct. 1079, 93 L.Ed. 1337 (1949).

exposure and perhaps in public masturbation as well. But Judge Bazelon, writing for the court, held that the defendant was not a "sex psychopath" as defined above:

> The unanimous testimony of all the expert witnesses that serious psychological harm would result from public exposure only to unusually sensitive adult women and small children leads us to conclude that the future sexual misconduct of the appellant, if any, is not sufficiently likely to cause the sort of harm required by the statute to justify further commitment. The appellant did not, it is true, prove that no such "potential viewers" would view him in the course of any future exhibitionism. But having shown that he was unlikely to commit such acts with great or uncontrollable frequency, and that in the event of such misconduct harm would be produced in only a small proportion of the population, the appellant could fairly demand of the Government that it show that the members of these restricted classes were not merely "potential viewers," but likely viewers. This the Government wholly failed to do. And without the assistance of any evidence adduced on this score, we cannot conclude that supersensitive women and small children are likely to suffer serious harm from isolated instances of exhibitionism. "Very seclusive, withdrawn, shy, sensitive" women are a minority. While the law must and does protect them like other citizens, there are limits on the extent to which the law can sweep the streets clear of all possible sources of occasional distress to such women. Small children present a different problem. But the expert testimony was not that the typical small child would be injured by witnessing an isolated act of exposure on the part of a stranger, but rather that psychological danger to their development was likely from repeated exposure to such abnormal adult sexual behavior. We therefore conclude that the likelihood of serious injury to a child happening to see the appellant expose himself in public is too remote to justify commitment. As for harm to the appellant's own children, we have already adverted in passing to the questionable nature of the sole evidence that the appellant ever did expose himself in his home before them. Even if we accept this evidence, however, and assume that the appellant might expose himself in his home if released, his children can be protected from the harm which might follow from repeated exposure by other means than his involuntary hospitalization. His wife need not permit the appellant to so abuse his children, and other legal remedies are available to her to insure that he does not inflict such harm on his children.

Id. at 698. The appellant conceded that he had been receiving treatment at St. Elizabeth's hospital; he was merely arguing that he was not a "sex psychopath." Id. at 966. Do you agree with the court's decision? Should this type of case be handled through the "criminal" process, or is it more properly a civil commitment case?

More fundamentally, are MDSO statutes and similar criminal laws a useful "hybrid" or should the criminal justice system focus on retribution and deterrence and leave treatment-oriented incapacitation to the civil commitment system?

Chapter Eight

CIVIL COMMITMENT

I. INTRODUCTION

History.[a] Involuntary treatment or care of the mentally disabled, outside the criminal setting, is usually called civil commitment. For many years, the United States did not have a "commitment system" as such. Once a method for committing the mentally disabled did develop, the dominant approach varied considerably over time, tending toward either a purely "libertarian" model—which is aimed at limiting the impact of commitment to those who will otherwise harm society—or a purely "paternalistic" model—which seeks to commit anyone who may benefit from state intervention.

In colonial America, the mentally disabled were the responsibility of their family or friends. For those unfortunate persons who lacked such support, the town sometimes would provide money to a designated individual for their care, but more frequently would banish them; thus they would often end up in bands of "drifters" which roamed the countryside. If a "madd" person became violent, he or she might be punished as a criminal. If not, the person was subjected to restraint and perhaps whipping; no treatment was provided, since none existed. In most locales, it is doubtful any explicit legal authority existed for such non-criminal detention. One exception was Massachusetts which, in 1676, enacted a statute ordering the selectmen of towns which had "dangerously distracted persons" to restrain them "that they do not damify others."

During the last half of the eighteenth century, the community became considerably more involved in dealing with the mentally disabled. In 1752, the Pennsylvania Assembly, in response to a petition drawn by Benjamin Franklin, authorized establishment of the first hospital to receive the sick poor, including the poverty-stricken mentally ill. The first hospital devoted exclusively to the mentally disabled was constructed at Williamsburg, Virginia in 1773. Also during this period, state legislatures began enacting statutes which expressly provided authority for confining the mentally disabled in community institutions. For instance, in 1788, the New York legislature passed a statute which permitted constables, after procuring a warrant from two or more justices, to apprehend and lock up the "furiously madd" or those "so far disordered in their senses that they may be dangerous to be permitted to go abroad." Confinement was permitted for the duration of the individual's dangerous condition, although the statute also provided that it should not be construed to prevent friends or relatives from assuming custody of the individual. Thus, this statute appeared to be aimed primarily at people who were violent and who could not be cared for privately; those disordered individuals who were non-threat-

a. The following historical account through the 1960's is taken from Brakel, Parry and Weiner, The Mentally Disabled and the Law 12–15 (1986); A. Deutsch, The Mentally Ill in America: A History of the Their Care and Treatment from Colonial Times (2d ed. 1949).

ening or who could be controlled by private citizens were not the principal targets of the law.

By the middle of the nineteenth century, some evidence suggests that detention of these latter two groups of individuals may have become more commonplace. For example, a 1842 New York statute *required* the confinement of *all* "lunatics", not just dangerous ones who were at large. It commissioned "assessors" to search for such people and allowed commitment, upon the authority of two assessors, for a *minimum* of six months. Another example of the loosening standards for commitment is furnished by the case of Josiah Oakes. In 1845, Oakes was detained in a hospital, not because he was violent, but on the ground that he suffered from hallucinations and had incompetently conducted his business affairs, as evidenced by the fact that he became engaged to a young woman of "unsavory" character a few days after the death of his wife. Oakes sought release via a writ of habeas corpus, alleging he had been illegally committed. In rejecting this claim, the Massachusetts Supreme Court stated:

> The right to restrain an insane person of his liberty is found in that great law of humanity, which makes it necessary to confine those whose going at large would be dangerous to themselves or others. . . . And the necessity which creates the law, creates the limitation of the law. The question must then arise in each particular case, whether a patient's own safety, or that of others, requires that he should be restrained for a certain time, and whether restraint is necessary for his restoration, or will be conducive thereto. The restraint can continue as long as the necessity continues.

Although the court recognized that limitations should be placed on the state's authority, it explicitly permitted indeterminate detention not only for those who demonstrated a proneness to harm others but also for those who might harm themselves.

The reasons for this "expansion"[b] of commitment authority are undoubtedly complex, but two explanations stand out. First, as society became more interdependent and government more pervasive, the traditional view that the family was obligated to take care of its own became outmoded. Second, a perception developed that techniques for caring for the disabled had improved. The American Psychiatric Association was founded in 1844. Many of its members, including Benjamin Rush and Isaac Ray, advocated and tried to develop a scientific approach to the treatment of the mentally disabled. These apparent advances in medicine meant that commitment could be char-

---

b. Some authors, see, e.g., Myers, "Involuntary Civil Commitment of the Mentally Ill: A System in Need of Change," 29 Vill.L.Rev. 367, 380 n. 62, 386 n. 102 (1983), have suggested that *Oakes* was merely a restatement of law that had existed for centuries, permitting the state to intervene when a person's mental disability might lead to dissipation of his or her estate. (For a description of this law, see the introduction to guardianship in Chapter Nine). Assuming this is so, *Oakes* still marks one of the first times a court explicitly permitted involuntary *commitment* of a nondangerous person.

acterized not merely as detention but as a means of providing treatment, or "restoration", as the *Oakes* court put it.

Nonetheless, for a time after the Civil War, a movement aimed at curtailing the reach of commitment law flourished, motivated in large part by a former mental hospital patient named Mrs. Packard. Packard was committed in 1860 under the following statute: "Married women and infants, who in the judgment of the medical superintendent are evidently insane or distracted, may be received and detained in the hospital at the request of the husband, . . . or [the] guardian of the infants, without the evidence of insanity or distraction required in other cases." Apparently, the primary evidence supporting Packard's commitment under this statute was provided by two doctors, one of whom stated she was rational but was a "religious bigot like Henry Ward Beecher and Horace Greeley," and the second of whom opined that her ideas were "novel." After her release three years later, Packard campaigned against laws and practices which permitted hospitalization solely on the basis of a person's opinions, with no attempt to gauge moral accountability. Her efforts were aided by the publication of "muckraking" books describing pitiful hospital conditions. By the 1890's, many states had adopted statutes which required a jury determination of the commitment issue, authorized the presence of counsel at the hearing, and penalized criminally anyone who knowingly sought the illegal commitment of another.

The movement toward a more legalized commitment process was relatively short-lived, however. From the "Packard era" until the 1970's, most changes in civil commitment law aimed at making commitment easier rather than more difficult, again in large part due to medical advances that increased optimism about treatment efficacy. By the early years of the twentieth century, in response to the ceaseless efforts of Dorothea Dix and others, at least 20 states established mental hospitals or enlarged or improved those in existence. Through the middle of this century, the construction of mental hospitals continued apace, and medical science developed several new treatment modalities, including modern psychotherapy, electro-convulsive therapy, psychosurgery and, probably most importantly, chemical therapy. Concurrent with these developments, many states "medicalized" the procedural requirements associated with commitment. Judges and juries were replaced by physicians or "lunacy commissions" and dangerousness almost disappeared as a criterion for commitment. By 1970, 31 states provided for hospitalization based simply on the certification of one or more physicians that the individual suffered from mental illness and needed treatment.

In the early 1970's, the pendulum swung once again. Influenced by the civil rights movement of the 1960's, by exposés of poor hospital conditions and commitment abuses, and by a growing distrust of psychiatric expertise and the medical model of mental illness upon which it is based, groups of lawyers, mental health professionals and patients successfully exerted pressure for legal reform. The leading statutory indication of the shift was the adoption of the Lanterman–Petris–Short Act in California. Passed in 1969, this statute made dangerousness to self or others the core criteria for commitment, defined these criteria relatively narrowly, and provided extensive procedural protections. It provided a model for many other state statutes. On the judicial front, the most important decision was handed down in 1973 by the federal district court for the Eastern District of Wisconsin. In *Lessard v. Schmidt*, infra, that court found the Wisconsin civil commitment statute unconstitutional "insofar as it . . . permits commitment without proof . . . that the patient is both 'mentally ill' and dangerous." *Lessard* also mandated procedural changes similar to those available in the criminal context. Several other federal and state courts followed *Lessard's* lead.

More recently, there have been signs of retrenchment. In 1979, the United States Supreme Court refused to hold that the criminal reasonable doubt standard is constitutionally required in the civil commitment context. *Addington v. Texas,* infra. The same year, it also found that the right to counsel and a judicial tribunal were not necessary attributes of a system for hospitalizing minors. *Parham v. J.R.,* infra. With the refinement of the American Psychiatric Association's Diagnostic and Statistical Manual, the advent of new chemical therapies, and the creation of Professional Standards Review Organizations (PSRO), some have claimed—as has been claimed in the past—that psychiatric science has improved substantially and the danger of overcommitment and improper treatment accordingly reduced. See, e.g., Stone, Mental Health and Law: A System in Transition 20–21, 65–76 (1975). Some states have returned to broad commitment criteria. Whether the pendulum will continue to swing back toward a more paternalistic model and, if so, how far it will go, remains to be seen.

Modern Commitment Statutes. There are three general diagnostic populations subject to today's civil commitment laws: the mentally ill, the developmentally disabled (including the mentally retarded), and persons addicted to drugs and alcohol. Many states have separate commitment laws for each. Commitment statutes may also vary depending upon the legal context. For instance, most states distinguish between adults and minors in establishing criteria and procedures for commitment of the mentally disabled. Most states also have separate statutes for commitment of those persons acquitted by reason of insanity and prisoners transferred to mental hospitals for treatment. The first four sections of this chapter examine the laws dealing with commitment of the adult mentally ill who have not been processed by the criminal system, because these laws have served as the model for other commitment laws. The final section examines commitment of insanity acquittees, prisoners, the developmentally disabled, substance abusers, and minors.

Modern statutes governing the commitment of the adult mentally ill are relatively uniform. At the present time (1990), virtually no state still adheres to the "mental illness plus need for treatment" standard of commitment; typically a person may not be involuntarily hospitalized unless the government can show that, as a result of mental illness, the person is "dangerous to others or to self." About 25 states also permit commitment of a mentally ill person who is shown to be, as a result of mental illness, "unable to provide for his or her basic needs," "gravely disabled" or "likely to deteriorate". Even if the proper criteria are met, virtually all statutes prohibit institutionalization if there is a less restrictive alternative available in the community. Every state also provides for a commitment hearing, with notice and counsel, and requires periodic reviews of the legal status of committed persons. Additionally, most states have enacted statutes which provide those who have been hospitalized with various rights, including the right to a treatment plan, the right to a safe, clean environment, and the right to communicate with the outside world. The various issues raised by these statutes will be treated in this and subsequent chapters.

The Context of Civil Commitment Law: Deinstitutionalization and Reinstitutionalization. In evaluating and interpreting civil commitment laws, it is important to have some sense of the context in which they operate—the public mental health system. Providing a full description of this context is not attempted here. But the following remarks should be sufficient to set the stage for an intelligent assessment of civil commitment law.

Probably the most significant historical fact connected with the public mental health system is that the census of public mental hospitals has dropped dramatically since the mid–1950's. In 1956, the number of patients in such institutions on an average day was 551,390. By 1980, one estimate indicated that the average daily population had dropped to 132,000. During the same time period, however, the annual admission rate for public mental hospitals almost doubled, from 185,597 to 390,000. S. Brakel, J. Parry & B. Weiner, The Mentally Disabled and the Law 47 (1986).

There are several explanations for this process of "deinstitutionalization", as it has come to be called, and the accompanying surge in admissions rates. It is tempting to ascribe most of these changes to the legal reforms of the 1960's and 70's. Certainly, to some extent, changes in civil commitment laws had an effect. In a number of states, narrowed commitment criteria, the least restrictive alternative doctrine, and additional procedural protections helped reduce the number of people sent to hospitals, at the same time shortened commitment terms made possible recommitments within the same year and thus increased the annual admission rate.[c] However, a number of studies also concluded that the "libertarian" reforms of the 1970's had only a

c. See Peters, et al., "The Effects of Statutory Change on the Civil Commit- ment of the Mentally Ill," 11 Law & Hum. Beh. 73 (1987) for a survey of the research.

minimal impact on the number or type of people hospitalized, largely because the new statutory language is still broad enough to be flexibly applied.[d] This research suggests that factors other than legal reform were responsible for much of the change in the hospital population and the admission rate.

One important such factor was the advent of psychotropic medication, first introduced as a treatment option in the mid–1950's. Because the various types of medication which fall under this rubric tend to suppress the symptomatology of persons diagnosed as suffering from schizophrenia, manic-depressive psychosis, depression and other major illnesses,[e] they offered, for the first time, an inexpensive, relatively quick treatment which could be made available to a large number of mentally ill people. Hospital beds could be emptied at a faster rate, allowing more admissions but also, in the long run, reducing the overall population.

Working in tandem with the medication revolution was the community treatment movement. In 1963, Congress passed the Community Mental Health Centers Act, which provided funding for the establishment of outpatient treatment centers. The CMHC Act was representative of a widespread effort to move the locus of treatment from isolated hospitals to the patients' communities, where they could be closer to support groups and employment opportunities. It reflected a perception that community treatment is at least as effective as confinement in a hospital, which many patient advocates thought aggravated rather than ameliorated patients' symptomatology. The Act and related federal laws also allowed state legislatures to reduce funding by closing state hospitals and shifting much of the financial burden to federal programs. Indeed, some have argued that the *primary* impetus behind deinstitutionalization actions taken by the states was fiscal. See C. Warren, The Court of Last Resort: Mental Illness and the Law 21–24 (1982). The community mental health centers and other community treatment programs, both outpatient and inpatient, which came into being as a result of this effort to offer an alternative to the traditional public mental hospital undoubtedly contributed to the reduction in the hospital population. However, the admission rate continues to increase because many communities still have not developed adequate aftercare programs for all types of patients; thus perhaps half of the patients who are discharged from the hospital as "stabilized" return within the year because no one monitors their post-discharge

d. Luckey & Berman, "Effects of a New Commitment Law on Involuntary Admissions and Service Utilization Patterns," 3 Law & Hum.Behav. 149 (1979) (Nebraska); Stier & Stoebe, "Involuntary Hospitalization of the Mentally Ill in Iowa: The Failure of the 1975 Legislation," 64 Iowa L.Rev. 1284, 1371–90 (1979); Faulkner, et al., "Effects of a New Involuntary Commitment Law: Expectations and Reality," 10 Bull.Am.Acad.Psychiat. & L. 249 (1982);

Cleveland, et al., "Do Dangerousness–Oriented Commitment Laws Restrict Hospitalization of Patients Who Need Treatment? A Test," 40 Hosp. & Comm.Psychiat. 266 (1989) (Pennsylvania).

e. The treatment of choice for manic-depressive psychosis is lithium, which is not technically an anti-psychotic drug. For further discussion of these medications, see pp. 848–870.

treatment or because post-discharge treatment is inadequate. See generally, "The New Snake Pits," Newsweek, May 15, 1978, at 93.

Other factors that have influenced the public hospital census are the increased use of private and veterans hospitals as a result of improved insurance coverage, and the advent of Medicaid and Medicare funding, which made possible largescale release of chronic patients to community nursing homes. Additionally, hospital population was reduced significantly by the death of elderly patients, a factor which accounted for 20 to 40 percent of all "releases" until the early 1960's, when community placement became available. See Goldman, Adams & Taube, "Deinstitutionalization: The Data Dymythologized," 34 Hosp. & Comm.Psych. 129 (1983).

Despite the many forces pushing for deinstitutionalization, there are some indications that a process of "reinstitutionalization" is beginning. Again, changes in the law may be partially responsible for this trend. See, e.g., Durham & LaFond, "The Empirical Consequences and Policy Implications of Broadening the Statutory Criteria for Civil Commitment," 3 Yale Law & Policy Rev. 395 (1985). But other factors seem to play a bigger role. For instance, civil commitments increased in New York City in the late 1980's, not because of a change in statutory language, but because the city administration decided to take aggressive action against the growing number of homeless individuals in the streets. See Fisher, Pierce & Appelbaum, "How Flexible Are our Civil Commitment Statutes?," 39 Hosp. & Comm.Psychiat. 711, 712 (1988).

At least some increase in the hospital census, independent of increases in the general population, is predictable. There is a growing realization that treatment in the community is an elaborate and expensive proposition. Probably no more than half of the projected 2,000 community mental centers have become operational. Moreover, community resources that are available are not always effective, at least for certain classes of people. As described by Scull: "Quite apart from the [community mental health] centers' uneven geographical distribution and their current fiscal problems, 'both their ideology and their most common services are not directed at the needs of those who have traditionally resided in state psychiatric institutions.'" Scull, "A New Trade in Lunacy: The Recommodification of the Mental Patient," 24 Amer.Behav. Scientist 724, 743–44, 748–49 (1981). See also Lamb, "Deinstitutionalization at the Crossroads," 39 Hosp. & Comm.Psychiat. 941 (1988). Given these facts, some degree of reinstitutionalization was probably inevitable.

The relationship of the public mental health system to the criminal system must also be noted. Clearly, some of the individuals who in the past were hospitalized are now being processed through the criminal justice system—often on misdemeanor charges akin to "vagrancy" violations—in an effort to remove them from the community. A debate has raged over whether this development represents the "criminaliza-

tion of mentally disordered behavior" or whether, instead, deinstitutionalization and commitment law reforms have prevented further
"psychiatrization of criminal behavior." See Abramson, "The
Criminalization of Mentally Disordered Behavior: Possible Side–Effect
of a New Mental Health Law," 23 Hosp. & Comm.Psychiat. 101 (1972)
and Monahan, "The Psychiatrization of Criminal Behavior: A Reply,"
24 Hosp. & Commun.Psychiat. 105 (1973). Whatever the outcome of
this debate, the key point for present purposes is that changes in one
system have usually brought about changes in the other, much like
squeezing a balloon and rearranging the air inside. Although the most
recent reforms have been of the public mental health system, one would
expect that if legislatures were to narrow the misdemeanor jurisdiction
of the criminal courts, the population subject to civil commitment
would expand.

In short, while attempting to understand the theoretical underpinnings of commitment and formulate appropriate commitment standards
and procedures is important, it should be recognized that commitment
law is just one of many variables affecting the numbers and types of
individuals who are subject to involuntary commitment. The implementation of the legal doctrines discussed in this chapter is likely to be
heavily influenced by factors only tangentially related to the language
found in civil commitment statutes.

II. THE BASIS FOR STATE INTERVENTION

A. INTRODUCTION

CASE ILLUSTRATIONS

The following descriptions of thirty individuals who were hospitalized in a psychiatric facility are taken from 45 cases reported in Dix,
"Acute Psychiatric Hospitalization of The Mentally Ill in the Metropolis: An Empirical Study", 1968 Wash.U.L.Q. 485, 504–47. Each of
these individuals was admitted to the St. Louis Acute Facility, as either
a voluntary or involuntary patient. In about one-fifth of the 45 cases
the patient "presented" him or herself. In another fifth the police
brought the patient. In the rest of the cases, family members, relatives
or members of the community were responsible for bringing the individual to the attention of the facility. Id. at 503.

Illustration 1. The patient, a 32 year old woman, worked as a
stenographer in a law office. On the day of admission she had experienced difficulty in concentrating on her work and had made numerous
mistakes. At noon she left to return home but instead checked into a
hotel. She reported hearing the sounds of a train depot and the voices
of old friends. Later in the afternoon, she presented herself to the
Acute Facility.

Illustration 2. The patient was observed by police wandering on
the street wearing hospital pajamas and a surgical cap. He did not
respond to attempts to elicit information from him. Several hospitals

in the vicinity were contacted but reported that they were not missing any patients. The patient was then taken to the Acute Facility.

Illustration 3. A neighbor of the patient called police and reported that the patient had chased her with a hatchet. The patient, when approached, stated, "This is the hatchet Mr. Robinson used to kill me. I died once. I do not know how I came back into this world."

Illustration 4. The patient, a middle aged woman who lived alone, was observed walking nude in the street late at night. Officers contacted her brother who requested that they take him and the patient to the Acute Facility. They did so.

Illustration 5. The patient believed that he was an F.B.I. agent, and he carried at least one weapon. He had accused his wife of being a "spy" and his mother-in-law of poisoning him. Three weeks before presentation he had been arrested for carrying a concealed weapon. Although it is extremely likely that he was exhibiting these symptoms at that time, he was not presented until several days before his preliminary hearing, when his wife called police and asked that they assist in presentation.

Illustration 6. The patient reportedly drank one pint of whiskey and, becoming irritated at a group of children, shook one of them. Police were called and the child was taken to a hospital where it was determined that she had suffered no significant harm. The officers then took the patient to the Acute Facility and told the resident that if the patient were not admitted he would be released, as there were no charges against him. The patient exhibited no symptoms of present mental illness. When the decision to admit was made, one officer called his superior and reported in a relieved tone, "They'll take him."

Illustration 7. The family reported that for the last two months the patient had been sleeping poorly and his general level of activity had increased. He spent money freely and the family was consequently forced into debt. Recently he had attempted to open several new charge accounts. The family also complained of the patient's argumentativeness and "resentfulness" at home and repeated complaints of his irritability at work.

Illustration 8. A woman who had been discharged from psychiatric hospitalization during which she had been diagnosed as paranoid schizophrenic began to exhibit symptoms again. She was "abusive," paraded around her home in the nude in front of her children and charged her husband with drugging her and inviting neighbors to have sexual relations with her. She also accused her neighbors of "wanting to get rid of her." She was not presented to the Acute Facility, however, until the landlord, in response to complaints made by neighbors, threatened to evict the family unless she was rehospitalized.

Illustration 9. The patient, a nineteen year old youth, had dropped out of high school because of a "nervous condition." He had been employed in a bakery but his employer called the family to take him home because he had been "acting strangely." The patient then became withdrawn and frequently paced the floor all night. Occasionally he would strike his brothers and sisters. Two days before presentation he swung at his mother with an iron bar and attempted to strangle his sister. No outside help was sought, however. On the day of presentation, he barricaded himself in the cellar and covered himself with soot and cobwebs. No attempt was made to obtain help until he left the cellar and ran out of the house. At this point, the police were called and the patient was apprehended and presented by the mother and police officers to the Acute Facility.

Illustration 10. The patient had been depressed for a period of time and had considered attempting suicide for two weeks. He had specifically threatened to kill himself, but no attempt was made to present him to the Acute Facility until his wife happened to notice an apparatus apparently designed by the patient to hang himself.

Illustration 11. The patient had been observed by police officers for three weeks. He wandered through the downtown area with a picture of Christ around his neck and carried a wooden staff. No pressure to present existed, however, until the patient walked into a store, selected a suit of clothing, identified himself as Jesus Christ and asked that the clothing be charged to God. The store owner complained to police, who presented the patient to the Acute Facility.

Illustration 12. Police officers presented a 36 year old man to the Acute Facility and reported that he had become irritated at a group of children and had shaken a small girl. A medical examination of the girl revealed no significant harm, and the officers reported that they had no charges against the pre-patient. The resident, who wanted to admit the pre-patient because of the potential for violence on his part, indicated that the patient signed a voluntary admission because he believed this was the only alternative to jail.

Illustration 13. A woman diagnosed as paranoid schizophrenic was referred to the Acute Facility from another hospital. She was actively hostile but admitted herself. The resident believed that this was because the patient's sister was already hospitalized in the Acute Facility and the patient wanted to be near her and felt the facility was beneficial for her sister and therefore would also be for her.

Illustration 14. A 24 year old unemployed musician presented himself at the Acute Facility. He reported that he had been depressed for a week, had experienced crying spells, and had observed an impairment in his ability to concentrate. He admitted having had suicidal thoughts and having specifically considered the use of sleeping pills as a means of taking his life. The resident admitted him.

Illustration 15. The patient, a 44 year old woman, was brought to the Acute Facility by her husband who was 85 years old. He reported that she suffered from insomnia and sometimes locked herself in the bathroom. During the interview with the resident, the patient talked to the empty emergency room. Among the factors influencing the decision to admit her on an involuntary basis was the resident's observation that in her neighborhood "people were robbing and raping all the time" and that she would be particularly subject to such attacks.

Illustration 16. The patient, a 32 year old woman, was seen in the emergency room on the 6th. She was given medication and the social service staff began to assist her in challenging the actions of the welfare office in terminating her AFDC payments. On the 23rd, the patient was returned to the facility by her sister. The sister reported that the patient had been depressed but had not taken her medication, had stated that she wished her children were dead and had given the children some unidentified medicine. The sister evidenced a great deal of concern over the safety of the children. The patient was admitted on a nonvoluntary basis; the admissions note stated that she could not be treated "safely" on an outpatient basis, principally because there was no adult member of the family to see that she took her medication and returned periodically to the clinic.

Illustration 17. The patient had been given a ride by a truck driver who found him hitchhiking along a highway. When the truck driver noticed that the patient had a gun, he took him to the police station. The police brought him to the Acute Facility where he refused to divulge anything other than the pronunciation of his name. He was admitted on a nonvoluntary basis.

Illustration 18. A young man who had broken up with his girl friend became intoxicated and threatened to kill her. This threat was communicated to the police. The young man presented himself to the Acute Facility after release from jail on a peace disturbance charge. The resident indicated that he did not believe the patient had the "guts" to harm anyone but that he admitted him because the threats which the patient had made had been so widely dispersed.

Illustration 19. A 26 year old woman had reportedly been "imagining things" since her marriage six months before presentation. She had accused her husband of spying on other men in public washrooms and believed that he had holes in the wall of their home through which he spied on her. She was presented at the facility by her husband and police officers after she called police and reported that her husband, in an attempt to kill her, had filled the apartment with gas. When police arrived they observed no gas and found the husband asleep. When the patient returned to her home, she was taken to the Acute Facility. In explaining her nonvoluntary admission, the resident emphasized her symptoms of psychosis.

Illustration 20. A medical report submitted to the probate court contained the following assertion offered to support the conclusion that the patient's judgment and insight were "poor": "He still sees no harm in the fact that he lived with a sixteen year old girl as husband and wife . . . [H]is reasoning at the present time is that his wife was not satisfactory at that time so why not have the girl . . ."

Illustration 21. The patient was presented to the Acute Facility after he had caused an auto accident while responding to hallucinations. He was diagnosed as a schizophrenic, paranoid type. The staff concluded on the basis of their experience with him after earlier hospitalizations that he would not continue to take medication after his release. The alternative course of treatment was seen as retaining him for about a week while a series of electroshock treatments were administered. But the staff also concluded that if his employer discovered that this was the reason for his absence from his job, he would be discharged. The tentative decision was to retain him in the facility but to give him a daily gate pass to go to his job; medication would be administered during this time and its effectiveness would be later evaluated.

Illustration 22. An 18 year old youth was admitted after being in an auto accident while under the influence of a drug. He denied taking amphetamines in addition to the drug which he had taken prior to the accident, but the staff psychiatrist indicated that he would be retained, involuntarily if necessary, for a week, because it was believed that he was in fact taking amphetamines and the psychiatrist expected withdrawal symptoms to develop.

Illustration 23. The patient, a 32 year old woman, was presented by her husband because he had returned after a week away to find that she had wandered to the home of an occasional acquaintance six miles away. The husband also reported that the patient had not been eating or sleeping properly and had gone to taverns alone the past three weekends. The patient reportedly told her husband that she had relations with another man and informed the resident that she was under the spell of a "wise old man." The resident indicated that a major factor in his decision to admit her as an involuntary patient was the fact that this was her first psychotic episode and that he desired an opportunity to diagnose her psychopathology.

Illustration 24. The patient, a 61 year old woman, lived alone. She had a history of persecutory delusions extending back over fifteen years. On a number of previous occasions, she had screamed at the neighbors; they finally responded by calling the police. On the occasion preceding her presentation, the neighbors specifically demanded that the police secure the patient's hospitalization. When examined at the Acute Facility, the patient indicated that she believed spirits came to her home and attempted to have "spiritual sex" with her. The resident, who admitted her on a nonvoluntary basis, indicated that a major factor in his decision was that he was not certain "how much the neighbors could take."

Illustration 25. The patient, a 33 year old man, had a history of amphetamine abuse and for two years had exhibited paranoid ideas. He had reportedly made certain threats, but his family did not believe he was capable of carrying them out. He had been seen several times in the emergency room and an administrative official of the Acute

Facility suggested that the next time he was seen in the emergency room he be admitted. Subsequently, the patient's car was stopped by police and he was discovered to be driving without a license. The officers found an out-patient clinic card in the patient's wallet, and they then called the Acute Facility. They were instructed to bring him to the emergency room; upon arrival, he represented himself as an Internal Revenue Agent and showed significant thought disorder. He was admitted.

Illustration 26. The patient, a 53 year old woman, was brought to the Acute Facility as a referral from another facility. She exhibited significant thought disassociation, a classical symptom of schizophrenia. The admitting resident indicated she had no insight at all, citing her statement, "If you take a drive in the city, you'll find lots of people crazier than I am." Curiously, the patient had functioned in her employment up to the time of admission. Little information was available as to the patient's home situation. The patient maintained that she had to return home to take care of her daughters, but the admitting resident believed that three of her daughters were married and the fourth was engaged. She was admitted despite her objections. The resident indicated that he felt she might well have been able to remain in the community if some supporting person had been available, but he had concluded that no one was available.

Illustration 27. The patient was a 38 year old woman who had been having severe marital difficulties. After receiving unexpected doctor bills, she took an overdose of sleeping medication and immediately informed her husband of what she had done. When, at the emergency room of a general hospital, she became abusive, she was taken to the Acute Facility. The resident, after determining that the dosage taken was not enough to be dangerous, was about to release her to "sleep it off." He indicated that he hospitalized her because the family was disrupted by the patient's insistence that she was unhappy with her marriage and desired to terminate it, and had been particularly shaken by the events of the evening. One son, the resident related, had been reported at home hiding in the bathroom from fright.

The patient . . . was staffed the morning following her admission. During the staffing she was belligerent but revealed no thought disorganization or loss of contact with reality. She maintained that she was unhappy with her husband and wanted to leave him but that he would not "let her go." She avoided responding to questions directed at determining why she did not simply leave. The staff concluded that her actions in taking the pills had not been a serious attempt to end her life; the fact that she called her husband's attention to her actions immediately after taking the pills suggested that she was using this as a weapon against him. No significant depression was observed, and it was agreed that the action was impulsive rather than symptomatic of serious depression. She was diagnosed as having "personality disorder" and it was decided to retain her for about eight days and then reevaluate her situation. During this time, she was to be given no medication but would be seen by the staff psychologist and an attempt to smooth out her marital discord would be made. It was also agreed that the possibility of a divorce would be raised.

Illustration 28. The medical report asserted that the patient had "jumped on his sister's son with intention to do great bodily harm." The patient's mother (who agreed that her son was sick and needed hospitalization) denied that the patient had ever assaulted or even threatened her grandchild. (The medical report also stated, "He remains withdrawn, suspicious, guarded, antisocial, hostile, defiant and it seems he is dangerous to himself and others.")

Illustration 29. The patient, who lived with her sister's family, reportedly threatened the members of the family. On the morning of her presentation to the Acute Facility, she threw a cup of hot coffee on her sister; this stimulated her presentation.

Illustration 30. The patient was a young woman who had voluntarily entered the Acute Facility but subsequently demanded her release. The medical report stated:

> The patient came to the emergency room . . . and was diagnosed as Anxiety Reaction. The patient went to New York . . . and lived there for three years. Her father went after her because he stated the patient had a nervous breakdown. No other factors are known. The patient was [previously] in . . . [a local private hospital] and received shock treatments. After her discharge she refused to go to the clinic and returned to New York. She called her father for money to pay her hotel bills while in New York. . . . [S]he came back to St. Louis but did not work. She made trips to Chicago and Detroit and kept calling her father for money. She lived in [an apartment hotel] . . . and when asked to pay the rent would cry. The patient had threatened to kill her sister and her brother-in-law. She had been moody, having nightmares, will sit and stare, will not talk and says she hates everybody.
>
> The patient . . . refused to answer any questions and showed poor insight into her problems. Her affect was shallow but there was no evidence of hallucinations and no evidence of delusions could be brought out . . . The patient remains hostile, unfriendly and uncooperative.

At the hearing the patient's father testified. He indicated obvious concern over the inconvenience and expense of getting the patient back to St. Louis after her trips. He also testified that he "had been told" that the patient had threatened to take her brother-in-law's gun and shoot his family (with whom she lived at the time) and to burn their house down. He also stated that she had once violently resisted the family's attempts to force her into a car to go to a psychiatric outpatient clinic. The patient's employment history was irregular; the father testified that he had been told that there were few hospitals in New York City where the patient had not worked.

The patient herself testified that she felt that she did not need further full time hospitalization and that she could—and would—take outpatient treatment. She emphatically indicated that she did not want additional electroshock treatments. When asked about her plans regarding what she would do if released, she was vague. She was not asked about the alleged threats to her brother-in-law's family, nor was any inquiry into her employment history made. The court ordered her committed.

NOTE: GOVERNMENT AND INDIVIDUAL INTERESTS

Whether in its libertarian or paternalistic guise, civil commitment law is usefully contrasted to the criminal law. Theoretically, the primary purpose of the criminal law is to punish; entry into the criminal justice system depends upon whether a person has engaged in behavior that is considered blameworthy enough, and sufficiently costly to society, that harsh sanctions are deserved, as well as necessary to deter others from engaging in similar behavior. The primary purpose of civil commitment, on the other hand, is not to punish for past acts but to control future ones: the impetus for a civil commitment system does not stem from retributive or deterrence concerns but rather is based on a perceived need for incapacitation or treatment, or both. This is not to say that civil commitment has never been used as a sanctioning device, or that the criminal law does not perform a control function. But, in theory at least, punishment is the preserve of the criminal system, while civil commitment is reserved for those who the state cannot, or will not, punish but who nonetheless need to be controlled for their own good or the good of others. As a result, the criminal law focuses on already committed conduct, while the civil commitment system relies on predictions of conduct.

The criminal justice system is justified as an exercise of the state's "police power," the power to act in furtherance of the general welfare and public safety. In *Jacobson v. Massachusetts*, 197 U.S. 11, 25 S.Ct. 358, 49 L.Ed. 643 (1905), the Supreme Court upheld a Massachusetts provision which permitted fines or imprisonment to be imposed on those who refused or neglected to be vaccinated for smallpox. In support of this decision, the Court described as a "fundamental princi-ple" the idea that

> persons and property [can be] subjected to all kinds of restraints and burdens, in order to secure the general comfort, health, and prosperity of the State[.] . . . The possession and enjoyment of all rights are subject to such reasonable conditions as may be deemed by the governing authority of the country essential to the safety, health, peace, good order and morals of the community. Even liberty itself, the greatest of all rights, is not unrestricted license to act according to one's will.

Clearly, when someone has committed a crime the state has the authority to deprive that person of liberty under the police power described in *Jacobson*.

The justification advanced for civil commitment depends upon the reason for commitment. When the government commits a mentally disabled person on the ground that he or she is "dangerous to others," the usual justification advanced for this deprivation of liberty is, as with criminal punishment, the police power. Confining a dangerous person is permissible to protect the public. On the other hand, when a person is committed for reasons other than potential harmfulness to others, the government's action is usually justified on a different ground: the parens patriae, or "parental", authority of the state. With respect to this second governmental power, the Supreme Court has stated:

> The concept of *parens patriae* is derived from the English constitutional system. As the system developed from its feudal beginnings, the King retained certain duties and powers, which were referred to as the 'royal prerogative.' . . . These powers and duties were said to be exercised by the King in his capacity as guardian of persons under legal disabilities to act for themselves. For example, Blackstone refers to the sovereign or his representative as 'the general guardian of all infants, idiots and lunatics,' and as the superintendent of all 'charitable uses in the kingdom.' In the United States, the 'royal prerogative' and the 'parens patriae' function of the King passed to the States.

Hawaii v. Standard Oil, 405 U.S. 251, 92 S.Ct. 885, 31 L.Ed.2d 184 (1972).

Accepting that both the police power and the parens patriae power are inherent attributes of sovereignty does not necessarily justify civil commitment, however. As the Supreme Court has recognized (in dictum), civil commitment results in a "massive deprivation of liberty." Humphrey v. Cady, 405 U.S. 504, 509, 92 S.Ct. 1048, 1052, 31 L.Ed.2d 394 (1972). One commentary described the impact of commitment as follows:

> The most basic deprivation caused by civil commitment is the restriction of liberty—the interest of "transcending value"—for a possibly indefinite period. When a patient is hospitalized, not only are his movements restricted to the confines of the institution, but his freedom to move about within the institution itself may also be regulated or completely deprived for safety or disciplinary reasons. Even if the individual is committed to a community mental health center, he will probably be required to report to the center periodically, a restriction quite similar to that involved in parole from a penal institution.

> Equally important, although a physically ill individual is ordinarily permitted to choose whether to seek medical attention and is protected in this right by common law tort doctrines, an involuntarily committed patient may not have the right to refuse treatment. This refusal to allow a committed individual to decline unwanted medical examination and treatment might, in the absence of a compelling state interest,

infringe a constitutional right to bodily privacy which has been adumbrated in various judicial statements. Moreover, hospitalization itself interferes with privacy, since the patient cannot shield himself from constant observation by both his fellow patients and the staff of the institution. Furthermore, patients in hospitals risk brutality at the hands of their fellow residents and even their attendants, and may be subjected to life in an institution which is overcrowded, inadequately staffed, poorly maintained, and unsanitary.

Compounding all of these deprivations is the fact that most persons are currently committed for an indefinite period of time. While statistics reveal that the average length of stay in mental institutions is relatively short, in most states an individual facing civil commitment is potentially exposed to lifelong deprivation of many of his most basic civil rights.

Individuals face further legal and social deprivations as a result of commitment. . . . [I]n a few states, commitment undermines a patient's legal competency, thereby affecting the exercise of his civil rights. [In these states, c]ivil commitment may result in loss of custody of one's children, and loss of the rights to vote, be a candidate for or retain public office, serve on a jury, practice a profession, obtain a driver's license, and make a contract or a will. Law enforcement officials might view a prior commitment as reason for viewing otherwise innocuous behavior with suspicion, and the entry of the patient's fingerprints and photographs in official records might have an impact similar to that of a criminal record. Finally, a patient whose release from commitment is conditional may be subject to summary recommitment, mandatory psychiatric tests, prior approval of his choice of home or job, and other deprivations of his civil rights.

Along with these official deprivations, a former mental patient may suffer from the social opprobrium which attaches to treatment for mental illness and which may have more severe consequences than do the formally imposed disabilities. Many people have an "irrational fear of the mentally ill." The former mental patient is likely to be treated with distrust and even loathing; he may be socially ostracized and victimized by employment and educational discrimination. Finally, the individual's hospitalization and posthospitalization experience may cause him to lose self-confidence and self-esteem.

Developments in the Law—Civil Commitment of the Mentally Ill, 87 Harv.L.Rev. 1190, 1193–1201 (1974). Given the consequences of involuntary commitment on a person's liberty, privacy, association and movement interests, it remains a matter of some controversy whether the state should be able to exercise its police and parens patriae powers through civil commitment and, if so, under what limitations.

B. POLICE POWER COMMITMENT

1. Rationale

Preventive detention—confinement based on a prediction of antisocial behavior rather than conviction of crime—has been condemned on two grounds. The first is that predicting behavior is much more difficult than ascertaining whether certain behavior has occurred and therefore should not normally form the basis for state intervention. As John Stuart Mill stated:

> The preventive function of government . . . is far more liable to be abused, to the prejudice of liberty, than the punitory function, for there is hardly any part of the legitimate freedom of action of a human being which would not admit of being represented, and fairly too, as increasing the facilities for some form or other of delinquency. [I]f a public authority, or even a private person, sees any one evidently preparing to commit a crime, they are not bound to look on inactive. . . . . Nevertheless, when there is not a certainty, but only a danger of mischief, no one but the person himself can judge of the sufficiency of the motive which may prompt him to incur the risk. . . .

Mill, On Liberty. In: The Philosophy of John Stuart Mill 197, 196 (1961).

Even if the requisite certainty of harm to society is present, preventive detention may be repugnant for a second reason. In describing why the criminal law requires proof of an act prior to criminal conviction, Packer wrote:

> It is important, especially in a society that likes to describe itself as 'free' and 'open,' that a government should be empowered to coerce people only for what they do and not for what they are. . . . Now, this self-denying ordinance can be and often is attacked as being inconsistent with the facts of human nature. People may in fact have little if any greater capacity to control their conduct . . . than their emotions or their thoughts. It is therefore unrealistic or hypocritical, so the argument runs, to deal with conduct as willed or to treat it differently from personality and character. This attack is, however, misconceived. . . . The idea of free will in relation to conduct is not, in the legal system, a statement of fact, but rather a value preference having very little to do with the metaphysics of determinism and free will. . . .

Packer, The Limits of the Criminal Sanction 74–75 (1968).

For these reasons, it is possible that imposing *criminal punishment* in the absence of an act violates the eighth amendment's prohibition against cruel and unusual punishment. In *Robinson v. California,* 370 U.S. 660, 82 S.Ct. 1417, 8 L.Ed.2d 758 (1962), the Supreme Court held that the eighth amendment was violated by a statute which criminalized narcotics addiction, as opposed to possession or sale of narcotics. In *Powell v. Texas,* 392 U.S. 514, 532, 88 S.Ct. 2145, 2154, 20 L.Ed.2d 1254 (1968), four members of the Supreme Court explained this holding in the following words:

> Evidence of propensity can be considered relatively unreliable and more difficult for a defendant to rebut; the requirement of a specific act thus provides some protection against false charges. . . . Perhaps more fundamental is the difficulty of distinguishing, in the

absence of any conduct, between desires of the day-dream variety and fixed intentions that may pose a real threat to society; extending the criminal law to cover both types of desire would be unthinkable, since '[t]here can hardly be anyone who has never thought evil'. When a desire is inhibited it may find expression in fantasy; but it would be absurd to condemn this natural psychological mechanism as illegal.

As the following case suggests, punishment in the absence of proof beyond a reasonable doubt that a crime has been committed may not only violate the eighth amendment but also infringe substantive due process. The implications of these notions for *commitment* are explored in the materials that follow *Salerno.*

UNITED STATES v. SALERNO

Supreme Court of the United States, 1987.
481 U.S. 739, 107 S.Ct. 2095, 95 L.Ed.2d 697.

* * *

CHIEF JUSTICE REHNQUIST delivered the opinion of the Court.

The Bail Reform Act of 1984 allows a federal court to detain an arrestee pending trial if the government demonstrates by clear and convincing evidence after an adversary hearing that no release conditions "will reasonably assure . . . the safety of any other person and the community." The United States Court of Appeals for the Second Circuit struck down this provision of the Act as facially unconstitutional, because, in that court's words, this type of pretrial detention violates "substantive due process."

* * *

The court concluded that the Government could not, consistent with due process, detain persons who had not been accused of any crime merely because they were thought to present a danger to the community. It reasoned that our criminal law system holds persons accountable for past actions, not anticipated future actions.

* * *

We [reject] these contentions. . . .

A

The Due Process Clause of the Fifth Amendment provides that "No person shall . . . be deprived of life, liberty, or property, without due process of law . . . ." This Court has held that the Due Process Clause protects individuals against two types of government action. So-called "substantive due process" prevents the government from engaging in conduct that "shocks the conscience," Rochin v. California, 342 U.S. 165, 172, 72 S.Ct. 205, 209, 96 L.Ed. 183 (1952), or interferes with rights "implicit in the concept of ordered liberty," Palko v. Connecticut, 302 U.S. 319, 325–326, 58 S.Ct. 149, 152, 82 L.Ed. 288 (1937). When government action depriving a person of life, liberty, or property survives substantive due process scrutiny, it must still be implemented in a fair manner. Mathews v. Eldridge, 424 U.S. 319, 335, 96 S.Ct. 893,

903, 47 L.Ed.2d 18 (1976). This requirement has traditionally been referred to as "procedural" due process.

Respondents first argue that the Act violates substantive due process because the pretrial detention it authorizes constitutes impermissible punishment before trial. The Government, however, has never argued that pretrial detention could be upheld if it were "punishment." The Court of Appeals assumed that pretrial detention under the Bail Reform Act is regulatory, not penal, and we agree that it is.

As an initial matter, the mere fact that a person is detained does not inexorably lead to the conclusion that the government has imposed punishment. To determine whether a restriction on liberty constitutes impermissible punishment or permissible regulation, we first look to legislative intent. Unless Congress expressly intended to impose punitive restrictions, the punitive/regulatory distinction turns on " 'whether an alternative purpose to which [the restriction] may rationally be connected is assignable for it, and whether it appears excessive in relation to the alternative purpose assigned [to it].' "

We conclude that the detention imposed by the Act falls on the regulatory side of the dichotomy. The legislative history of the Bail Reform Act clearly indicates that Congress did not formulate the pretrial detention provisions as punishment for dangerous individuals. Congress instead perceived pretrial detention as a potential solution to a pressing societal problem. There is no doubt that preventing danger to the community is a legitimate regulatory goal.

Nor are the incidents of pretrial detention excessive in relation to the regulatory goal Congress sought to achieve. The Bail Reform Act carefully limits the circumstances under which detention may be sought to the most serious of crimes. See 18 U.S.C. § 3142(f) (detention hearings available if case involves crimes of violence, offenses for which the sentence is life imprisonment or death, serious drug offenses, or certain repeat offenders). The arrestee is entitled to a prompt detention hearing, *ibid.*, and the maximum length of pretrial detention is limited by the stringent time limitations of the Speedy Trial Act.[4] Moreover, as in *Schall v. Martin,* [467 U.S. 253, 104 S.Ct. 2403 (1984) (which upheld preventive detention of juveniles charged with delinquency offenses)] the conditions of confinement envisioned by the Act "appear to reflect the regulatory purposes relied upon by the" government. As in *Schall,* the statute at issue here requires that detainees be housed in a "facility separate, to the extent practicable, from persons awaiting or serving sentences or being held in custody pending appeal." 18 U.S.C. § 3142(i)(2). We conclude, therefore, that the pretrial detention contemplated by the Bail Reform Act is regulatory in nature, and

---

4. We intimate no view as to the point at which detention in a particular case might become excessively prolonged, and therefore punitive, in relation to Congress' regulatory goal.

[The Speedy Trial Act requires that trial take place within 100 days of arrest, 18 U.S.C.A. § 1361, although this period may be extended on a number of different grounds. Eds.]

does not constitute punishment before trial in violation of the Due Process Clause.

The Court of Appeals nevertheless concluded that "the Due Process Clause prohibits pretrial detention on the ground of danger to the community as a regulatory measure, without regard to the duration of the detention." Respondents characterize the Due Process Clause as erecting an impenetrable "wall" in this area that "no governmental interest—rational, important, compelling or otherwise—may surmount."

We do not think the Clause lays down any such categorical imperative. We have repeatedly held that the government's regulatory interest in community safety can, in appropriate circumstances, outweigh an individual's liberty interest. For example, in times of war or insurrection, when society's interest is at its peak, the government may detain individuals whom the government believes to be dangerous. Even outside the exigencies of war, we have found that sufficiently compelling governmental interests can justify detention of dangerous persons. Thus, we have found no absolute constitutional barrier to detention of potentially dangerous resident aliens pending deportation proceedings. We have also held that the government may detain mentally unstable individuals who present a danger to the public, *Addington v. Texas,* 441 U.S. 418, 99 S.Ct. 1804, 60 L.Ed.2d 323 (1979), and dangerous defendants who become incompetent to stand trial, *Jackson v. Indiana,* 406 U.S. 715, 731–739, 92 S.Ct. 1845, 1854–1858, 32 L.Ed.2d 435 (1972). We have approved of postarrest regulatory detention of juveniles when they present a continuing danger to the community. *Schall v. Martin, supra.* Even competent adults may face substantial liberty restrictions as a result of the operation of our criminal justice system. If the police suspect an individual of a crime, they may arrest and hold him until a neutral magistrate determines whether probable cause exists. *Gerstein v. Pugh,* 420 U.S. 103, 95 S.Ct. 854, 43 L.Ed.2d 54 (1975). Finally, respondents concede and the Court of Appeals noted that an arrestee may be incarcerated until trial if he presents a risk of flight, see *Bell v. Wolfish,* 441 U.S., at 534, 99 S.Ct., at 1871, or a danger to witnesses.

Respondents characterize all of these cases as exceptions to the "general rule" of substantive due process that the government may not detain a person prior to a judgment of guilt in a criminal trial. Such a "general rule" may freely be conceded, but we think that these cases show a sufficient number of exceptions to the rule that the congressional action challenged here can hardly be characterized as totally novel. Given the well-established authority of the government, in special circumstances, to restrain individuals' liberty prior to or even without criminal trial and conviction, we think that the present statute providing for pretrial detention on the basis of dangerousness must be evaluated in precisely the same manner that we evaluated the laws in the cases discussed above.

The government's interest in preventing crime by arrestees is both legitimate and compelling. In *Schall,* we recognized the strength of the State's interest in preventing juvenile crime. This general concern with crime prevention is no less compelling when the suspects are adults. Indeed, "[t]he harm suffered by the victim of a crime is not dependent upon the age of the perpetrator." The Bail Reform Act of 1984 responds to an even more particularized governmental interest than the interest we sustained in *Schall.* The statute we upheld in *Schall* permitted pretrial detention of any juvenile arrested on any charge after a showing that the individual might commit some undefined further crimes. The Bail Reform Act, in contrast, narrowly focuses on a particularly acute problem in which the government interests are overwhelming. The Act operates only on individuals who have been arrested for a specific category of extremely serious offenses. Congress specifically found that these individuals are far more likely to be responsible for dangerous acts in the community after arrest. Nor is the Act by any means a scattershot attempt to incapacitate those who are merely suspected of these serious crimes. The government must first of all demonstrate probable cause to believe that the charged crime has been committed by the arrestee, but that is not enough. In a full-blown adversary hearing, the government must convince a neutral decisionmaker by clear and convincing evidence that no conditions of release can reasonably assure the safety of the community or any person. While the government's general interest in preventing crime is compelling, even this interest is heightened when the government musters convincing proof that the arrestee, already indicted or held to answer for a serious crime, presents a demonstrable danger to the community. Under these narrow circumstances, society's interest in crime prevention is at its greatest.

On the other side of the scale, of course, is the individual's strong interest in liberty. We do not minimize the importance and fundamental nature of this right. But, as our cases hold, this right may, in circumstances where the government's interest is sufficiently weighty, be subordinated to the greater needs of society. We think that Congress' careful delineation of the circumstances under which detention will be permitted satisfies this standard. When the government proves by clear and convincing evidence that an arrestee presents an identified and articulable threat to an individual or the community, we believe that, consistent with the Due Process Clause, a court may disable the arrestee from executing that threat. Under these circumstances, we cannot categorically state that pretrial detention "offends some principle of justice so rooted in the traditions and conscience of our people as to be ranked as fundamental."

Finally, we may dispose briefly of respondents' facial challenge to the procedures of the Bail Reform Act. To sustain them against such a challenge, we need only find them "adequate to authorize the pretrial detention of at least some [persons] charged with crimes," whether or not they might be insufficient in some particular circumstances. We think they pass that test. As we stated in *Schall,* "there is nothing inherently unattainable about a prediction of future criminal conduct."

Under the Bail Reform Act, the procedures by which a judicial officer evaluates the likelihood of future dangerousness are specifically designed to further the accuracy of that determination. Detainees have a right to counsel at the detention hearing. They may testify in their own behalf, present information by proffer or otherwise, and cross-examine witnesses who appear at the hearing. *Ibid.* The judicial officer charged with the responsibility of determining the appropriateness of detention is guided by statutorily enumerated factors, which include the nature and the circumstances of the charges, the weight of the evidence, the history and characteristics of the putative offender, and the danger to the community. The government must prove its case by clear and convincing evidence. Finally, the judicial officer must include written findings of fact and a written statement of reasons for a decision to detain. The Act's review provisions, provide for immediate appellate review of the detention decision.

We think these extensive safeguards suffice to repel a facial challenge. The protections are more exacting than those we found sufficient in the juvenile context, see *Schall,* and they far exceed what we found necessary to effect limited postarrest detention in *Gerstein v. Pugh,* 420 U.S. 103, 95 S.Ct. 854, 43 L.Ed.2d 54 (1975). Given the legitimate and compelling regulatory purpose of the Act and the procedural protections it offers, we conclude that the Act is not facially invalid under the Due Process Clause of the Fifth Amendment.

[The Court also rejected a challenge to the statute under the eighth amendment's clause prohibiting excessive bail.]

* * *

JUSTICE MARSHALL, with whom JUSTICE BRENNAN joins, dissenting.

* * *

Let us apply the majority's reasoning to a similar, hypothetical case. After investigation, Congress determines (not unrealistically) that a large proportion of violent crime is perpetrated by persons who are unemployed. It also determines, equally reasonably, that much violent crime is committed at night. From amongst the panoply of "potential solutions," Congress chooses a statute which permits, after judicial proceedings, the imposition of a dusk-to-dawn curfew on anyone who is unemployed. Since this is not a measure enacted for the purpose of punishing the unemployed, and since the majority finds that preventing danger to the community is a legitimate regulatory goal, the curfew statute would, according to the majority's analysis, be a mere "regulatory" detention statute, entirely compatible with the substantive components of the Due Process Clause.

The absurdity of this conclusion arises, of course, from the majority's cramped concept of substantive due process. The majority proceeds as though the only substantive right protected by the Due Process Clause is a right to be free from punishment before conviction. The majority's technique for infringing this right is simple: merely redefine any measure which is claimed to be punishment as "regulation," and, magically, the Constitution no longer prohibits its imposition.

* * *

Questions and Comments

1. *Regulatory confinement.* Note that the Court uses its decision in *Addington v. Texas,* dealing with civil commitment, as an illustration of a situation in which regulatory confinement is permissible. The specific holding of *Addington,* which is reprinted in full later in this chapter, was that the due process clause requires only a clear and convincing showing, as opposed to proof beyond a reasonable doubt, that the criteria for commitment are met in order to justify confinement. Underlying this holding, at least according to the majority in *Salerno,* was the finding that commitment is a constitutional exercise of state power. Assuming for the moment that this is the case, does the Court's opinion in *Salerno* suggest any constitutional limitations on civil commitment when that process is used to confine persons thought to be dangerous to others?

2. *Treating the mentally ill specially.* The foregoing assumption—that involuntary commitment of the dangerous mentally ill is constitutionally permissible—can be challenged. Although, as *Salerno* makes clear, other groups besides the mentally disabled may be preventively detained, only the mentally disabled may be subjected to prolonged, indeterminate confinement based solely on a finding of dangerousness to others. Why are the mentally disabled singled out in this way? Can one fashion an equal protection type argument that police power commitment is unconstitutional? Consider the following excerpts.

NOTE, CIVIL COMMITMENT OF THE MENTALLY ILL: DEVELOPMENTS IN THE LAW
87 Harvard Law Rev. 1190, 1230.
(1974).

. . . One potential justification for the restriction of preventive detention to the mentally ill might be that the mentally ill, solely by reason of their condition, are substantially more dangerous than other groups. Although there is evidence that this belief is commonly held, studies indicate that the mentally ill as a class are at most slightly more dangerous, and quite possibly less dangerous, than their fellow citizens. Society would therefore obtain roughly similar protection against antisocial conduct if involuntary commitment were limited to the mentally healthy or were employed randomly. Since the vast majority of mentally ill individuals will not engage in dangerous behavior if they are permitted to retain their freedom, preventive detention based solely on mental illness would not appear to be even rationally related to the state's police power interest in protecting society. . . . .

A second possible rationale for limiting preventive detention of the dangerous to the mentally ill is premised on the ability of society to provide treatment which benefits them. However, to the extent that the state relies on the benefit which the individual will derive from treatment to support his commitment, it confuses the *parens patriae* and police power justifications for commitment. Requiring a competent individual to accept treatment for his own benefit should be viewed as an additional deprivation of liberty rather than as a benefit which justifies confinement for the protection of others.

Nevertheless, the state might argue that only the dangerous mentally ill are preventively detained because the ability to cure their illness enables the state to safeguard society's interests without indefinite deprivation of their liberty. However, since some mental illnesses are presently untreatable and others cannot be readily cured, many of the dangerous mentally ill face indefinite institutionalization as a result of commitment. Moreover, dangerousness, the link between preventive detention and the police power, may be treated through behavior conditioning which is applicable to the mentally ill and nonmentally ill alike.

A final justification for limiting involuntary police power commitments to the mentally ill can be derived from the reasons apparently underlying the decision not to authorize preventive detention of other dangerous individuals. By requiring a conviction before depriving persons who are not mentally ill of their liberty, the criminal law system relies on deterrence to reduce antisocial behavior. A state could argue that this punishment-deterrence approach fosters personal autonomy by allowing its citizens to choose whether to obey the law. The state's interest in employing a deterrence system that recognizes individual autonomy furnishes a rationale for excluding criminally responsible individuals—those able to appreciate the sanctions imposed for criminal activity and capable of conforming their actions to the dictates of the criminal law—from a prediction-prevention approach to harmful conduct. This justification would seem to provide a distinction between equally dangerous groups of mentally healthy and criminally insane individuals sufficient to satisfy the demands of equal protection. The latter group contains individuals whose mental condition excludes them from the operation of the traditional punishment-deterrence system, because they are both unable to make autonomous decisions about their antisocial behavior and unaffected by the prospect of punishment. . . .

MORSE, A PREFERENCE FOR LIBERTY: THE CASE AGAINST INVOLUNTARY COMMITMENT OF THE MENTALLY DISORDERED

70 Cal.L.R. 54, 59–65.
(1982).

The belief that disordered persons particularly lack competence or behavioral control is a strongly ingrained social dogma that underlies the special legal treatment accorded mentally disordered persons.

* * *

But the assertion that the crazy behavior of mentally disordered persons is compelled, in contrast to the freely chosen behavior of normal persons, is a belief that rests on commonsense intuitions and not on scientific evidence. Indeed, the degree of lack of behavioral control necessary to justify involuntary commitment is fundamentally a moral, social, and legal question—not a scientific one. Social and behavioral scientists can only provide information about the pressures affecting an actor's freedom of choice. The law must determine for itself when the actor is no longer to be treated as autonomous.

In fact, empirical evidence bearing on the question of the control capacity of mentally disordered persons would seem to indicate that mentally disordered persons have a great deal of control over their crazy behavior and legally relevant behavior related to it; indeed, often they may have as much control over their behavior as normal persons do.

* * *

For comparison, imagine the case of a habitually hot-tempered person who takes offense at something his doctor says and threatens to harm the doctor. Is this person more in control or rational than the delusional person? Or, consider the case of a severely ill cardiac patient who refuses to modify dietary, exercise, or smoking habits because the person prefers his or her habitually unhealthy lifestyle. The person's behavior can disrupt the well-being of the family, help drive up health care and insurance costs, and, if the result is an untimely death, impoverish the family. Is this person more in control or rational than the delusional person, and if so, in what sense? Of course, we all "understand" the behavior of the hot-tempered person and the cardiac patient, while the behavior of the delusional person makes no sense whatsoever. Still, there is no conclusive means to prove that any of these persons has greater or lesser control than any of the others.

* * *

Questions and Comments

1. *The mentally ill and dangerousness.* The Developments piece asserts that the mentally ill are no more dangerous as a class than the general population. Research since 1974 confirms this conclusion, *if* mental illness is equated with the psychoses. However, there is a high correlation between dangerousness and some personality disorders, in particular the antisocial personality disorder. And within the psychoses, there may be subgroups which tend to be more violence-prone than others.[f] At the same time, there are clearly groups which are more dangerous than the mentally ill. As Ennis & Emery point out:

f. The research on these points is summarized in detail at pages 429–431 of this book.

Probably 50 to 80 percent of all ex-felons will commit crimes after release from prison. But when their sentences expire, we let them go, and do not 'civilly commit' them as dangerous. Ghetto residents and teenage males are also much more likely to commit dangerous acts than the 'average' citizen, but we do not confine them.

Ennis & Emery, The Rights of Mental Patients 45 (1978). What implications does this information have for civil commitment of the mentally ill?

2. *The mentally ill and treatability.* The Development authors' assertion that some mental disorders are difficult or impossible to treat also retains validity. However, as noted in the introduction to this chapter, many of the psychoses (e.g., schizophrenia, manic-depressive psychosis) and depression are responsive to medication. See also, Tupin, et. al., "The Long–Term Use of Lithium in Aggressive Prisoners," 14 Comprehensive Psychiatry 311 (1973) (after being put on lithium, 21 our of 23 subjects had a statistically significant decrease in disciplinary actions for violence and 14 improved substantially). Thus, a person whose dangerousness stems from one of these mental disorders *may* be more "treatable" (with respect both to efficacy and to necessary duration of confinement) than a person whose dangerousness can only be treated through the behavioral therapy mentioned in the excerpt. Does this possibility justify treating the mentally ill differently?

If the person who is dangerous to others is not treatable or no treatment is available should commitment be barred? Consider the following excerpt from *Lynch v. Baxley,* 386 F.Supp. 378, 391–2 (M.D.Ala.1974):

An exception to this general requirement of due process [that commitment occur only when treatment is available] is recognized in the case of a presently and seriously dangerous person for whose illness there is no known cure or treatment. In such instances, the state may well have an obligation under the police power to restrain the liberty of the threatening individual, even though his condition is not amenable to any currently available treatment. Since the involuntary commitment of an untreatable person is an exception to the general due process requirement that treatment be available and afforded, the committing court must make a finding, based upon clear and convincing evidence, that confinement even without a proposed treatment program is necessary for the safety and well-being of the community and of the person to be committed. Such orders of commitment, when granted, shall provide that, should treatment for the patient's illness become available at any time during the period of his confinement, such treatment shall be made available to him immediately.

3. *The mentally ill and rational control.* As to the assertion made by Morse that the mentally disabled "often . . . have as much control over their behavior as normal persons do," considerable research supports his conclusion. A survey of studies of people diagnosed as suffering from schizophrenia concluded that "it is abundantly clear that most persons identified as schizophrenics do not function differently from most persons identified as nonschizophrenics". Sarbin & Mancuso, Schizophrenia: Medical Diagnosis or Moral Verdict? 22–51 (1980). Even more relevant are studies which show that the hospitalized mentally ill respond to rewards

and disincentives in a way that is consistent with rationally controlled behavior. Fisher, et. al. "Implications for Concepts of Psychopathology of Studies of Economic Principles in Behavior Therapy," 166 J. Nervous & Mental Disease 187, 191–93 (1978). However, none of these studies permit the conclusion that all mentally ill people behave as rationally as others. As Morse stated in another article:

> Again, I do not mean to make an absurd claim. A chronically disabled, hallucinating, and delusional person who wanders the streets in rags speaking gibberish is not 'like' normal persons, and the law should probably treat this person specially. Nevertheless, the law should be far more cautious before concluding that large numbers of crazy people are so incapable of responsible behavior that deprivation of liberty is justified.

Morse, "Treating Crazy People Less Specially," 90 W.Va.L.Rev. 353, 370 (1988).

4. *Predicting danger to others.* A final attack on the police power commitment authority asserts that it cannot be effectively implemented. That is, even if preventive detention of the dangerously mentally ill is justifiable theoretically, it should not be sanctioned because we are unable to determine accurately who among the mentally ill is dangerous. The commonly accepted wisdom is that a prediction of dangerousness to others is likely to be wrong two out of three times. See Monahan, The Clinical Prediction of Violent Behavior 60 (1980). How does the *Salerno* decision deal with this type of contention? Should difficulties in prediction preclude anticipatory confinement?

Recent scholarship has questioned the conclusion that predictions of violence-proneness are more often wrong than right. After a meticulous review of the literature, Litwack and Schlesinger asserted that few if any of the existing studies have tested the accuracy of explicit predictions of dangerousness for people who are subsequently released in the community rather than confined and treated.[g] Thus, they "suggest",

> clear and convincing evidence exists whenever any of the following indicia of future violence are evident: (1) a recent history of repeated violence (absent treatment or evidence of significant changes in the circumstances or attitudes that led to violence in the past); (2) a more distant history of violence together with clear and convincing evidence that the complex of attitudes and personality traits (and physical abilities) that led to violence in the past still exist and that there is a likelihood that the circumstances (or like circumstances) that led to violence in the past will recur in the foreseeable future (or, in any event, before the individual's violence-tending attitudes are likely to change); (3) unequivocal threats or other like evidence of serious intentions to commit violence, especially when based on delusional thinking; and (4) other clear and convincing evidence that the individual whose violence is being predicted is on the brink of violence. One example of this latter criteria would be that of a man who sat incessantly at the edge of his bed with a loaded rifle vigilantly waiting,

g. See pp. 427–429 for a more detailed treatment of this research.

because of his paranoid delusions, for his home to be attacked. Other examples would include individuals with a history of violence who express paniclike fears of losing control over violent impulses or who feel driven toward violence (e.g., by command hallucinations).

[W]e note again that while research has yet to establish the predictive power of these indices—and because of the practical and ethical problems involved may never do so—neither (to our knowledge) is there any evidence that refutes the legitimacy of relying on these indices to establish 'clear and convincing' evidence of 'dangerousness'. On the other hand, we question, again, whether 'clear and convincing' evidence of dangerousness can be had without any of these or similar indicia.

Litwack & Schlesinger, "Assessing and Predicting Violence: Research, Law, and Applications," in Handbook of Forensic Psychology (Weiner, Hess, eds.) 205, 224 (1987).

Moreover, Monahan has suggested that *short-term* predictions—i.e., predictions of future behavior in the immediate future—are likely to be more valid than the long-term predictions studied in most of the research to date, given the "small situational and temporal 'gap' between the behavior used as a predictor and the outcome that is being predicted." Monahan, The Clinical Prediction of Violent Behavior 59 (1980). See also McNeil & Binder, "Judgments of Dangerousness in Emergency Civil Commitment," 144 Am.J.Psychiat. 197 (1987) (those committed as dangerous to others much more likely than others to be assaultive in first 24 hours after prediction). Predictions made at civil commitment—unlike those made at criminal sentencing or after acquittal by reason of insanity—often focus on short-term prediction.

2. Implementing the Police Power

a. Defining Mental Illness.

DODD v. HUGHES

Supreme Court of Nevada, 1965.
81 Nev. 43, 398 P.2d 540.

THOMPSON, JUSTICE.

By a habeas corpus application addressed to the Second Judicial District Court, Dodd sought his release from the Nevada State Hospital (NRS 433.040). He had been committed to that institution as a mentally ill person by order of the Fourth Judicial District Court. At the habeas hearing, the Superintendent of the Nevada State Hospital gave his opinion that Dodd, though a sociopath, was not psychotic, and therefore not "mentally ill" within the meaning of NRS 433.200. He suggested that Dodd be released from his confinement. Another doctor was of a different view. Though he agreed that Dodd was not psychotic, he believed that a sociopathic personality may be considered "mentally ill" as that term is used in the state. Additionally, he stressed Dodd's high potential for homicidal activity. At the conclusion of the hearing, the court directed the superintendent to apply to the board of the state prison commissioners for that board's consent to confine Dodd at the Nevada State Prison. The superintendent did as directed. The prison commissioners consented, and Dodd was delivered to the Nevada State Prison for confinement until further order of the court (NRS 433.310).[a]

The legislature did not define "mentally ill" when it passed the law governing the Nevada State Hospital (NRS 433.010–433.640). Its failure to do so supplies the basis for Dodd's appeal. It is his position that a person must exhibit one of the psychotic reactions as classified by the American Psychiatric Association before he may be considered mentally ill. Absent a classified psychosis, one may not be committed and confined. A sociopath (defined in the testimony as a disorder of personality affecting the ethical and moral senses) like Dodd, (and all the evidence is in accord that Dodd is, indeed, a sociopath), does not fall within any of the classified psychotic reactions and, therefore, may not be institutionalized. So it is that we are urged to fashion a definition for the words "mentally ill" and thereby fill the void in the statutory hospital law. It is suggested that we confine mental illness to the psychotic reactions as classified by the American Psychiatric Association. We are wholly unable to follow that suggestion. The record before us shows that the psychiatrists who testified do not agree on the statutory meaning of "mentally ill." Further, the record reflects that psychiatrists in general are at war over the propriety of the classifications of psychosis as specified by the American Psychiatric Association. We seriously doubt that the legislature ever intended medical classifications to be the sole guide for judicial commitment. The judicial inquiry is not to be limited so as to exclude the totality of circumstances involved in the particular case before the court. Recidivism, repeated acts of violence, the failure to respond to conventional penal and rehabilitative measures, and public safety, are additional and relevant considerations for the court in deciding whether a person is mentally ill. The assistance of medical examination and opinion is a necessary concomitant of the court hearing, but the court alone is invested with the power of decision. That power is to be exercised within the permissible limits of judicial discretion.

Here the record demonstrates a combination of things which should, and did, unquestionably, influence the lower court to enter the order it did. Dodd, an 18 year old, was shown, by testing, to have the intelligence quotient of a high grade moron. All agree that he is a sociopath almost devoid of moral sense. He has been proven, at least to

a. NRS 433.310 provides:

"1. Whenever a person legally adjudged to be mentally ill is deemed by the court or the superintendent to be a menace to public safety, and the court is satisfied that the facilities at the hospital are inadequate to keep such mentally ill person safely confined, the court may, upon application of the superintendent, commit such person to the Nevada state prison. The person shall be confined in the Nevada state prison until the further order of the committing court either transferring him to the hospital or declaring him to be no longer mentally ill.

date, wholly unresponsive to either penal or rehabilitative measures,[b] nor does he give promise of response to available probation services or psychiatric treatment. He possesses homicidal tendencies, and is dangerous. Finally, one of the testifying psychiatrists stated that Dodd is mentally ill within the intendment of the statute. In these circumstances the lower court did not abuse its discretion in denying habeas relief and ordering that Dodd be transferred to the Nevada State Prison for confinement.

Affirmed.

Questions and Comments

1. *Mental illness and police power commitments.* Aside from provisions excluding mental retardation and conditions resulting from drug or alcohol abuse, few civil commitment statutes are very precise in their definitions of mental illness. None of the definitions distinguish between police power and parens patriae commitment. Some, like Alabama and Arkansas, do not define mental illness at all. Many provide a definition which is almost tautological. Under Texas' civil commitment statute, for instance, a mentally ill person is "a person whose mental health is substantially impaired." Vernon's Ann. Texas Civ.Stat. § 5547–4(k). Similarly, Florida defines mental illness as a "mental, emotional or behavioral disorder which substantially impairs the person's mental health." West's Fla.Stat.Ann. § 394.455(3). Most state laws contain language similar to that found in New Mexico's statute: "Mental disorder means the substantial disorder of the person's emotional processes, thought or cognition which grossly impairs judgment, behavior or capacity to recognize reality." N.M.Stat.Ann. 1979, § 43–1–3(N).

Judicial interpretation of these standards varies. Probably the most controversial issue connected with the definition of mental illness in police power commitment is that posed in *Dodd*—whether the definition should include sociopathy (also known as antisocial personality disorder). What are the implications of the holding in *Dodd?* Why do you think the superintendent of the Nevada State Hospital was arguing that Dodd was *not* mentally ill? Assuming Dodd was mentally ill, should it be permissible to transfer him from the hospital to the state prison, as provided by NRS 433.310?

The Supreme Court of Minnesota has held that an antisocial personality is not within the definition of mental illness unless the individual has "lost the ability to control his actions." *Johnson v. Noot,* 323 N.W.2d 724, 727 (Minn.1982). Arizona's statute excludes from the definition of mental disorder "[c]haracter and personality disorders characterized by lifelong and deeply ingrained anti-social behavior patterns, including sexual behaviors which are abnormal and prohibited by statute unless the behavior

---

b. He experienced trouble with the police when eight years old. He was placed in the Elko Boys School from 1960–1962. While there he fought frequently. He escaped. While loose he hit an elderly man on the head with a crowbar, covered him with kerosene or gas, and set him on fire. He was then sent to Preston, California, a prison for hardcore youth criminals. In 1963 he was committed to the Nevada State Hospital, from which he "eloped" on four separate occasions.

results from a mental disorder." Ariz.Rev.Stat. § 36–501(1)(c). Is either of these a better approach than *Dodd's?* In general, how should mental illness be defined for police power commitments? If the only referent of mental illness is behavior, why should statutes make *any* explicit reference to mental illness?

2. *Incapacity and police power commitment.* The American Psychiatric Association's Model Law for civil commitment permits commitment of the dangerous mentally ill but only upon a showing that the person lacks "capacity to make an informed decision concerning treatment." Stromberg & Stone, "A Model State Law on Civil Commitment of the Mentally Ill," 20 Harv.J.Leg. 275, 301 (1982). A few states also appear to have adopted such a requirement. See, e.g., Wyo.Stat. 1977, 25–10–101(a)(viii). Is this type of restriction on the effect of mental illness required in the context of police power commitments? Advisable?

3. *Causation.* Most state statutes require proof that the person's dangerousness is "caused by" or is "the result of" mental illness before commitment may occur. Does this requirement follow from the purported rationales of police power commitment? If so, is the Nevada statute under which Dodd was committed invalid on its face? Assuming sociopathy is a mental illness for purposes of civil commitment, was Dodd's dangerousness "caused" by his mental illness?

b. *Defining Danger to Others.*

LESSARD v. SCHMIDT

United States District Court, E.D. Wisconsin, 1972.
349 F.Supp. 1078.

SPRECHER, CIRCUIT JUDGE.

* * *

Wisconsin defines "mental illness" as "mental disease to such extent that a person so afflicted requires care and treatment for his own welfare, or the welfare of others, or of the community." Wis.Stat. Ann. § 51.75, Art. II(f) (1971 Supp.). Interpreting § 51.02(5) in the light of this provision in Humphrey v. Cady, 405 U.S. 504, 509, 92 S.Ct. 1048, 1052, 31 L.Ed.2d 394 (1972), the Supreme Court noted (in dicta) that implicit in this definition is the requirement that a person's "potential for doing harm, to himself or to others, is great enough to justify such a massive curtailment of liberty." In other words, the statute itself requires a finding of "dangerousness" to self or others in order to deprive an individual of his or her freedom. The Court did not directly address itself to the degree of dangerousness that is constitutionally required before a person may be involuntarily deprived of liberty. However, its approval of a requirement that the potential for doing harm be "*great enough* to justify such a *massive curtailment* of liberty" implies a balancing test in which the state must bear the burden of proving that there is an extreme likelihood that if the person is not confined he will do immediate harm to himself or others. Although attempts to predict future conduct are always difficult, and confinement based upon such a prediction must always be viewed with suspicion, we believe civil confinement can be justified in some cases if the proper burden of proof is satisfied and dangerousness is based upon a finding of a recent overt act, attempt or threat to do substantial harm to oneself or another.

* * *

ALEXANDER BROOKS, DANGEROUSNESS DEFINED IN LAW, PSYCHIATRY & MENTAL HEALTH SYSTEMS 680.
(1974).

* * *

Definitions of what is "dangerous" tend to be as diverse as the views of individual judges, courts, and jurisdictions. It may be that persons committed on the basis that they are "dangerous" need not be, and would not be, if the term were more carefully defined and its component elements identified, even if those elements could not be evaluated with a high degree of accuracy or quantification. A more rigorous analysis, if not too cumbersome, might well result in more sophisticated judicial decision-making.

The term "dangerous" can be broken down into at least four component elements: (1) magnitude of harm; (2) probability that the harm will occur; (3) frequency with which the harm will occur; (4) imminence of the harm.

To call a person "dangerous" is to express a judgment in the form of a prediction about his potential behavior. A person can be characterized as "dangerous" or not, depending on a balancing of these four components. For example, a harm which is not likely to occur, but which is very serious, may add up to "dangerousness." By the same token, a relatively trivial harm which is highly likely to occur with great frequency might also add up to dangerousness. On the other hand, a trivial harm, even though it is likely to occur, might not add up to dangerousness.

* * *

MATTER OF GREGOROVICH [*]
Court of Appeal, First District, 1980.
89 Ill.App.3d 528, 44 Ill.Dec. 615, 411 N.E.2d 981.

LORENZ, JUSTICE:

This is an appeal by respondent from an order entered in the circuit court of Cook County, finding her to be a person subject to involuntary admission under the provisions of the Mental Health and Developmental Disabilities Code. (Ill.Rev.Stat.1979, ch. 91½, pars. 1–100 et seq., 1–119.) * * *

On May 9, 1979, respondent's mother, Celia Gregorovich filed a petition for involuntary judicial admission, alleging that respondent was reasonably expected to inflict serious physical harm upon herself or another in the near future and was unable to provide for her basic physical needs so as to guard herself from serious harm and that she was in need of immediate admission for the prevention of such harm. The petition alleged that respondent had threatened to harm herself and her mother after she had cut all the cords to the electrical lamps and television.

The following pertinent evidence was adduced at the hearing on May 9, 1979.

Celia Gregorovich

Her husband, respondent's father, had been sick for 7 years with Parkinson's Disease and had been hospitalized since January 1979. Respondent, who was 21 years of age, blamed her mother for her father's illness, started talking to herself and would not eat. About a month earlier, when respondent cursed her, she struck respondent with a broom, and respondent then scratched her hand with her nails. The scratch marks took 3 weeks to heal. When she asked respondent to lower the television volume, respondent cut the television wires with scissors. Respondent then held the scissors in her fist, with the point sticking out, and pointed them at her mother, who was about 2 or 3 feet away. When respondent put down the scissors, Mrs. Gregorovich called the police. On cross-examination, she testified she did not have to seek medical attention when respondent scratched her hands, and respondent had never physically harmed her before this or tried to hurt herself. She further indicated respondent took care of herself at home and was very clean and neat about herself.

Gregory Nooney, mental health worker at Northwestern Hospital

Respondent, who was hospitalized at Northwestern, said she would not change her clothes until she went to court because that would prove she was not crazy; she slept in her clothes and had not bathed although she was eating. Respondent told him she knew that mental patients often had symptoms similar to ESP and she wanted to prove that she had ESP and that she was not crazy. On cross-examination, he testified respondent had never attacked any other patient on the hospital unit or caused any physical harm to anyone.

Dr. David Altman, a Board Certified Psychiatrist

He examined respondent on May 4, 1979. Respondent was sitting on the couch, moving her mouth and gesturing toward the television set which was turned on. When he was introduced to her, respondent yelled at him, then turned back toward the television set and continued to gesture toward it. When he attempted to engage her in a conversation, she moved to another part of the room and continued to face the television and gesture toward it. When he saw that respondent was becoming more upset, he told her he would stop, and respondent became calm and laughed in the direction of the television set. This process was repeated during the day on May 4. He also observed respondent in front of the television on other occasions when she would at times be watching the television with other patients, moving her mouth and occasionally making gestures. He spoke to her again the morning of the hearing, May 9, when respondent was again in front of the television set. She told him she did not want to talk to him, and the only information he was able to obtain from the interview was that respondent believed that it was dangerous for her to be in the hospital and that she would gain more ESP power from other patients and this would be dangerous. When he asked her to elaborate, respondent said that she would explain it to the judge.

In his opinion, based on information he received from other members of the staff and based on his contact with respondent, she was suffering from an acute schizophrenic episode, a mental illness involving auditory and visual hallucinations. He believed she was under a delusion, a fixed false belief, since she thought she had the power to control peoples' minds and read other persons' minds. He concluded that respondent would be unable to take care of her basic physical needs and protect herself against physical injury based on the fact that she cut the electrical wires prior to admission, that she was quite hostile, that she refused a physical examination and routine laboratory work upon admission because it would somehow prejudice her case, that she thinks she has extra sensory powers rather than having a mental illness, and that she had not bathed and was "essentially not caring for herself in a manner which she would need to do in order to be released." He recommended that she continue to be hospitalized although she had not inflicted injury on herself or anyone else in the hospital.

* * *

Dr. Sydney Wright, licensed Physician and Psychiatric Resident at Northwestern Memorial Hospital

He examined respondent on May 3, 1979. Respondent told him she felt she was being brought into the hospital against her will. In an effort to demonstrate her dissatisfaction about being brought to the hospital, she kicked a police officer when she was being escorted to Northwestern Hospital. Respondent told this doctor that she had received ESP powers, but that people doubted that she had these powers. She said she had been involved in a power struggle with another person called Jeffery who had ESP and lived in Philadelphia and who had sent her ESP messages that he loved her; but she subsequently became aware of the fact that he wished to harm her and became involved in an ESP power struggle with him in which he attempted to kill her. She believed her ESP powers may have killed Jeffery since she had not recently heard from him.

Respondent also told him she had cut the television cord because God had told her to do so, and she became convinced that a university was "bugging" her house and was receiving information about her activities which would end if she cut the cord. She also stated that she was going to kill her mother.

In his opinion, respondent was suffering from a mental illness and would be unable to take care of her basic physical needs or protect herself against physical injury. Dr. Wright also noted that respondent showed gross disorganization of her thought processes characterized by concrete thinking, a looseness of association, and a marked pressure of speech. When asked if she might intentionally or unintentionally harm others, he answered, "I believe that is a possibility based on her statements to me." When asked if she was more likely than not to harm herself or others without further treatment, he related another episode which occurred the day following hospitalization. When the nurse assigned to work with respondent approached respondent, she told her she was a whore and would have nothing to do with her.

When he was again asked if it was more likely than not without further treatment that respondent might intentionally or unintentionally harm someone within a reasonable time, Dr. Wright responded: "Well, it is very difficult for me to predict the future. I would say there is a possibility she could harm someone." He recommended that respondent remain in the hospital for continued treatment. This course of action was based on respondent's statements to him that she believed her powers were sufficient to kill another individual, that she wanted to kill her mother and that she had an "aggressive and hostile stance toward specific staff members." He concluded, "I would say there is a possibility she could injure someone."

Respondent, on her own Behalf

She would get out-patient treatment if she were discharged. On cross-examination, when asked why she would not accept out-patient treatment at Northwestern Hospital, respondent explained that she was not told why she was there and that she was taken there forcibly even though she did not do anything violent. When asked if she needed any help from a mental point of view, she answered, "Possible, but I don't think so, I just need someone to talk to." She admitted she had "mental problems" in the past but had "got over it." When asked if there was anything currently wrong, she mentioned her mother saying, "but, if you knew my mother you would understand."

OPINION

Section 1–119 of the Mental Health and Developmental Disabilities Code (Ill.Rev.Stat.1979, ch. 91½, par. 1–119) defines persons subject to involuntary admission as:

    "(1) A person who is mentally ill and who because of his illness is reasonably expected to inflict serious physical harm upon himself or another in the near future; or

    (2) . . . who because of his illness is unable to provide for his basic physical needs so as to guard himself from serious harm."

The State is required to prove that respondent is a person subject to involuntary admission by clear and convincing evidence. Respondent argues she was not proven to be a person subject to involuntary commitment in that it was not established that she was unable to provide for her basic physical needs so as to guard herself from serious harm. The State does not address this argument in its brief; however, we do not consider the evidence establishes respondent was unable to take care of her basic physical needs so as to guard herself from physical harm.

Respondent also argues there was insufficient evidence that she was reasonably expected in the near future to inflict serious physical harm upon herself or another. For reasons set forth below we conclude that the evidence presented in this case was clear and convincing that respondent was mentally ill and because of this was reasonably expected to inflict serious physical harm upon another person in the near future.[1]

* * *

We first conclude that the uncontradicted expert medical evidence, which was supported by the lay testimony, clearly and convincingly established respondent was "mentally ill." Respondent's assertion that she merely had powers of extra sensory perception, given evidence to the contrary, is unconvincing.

In *People v. Sansone* (1974), 18 Ill.App.3d 315, 326, 309 N.E.2d 733, this court held that the State must prove the person is in need of mental treatment by means of a medical opinion which is clear and convincing and which is based upon facts which are established by clear and convincing evidence. Thus, we held both (1) that the facts upon which the medical opinion was based must be established by clear and convincing evidence, and (2) that the medical opinion, itself, must be clear and convincing. * * *

In this case, we find Dr. Wright's testimony, when considered along with the evidence of previous dangerous conduct, was sufficiently clear and convincing evidence that respondent was reasonably expected to inflict serious physical harm upon another in the near future. Respondent's actions including scratching her mother on the hand during an altercation and holding a pair of scissors a few feet from her mother on the occasion which led to her emergency hospitalization are supportive of this conclusion. The latter conduct was a serious threat which (apart from the issue of criminal intent), could constitute an aggravated assault.

Obviously, her mother felt threatened, since she immediately called police. Respondent, in cross-examining her mother through her attorney, attempted to show that although respondent at this time had the opportunity to harm her mother, she did not do so, and she repeats this argument here. However, the statute [does] not require the infliction of actual harm before commitment was authorized. Other evidence, including respondent's admissions and her own testimony, established respondent's continuing hostility, particularly toward her mother. Respondent in fact threatened to kill her mother following her hospitaliza-

1. We do not therefore, find it necessary to consider whether the evidence was sufficient to show she was likely to harm herself[.]

tion on an emergency basis, and it is apparent that respondent's hostility toward her mother increased following her hospitalization. Respondent in her testimony blamed her present difficulties on her mother. Respondent had the opportunity, when she testified, to explain the incident with the scissors, but she failed to do so.

* * *

Respondent would have us focus narrowly on Dr. Wright's use of the term "possibly" in evaluating his testimony, to show it was of an equivocal nature. A similar opinion was found not to be a clear and convincing medical opinion of the type required in *Sansone*. *People v. Bradley*. In *Bradley*, the expert witness phrased his opinion in terms of "conceivably," rather than "possibly." However, this requirement has been somewhat relaxed in subsequent cases especially when there is clear evidence of prior dangerous conduct or strong lay evidence. This court has upheld commitment orders under resembling circumstances in which there was no explicit medical opinion regarding the patient's future dangerous conduct, but where there was evidence of actual prior dangerous conduct and other evidence such as lay opinion. After considering the doctor's entire testimony together with the other evidence presented, we conclude that there was sufficient evidence in the present case to show respondent's dangerous propensities.

IN INTEREST OF NYFLOT
Supreme Court of North Dakota, 1983.
340 N.W.2d 178.

GIERKE, JUSTICE.

This is an appeal by the respondent, Cynthia Jewel Nyflot, from an Order for Hospitalization and Treatment Following Treatment Hearing entered in the County Court of Cass County on September 14, 1983. We affirm.

* * *

The respondent's fourth contention is that the facts do not support the conclusion that the respondent is a person requiring treatment because she did not present a serious risk of harm, as defined by § 25–03.1–02(11), N.D.C.C.

The court found as a fact that:

". . . on August 29 and September 2, 1983, the respondent started two separate fires in the women's bathroom at the dormitory and that on one of those occasions a great amount of smoke escaped from the bathroom causing personnel to check into the bathroom where the respondent was found by herself in her pajamas; . . ."

Respondent contends that because these fires amounted to little property damage, due to the fact that the bathrooms where the fires were started were virtually inflammable, there was no substantial likelihood that significant property damage or bodily harm could have resulted to the respondent or others as a result of the fires. The statute, however, is not concerned with harm which occurred in the past except as it establishes a potential for serious harm by future behavior of the respondent acting in conformity with previous conduct. The respondent testified that she started the fires to gain attention and to dramatize the fact that she did not want to be in the institution. She also testified that it was not her intent to harm anyone, including herself, and that she felt that there was no likelihood of such harm under the circumstances. Her subjective intentions and assessment of the likelihood of harm, however, do not alter the fact that she was willing to start fires to attract attention to herself. Absent compelling evidence to the contrary, it is a mere fortuity that more damage was not done or that the respondent suffered no ill effects from the smoke produced.

Other undisputed facts further support the conclusion that the respondent presented a serious risk of harm. She rolled lit cigarettes under the door of another patient's room. When the attendants attempted to take her cigarette lighter away from her, she concealed it in her vagina. She cut the screen on a window, using wire cutters which had been smuggled into the institution to her by a friend and, when discovered, she hid the wire cutters in her panties. We believe that these facts clearly support the court's determination that the respondent presented a serious risk of harm to herself, to others, and to property.

For the reasons stated in the opinion, the order of the county court is affirmed.

ERICKSTAD, C.J., and PEDERSON, VANDEWALLE and SAND, JJ., concur.

WHALEY v. JANSEN

District Court of Appeal, Fourth District, California, 1962.
208 Cal.App.2d 222, 25 Cal.Rptr. 184.

[Whaley brought a civil action against the city of San Diego, the police of that city, and two psychiatrists, among others, alleging false arrest and false imprisonment. According to the court]:

Plaintiff alleges generally that on May 29, 1959, while he was going from house to house in San Diego "exposing wrong-doers in government," he carried with him a letter entitled, "A MOST APPALLING CONDITION," which letter outlined his grievances and requested the use of the home to call in the neighbors and friends so he could deliver a lecture and obtain voluntary contributions from them to carry on his work; that about noon he was walking on the sidewalk in a residential district when defendant Officer Ludvigson stopped him and questioned him; that plaintiff told Officer Ludvigson what he had been doing and the officer asked him to get into the patrol car and talk and that plaintiff walked away; that the officer told him that if he walked away he would place him under arrest; that plaintiff continued walking away from the officer and the officer stated, "You're under arrest for vagrancy"; that plaintiff was forced into the car and literature was removed from his pocket with such titles as "A MOST APPALLING

CONDITION, KIDNAPPED AND RAILROADED TO THE BUG HOUSE," and "Earl Warren a Travesty of Equal Justice Under the Law"; that after reading the articles and talking to plaintiff, Officer Ludvigson transported plaintiff to the police station and plaintiff remained in the car while the officer went to the office; that Officer Ludvigson returned and asked plaintiff if he had a permit to solicit and plaintiff answered that he had none because he was not soliciting money; that the officer then went back and in a few minutes returned with another officer and they took plaintiff to the county psychiatric unit; that plaintiff told them that they had no right to do this and attempted to walk away from them and Officer Drake took him into the psychiatric unit; that he was there interviewed by Dr. Reed and plaintiff demanded of the doctor that he be released; that the doctor replied that he had no authority to do so and that plaintiff's release would have to be effected through defendants Dr. Wiend or Dr. Lengyel; that on June 1, 1959, these two doctors interviewed plaintiff and on June 3, 1959, without being formally charged with a crime or mental illness, he was released.

* * *

Sufficient facts are recited in the complaint to justify the officer's belief that plaintiff was so mentally ill as to be likely to cause injury to himself or others and to require medical care or restraint.

Questions and Comments

1. *Typical state statutes; vagueness doctrine.* Many state statutes, like *Lessard* and the California statute at issue in *Whaley*, do not identify the type of danger to others that must be manifested in order to justify commitment. For instance, Alaska requires a showing that the person be "likely to injure others." Alaska Code § 47.30.735. California's Lanterman-Petris-Short Act, enacted seven years after the *Whaley* decision, merely requires proof of a potential for "substantial, physical harm to others." Cal.Welf. & Inst.Code § 5304. Even the most elaborate statutes provide little more by way of definition. For example, in Massachusetts the relevant criterion permits commitment upon a showing of "a substantial risk of physical harm to other persons as manifested by evidence of homicidal or other violent behavior or evidence that others are placed in reasonable fear of violent behavior and serious physical harm to them." Mass.St., c. 356, § 3.

Should commitment statutes be more specific, as is usually the case with the criminal law? To answer this question, some understanding of the void-for-vagueness doctrine might be useful. The doctrine developed in the nineteenth century as a means of judicially monitoring the precision of the criminal law. Two rationales are advanced to support it. The first is that ambiguous language fails to give potential violators fair warning of the conduct that is criminal. The second, more important, rationale is that such language allows law enforcement officials, the jury and the courts, rather than duly elected legislators, to decide at their whim the type of conduct that will be defined as criminal.

Although the doctrine is potentially quite broad in its reach, given the imprecision found in many statutes, it has been applied sparingly. Most of the laws that the Supreme Court has found unconstitutional on vagueness grounds impinged upon "fundamental" interests, such as freedom of expression, or were perceived to be vehicles for harassment of minority groups or the poor. See, e.g., *N.A.A.C.P. v. Button*, 371 U.S. 415, 83 S.Ct. 328, 9 L.Ed.2d 405 (1963); *Coates v. City of Cincinnati*, 402 U.S. 611, 91 S.Ct. 1686, 29 L.Ed.2d 214 (1971); *Kolender v. Lawson*, 461 U.S. 352, 103 S.Ct. 1855, 75 L.Ed.2d 903 (1983). In *Papachristou v. City of Jacksonville*, 405 U.S. 156, 92 S.Ct. 839, 31 L.Ed.2d 110 (1972), for instance, the Supreme Court considered a municipal ordinance which classified as "vagrants," among others, "rogues and vagabonds, or dissolute persons who go about begging . . . common drunkards, . . . lewd, wanton and lascivious persons, . . . persons wandering or strolling around from place to place without any lawful purpose or object, habitual loafers, disorderly persons, [and] . . . persons able to work but habitually living upon the earnings of their wives or minor children. . . ." In striking down this statute on vagueness grounds, and reversing the convictions of two white women and two black men found driving on the main thoroughfare of Jacksonville, the Court stated:

> Those generally implicated by the imprecise terms of the ordinance—poor people, non-conformists, dissenters, idlers—may be required to comport themselves according to the lifestyle deemed appropriate by the Jacksonville police and the courts. Where, as here, there are no standards governing the exercise of the discretion granted by the ordinance, the scheme permits and encourages an arbitrary and discriminatory enforcement of the law. . . . It results in a regime in which the poor and the unpopular are permitted to "stand on a public sidewalk . . . only at the whim of any police officer." . . . Under this ordinance, "[I]f some carefree type of fellow is satisfied to work just so much, and no more, as will pay for one square meal, some wine, and a flophouse daily, but a court thinks this kind of living subhuman, the fellow can be forced to raise his sights or go to jail as a vagrant."

> . . . Of course, vagrancy statutes are useful to the police. Of course, they are nets making easy the roundup of so-called undesirables. But the rule of law implies equality and justice in its application. Vagrancy laws of the Jacksonville type teach that the scales of justice are so tipped that even-handed administration of the law is not possible. The rule of law, evenly applied to minorities as well as majorities, to the poor as well as the rich, is the great mucilage that holds society together.

When a statute does not "chill" fundamental rights or create the type of problem described in *Papachristou*, it is less likely to be found vague, even if the language is very ambiguous. See, e.g., *Nash v. United States*, 229 U.S. 373, 33 S.Ct. 780, 57 L.Ed. 1232 (1913) (upholding a provision in the Sherman Antitrust Act which makes illegal "[e]very contract, combination in the form of trust or otherwise, or conspiracy in restraint of trade or commerce," so long as it is interpreted to prohibit only "undue" restraints of trade). Moreover, the Supreme Court has indicated that a statute is less likely to be declared void for vagueness if more precise language would be difficult to produce. *United States v. Petrillo*, 332 U.S. 1, 67 S.Ct. 1538, 91 L.Ed. 1877 (1947).

In light of this caselaw, consider the following excerpt from Dershowitz, "Dangerousness as a Criterion for Confinement," 11 Bull.Amer.Acad. Psychiat. & Law 172 (1974):

> The initial and fundamental question which must be asked by any system authorizing incarceration is: which harms are sufficiently serious to justify resort to this rather severe sanction. This question is asked and answered in the criminal law by the substantive definitions of crime. Thus, homicide is a harm which justifies the sanction of imprisonment; miscegenation does not; and adultery is a close case about which reasonable people may, and do, disagree. It is difficult to conceive of a criminal process which did not make some effort at articulating these distinctions. Imagine, for example, a penal code which simply made it an imprisonable crime to cause injury to self or others, without defining injury. It is also difficult to conceive of a criminal process—at least in jurisdictions with an Anglo–American tradition—in which these distinctions were not drawn by the legislature or courts. It would seem beyond dispute that the question of which harms do, and which do not, justify incarceration is a legal— indeed a political decision, to be made not by experts, but by the constitutional authorized agents of the people. Again, try to imagine a penal code which authorized incarceration for anyone who performed an act regarded as injurious by a designated expert, say a psychiatrist or penologist.

> To be sure there are differences between the criminal and the civil commitment processes: the criminal law is supposed to punish people for having committed harmful acts in the past: whereas civil commitment is supposed to prevent people from committing harmful acts in the future. While this difference may have important implications in some contexts, it would seem entirely irrelevant in deciding which acts are sufficiently harmful to justify incarceration either as an after-the-fact punitive sanction or as a before-the-fact preventive sanction. The considerations which require clear definition of such harms in the criminal process would seem to be fully applicable to the civil commitment process.

Do you agree that the differences between the criminal law and civil commitment are "entirely irrelevant in deciding which acts are sufficiently harmful to justify" commitment? If so, why not draft a civil commitment statute which defines danger to others by incorporating the criminal code? A person would be considered dangerous to others if he or she is likely to commit an act that has been criminalized. Is the criminal code too narrow for this purpose? Too broad?

2. *Magnitude of harm.* Although Brooks' four-factor analysis of dangerousness (excerpted above) does not answer these questions, it is helpful and will be used as an organizing device in these notes, beginning with the first factor, magnitude of harm. Assuming the validity of police power commitment, homicide or serious bodily injury would presumably be a

harm the state may act to prevent. For what other types of predicted harms may the state deprive one of liberty?

Minor physical injury. Should the type of injury suffered by the mother of Gregorovich be sufficient to justify commitment, if we could predict accurately that it would occur again? Note that the assault statutes in most states require "bodily injury" for the result element of that crime. See, e.g., Model Penal Code § 211.1. Under the Model Penal Code, this term is defined as "physical pain, illness, or any impairment of physical condition." Model Penal Code § 210.0(2).

Non-physical danger to others. A few states explicitly permit commitment if the court finds that a person may cause "emotional" or "psychic" harm to others. For instance, the Iowa law authorizes commitment of a mentally ill individual who is "likely to inflict serious emotional injury on members of his or her family or others who lack reasonable opportunity to avoid contact with the afflicted person if the afflicted person is allowed to remain at liberty without treatment." Iowa Code Ann. § 229.1(2)(b).

The criminal law contains provisions that are analogous. For instance, the Model Penal Code includes a crime called "harassment" which is defined as follows:

> A person commits a petty misdemeanor if, with purpose to harass another, he: (a) makes a telephone call without purpose of legitimate communication; or (b) insults, taunts or challenges another in a manner likely to provoke violent or disorderly response; or (c) makes repeated communications anonymously or at extremely inconvenient hours, or in offensively coarse language; or (d) engages in any other course of harmful conduct serving no legitimate purpose of the actor.

Model Penal Code § 250.4. Professor Feinberg has tried to justify such criminal law provisions with reference to what he calls the "offense" principle, which he distinguishes from the "harm" principle, the latter being the primary justification for criminalizing behavior. In Feinberg's view, the state may penalize seriously offensive behavior, even though it does not cause physical harm. Borrowing from nuisance theory in tort, he attempts to provide some guidelines for evaluating the offensiveness of behavior:

> The seriousness of the offensiveness would be determined by (1) the intensity and durability of the repugnance produced, and the extent to which repugnance could be anticipated to be the general reaction of strangers to the conduct displayed or represented (conduct offensive only to persons with an abnormal susceptibility to offense would not count as *very* offensive); (2) the ease with which unwilling witnesses can avoid the offensive displays; and (3) whether or not the witnesses have willingly assumed the risk of being offended either through curiosity or the anticipation of pleasure. . . .

> These factors would be weighed as a group against the reasonableness of the offending party's conduct as determined by (1) its personal importance to the actors themselves and its social value generally, remembering always the enormous social utility of unhampered expression (in those cases where expression is involved); (2) the availabil-

ity of alternative times and places where the conduct in question would cause less offense; (3) the extent, if any, to which the offense is caused with spiteful motives.

Feinberg, Offense to Others 26 (1985). Should this type of analysis be applied to the civil commitment context? How would you apply it to *Whaley*? To Case 24 on p. 608?

Danger to property. Some states also include harm to "property" as a commitment criterion. In *Suzuki v. Yuen*, 617 F.2d 173 (9th Cir.1980), the Ninth Circuit Court of Appeals found such a provision in Hawaii's statute unconstitutionally broad. It stated:

> We need not decide whether a state may ever commit one who is dangerous to property. This statute would allow commitment for danger to any property regardless of value or significance. . . . Under the current Hawaii definition of 'danger to property,' a person could be committed if he threatened to shoot a trespassing dog. The state's interest in protecting animals must be outweighed by the individual's interest in personal liberty.

Do you agree? How can the state legislature retain danger to property as a criterion for commitment while avoiding the court's prohibition?

3. *Frequency of harm.* No state statute makes explicit a requirement that the factfinder assess the frequency of the anticipated harm, perhaps because, as the excerpt from Feinberg illustrates, frequency is an integral part of the magnitude-of-harm analysis. On the assumption that they are treatable, consider the committability of the persons in the following hypotheticals:

A: An "exhibitionist" who on several occasions has given in to difficult-to-resist urges to expose himself to others, but who never flashes the same person twice.

B: A person who suffers from Gilles La Tourette syndrome, which causes him to utter repeatedly obscenities such as "fuck, fuck, fuck" while walking down the street.

C: A man who, while muttering to himself, has masturbated on a bus on one occasion. The diagnosis is senile dementia.

4. *Probability of harm.* As noted earlier, the Supreme Court has held that, under the due process clause of the federal constitution, the criteria for civil commitment must be proven by clear and convincing evidence, a standard of proof below the criminal reasonable doubt standard and above the preponderance of the evidence standard used in most civil trials. A few states have opted for the higher reasonable doubt standard. See Superintendent Worcester State Hospital v. Hagberg, 374 Mass. 271, 372 N.E.2d 242 (1978); see also, Hawaii Rev.Stat. § 334–60(b)(4)(1); Lausche v. Commissioner of Public Welfare, 302 Minn. 65, 225 N.W.2d 366 (1974), cert. denied 420 U.S. 993, 95 S.Ct. 1430, 43 L.Ed.2d 674 (1975).

Also noted earlier was the debate over whether dangerousness to others can ever be proven by clear and convincing evidence, much less the reasonable doubt standard. Monahan and Wexler have contended that this debate misses the point, because it does not take into account the typical definition of dangerousness. Many statutes require only that the state prove the person is "likely" or "probable" or "more likely than not" dangerous to others. Quantifying the matter, these statutes could be said to define "dangerousness" as a 51% chance that the person will harm someone in the future. Assuming that proof by clear and convincing evidence correlates with a 75% degree of certainty, these states only require a showing of something like a 38% chance that the person will harm others in the future. Monahan & Wexler, "A Definite Maybe: Proof and Probability in Civil Commitment," 2 Law & Hum.Beh. 37 (1978). In those jurisdictions which use the "more-likely-than-not" standard, is commitment of a person based on a 38% chance of harmful behavior justifiable?

5. *Imminence requirement.* *Lessard* and the statutes of most states prohibit commitment as dangerous to others unless the danger is "imminent." Should this be a requirement? If so, should it be made more specific (e.g., within the next two weeks, within the next two days) or should its definition depend upon the other factors discussed above?

c. *The Overt Act Requirement.*

PEOPLE v. SANSONE

Appellate Court of Illinois, 1974.
18 Ill.App.3d 315, 309 N.E.2d 733.

STAMOS, JUSTICE.

* * *

Initially, respondent argues that to sustain a finding of likelihood of injury to respondent or others, proof of prior dangerous conduct must be adduced, and in the absence of such proof, civil commitment is preventive detention. Respondent asserts that, pursuant to the theory of Robinson v. California, 370 U.S. 660, 82 S.Ct. 1417, 8 L.Ed.2d 758, confinement based upon a prediction of future dangerous conduct is confinement based upon status. Respondent relies upon Cross v. Harris, 135 U.S.App.D.C. 259, 418 F.2d 1095 and Lessard v. Schmidt, 349 F.Supp. 1078 (E.D.Wis.) for the proposition that a prediction of future dangerousness must be based upon documented prior overt acts or threats.

* * *

In the area of mental health law, the State must balance the curtailment of liberty against the danger of harm to the individual or others. The paramount factor is the interest of society which naturally includes the interest of the patient in not being subjected to unjustified confinement. We agree with respondent that the "science" of predicting future dangerous behavior is inexact, and certainly is not infallible. We also agree that the mere establishment of a mental problem is not an adequate basis upon which to confine a person who has never harmed or attempted to harm either himself or another. However, we are of the opinion that a decision to commit based upon a medical opinion which clearly states that a person is reasonably expected to engage in dangerous conduct, and which is based upon the experience and studies of qualified psychiatrists, is a determination which properly can be made by the State.

Moreover, we cannot agree that commitment in the absence of evidence of prior harmful conduct is preventive detention based upon the patient's status as a mentally ill person. Again, we reiterate that a finding must be based upon an explicit medical opinion regarding the patient's future conduct, and cannot be based upon a mere finding of mental illness. Secondly, the purpose of the Mental Health Code is to provide treatment, and in fact, the Code affords every patient the right to treatment. This is a very different situation from that in Robinson v. California, supra, wherein the Court held that a law which imprisons a person afflicted with a disease inflicts cruel and unusual punishment. The Court in *Robinson* distinguished criminal punishment and detention from detention based upon laws which require medical treatment. 370 U.S. 660, 666, 82 S.Ct. 1417, 8 L.Ed.2d 758. Therefore, we hold that a finding of "in need of mental treatment," absent evidence of prior harmful conduct, is not *per se* violative of due process.

* * *

In the instant case, respondent's delusions regarding law enforcement and law enforcement officers were established without contradiction by the testimony of the psychiatrist and the social worker, both of whom interviewed respondent on two different occasions. The medical opinion was that respondent believed that persons were "after him," and that respondent could be dangerous to others. The psychiatrist testified that persons he had known with the same type of delusions had injured or attempted to injure others. Therefore, although the psychiatrist could not give any degree of probability of dangerousness, and although there was no evidence of prior dangerous conduct, the uncontradicted testimony established by clear and convincing evidence that respondent was in need of mental treatment.

IN MATTER OF MENTAL HEALTH OF D.R.S.

Supreme Court of Montana, 1986.
221 Mont. 245, 718 P.2d 335.

[D.R.S. was committed under a statute which required the state to show that he was "suffering from a mental disorder which has resulted in . . . injury to others or the imminent threat thereof. . . ." The statute defined injury to mean "physical injury," Mont.Code Ann. 53–21–102(14), and provided that imminent threat of injury to others "shall be evidenced by overt acts, sufficiently recent in time as to be material and relevant as to the respondent's present condition." Mont. Code Ann. 53–21–126(2). The sole overt act proven by the state was an armed robbery for which D.R.S. was not convicted. As described by the Montana Supreme Court, D.R.S. and another person "committed the robbery" on November 5, 1982. In the course of the robbery, they took the store clerk behind a woodpile by the store, taped him up, covered him with wood and left him in the cold. The clerk identified D.R.S. as the person who taped him and stated that the other person threatened to shoot him if he didn't tell them the combination to the safe. The clerk testified that both robbers frightened him and that he feared for his life.

D.R.S. was found incompetent to stand trial on the robbery charge and hospitalized for the purpose of restoration to competency. After almost two years in the hospital, he was found competent, but charges against him were dismissed on speedy trial grounds on January 8, 1985. On February 14, 1985, he was civilly committed. The Montana Supreme Court upheld the commitment against a challenge that the robbery was insufficiently recent. The court justified this decision as follows]:

The circumstances in the case at bar are such that a lapse of time between the overt act and the commitment proceedings do not preclude relying on the overt act [the robbery] as evidence of D.R.S.' mental condition.

Dr. James Deming, the psychologist who treated D.R.S. for the two-year period at Montana State Hospital testified that D.R.S.' condition was essentially unchanged from that in 1982. He testified that:

[D.R.S.] continued to exhibit symptoms of a significant mental illness, continued to be confused, continued to develop neologisms or new words, continued to be convinced of specific bizarre ideations, as an example, [D.R.S.] was convinced that his lawyer was my brother. On the basis of the information that both of us wore mustaches. He continued to have—to exhibit a significant thought disorder which renders him unpredictable, and in my judgment, imminently dangerous.

Dr. Deming relied on several factors in concluding that D.R.S. is dangerous. In addition to the primary element of the charges against D.R.S., Dr. Deming considered his statements of unwillingness to accept supervision in a community setting for his disorder, D.R.S.' stated intent to use alcohol when he leaves the hospital, and the deterioration of his condition while in the county jail. Dr. Deming explained that a small amount of alcohol would render D.R.S. confused and disoriented, resulting in dangerous behavior, and that he had not received medication during his stay in jail. The fact that D.R.S. had not exhibited dangerous or "acting-out" behavior in the hospital was due to the supervised environment and the control of his medication. If taken out of this supervised setting, Dr. Deming said that D.R.S. would become imminently dangerous within two months. Finally, the doctor expressed his opinion that D.R.S. is seriously mentally ill and imminently dangerous to himself and others due to his mental disease of paranoid schizophrenia.

D.R.S.' conduct during the robbery, under the circumstances presented here, is "sufficiently recent in time as to be material and relevant" to his present condition. The time lapse between the overt act and his commitment hearing was due to his serious mental illness.

The evidence showed his condition remained as it was at the time of the overt act. In addition, the psychiatric evaluation stated that D.R.S. would be imminently dangerous within two months of leaving the supervised hospital setting. We hold that the District Court had sufficient evidence to find D.R.S. is seriously mentally ill.

Questions and Comments

1. *The necessity for an overt act requirement.* The *Lessard* decision prohibited commitment unless the person is found to be dangerous "based upon a finding of a recent overt act, attempt or threat to do substantial harm." Approximately ten state statutes include a similar provision. A number of other states accomplish the same effect with wording like that found in the Montana statute recited in *D.R.S.* The rest, well over half of the states, do not require proof of an overt act.

What is the argument that the constitution mandates such a showing? Cf. *Robinson v. California,* supra; *United States v. Salerno,* supra. Are there other, "pragmatic", reasons for such a requirement? Under California's Lanterman–Petris–Short Act, those considered dangerous to others are potentially subject to three "stages" of commitment: a 72–hour emergency detention, a 14–day short-term detention, and a 180–day commitment. Proof of an overt act is required for the third-stage 180–day commitment, but not for the first and second stages of the commitment process. Cal.Code §§ 5150, 5200, 5250, 5300. Can you think of a rationale for this approach?

2. *The content of the overt act requirement.* If proof of an overt act is required, how should it be defined? Is a threat to harm another enough? Statements like those in *Sansone* that "people are out to get me?" Purchase of a weapon?

The criminal law has dealt with an analogous issue through definition of the actus reus for attempt crimes. Typically, "mere preparation" for a crime is considered insufficient conduct to impose liability for attempt. Various tests developed to capture this notion. For instance, one such test asked whether the person had committed the "last proximate act" of the offense in question. Thus, if a person fires a gun at the intended victim and misses, he can be found guilty of attempted murder. If he merely lies in wait for the victim but does not fire the gun, he cannot be. A second, less restrictive test, developed by Justice Holmes, focused on whether the person was in "dangerous proximity to success." See generally, Low, Jeffries, & Bonnie, Criminal Law: Cases and Materials 132–37 (2d ed. 1986). The Model Penal Code, which has heavily influenced many state legislatures, defines the actus reus for attempt as "an act of omission constituting a substantial step in a course of conduct planned to culminate in his commission of the crime." Model Penal Code § 5.01(1)(c). The Code then states:

> Conduct shall not be held to constitute a substantial step . . . unless it is strongly corroborative of the actor's criminal purpose. [T]he following, if strongly corroborative of the actor's criminal purpose, shall not be held insufficient as a matter of law:

a) lying in wait, searching for or following the contemplated victim of the crime;

b) enticing or seeking to entice the contemplated victim of the crime to go to the place contemplated for its commission;

c) reconnoitering the place contemplated for the commission of the crime;

d) unlawful entry of a structure, vehicle or enclosure in which it is contemplated that the crime will be committed;

e) possession of materials to be employed in the commission of the crime, which are specially designed for such unlawful use or which can serve no lawful purpose of the actor under the circumstances;

f) possession, collection or fabrication of materials to be employed in the commission of the crime, at or near the place contemplated for its commission, where such possession, collection or fabrication serves no lawful purpose of the actor under the circumstances;

g) soliciting an innocent agent to engage in conduct constituting an element of the crime.

Model Penal Code § 5.02. Should civil commitment statutes include this list or one like it? What effect would an overt act requirement have in Case 5 on p. 605? Case 17 on p. 607?

3. *Recency of the overt act.* The *Lessard* court also requires that the overt act be "recent", as does the Montana statute in *D.R.S.* Other states (e.g., California) do not explicitly include a recency requirement. What is the purpose of this requirement? Does it link with the imminence requirement? Do you agree with the holding in *D.R.S.* on this issue?

The Arizona commitment statute provides as follows:

§ 36–501(3). "Danger to others" means behavior which constitutes a danger of inflicting substantial bodily harm upon another person based upon a history of having inflicted or having attempted to inflict substantial bodily harm upon another person within twelve months preceding the hearing on court ordered treatment, except that:

(a) If the proposed patient has existed under conditions of being restrained by physical or pharmacological means, or of being confined, or of being supervised, which have deterred or tended to deter him from carrying out acts of inflicting or attempting to inflict bodily harm upon another person, the time limit of within twelve months preceding the hearing may be extended to a time longer than twelve months as consideration of the evidence indicates; or,

(b) If the bodily harm inflicted upon or attempted to be inflicted upon another person was grievous or horrendous, the time limit of within twelve months preceding the hearing may be extended to a time longer than twelve months as consideration of the evidence indicates.

4. *Standard of proof.* Although proof of dangerousness need only be by clear and convincing evidence, can an argument be made that proof of the overt act must be beyond a reasonable doubt? Montana's statute, at

issue in *D.R.S.*, is unique among the states, in that it requires proof beyond a reasonable doubt of any "physical facts or evidence" and clear and convincing proof "as to all other matters, except that mental disorders shall be evidenced to a reasonable medical certainty." Mont.Code Ann. 53–21–126(2). Is the Montana approach coherent? As applied to the criteria necessary to commit D.R.S., is the standard met?

C. PARENS PATRIAE COMMITMENTS

1. Rationale

The parens patriae authority is premised on the power of government to act as "parent" toward its citizens. This country has a strong tradition of anti-paternalism, based on strains of individualism dating back to the colonization of the eastern seaboard by dissidents and outcasts. John Stuart Mill provided one of the earliest and most forceful defenses of the anti-paternalism position.

> The only purpose for which power can be rightfully exercised over any member of a civilized community against his will, is to prevent harm to others. His own good, either physical or moral, is not a sufficient warrant. He cannot rightfully be compelled to do or forbear because it will be better for him to do so, because it will make him happier, because in the opinion of others to do so would be wise, or even right. These are reasons for remonstrating with him, or reasoning with him, or persuading him, or entreating him, but not for compelling him, or visiting him with any evil in case he do otherwise.

J.S. Mill, On Liberty, in The Philosophy of John Stuart Mill 197 (1961).

Yet, as Shapiro has pointed out, "if antipaternalism is the dominant strain, it has surely not won the day:"

> Defenders of paternalism, or at least of a more neutral stance, have argued forcefully for their position on both descriptive and normative grounds. Paternalist motives, they suggest, help to account for a vast range of present-day legislation and judicial doctrine (not to speak of the actions of individuals toward one another); failure to recognize these motives can only lead to confusion and hypocrisy. Moreover, paternalism has a legitimate place among human motivations—perhaps more legitimate than other, more selfish, reasons for action—since its regard for others is rooted in 'empathy or love.'

Shapiro, "Courts, Legislatures, and Paternalism," 74 Va.L.Rev. 519, 519–20 (1988). As Shapiro notes, paternalistic legislation has become an accepted feature of modern life. Laws regulating food quality and the environment, employment conditions (e.g., minimum wage and maximum hour laws), and transportation (e.g., seat-belt and motorcycle helmut statutes) are just a few examples of legislation that might be characterized as paternalistic in motivation.

Civil commitment remains the most dramatic example of state paternalism. Every state permits involuntary, prolonged hospitalization of someone found to be mentally ill and "dangerous to self", "unable to care" for themselves, "gravely disabled" or some combination thereof. The usual justification advanced for these provisions is that the mentally ill lack the capacity to make decisions about treatment and hospitalization; thus, the state has the authority to make those decisions for them. Note, "Civil Commitment of the Mentally Ill: Developments in the Law," 87 Harv.L.Rev. 1190, 1212 (1974). Even Mill recognized an exception to his general rule for those who are "incompetent," including youth and the mentally disabled, on the ground that one cannot exercise one's political rights unless one has the capacity to do so. See Waithe, "Why Mill Was For Paternalism," 6 Int'l J.L. & Psychiat. 101 (1983).

Several arguments against this use of state power can be advanced. The first, analogous to the argument against police power commitment of the mentally ill, is that the mentally ill as a class are no more incompetent than others and therefore should not be singled out for special treatment. Morse makes the argument most directly:

> Are the mentally disordered particularly incompetent? The question is crucial because involuntary commitment substitutes the state's judgment about the necessity for hospitalization (and often for treatment as well) for the judgment of the individual. Although commitment rarely includes a formal finding of legal incompetence at present, it at least implies the judgment that in some cases the person cannot cope or make decisions in his or her own best interest. * * *

> There is however, little empirical or theoretical justification for the belief that the mentally disordered as a class are especially incapable of managing their lives or deciding for themselves what is in their own best interests. Available empirical evidence demonstrates that the mentally disordered as a class are probably not more incompetent than normal persons as a class. Indeed, there is no necessary relationship between mental disorder and legal incompetence.

> * * * While some disordered persons are clearly incompetent according to any reasonable criteria, the social goal of reducing the consequences of incompetence is not well served by allowing involuntary hospitalization, guardianship, or treatment of only the mentally disordered.

Morse, "A Preference for Liberty: The Case Against Involuntary Commitment of the Mentally Disordered," 70 Cal.L.Rev. 54, 63–64 (1982).

The second argument against parens patriae commitment assumes the theoretical validity of committing the incompetent mentally ill (at least when incompetency causes serious dysfunction), but questions whether "reasonable criteria" for judging who is incompetent can be developed and applied. Szasz is particularly vigorous in advancing this view. In his most recent work, for instance, he stated:

> [W]henever one person, A, claims that another person, B, is incompetent, we are confronted with a situation from which we can draw two quite different inferences, one more probable than the other. The less probable inference is that A's assertion is true: in other words, that B is indeed incompetent. The more probable inference is that A's asser-

tion is untrue: in other words, that A wants to paternistically control or coerce B.

T. Szasz, Insanity: The Idea and Its Consequences 249–50 (1987). A more detailed investigation of this difficult issue is left until Chapter Nine, which deals with the question of competency generally. For now, the following definition of competency is offered:

> Since the purpose of the incapacity standard is to distinguish persons whose decisions to refuse treatment must be accepted as final from those whose choices may be validly overridden through *parens patriae* commitments, the standard should focus on the ability to engage in a decision-making process rather than the resulting decision. . . . [C]ommentary accompanying the National Institute of Mental Health's 1952 Draft Act Governing Hospitalization of the Mentally Ill appears to provide a workable definition of incapacity[:] an individual lacks capacity if, as a result of a mental disease or disorder, he has lost the 'power to make choices or become so confused . . . [that he cannot] make a decision having any relation to the factors bearing on his hospitalization.'

Developments, supra at 1217.

Even if one accepts that parens patriae commitment is theoretically justified and that the incompetent mentally ill can be accurately identified, the following question must also be answered: who among the incompetent mentally ill may be involuntarily hospitalized? This section addresses this question.

NOTE, CIVIL COMMITMENT OF THE MENTALLY ILL: DEVELOPMENTS IN THE LAW
87 Harvard L.R. 1190, 1218–19.
(1974).

* * *

Best Interest of the Individual: A Balancing Requirement.—After the threshold requirement of incapacity has been met, the state may act as *parens patriae* for the individual. Although the state ideally should attempt to duplicate the decision which its ward would have made, the need to ascertain each ward's value structure would make such a process highly impractical. Consequently, the state as substitute decision-maker should objectively evaluate alternatives and select the one which best serves the ward's interest. The propriety of a decision to require psychiatric treatment or to compel hospitalization will thus depend on whether either action constitutes the most desirable response to the individual's condition. The advisability of ordering commitment will naturally vary depending on such individual factors as the debilitating effect of the mental disorder, the prognosis with and without treatment, the expected duration of treatment, the need for and length of institutionalization, the institutional conditions, the legal disabilities resulting from commitment, and the disruptive effect on preexisting lifestyle.

Although the "best interest" test entails a flexible balancing of costs and benefits, the serious stigma and the interference with physical freedom produced by even short term commitment to a mental institution suggest that a substantial expected benefit should be required for involuntary commitment. Consequently, a mental disorder which does not pose a danger to the individual's physical health or substantially impair his ability to function in society should rarely result in forced institutional care. State commitment statutes which require that the individual be dangerous to himself or that his condition create a substantial risk of his physical injury can be viewed as expressing a legislative judgment that the likelihood that individuals who do not meet those standards would not benefit sufficiently to justify their confinement outweighs the possibility that commitment would sometimes be appropriate in such cases.

The potential of beneficial treatment is another possible limitation on *parens patriae* commitments derived from the best interest requirement. In *In re Ballay*, the District of Columbia Circuit contended in dictum that "[w]ithout some form of treatment the state justification for acting as *parens patriae* becomes a nullity." However, the court's belief that custodial care is an impermissible use of the *parens patriae* power seems unwarranted. As with other relevant factors, the untreatable patient's potential need for indefinite confinement for his own protection should be considered in balancing the costs and benefits of imposing various types of care. The danger of substantial physical harm created when an untreatable mental disorder impairs the individual's ability to provide for his basic needs might well be sufficient to justify action under the *parens patriae* power, although there are alternative modes of providing protective care which may be preferable to hospitalization of the untreatable. . . .

O'CONNOR v. DONALDSON

Supreme Court of the United States, 1975.
422 U.S. 563, 95 S.Ct. 2486, 45 L.Ed.2d 396.

* * *

MR. JUSTICE STEWART delivered the opinion of the Court.

The respondent, Kenneth Donaldson, was civilly committed to confinement as a mental patient in the Florida State Hospital at Chattahoochee in January 1957. He was kept in custody there against his will for nearly 15 years. The petitioner, Dr. J.B. O'Connor, was the hospital's superintendent during most of this period. Throughout his confinement Donaldson repeatedly, but unsuccessfully, demanded his release, claiming that he was dangerous to no one, that he was not mentally ill, and that, at any rate, the hospital was not providing treatment for his supposed illness. Finally, in February 1971, Donaldson brought this lawsuit under 42 U.S.C. § 1983, in the United States District Court for the Northern District of Florida, alleging that O'Connor, and other members of the hospital staff named as defendants, had intentionally and maliciously deprived him of his constitutional right to liberty. After a four-day trial, the jury returned a verdict assessing both compensatory and punitive damages against O'Connor and a codefendant. The Court of Appeals for the Fifth Circuit affirmed the judgment. We granted O'Connor's petition for certiorari, because of the important constitutional questions seemingly presented.

I

Donaldson's commitment was initiated by his father, who thought that his son was suffering from "delusions." After hearings before a county judge of Pinellas County, Fla., Donaldson was found to be suffering from "paranoid schizophrenia" and was committed for "care, maintenance, and treatment" pursuant to Florida statutory provisions that have since been repealed.[2] The state law was less than clear in specifying the grounds necessary for commitment, and the record is scanty as to Donaldson's condition at the time of the judicial hearing. These matters are, however, irrelevant, for this case involves no challenge to the initial commitment, but is focused, instead, upon the nearly 15 years of confinement that followed.

The evidence at the trial showed that the hospital staff had the power to release a patient, not dangerous to himself or others, even if he remained mentally ill and had been lawfully committed. Despite many requests, O'Connor refused to allow that power to be exercised in Donaldson's case. At the trial, O'Connor indicated that he had believed that Donaldson would have been unable to make a "successful adjustment outside the institution," but could not recall the basis for that conclusion. O'Connor retired as superintendent shortly before this suit was filed. A few months thereafter, and before the trial, Donaldson secured his release and a judicial restoration of competency, with the support of the hospital staff.

The testimony at the trial demonstrated, without contradiction, that Donaldson had posed no danger to others during his long confinement, or indeed at any point in his life. O'Connor himself conceded that he had no personal or secondhand knowledge that Donaldson had ever committed a dangerous act. There was no evidence that Donald-

---

2. The judicial commitment proceedings were pursuant to § 394.22(11) of the State Public Health Code, which provided:

"Whenever any person who has been adjudged mentally incompetent requires confinement or restraint to prevent self-injury or violence to others, the said judge shall direct that such person be forthwith delivered to a superintendent of a Florida state hospital, for the mentally ill, after admission has been authorized under regulations approved by the board of commissioners of state institutions, for care, maintenance, and treatment, . . .

* * *

Donaldson had been adjudged "incompetent" several days earlier under § 394.22(1), which provided for such a finding as to any person who was "incompetent by reason of mental illness, sickness, drunkenness, excessive use of drugs, insanity, or other mental or physical condition, so that he is incapable of caring for himself or managing his property, or is likely to dissipate or lose his property or become the victim of designing persons, or inflict harm on himself or others . . . .." Fla.Gen.Laws 1955, c. 29909, § 3, p. 831.

* * *

son had ever been suicidal or been thought likely to inflict injury upon himself. One of O'Connor's codefendants acknowledged that Donaldson could have earned his own living outside the hospital. He had done so for some 14 years before his commitment, and immediately upon his release he secured a responsible job in hotel administration.

Furthermore, Donaldson's frequent requests for release had been supported by responsible persons willing to provide him any care he might need on release. In 1963, for example, a representative of Helping Hands, Inc., a halfway house for mental patients, wrote O'Connor asking him to release Donaldson to its care. The request was accompanied by a supporting letter from the Minneapolis Clinic of Psychiatry and Neurology, which a codefendant conceded was a "good clinic." O'Connor rejected the offer, replying that Donaldson could be released only to his parents. That rule was apparently of O'Connor's own making. At the time, Donaldson was 55 years old, and, as O'Connor knew, Donaldson's parents were too elderly and infirm to take responsibility for him. Moreover, in his continuing correspondence with Donaldson's parents, O'Connor never informed them of the Helping Hands offer. In addition, on four separate occasions between 1964 and 1968, John Lembcke, a college classmate of Donaldson's and a longtime family friend, asked O'Connor to release Donaldson to his care. On each occasion O'Connor refused. The record shows that Lembcke was a serious and responsible person, who was willing and able to assume responsibility for Donaldson's welfare.

The evidence showed that Donaldson's confinement was a simple regime of enforced custodial care, not a program designed to alleviate or cure his supposed illness. Numerous witnesses, including one of O'Connor's codefendants, testified that Donaldson had received nothing but custodial care while at the hospital. O'Connor described Donaldson's treatment as "milieu therapy." But witnesses from the hospital staff conceded that, in the context of this case, "milieu therapy" was a euphemism for confinement in the "milieu" of a mental hospital.[4] For substantial periods, Donaldson was simply kept in a large room that housed 60 patients, many of whom were under criminal commitment. Donaldson's requests for ground privileges, occupational training, and an opportunity to discuss his case with O'Connor or other staff members were repeatedly denied.

At the trial, O'Connor's principal defense was that he had acted in good faith and was therefore immune from any liability for monetary damages. His position, in short, was that state law, which he had believed valid, had authorized indefinite custodial confinement of the "sick," even if they were not given treatment and their release could harm no one.

---

4. There was some evidence that Donaldson, who is a Christian Scientist, on occasion refused to take medication. The trial judge instructed the jury not to award damages for any period of confinement during which Donaldson had declined treatment.

The trial judge instructed the members of the jury that they should find that O'Connor had violated Donaldson's constitutional right to liberty if they found that he had

> "confined [Donaldson] against his will, knowing that he was not mentally ill or dangerous or knowing that if mentally ill he was not receiving treatment for his alleged mental illness.

> * * *

> "Now, the purpose of involuntary hospitalization is treatment and not mere custodial care or punishment if a patient is not a danger to himself or others. Without such treatment there is no justification from a constitutional stand-point for continued confinement unless you should also find that [Donaldson] was dangerous to either himself or others." [6]

The trial judge further instructed the jury that O'Connor was immune from damages if he

> "reasonably believed in good faith that detention of [Donaldson] was proper for the length of time he was so confined. . . .

> "However, mere good intentions which do not give rise to a reasonable belief that detention is lawfully required cannot justify [Donaldson's] confinement in the Florida State Hospital."

The jury returned a verdict for Donaldson against O'Connor and a codefendant, and awarded damages of $38,500, including $10,000 in punitive damages.

The Court of Appeals affirmed the judgment of the District Court in a broad opinion dealing with "the far-reaching question whether the Fourteenth Amendment guarantees a right to treatment to persons involuntarily civilly committed to state mental hospitals." The appellate court held that when, as in Donaldson's case, the rationale for confinement is that the patient is in need of treatment, the Constitution requires that minimally adequate treatment in fact be provided. The court further expressed the view that, regardless of the grounds for involuntary civil commitment, a person confined against his will at a state mental institution has "a constitutional right to receive such individual treatment as will give him a reasonable opportunity to be cured or to improve his mental condition." Conversely, the court's opinion implied that it is constitutionally permissible for a State to

---

6. The District Court defined treatment as follows:

"You are instructed that a person who is involuntarily civilly committed to a mental hospital does have a *constitutional right to receive such treatment as will give him a realistic opportunity to be cured or to improve his mental condition.*" (Emphasis added.) O'Connor argues that this statement suggests that a mental patient has a right to treatment even if confined by reason of dangerousness to himself or others. But this is to take the above paragraph out of context, for it is bracketed by paragraphs making clear the trial judge's theory that treatment is constitutionally required only if mental illness alone, rather than danger to self or others, is the reason for confinement. If O'Connor had thought the instructions ambiguous on this point, he could have objected to them and requested a clarification. He did not do so. We accordingly have no occasion here to decide whether persons committed on grounds of dangerousness enjoy a "right to treatment."

* * *

confine a mentally ill person against his will in order to treat his illness, regardless of whether his illness renders him dangerous to himself or others.

II

We have concluded that the difficult issues of constitutional law dealt with by the Court of Appeals are not presented by this case in its present posture. Specifically, there is no reason now to decide whether mentally ill persons dangerous to themselves or to others have a right to treatment upon compulsory confinement by the State, or whether the State may compulsorily confine a non-dangerous, mentally ill individual for the purpose of treatment. As we view it, this case raises a single, relatively simple, but nonetheless important question concerning every man's constitutional right to liberty.

The jury found that Donaldson was neither dangerous to himself nor dangerous to others, and also found that, if mentally ill, Donaldson had not received treatment. That verdict, based on abundant evidence, makes the issue before the Court a narrow one. We need not decide whether, when, or by what procedures, a mentally ill person may be confined by the State on any of the grounds which, under contemporary statutes, are generally advanced to justify involuntary confinement of such a person—to prevent injury to the public, to ensure his own survival or safety, or to alleviate or cure his illness. For the jury found that none of the above grounds for continued confinement was present in Donaldson's case.[10]

Given the jury's findings, what was left as justification for keeping Donaldson in continued confinement? The fact that state law may have authorized confinement of the harmless mentally ill does not itself establish a constitutionally adequate purpose for the confinement. Nor is it enough that Donaldson's original confinement was founded upon a constitutionally adequate basis, if in fact it was, because even if his involuntary confinement was initially permissible, it could not constitutionally continue after that basis no longer existed.

A finding of "mental illness" alone cannot justify a State's locking a person up against his will and keeping him indefinitely in simple custodial confinement. Assuming that that term can be given a reasonably precise content and that the "mentally ill" can be identified with

---

10. O'Connor argues that, despite the jury's verdict, the Court must assume that Donaldson was receiving treatment sufficient to justify his confinement, because the adequacy of treatment is a "nonjusticiable" question that must be left to the discretion of the psychiatric profession. That argument is unpersuasive. Where "treatment" is the sole asserted ground for depriving a person of liberty, it is plainly unacceptable to suggest that the courts are powerless to determine whether the asserted ground is present. See Jackson v. Indiana, 406 U.S. 715, 92 S.Ct. 1845, 32 L.Ed.2d 435. Neither party objected to the jury instruction defining treatment. There is, accordingly, no occasion in this case to decide whether the provision of treatment, standing alone, can ever constitutionally justify involuntary confinement or, if it can, how much or what kind of treatment would suffice for that purpose. In its present posture this case involves not involuntary treatment but simply involuntary custodial confinement.

reasonable accuracy, there is still no constitutional basis for confining such persons involuntarily if they are dangerous to no one and can live safely in freedom.

May the State confine the mentally ill merely to ensure them a living standard superior to that they enjoy in the private community? That the State has a proper interest in providing care and assistance to the unfortunate goes without saying. But the mere presence of mental illness does not disqualify a person from preferring his home to the comforts of an institution. Moreover, while the State may arguably confine a person to save him from harm, incarceration is rarely if ever a necessary condition for raising the living standards of those capable of surviving safely in freedom, on their own or with the help of family or friends. See Shelton v. Tucker, 364 U.S. 479, 488–490, 81 S.Ct. 247, 252–253, 5 L.Ed.2d 231.

May the State fence in the harmless mentally ill solely to save its citizens from exposure to those whose ways are different? One might as well ask if the State, to avoid public unease, could incarcerate all who are physically unattractive or socially eccentric. Mere public intolerance or animosity cannot constitutionally justify the deprivation of a person's physical liberty.

In short, a State cannot constitutionally confine without more a nondangerous individual who is capable of surviving safely in freedom by himself or with the help of willing and responsible family members or friends. Since the jury found, upon ample evidence, that O'Connor, as an agent of the State, knowingly did so confine Donaldson, it properly concluded that O'Connor violated Donaldson's constitutional right to freedom.

MR. CHIEF JUSTICE BURGER, concurring.

Although I join the Court's opinion and judgment in this case, it seems to me that several factors merit more emphasis than it gives them. I therefore add the following remarks. * * *

There can be no doubt that involuntary commitment to a mental hospital, like involuntary confinement of an individual for any reason, is a deprivation of liberty which the State cannot accomplish without due process of law. Commitment must be justified on the basis of a legitimate state interest, and the reasons for committing a particular individual must be established in an appropriate proceeding. Equally important, confinement must cease when those reasons no longer exist.

The Court of Appeals purported to be applying these principles in developing the first of its theories supporting a constitutional right to treatment. It first identified what it perceived to be the traditional bases for civil commitment—physical dangerousness to oneself or others, or a need for treatment—and stated:

> "[W]here, as in Donaldson's case, the rationale for confinement is the 'parens patriae' rationale that the patient is in need of treatment, the due process clause requires that minimally adequate treatment be

in fact provided. . . . 'To deprive any citizen of his or her liberty upon the altruistic theory that the confinement is for humane therapeutic reasons and then fail to provide adequate treatment violates the very fundamentals of due process.'"

The Court of Appeals did not explain its conclusion that the rationale for respondent's commitment was that he needed treatment. The Florida statutes in effect during the period of his confinement did not require that a person who had been adjudicated incompetent and ordered committed either be provided with psychiatric treatment or released, and there was no such condition in respondent's order of commitment.   More important, the instructions which the Court of Appeals read as establishing an absolute constitutional right to treatment did not require the jury to make any findings regarding the specific reasons for respondent's confinement or to focus upon any rights he may have had under state law.   Thus, the premise of the Court of Appeals' first theory must have been that, at least with respect to persons who are not physically dangerous, a State has no power to confine the mentally ill except for the purpose of providing them with treatment.

That proposition is surely not descriptive of the power traditionally exercised by the States in this area.   Historically, and for a considerable period of time, subsidized custodial care in private foster homes or boarding houses was the most benign form of care provided incompetent or mentally ill persons for whom the States assumed responsibility. Until well into the 19th century the vast majority of such persons were simply restrained in poorhouses, almshouses, or jails.   The few States that established institutions for the mentally ill during this early period were concerned primarily with providing a more humane place of confinement and only secondarily with "curing" the persons sent there.

As the trend toward state care of the mentally ill expanded, eventually leading to the present statutory schemes for protecting such persons, the dual functions of institutionalization continued to be recognized.   While one of the goals of this movement was to provide medical treatment to those who could benefit from it, it was acknowledged that this could not be done in all cases and that there was a large range of mental illness for which no known "cure" existed.   In time, providing places for the custodial confinement of the so-called "dependent insane" again emerged as the major goal of the States' programs in this area and remained so well into this century.

In short, the idea that States may not confine the mentally ill except for the purpose of providing them with treatment is of very recent origin, and there is no historical basis for imposing such a limitation on state power.   Analysis of the sources of the civil commitment power likewise lends no support to that notion.   There can be little doubt that in the exercise of its police power a State may confine individuals solely to protect society from the dangers of significant antisocial acts or communicable disease. Jacobson v. Massachusetts, 197 U.S. 11, 25–29, 25 S.Ct. 358, 360–362, 49 L.Ed. 643 (1905). Additionally, the States are vested with the historic *parens patriae* power, including the duty to protect "persons under legal disabilities to act for themselves." The classic example of this role is when a State undertakes to act as " 'the general guardian of all infants, idiots, and lunatics.' "

Of course, an inevitable consequence of exercising the *parens patriae* power is that the ward's personal freedom will be substantially restrained, whether a guardian is appointed to control his property, he is placed in the custody of a private third party, or committed to an institution. Thus, however the power is implemented, due process requires that it not be invoked indiscriminately. At a minimum, a particular scheme for protection of the mentally ill must rest upon a legislative determination that it is compatible with the best interests of the affected class and that its members are unable to act for themselves. Moreover, the use of alternative forms of protection may be motivated by different considerations, and the justifications for one may not be invoked to rationalize another.

However, the existence of some due process limitations on the *parens patriae* power does not justify the further conclusion that it may be exercised to confine a mentally ill person only if the purpose of the confinement is treatment. Despite many recent advances in medical knowledge, it remains a stubborn fact that there are many forms of mental illness which are not understood, some which are untreatable in the sense that no effective therapy has yet been discovered for them, and that rates of "cure" are generally low. There can be little responsible debate regarding "the uncertainty of diagnosis in this field and the tentativeness of professional judgment." Similarly, as previously observed, it is universally recognized as fundamental to effective therapy that the patient acknowledge his illness and cooperate with those attempting to give treatment; yet the failure of a large proportion of mentally ill persons to do so is a common phenomenon. It may be that some persons in either of these categories,[6] and there may be others, are unable to function in society and will suffer real harm to themselves unless provided with care in a sheltered environment. At the very least, I am not able to say that a state legislature is powerless to make that kind of judgment.

* * *

6. Indeed, respondent may have shared both of these characteristics. His illness, paranoid schizophrenia, is notoriously unsusceptible to treatment, see Livermore, Malmquist, & Meehl, On the Justifications for Civil Commitment, 117 U.Pa.L.Rev. 75, 93, and n. 52 (1968), and the reports of the Florida State Hospital staff which were introduced into evidence expressed the view that he was unwilling to acknowledge his illness and was generally uncooperative.

STATE ex rel. HAWKS v. LAZARO

Supreme Court of West Virginia, 1974.
157 W.Va. 417, 202 S.E.2d 109.

* * *

There is persuasive evidence that the alleged improvement in treatment in modern state facilities from medieval times to our own is more myth than reality, and that at the current low level of sociological and psychological knowledge, combined with the current parsimonious level of governmental support for state institutions, the state and its officers have a limited therapeutic role and a predominantly custodial role.

In recognition of the conditions which exist at state institutions, numerous courts have recently required the state to demonstrate a reasonable relationship between the alleged harm which a person is likely to do to himself and the treatment designed to ameliorate the illness which may cause that harm. [T]he ancient doctrine of *parens patriae* is in full retreat on all fronts except in those very narrow areas where the state can demonstrate, as a matter of fact, that its care and custody is superior to any available alternative. Therefore, in determining whether there is any justification under the doctrine of *parens patriae* for deviation from established due process standards, it is appropriate for this Court to consider that the State of West Virginia offers to those unfortunates who are incarcerated in mental institutions Dickensian squalor of unconscionable magnitudes.

In 1970 West Virginia spent $7.19 per day per patient in public mental hospitals, thus ranking 49th among the states. * * * The dry facts concerning financial support are hardly as persuasive as the narrative description of the physical conditions reported by members of the West Virginia Legislature in 1972.

"The Committee was thoroughly disgusted at the deplorable conditions existing at this facility. Dirt and filth and foul odors were everywhere. Daily housekeeping and routine maintenance were not being performed. There was a need for screens, flies were swarming and garbage cans were uncovered and overflowing. While the hospital could undoubtably (sic) use additional housekeeping and maintenance people, the present personnel have become dilatory in their work. . . .

"Security is a problem at several state hospitals, but is particularly acute at Weston. . . . There were 91 elopements from the hospital in 1971 and 35 during 1972 up to the time of inspection.

"At the time of inspection, the Committee observed patients administering drugs to patients. . . ."

The parsimonious level of financial support is again reflected in the rate of rehabilitation of mental patients. In 1972–73 the average length of stay for involuntarily committed resident patients in West Virginia mental institutions was 15.91 years, and as of June 30, 1973, of

1,873 involuntarily committed patients, 1,119 patients had been institutionalized for over ten years. In West Virginia as of 1969, only 9.8 percent of total rehabilitations achieved in federal-state programs were rehabilitated mental illness clients, which ranked West Virginia 45th among the states in this category. Recent research demonstrates that institutionalization is frequently the worst treatment which can be provided a person suffering from mental problems. All of these statistics and observations give persuasive support to the following observations of Albert Deutsch, which suggest that the hospitalization of the mentally ill under current conditions may inflict positive harm on the patients:

> "The enormous disability associated with mental illness is, to a large extent, superimposed, preventable, and treatable. . . . Disability is superimposed by rejection mechanism stemming from cultural attitudes. . . . Hospitalization as such is an important cause of disability. . . . The best treatment-minded state hospitals perform a disabling function.
>
> "We can no longer tolerate the paradox of depriving mental patients of their civil rights in the name of hospital treatment when we know that it is not only unnecessary for security but harmful to potential recovery. . . ."

* * *

For the foregoing reasons, we hold unconstitutional the standard enunciated in Code, 27–5–4(2), as amended, which permits involuntary hospitalization if the individual:

"(2) Is in need of custody, care or treatment in a hospital and, because of his illness or retardation lacks sufficient insight or capacity to make responsible decisions with respect to his hospitalization. . . ."

* * *

Society abounds with persons who should be hospitalized, either for gallbladder surgery, back operations, corrective orthopedic surgery, or other reasons; yet, in these areas society would not contemplate involuntary hospitalization for treatment. As Code, 27–5–4, as amended, permits incarceration, due process as developed with regard to criminal statutes mandates that the grounds for incarceration be stated with specificity. The standard of hospitalization for the benefit of the individual leaves an entirely subjective determination for the committing authority which violates due process because it forecloses a meaningful appeal and places the individual in jeopardy of losing his freedom without providing an objective standard against which the committing authority's determination can be measured.

* * *

Modern welfare programs, community mental health facilities and private social service agencies have eliminated the problems of actual starvation and persecution of the mentally disturbed which were prevalent in the latter half of the Nineteenth Century. Accordingly, it is possible for many nonviolent people, even those who suffer from a mental disease or retardation to such an extent that they are unable to earn a living, to live outside of an institution, and when these people prefer to do so, regardless of the wisdom of their decision, or the strength of their reasoning powers, the constitution guarantees them the right to follow their own desires.

Notwithstanding the invalidity of Code, 27–5–4(2), as amended, we hold that Code, 27–5–4(1), as amended, does establish reasonable and definite criteria for involuntary hospitalization when it permits the State to hospitalize an individual if:

"(1) Because of his illness or retardation [he] is likely to injure himself or others if allowed to remain at liberty. . . ."

Society is entitled to protect itself against predatory acts on the part of anti-social people, regardless of the cause of their anti-social actions. Therefore, if the State can prove that an individual is likely to injure others if left at liberty, it may hospitalize him. The State is also entitled to prevent a person from injuring himself in the very specific sense of doing physical damage to himself, either actively or passively. Therefore, when it can be demonstrated that an individual has a self-destructive urge and will be violent towards himself, or alternatively that he is so mentally retarded or mentally ill that by sheer inactivity he will permit himself to die either of starvation or lack of care, then the State is entitled to hospitalize him. The State would also be permitted, under the Constitution, to hospitalize a person who suffers from a mental illness or retardation which is likely to produce some form of injury other than direct physical injury, if the type of injury were definitely ascertainable, and if the State had a treatment program which it could be demonstrated offered a reasonable likelihood of ameliorating the illness or condition.

Questions and Comments

1. *The meaning of* Donaldson. As presented to the Supreme Court, *Donaldson* was in part a "right to treatment" case. The Fifth Circuit Court of Appeals had decided that all civilly committed patients are entitled to treatment. Clearly, the Supreme Court avoided deciding this issue; what is not clear is what the Court did establish. The key sentence in *Donaldson* is usually thought to be the following: "In short, a State cannot constitutionally confine without more a nondangerous individual who is capable of surviving safely in freedom by himself or with the help of willing and responsible family members or friends." From the rest of the opinion, are you able to discern the conditions under which a person might be considered incapable "of surviving safely"? Does the incapacity have to be the result of mental illness, or can it merely result from physical, financial or motivational limitations? Does use of the phrase "surviving *safely*" mean that people who can "survive" outside the hospital may nonetheless be committable under certain circumstances? What circumstances? Even if a person is shown to be nondangerous and capable of surviving safely without hospitalization, the Court apparently would per-

mit confinement if "more" than mere confinement is provided. Is the "more" to which the Court refers treatment or, as Chief Justice Burger's concurring opinion contends, is "custodial care" sufficient under some circumstances? If treatment is required, precisely what must the treatment accomplish?

Do you agree with the answers to these questions provided by the West Virginia Supreme Court's opinion in *Lazaro?* If the hospital conditions described in *Lazaro* were substantially improved (as they have been in many states), should those answers change?

2. *Treatment efficacy.* As the preceding material makes clear, crucial to an assessment of the validity of parens patriae commitment is a showing that commitment will confer some benefit on, or at least not harm, the potential patient. Research and practice suggest that to the extent suicide or self-neglect is caused by psychosis or depression, various types of treatment can, by treating the underlying condition, reduce the potential for self-harm. A review of the effectiveness of antipsychotic medication, for instance, indicated that the drugs were more effective than a placebo in 73% of the 125 studies reviewed. Davis, "Efficacy of Tranquilizing and Anti–Depressant Drugs," 13 Arch.Gen.Psychiat. 552 (1965). A review of research on the efficacy of antidepressant drugs concluded that the average treated person is better off than 70% of the otherwise comparable but untreated group. Smith, Glass, & Miller, Benefits of Psychotherapy 56 (1980). Similar results have been obtained in studies of electroconvulsive therapy. Burke, Rutherford, Zorumbski, "Electroconvulsive Therapy and the Elderly," 26 Comp.Psychiat. 480 (1985) (reporting an improvement in symptoms in over 90% of the patients—elderly persons diagnosed as manic or schizoaffective—who received ECT). Additionally, vocational training, "socialization" programs, and simulation of community environments can help mentally ill people to learn survival skills even if they have spent long periods of time dependent upon others. Farkas, Rogers, & Thurer, "Rehabilitation Outcome of Long–Term Hospital Patients Left Behind by Deinstitutionalization," 38 Hosp. & Comm.Psychiat. 864 (1987).

But findings such as these do not establish that involuntary hospitalization is beneficial for all mentally ill individuals. According to Durham & LaFond, who conducted an extensive review of research on the efficacy of various treatment modalities:

> [P]sychotherapy and drugs are the treatment of choice for non-dangerous mentally ill patients committed involuntarily to hospitals for treatment. The best available evidence shows only that, at a very general level, providing these therapies to mentally ill individuals is better than doing nothing at all. However, the vast majority of studies generally focused on patients who were: (1) not seriously ill; (2) not being treated as inpatients in public institutions; (3) seeking treatment voluntarily. Unfortunately, the evidence simply does not establish that these treatment modalities are effective in treating non-dangerous mentally ill patients confined against their will to hospitals. Perhaps as important, outpatient programs have been shown to offer outcomes which are as good or better than hospital-based treatment and at lower cost.

Durham & LaFond, "A Search for the Missing Premise of Involuntary Therapeutic Commitment: Effective Treatment of the Mentally Ill," 40 Rutgers L.Rev. 303, 356 (1988). With respect to drug therapy, they also point out that the studies have not established when medication will be effective for a *particular* patient, and that "some 40% of all schizophrenics who are discharged from hospitals suffer relapses within two years, even with continued drug treatment (although the number may increase to 80% if drugs are discontinued)." Id. at 347–48.

The possible harmful effects of involuntary treatment must also be considered. For instance, as developed further at pp. 854–859, virtually all of the drug therapies have side effects, some of them quite potent and most of them annoying. Additionally, even assuming the conditions of squalor described in *Lazaro* are eliminated, hospitalization itself may be detrimental. Focusing on suicide prevention, Greenberg makes the following assertions:

> Commitment to a mental institution, especially if involuntary, may create additional problems for the patient without alleviating old ones. While some problems may be attenuated by a temporary absence from the scene, others may be exacerbated. The high rate of suicides among hospitalized mental patients in the period just after release has, in fact, led some suicide researchers to stress the need for supportive aftercare services to help the released patient cope with the stresses of life outside the institution. The possibility should not be overlooked, however, that institutionalization contributed to these stresses, and that the provision of social services on a voluntary basis might have rendered hospitalization unnecessary.

> An additional dynamic may also be at work—that of the self-fulfilling prophecy. To adopt so drastic a measure as incarceration may be to convey to the prisoner-patient that both 'experts' and the court concur in the belief that a suicide is both likely and difficult or impossible to prevent. Precautions taken to prevent a hospitalized patient from killing himself within the institution may further help the patient to construct for himself an identity as someone who is likely to commit suicide. This construction and the sense of hopelessness engendered by commitment proceedings might well increase the suicide rate from what it would have been had a less drastic and dramatic alternative been chosen. Some clinical evidence suggests that this process does take place. One may also plausibly conjecture that the degradation ceremonies attendant on admission to mental institutions, by stripping away the patient's former social identity, denigrating dignity and enhancing or creating feelings of worthlessness in the patient may contribute further to the likelihood of future suicide attempts.

> A related matter concerns the suicide rates *within* mental institutions. We have no current data concerning in-hospital suicide rates. Two decades ago, Albert Rosen estimated that the in-hospital suicide rate was about ⅓ of 1%. There is reason to believe, however, that the rate has gone up dramatically since Rosen wrote; and it is not inconceivable that the in-hospital rate by now equals or exceeds the outpatient rate [which is about 1%].

Greenburg, "Involuntary Psychiatric Commitments to Prevent Suicide," 49 N.Y.U.L.Rev. 227, 257–58 (1974).

Similarly, as *Lazaro* points out, there is evidence suggesting that hospitalization can accentuate a *non* -suicidal person's difficulties in coping with the demands of living. At least when institutionalization is prolonged, some patients become dependent upon the hospital and lose whatever survival skills they once had. Goffman, Asylum (1961); Durham & LaFond, "The Empirical Consequences and Policy Implications of Broadening the Statutory Criteria for Civil Commitment," 3 Yale L. & Pol'y Rev. 395, 428–31 (1985).

Assuming that hospitalization may actually cause some harm to a patient, should it nonetheless be allowed if that harm is less than the harm that would occur if the person were allowed to remain at liberty? Consider the following comment from Klein, arguing for laws which permit involuntary commitment for those in need of treatment who are unlikely to seek it.

> For example, some depressed people believe they are unworthy of help. There are also paranoids who reject treatment on such grounds as that the psychiatrist 'is a CIA agent who will plant a tape recorder in my head.' And, perhaps most significantly, there are numerous extremely passive people, including many elderly, who simply will not seek treatment on their own. If they are not treated involuntarily—and here I think the concept of 'involuntariness' is largely metaphysical— we know by recent experience that many of them will wander aimlessly through our blighted inner cities, subject to a host of dangers.

Klein, "Legal Doctrine at the Crossroads," Mental Health Law Project Summary of Activities 7, 8 (Mar. 1976) (quoted in Hermann, "Barriers to Providing Effective Treatment: A Critique of Revisions in Procedural, Substantive, and Dispositional Criteria in Involuntary Civil Commitment," 39 Vand.L.Rev. 83, 95 n. 63 (1986)).

3. *Predictions of self-harming behavior.* As with police power commitments, parens patriae commitments usually require a prediction of harm—that the person will commit suicide, starve, or otherwise fare poorly without state intervention. Research on our ability to make predictions of suicidal behavior is voluminous; in general the accuracy rate seems to be quite low. See, e.g., MacKinnon & Farberow, "An Assessment of the Utility of Suicide Prevention," 6 Suicide & Life Threatening Beh. 86 (1976) (prediction devices yield false positive rate of 80%); see generally, Beck, Resnick & Lettieri, The Prediction of Suicide (1974). However, as with violence-proneness prediction research, studies of predictive validity in this area are usually compromised by the fact that once such a prediction is made, intervention takes place, thereby presumably reducing the potential for harm. Research on the other types of predictions required for parens patriae commitment is not as well developed. See generally, Morse, "Crazy Behavior, Morals and Science: An Analysis of Mental Health Law," 51 S.Cal.L.Rev. 527, 596 n. 133 (1978).

4. *Revisiting the incapacity-as-threshold requirement.* Assume that the state can establish by clear and convincing evidence that a particular individual is more likely than not unable to survive "safely" outside the hospital and that short-term treatment or custodial care in a hospital

would enable him to do so. Should it also have to show—as traditional theory has posited and we have assumed up to now—that the person is "incompetent" to make a decision about the advisability of hospitalization in order to justify involuntary commitment under the parens patriae authority? This type of issue is most starkly raised when the state seeks commitment of a person who has tried to commit suicide for reasons that cannot clearly be labelled "irrational." Consider the following excerpt:

> Obviously, paternalistic measures taken on behalf of a person *with* his or her consent are ordinarily unobjectionable. Furthermore, as the contemporary philosopher Gerald Dworkin has demonstrated in his essay "Paternalism", there are instances where paternalistic interference can be justified by the doctrine of consent even though, at the precise time of the paternalistic intervention, the affected individual might object to the action[.] . . . Dworkin . . . gives an example:
>
>> [I]t is very difficult for a child to defer gratification for any considerable period of time. . . . [G]iven the very real and permanent dangers that may befall the child it becomes not only permissible but even a duty of the parent to restrict the child's freedom in various ways. There is however an important moral limitation on the exercise of such parental power which is provided by the notion of the child eventually coming to see the correctness of his parent's interventions. Parental paternalism may be thought of as a wager by the parent on the child's subsequent recognition of the wisdom of the restrictions. There is an emphasis on what could be called future-oriented consent—on what the child will come to welcome, rather than on what he does welcome.
>
> 'Future-oriented' consent, while used in the above example to justify interference with a legally incompetent subject, need not necessarily be restricted to instances of incompetency. Persons who attempt suicide are by no means always mentally incompetent at the time of the attempt. Of the competent ones, some may have rationally wanted to die, while others, though perhaps sincere in their desire to die, may have been 'wrong.' If all persons who attempted suicide were somehow saved by society's suicide prevention efforts, the saved persons would presumably have differing reactions concerning society's paternalistic efforts. The incompetent ones, if and when they regained competency, might well appreciate society's efforts, as might those who were competent but 'wrong' about their decision to die. Only those who were competent and arguably rational about their attempted suicide (for instance, terminally ill persons, etc.) might strongly object to society's 'benevolent' action in saving them.
>
> If we wanted to be philosophically pure in our paternalistic suicide prevention efforts—and if we were practically equipped to make the necessary subtle distinctions—we might well let the competent but 'correct' persons die, but might save the others in the expectation of receiving their future consent. Surely, if future consent were to be actually given, we would doubtless feel justified in our earlier paternalistic invasions. And because we cannot in practice determine at the critical time of rescue which persons would give future consent to the

rescue efforts and which would not, we feel justified in saving them all, presumably on the assumption—and this is an empirical matter—that not an insubstantial number would be belatedly appreciative.

Wexler, Mental Health Law: Major Issues 45–7 (1981). Cf. Choron, Suicide 50 (1972) (citing several studies from different countries in which 90% to 100% of rescued suicide attempters reported they were glad they had been saved); Rubinstein, Moses & Lidz, "On Attempted Suicide," 79 A.M.A. Archives Neurol. & Psychiat. 103, 111 (1958) ("[W]e have come to regard attempted suicide not as an effort to die but rather as a communication to others in an effort to improve one's life.")

Do you agree with Wexler's suggestion that the degree of incompetency is irrelevant when deciding whether to commit potential suicides? Should this reasoning be extended to those who are not suicidal but merely have trouble subsisting?

2. Implementing the Parens Patriae Authority

MAYOCK v. MARTIN

Supreme Court of Errors of Connecticut, 1968.
157 Conn. 56, 245 A.2d 574, cert. denied 393 U.S. 1111, 89 S.Ct. 924,
21 L.Ed.2d 808 (1969).

RYAN, ASSOCIATE JUSTICE. In this application for a writ of habeas corpus, the plaintiff claims that his confinement in the Norwich State Hospital is illegal because his present mental condition does not require, nor does it legally justify, his involuntary confinement or custodial care. From the judgment dismissing the writ, the plaintiff has appealed.

The few corrections to which the plaintiff has shown himself entitled are incorporated in the following statement of facts found by the trial court: The plaintiff was first confined to the Norwich State Hospital in October, 1943, and was released in January, 1944. On July 23, 1944, the plaintiff removed his right eye and was recommitted but was released subsequently for a probationary period. On July 20, 1947, the last day of the probationary period, the plaintiff, after examination by a staff physician, was unconditionally discharged from the hospital. Three days later, on July 23, 1947, the plaintiff removed his right hand. Shortly thereafter, he was again committed to the state hospital, where he is still confined. The plaintiff runs the newsstand in the hospital's administration building, where he sells newspapers and magazines to employees and to patients of the hospital. In this operation, he has been entrusted with the handling of financial matters. He has been placed in charge of a recreation center for parole-privileged patients which is operated by a committee of patients for group-recreational activity on weekends and which also serves coffee and performs other functions for patients. He believes sincerely that he is a prophet or revelator with a divine message. He believes in God and in doing what God wants us to do on earth. He also believes that society is trying to establish world peace by force but that God's way is by a brotherhood which seeks through the commandment of God to make people love one another; that world peace and brotherhood will be established by a certain church of God which the Old Testament refers to as being established by God in the latter days in the Holy Mountain; that, if the world continues in the present direction, many lives will be lost and that he has a responsibility in this matter; that he has a key role to fulfil in establishing world peace through the revelation and disclosure of the divine message; that he was not born into the country without a reason and that he was not born left-handed without a reason; that God has intended that one man shall be called to make a peace offering to God; that it is far better for one man to believe and accept an appropriate message from God to sacrifice an eye or a hand according to the sacred scriptures rather than for the present course of the world to cause even greater loss of human life; that the removal of his eye in July, 1944, was an offer of thanks to God for a revelation which he received and that it was God's command that he remove it; that the removal of his right hand in July, 1947, was an offering to God as a covenant between God and him as the person selected; that in each of these acts he has complied properly with sacred scripture; and that he is the one man called upon by God to make such spiritual sacrifices. The plaintiff has a strong belief in the Bible. Although he does not plan to cut off either of his feet or any other part of his body, he admits that he would cut off his foot either as a freewill offering or in response to a revelation from the Lord. The plaintiff wants to be released from the hospital so that he can better express his divine message to our people and our policy makers.

The court also found as facts the following: When the plaintiff first entered the state hospital on October 2, 1943, his mental condition was diagnosed as dementia praecox, paranoid type, and this continued to be the diagnosis to the time of trial. This condition is manifested by what psychiatrists term the plaintiff's false beliefs regarding his role as a prophet, his divine message and the meaning of sacred scripture. These beliefs and the fact that he acted upon them by the removal of his eye and the amputation of his hand are the only factors which entered into the diagnosis that the plaintiff is mentally ill. Such beliefs were held by the plaintiff not only before these incidents but ever since then. Because of his persistent false beliefs without any observable improvement, it is expected that these beliefs will remain for a foreseeable period of time, and the possibility of a further self-injurious act cannot be ruled out. Although the possibility of suicide is ruled out, there is a possibility that the plaintiff might receive further communications from God and might respond by removing a foot. The mere medical diagnosis of dementia praecox, paranoid type, would not in itself require the plaintiff's confinement in a hospital for the mentally ill. In the opinion of the psychiatrist from the staff of the state hospital, the plaintiff is not dangerous to anyone other than himself. He has not done any self-injurious act in twenty years. The plaintiff's mental condition has remained about the same since 1947, but there is no evidence of gross worsening of this condition. The fact that the plaintiff currently needs further confinement in a hospital for the mentally ill is based on the opinion of the psychiatrist that there is a possibility that the plaintiff might cut off his right foot. The plaintiff's religious beliefs are considered by the psychiatrist as "grandiose" and "grossly false" and represent a fantasy which is one of the primary symptoms of schizophrenic reaction, paranoid type. The plaintiff's removal of his right eye in 1944 and his right hand in 1947 were not the manifestations of a religious belief but indications of a mental illness. The mental illness from which the plaintiff suffered in 1947 still persists, and he is currently in need of further confinement in a hospital for the mentally ill.

* * *

The plaintiff's basic claim is that he is being illegally confined because of his religious beliefs in violation of the first and fourteenth amendments to the United States constitution and of article first, §§ 3 and 20, of the Connecticut constitution. He urges that he is not likely to injure any other person; that, at the very worst, the state is concerned with a mere possibility that he will remove a foot; and that even if he did remove a foot, there is no evidence that the removal would prevent him from leading a useful and productive life. * * * A "mentally ill person" includes "each person afflicted by mental disease to such extent that he requires care and treatment for his own welfare or the welfare of others or of the community." General Statutes § 17–176. The claim of the plaintiff that he is being confined solely because of his religious beliefs is not supported by the finding. It is common knowledge that the mental illness of many persons is associated with apparently fervent religious beliefs. The court found, on the basis of expert psychiatric evaluation, that the incidents wherein the plaintiff removed his eye and his hand were not manifestations of a religious belief but were symptoms of mental illness which continued to exist to the date of trial.

* * *

Although the psychiatrist who examined the plaintiff had never heard of anyone else having a religious belief which caused the believer to do this kind of damage to himself, and the trial court so found, the plaintiff insists that his confinement discriminates against him because of his religious belief. "The First Amendment declares that Congress shall make no law respecting an establishment of religion or prohibiting the free exercise thereof. * * * No one would contest the proposition that a State may not, by statute, wholly deny the right to preach or to disseminate religious views. Plainly such a previous and absolute restraint would violate the terms of the guarantee. It is equally clear that a State may * * * safeguard the peace, good order and comfort of the community, without unconstitutionally invading the liberties protected by the Fourteenth Amendment." Cantwell v. State of Connecticut, 310 U.S. 296, 303, 60 S.Ct. 900, 903, 84 L.Ed. 1213.

The conclusions of the trial court that the continued confinement for treatment of the plaintiff in accordance with statute is not illegal and that there has been no infringement of the rights accorded him by the constitution of the United States and the constitution of Connecticut cannot be disturbed.

There is no error.

* * *

SHEA, ACTING JUSTICE (dissenting).

* * *

The opinion of the psychiatrist that there is a possibility that the plaintiff might cut off his right foot is the sole basis for the conclusion that further confinement of the plaintiff is needed. The finding states also that "the plaintiff is not dangerous to anyone other than himself, and the latter danger is not a definite thing, in that it is only a possibility in the plaintiff's mind."

* * *

To warrant a conclusion under the statute that the welfare of the plaintiff requires continued treatment in a mental institution, the risk of self-inflicted mayhem on his part ought to be substantially greater than for normal citizens engaged in the many hazardous pursuits of modern life. Perhaps the subordinate facts found, relating to acts performed by the plaintiff twenty years ago, would support such an inference, if it had been drawn by the trial court. A court of review, however, is limited to the finding, and here it is explicitly stated that the need for confinement is based solely on the possibility that the plaintiff may harm himself upon release.

As between the possibility that the plaintiff may amputate his foot and the certainty that, under this judgment, he must remain incarcerated against his will indefinitely, I choose the former.[h]

Accordingly, I dissent.

BOGGS v. N.Y. CITY HEALTH & HOSP. CORP.

Supreme Court, Appellate Division, First Department, 1987.
132 A.D.2d 340, 523 N.Y.S.2d 71.

* * *

Ms. Billie Boggs (Ms. Boggs) is a forty year old woman, whose real name is Ms. Joyce Brown. She chooses to use the name Ms. Billie Boggs, since she admires a television personality of that name, and she desires to thwart her family's efforts to locate her. For the past year,

---

h. According to Frances, "The Borderline Self–Mutilator: Introduction," 29 Comp.Psychiat. 259 (1987), "of all disturbing patient behaviors, self-mutilation is the most difficult for clinicians to understand and treat. . . . Many times an otherwise promising treatment reaches a stalemate or ends because of the inability of the patient and the clinician to manage the self-mutilation in a fashion that will reduce or eliminate it." Another article states: "With the possible exception of patients who are severely mentally retarded or who have diseases with an overwhelming biological component, deviant self-mutilation is best thought of as a purposeful, if morbid, act of self-help." Favazza, "Why Patients Mutilate Themselves," 40 Hosp. & Comm.Psychiat. 137, 143 (1989). [Footnote by eds.]

Ms. Boggs has lived on the public sidewalk in front of a restaurant, located on 65th Street and Second Avenue, in New York County, and she has used this location as her bedroom, toilet and living room.

Over the course of the subject year, Ms. Boggs has been observed on an almost daily basis by persons affiliated with Project Help, which is an emergency psychiatric service for allegedly mentally ill homeless persons, who live on the streets in New York City. The personnel of this organization are comprised of a clinical team of psychiatrists, nurses and social workers, who travel around New York City, for the purpose of identifying persons, who live in the street, and who appear to be particularly in need of immediate psychiatric hospital treatment, due to the fact that those persons appear to be in danger of doing serious harm to themselves or others.

On October 28, 1987, Dr. Lincoln Robert Asher Hess, who is a psychiatrist with Project Help, determined, after a number of observations of Ms. Boggs, at her location on the pavement, that Ms. Boggs was severely mentally ill, and that she needed *immediate hospitalization*, since she posed a danger of serious harm to herself. Thereafter, Project Help arranged for Ms. Boggs' transportation, against her will, to Bellevue Hospital (Bellevue), pursuant to § 9.39 of the Mental Hygiene Law (MHL). In pertinent part, subdivision (a) of § 9.39 of the MHL authorizes a hospital to receive and retain as a patient, for a period of fifteen days, any person "alleged to have a mental illness for which immediate observation, care, and treatment in a hospital is appropriate and which is likely to result in serious harm to . . . [herself] or others . . . ." [material in brackets added].

* * *

On October 30, 1987, a hearing was conducted, and both the petitioner and respondents presented evidence.

* * *

The respondents presented their case first, in opposition to Ms. Boggs' release.

* * *

On direct examination, Dr. Hess, after his qualification as an expert by the Court, testified, that he works as a psychiatrist with Project Help three days a week; in the course of his duties with Project Help, he first saw Ms. Boggs in the street on July 23, 1987; on that occasion, he approached her, with the knowledge that Ms. Boggs had exhibited hostility to Project Help's staff in the past; he observed that Ms. Boggs was dressed in disheveled clothing; although, it was not raining, Ms. Boggs was twirling an open umbrella to avoid eye contact with him and the persons passing by; at that time, Dr. Hess heard Ms. Boggs speaking in rhymes, and, according to the witness, the content of these rhymes was sexual, and related to Dr. Hess' and Ms. Boggs' genitals; in the witness' professional opinion this type of verbalization is referred to as "Clanging", and is indicative of a thought disorder, in which a person transfers their thinking from one thought to another without any logical sequence.

The second time Dr. Hess observed Ms. Boggs in the street was five days later, on July 28, 1987. Since the first time that he had seen her, Dr. Hess testified, in substance, that Ms. Boggs' clothing had become more disheveled, dirty and torn, and she was barefoot. When Dr. Hess attempted to speak to Ms. Boggs, she cursed him, flipped open her skirt and exposed her nude buttocks, and made references to his genitals. In Dr. Hess' professional opinion, on July 28th, Ms. Boggs appeared to be flat, and disordered, which he testified is characteristic of schizophrenia.

Dr. Hess made his third street observation of Ms. Boggs on September 22, 1987. As before, Dr. Hess found Ms. Boggs at the same location, which was the sidewalk at Second Avenue near 65th Street. In pertinent part, Dr. Hess testified that Ms. Boggs' clothes were even dirtier than before, and torn to the point that large portions of her torso were exposed, and her clothing was inadequate for the weather; her hair was matted; he noticed the smell of urine and feces emanating from her; he saw pieces of United States currency, which had been torn up in neat pieces stuck to the sidewalk near Ms. Boggs, upon which she appeared to have urinated; Ms. Boggs cursed and shouted obscenities at him; nevertheless, Ms. Boggs did accept food from him, after first refusing it, but, after accepting same, she then threw the contents of this lunch at Dr. Hess, and chased him around the corner. On this occasion of September 22nd, Dr. Hess evaluated Ms. Boggs as having angry, threatening, and intensely hostile feelings, and "again there was a sign of throatiness in the sense there was no modulation . . . .".

In evaluating Ms. Boggs, Dr. Hess considered his personal observations, her history, and information he received from other Project Help members, such as psychiatrists, nurses and social workers. As a result of this data, Dr. Hess was of the opinion that Ms. Boggs exhibited a deteriorating psychosis and a deteriorating ability to care for herself. For example, he had received information that Ms. Boggs had run out into the traffic to throw away warm clothing that she had received from personnel representing Project Help.

Finally, on October 28th, Dr. Hess observed Ms. Boggs lying at her location with her head resting on a cardboard box. She smelled strongly of feces, and Dr. Hess again saw torn currency stuck to the pavement and stained by urine. The currency was very neatly torn and urinated upon, and Dr. Hess testified that this was a ritualistic tearing, which suggested magical thinking or delusion. She said repeatedly to Dr. Hess, "What is my name?", which is also indicative of a thought disorder.

* * *

Ms. Putnam was a psychiatric social worker, who had been the coordinator of Project Help for five years and she was qualified by the Court as an expert psychiatric social worker. [A]ccording to Ms.

Putnam, as Project Help observed Ms. Boggs, over the course of the year, her behavior changed for the worse. In the winter of 1986–87, Ms. Boggs appeared to be passive, but by the Spring, Ms. Boggs became more aggressive.

On May 8th, 1987, Ms. Putnam personally observed an incident, involving Ms. Boggs' hostile reaction to some delivery men, who were across the street from her location. These men were gathered outside a restaurant, apparently making a delivery. Suddenly, according to Ms. Putnam, Ms. Boggs began screaming racial epithets at these men, calling them f...... n....., b...... s...." shouting at them to get away from her, and cursing at them. As a result of this incident, Ms. Putnam became concerned that Ms. Boggs might be assaulted, due to her provocative behavior, and Ms. Putnam perceived that Ms. Boggs might have delusions regarding black men, whom she believed treated her as a prostitute. Also, Ms. Putnam reported her May 8th, 1987 observation about Ms. Boggs' reaction to the delivery men, to Project Help psychiatrists.

* * *

The next witness, for the respondents, was Dr. Mahon, who was Ms. Boggs' treating psychiatrist at respondent Bellevue. Before testifying, Dr. Mahon was qualified by the Court as an expert in psychiatry.

* * *

Dr. Mahon, . . . first saw Ms. Boggs on October 29th; at that time, Dr. Mahon did not speak with Ms. Boggs, since Ms. Boggs' was hostile, angry, and used threatening gestures; verbally, Ms. Boggs was obscene and loud. Thereafter, Dr. Mahon, saw Ms. Boggs on October 30th; and, on that date, Ms. Boggs appeared to be less angry and Dr. Mahon spent about 30 minutes with her. [T]he third time Dr. Mahon saw Ms. Boggs was on October 31st. Dr. Mahon noted that on each encounter, Ms. Boggs and Dr. Mahon established more of a relationship.

Finally, on November 2nd, the morning of the Hearing, Dr. Mahon saw Ms. Boggs again, and found her to be bright, verbal and oriented, as to time and place. Furthermore, that morning, Ms. Boggs was more cooperative than ever, even allowing Dr. Mahon to ask her to interpret certain proverbs.

In her diagnosis, Dr. Mahon found Ms. Boggs to be a chronic schizophrenic, axis one, paranoid type. Moreover, Dr. Mahon stated that Ms. Boggs' mental condition had improved during her hospitalization at Bellevue, and that it was very common for a patient like Ms. Boggs to stabilize in a structured setting. Furthermore, Dr. Mahon thought that some of Ms. Boggs' improvement may have been due to a dose of medication, "Heloperidol", which she received when she was first admitted to the hospital.

* * *

[T]he Court asked if Ms. Boggs' mental status could change markedly in three weeks, from the time Ms. Boggs was seen at Metropolitan

Hospital, until she was admitted to Bellevue. Dr. Mahon answered that question, in substance, as follows:

> "I think Miss Boggs shows remarkable ability, as is not uncommon with some psychiatric patients, to adapt and to regroup and organize herself temporarily in settings such [as] psychiatric emergency rooms, such as the inpatient service here at Bellevue and appear to be very rational and appear not to have any severe psychosis.

> "However, as a psychiatrist what I have to do is make sure I evaluate not only what I am seeing now and on a daily basis with Miss Boggs, but look at the history, and running in front of traffic and saying she has a right to endanger her life is suicidal and as a psychiatrist, I have to call that suicidal behavior and I have to treat it as a clinician . . . .". [material in brackets added]

* * *

Ms. Boggs, the petitioner, then presented her case.

* * *

One psychiatrist who testified for Ms. Boggs was Dr. Gould, who was a professor of psychiatry at New York Medical College, and an attending psychiatrist at Metropolitan Hospital. Respondents stipulated that he is an expert in psychiatry.

In substance, on direct examination, Dr. Gould testified, as follows: four days after Ms. Boggs was admitted to Bellevue, on November 1st, 1987, he first examined Ms. Boggs, and found her to be "warm and open, spoke without any pressure spontaneously, coherently, logically, without any tangential thinking . . ."; he had never seen Ms. Boggs on the street; he found no suicidal or homicidal ideation and no delusions or hallucinations concerning Ms. Boggs; and, upon this basis he concluded that Ms. Boggs was not psychotic.

Furthermore, Dr. Gould noted that Ms. Boggs' judgment "was the only thing that was slightly impaired in a sense that she was not aware socially of the kind of troubles ensue from her behavior. [Her] insight was somewhat impaired along the same lines, but by no means nil . . . ." In the witness' professional opinion, Ms. Boggs is not schizophrenic; he discussed with Ms. Boggs the incidents reported by other doctors, and, that she explained her reasons for her actions; he indicated that Ms. Boggs has no delusions about money, rather, he explained, that when someone threw paper money at Ms. Boggs and she found it insulting or degrading, she would destroy it; with respect to her urinating and defecating on the street, the witness thought that it was not delusional because Ms. Boggs, according to him, had no alternative; he did not believe Ms. Boggs was either suicidal or dangerous to herself; when Ms. Boggs ran in front of traffic, the witness testified "there was no indication, in my questioning her about this, that she was interested in having herself killed . . .."; he further noted "the fact that she has never been hurt and she's never hurt herself is strong indication that she has very good survival skills"; he believed Ms. Boggs' verbal abuse of others presented no danger, since he explained that Ms. Boggs simply did not wish to be disturbed by some individuals who invaded her privacy and she cursed at them to go away; he stated that Ms. Boggs was congenial to those people she liked, even though he had never observed her in the street; when asked if her verbal response to those she disliked presented a danger, the witness responded "I think that comes under the old cliche of sticks and stones may break my bones, but words can never hurt me. That is all she's ever done, being verbally abusive . . ."; he rejected the testimony of respondents' experts that a paranoid schizophrenic could stabilize within a few days of an involuntary admission to a hospital; in fact, in his opinion, rather than stabilized, he believed that Ms. Boggs would become more angry; he indicated that, in his opinion, the small amount of medication Ms. Boggs had been given could not account for the change in her behavior following her admission to Bellevue; with respect to predictions of future dangerousness, he found them suspect, in view of the fact that to diagnose someone who is suicidal, there must be a history of severe depression and usually suicide attempts; with respect to violent behavior towards others, it would be necessary, in his opinion, to show violence in the past, "that she may have been carrying weapons or using weapons at times . . ."; he found no evidence of deterioration in Ms. Boggs mental or physical condition; he believed she provided for herself quite well, by eating every day from a nearby deli; and he found that her only deterioration was in the state of her clothing.

* * *

Ms. Boggs testified in her own behalf. She lives next to a restaurant on Second Avenue, between 65th and 66th Streets and she stays at that location, since there is a hot air vent, although she lived on the streets during the winter of 1986, she indicated that she had never been cold; she panhandles money for food, and, in that fashion, she makes between eight and ten dollars a day; she needs allegedly about seven dollars a day to buy her food; she admitted to urinating and defecating on the street, she denied defecating on herself or in her clothes; . . . she admitted . . . that she did defecate and urinate in her clothes; she claims she has adequate clothes, and that when she needed more she had "friends" who would supply them to her; she used profanity in order to make the staff of Project Help go away; she claims that her umbrella serves the purpose of protecting her from the sun; she claimed that she had never run in traffic, but, on one occasion, when Project Help tried to offer her a pair of slacks, she stepped between two cars and threw the slacks into the street; she destroys paper money, if it is thrown at her or given to her in an allegedly offensive manner; she has no delusions about black persons giving her money for sex; and, she never hurt anyone on the street or threatened anyone, and no one ever threatened her for using profanity.

Furthermore, Ms. Boggs testified that she would go back to the streets, if released.

* * *

It is well-established in this State that a person may be involuntarily confined for care and treatment, where his or her mental illness manifests itself in neglect or refusal to care for themselves to such an extent that there is presented "serious harm" to their own well-being. . . .

* * *

We find that the Hearing Court erred in placing "great weight on the demeanor, behavior and testimony" of Ms. Boggs, since the Hearing Court does not claim that the demeanor and behavior of Ms. Boggs, when she appeared before it, remotely resembled the demeanor and behavior she exhibited when she lived on the streets, and was involuntarily committed to Bellevue on October 28, 1987.

It is hardly surprising that the Hearing Court stated, "Throughout her testimony, . . . [Ms. Boggs] was rational, logical, coherent. Her use of English, both in syntox (sic) and vocabulary, is very good and bespeaks an educated, intelligent person. She displayed a sense of humor, pride, a fierce independence of spirit, quick mental reflexes . . .", in view of the fact that, when Ms. Boggs was in the courtroom, she had recently been bathed, was dressed in clean clothes, and had just received approximately a week of hospital treatment.

* * *

We reject, as against the weight of the evidence, the Hearing court's conclusion that, in substance, Ms. Boggs' homelessness is not a result of serious mental illness, but, rather, is the result of New York's lack of housing for the poor.

* * *

Accordingly, order, Supreme Court, New York County (Robert D. Lippmann, J.), entered November 12, 1987, which granted the petition of Ms. Billie Boggs, and directed her release from respondent Bellevue Hospital by 6:00 P.M. on November 12, 1987, is reversed, on the law and on the facts, petition is denied and the proceeding is dismissed, without costs.

* * *

MILONAS, JUSTICE (dissenting).

* * *

All of respondents' psychiatrists specifically deny that Brown has suicidal ideation. She has certainly never physically harmed herself, and respondents do not really advance the proposition that she is apt to do so in the future. The record does not show a single instance in which petitioner has ever hurt herself.

* * *

In the end, respondents' effort to institutionalize petitioner can be narrowed down to one claim: she is dangerous to herself because, as a result of her abusive and obscene speech and generally obnoxious behavior, she is likely to provoke others to do injury to her. Respondents contend that Brown has been living on the streets for some time, cursing and shouting and engaging in various bizarre behavior. Yet no one has assaulted her.

* * *

Petitioner's conduct on the street is understandable if we appreciate her obvious pride in her independence and in her ability to survive on her own. She derives a unique sense of success and accomplishment in her street life. In petitioner's words, when poignantly describing her ability to endure on the streets, she has called herself a "professional". Now in the face of petitioner's assessment of herself, and in her own view, Project HELP has been endeavoring to compel her to accept assistance and be dependent. Moreover, on at least five occasions, Project HELP forced her, while handcuffed, to be transported to Metropolitan Hospital, where various physicians always refused to admit her since she was deemed to be not dangerous. In fact, she was taken to Metropolitan Hospital under restraint shortly after both incidents considered significant by respondents—her running into the street and her shouting at the delivery men. Both times she was observed by different doctors while she was at her worst and still determined not to be dangerous to herself or others. Petitioner's explanation for her street conduct is that she has learned that by employing her "profanity" and assorted bag of obnoxious tricks, she was always able to induce Project HELP to retreat.

* * *

It is a tragedy that in our wealthy society so many people have been driven to homelessness, and those of us who are more fortunate must helplessly witness and feel their misery on a daily basis. Regrettably, our affluent, sophisticated and medically advanced society has not developed a more rational, effective and humane way of dealing with the mentally disturbed homeless than in a manner other than what appears to be revolving door mental health—that is, forcibly institutionalize, forcibly medicate, stabilize, discharge back into the same environment, and then repeat the cycle. These ill and unfortunate citizens especially deserve our sympathy since they are not only homeless, but hopeless. Yet, they have shown extraordinary courage, strength and resourcefulness in their ability to survive in conditions where the "normal" person would be unable to endure.

Questions and Comments

1. *Mental illness and parens patriae commitment.* Although incapacity to make treatment decisions has traditionally been thought to be the necessary predicate for parens patriae commitment, only a few states specifically require such a finding; most merely require proof that "mental illness" is causing the self-harming condition. As suggested in the previous materials, there may be theoretical justification for the latter approach. In light of *Mayock* and *Boggs,* do you think an incapacity requirement would make a difference in practice?

2. *Defining the bases for intervention.* A perusal of judicial decisions reveals several separate grounds for intervention under the parens patriae

authority. They might be classified generally under two categories: direct physical harm to self and self-neglecting behavior. Under the first category would fall (1) suicide; (2) "self-mayhem", as illustrated by *Mayock;* and (3) harm to self caused by provocation of others (as argued by the state in *Boggs*). Self-neglect might be subdivided into (4) an inability to provide for one's survival needs; (5) a present ability to survive, but an inattention to deteriorating mental and physical health; or, most broadly, (6) a need for treatment.

Most state statutes do not explicitly differentiate between these various bases for commitment. For instance, in several states, the only parens patriae ground for commitment is "danger to self." This language clearly encompasses suicidal behavior but is also, as *Boggs* illustrates, often meant to cover other self-harming conduct as well, including at least some versions of self-neglectful behavior. Cf. *Lazaro,* supra. Most other statutes divide parens patriae commitment into two categories: danger to self and inability to care for self. The latter standard is framed in a number of different ways. Many states just use the inability to care language. California permits commitment when a person is "gravely disabled," which is defined to mean "[a] condition in which a person, as a result of a mental disorder, is unable to provide for his basic personal needs for food, clothing, or shelter." Cal.Code § 5008(h)(1). Michigan's statute is more specific, requiring proof that the person "is unable to attend to those of his basic physical needs such as food, clothing, or shelter that must be attended to in order for him to avoid serious harm in the near future, and who has demonstrated that inability by failing to attend to those basic physical needs." Mich.Comp.Laws Ann. § 330.1401.

A few states explicitly permit commitment on "potential-for-deterioration" grounds, a standard which has been forcefully recommended by the American Psychiatric Association. The APA's Model Act would permit commitment when the person "will if not treated suffer or continue to suffer severe and abnormal mental, emotional, or physical distress, and this distress is associated with significant impairment of judgement, reason or behavior causing a substantial deterioration of his previous ability to function on his own." Stromberg & Stone, "A Model State Law on Civil Commitment of the Mentally Ill," 20 Harv.J.Legis. 275, 330 (1983). The APA states that this provision is meant to permit commitment "of severely mentally ill individuals who are moving toward sudden collapse," id. at 305, and that it applies to a group of people "commonly excluded from the mental health system by current legal standards [such as grave disability]." Id. at 304, 335.

Research seems to bear this latter assertion out. In 1979, Washington amended its definition of grave disability to include not only a mentally ill individual who "is in danger of harm resulting from a failure to provide for essential human needs of health or safety," but also one who "manifests severe deterioration in routine functioning evidenced by repeated and escalating loss of cognitive or volitional control over his or her actions and [who] is not receiving such care as is essential for his or her health or safety." West's Rev.Code Wash.Ann. 71.05.020(1). A study comparing commitment records for the two years prior to passage of this amendment to the two years after passage found that the amendment had a significant impact on the hospital population. Among its findings were the following:

> 2) the number of patients committed involuntarily increased significantly, and many patients who had had no previous contact with state hospitals were committed to psychiatric facilities; 3) these new patients stayed in hospitals longer than other patients and became chronic users of the state mental hospitals; 4) the major state mental hospital became extremely overcrowded and tried unsuccessfully to put a limit on new admissions; 5) voluntary patients were virtually excluded from state hospitals . . .

Durham & LaFond, "The Empirical Consequences and Policy Implications of Broadening the Statutory Criteria for Civil Commitment, 3 Yale Law & Policy Review, 395, 401 (1985); see also, Hasebe & McRae, "A Ten–Year Study of Civil Commitments in Washington State," 38 Hosp. & Comm. Psychiat. 983 (1987). Particularly interesting is the authors' conclusion that the broadened criteria have created a new class of chronic patients. Wexler has suggested a reason why this might be the case. Noting that "the very process of gathering evidence of a person's committability under a [law which requires specific indicia of inability to care] may operate therapeutically to render commitment unnecessary," he suggests, in contrast, that laws which do not require such indicia may countertherapeutically encourage a failure to assert oneself and test one abilities, thus ultimately creating a dependence upon state institutions. Wexler, "Grave Disability and Family Therapy: The Therapeutic Potential of Civil Libertarian Commitment Codes," 9 Int'l J.Law & Psychiat. 39, 54 (1986).

The final variation of parens patriae commitment is simply a standard which permits involuntary hospitalization if a person needs treatment as a result of mental illness. Although prior to 1970 many statutes used this precise language, today no state does. However, a few statutes permit commitment for the "welfare" of the person. See, e.g., Md.Ann.Code 59 § 3(g); N.J.Stat.Ann. 30:4–23.

Under which of these formulations, if any, would Mayock or Brown be committable? The persons described in Cases 2, 19 and 22, on pp. 604–608?

3. *Vagueness doctrine.* Some courts have held that particular language implementing the parens patriae authority is so vague that it violates the due process clause of the United States Constitution.[i] *Lazaro*, supra, is one example. Another is Commonwealth ex rel. Finken v. Roop, 234 Pa.Super. 155, 339 A.2d 764 (1975), in which the court struck down a Pennsylvania statute which permitted commitment of any person who "is believed to be mentally disabled and in need of care or treatment of such mental disability." The court stated: " 'In need of care' is so broad as to be virtually meaningless. Furthermore, once a finding of mental illness is made, it would be impossible not to find that the individual is in need of

---

i. Statutory language authorizing state intervention on dangerousness to others grounds has also been challenged on vagueness grounds, see, e.g., Jurek v. Texas, 428 U.S. 262, 96 S.Ct. 2950, 49 L.Ed.2d 929 (1976), but most, if not all, *successful* vagueness challenges of civil commitment statutes have focused on parens patriae provisions.

care." Is the vagueness doctrine the appropriate vehicle for such a decision? See pp. 636–638. If so, might it not also be used to strike down statutes which permit commitment of those who are "dangerous to self"?

4. *Parens patriae and guardianship.* In several states, procedures exist for appointing a guardian for individuals who are committed for self-neglecting behavior. For instance, in California, a "conservator" may be appointed to make decisions about treatment and other personal matters for anyone who is found to be gravely disabled (but not for those who are committed as suicidal). Cal.Code § 5350. In many jurisdictions, the process may be reversed; that is, a person may be adjudicated incompetent to handle his or her affairs and thus in need of a guardian, who might then seek court authorized institutionalization. Guardianship will be discussed in more detail in Chapter Nine. For present purposes, the following questions about guardianship and its relationship to commitment can be posed. If commitment is under the parens patriae authority, is there some value in having a guardian make the ultimate decisions about treatment or care, rather than the patient or the treatment staff? If so, should a guardian be appointed for every person committed under the parens patriae authority? Or, as is true in California, should a guardian be appointed only for those who fall under certain categories of parens patriae commitment?

5. *Comparing parens patriae and police power commitment.* Setting aside the obvious differences concerning the harms focused upon, provisions implementing the parens patriae and police power authority tend to be consistent. For instance, as already noted, the same definition of mental illness is used in both contexts. Yet arguably the type of mental illness contemplated by each type of commitment is significantly different. Other aspects of the parens patriae and police power perspectives worth comparing are considered below.

The Overt Act and Imminence Requirements. Typically, a state statute which requires a recent overt act and a prediction of imminent danger when defining the police power also does so when defining danger to self; likewise, if these requirements are not present in the definition of danger to others, they are absent when defining danger to self as well. Are the theoretical and practical justifications for the overt act and imminence requirements in police power commitment present when committing someone thought to be suicidal? In this regard, consider that only "one quarter to one half of all completed suicides have a history of prior suicide attempts" and that "the majority of patients who attempt suicide do not go on to commit suicide." Hirschfeld & Davidson, "Clinical Risk Factors for Suicide," 18 Psychiatric Annals 628, 632 (1988).

In connection with the inability to care criterion, most state statutes do not require an overt act in so many words but, as the examples given above illustrate, they do require a showing that the person is unable to provide for basic needs, which may be equivalent. On the other hand, some versions of the deterioration standard (see language from APA Act, supra) do not seem to contemplate any explicit overt act requirement. Moreover, the imminence requirement is rarely associated with either criterion. Is this appropriate? Consider this example from Treffert, "The Practical Limits of Patients' Rights," 5 Psychiat. Annals 4 (1975).

A 49 year-old woman with anorexia nervosa, admitted to a medical unit in a general hospital because of profound weight loss, steadfastly refused to eat. She presented a life-threatening situation, albeit not an imminent one. This was her response to a family struggle in which she was deeply enmeshed, but she was in good general contact with reality and was not flagrantly psychotic. She refused voluntary psychiatric intervention and, in spite of her frail and deteriorating condition, insisted on leaving the hospital. Her family and physician petitioned the court for psychiatric observation of the patient. The judge believed, however, that the situation lacked dangerousness in an *immediate or imminent sense,* and the patient therefore failed to qualify for involuntary commitment. She was sent home, as she desired, and three weeks later she died from inanition.

[Emphasis in original].

Durational Limitations. Most states also do not differentiate between the length of commitment authorized for police power and parens patriae commitment. California's statute, on the other hand, provides several different durational limits. All patients are subject to an initial 72–hour emergency detention period and a 14 day "intensive treatment" period. But if further commitment is necessary the statute distinguishes between categories. It limits confinement of suicidal individuals to 14 additional days, while authorizing confinement of those considered dangerous to others for up to 180 days (with additional 180–day extensions, if an overt act occurs during confinement). For those who are found to be gravely disabled, after a 30 day investigation period commitment is authorized for up to one year (with continuous one-year extensions permitted). Cal.Code §§ 5260, 5300, 5361.

Overlap. Ultimately, how meaningful is the distinction between the two grounds for intervention when applied to individual cases? Cannot an argument be made that both Mayock and Brown are dangerous to others, at least under the broader definitions of that term? Cannot one say that Nyflot, Sansone and D.R.S. acted in "self-harming" ways? Is there a reason for avoiding such characterizations (perhaps by saying we're only interested in the behavior that is "proximately caused" by mental illness), or should we be willing to classify individuals under both categories if we can possibly do so?

III. THE LEAST RESTRICTIVE ALTERNATIVE DOCTRINE

Whether the basis of state intervention is the police power or *parens patriae,* almost all state statutes require the committing authority to consider dispositions other than hospitalization in a mental institution. This requirement has come to be known as the least restrictive alternative doctrine. Least restrictive alternative analysis has also played a significant role in two other contexts associated with mental disability law. First, it has been used as a device for regulating treatment imposed on persons *after* they have been committed or otherwise subjected to state intervention. Second, it has been relied upon in asserting that the government has an *obligation to create* community-based services. These second and third variants of the doctrine are considered in Chapter Ten. Here the focus will be on how the least restrictive alternative doctrine regulates the "front-end" dispositional decision made by the committing authority.

LAKE v. CAMERON

United States Court of Appeals, District of Columbia Circuit, 1966.
364 F.2d 657.

BAZELON, CHIEF JUDGE:

Appellant is confined in Saint Elizabeths Hospital as an insane person and appeals from denial of release in habeas corpus. On September 29, 1962, when she was sixty years old, a policeman found her wandering about and took her to the D.C. General Hospital. On October 11, 1962, she filed in the District Court a petition for a writ of habeas corpus. The court transferred her to St. Elizabeths Hospital for observation in connection with pending commitment proceedings, allowed her to amend her petition by naming the Superintendent of Saint Elizabeths as defendant, and on November 2, 1962, dismissed her petition without holding a hearing or requiring a return.

After she filed her appeal from denial of habeas corpus, she was adjudged "of unsound mind" and committed to Saint Elizabeths. At the commitment hearing two psychiatrists testified that she was mentally ill and one of them that she was suffering from a "chronic brain syndrome" associated with aging and "demonstrated very frequently difficulty with her memory * * *. Occasionally, she was unable to tell me where she was or what the date was." Both psychiatrists testified to the effect that she could not care for herself adequately. She did not take a timely appeal from the commitment order. We heard her appeal from the summary dismissal of her petition for habeas corpus and remanded the case to the District Court with directions to require a return and hold a hearing.

At the hearing on remand, the sole psychiatric witness testified that appellant was suffering from a senile brain disease, "chronic brain syndrome, with arteriosclerosis with reaction." The psychiatrist said she was not dangerous to others and would not intentionally harm herself, but was prone to "wandering away and being out exposed at night or any time that she is out." This witness also related that on one occasion she wandered away from the Hospital, was missing for about thirty-two hours, and was brought back after midnight by a police officer who found her wandering in the streets. She had suffered a minor injury which she attributed to being chased by boys. She thought she had been away only a few hours and could not tell where she had been. The psychiatrist also testified that she was "confused and agitated" when first admitted to the Hospital but became "comfortable" after "treatment and medication."

At both the commitment hearing and the habeas corpus hearing on remand, appellant testified that she felt able to be at liberty. At the habeas corpus hearing her husband, who had recently reappeared after a long absence, and her sister said they were eager for her release and would try to provide a home for her. The District Court found that she "is suffering from a mental illness with the diagnosis of chronic brain syndrome associated with cerebral arteriosclerosis"; that she "is in need of care and supervision, and that there is no member of the family able to give the petitioner the necessary care and supervision; and that the family is without sufficient funds to employ a competent person to do so"; that she "is a danger to herself in that she has a tendency to wander about the streets, and is not competent to care for herself." The District Court again denied relief in habeas corpus, but noted appellant's right "to make further application in the event that the patient is in a position to show that there would be some facilities available for her provision." The court thus recognized that she might be entitled to release from Saint Elizabeths if other facilities were available, but required her to carry the burden of showing their availability.

Appellant contends in written and oral argument that remand to the District Court is required for a consideration of suitable alternatives to confinement in Saint Elizabeths Hospital in light of the new District of Columbia Hospitalization of the Mentally Ill Act, which came into effect after the hearing in the District Court. Indeed, her counsel appointed by this court, who had interviewed appellant, made clear in answer to a question from the bench on oral argument that although appellant's formal pro se pleading requests outright release, her real complaint is total confinement in a mental institution; that she would rather be in another institution or hospital, if available, or at home, even though under some form of restraint.

* * *

We are not called upon to consider what action we would have taken in the absence of the new Act, because we think the interest of justice and furtherance of the congressional objective require the application to the pending proceeding of the principles adopted in that Act. It provides that if the court or jury finds that a "person is mentally ill and, because of that illness, is likely to injure himself or other persons if allowed to remain at liberty, the court may order his hospitalization for an indeterminate period, or order any other alternative course of treatment which the court believes will be in the best interests of the person or of the public." D.C.Code § 21–545(b) (Supp. V, 1966). This confirms the view of the Department of Health, Education and Welfare that "the entire spectrum of services should be made available, including outpatient treatment, foster care, halfway houses, day hospitals, nursing homes, etc." The alternative course of treatment or care should be fashioned as the interests of the person and of the public require in the particular case. Deprivations of liberty solely because of dangers to the ill persons themselves should not go beyond what is necessary for their protection.

The court's duty to explore alternatives in such a case as this is related also to the obligation of the state to bear the burden of exploration of possible alternatives an indigent cannot bear. This appellant, as appears from the record, would not be confined in Saint Elizabeths if her family were able to care for her or pay for the care she needs. Though she cannot be given such care as only the wealthy can afford, an earnest effort should be made to review and exhaust available resources of the community in order to provide care reasonably suited to her needs.

At the habeas corpus hearing, the psychiatrist testified that appellant did not need "constant medical supervision," but only "attention"; that the psychiatrist would have no objection if appellant "were in a nursing home, or a place where there would be supervision." At the commitment hearing one psychiatrist testified that "Mrs. Lake needs care, whether it be in the hospital or out of the hospital," and did not specify what, if any, *psychiatric* care she needs. The second psychiatrist testified that she "needs close watching. She could wander off. She could get hurt and she certainly needs someone to see that her body is adequately cared for * * *. [She] needs care and kindness * * *." It does not appear from this testimony that appellant's illness required the complete deprivation of liberty that results from commitment to Saint Elizabeths as a person of "unsound mind."

* * *

We remand the case to the District Court for an inquiry into "other alternative courses of treatment." The court may consider, *e.g.,* whether the appellant and the public would be sufficiently protected if she were required to carry an identification card on her person so that the police or others could take her home if she should wander, or whether she should be required to accept public health nursing care, community mental health and day care services, foster care, home health aide services, or whether available welfare payments might finance adequate private care. Every effort should be made to find a course of treatment which appellant might be willing to accept.

* * *

We express no opinion on questions that would arise if on remand the court should find no available alternative to confinement in Saint Elizabeths.

* * *

Remanded for further proceedings in accordance with this opinion.

[The concurring opinion of J. Skelly Wright is omitted.]

BURGER, CIRCUIT JUDGE, with whom DANAHER and TAMM, CIRCUIT JUDGES, join (dissenting).

We disagree with remanding the case to require the District Court to carry out an investigation of alternatives for which Appellant has never indicated any desire. The only issue before us is the legality of

Mrs. Lake's confinement in Saint Elizabeths Hospital and the only relief she herself has requested is immediate unconditional release. The majority does not intimate that Appellant's present confinement as a patient at Saint Elizabeths Hospital is illegal, or that there is anything wrong with it except that she does not like it and wishes to get out of any confinement. Nevertheless, this Court now orders the District Court to perform functions normally reserved to social agencies by commanding search for a judicially approved course of treatment or custodial care for this mentally ill person who is plainly unable to care for herself. Neither this Court nor the District Court is equipped to carry out the broad geriatric inquiry proposed or to resolve the social and economic issues involved.

* * *

If Appellant were to receive precisely the same care she is presently receiving in the geriatrics ward of St. Elizabeths at an institution elsewhere with a name like Columbia Rest Haven, it does not appear that there would be much disagreement over the propriety of her confinement. However, a person's freedom is no less arrested, nor is the effect on him significantly different, if he is confined in a rest home with a euphemistic name rather than at St. Elizabeths Hospital.

* * *

We can all agree in principle that a series of graded institutions with various kinds of homes for the aged and infirm would be a happier solution to the problem than confining harmless senile ladies in St. Elizabeths Hospital with approximately 8000 patients, maintained at a great public expense. But it would be a piece of unmitigated folly to turn this appellant loose on the streets with or without an identity tag; and I am sure for my part that no District Judge will order such a solution. This city is hardly a safe place for able-bodied men, to say nothing of an infirm, senile, and disoriented woman to wander about with no protection except an identity tag advising police where to take her. The record shows that in her past wanderings she has been molested, and should she be allowed to wander again all of her problems might well be rendered moot either by natural causes or violence. * * *

Questions and Comments

1. *The constitutional status of the least restrictive alternative doctrine.* The court in *Lake* based its holding on an interpretation of the District of Columbia's commitment statute. Still unresolved, at least by the United States Supreme Court, is whether the least restrictive alternative doctrine has constitutional status. As a theoretical matter, limiting state intervention to that necessary to achieve the government's objective might seem an important goal; indeed, the Supreme Court has applied this idea in a number of individual cases, most notably those involving the first amendment. In Shelton v. Tucker, 364 U.S. 479, 81 S.Ct. 247, 5 L.Ed.2d 231 (1960), the most widely cited case of this type, the Court stated:

In a series of decisions this Court has held that, even though the governmental purpose be legitimate and substantial, that purpose cannot be pursued by means that broadly stifle fundamental personal liberties when the end can be more narrowly achieved. The breadth of legislative abridgement must be viewed in light of less drastic means for achieving the same basic purpose.

Id. at 488, 81 S.Ct. at 252. But the Court has been unwilling to adopt the "least drastic means" principle as a mandatory aspect of judicial review in any area of the law. See generally, Chambers, "Alternatives to Civil Commitment of the Mentally Ill: Practical Guides and Constitutional Imperatives," 70 Mich.L.Rev. 1107, 1146–1151 (1972).

This ambivalence toward less drastic means analysis has carried over into civil commitment. In *Sanchez v. New Mexico,* 396 U.S. 276, 90 S.Ct. 588, 24 L.Ed.2d 469 (1969), the Supreme Court dismissed "for want of a substantial federal question" a New Mexico supreme court decision rejecting the argument that *Shelton* and other cases required the committing authority to consider alternatives to hospitalization. However, in *O'Connor v. Donaldson,* supra, the Court cited *Shelton* in support of the following statement: "[W]hile the State may arguably confine a person to save him from harm, incarceration is rarely if ever a necessary condition for raising the living standards of those capable of surviving safely in freedom, on their own or with the help of family or friends." In a more recent case, *Youngberg v. Romeo,* 457 U.S. 307, 321, 102 S.Ct. 2452, 2461, 73 L.Ed.2d 28 (1982), the Supreme Court had occasion to consider the minimal conditions that the due process clause requires the state to provide to hospitalized mental patients. There it expressly adopted the following statement made by a judge in the lower court:

> [T]he Constitution only requires that the courts make certain that professional judgment in fact was exercised. It is not appropriate for the courts to specify which of several professionally acceptable choices should have been made.

While *Youngberg,* which is discussed in detail in Chapter Ten, did not directly address the constitutionality of the least restrictive alternative doctrine, some courts have relied on this language in questioning whether the doctrine is constitutionally required. Other lower courts, however, have held that *Youngberg* does not foreclose such a finding. See generally, Costello & Preis, "Beyond Least Restrictive Alternative: A Constitutional Right to Treatment for Disabled Persons in the Community," 20 Loyola L.A.L.Rev. 1527, 1545–52 (1987).

For the purpose at issue here—that is, evaluating the impact of the doctrine on the dispositional decision made by the committing authority— the constitutional status of the doctrine may not be an important issue. As of 1985, at least forty-seven states required that involuntary patients be committed to treatment in the least restrictive setting. Keilitz, Conn, & Giampetro, "Least Restrictive Treatment of Involuntary Patients: Translating Concepts Into Practice," 29 St. Louis Univ.L.Rev. 691, 708 (1985).

2. *The meaning of the doctrine.* As Hoffman and Foust point out, Hoffman & Foust, "Least Restrictive Treatment of the Mentally Ill: A Doctrine in Search of Its Senses," 14 San Diego L.Rev. 1100, 1139–43 (1977),

neither the purpose of the least restrictive alternative doctrine nor the manner in which it is supposed to operate are clear.

The [least restrictive alternative] doctrine's current conceptualization and application to the involuntary treatment of the mentally ill . . . raises serious questions about its implementation, definition and fundamental purpose. As applied at the outset of the commitment process, for example, the least restrictive alternative concept makes little practical sense. Virtually all jurisdictions relying upon mandatory application of the doctrine prior to court-ordered hospitalization foresee this application as an additional safeguard to prevent unnecessarily coercive treatment. It is as if no one prior to the commitment hearing had examined or even entertained the possibility of alternatives to hospitalization. But in the majority of cases this is patently absurd. Civil commitment proceedings more often *follow* trials of less restrictive alternatives than trigger them. The competent clinician treating a patient as an outpatient, for example, tries to avoid hospitalization until virtually no other alternative offers sufficient therapeutic promise or safety for the patient and others. Family members and friends of the patient also seek alternatives to involuntary hospitalization even if for no other reason than to avoid the personal discomfort and stigma of formal commitment proceedings. The unworkability of less restrictive alternatives, and not the failure to consider them, ultimately leads to most commitment proceedings. It is little wonder, therefore, that many judges . . . believe the requirement to find less restrictive alternatives inappropriate before ordering involuntary hospitalization to be a mere formality.

Even assuming a serious judicial interest in less restrictive alternatives, current statutory construction of the doctrine does not designate who will search for or assess the relative merits of less restrictive treatment alternatives. Moreover, the judiciary's attempts to assign these responsibilities to itself, the state, the clinician, or the patient have failed to achieve meaningful results because these parties have been incapable or unwilling to assume the tasks. . . .

The confusion apparent in the administration of the doctrine is compounded by current legislative and judicial constructions which rely upon simple definitions of its critical elements. . . . [T]he doctrine's exclusive reliance upon physical restrictiveness is untenable on its face. The psychic intrusiveness of chemical or biological treatments, for instance, which are administered in a variety of therapies may be no less important than the physical aspects of the treatment facility. In addition to the nature of treatment and the setting in which it occurs, the duration of coerced treatment may be relevant to considerations of its restrictiveness.

However slippery its definition of restrictiveness, the doctrine's conceptualization of effectiveness seems even more elusive. Presumably the doctrine contemplates a consensus—medical, legal, and preferably both—about how treatment effectiveness will be measured, and what should be the minimum goals attained by the patient before the state's interest in coerced treatment will no longer prevail. Yet historically,

the absence of consensus about the goals of treatment has characterized the endless debates over involuntary treatment of the mentally ill.
[Moreover], the clinician is often unable to predict the outcome of a
treatment alternative without an adequate trial of that therapeutic
option and an empirical assessment of its results.

If there can be no immediate agreement about the goals of treatment,
or even about the threshold below which the state will not coerce
treatment, perhaps the doctrine would at least presume some relationship between the variables of restrictiveness and treatment effectiveness. Of course, there may be no relationship between these variables,
but restrictiveness might vary inversely with effectiveness so that least
restrictive treatment provides the least effective care. Finally, a third
relationship might exist in which the variables are directly related,
rather than inversely, and the most effective treatment is unfortunately also the most restrictive. . . .

This problem arises frequently in decisions to commit patients to the
hospital for acute and intensive care in lieu of providing treatment
within the community. The acutely psychotic patient, for example,
who is out of touch with reality, suffers generally from severe environmental over-stimulation.[118] Literally flooded with confusing sensations
and thoughts, these patients frequently benefit from and even request
physical isolation or seclusion from other persons to better organize
their thoughts and perceptions.[119] Indeed, for these patients, institutions during the pre-phenothiazine era functioned as true "asylums"
for the insane. In the alternative, certain adolescent patients locked
in destructive conflicts with their parents or other authorities may
consciously or unconsciously seek restrictions on their behavior. A
consistent, fair, and even restrictive parent (or parent-substitute) may
provide the adolescent with an essential model of human behavior to
emulate in later years. To the extent that such goals are thought to be
desirable, appropriate treatment may be more restrictive. . . .

Obviously, when effective treatment is also the most restrictive, a
balance must be struck between the interests of liberty on the one
hand and therapy on the other. Moreover, the balance will be different for individual patients according to their idiosyncrasies. Yet even
as a normative statement, the doctrine does not establish a sufficiently
precise theoretical basis for making these difficult clinical judgments.
Instead, all too often it finds expression in inarticulate statutory
construction and simple judicial notions of "need for treatment," and
"restrictiveness.". . . .

Hoffman and Foust suggest that, at the initial commitment proceeding,
the most effective treatment should be sought; the physical restrictiveness
of the therapy should be a secondary concern. Only after "the maximum

---

118. So desperate may be the need of
such patients for less, rather than more
stimulation, that some authors question
whether the normal hospital environment
is sufficiently tranquil. See Van Putten,
"Milieu Therapy: Contraindications?"
130 Arch. Gen. Psych. 52 (1973).

119. Not only do certain patients seek
isolation from others, but they improve
with such "treatment." See Goldberg &
Rubin, "Recovery of Patients During Periods of Supposed Neglect," 37 Brit. J. Med.
Psychiat. 265 (1964).

benefits of care have already accrued, or the patient has not responded to the institution and is untreatable in that setting" should "the importance of patient treatability diminish . . . [and] that of treatment restrictiveness emerge. . . ." Id. at 1146. Is the approach suggested by Hoffman and Foust consistent with the premise of the least restrictive alternative doctrine?

3. *Effectiveness of community treatment.* As Hoffman and Foust note, whether or not it is the primary consideration, treatment efficacy should presumably at least be considered in deciding between hospitalization and some community alternative, such as a nursing home, a halfway house, or outpatient treatment. Probably the best survey of studies comparing hospital and community treatment is found in Kiesler & Sibulkin, Mental Hospitalization 152–180 (1987). After looking at all the available studies involving random assignment of patients to either hospital or alternative care, these authors concluded that "the most general conclusion one can draw . . . is that alternative care is more effective and less costly than mental hospitalization." Id. at 179. In another summary of basically the same data, Kiesler stated:

> It seems quite clear from these studies that for the vast majority of patients now being assigned to inpatient units in mental institutions, care of at least equal impact could be otherwise provided. There is not an instance in this array of studies in which hospitalization had any positive impact on the average patient care investigated in this study. In almost every case, alternative care had more positive outcomes. There were significant and powerful effects on such life-related variables as employment, school attendance, and the like. There were significant and important effects on the probability of subsequent readmission. Not only did the patients in the alternative care not undergo the initial hospitalization but they were less likely to undergo hospitalization later, as well.

Kiesler, "Mental Hospitals and Alternative Care: Noninstitutionalization as Potential Public Policy for Mental Patients," 37 Am.Psychol. 349, 350 (1982).

Other research which looks at the efficacy of community treatment in isolation (that is, without a hospital control group) indirectly confirms these findings, even with those groups, such as the "chronically" mentally ill, which were formerly thought to require constant inpatient care. One review of this second type of research found, for instance, that if a full range of comprehensive community services is provided to such people:

> [h]ospitalization can be virtually eliminated for all but 15% to 25% of these [chronically mentally ill] individuals. Psychotic symptomatology can be dramatically reduced. Client satisfaction with life can be somewhat increased, social functioning can be maintained or restored to pre-morbid levels and in some cases improved. While many of these persons will be unable to sustain normal work and social roles, most will be able to participate in employment and social activities if ongoing supportive or some semi-sheltered environments in these areas are provided.

Test, "Effective Treatment of the Chronically Mentally Ill: What is Necessary", 37 J. Social Issues 71, 82 (1981).

However, as Kiesler and Sibulkin admit, the research consensus that alternative care is more effective than hospital treatment may not apply to *all* potential patients. While they note that most of the studies involved treatment of the severely disabled, they also state that their generalization about the superior quality of community care "may not be true for all disorders, age groups, etc. Insufficient detail is provided in these studies to assess such questions even preliminarily." Id. at 177. Indeed, none of the studies reviewed by Kiesler and Silbulkin appear to involve patients considered imminently dangerous to self or others. Given current perceptions about the mentally disabled, it would be difficult, if not impossible, to arrange a study randomly assigning, as all of Kiesler's studies did, half the subjects to community treatment, if the subject population were composed of people who were thought to be on the verge of harming themselves or others.

Assuming that alternative care would be more effective for a particular patient, a second problem with generalizing the research is that many communities lack the types of innovative programs reported in the reviews mentioned above; instead, they offer only mediocre inpatient care in a local facility. This phenomenon, which has been dubbed "*trans*institutionalization", may result in care that is neither more efficacious nor less physically restrictive than care in the hospital. See Bachrach, "Is the Least Restrictive Environment Always the Best? Sociological and Termantic Implications," 31 Hosp.Com.Psychiat. 97 (1980). If the dispositional choice is between a hospital and one of these community inpatient units, is there still an argument to be made in favor of choosing the latter?

4. *Outpatient commitment.* As of 1985, twenty-six states had enacted statutes explicitly authorizing commitment on an out-patient basis, and virtually all other states implicitly allow such commitment by requiring that treatment be provided in the least restrictive environment. Keilitz & Hall, "State Statutes Governing Involuntary Outpatient Civil Commitment," 9 Mental and Phys.Dis.L.Rep. 378 (1985). Statutes which explicitly authorize outpatient commitment differ significantly, but three general models can be posited. The first permits outpatient commitment only after some form of inpatient commitment, either in a hospital or in the community. Under this model, outpatient commitment functions somewhat like parole; the patient is permitted to leave the hospital so long as he or she continues to follow a certain treatment regimen on an outpatient basis. This approach might be especially useful for those patients who tend to go off their medication. The second model, more relevant to the present discussion, authorizes outpatient commitment to a community facility at the "front end" of the commitment process if the traditional commitment criteria are met, without any preliminary requirement of inpatient treatment. Presumably this model is an explicit statutory effort to implement the least restrictive alternative doctrine. The third model—sometimes called preventive commitment—also permits outpatient commitment at the front end, but under commitment standards which are significantly different from typical "libertarian" commitment standards: they require only a

showing that the individual will *soon meet* the traditional standards for institutionalization (and thus are very similar if not identical to the "deterioration" standard described in the previous section). Apparently this type of outpatient commitment is a response to a number of factors, including "concerns about . . . a growing number of mentally disordered people in shelters and on the streets, resistant to treatment and in various stages of decompensation, who cannot be hospitalized under the strict commitment criteria; a backlash among psychiatrists and mental health professionals to what is perceived as over-legalization of the mental health system; and advocacy by increasingly vocal parents' groups, particularly the National Alliance for the Mentally Ill, who are demanding treatment for their family members and increasingly allying themselves with mental health professionals to press for the easing of commitment standards." Stefan, "Preventive Commitment: The Concept and Its Pitfalls," 11 Men. Dis.L.Rep. 288 (1987). About five states have enacted preventive outpatient commitment statutes. The rest authorize either the first or second types of outpatient commitment or, most commonly, authorize both.

The implementation of any of these models can present significant obstacles. Schwartz and Costanzo, "Compelling Treatment in the Community: Distorted Doctrines and Violated Values," 20 Loyola L.A.L.Rev. 1329, 1377 (1987), state:

> While outpatient commitment has been an available option in most jurisdictions for many years, several factors have precluded states from relying extensively on what is arguably a more desirable alternative. These operational barriers include: (1) the lack of appropriate community mental health programs; (2) the difficulty of compelling committed individuals to comply with treatment plans; (3) the probability that few persons would comply with court-ordered treatment and yet be unwilling to voluntarily participate in a community program; (4) the reluctance of mental health providers to treat their clients involuntarily and subject themselves to judicial supervision; (5) the absence of judicial mechanisms and personnel to adequately supervise outpatient care; (6) the resistance of neighbors and public officials to accept committed persons in their community; (7) the fears of professionals concerning liability for inadequate treatment or foreseeable harm; and (8) the potential creation of a governmental obligation to fund a comprehensive system of community services for individuals subject to outpatient commitment.

There is a fair amount of research supporting many of these assertions. First, Schwartz and Costanzo are correct in contending that outpatient commitment is not widely used. A nationwide survey found that, in those jurisdictions which permit such commitment, it is chosen as the proper disposition less than five percent of the time. Miller, "Commitment to Outpatient Treatment: A National Survey," 36 Hosp. & Comm.Psychiat. 265 (1985). Other research suggests that this reluctance to use outpatient commitment is due in part to the types of reasons advanced by Schwartz and Costanzo. One such study looked at an outpatient commitment system in North Carolina which combined the first two models noted above. It described the results of outpatient commitment both before and after a

1979 statutory change designed to improve the system by requiring that proposed outpatient treatment be shown to be available in the community and by providing for specific procedures for dealing with treatment non-compliance. The study found that treatment experiences of patients before and after passage of the statute changed very little. Indeed, after passage, the percentage of patients who complied with their court-ordered treatment plans actually dropped from 77% to 50% and the community staff continued to evaluate outpatient commitment treatment as effective in only 46% of the cases, the same percentage obtained prior to passage. The authors of the study speculated, based in part on a survey of the relevant treatment professionals, that these results stemmed from several factors, including: (1) the fact that a significant proportion of the commitments were the result of "plea bargaining" which often ignored the wishes of the patient and the clinical recommendations of the treatment staff; (2) the ideological resistance of community-based clinicians to involvement in the provision of involuntary treatment and their fear of liability; (3) the difficulty of communicating between hospitals and community mental health centers. Miller and Fiddleman, "Outpatient Commitment: Treatment in the Least Restrictive Environment?" 35 Hosp. & Comm. Psychiat. 147 (1984). A review of the few studies of preventive commitment also concluded that the programs were "underfunded, underutilized and generally ineffective." Stefan, supra at 291. The most successful outpatient commitment programs appear to be those adopting the first model rather than the second or third, and even these have experienced serious implementation problems. See studies collected in American Psychiatric Association Task Force Report on Outpatient Commitment (1982).

As a counter to this research, the reader is again referred to the studies reviewed by Kiesler and Sibulkin, many of which compared outpatient care in the community to hospital care; these studies suggest that certain types of outpatient treatment are more effective than inpatient commitment for at least *some* groups of people. Is outpatient commitment an idea worth pursuing or, as Schwartz and Costanzo argue, ibid. at 1404, is it neither feasible nor necessary?

5. *The effect of the doctrine on commitment criteria.* If the least restrictive alternative doctrine is implemented aggressively—by endorsing a preference for community treatment in most cases and outpatient commitment in many—what will be the likely impact on the criteria for commitment? If an expansion of the commitment net were to occur as a result of more aggressive application of the doctrine, could it be justified on the ground that the deprivation of liberty which results is less intrusive? On any other grounds?

IV. PROCEDURES

A. GENERAL CONSIDERATIONS

As recounted at the beginning of this chapter, until the 1970's the civil commitment proceedings of many states were extremely informal. Because they were perceived to be medical rather than legal, commitment decisions were often made by mental health professionals, with little or no input by lawyers and few procedural rules. Today, however, every state requires more legalistic procedures. The model for these reforms has been the criminal justice system, which grants the accused a number of rights, including the right to a public trial in front of a judge and jury, the right to notice of the charges, the rights to an opportunity to confront accusers and subpoena witnesses, the right to the assistance of counsel and the right to remain silent in response to government questions. This section examines the extent to which the criminal process model is an appropriate one for civil commitment.

LESSARD v. SCHMIDT

United States District Court, E.D.Wisconsin, 1972.
349 F.Supp. 1078.

* * *

[T]he lifting of procedural safeguards in [civil commitment proceedings] appears to rest in part on the realities of better treatment for the person subjected to incarceration in a civil proceeding. In Kent v. United States, the Supreme Court, discussing the issue in the context of juvenile courts, observed:

> "The objectives are to provide measures of guidance and rehabilitation for the child and protection for society, not to fix criminal responsibility, guilt and punishment. The State is *parens patriae* rather than prosecuting attorney and judge. But the admonition to function in a 'parental' relationship is not an invitation to procedural arbitrariness.

> "2. Because the State is supposed to proceed in respect of the child as *parens patriae* and not as adversary, courts have relied on the premise that the proceedings are 'civil' in nature and not criminal, and have asserted that the child cannot complain of the deprivation of important rights available in criminal cases. It has been asserted that he can claim only the fundamental due process right to fair treatment. . . .

> "While there can be no doubt of the original laudable purpose of juvenile courts, studies and critiques in recent years raise serious questions as to *whether actual performance measures well enough against theoretical purpose to make tolerable the immunity of the process from the reach of constitutional guaranties applicable to adults.* There is much evidence that some juvenile courts, . . . lack the personnel, facilities and techniques to perform adequately as representatives of the State in a *parens patriae* capacity, at least with respect to children charged with law violation. There is evidence, in fact, that there may be grounds for concern that the child receives the worst of both worlds: that he gets neither the protections accorded to adults nor the solicitous care and regenerative treatment postulated for children."

(Emphasis added). Few persons familiar with the mental health field will question the applicability of much of the above to persons subjected to involuntary commitment in state institutions.

In any event, the argument in favor of relaxed procedures on the basis of a subsequent right to treatment ignores the fact that unless constitutionally prescribed procedural due process requirements for involuntary commitment are met, no person should be subjected to "treatment" against his will. The argument also ignores the fact that many mental illnesses are untreatable, and the substantial evidence that any lengthy hospitalization, particularly where it is involuntary, may greatly increase the symptoms of mental illness and make adjustment to society more difficult.

* * *

A second justification for less stringent safeguards in civil commitment proceedings is simply that the proceedings are "civil" and not "criminal." That argument should have been laid to rest following the Supreme Court's decision in In re Gault, in which the Court found the distinction unpersuasive as an excuse for providing lesser safeguards for juveniles in delinquency proceedings than were given adults charged with violations of the criminal law.

* * *

Even a brief examination of the effects of civil commitment upon those adjudged mentally ill shows the importance of strict adherence to stringent procedural requirements and the necessity for narrow, precise standards.

An individual committed to a mental institution loses numerous civil rights. In Wisconsin, hospitalization for mental illness, whether by voluntary admission or involuntary commitment, raises a rebuttable presumption of incompetency. The presumption continues as long as the patient is under the jurisdiction of hospital authorities. An individual adjudged mentally ill in Wisconsin also faces restrictions on making contracts and limitations on the right to sue and be sued. Restrictions on licenses required to engage in certain professions also accompany an adjudication of mental illness in Wisconsin. Wis.Stat.Ann. § 441.07 (1972 Supp.) (registered and practical nurses), § 447.07(7) (1972 Supp.) (dentists and dental hygienists), § 256.286 (attorneys). Persons found mentally ill in Wisconsin are, like felons, unable to vote. The mentally ill are also prohibited from driving a car and serving on juries. No person found to be "insane, imbecile, or feeble-minded" may participate in a marriage contract.

It is obvious that the commitment adjudication carries with it an enormous and devastating effect on an individual's civil rights. In some respects, such as the limitation on holding a driver's license, the civil deprivations which follow civil commitment are more serious than the deprivations which accompany a criminal conviction.

In addition to the statutory disabilities associated with an adjudication of mental illness, and just as serious, are the difficulties that the committed individual will face in attempting to adjust to life outside the institution following release. Evidence is plentiful that a former mental patient will encounter serious obstacles in attempting to find a job, sign a lease or buy a house. One commentator, noting that "former mental patients do not get jobs," has insisted that, "[i]n the job market, it is better to be an ex-felon than ex-patient."

In summary, an adjudication of mental illness in Wisconsin carries with it loss of basic civil rights and loss of future opportunities. The damage done is not confined to a small number among the population. * * * It would thus appear that the interests in avoiding civil commitment are at least as high as those of persons accused of criminal offenses. The resulting burden on the state to justify civil commitment must be correspondingly high.

Questions and Comments

1. *Procedural due process analysis.* Two years after *Lessard* the United States Supreme Court formulated what has become the standard analysis for determining how much process is due when a particular government action is contemplated. In *Mathews v. Eldridge,* 424 U.S. 319, 335, 96 S.Ct. 893, 903, 47 L.Ed.2d 18 (1976), involving the administration of social security benefits, the Court outlined three basic factors that must be considered: (1) the private interest that will be affected by the official action; (2) the risk of an erroneous deprivation of such interest through the procedures used, and the probable value, if any, of additional or substitute procedural safeguards; and (3) the government's interest, including the function involved and the fiscal and administrative burdens that the additional or substitute requirements would entail. *Mathews* is usually cited by courts considering the process due in civil commitment cases.

2. *Changes since* Lessard. Although true at the time of *Lessard,* few states today link involuntary hospitalization with incompetency. Most jurisdictions abide by the holding in *Wyatt v. Stickney,* 344 F.Supp. 373 (M.D.Ala.1972), that "[n]o person shall be deemed incompetent to manage his affairs, to contract, to hold professional or occupational or vehicle operator's licenses, to marry and obtain a divorce, to register and vote, or to make a will *solely* by reason of his admission or commitment to the hospital." Id. at 379. (Emphasis in original). Thus, until the person is adjudicated incompetent and has a guardian appointed, these privileges are not forfeited.[j] In many states, however, the hospitalized person does lose the right to refuse treatment; control over personal funds may also be circumscribed to some extent. S. Brakel, J. Parry & B. Weiner, The Mentally Disabled and the Law 258–59 (1985). How do these developments affect the analysis in *Lessard*?

3. *Juvenile justice analogy.* As *Lessard* indicates, presaging the reform of the civil commitment process was an analogous movement in the juvenile justice system. Prior to the mid–1960's, hearings to determine whether a child was "delinquent" (i.e., had committed an act which would be a crime if the child had been an adult) were very informal, often presided over by "judges" who were not legally trained; lawyers were either not present or acted perfunctorily. As with civil commitment, the

j. These issues are addressed further in Chapter Nine.

premise of this system was paternalistic. Intervention by the state was for
the purpose of setting the child on the right track, not to punish. According to proponents of the system, therefore, delinquency hearings did not
need the trappings and procedural ridigity of the adult criminal system.

In a series of decisions between 1966 and 1975, the Supreme Court
seriously undermined this position. It revamped procedures for transferring children to adult court in *Kent v. United States,* 383 U.S. 541, 86 S.Ct.
1045, 16 L.Ed.2d 84 (1966), mandated that notice, counsel, confrontation
rights and the right to remain silent be provided children alleged to be
delinquent in *In re Gault,* 387 U.S. 1, 87 S.Ct. 1428, 18 L.Ed.2d 527 (1967)
and, in *In re Winship,* 397 U.S. 358, 90 S.Ct. 1068, 25 L.Ed.2d 368 (1970),
held that the reasonable doubt standard of proof applied in such proceedings. The essential rationale of these decisions was the minimal difference
between criminal proceedings against adults and delinquency proceedings
against children. By 1975, Chief Justice Burger was able to state, in the
course of holding that the double jeopardy clause applies to delinquency
proceedings, that "it is simply too late in the day to conclude . . . that a
juvenile is not put in jeopardy at a proceeding whose object is to determine
whether he has committed acts that violate a criminal law and whose
potential consequences include both the stigma inherent in such a determination and the deprivation of liberty for many years." *Breed v. Jones,* 421
U.S. 519, 95 S.Ct. 1779, 44 L.Ed.2d 346 (1975).

As *Lessard* illustrates, these cases were viewed as precedent for reform-
minded courts deliberating on the proper procedures for civil commitment.
In particular, note the court's use of *Kent* and *Gault* to rebut the two
arguments usually advanced for relaxing procedures in the civil commitment context: the therapeutic goals of civil commitment and its "civil"
label. But the comparison between the juvenile system and civil commitment is not necessarily as compelling as *Lessard* suggests. While rehabilitation remains an important goal of juvenile justice, the clear recent trend,
triggered in part by the Court's decisions, has been to recognize that
dispositions in juvenile delinquency cases have a significant punitive element. See W. Wadlington, C. Whitebread, & S. Davis, Children in the
Legal System 198–99 (1983). One consequence of this recognition is that
many states have moved away from indeterminate sentences—designed to
provide flexibility for juvenile treatment authorities—toward strictly limited dispositions based on culpability. See e.g., the Uniform Juvenile Court
Act § 36 (limiting disposition to two years). The explicit punishment
orientation of the "new" juvenile court obviously distinguishes it from civil
commitment. Should this difference make a difference in terms of procedures used in the two systems? Might the answer to this question depend
upon whether the basis for commitment is the police power or parens
patriae?

A second point worth considering in trying to draw analogies between
the two types of proceedings is that, despite the new punishment orientation of the juvenile system, many policymakers remain ambivalent about
imposing adult procedures in their entirety. This ambivalence was evident
in the Supreme Court's decision in *McKeiver v. Pennsylvania,* 403 U.S. 528,
91 S.Ct. 1976, 29 L.Ed.2d 647 (1971), which refused to apply the right to

jury trial in the juvenile delinquency context. In justifying this decision (the only Court holding that failed to equate adult and juvenile procedures), the Court stated that applying the right to jury trial would "remake the juvenile proceeding into a fully adversary process and . . . put an effective end to what has been the idealistic prospect of an intimate, informal protective proceeding." The jury trial right would not necessarily lead to more accurate factfinding, while it "would tend once again to place the juvenile squarely in the routine of the criminal process" with the attendant "traditional delay, the formality, and the clamor of the adversary system." Imposing the right would also forbid the states "to experiment further and to seek in new and different ways the elusive answers to the problems of the young." The notions suggested by this language in *McKeiver* are worth noting because they resurface in some of the Court's later civil commitment cases.

4. *The impact of reform.* Do criminal-type procedural rules have any effect on outcome? Empirical research on the issue is ambiguous. Some studies show that reforms of both the substantive criteria and procedural rules have reduced hospital admissions. But a number of studies indicate little change in outcome. Most importantly for purposes of the topic at hand, the research indicates that commitment hearings are usually adversarial in name only even in the most legalistic states.[k]

Representative are the findings of Stier & Stoebe, in "Involuntary Hospitalization of the Mentally Ill in Iowa: The Failure of the 1975 Legislation," 64 Iowa L.Rev. 1284 (1979). They concluded that, despite being highly "legalized" on paper, the Iowa commitment process was in fact very informal. They found that three-fourths of the referees (judges) and clerks of court admitted that commitment hearings were usually not conducted in an adversary manner. Defense attorneys requested an independent mental health evaluation (available by right under the statute) in fewer than 1% of cases, and they rarely called more than two witnesses (often none). The majority of attorneys failed to put the respondents on the stand. One attorney even reasoned that to do so would risk the respondents persuading the referee that they were not mentally ill. Consistent with their lack of active participation in the hearings, the attorneys uniformly spent less than two hours in preparation of these cases.

For their part, the referees encouraged passivity on the part of defense attorneys. Some referees expressly discouraged cross-examination of witnesses; if questions were to be asked, the referees themselves would ask them. The result was that commitment hearings were little more than a stamp of approval for the attending physician's opinion. In fact, a change in treatment plan from that which the hospital physician had recommended was observed in fewer than 1% of cases. Referees and attorneys generally agreed that clinicians should decide whether the elements of the standard for civil commitment had been met, and, if so, what the conditions of treatment should be.

k. See articles cited in footnotes c and d of this chapter. See also, Hiday, "Reformed Commitment Procedures: An Empirical Study in the Courtroom," 11 Law Soc'y Rev. 651 (1977); Andalman & Chambers, "Effective Counsel for Persons Facing Civil Commitment: A Survey, a Polemic, and a Proposal," 45 Miss.L.J. 43 (1974).

Finally, with respect to the meaningfulness of reform, consider the following excerpt from S. Brakel, J. Parry & B. Weiner, The Mentally Disabled and the Law 27–28 (1985):

The erection of . . . legal safeguards [in civil commitment] is based on at least two basic assumptions about "involuntary" commitment: (1) that without the safeguards people who do not belong in mental institutions will be railroaded there and (2) that involuntary commitment is a real contest between parties with opposite interests—the party who applies for institutionalization (the state, the institution, or the family) versus the individual who does not want to be institutionalized. It is the wholesale unreality of these assumptions that threatens to make their implements, the procedural safeguards, inapposite or worse. And once the procedures are enacted, their effects are difficult to avoid: the prospect of being able to apply them with proper selectivity only to those relatively few cases in which they are useful is dim, and the price of such selectivity, as mentioned, is high.

The real nature of the commitment process has been more accurately described by scholars such as Ralph Slovenko, who reports that "[a]pproximately two-thirds of [involuntarily] committed patients are passive, stuporous, or uncommunicative, or in perfect agreement with the physician's recommendation. The others protest initially, but after a few days of hospitalization they have a change of mind." [40] The real problem with institutionalization, according to Slovenko, is not the railroading of unwilling individuals but almost the opposite. In 1971, for example, although around four million Americans received treatment for mental illness in state hospitals, general hospitals, outpatient clinics, and private offices, another two million were turned away because of the lack of treatment personnel to handle them. From this perspective, the legalization and criminalization of civil commitment are an exercise in irrelevance at best. The procedure is dysfunctional—overprotective and overly technical when observed, a block to achieving generally desired results in some cases, mere wasteful and empty ritual in others. But most often, of course, it is simply not followed. Slovenko notes that commitment statutes are ignored for essentially two reasons: "they are overly complicated, and they are for the most part unnecessary."

Psychiatrists have bemoaned their plight of being part of "belegaled" profession. They have a case, and they are not alone in our belegaled society. Slovenko has written derisively of the "junk pile theory" of law: among all the legal garbage that exists to address mental health problems there must be something of use or value. The same intricate legal structure surrounding commitment that is hailed by legal reform-

---

40. There are also patients, however, who come willingly (i.e., voluntarily) to the hospital first but then after a week or two when the worst of their anxiety has passed (though they may still be "ill" and in need of treatment) decide they want out. In a recent medical journal, such patients were described as an identifiable group of "re-volving door type" patients who have slipped into a form of sociopathy that makes them unable to deal either with the freedom of life outside the hospital or with the dependency within it. Geller, The "Revolving Door": A Trap or A Life Style? 33 Hosp. & Community Psychiatry 388 (1982).

ers as crowning testimony to the law's concern for the unprotected appears to the psychiatric practitioner and others as an unwieldy, obstructionist mass of procedural "junk" that only inhibits the effort to protect.[1]

5.) *The therapeutic effect of adversarial procedures.* A common argument against adversarial procedures, alluded to in the foregoing passage, is that, if they *are* effectively implemented, they will be antitherapeutic. Ensminger and Liguori, in "The Therapeutic Significance of the Civil Commitment Hearing: An Unexplored Potential," 6 J. Psychiat. & L. 5 (1978), provide the following summary of such arguments:

[The] belief in the antitherapeutic effect of the civil commitment hearing appears to be almost as old as the institutions into which such involuntary confinement can be made. Reasons suggested in support of this belief include the following.

1. time being lost in the courtroom which can be used to better advantage in treating the prospective patient;

2. revelation in a public setting of embarrassing material, such as hostility toward parents or homosexuality;

3. revelation to the prospective patient of the physician's opinion of a serious diagnosis or poor prognosis;

4. creation of overly optimistic hopes of cure in the patient;

5. confirmation of delusions of persecution, particularly in paranoid types;

6. impairment of the psychiatrist's ability to work due to the impact of directives given by the courts;

7. trauma and exasperation resulting from the length of the hearing;

8. revelation by the therapist of statements made by the patient in sessions, the true significance of which may not yet be apparent;

9. revelation to the prospective patient of opinions of close family members;

10. disclosure of material which the patient justifiably believed was revealed in confidence;

11. rejection of any further attempts at treatment by a patient who refuses to accept suggestion that he is mentally ill;

12. traumatic effect on family members upon hearing testimony concerning their relative.

Ensminger and Liguori contest these assertions, arguing on the basis of empirical research and their own experiences in a mental health advocacy unit that "the civil commitment process has considerable potential for therapeutic effect." First, they note that the hearing, if properly conducted, represents an open acknowledgement that the patient's hospitalization

---

1. Actually, a review of psychiatrists' attitudes toward issues related to involuntary civil commitment concluded that a substantial majority of psychiatrists favor the adoption of legal procedures such as a right to notice, counsel, confrontation, and independent experts. Kahle, et al. "On Unicorns Blocking Commitment Law Reform," 6 J. Psychiat. & L. 89 (1978). [Footnote by eds.]

is involuntary. Without such acknowledgement, they assert, a double message may be conveyed by professionals who act as if they care only about the patient's well-being but nonetheless refuse to let the patient leave and restrict behavior in other ways as well. This conflicting message may be countertherapeutic to the extent the patient feels deceived—his or her response may even be "schizophrenic" if the patient feels unable to comment on the feeling of deception.

Relatedly, the authors assert that the hearing can improve the treatment of the patient and his or her relationship with the treatment staff. They contend that "the introduction of commitment hearings leads to better documentation and earlier staffing for involuntarily committed patients" and that this improvement in preparation "has led to a greater tendency to release patients, when the hospital physicians have that authority, in cases where the case for committability appears to be marginal." They also believe that "the commitment hearing should provide an opportunity for the therapist to clarify his role" and that the therapist's testimony at the hearing "can operate as something close to a reinforcement mechanism." Additionally:

> The members of the hospital staff could analyze the hearing as a group process of considerable significance for the patient. . . . For instance, the "therapeutic community" concept suggests that crisis resolution should involve (1) a face-to-face confrontation involving all major participants in the crisis situation; (2) occurring as soon as possible after the crisis arises; (3) under skilled neutral leadership; (4) allowing for open communication without fear of reprisal; and (5) with an appropriate level of feeling, neither too little nor too much. The analogies to the commitment process are evident.

Finally, the authors note that the hearing can improve the patient's relationship with the family and assist in understanding that relationship.

> Several of the arguments for the deleterious effect of commitment hearings involve notions of their effect on family relationships—that the patient will be harmed by learning what his relatives think or that they will be disturbed learning about the patient's condition. Neither of these arguments can receive much scientific support. When the patient does not know of the true feelings of his relatives, it will frequently be because they have expressed something else to him. If the hearing exposes this duplicity, it can serve the function of eliminating yet another "double bind" situation. If there is a possibility of embarrassing material being revealed, another reason suggested earlier as to why hearings are harmful, the general public can be excluded to protect the patient and the family members.

> Certain trends in psychological research and practice are beginning to view taking into account the family system as vital to the effective treatment of some cases. Indeed, the patient may just be the individual manifesting the most bizarre behavior of a maladaptation of the whole family unit. It is our opinion that the increased acceptance of this approach must involve radical restructuring of present notions of rights and duties in mental health law, if not also criminal law and jurisprudence generally.

* * *

In some states, notice of the hearing must be given to family members. It has been noted that some judges send patients out of the room while they interrogate the relatives. Aside from the infringement of the defendant's right of confrontation, it is our opinion that this deprives the therapist (who, it is asserted, should not be excluded for such testimony) of an exceptional opportunity to view the family dynamics in action. The hearing may, in fact, provide a mechanism for educating the family as to the needs of a particular member caught in the commitment process. The judge, even though he may not be able to extend his authority to other members of the family, may be able to impress upon them, in a way that doctors cannot, their responsibilities in the matter.

6. *Procedure as surrogate.* In thinking about how much procedure is due in civil commitment proceedings, the following questions, paraphrased from Cover, Fiss & Resnik, Procedure 133–134 (1988), might be usefully kept in mind. Are your views on the proper level of procedural formality "outcome-driven?" In other words, are you an advocate for more procedural formality because you hope that, under such a regime, fewer people will be committed? Or an opponent because you believe that too many will not be? At a more general level, are you concerned about restraining government power because you have concerns about the likelihood it will be abused? In what sense other than these general outcome measures might increased procedural formality improve the commitment decision? Do you believe it will improve the "accuracy" of the results reached in commitment hearings? Or, believing "accuracy" to be a loaded term, are you more influenced by the degree of participation or "sense of fairness" that various types of procedures produce?

B. EMERGENCY DETENTION AND SCREENING MECHANISMS

The focus of most litigation concerning the process of commitment has been on the procedural accoutrements of the "adjudicatory" commitment hearing, at which a determination is made about long-term commitment. Perhaps more important, however, are the procedures connected with emergency admission, which is the mechanism by which most individuals become enmeshed in the civil commitment system. According to the National Center for State Courts in "Guidelines for Involuntary Civil Commitment," 10 Men.Dis. Law Rep. 409, 427 (1986):

> The greatest activity in involuntary civil commitment proceedings occurs not in the court hearing—inaccurately considered by many to be the centerpiece of involuntary civil commitment—but rather during events before any formal judicial involvement. A person initially may become subject to involuntary civil commitment by one of several ways: by being apprehended by police; by being brought to a hospital by relatives or friends; by being converted from a voluntary patient to an involuntary patient when, after entering a mental health facility voluntarily, the person attempts to leave against the advice of the facility staff; or, finally, by being taken into custody as a result of a

legal petition submitted to and validated by a court.[m] In most jurisdictions, very little screening, early diversion of persons from involuntary mental health care, and placement in appropriate voluntary care occurs except when a formal petition has been filed with and reviewed by a court. For the most part, persons become involuntary patients by means of "emergency" commitments resulting from apprehension by police or by simply appearing on the doorstop of a mental health facility.

All states permit, under appropriate circumstances, the emergency admission of an individual without any prior formal legal hearing. In California, for instance, either a police officer or a clinician may authorize emergency admission. Cal.Code § 5150. In New York, the decision is made by a clinician at the admitting facility or by the county director of mental health. N.Y.Code §§ 9.37, 9.39. In Virginia a judge or magistrate makes the emergency detention decision, but he or she need not actually see the patient and in fact may make the decision based on information received over the phone. Va.Code 1950, § 37.1–67.1. The standard of proof to be applied by these decisionmakers is either not stated or minimal. Neither New York nor Virginia require any particular standard of proof; California requires that the decisionmaker find that "probable cause" exists to believe that the person is mentally disordered and, as a result, gravely disabled or a danger to self or others. Cal.Code § 5150.

The lack of process associated with the initial emergency admission has rarely been challenged, since most agree that a more formal process would be counterproductive.[n] A more difficult question has been whether a subsequent "detention" hearing, separate and apart from the ultimate "adjudicatory" hearing at which commitability is decided, should be held to determine whether the initial admission was appropriate and, if so, how soon and with what procedural requirements. As the next case indicates, such a preliminary hearing is required in the criminal process under certain circumstances.

GERSTEIN v. PUGH

Supreme Court of the United States, 1975.
420 U.S. 103, 95 S.Ct. 854, 43 L.Ed.2d 54.

* * *

II

As framed by the proceedings below, this case presents two issues: whether a person arrested and held for trial on an information is

---

m. This last method of initiating the commitment process, analogous to an arrest warrant, is apparently rarely used in any jurisdiction. [Eds.]

n. One corollary issue which has been raised has to do with police authority to arrest mentally disordered individuals. Under the common law, the traditional rule was that a police officer could not, absent a warrant, arrest someone for a misdemeanor (as opposed to a felony) unless the officer witnessed the misdemeanor occurring. However, at least one court has held that, if the consequence of the arrest is commitment, this rule need not be followed. *McKinney v. George*, 556 F.Supp. 645 (N.D.Ill.1983).

entitled to a judicial determination of probable cause for detention, and if so, whether the adversary hearing ordered by the District Court and approved by the Court of Appeals is required by the Constitution.

A

Both the standards and procedures for arrest and detention have been derived from the Fourth Amendment and its common-law antecedents. . . . The standard for arrest is probable cause, defined in terms of facts and circumstances "sufficient to warrant a prudent man in believing that the [suspect] had committed or was committing an offense." Beck v. Ohio, 379 U.S. 89, 91, 85 S.Ct. 223, 225, 13 L.Ed.2d 142 (1964). . . . This standard, like those for searches and seizures, represents a necessary accommodation between the individual's right to liberty and the State's duty to control crime. . . .

To implement the Fourth Amendment's protection against unfounded invasions of liberty and privacy, the Court has required that the existence of probable cause be decided by a neutral and detached magistrate whenever possible. The classic statement of this principle appears in Johnson v. United States, 333 U.S. 10, 13–14, 68 S.Ct. 367, 369, 92 L.Ed. 436 (1948):

> "The point of the Fourth Amendment, which often is not grasped by zealous officers, is not that it denies law enforcement the support of the usual inferences which reasonable men draw from evidence. Its protection consists in requiring that those inferences be drawn by a neutral and detached magistrate instead of being judged by the officer engaged in the often competitive enterprise of ferreting out crime."

* * *

Maximum protection of individual rights could be assured by requiring a magistrate's review of the factual justification prior to any arrest, but such a requirement would constitute an intolerable handicap for legitimate law enforcement. Thus, while the Court has expressed a preference for the use of arrest warrants when feasible, . . . it has never invalidated an arrest supported by probable cause solely because the officers failed to secure a warrant. . . .

Under this practical compromise, a policeman's on-the-scene assessment of probable cause provides legal justification for arresting a person suspected of crime, and for a brief period of detention to take the administrative steps incident to arrest. Once the suspect is in custody, however, the reasons that justify dispensing with the magistrate's neutral judgment evaporate. There no longer is any danger that the suspect will escape or commit further crimes while the police submit their evidence to a magistrate. And, while the State's reasons for taking summary action subside, the suspect's need for a neutral determination of probable cause increases significantly. The consequences of prolonged detention may be more serious than the interference occasioned by arrest. Pretrial confinement may imperil the suspect's job, interrupt his source of income, and impair his family relationships. . . . Even pretrial release may be accompanied by burdensome conditions that effect a significant restraint of liberty. See, e.g., 18 U.S.C. §§ 3146(a)(2), (5). When the stakes are this high, the detached judgment of a neutral magistrate is essential if the Fourth Amendment is to furnish meaningful protection from unfounded interference with liberty. Accordingly, we hold that the Fourth Amendment requires a judicial determination of probable cause as a prerequisite to extended restraint of liberty following arrest.

* * *

B

Under the Florida procedures challenged here, a person arrested without a warrant and charged by information may be jailed or subjected to other restraints pending trial without any opportunity for a probable cause determination. Petitioner defends this practice on the ground that the prosecutor's decision to file an information is itself a determination of probable cause that furnishes sufficient reason to detain a defendant pending trial. Although a conscientious decision that the evidence warrants prosecution affords a measure of protection against unfounded detention, we do not think prosecutorial judgment standing alone meets the requirements of the Fourth Amendment.

* * *

III

Both the District Court and the Court of Appeals held that the determination of probable cause must be accompanied by the full panoply of adversary safeguards—counsel, confrontation, cross-examination, and compulsory process for witnesses.

These adversary safeguards are not essential for the probable cause determination required by the Fourth Amendment. The sole issue is whether there is probable cause for detaining the arrested person pending further proceedings. This issue can be determined reliably without an adversary hearing. The standard is the same as that for arrest. That standard—probable cause to believe the suspect has committed a crime—traditionally has been decided by a magistrate in a nonadversary proceeding on hearsay and written testimony, and the Court has approved these informal modes of proof.

The use of an informal procedure is justified not only by the lesser consequences of a probable cause determination but also by the nature of the determination itself. It does not require the fine resolution of conflicting evidence that a reasonable-doubt or even a preponderance standard demands, and credibility determinations are seldom crucial in deciding whether the evidence supports a reasonable belief in guilt. . . . This is not to say that confrontation and cross-examination might not enhance the reliability of probable cause determinations in some cases. In most cases, however, their value would be too slight to justify holding, as a matter of constitutional principle, that these formalities and safeguards designed for trial must also be employed in making the Fourth Amendment determination of probable cause.

* * *

Although we conclude that the Constitution does not require an adversary determination of probable cause, we recognize that state systems of criminal procedure vary widely.

* * *

Whatever procedure a State may adopt, it must provide a fair and reliable determination of probable cause as a condition for any significant pretrial restraint of liberty,[1] and this determination must be made by a judicial officer either before or promptly after arrest.

* * *

Questions and Comments

1. *Applicability of* Gerstein *to commitment.* What implications, if any, does *Gerstein* have for the emergency admission process? Is emergency admission a "seizure" as that word is used in the Fourth Amendment? Should there be a hearing, presided over by a judicial officer, to check the emergency admission decision? Should a showing of probable cause be required? How formal should such a proceeding be in other respects? Should there be a right to be present? The right to an attorney?

Most states require some kind of post-admission check after emergency admission of a person thought to be mentally disabled, but the procedures vary widely. In Virginia, for instance, a hearing presided over by a judge, with the respondent and an attorney for the respondent present, must take place within 48 hours of admission (usually the full-fledged adjudicatory hearing takes place at this time as well). Va.Code 1950, § 37.1–67.3. In California, "certification" must take place within 72 hours, but requires only that two professionals, one of them a physician, sign a notice of certification finding that the person meets the commitment criteria. Once certified, a person may be detained for up to 14 days before a full judicial hearing. Moreover, the patient may be detained for a further 14 days without such a hearing if two professionals find that the patient "threatened or attempted to take his own life or . . . was detained for evaluation and treatment because he threatened or attempted to take his own life and . . . continues to present an imminent threat of taking his own life." Cal. Code §§ 5250, 5251, 5260, 5261. In New York, the individual may be detained up to 15 days if a mental health professional other than the admitting clinician has examined the person within 48 hours of admission and finds that the individual is mentally ill and dangerous to self or others. New York Code § 9.39(a). Confinement for a further *60* days is permitted if two physicians certify that the individual meets the commitment standards and a third physician, at the admitting institution, agrees after examining the patient and considering alternatives. N.Y.Code §§ 9.27; 9.31. In all states, judicial review (via habeas corpus) is available during the initial detention period, but only upon the patient's request and usually only after some delay (in New York, for instance, review need not take

1. Because the probable cause determination is not a constitutional prerequisite to the charging decision, it is required only for those suspects who suffer restraints on liberty other than the condition that they appear for trial. There are many kinds of pretrial release and many degrees of conditional liberty. . . . We cannot define specifically those that would require a prior probable cause determination, but the key factor is significant restraint on liberty.

place until five days from the request date). Additionally, in New York, the Mental Hygiene Legal Service, a legal advocacy organization, is located on the grounds of most facilities and monitors the patients who are admitted. N.Y.Code § 9.39(a).

2. *Procedural timeframes. Gerstein* does not set any time limits for the criminal probable cause hearing, merely stating that it should be soon after arrest and prior to subjecting the accused to release conditions such as bail. Most states, however, mandate a *"Gerstein* hearing" within 48 to 72 hours of a warrantless arrest. The time period between the *Gerstein* hearing and trial can vary immensely, limited only by statutory speedy trial provisions (rarely requiring trial less than 100 days from arrest) and the guarantee of a speedy trial in the Sixth Amendment.

In civil commitment, as the foregoing statutory illustrations indicate, the analogous time periods between detention and the detention hearing (if there is one), and between the latter hearing and the adjudicatory hearing also vary significantly, although the latter hearing always occurs much earlier, relatively speaking, than the typical criminal trial. What considerations should govern the duration of these timeframes? In *Lynch v. Baxley,* 386 F.Supp. 378, 388 (M.D.Ala.1974), the court stated:

> Just as emergency detention is justified only until a probable cause hearing can be conducted, temporary detention following a finding of probable cause to believe that confinement is necessary can be justified only for the length of time required to arrange a full hearing on the need for commitment. Due process requires that such hearing be held within a reasonable time following initial detention, but in no event sooner than will permit adequate preparation of the case by counsel or later than thirty (30) days from the date of the initial detention.

The United States Supreme Court is perhaps willing to stretch the pre-hearing periods considerably further. In the 1970's, it summarily affirmed[o] both *French v. Blackburn,* 428 F.Supp. 1351 (M.D.N.C.1977), affirmed 443 U.S. 901, 99 S.Ct. 3091, 61 L.Ed.2d 869 (1979), and *Logan v. Arafeh,* 346 F.Supp. 1265 (D.Conn.1972), affirmed sub nom., *Briggs v. Arafeh,* 411 U.S. 911, 93 S.Ct. 1556, 36 L.Ed.2d 304 (1973). The three-judge district court in *Blackburn* had found a statute permitting a ten-day period between detention and the "probable cause" hearing constitutional. In *Arafeh,* a three-judge court had upheld a statute under which a hearing could be delayed for up to 45 days, so long as a physician certified that the person met the commitment criteria and a "complaint" was filed within fifteen days. Although the Supreme Court did not issue an opinion in connection with its affirmance of these decisions, both lower court opinions relied on the same two grounds, which are concisely summarized by this language from *Blackburn:* "During [the pre-hearing] period the respondent is receiving treatment which may not only aid his health, but which also may be necessary to an adequate and informed hearing on the necessity of

o. A summary affirmance is considered binding precedent. Hicks v. Miranda, 422 U.S. 332, 95 S.Ct. 2281, 45 L.Ed.2d 223 (1975). However, "finding the precise limits of a summary affirmance has proven to be no easy task." Hardwick v. Bowers, 760 F.2d 1202, 1207 (11th Cir.1985). Without analyzing the ultimate precedential significance of *Blackburn* and *Arafeh,* it is important to note that their weight as precedent is somewhat suspect.

his commitment." 428 F.Supp. at 1355. See also, *Arafeh*, 346 F.Supp. at 1268–69.

Are the courts' assumptions accurate about how much time is needed for lawyers and clinicians to develop information relevant to commitment issues? Good clinical practice dictates that decisions about treatment be predicated on careful observation and a trial of treatment. According to a basic psychiatric text, for instance:

> When there is no acute problem (such as severe agitation or life-threatening behavior) that requires use of medication, it is helpful to observe the patient in a drug-free state for several days (or even several weeks) to see how symptoms change over time. This is particularly useful if there is some question about whether medication is likely to be helpful, or when there is confusion about the diagnosis. For example, a patient admitted to the hospital with a psychotic episode might not reveal to you that he has abused drugs. If you immediately administer an antipsychotic, you may erroneously believe that the medication alleviated a psychosis that would have abated of its own accord when the abused substance was cleared from the patient's body. Or an outpatient's depressive symptoms might improve dramatically after one or two meetings with a concerned therapist. If this patient had been given antidepressants immediately, the effect would have been attributed to the medication, and the patient's anxiety might be maintained on the drug unnecessarily. Another patient's anxiety might mask an underlying psychosis. Such a patient could easily be medicated incorrectly with an antianxiety agent before the disordered thinking became apparent.

American Psychiatric Press, Psychiatry for Medical Students (1984). The same source suggests that, before medication is administered, the psychiatrist take a careful history, and perform a routine physical examination and routine laboratory tests to rule out organic causes. Once a patient is on a particular drug, further time is necessary to gauge the patient's response, possible side effects, and the appropriate dosage, a process which can take up to six weeks. Id.

3. *Justice Brennan's* Parham *dissent*. In *Parham v. J.R. et al.*, 442 U.S. 584, 99 S.Ct. 2493, 61 L.Ed.2d 101 (1979), the Supreme Court deliberated upon the proper procedural protections for the commitment of juveniles. This decision, reprinted at pp. 788–799, has several possible implications for adult commitment procedures as well, all of which will be explored in this section. Of concern here is Justice Brennan's opinion in *Parham*, concurring in part and dissenting in part, because it suggests still other considerations in deciding whether and when to hold a formal legal hearing. The majority in *Parham* held that juveniles could be admitted initially to a mental institution based on the authority of their parents and the treating professionals, without benefit of legal counsel; it did not directly address whether the constitution requires, at some later point in time, more formal procedures to determine whether continuing commitment is justified (although it suggested strongly that it did not). Brennan argued that procedures akin to those provided adults should be required before long-term detention. However, he also stated the following:

. . . While as a general rule due process requires that commitment hearings precede involuntary hospitalization, when parents seek to hospitalize their children special considerations militate in favor of postponement of formal commitment proceedings and against mandatory adversarial preconfinement commitment hearings.

First, the prospect of an adversarial hearing prior to admission might deter parents from seeking needed medical attention for their children. Second, the hearings themselves might delay treatment of children whose home life has become impossible and who require some form of immediate state care. Furthermore, because adversarial hearings at this juncture would necessarily involve direct challenges to parental authority, judgment or veracity, preadmission hearings may well result in pitting the child and his advocate against the parents. This, in turn, might traumatize both parent and child and make the child's eventual return to his family more difficult.

Because of these special considerations I believe that States may legitimately postpone formal commitment proceedings when parents seek in-patient psychiatric treatment for their children. Such children may be admitted, for a limited period, without prior hearing, so long as the admitting psychiatrist first interviews parent and child and concludes that short term in-patient treatment would be appropriate.

442 U.S. at 632–633, 99 S.Ct. at 2519–2520. To what extent is this passage applicable to adult commitment?

4. *Pre-hearing screening.* Beginning in the 1980's, a number of states established, by statute, "screening" organizations at the community level that are charged with referring mentally disabled people to the most effective treatment program available. National Center for State Courts, "Guidelines for Involuntary Civil Commitment," 10 Men.Dis.Law Rep. 409, 429–433 (1986). A number of other jurisdictions have set up equivalent systems through local custom. Id. at 429.

In jurisdictions which have institutionalized such programs, the number of people subjected to the involuntary commitment process—including the emergency detention hearing—may be reduced considerably. According to one report, in these localities, "the great majority of persons entering the mental health-judicial system never see the inside of a courthouse, and many persons are screened and diverted to more suitable alternatives, many elect to enter mental health treatment and care programs voluntarily, and some are discharged shortly after arrival at a mental health facility." Id. at 427. For instance, Arizona requires that screening agencies—usually the local community mental health center—complete a "prepetition screening" within forty-eight hours of initial contact with an individual alleged to be disordered, designed to determine the best possible disposition. Ariz.Stat. § 36–529. Although "emergency" cases are specifically exempted from this procedure, it nonetheless appears to have enabled a significant number of individuals who would have been "emergency admissions" under the old system to avoid the involuntary commitment process altogether. In Tucson, about three times as many individuals are diverted through screening—to voluntary care, to halfway houses, and to other social agencies—than proceed through the involuntary petition process. Institute on Mental Disability and the Law, National Center for State Courts, "A Model for the Application of the Least Restrictive Alternative Doctrine in Involuntary Civil Commitment" 291–323 (1984).

Many commentators argue that such pre-hearing diversion is highly beneficial and should be encouraged. For instance, the National Task Force on Guidelines for Involuntary Civil Commitment asserted the following:

> Screening should begin as early as possible in the involuntary civil commitment process in order to avoid unnecessary infringement of liberty, to ensure that persons are guided quickly and effectively toward the placement and treatment indicated by their presenting problems, and to minimize needless waste of limited resources. Initial processing decisions are based not merely on whether the legal criteria for involuntary civil commitment are met. The threshold question may be whether the person who is considered a candidate for involuntary civil commitment is indeed mentally disordered. If so, are there alternative forms of treatment and care, other than involuntary civil commitment? Even if the person is not considered to be mentally disordered, he or she may require social services of some type. Is mandatory hospitalization necessary? Will the person consider seeking mental health treatment voluntarily? Answers to these questions require intervention and decisions long before a candidate for involuntary civil commitment has a judicial hearing.

> Such early intervention may entail no more than a mental health worker answering a telephone call from a distraught individual who is seeking help for a family member. Referral to a community mental health center or a family support group may divert a person who may otherwise become subject to formal involuntary civil commitment proceedings. These early interventions should be based on knowledge of the mental health services delivery in the area and should take into account such factors as the range of treatment and services available, the criteria for admission to various facilities, the security of particular mental health facilities, and the conditions within facilities. Good initial processing decisions also require an understanding of the linkages between the agencies.

Id. at 428.

As this excerpt suggests, in a sense the pre-hearing screening programs function as the procedural facet of the least restrictive alternative doctrine. One possible problem with such programs is that they encourage "voluntary" dispositions which are in fact not voluntary at all. This issue is addressed in detail in the materials on voluntary treatment, at pp. 745–755.

C. ADJUDICATORY HEARING PROCEDURES

1. *Standard of Proof*

ADDINGTON v. TEXAS

Supreme Court of the United States, 1979.
441 U.S. 418, 99 S.Ct. 1804, 60 L.Ed.2d 323.

MR. CHIEF JUSTICE BURGER delivered the opinion of the Court.

The question in this case is what standard of proof is required by the Fourteenth Amendment to the Constitution in a civil proceeding brought under state law to commit an individual involuntarily for an indefinite period to a state mental hospital.

* * *

II

The function of a standard of proof, as that concept is embodied in the Due Process Clause and in the realm of factfinding, is to "instruct the factfinder concerning the degree of confidence our society thinks he should have in the correctness of factual conclusions for a particular type of adjudication." The standard serves to allocate the risk of error between the litigants and to indicate the relative importance attached to the ultimate decision.

Generally speaking, the evolution of this area of the law has produced across a continuum three standards or levels of proof for different types of cases. At one end of the spectrum is the typical civil case involving a monetary dispute between private parties. Since society has a minimal concern with the outcome of such private suits, plaintiff's burden of proof is a mere preponderance of the evidence. The litigants thus share the risk of error in roughly equal fashion.

In a criminal case, on the other hand, the interests of the defendant are of such magnitude that historically and without any explicit constitutional requirement they have been protected by standards of proof designed to exclude as nearly as possible the likelihood of an erroneous judgment. In the administration of criminal justice, our society imposes almost the entire risk of error upon itself. This is accomplished by requiring under the Due Process Clause that the state prove the guilt of an accused beyond a reasonable doubt.

The intermediate standard, which usually employs some combination of the words "clear," "cogent," "unequivocal," and "convincing," is less commonly used, but nonetheless "is no stranger to the civil law." One typical use of the standard is in civil cases involving allegations of fraud or some other quasi-criminal wrongdoing by the defendant. The interests at stake in those cases are deemed to be more substantial than mere loss of money and some jurisdictions accordingly reduce the risk to the defendant of having his reputation tarnished erroneously by increasing the plaintiff's burden of proof. Similarly, this Court has used the "clear, unequivocal and convincing" standard of proof to protect particularly important individual interests in various civil cases [*i.e.,* deportation and denaturalization].

Candor suggests that, to a degree, efforts to analyze what lay jurors understand concerning the differences among these three tests on the nuances of a judge's instructions on the law may well be largely an academic exercise; there are no directly relevant empirical studies. Indeed, the ultimate truth as to how the standards of proof affect decisionmaking may well be unknowable, given that factfinding is a process shared by countless thousands of individuals throughout the country. We probably can assume no more than that the difference between a preponderance of the evidence and proof beyond a reasonable doubt probably is better understood than either of them in relation to the intermediate standard of clear and convincing evidence. Nonetheless, even if the particular standard-of-proof catchwords do not always make a great difference in a particular case, adopting a "standard of proof is more than an empty semantic exercise."

III

In considering what standard should govern in a civil commitment proceeding, we must assess both the extent of the individual's interest in not being involuntarily confined indefinitely and the state's interest in committing the emotionally disturbed under a particular standard of proof. Moreover, we must be mindful that the function of legal process is to minimize the risk of erroneous decisions.

A

This Court repeatedly has recognized that civil commitment for any purpose constitutes a significant deprivation of liberty that requires due process protection. Moreover, it is indisputable that involuntary commitment to a mental hospital after a finding of probable dangerousness to self or others can engender adverse social consequences to the individual. Whether we label this phenomena "stigma" or choose to call it something else is less important than that we recognize that it can occur and that it can have a very significant impact on the individual.

The state has a legitimate interest under its *parens patriae* powers in providing care to its citizens who are unable because of emotional disorders to care for themselves; the state also has authority under its police power to protect the community from the dangerous tendencies of some who are mentally ill. Under the Texas Mental Health Code, however, the State has no interest in confining individuals involuntarily if they are not mentally ill or if they do not pose some danger to themselves or others. Since the preponderance standard creates the risk of increasing the number of individuals erroneously committed, it is at least unclear to what extent, if any, the state's interests are furthered by using a preponderance standard in such commitment proceedings.

The expanding concern of society with problems of mental disorders is reflected in the fact that in recent years many states have enacted statutes designed to protect the rights of the mentally ill. However, only one state by statute permits involuntary commitment by a mere preponderance of the evidence, Miss.Code Ann. § 41–21–75 (1978 Supp.), and Texas is the only state where a court has concluded that the preponderance-of-the-evidence standard satisfies due process. We attribute this not to any lack of concern in those states, but rather to a belief that the varying standards tend to produce comparable results. As we noted earlier, however, standards of proof are important for their symbolic meaning as well as for their practical effect.

At one time or another every person exhibits some abnormal behavior which might be perceived by some as symptomatic of a mental or emotional disorder, but which is in fact within a range of conduct that is generally acceptable. Obviously, such behavior is no basis for compelled treatment and surely none for confinement. However, there is the possible risk that a factfinder might decide to commit an individual based solely on a few isolated instances of unusual conduct. Loss of liberty calls for a showing that the individual suffers from something more serious than is demonstrated by idiosyncratic behavior. Increasing the burden of proof is one way to impress the factfinder with the importance of the decision and thereby perhaps to reduce the chances that inappropriate commitments will be ordered.

The individual should not be asked to share equally with society the risk of error when the possible injury to the individual is significantly greater than any possible harm to the state. We conclude that the individual's interest in the outcome of a civil commitment proceeding is of such weight and gravity that due process requires the state to justify confinement by proof more substantial than a mere preponderance of the evidence.

B

Appellant urges the Court to hold that due process requires use of the criminal law's standard of proof—"beyond a reasonable doubt."

* * *

There are significant reasons why different standards of proof are called for in civil commitment proceedings as opposed to criminal prosecutions. In a civil commitment state power is not exercised in a punitive sense. Unlike the delinquency proceeding in *Winship*, a civil commitment proceeding can in no sense be equated to a criminal prosecution.

In addition, the "beyond a reasonable doubt" standard historically has been reserved for criminal cases. This unique standard of proof, not prescribed or defined in the Constitution, is regarded as a critical part of the "moral force of the criminal law," and we should hesitate to apply it too broadly or casually in noncriminal cases.

The heavy standard applied in criminal cases manifests our concern that the risk of error to the individual must be minimized even at the risk that some who are guilty might go free. The full force of that idea does not apply to a civil commitment. It may be true that an erroneous commitment is sometimes as undesirable as an erroneous conviction * * *. However, even though an erroneous confinement should be avoided in the first instance, the layers of professional review and observation of the patient's condition, and the concern of family and friends generally will provide continuous opportunities for an erroneous commitment to be corrected. Moreover, it is not true that the release of a genuinely mentally ill person is no worse for the individual than the failure to convict the guilty. One who is suffering from a debilitating mental illness and in need of treatment is neither wholly at liberty nor free of stigma. It cannot be said, therefore, that it is much better for a mentally ill person to "go free" than for a mentally normal person to be committed.

Finally, the initial inquiry in a civil commitment proceeding is very different from the central issue in either a delinquency proceeding or a criminal prosecution. In the latter cases the basic issue is a straightforward factual question—did the accused commit the act alleged? There may be factual issues to resolve in a commitment proceeding, but the factual aspects represent only the beginning of the inquiry. Whether the individual is mentally ill and dangerous to either himself or others and is in need of confined therapy turns on the *meaning* of the facts which must be interpreted by expert psychiatrists and psychologists. Given the lack of certainty and the fallibility of psychiatric diagnosis, there is a serious question as to whether a state could ever prove beyond a reasonable doubt that an individual is both mentally ill and likely to be dangerous.

The subtleties and nuances of psychiatric diagnosis render certainties virtually beyond reach in most situations. The reasonable-doubt standard of criminal law functions in its realm because there the standard is addressed to specific, knowable facts. Psychiatric diagnosis, in contrast, is to a large extent based on medical "impressions" drawn from subjective analysis and filtered through the experience of the diagnostician. This process often makes it very difficult for the expert physician to offer definite conclusions about any particular patient. Within the medical discipline, the traditional standard for "factfinding" is a "reasonable medical certainty." If a trained psychiatrist has difficulty with the categorical "beyond a reasonable doubt" standard, the untrained lay juror—or indeed even a trained judge—who is required to rely upon expert opinion could be forced by the criminal law standard of proof to reject commitment for many patients desperately in need of institutionalized psychiatric care. Such "freedom" for a mentally ill person would be purchased at a high price.

* * *

That some states have chosen—either legislatively or judicially—to adopt the criminal law standard gives no assurance that the more stringent standard of proof is needed or is even adaptable to the needs of all states. The essence of federalism is that states must be free to develop a variety of solutions to problems and not be forced into a common, uniform mold. As the substantive standards for civil commitment may vary from state to state, procedures must be allowed to vary so long as they meet the constitutional minimum. We conclude that it is unnecessary to require states to apply the strict, criminal standard.

C

Having concluded that the preponderance standard falls short of meeting the demands of due process and that the reasonable-doubt standard is not required, we turn to a middle level of burden of proof that strikes a fair balance between the rights of the individual and the legitimate concerns of the state. We note that 20 states, most by statute, employ the standard of "clear and convincing" evidence; 3 states use "clear, cogent and convincing" evidence; and 2 states require "clear, unequivocal and convincing" evidence.

We have concluded that the reasonable-doubt standard is inappropriate in civil commitment proceedings because, given the uncertainties of psychiatric diagnosis, it may impose a burden the state cannot meet and thereby erect an unreasonable barrier to needed medical treatment. Similarly, we conclude that use of the term "unequivocal" is not constitutionally required, although the states are free to use that standard. To meet due process demands, the standard has to inform the factfinder that the proof must be greater than the preponderance-of-the-evidence standard applicable to other categories of civil cases.

*   *   *

Vacated and remanded.

MR. JUSTICE POWELL took no part in the consideration or decision of this case.

Questions and Comments

1. *Implications of* Addington. The selection of the proper standard of proof is really a "substantive" issue, not a "procedural" one. See Jeffries & Stephan, "Defenses, Presumptions, and Burden of Proof in the Criminal Law," 88 Yale L.J. 1325 (1979). In civil commitment, as previous sections made clear, whether someone is committed should depend upon whether the state can establish by a given *probability,* designated by the standard of proof, that he or she will commit a harmful act or that he or she is gravely disabled.[p] But *Addington* is usefully considered in a discussion of procedu-

---

p. It should be remembered that the standard of proof may interact with the statutory definition of the criteria to produce a lower burden of proof overall.

Thus, if the state defines "danger to others" as a likelihood that a person will harm others, and this likelihood is to be proven by clear and convincing evidence,

ral issues as well because of the insight it gives into the Court's general perception of the competing interests involved in civil commitment. In this regard, several aspects of the Court's justification for adopting the clear and convincing standard rather than the reasonable doubt standard are worth noting: (1) the Court's insistence that the decisions made at a civil commitment hearing are primarily "medical" in nature; (2) its implicit conclusion that civil commitment is unlike juvenile delinquency proceedings, as evidenced by its refusal to follow *Winship,* the decision which imposed the reasonable doubt standard in such proceedings; and (3) its statement that "[i]t cannot be said . . . that it is much better for a mentally ill person to 'go free' than for a mentally normal person to be committed." Do you agree with these perceptions?

2. *The basis of intervention.* Should the Court have considered whether the standard of proof should vary depending upon whether the basis for intervention is the police power or the parens patriae authority?

2. The Decisionmaker

In criminal proceedings, the accused is guaranteed a right to a jury trial by the Sixth Amendment. This right may be waived, in which case the trial is presided over by a judge. At the adjudicatory hearing stage of civil commitment, at least four different types of ultimate decisionmakers have been authorized by state statutes: (1) a judicial officer (very often a "special judge" or a probate judge); (2) a jury (usually six strong); (3) an administrative board which does not include a judicial officer (in Nebraska, for instance, the administrative board consists of a lawyer, a mental health professional and a third person who is either a mental health professional or a layperson. Neb.Rev. Stat. § 83–325); and (4) a psychiatric board. Today almost every state relies upon a legally trained judicial officer to make the long-term commitment decision. However, several provide the respondent with the right to jury trial, if a jury is requested. A small number in addition to Nebraska permit commitment based on the decision of an administrative board. See, e.g., R.I.Gen.Laws 1956, § 40.1–5.1–9. None currently authorizes the fourth option, although it was the dominant method of decisionmaking prior to 1970. The closest any state comes to a psychiatric board is New York, which permits involuntary hospitalization for up to 60 days based on the authority of three mental health professionals, after which time a judicial hearing must take place. N.Y.Code § 9.31.

Questions and Comments

1. *Jury trial.* As noted earlier, the United States Supreme Court held in *McKeiver v. Pennsylvania,* 403 U.S. 528, 91 S.Ct. 1976, 29 L.Ed.2d 647 (1971), that there is no right to jury trial in juvenile delinquency proceedings, citing in particular the need to maintain the "intimacy" of the proceeding and to avoid the "clamor" of the adversary process. Most

the state need only show something like a
38% chance of harm to others. See discussion on pp. 640–641.

courts have relied on *McKeiver* in deciding that the right is not required at commitment proceedings either. See, e.g., *Lynch v. Baxley,* 386 F.Supp. 378 (M.D.Ala.1974); *Markey v. Wachtel,* 164 W.Va. 45, 264 S.E.2d 437 (1979). In the latter case the court stated:

> The heart of the adversarial issue is the mental condition of the individual which, as *Addington* recognizes, is a technically complex question based on the testimony of experts which a lay jury has difficulty understanding. We are unwilling to hold as a constitutional principle that the resolution of this issue can only be accomplished by a jury. Neither historical precedent nor the requisite due process procedural balance mandates such a conclusion.

Id. at 443.

Duncan v. Louisiana, 391 U.S. 145, 88 S.Ct. 1444, 20 L.Ed.2d 491 (1968), is the Supreme Court decision which held that the right to jury trial is a fundamental right guaranteed to state criminal defendants through the fourteenth amendment. *Duncan* stressed that the jury trial tradition resulted from "a reluctance to entrust plenary powers over the life and liberty of the citizen to one judge or a group of judges" and that the jury "in serious criminal cases is a defense against arbitrary law enforcement." It also pointed to the role of the jury as a means of providing decisionmaking by representatives of the community and promoting a sense of citizen participation. The Court rejected the argument that juries cannot be trusted to reach accurate conclusions. It stated that if juries occasionally reach a different decision than a judge in a particular case, "it is usually because they are serving some of the very purposes for which they were created and for which they are now employed."

Are these same points as valid when applied to civil commitment? To what extent does the jury's traditional role as a group of "peers" affect its usefulness in civil commitment? To what extent, independent of its "accuracy" as a decisionmaker, would the presence of a jury as the decisionmaker affect the "image" of civil commitment? How would it affect the mental state of the respondent? Note that the Supreme Court later limited the jury trial right in criminal proceedings to those cases involving a crime carrying a sentence of more than six months, on the ground that the "disadvantages, onerous though they may be", of imprisonment for six months or less are "outweighed by the benefits that result from speedy and inexpensive nonjury adjudication." Baldwin v. New York, 399 U.S. 66, 90 S.Ct. 1886, 26 L.Ed.2d 437 (1970).

2. *Administrative boards.* In *Doremus v. Farrell,* 407 F.Supp. 509, 516 (N.D.Neb.1975), the court held that the Nebraska administrative board (at that time composed of a lawyer, a psychiatrist and the clerk of the court) did not violate the constitution:

> Although a judicial determination would be desirable, since courts can more effectively preserve procedural due process and constitutional rights, as well as rule more proficiently on evidentiary questions, we do not believe that due process or equal protection mandates a judicial hearing. The Supreme Court has recognized the power of administrative boards to revoke parole and probation. Gagnon v. Scareplli, 411 U.S. 778, 93 S.Ct. 1756, 36 L.Ed.2d 636 (1973); Morrissey v. Brewer, 408

U.S. 471, 92 S.Ct. 2593, 33 L.Ed.2d 484 (1972). The deportation of aliens has long been considered a proper function for executive commissions. The procedural safeguards guaranteed by due process, the standards for commitment and the availability of prompt de novo review by the district court after the finding of mental illness by the county board, convinces the Court that an administrative determination is not constitutionally objectionable.

Whether the court would have arrived at the same conclusion had there been no provision for de novo review by a court is unclear. The court also found that using the board did violate the constitution if—as was apparently quite frequently the case in Nebraska—the psychiatrist who examined the respondent for purposes of the commitment proceeding also sat on the board. The court stated that "combin[ing] the investigative, prosecutorial and adjudicative functions in one authority . . . denies the subject due process of law." Id. at 516.

While the Supreme Court has not directly addressed the decisionmaker issue, at least two of its opinions are relevant. The first is *Vitek v. Jones,* 445 U.S. 480, 100 S.Ct. 1254, 63 L.Ed.2d 552 (1980), in which the Court considered the proper procedures for transferring prisoners alleged to need psychiatric care from correctional facilities to psychiatric facilities. Despite the fact that such prisoners are already confined at the time of transfer, the Court found that some process is due prior to such transfers because they occasion "adverse social consequences", including the stigma of being labelled mentally ill, and may involve exposure to mandatory behavior modification. But the Court was unwilling to require that a judicial officer preside over such hearings; rather it mandated only that an "independent decisionmaker" fulfill this role. Moreover, the independent decisionmaker need not come from outside the prison or hospital administration; to hold otherwise would cause "unnecessary intrusion into either medical or correctional judgments."

The second relevant Supreme Court decision is *Parham v. J.R.,* 442 U.S. 584, 99 S.Ct. 2493, 61 L.Ed.2d 101 (1979), in which the Court held that the decision to admit a child to a mental facility may be made by a mental health professional, even, apparently, if that professional is the evaluating clinician. In justifying this decision, the Court stated:

> Due process has never been thought to require that the neutral and detached trier of fact be law-trained or a judicial or administrative officer. Surely, this is the case as to medical decisions for 'neither judges nor administrative hearing officers are better qualified than psychiatrists to render psychiatric judgments.' Thus, a staff physician will suffice, so long as he or she is free to evaluate independently the child's mental and emotional condition and need for treatment.

> * * *

> What process is constitutionally due cannot be divorced from the nature of the ultimate decision that is being made. . . . Here, the questions are essentially medical in character: whether the child is mentally or emotionally ill and whether he can benefit from the treatment that is provided by the state. While facts are plainly necessary for a proper resolution of those questions, they are only a

first step in the process. In an opinion for a unanimous Court, we recently stated in *Addington v. Texas* that the determination of 'whether [a person] is mentally ill turns on the *meaning* of the facts which must be interpreted by expert psychiatrists and psychologists.'

Although we acknowledge the fallibility of medical and psychiatric diagnosis, we do not accept the notion that the shortcomings of specialists can always be avoided by shifting the decision from a trained specialist using the traditional tools of medical science to an untrained judge or administrative hearing officer after a judicial-type hearing. Even after a hearing, the nonspecialist decisionmaker must make a medical-psychiatric decision. Common human experience and scholarly opinions suggest that the supposed protections of an adversary proceeding to determine the appropriateness of medical decisions for the commitment and treatment of mental and emotional illness may well be more illusory than real. [Here the Court cited studies showing the informality of supposedly "legalized" proceedings].

Id. at 606–09, 99 S.Ct. at 2506–07. The primary state interests the Court identified in support of this decision were "a significant interest in not imposing unnecessary procedural obstacles that may discourage the mentally ill or their families from seeking needed psychiatric assistance" and a "genuine interest in allocating priority to the diagnosis and treatment of patients as soon as they are admitted to a hospital rather than to time-consuming procedural minuets before the admission." Id. at 605, 99 S.Ct. at 2505. Although, as noted earlier, the Court's decision focused on the process for reviewing the initial admission decision rather than on periodic review procedures, it also stated, in dictum, that the "child's continuing need for commitment" need only be reviewed "by a similarly independent procedure." Id. at 607, 99 S.Ct. at 2506.

Do you think the Court would uphold Nebraska's administrative board as a decisionmaking body for civil commitment? A psychiatric board? Should it? With respect to the last question, consider the following excerpt from Bazelon, "Institutionalization, Deinstitutionalization and the Adversary Process," 75 Colum.L.Rev. 897, 910–911 (1975).

There is a central but limited role for courts in [the system for involuntarily hospitalizing disturbed or disturbing individuals]—that role is to guide professional decisionmaking, and may be best described by the familiar model of judicial review of administrative decisionmaking. Courts must determine whether there has been a full exploration of all relevant facts, opposing views and possible alternatives, whether the results of the exploration relate rationally to the ultimate decision, and whether constitutional and statutory procedural safeguards have been faithfully observed. Our function is thus not to determine whether the decisions taken by those charged with handling disturbed or disturbing individuals are correct or wise—but whether they are rational in the manner I have just described.

There are some who still say that we should leave these delicate questions of state intervention to the behavioral experts. But I would remind those who suggest this—both outside and within the legal profession—that state intervention involves a serious compromise of individual rights and hence a difficult balancing of power between the state and the individual, where the stakes are highest for human and personal rights. Courts have traditionally been the protector of individual rights against state power, and there is no reason why the particularly difficult problems in the area of state intervention are any different. We cannot delegate this responsibility to the medical professions. Those disciplines are, naturally enough, oriented toward helping people by treating them. Their value system assumes that disturbed and disturbing individuals need treatment, that medical disciplines can provide it, and that attempts to resist it are misguided or delusionary. The medical disciplines can no more judge the legitimacy of state intervention into the lives of disturbed or disturbing individuals than a prosecutor can judge the guilt of a person he has accused.

Finally, it is interesting to note that some research indicates that judges are more likely than psychiatrists to believe that commitment is required. Simon & Cockerham, "Civil Commitment, Burden of Proof, and Dangerous Acts: A Comparison of the Perspectives of Judges and Psychiatrists," 5 J. Psychiat. & L. (1977).

3. The Adversary Process: Notice, Public Trial and Confrontation Rights

The notion of an "adversary process" is relatively easy to visualize: the relevant parties confront each other with their version of the facts, after which an impartial decisionmaker decides who wins. The specific means by which this process is implemented in criminal trials in the United States derive primarily from the Sixth Amendment, which states in pertinent part:

> In all criminal prosecutions, the accused shall enjoy the right to a . . . public trial . . . and to be informed of the nature and cause of the accusation; to be confronted with the witnesses against him; to have compulsory process for obtaining witnesses in his favor, and to have the Assistance of Counsel for his defence.

The right to notice of one's charges is essential as a means of initiating the adversary process. As Justice Frankfurter stated in *Joint Anti–Fascist Refugee Committee v. McGrath*, 341 U.S. 123, 171–72, 71 S.Ct. 624, 648–49, 95 L.Ed. 817 (1951), "No better instrument has been devised for arriving at truth than to give a person in jeopardy of serious loss notice of the case against him and opportunity to meet it." Notice is considered so important that, as a matter of due process, it has been required prior to virtually all proceedings in which the government is a party, not just prior to the "criminal prosecutions" to which the Sixth Amendment refers. See, e.g., *Vitek v. Jones*, 445 U.S. 480, 100 S.Ct. 1254, 63 L.Ed.2d 552 (1980); *In re Gault*, 387 U.S. 1, 87 S.Ct. 1428, 18 L.Ed.2d 527 (1967).

Although perhaps not theoretically necessary to a well-functioning adversary process, ensuring that the public can observe that process at work has always been considered a second important attribute of the system. The Sixth Amendment's public trial provision was meant to deter the government from engaging in "Star Chamber" proceedings which ignore or merely mimic procedural formality; it thus encourages proceedings which are truly adversarial. In *In re Oliver,* 333 U.S. 257, 68 S.Ct. 499, 92 L.Ed. 682 (1948), the Supreme Court stated that the right "has always been recognized as a safeguard against any attempt to employ our courts as instruments of persecution. The knowledge that every criminal trial is subject to contemporaneous review in the forum of public opinion is an effective restraint on possible abuse of judicial power." Id. at 270. The Court explained further that "the presence of interested spectators may keep [the accused's] triers keenly alive to a sense of their responsibility and to the importance of their functions." Id. at 270 n. 25, 68 S.Ct. at 506 n. 25.

The third and most obviously "adversarial" attribute of the adversary process is the right to confront one's accusers and the associated right to subpoena witnesses to rebut one's accusers (the right to "compulsory process"). For reasons that should be apparent, the right to confrontation incorporates the right to be present at trial and the right to cross-examine one's accusers. The Supreme Court has termed the right to be present "one of the most basic of the rights guaranteed by the Confrontation Clause . . ." *Illinois v. Allen,* 397 U.S. 337, 90 S.Ct. 1057, 25 L.Ed.2d 353 (1970). And in *Pointer v. Texas,* 380 U.S. 400, 85 S.Ct. 1065, 13 L.Ed.2d 923 (1965), the decision which applied the confrontation clause to the states, the Court stated "probably no one, certainly no one with experience in the trial of lawsuits, would deny the value of cross-examination in exposing falsehood and bringing out the truth in the trial of a criminal case."

The following notes discuss application of these rights to civil commitment. Discussion of the right to counsel, probably the most important method of ensuring a truly adversary process, is deferred until the next subsection.

Questions and Comments

1. *Notice.* The most fundamental issue connected with the right to notice in civil commitment is whether the state can forego such notice to protect the putative patient or a third party (such as the person who brought the petition). This topic is closely connected with the right to be present, discussed below. For now, it should be noted that some states provide for special methods of giving notice to allegedly mentally disabled individuals. For instance, Vermont's statute states: "If the court has reason to believe that notice to the proposed patient will be likely to cause injury to the proposed patient or others, it shall direct the proposed patient's counsel to give the proposed patient oral notice prior to written notice under circumstances most likely to reduce likelihood of injury." Vt. Stat.Ann. tit. 18, § 7613(c).

A second issue raised by the cases has to do with the type of information that must be included in the notice. The Supreme Court has held that

constitutional requirements are satisfied if the notice "is reasonably calculated to inform the person to whom it is directed of the nature of the
proceeding." *Mullane v. Central Hanover Bank & Trust Co.,* 339 U.S. 306,
70 S.Ct. 652, 94 L.Ed. 865 (1950). In *Doremus v. Farrell,* 407 F.Supp. 509
(N.D.Neb.1975), the court explained that this rule, when applied to civil
commitment, meant the following:

> The notice prior to the preliminary inquiry for the emergency deten-
> tion must inform the person of the nature of grounds, reasons and
> necessity for the emergency detention, in addition to notice of the time
> and location of the hearing. The notice should also inform the subject
> of his right to counsel. The notice prior to the formal hearing must
> include, in addition to notice of the time and location of the hearing,
> notice to the individual of the reasons for his detention, the standards
> for commitment, and the petition itself . . .

In *French v. Blackburn,* 428 F.Supp. 1351 (M.D.N.C.1977), affirmed 443 U.S.
901, 99 S.Ct. 3091, 61 L.Ed.2d 869 (1979), however, the court held that
notice need not include the reasons for detention, the standards for commitment, nor the petition itself. The court found that the statute before it,
which provided for notice of the purpose of the hearing, the right to
counsel, the right to present evidence, and the possible consequences of the
hearing, was sufficient. It further stated:

> At first blush it would appear that it might be better to serve the
> respondent with a copy of the petition or affidavit forming the basis of
> his custody. This would parallel the service of a copy of the complaint
> in a traditional civil action and a copy of the indictment or information
> in a criminal proceeding. However, . . . [a]s was the case here, the
> petitions may have been filed by members of the respondent's family
> and service of such might possibly cause more harm to such a respon-
> dent than nonservice.

Id. at 1357 n. 10.

A third issue associated with notice is when it should be given. The
general rule is that it be given "sufficiently in advance of the proceeding to
afford one a reasonable opportunity to prepare." *In re Gault,* 387 U.S. 1,
33, 87 S.Ct. 1428, 1446, 18 L.Ed.2d 527 (1967). In *Blackburn,* the court held
that 48 hour notice is sufficient. 428 F.Supp. at 1357. In many states,
given the timeframe between initial admission and the detention hearing,
this approximates the maximum time available (though under the statute
at issue in *Blackburn* the hearing did not take place until ten days after
admission). Of course, if a detention hearing is held, notice of the adjudicatory hearing can be, and often is, given at that time.

A final issue which may arise is whether notice should be given to
anyone other than the respondent and the attorney. Many states also
provide for notice to the parents, guardian, spouse or next-of-kin of the
patient. See, e.g., Tenn.Code § 33–604(b). Do these latter parties have a
right to notice?

2. *Public trial.* Commitment hearings are likely to canvass very
intimate, personal information. Thus, even assuming that respondents
have a right to a public hearing, they may often want to waive the right.

The state may also want to exclude the public, to protect "confidential" information and to expedite the process. Most state statutes which address the issue express a preference for private proceedings. Some, like North Dakota, simply close all hearings to the public. § 25–03.1–19. In Iowa, the hearing is closed, "except that the court may admit persons having a legitimate interest in the hearing." Iowa Code Ann. § 229.12(2). Ohio is representative of many states in keeping the hearing closed unless the patient and counsel request it to be open. § 5122.15–(a)(5). Finally, a number of states leave the question to the court's discretion. See, e.g., Kansas Stat.Ann. 59–2914(a); 59–2917.

If the general public or the press want to witness a particular proceeding, should the respondent be able to keep it closed? May the *state*, by statute, keep the public from attending commitment proceedings? These issues have seldom been raised, probably because most commitment hearings are of little interest to the public and are not widely publicized.

However, there has been considerable litigation over analogous issues in the criminal and juvenile delinquency contexts. While the Supreme Court has made it clear that a criminal defendant can waive his Sixth Amendment right to a public proceeding, *Gannett Co., Inc. v. DePasquale,* 443 U.S. 368, 99 S.Ct. 2898, 61 L.Ed.2d 608 (1979), it has also vigorously upheld, even over the defendant's objection, the *public's* right of access to trial, based on the First Amendment. In *Richmond Newspapers, Inc. v. Virginia,* 448 U.S. 555, 100 S.Ct. 2814, 65 L.Ed.2d 973 (1980), the Court held that the right of the public and the press to attend criminal trials, which it called "implicit in the guarantees of the First Amendment" rights to free speech and press, would normally outweigh any interest the defendant might have in closing the trial. Only if making the trial public creates problems "beyond the realm of the manageable"—by which the Court seemed to mean problems having to do with maintaining court decorum—can the trial be closed. Id. at 581. See also *Press–Enterprise Co. v. Superior Court,* 478 U.S. 1, 106 S.Ct. 2735, 92 L.Ed.2d 1 (1986).

On the other hand, in the juvenile delinquency context, the clear tendency is to allow closure. All 50 states have statutes which protect the confidentiality of such proceedings. See McNulty, "First Amendment Versus Sixth Amendment: A Constitutional Battle in the Juvenile Courts," 10 N.M.L.Rev. 311 (1980). In *In re J.S.,* 140 Vt. 458, 438 A.2d 1125 (1981), the Vermont Supreme Court held that *Richmond Newspapers* does not apply to juvenile proceedings. In the course of its opinion, it quoted from Justice Rehnquist's opinion in *Smith v. Daily Mail Publishing Co.,* 443 U.S. 97, 107, 99 S.Ct. 2667, 2673, 61 L.Ed.2d 399 (1979):

> It is a hallmark of our juvenile justice system in the United States that virtually from its inception at the end of the last century its proceedings have been conducted ouside of the public's full gaze and the youths brought before our juvenile courts have been shielded from publicity. This insistence on confidentiality is born of a tender concern for the welfare of the child, to hide his youthful errors and 'bury them in the graveyard of the forgotten past.' The prohibition of publication of a juvenile's name is designed to protect the young person from the

stigma of his misconduct and is rooted in the principle that a court concerned with juvenile affairs serves as a rehabilitative and protective agency of the State.

Most courts do, however, permit the delinquency proceeding to be open if the child so requests. In *RLR v. State*, 487 P.2d 27 (Alaska 1971), for instance, the court stated:

> Delinquency proceedings as much as adult criminal prosecutions can be used as instruments of persecution, and may be subject to judicial abuse. The appellate process is not a sufficient check on juvenile courts, for problems of mootness and the cost of prosecuting an appeal screen most of what goes on from appellate court scrutiny. We cannot help but notice that children's cases appealed to this court have often shown much more extensive and fundamental error than is generally found in adult criminal cases, and wonder whether secrecy is not fostering a judicial attitude of casualness toward the law in children's proceedings. . . .

> Therefore, we hold that children are guaranteed the right to a public trial by the Alaska Constitution.

> . . . It is an abuse of discretion for the court to refuse admittance to individuals whose presence is favored by the child, except in special circumstances such as the unavailability of a courtroom sufficiently large to hold all the individuals whose presence is sought. If a child or his guardian ad litem wants the press, friends, or others to be free to attend, then the hearing must be open to them. The area of discretion in the rule, where the court may refuse to open the hearing, involves persons whose presence is not desired by the child.

3. *Presence of respondent.* The right to be present at one's criminal trial can be abridged if the defendant is so disruptive that an orderly proceeding cannot take place. *Illinois v. Allen*, 397 U.S. 337 (1970). The right may also be waived, if the waiver is "knowing and intelligent". *Tacon v. Arizona*, 410 U.S. 351 (1973). Otherwise, the accused's right to be present at trial is sacrosanct. In contrast, a large number of state commitment statutes grant the right to be present at the commitment hearing only if presence will not "harm" the patient. See, e.g., Alas.Stat. § 47.30.735(b)(1); Okla.Stat. 43A § 54.41 (requiring clear and convincing proof that having the patient appear at the hearing would be "improper and unsafe" and that alternatives to exclusion have been "attempted").

In *Stamus v. Leonhardt*, 414 F.Supp. 439 (S.D.Iowa 1976), the court found such a provision in the Iowa commitment statute unconstitutional.

> Section 229.4 of the Code accorded the subject the right to be present at hearings unless the hospitalization commission found that the subject's presence would 'probably be injurious' to the subject 'or attended with no advantage.' Pursuant to this provision, Dorothy Stamus was taken before the hospitalization commission during her hearing and questioned. However, as was the general practice in Polk County, she was excluded from the hearing room preceding and after the questioning period. This restriction on the plaintiff's right to be present was an unconstitutional deprivation of her right to due process.

* * *

. . . . The same purposes for requiring the person's presence exist in both the civil and criminal context: to allow the individual to assure that his or her interests are being protected and to give the fact-finder an opportunity to speak with the person and observe his or her demeanor. The results of the hearings, confinement in an institution and a loss of personal liberty, are often the same in the civil commitment and criminal context. Thus, there must be a right for the individual under discussion to be present at all proceedings for civil commitment. . . .

What is the impact of an adversary hearing on the typical person alleged to be mentally disabled? Recall the assertion by Ensminger and Liguori in the introduction to this section that confronting one's family and the treating professionals can often be "therapeutic." Consider also, however, the following passage:

> The patient who has his 'day in court' may be subjected to anguish, humiliation, suspicion, alienation from family, self-depreciation, and anxiety. Consider patient A, a paranoid person who thinks people are against him; patient B, a manic who has all kinds of funny, grandiose ideas; patient C, a depressed person who feels nobody loves him or wants him. Suppose each of these patients were to insist on his day in court. Patient A would hear neighbors say why he ought to be hospitalized. What would that do to his paranoid ideas? Patient B would provide an unroariously good time for spectators as he made a clown of himself. What would that do to his loved ones? Patient C would hear his nearest and dearest swear that he ought to be hospitalized. What would this do to his self-evaluation?

Davidson, "Mental Hospitals and the Civil Liberties Dilemma," 51 Mental Hygiene 371, 374 (1967).

According to the Supreme Court, the right to be present in criminal proceedings incorporates not only the right to be physically present but the right to be "mentally present," i.e., competent to stand trial. *Pate v. Robinson,* 383 U.S. 375, 86 S.Ct. 836, 15 L.Ed.2d 815 (1966). Defendants must have a minimal understanding of the proceedings against them and be able to assist the attorney in confronting their accusers, or the state may not try them. Should the right to avoid trial while incompetent be extended to civil commitment respondents? Note that in the criminal system, a person found incompetent to stand trial may be involuntarily treated until restored to competency. See pp. 912–923.

4. *Cross-examination and hearsay.* The principal issue connected with the right to cross-examine accusers at civil commitment proceedings is the extent to which hearsay is admissible. Since hearsay, by definition, involves out-of-court statements by persons who are not present in the courtroom, the confrontation clause could be construed to exclude all hearsay. However, even in the criminal context, the Supreme Court has held that many types of hearsay are admissible, especially when a "firmly rooted" common law exception to the hearsay rule is applicable. *Ohio v. Roberts,* 448 U.S. 56, 100 S.Ct. 2531, 65 L.Ed.2d 597 (1980). Such exceptions include the party admission rule, which would permit description of the

respondent's out-of-court statements about his or her mental state or intended actions by the person who heard them, and the "business records" exception, which would admit virtually all observations of the respondent's mental state made by clinicians and recorded as a routine matter in medical and psychiatric records. See Fed.R.Evid. 801(d)(2); 803(6).

An example of testimony that would not fit any well-accepted hearsay exception would be a description of an out-of-court declaration by a third-party about what the respondent did or said on a particular day (so-called "double hearsay" because the person who observed or heard the respondent is not in court). For instance, the hearsay rule would probably bar a mental health professional's testimony that a family member had told him two days before the hearing that the respondent had threatened to hurt the family member.[q] Similarly, the rule would prohibit the respondent's mother from testifying that the respondent's friend had told her the respondent had attempted suicide on several occasions.

Should such testimony be admissible in any event? Or should the state be required to present the people who heard the respondent's statements first-hand, if they are available? Several courts have held that the rules of evidence, including the hearsay rule, should apply in commitment proceedings. See, e.g., *State ex rel. Hawks v. Lazaro,* 202 S.E.2d 109, 125 (W.Va.1973); *Lessard v. Schmidt,* 349 F.Supp. 1078 (E.D.Wis.1972). Some state statutes take this stance as well; many others are simply silent about the issue, and some provide, as does Utah, that the hearing "shall be conducted in as informal a manner as may be consistent with orderly procedure." Utah Code § 64–7–36(9). The American Psychiatric Association's Model Law provides that "[h]earsay evidence may be received, and experts and other witnesses may, consistent with law, testify to any relevant and probative facts at the discretion of the court." Stromberg & Stone, "A Model State Law on Civil Commitment of the Mentally Ill," 20 Harv.J.Legis. 275, 340 (1983). In support of this position, the commentary states, id. at 340–41:

> [H]earsay evidence may be especially necessary in some civil commitment cases because the facts sought to be established include the elusive datum of mental status, not just physical events as in most criminal trials. Especially where the issues are tried before a judge, who can weigh the probative value of the evidence, such hearsay need not be excluded. It also may be proper to afford a broader ambit to psychiatric opinion evidence. Similarly, the interests that underlie the privilege against spousal testimony in criminal cases may not be served by invoking such a privilege in civil commitment. There may be proper exceptions to other privileges as well, such as the psychotherapist-patient privilege.

5. *Compulsory process.* Of course, if the respondent in a civil commitment proceeding has a wide-open right to subpoena witnesses, then he or she can circumvent any attempt by the state to rely on hearsay by serving process on the relevant out-of-court declarants. Some states statutes ex-

---

q. Note, however, that under Federal Rule of Evidence 703 and equivalent state rules such testimony, although hearsay, would still be admissible if of the type "reasonably relied upon" by experts in the field. See pp. 479–484.

plicitly grant the respondent subpoena authority for persons and documents, but whether such a right is constitutionally required and the extent to which it can be exercised as a discovery mechanism is unclear. Perhaps of relevance here is *Vitek v. Jones,* 445 U.S. 480, 100 S.Ct. 1254, 63 L.Ed.2d 552 (1980), the case involving the process due prisoners who are transferred to psychiatric facilities. In *Vitek,* the Supreme Court held that the state must give the prisoner the "opportunity . . . to present testimony of witnesses . . . and to confront and cross-examine witnesses called by the state, *except* upon a finding, not arbitrarily made, of good cause for not permitting such presentation, confrontation or cross-examination." [emphasis added] The Court held that such a limitation was permissible because it recognized "[t]he interests of the State in avoiding disruption." Id. at 495–96.

Another limitation on the respondent's compulsory process right may arise from the by-now familiar concern that the information thereby obtained will harm either the respondent or third parties who have revealed information about the respondent. Of possible relevance here is the Supreme Court's decision in *Pennsylvania v. Ritchie,* 480 U.S. 39, 107 S.Ct. 989 94 L.Ed.2d 40 (1987), in which the Court held that even a criminal defendant's "right to discover exculpatory evidence does not include the unsupervised authority to search through the Commonwealth's files." At most, the Court held, the defense may ask the trial court to review the files *in camera* to determine what information, if any, is material to the defendant's case; even this limited right is conditioned upon the defendant "first establishing a basis for his claim that it contains material evidence." Thus, the state may be able to stymie a respondent's attempt, prior to a civil commitment hearing, to subpoena evidence possessed by the state (e.g., in hospital records) by requiring a showing of materiality and a judicial determination that the records should be disclosed.

4. *The Right to Counsel*

The Supreme Court has clearly established a right to counsel at trial—and a concomitant duty on the part of the state to provide counsel to indigents who cannot afford one—for both the criminal accused, *Argersinger v. Hamlin,* 407 U.S. 25, 92 S.Ct. 2006, 32 L.Ed.2d 530 (1972), and juveniles alleged to be delinquent, *In re Gault,* 387 U.S. 1, 87 S.Ct. 1428, 18 L.Ed.2d 527 (1967). Endorsement of a right to counsel in civil commitment proceedings has been less firm. While virtually every modern court which has considered the issue has held that the due process clause requires counsel at the commitment hearing, a few state statutes still apparently do not provide indigent individuals with counsel at any point in the process. See Elkins, "Legal Representation of the Mentally Ill," 82 W.Va.L.Rev. 157 (1979). Moreover, it is not entirely free from doubt that the Supreme Court would agree with the lower courts on this matter. In both *Parham v. J.R.* and *Vitek v. Jones* the Court refused to find a right to legally trained counsel for persons subjected to a proceeding to determine the existence and extent of their mental disability. The language of Justice Powell's concurring opinion in *Vitek,* which controlled the disposition of the right to counsel issue in that case, is worth looking at in full:

VITEK v. JONES

Supreme Court of the United States, 1980.
445 U.S. 480, 100 S.Ct. 1254, 63 L.Ed.2d 552 (1981).

MR. JUSTICE POWELL, concurring in part.

* * *

I

In *Gagnon v. Scarpelli,* 411 U.S. 778, 93 S.Ct. 1756, 36 L.Ed.2d 656 (1973), my opinion for the Court held that counsel is not necessarily required at a probation revocation hearing. In reaching this decision the Court recognized both the effects of providing counsel to each probationer and the likely benefits to be derived from the assistance of counsel. "The introduction of counsel into a revocation proceeding [would] alter significantly the nature of the proceeding," because the hearing would inevitably become more adversarial. We noted that probationers would not always need counsel because in most hearings the essential facts are undisputed. In lieu of a *per se* rule we held that the necessity of providing counsel should be determined on a case-by-case basis. In particular, we stressed that factors governing the decision to provide counsel include (i) the existence of factual disputes or issues which are "complex or otherwise difficult to develop or present," and (ii) "whether the probationer appears to be capable of speaking effectively for himself."

Consideration of these factors, and particularly the capability of the inmate, persuades me that the Court is correct that independent assistance must be provided to an inmate before he may be transferred involuntarily to a mental hospital. The essence of the issue in an involuntary commitment proceeding will be the mental health of the inmate. The resolution of factual disputes will be less important than the ability to understand and analyze expert psychiatric testimony that is often expressed in language relatively incomprehensible to laymen. It is unlikely that an inmate threatened with involuntary transfer to mental hospitals will possess the competence or training to protect adequately his own interest in these state-initiated proceedings. And the circumstances of being imprisoned without normal access to others who may assist him places an additional handicap upon an inmate's ability to represent himself. I therefore agree that due process requires the provision of assistance to an inmate threatened with involuntary transfer to a mental hospital.

II

I do not believe, however, that an inmate must always be supplied with a licensed attorney. "[D]ue Process is flexible and calls for such procedural protections as the particular situation demands." *Morrissey v. Brewer,* 408 U.S. 471, 481, 92 S.Ct. 2593, 2600, 33 L.Ed.2d 484 (1972).

Our decisions defining the necessary qualifications for an impartial decisionmaker demonstrate that the requirements of due process turn on the nature of the determination which must be made. "Due Process has never been thought to require that the neutral and detached trier of fact be law-trained or a judicial or administrative officer." *Parham v. J.L.*, 442 U.S. 584, 607, 99 S.Ct. 2493, 2506, 61 L.Ed.2d 101 (1979). In that case, we held that due process is satisfied when a staff physician determines whether a child may be voluntarily committed to a state mental institution by his parents. That holding was based upon recognition that the issues of civil commitment "are essentially medical in nature," and that " 'neither judges nor administrative hearing officers are better qualified than psychiatrists to render psychiatric judgments.' "

In my view, the principle that due process does not always require a law-trained decisionmaker supports the ancillary conclusion that due process may be satisfied by the provision of a qualified and independent advisor who is not a lawyer. As in *Parham v. J.L.*, the issue here is essentially medical. Under state law, a prisoner may be transferred only if he "suffers from a mental disease or defect" and "cannot be given proper treatment" in the prison complex. Neb.Rev.Stat. § 83–180(1). The opinion of the Court allows a non-lawyer to act as the impartial decisionmaker in the transfer proceeding.

The essence of procedural due process is a fair hearing. I do not think that the fairness of an informal hearing designed to determine a medical issue requires participation by lawyers. Due process merely requires that the State provide an inmate with qualified and independent assistance. Such assistance may be provided by a licensed psychiatrist or other mental health professional. Indeed, in view of the nature of the issue involved in the transfer hearing, a person possessing such professional qualifications normally would be preferred. As the Court notes, "[t]he question whether an individual is mentally ill and cannot be treated in prison 'turns on the meaning of the facts which must be interpreted by expert psychiatrists and psychologists.' " *Ante,* at 1265, quoting *Addington v. Texas*. I would not exclude, however, the possibility that the required assistance may be rendered by competent laymen in some cases. The essential requirements are that the person provided by the State be competent and independent, and that he be free to act solely in the inmate's best interest.

In sum, although the State is free to appoint a licensed attorney to represent an inmate, it is not constitutionally required to do so. Due process will be satisfied so long as an inmate facing involuntary transfer to a mental hospital is provided qualified and independent assistance.

Questions and Comments

1. *Implications of the Court's cases.* What are the implications of *Vitek* and *Parham* for the civil commitment process? Note that Justice

Powell relied heavily on *Gagnon v. Scarpelli* and *Morrissey v. Brewer* in reaching his conclusions. Consider this fuller excerpt from *Scarpelli:*

The introduction of counsel into a revocation proceeding will alter significantly the nature of the proceeding. If counsel is provided for the probationer or parolee, the State in turn will normally provide its own counsel; lawyers, by training and disposition, are advocates and bound by professional duty to present all available evidence and arguments in support of their clients' positions and to contest with vigor all adverse evidence and views. The role of the hearing body itself, aptly described in *Morrissey* as being "predictive and discretionary" as well as fact finding, may become more akin to that of a judge at a trial, and less attuned to the rehabilitative needs of the individual probationer or parolee. In the greater self-consciousness of its quasi-judicial role, the hearing body may be less tolerant of marginal deviant behavior and feel more pressure to reincarcerate than to continue nonpunitive rehabilitation. Certainly, the decisionmaking process will be prolonged, and the financial cost to the State—for appointed counsel, counsel for the State, a longer record and the possibility of judicial review—will not be insubstantial.

In some cases, these modifications in the nature of the revocation hearing must be endured and the costs borne because, as we have indicated above, the probationer's or parolee's version of a disputed issue can fairly be represented only by a trained advocate. But due process is not so rigid as to require that the significant interests in informality, flexibility, and economy must always be sacrificed.

Is *Scarpelli* authority for or against a right to counsel at civil commitment?

2. *The role of counsel.* Assuming the person subjected to commitment proceedings has an advocate, should the advocate "act like a lawyer"? Or, as suggested by Justice Powell's reasoning in *Scarpelli,* might the nature of the commitment process justify a different, less adversarial approach? At least three possible advocacy roles can be envisioned. The first is the adversarial role traditionally taken by lawyers, in which it is assumed that the client knows best and the advocate makes the most persuasive arguments available in support of the client's wishes. The second role might be called the "guardian ad litem" stance, in which the advocate acts in the "best interests" of the client, after assessing all the circumstances. Although the client's wishes are taken into account, they are not dispositive; thus, under this model, it is assumed that the lawyer, rather than the client, knows best. Finally, there is a cooperative role in which the advocate assumes that the "doctor knows best." Under this model, the advocate may help develop facts for the expert's consideration, but does not dispute the expert's final decision.

The Model Code of Professional Responsibility is not particularly helpful in deciding, from a professional ethics standpoint, which role may or should be followed. Canon 7 of the Code states: "A lawyer should represent a client zealously within the bounds of the law." Consider the following "Ethical Considerations" (EC) designed to flesh out this Canon:

EC 7–7 In certain areas of legal representation not affecting the merits of the cause or substantially prejudicing the rights of a client, a lawyer is entitled to make decisions on his own. But otherwise the authority to make decisions is exclusively that of the client and, if made within the framework of the law, such decisions are binding on his lawyer. As typical examples in civil cases, it is for the client to decide whether he will accept a settlement offer or whether he will waive his right to plead an affirmative defense. A defense lawyer in a criminal case has the duty to advise his client fully on whether a particular plea to a charge appears to be desirable and as to the prospects of success on appeal, but it is for the client to decide what plea should be entered and whether an appeal should be taken.

EC 7–8 A lawyer should exert his best efforts to insure that decisions of his client are made only after the client has been informed of relevant considerations. A lawyer ought to initiate this decision-making process if the client does not do so. Advice of a lawyer to his client need not be confined to purely legal considerations. . . . He may emphasize the possibility of harsh consequences that might result from assertion of legally permissible positions. In the final analysis, however, the lawyer should always remember that the decision whether to forego legally available objectives or methods because of non legal factors is ultimately for the client and not for himself. In the event that the client in a non-adjudicatory matter insists upon a course of conduct that is contrary to the judgment and advice of the lawyer but not prohibited by Disciplinary Rules, the lawyer may withdraw from the employment.

* * *

EC 7–12 Any mental or physical condition of a client that renders him incapable of making a considered judgment on his own behalf casts additional responsibilities upon his lawyer. Where an incompetent is acting through a guardian or other legal representative, a lawyer must look to such representative for those decisions which are normally the prerogative of the client to make. If a client under disability has no legal representative, his lawyer may be compelled in court proceedings to make decisions on behalf of the client. If the client is capable of understanding the matter in question or of contributing to the advancement of his interests, regardless of whether he is legally disqualified from performing certain acts, the lawyer should obtain from him all possible aid. If the disability of a client and the lack of a legal representative compel the lawyer to make decisions for his client, the lawyer should consider all circumstances then prevailing and act with care to safeguard and advance the interests of his client. But obviously a lawyer cannot perform any act or make any decision which the law requires his client to perform or make, either acting for himself if competent, or by a duly constituted representative if legally incompetent.

Assume that you are representing a client who appears to be imminently suicidal and treatable, but who adamantly refuses to consent to any type of treatment or hospitalization because "the hospital is Hell and if I kill myself I'll go to Heaven." Alternatively, assume your client is extremely malnourished and disheveled, murmuring incoherently, smearing feces on the wall, and able only to nod negatively when asked if he is willing to go to the hospital. Under the Code, what options are available to you? Should you follow the clients' direction? Seek appointment of a guardian? Withdraw? Disregard the clients' wishes because you believe that treatment would be in the client's best interests? The last sentence of the above excerpt prohibits attorneys from performing any act or making any decision "which the law requires his client to perform or make." In the hypothetized situations, what does "the law" leave up to the client? Would your approach to these situations be different if, as is true in many states, the government is "represented" solely by a mental health professional because no provision is made for state attorneys to appear in commitment hearings?

Several commentators have emphasized that, whatever role the advocate assumes—adversarial, guardian ad litem, or cooperative—at the least he or she should perform an investigative function. Cohen, "The Function of the Attorney and the Commitment of the Mentally Ill," 44 Tex.L.Rev. 424, 452 (1966), states:

> Prior to the hearing the attorney must make a thorough study of all the records that are available to him through the court, the hospital, and, at times, social agencies. He must always communicate with the proposed patient and, where possible, family and friends. The attorney should work toward an understanding of the events that led up to and contributed to the filing of the petition. Only in this way can he attempt to develop possible alternatives to hospitalization.

Armed with this knowledge, the advocate may be able to bargain for a less restrictive disposition and will be able to conduct more effective questioning of witnesses. The advocate can also make sure the proper procedures are followed at the hearing, both through objections and through appealing various rulings, if appeal is available. See also, "Preparation and Trial of a Civil Commitment Case," 5 Men.Dis.L.Rep. 201, 281 (1981).

3. *Ineffective assistance of counsel.* Most commitment attorneys do not undertake even the modest tasks just outlined. As noted earlier, numerous studies have documented that attorneys rarely spend more than a few minutes preparing for the hearing, seldom call witnesses, and usually fail to engage in vigorous cross-examination of the experts. To some extent, this state of affairs may be due to their unfamiliarity with psychiatric issues or the low fees provided by the state for defending commitment respondents. But one study suggests that, even when these factors are not present, many attorneys continue to be passive. Poythress found that lawyers who were specifically trained to adopt a more adversarial stance and who were provided with information about the inadequacies of testimony by mental health professionals persisted in avoiding careful cross-examination of expert witnesses, apparently because of a belief that to do so was in the best interests of their clients. Poythress, "Psychiatric Expertise in Civil Commitment: Training Attorneys to Cope with Expert Testimony," 2 Law Hum.Behav. 1 (1978).

One possible remedy for this situation, if a remedy is thought to be worthwhile, is to require legislatively that the attorneys perform certain duties. For instance, Arizona has granted the commitment court the power to hold attorneys in contempt unless they perform several listed tasks prior to and during the hearing. Ariz.Stat. § 36–537. A second possible approach is to import Sixth Amendment ineffective assistance of counsel analysis into the commitment context. In *Strickland v. Washington*, 466 U.S. 668, 104 S.Ct. 2052, 80 L.Ed.2d 674 (1984), the Supreme Court established a two-prong test for determining whether defense counsel was ineffective under the Sixth Amendment. The defendant must show both that "counsel's performance was deficient" and that "the deficient performance prejudiced the defense." Performance is "deficient" if the attorney fails "to advocate the defendant's cause[,] . . . consult with the defendant on important decisions, [or] . . . keep the defendant informed of important developments." The attorney must also "bring to bear such skill and knowledge as will render the trial a reliable adversarial testing process" and "make reasonable investigations or . . . make a reasonable decision that makes particular investigations unnecessary." Proof of "prejudice" exists if "there is a reasonable probability that, but for counsel's unprofessional errors, the result of the proceeding would have been different." If both prongs are met, the defendant's conviction must be reversed. Would application of *Strickland's* standards to civil commitment (through the due process clause, since the sixth amendment applies only to "criminal prosecutions") provide a realistic remedy for attorney passivity?

4. *The right to an independent expert evaluation.* To what extent does the effective assistance of counsel notion require that the advocate seek consultation with a mental health professional? For the wealthy respondent such consultation is easily arranged, but for the indigent (and typical) person subjected to civil commitment, the only expertise available in most jurisdictions is provided by those mental health professionals who testify for the government. Only a few states have authorized the appointment of an independent expert if the defendant so requests. See, e.g., Cal. Code §§ 5251, 6507.

Some courts have held that the latter type of provision is constitutionally required. In *In re Gannon*, 123 N.J.Super. 104, 301 A.2d 493, 494 (1973), the court stated:

> Commitment to a psychiatric hospital obviously entails a significant loss of liberty which, as in a criminal proceeding, must be under due process of law. It is the opinion of this court that in a commitment proceeding due process of law includes the right to an independent psychiatric examination.
>
> The right of an indigent to have counsel appointed has already been established, but the presence of a lawyer at the commitment hearing is not a sufficient safeguard for the patient's rights. No matter how brilliant the lawyer may be, he is in no position to effectively contest the commitment proceedings because he has no way to rebut the testimony of the psychiatrist from the institution who has already certified to the patient's insanity. . . .
>
> This court has had enough experience to know that psychiatrists differ very definitely in their evaluations and diagnoses of mental illness. In a commitment proceeding where the court is in effect bound by the expertise of the psychiatrist, the right to counsel is of little value without a concurrent right to an independent psychiatric examination.

However, the court limited the right to an independent evaluation in the following manner:

> The right to counsel has not been construed to allow an indigent to choose his own lawyer. Similarly, an indigent in a commitment proceeding should not have the right to 'shop around' for a psychiatrist who agrees with him. The independent psychiatrist is to assist the court, not the patient; all he need do is render his best judgment and make all relevant information available both to the court and to the defense.

Id. at 494.

Does the court's conclusion follow from its analogy between choosing a lawyer and choosing an expert? Note that in *Ake v. Oklahoma,* 470 U.S. 68, 105 S.Ct. 1087, 84 L.Ed.2d 53 (1985), reprinted at pp. 450–459, the Supreme Court held, using reasoning similar to that used by the *Gannon* court, that the due process clause entitles the indigent criminal defendant to a psychiatric consultant when sanity at the time of the offense is "a significant factor at trial" and, in capital cases, when dangerousness is a factor to be considered at sentencing. More specifically, on the insanity expert issue, the Court held:

> We therefore hold that when a defendant demonstrates to the trial judge that his sanity at the time of the offense is to be a significant factor at trial, the State must, at a minimum, assure the defendant access to a competent psychiatrist who will conduct an appropriate examination and assist in evaluation, preparation, and presentation of the defense. This is not to say, of course, that the indigent defendant has a constitutional right to choose a psychiatrist of his personal liking or to receive funds to hire his own. Our concern is that the indigent defendant have access to a competent psychiatrist for the purpose we have discussed, and as in the case of the provision of counsel we leave to the State the decision on how to implement this right.

470 U.S. at 83, 105 S.Ct. at 1096. To what extent does *Ake* support the result in *Gannon?*

5. *The Privilege Against Self–Incrimination*

ALLEN V. ILLINOIS

Supreme Court of the United States, 1986.
478 U.S. 364, 106 S.Ct. 2988, 92 L.Ed.2d 296.

JUSTICE REHNQUIST delivered the opinion of the Court.

The question presented by this case is whether the proceedings under the Illinois Sexually Dangerous Persons Act (Act), Ill.Rev.Stat., ch. 38, ¶ 105–1.01 *et seq.* (1985),[r] are "criminal" within the meaning of the Fifth Amendment's guarantee against compulsory self-incrimination.

* * *

r. For a full discussion of sex offender statutes, see pp. 586–595.

The Self–Incrimination Clause of the Fifth Amendment, which applies to the States through the Fourteenth Amendment, *Malloy v. Hogan,* 378 U.S. 1, 84 S.Ct. 1489, 12 L.Ed.2d 653 (1964), provides that no person "shall be compelled in any criminal case to be a witness against himself." This Court has long held that the privilege against self-incrimination "not only permits a person to refuse to testify against himself at a criminal trial in which he is a defendant, but also 'privileges him not to answer official questions put to him in any other proceeding, civil or criminal, formal or informal, where the answers might incriminate him in future criminal proceedings.'" In this case the Illinois Supreme Court ruled that a person whom the State attempts to commit under the Act is protected from use of his compelled answers in any subsequent criminal case in which he is the defendant. What we have here, then, is not a claim that petitioner's statements to the psychiatrists might be used to incriminate him in some future criminal proceeding, but instead his claim that because the sexually dangerous person proceeding is itself "criminal," he was entitled to refuse to answer any questions at all.

The question whether a particular proceeding is criminal for the purposes of the Self–Incrimination Clause is first of all a question of statutory construction. Here, Illinois has expressly provided that proceedings under the Act "shall be civil in nature," ¶ 105–3.01, indicating that when it files a petition against a person under the Act it intends to proceed in a nonpunitive, noncriminal manner, "without regard to the procedural protections and restrictions available in criminal prosecutions." As petitioner correctly points out, however, the civil label is not always dispositive. Where a defendant has provided "the clearest proof" that "the statutory scheme [is] so punitive either in purpose or effect as to negate [the State's] intention" that the proceeding be civil, it must be considered criminal and the privilege against self-incrimination must be applied. We think that petitioner has failed to provide such proof in this case.

The Illinois Supreme Court reviewed the Act and its own case law and concluded that these proceedings, while similar to criminal proceedings in that they are accompanied by strict procedural safeguards, are essentially civil in nature. We are unpersuaded by petitioner's efforts to challenge this conclusion. Under the Act, the State has a statutory obligation to provide "care and treatment for [persons adjudged sexually dangerous] designed to effect recovery," ¶ 105–8, in a facility set aside to provide psychiatric care, *ibid.* And "[i]f the patient is found to be no longer dangerous, the court shall order that he be discharged." ¶ 105–9. While the committed person has the burden of showing that he is no longer dangerous, he may apply for release at any time. *Ibid.* In short, the State has disavowed any interest in punishment, provided for the treatment of those it commits, and established a system under which committed persons may be released after the briefest time in confinement. The Act thus does not appear to promote either of "the traditional aims of punishment—retribution and deterrence." Cf. *Addington v. Texas,* 441 U.S. 418, 428, 99 S.Ct. 1804, 1810, 60 L.Ed.2d 323 (1979) (in Texas "civil commitment state power is not exercised in a punitive sense"); *French v. Blackburn,* 428 F.Supp. 1351, 1358–1359 (MDNC (1977)), summarily aff'd, 443 U.S. 901, 99 S.Ct. 3091, 61 L.Ed.2d 869 (1979) (state need not accord privilege against self-incrimination in civil commitment proceeding).

Petitioner offers several arguments in support of his claim that despite the apparently nonpunitive purposes of the Act, it should be considered criminal as far as the privilege against self-incrimination is concerned. He first notes that the State cannot file a sexually-dangerous-person petition unless it has already brought criminal charges against the person in question. ¶ 105–3. In addition, the State must prove that the person it seeks to commit perpetrated "at least one act of or attempt at sexual assault or sexual molestation." 107 Ill.2d, at 105, 89 Ill.Dec., at 954, 481 N.E.2d, at 697. To petitioner, these factors serve to distinguish the Act from other civil commitment, which typically is not tied to any criminal charge and which petitioner apparently concedes is not "criminal" under the Self–Incrimination Clause. We disagree. That the State has chosen not to apply the Act to the larger class of mentally ill persons who might be found sexually dangerous does not somehow transform a civil proceeding into a criminal one. And as the State points out, it must prove more than just the commission of a sexual assault: the Illinois Supreme Court, as we noted above, has construed the Act to require proof of the existence of a mental disorder for more than one year and a propensity to commit sexual assaults, in addition to demonstration of that propensity through sexual assault.

The discussion of civil commitment in *Addington, supra,* in which this Court concluded that the Texas involuntary-commitment scheme is not criminal insofar as the requirement of proof beyond a reasonable doubt is concerned, fully supports our conclusion here:

> "[T]he initial inquiry in a civil commitment proceeding is very different from the central issue in either a delinquency proceeding or a criminal prosecution. In the latter cases the basic issue is a straightforward factual question—did the accused commit the act alleged? There may be factual issues to resolve in a commitment proceeding, but the factual aspects represent only the beginning of the inquiry. Whether the individual is mentally ill and dangerous to either himself or others and is in need of confined therapy turns on the *meaning* of the facts which must be interpreted by expert psychiatrists and psychologists." 441 U.S., at 429, 99 S.Ct., at 1811 (emphasis in original).

While here the State must prove at least one act of sexual assault, that antecedent conduct is received not to punish past misdeeds, but primarily to show the accused's mental condition and to predict future behavior.

In his attempt to distinguish this case from other civil commitment, petitioner places great reliance on the fact that proceedings under the Act are accompanied by procedural safeguards usually found in criminal trials. In particular, he observes that the Act provides an accused with the right to counsel, ¶ 105–5, the right to demand a jury trial, *ibid.,* and the right to confront and cross-examine witnesses. At the conclusion of the hearing, the trier of fact must determine whether the prosecution has proved the person's sexual dangerousness beyond a reasonable doubt. ¶ 105–3.01. But as we noted above, the State has indicated quite clearly its intent that these commitment proceedings be civil in nature; its decision nevertheless to provide some of the safeguards applicable in criminal trials cannot itself turn these proceedings into criminal prosecutions requiring the full panoply of rights applicable there.

Relying chiefly on *In re Gault,* 387 U.S. 1, 87 S.Ct. 1428, 18 L.Ed.2d 527 (1967), petitioner also urges that the proceedings in question are "criminal" because a person adjudged sexually dangerous under the Act is committed for an indeterminate period to the Menard Psychiatric Center, a maximum security institution that is run by the Illinois Department of Corrections and that houses convicts needing psychiatric care as well as sexually dangerous persons. Whatever its label and whatever the State's alleged purpose, petitioner argues, such commitment is the sort of punishment—total deprivation of liberty in a criminal setting—that *Gault* teaches cannot be imposed absent application of the privilege against self-incrimination. We believe that *Gault* is readily distinguishable.

First, *Gault's* sweeping statement that "our Constitution guarantees that no person shall be 'compelled' to be a witness against himself when he is threatened with deprivation of his liberty" is plainly not good law. Although the fact that incarceration may result is relevant to the question whether the privilege against self-incrimination applies, *Addington* demonstrates that involuntary commitment does not itself trigger the entire range of criminal procedural protections. Indeed, petitioner apparently concedes that traditional civil commitment does not require application of the privilege. * * *

The Court in *Gault* was obviously persuaded that the State intended to *punish* its juvenile offenders, observing that in many States juveniles may be placed in "adult penal institutions" for conduct that if committed by an adult would be a crime. Here, by contrast, the State serves its purpose of *treating* rather than punishing sexually dangerous persons by committing them to an institution expressly designed to provide psychiatric care and treatment. That the Menard Psychiatric Center houses not only sexually dangerous persons but also prisoners from other institutions who are in need of psychiatric treatment does not transform the State's intent to treat into an intent to punish. Nor does the fact that Menard is apparently a maximum security facility affect our analysis:

> "The state has a legitimate interest under its *parens patriae* powers in providing care to its citizens who are unable because of

emotional disorders to care for themselves; the state also has authority under its police power to protect the community from the dangerous tendencies of some who are mentally ill." *Addington,* 441 U.S., at 426, 99 S.Ct., at 1809.

Illinois' decision to supplement its *parens patriae* concerns with measures to protect the welfare and safety of other citizens does not render the Act punitive.

Petitioner has not demonstrated, and the record does not suggest, that "sexually dangerous persons" in Illinois are confined under conditions incompatible with the State's asserted interest in treatment. Had petitioner shown, for example, that the confinement of such persons imposes on them a regimen which is essentially identical to that imposed upon felons with no need for psychiatric care, this might well be a different case. But the record here tells us little or nothing about the regimen at the psychiatric center, and it certainly does not show that there are no relevant differences between confinement there and confinement in the other parts of the maximum-security prison complex. Indeed, counsel for the State assures us that under Illinois law sexually dangerous persons must not be treated like ordinary prisoners. We therefore cannot say that the conditions of petitioner's confinement themselves amount to "punishment" and thus render "criminal" the proceedings which led to confinement.

Our conclusion that proceedings under the Act are not "criminal" within the meaning of the Fifth Amendment's guarantee against compulsory self-incrimination does not completely dispose of this case. Petitioner rather obliquely suggests that even if his commitment proceeding was not criminal, the Fourteenth Amendment's guarantee of due process nonetheless required application of the privilege. In particular, petitioner contends that the Illinois Supreme Court "grossly miscalculated" in weighing the interests set out in *Mathews v. Eldridge,* 424 U.S. 319, 96 S.Ct. 893, 47 L.Ed.2d 18 (1976). This Court has never held that the Due Process Clause of its own force requires application of the privilege against self-incrimination in a noncriminal proceeding, where the privilege claimant is protected against his compelled answers in any subsequent criminal case. We decline to do so today.

We think that the parties have in their reliance on *Mathews v. Eldridge* misconceived that decision. *Mathews* dealt with the procedural safeguards required by the Due Process Clause of the Fifth Amendment before a person might be deprived of property, and its focus was on such safeguards as were necessary to guard against the risk of erroneous deprivation. As the Supreme Court of Illinois and the State have both pointed out, it is difficult, if not impossible, to see how requiring the privilege against self-incrimination in these proceedings would in any way advance reliability. Indeed, the State takes the quite plausible view that denying the evaluating psychiatrist the opportunity to question persons alleged to be sexually dangerous would *decrease* the reliability of a finding of sexual dangerousness. As in *Addington,* "to adopt the criminal law standard gives no assurance" that States will reach a "better" result.

The privilege against self-incrimination enjoined by the Fifth Amendment is not designed to enhance the reliability of the fact-finding determination; it stands in the Constitution for entirely independent reasons. Just as in a "criminal case" it would be no argument against a claim of the privilege to say that granting the claim would decrease the reliability of the fact-finding process, the privilege has no place among the procedural safeguards discussed in *Mathews v. Eldridge,* which are designed to enhance the reliability of that process.

For the reasons stated, we conclude that the Illinois proceedings here considered were not "criminal" within the meaning of the Fifth Amendment to the United States Constitution, and that due process does not independently require application of the privilege. * * * The judgment of the Supreme Court of Illinois is therefore

Affirmed.

Questions and Comments

1. *The right to remain silent and civil commitment.* Because it limits application of the right to remain silent to criminal proceedings, *Allen* presumably forecloses a court from finding, under the federal constitution, that the right applies in civil commitment proceedings. See also, *French v. Blackburn,* 428 F.Supp. 1351, 1358–9 (M.D.N.C.1977), affirmed mem. 443 U.S. 901, 99 S.Ct. 3091, 61 L.Ed.2d 869 (1979). In fact, prior to *Allen,* only a few courts had so held. See, e.g., *Lessard v. Schmidt,* 349 F.Supp. 1078 (E.D.Wis.1972). Most decisions, even those which were otherwise sympathetic to constitutional claims in the civil commitment context, presaged *Allen* and found no right to remain silent at any point in the commitment process. See, e.g., *State ex rel. Hawks v. Lazaro,* 157 W.Va. 417, 202 S.E.2d 109, 126 (1974); *Suzuki v. Yuen,* 617 F.2d 173, 177–78 (9th Cir.1980); *Tippett v. Maryland,* 436 F.2d 1153 (4th Cir.1971).

However, some states, including Illinois, require that persons who are the subject of civil commitment proceedings be advised that they may refuse to talk to examining experts. See Ill.Stat. ch. 91½ § 3–208. Moreover, statements that are "compelled" by the state during the commitment process are probably not admissible in a subsequent criminal proceeding; at least, *Allen* strongly implied as much with respect to statements made in the course of sex offender proceedings.

2. *Evaluating* Allen. In deciding that the privilege against self-incrimination does not apply to sex offender proceedings, the Court rejected a "deprivation of liberty" analysis and focused instead on whether the objective of such proceedings is punishment or treatment. Accepting this change in analysis, can it be said that the objective of criminal or civil commitment is *always* treatment?

Perhaps, as its rejection of the petitioner's due process claim suggests, the Court was also concerned about the practical consequences of a contrary decision. Consider the commentary to the American Psychiatric Association's "model" provision recommending that the respondent in civil commitment proceedings not be accorded a right to remain silent:

> Many cases that discuss whether the privilege should apply focus on the metaphysical issue of whether commitment is 'essentially' a civil or criminal proceeding. This analysis misses the point. Advising a patient—who may well have an emergency psychiatric condition—at the beginning of an interview about his right to remain silent would be fundamentally inconsistent with the therapeutic purposes of the process. It might bewilder and alarm the patient. It might make it impossible to ascertain the patient's mental state, thereby preventing the assessment both of his need for treatment and his potential dangerousness.

> Commitment decisions would be transformed into judgments based solely on overt acts, becoming virtually indistinguishable from decisions made in the criminal process. Granting the Fifth Amendment privilege would establish a bootless procedural right—in some cases forcing the state to instigate criminal proceedings and in many cases depriving seriously mentally ill persons of needed treatment.[226]

Stromberg & Stone, "A Model State Law on Civil Commitment of the Mentally Ill," 20 Harv.J.Legis. 274, 342–43 (1983).

Would the right to remain silent make it "impossible" to garner evidence about a mentally disabled person's mental state, as the APA commentary suggests might be true in some cases? Note that even in criminal cases, only 10 to 20% of the defendants who are told they have a right to remain silent assert that right. Seeburger & Wettick, "Miranda in Pittsburgh: A Statistical Study," 29 U.Pitt.L.Rev. 1, 23–6 (1967). In any event, how important is it to have access to the subject of the proceeding when the issue is dangerousness or treatability (as compared, for instance, to sanity at the time of the offense)? Would it not be useful, through recognition of the right to remain silent, to encourage the state to develop alternative sources of information?

3. *Consequences of* Allen. If there is no right to remain silent in civil commitment proceedings, then the state may not only compel the respondent to answer questions during a psychiatric examination (as was the case in *Allen*), but may also compel testimony in court. What sanction may be imposed on the person who refuses to speak to the examiner or in court? In the analogous situations in criminal proceedings, the court has several options: (1) a contempt citation; (2) an instruction that the jury may infer guilt from the defendant's silence; and (3) prohibition of the defendant's expert testimony, at least in cases where the defendant has refused to talk to the state's expert. Will any of these sanctions "work" in the civil commitment context? With respect to the first sanction, what "punishment" should be imposed once the respondent is found in contempt? In regard to the second sanction, what inferences can be drawn from the

---

226. ". . . It would do a great disservice to individuals to make the procedural requirements so cumbersome that suicidal and maniacal individuals could never be hospitalized until they had injured themselves or others." State *ex rel. Hawks v. Lazaro,* 157 W.Va. 417, 443–44, 202 S.E.2d 109, 126 (1974).

respondent's silence? As to the third sanction, is it fair if the respondent is willing to talk in court?

Another issue associated with the right to remain silent is whether the respondent's attorney may observe the pre-hearing examination process. If the fifth amendment applied, then by analogy to the Supreme Court's opinion in *Miranda v. Arizona*, 384 U.S. 436 (1966), the respondent should be told not only of the right to remain silent but also of the right to have counsel present during the examination. Is this a good idea? Even if there is no fifth amendment right to have counsel present during the evaluation, can one construct a sixth amendment argument in support of that right?

D. RELEASE PROCEDURES

FASULO v. ARAFEH

Supreme Court of Connecticut, 1977.
173 Conn. 473, 378 A.2d 553.

LONGO, ASSOCIATE JUSTICE.

The plaintiffs, Ann Fasulo and Marie Barbieri, alleging that they were illegally confined in the Connecticut Valley Hospital by the defendant superintendent, petitioned the Superior Court for writs of habeas corpus. The court denied the writs and the plaintiffs appealed.

Ann Fasulo was civilly committed to Connecticut Valley Hospital in 1951, as was Marie Barbieri in 1964. * * * They claim that because their commitments are of indefinite duration and there is no procedure for periodic court review of the necessity for their confinement, their confinement is in violation of the due process guarantee of article first, § 8, of the Connecticut constitution.

* * *

As the United States Supreme Court has recognized, "At the least, due process requires that the nature and duration of commitment bear some reasonable relation to the purpose for which an individual is committed." *Jackson v. Indiana*, 406 U.S. 715, 738. Once the purpose of the commitment no longer exists, there is no constitutional basis for the state to continue to deprive the individual of his liberty. To satisfy due process, the procedure for releasing a civilly committed patient must be adequate to assure release of those who may no longer constitutionally be confined.

These plaintiffs have been deprived of their liberty. Their loss is already great, but can be initially justified as a result of the legitimate exercise of the parens patriae power of the state. The plaintiffs, however, have been committed indefinitely and confined for periods of twenty-six and thirteen years respectively, thus requiring us to heed the warning of the United States Supreme Court that the longer the commitment, the greater the safeguards which are required to ensure that no one is deprived of liberty without due process. We must, therefore, review the plaintiffs' claims in light of the important interest at stake—liberty—and the great loss which its extended deprivation constitutes.

Any procedure to allow the release of involuntarily confined civilly committed individuals must take account of the controlled and often isolated environment of the mental hospital from which the confined individuals will seek release. It must calculate the possible incompetence of those confined, their limited knowledge of release procedures, the cost of pursuing review and the amount of effort necessary to pursue review. Further, the procedure must be adapted to the possible effect of drugs or other treatment on the patient's capacity and must be formulated with consideration of institutional pressures to rely on the *medical* judgments of the hospital staff rather than to pursue extrainstitutional *legal* remedies. See note, "Civil Commitment of the Mentally Ill," 87 Harv.L.Rev. 1190, 1398.

At present, Connecticut provides several routes by which a mental patient can challenge his confinement. General Statutes § 17–192 allows for release (1) by order of the Probate Court "upon application and satisfactory proof that such person has been restored to reason," or (2) "[i]f the officers, directors or trustees of a state hospital for mental illness are notified by the superintendent or other person in a managerial capacity of such institution that he has reason to believe that any person committed thereto by order of a probate court is not mentally ill or a suitable subject to be confined in such institution, such officers, directors or trustees may discharge such person." Under the second method the patient runs the risk of having his release prevented by a superintendent whose determination may later be found by a court to have been erroneous. Furthermore, the second procedure disregards the fundamental fact that the state's power legitimately to confine an individual is based on a legal determination under General Statutes § 17–178 "that the person complained of is mentally ill and dangerous to himself or herself or others or gravely disabled" and that the commitment shall only continue "for the period of the duration of such mental illness or until he or she is discharged in due course of law." The state's power to confine terminates when the patient's condition no longer meets the legal standard for commitment. Since the state's power to confine is measured by a legal standard, the expiration of the state's power can only be determined in a judicial proceeding which tests the patient's present mental status against the legal standard for confinement. That adjudication cannot be made by medical personnel unguided by the procedural safeguards which cushion the individual from an overzealous exercise of state power when the individual is first threatened with the deprivation of his liberty.

* * *

We also find the first method of release provided for in General Statutes § 17–192 constitutionally deficient. The method allows release of a patient after he has applied to the Probate Court for discharge and has proved that he has been "restored to reason." We find this procedure inadequate on two grounds. First, it places the burden of initiating review of his status on the patient, a requirement which suffers from conceptual as well as serious practical deficiencies. As we stated previously, since the state's power to confine is premised on the individual's present mental status, the original involuntary commitment proceeding can only establish that the state may confine the individual at the time of the hearing and for the foreseeable period during which that status is unlikely to change. Upon the expiration of that period, the state's power to deprive the patient of his liberty lapses and any further confinement must be justified anew. The state, therefore, must bear the burden of initiating recommitment proceedings.

This same reasoning applies to the burden of proof at the recommitment hearing. The burden should not be placed on the civilly committed patient to justify his right to liberty. Freedom from involuntary confinement for those who have committed no crime is the natural state of individuals in this country. The burden must be placed on the state to prove the necessity of stripping the citizen of one of his most fundamental rights, and the risk of error must rest on the state.

* * *

Furthermore, to require a patient to initiate judicial review of his confinement and to bear the burden of proving the nonexistence of the necessity for that confinement ignores the practical considerations discussed above which are inherent in the mental patient's situation. Briefly, these include the difficulties of overcoming an isolated environment to initiate and coordinate a challenge to one's confinement. For instance, we cannot assume that friends and allies will always be available to secure counsel and marshal evidence on the patient's behalf. Nor can we assume that even if a patient is notified of his right to pursue any of the available remedies, he will be adequately protected. [Merely giving the patient notice] ignores the practical difficulties of requiring a mental patient to overcome the effects of his confinement, his closed environment, his possible incompetence and the debilitating effects of drugs or other treatment on his ability to make a decision which may amount to the waiver of his constitutional right to a review of his status.

* * *

We, therefore, hold that these plaintiffs have been denied their due process rights under the Connecticut constitution by the state's failure to provide them with periodic judicial review of their commitments in the form of state-initiated recommitment hearings replete with the safeguards of the initial commitment hearings at which the state bears the burden of proving the necessity for their continued confinement.

* * *

It is, therefore, ordered that the writs be granted and that the plaintiffs be afforded a hearing at which the state must justify their continued confinement.

There is error, and the case is remanded with direction to grant the writs in accordance with this opinion.

In this opinion SPEZIALE, J., concurs.

BOGDANSKI, ASSOCIATE JUSTICE (concurring).

* * *

[The dissenting opinion of Justice Loiselle in which Chief Justice House concurred is omitted.]

Questions and Comments

1. *Current status of periodic review.* Although at one time commitment in many states was truly indeterminate, most states now require, in line with the holding in *Fasulo,* that a review hearing be held after a certain period of involuntary treatment. Typically, a hearing similar in kind to the initial adjudicatory hearing must be held within six months of the previous commitment; other fairly common review periods are three months and a year. West Virginia and Ohio do not require review until two years have elapsed, and a few states appear still to permit indefinite confinement. See S. Brakel, J. Parry & B. Weiner, The Mentally Disabled and the Law 122–126 (1985) (statute chart).

Of course, judicial review through a writ of habeas corpus is always available if the patient requests it. Moreover, most patients are released prior to the first review hearing. The average length of stay in the hospital for the majority of patients is probably well under 90 days. See Gove & Fain, "A Comparison of Voluntary and Committed Mental Patients," 34 Arch.Gen.Psychiat. 669, 673 (1977) (67% of involuntary patients discharged within 38 days); Tomellieri, Lakshminanayanan & Herjanic, "Who are the Committed," 165 J. Nervous & Mental Dis. 288, 291 (1977) (63% of committed patients discharged within 90 days). Nonetheless, a substantial number of patients are still *not* voluntarily discharged by the hospital within a short period of time. And relief via habeas corpus is hampered not only by the requirement that the patient initiate such proceedings but also because the petitioner bears the burden of proving the challenged detention is illegal.

2. *Timing of review. Fasulo* does not indicate when the judicial review it mandates must take place. However, it does quote the Supreme Court's statement in Jackson v. Indiana, 406 U.S. 715, 92 S.Ct. 1845, 32 L.Ed.2d 435 (1972), that "due process requires that the nature and duration of commitment bear some reasonable relation to the purpose for which the individual is committed." [s] With this language in mind, of what relevance is research that shows that the vast majority of civilly committed patients can be treated effectively within 100 days? Klerman, "National Trends in Hospitalization," 30 Hosp. & Comm. Psychiat. 110 (1979). If this research is substantiated, should a hearing be constitutionally mandated at the end of this period? Alternatively, given the possibility that no further treatment will be effective, should all patients simply be released at the

[s] *Jackson* held that hospitalization of those found incompetent to stand trial may last only so long as there is a substantial probability that the patient will attain competency in the foreseeable future. See pp. 912–919.

expiration of 100 days? In arguing in favor of such a rule, Stromberg and Stone cite the above-mentioned research and state:

> We believe that after a certain period of treatment and involuntary confinement, society must give patients a chance on their own. We might agree that this should not apply to an imminently suicidal person if it would be predicted that some finite further period of treatment would likely end the person's suicidal impulses. Unfortunately, this is rarely possible.

Stromberg & Stone, "A Model State Law on Civil Commitment of the Mentally Ill," 20 Harv.J.Leg. 275, 380 (1983). Might agreement with the Stromberg and Stone proposal depend upon whether the commitment is for parens patriae or police power purposes?

3. *Formality of review.* Are there any differences between the initial commitment and the review process that merit additional (or fewer) procedural protections at the latter proceeding? Should the state have to meet a heavier burden if it seeks continued commitment? Might a public jury decision be more useful in the review process than at the initial commitment?

4. *Waiver of review hearing.* The *Fasulo* court suggested that allowing the patient to decide whether a hearing should take place is unconstitutional. Does this mean that the majority would reject a provision allowing a waiver of the right to a hearing? Consider the following, from Wexler, "The Waivability of Recommitment Hearings," 20 Ariz.L.Rev. 175, 184–86 (1978).

> Clearly, if mechanisms could be devised to eliminate the need for those, and only those, recommitment hearings that are truly unnecessary and truly unwanted by the patients, a host of considerations would favor a rule of waivability. A number of such considerations come quickly to mind.

> There is, of course, the sheer economic consideration involving the depletion of judicial, mental health, and related resources. Courts sitting in the vicinity of state hospitals have terribly heavy commitment calendars. They assuredly would wish to be spared the time and expense of conducting unnecessary and unwanted recommitment hearings.

> The judicial time-and-cost saving interest would be particularly evident, of course, if an appreciable number of patients wished to waive such hearings. At the moment, the percent of patients desiring waiver is an empirical unknown. It would not be at all surprising, however, for a rather large number of patients to desire waiver. The depressed and suicidal might well constitute one such patient category. So too, many elderly, "gravely disabled" patients might opt for waiver, were it available, rather than attend hearings only to learn what they already know: that their clinical and family situation is unchanged or has worsened, and that no facilities less restrictive than full-time hospitalization can yet be found for their placement.

> Needless to say, physicians, nurses, and ward attendants would also prefer to treat than to testify. To the extent that they are called upon

to testify in unnecessary and unwanted hearings, the patients and the public would be best served by those mental health witnesses playing instead a therapeutic role.

* * *

The interests of psychotherapists and of certain patients converge in their concern over the possible traumatic and anti-therapeutic effects of recommitment hearings. Unlike initial hearings, where the possible trauma to the patient is probably outweighed by the feedback to him of the impropriety of his behavior and by the presentation of convincing evidence that commitment is called for, the interests deserve to be balanced differently in the framework of recommitment.

By the time of recommitment, a patient may well be quite aware of what is objectionable about his behavior or of why alternative placement seems unsuitable. Moreover, whether hearing adverse testimony will prove traumatic or anti-therapeutic is no longer a matter of enormous abstract speculation: the patient will have already experienced one commitment hearing and may now be in a fairly good position to assess the relative costs and benefits of contesting recommitment. If recommitment is in any event likely, a number of patients may wish to avoid hearings at which testimony will be given regarding, for example, the persistence of their depressed and suicidal state, or the continuing unwillingness of families or of nursing homes to accept patients who act out conflicts or who are sometimes assaultive.

* * *

. . . Waivability—consent to recommitment for up to a specified period—should probably be authorized if a lawyer playing an adversary role certifies to the court that he has investigated the case and has consulted with his client, that he has explained to the client the options and the right to consent recommitment, and that he has concluded that the client desires to consent to recommitment.

5. *Conditional release.* One reason for the short hospitalization periods of many patients described in note 1 is the development of conditional release programs. Theoretically, these programs function somewhat like parole. A patient is released on "conditional" or "convalescent" status to a community mental health center, halfway house, or other community service in an effort to ease the transition to normal life, on the condition that the patient adheres to a particular treatment regimen (e.g., periodic medication, attendance at group therapy sessions) and remains stable. Immediate rehospitalization is permissible, however, if the patient is shown to require it. In practice, these programs have been hampered by lack of adequate community resources and poor communication between hospitals and community service providers. See generally, Note, "Constitutional Law: The Summary Revocation of an Involuntary Mental Patient's Convalescent Leave—Is It Unconstitutional?" 33 Okla.L.Rev. 366, 369 (1980).

A preliminary question with respect to conditional release is whether such programs are permissible exercises of state power. Most statutes imply, if they do not state explicitly, that those patients who are conditionally released no longer meet commitment standards. See Application of True v. Department of Health and Welfare, 103 Idaho 151, 645 P.2d 891,

898 (1982). If so, under what authority may the state continue to maintain
any control over the patient? Perhaps, as discussed in the materials on the
least restrictive alternative doctrine, the justification for such continued
interference is that it contemplates a lesser deprivation of liberty and thus
is permissible on a lesser showing than that demanded by the commitment
standards. There may be other justifications as well. Cf. American Bar
Association Criminal Justice Mental Health Standard 7–7.4 (permitting
continued confinement of an insanity acquittee who no longer meets the
commitment criteria if the state can show that the only reason the criteria
are not met is that the patient is undergoing treatment that is likely to end
unless commitment continues).

In any event, the most significant litigation with respect to conditional
release programs has assumed their constitutionality and focused instead
on procedural questions. In particular, courts have been concerned with
provisions that permit conditional release to be revoked on the authority of
the hospital director, with no requirement of judicial supervision other
than, in some states, an ex parte order. Not surprisingly, given the
similarity between conditional release and parole, these courts have focused on the Supreme Court's decision in *Morrissey v. Brewer,* 408 U.S. 471,
92 S.Ct. 2593, 33 L.Ed.2d 484 (1972), which held that the "conditional
liberty" of paroled criminals entitles them to preliminary and final parole
revocation hearings, notice and confrontation rights and, in "complex"
revocation proceedings, the right to counsel as well.

In *Dietrich v. Brooks,* 27 Or.App. 821, 558 P.2d 357 (1976), the court
found that there are "profound differences of nature, degree and function"
between conditional hospital release and parole. Specifically, the court
noted three distinctions: (1) the underlying nature of imprisonment and
parole is penal, while conditional release is a therapeutic device; (2) the
length of the deprivation of liberty differs; and (3) there is a closer
relationship between the conditional liberty and the institutional program
with conditional release than with parole. Thus, the court held, summary
revocation of conditional release is adequate under the due process clause.

Other courts have decided that more process is due patients whose
conditional release is revoked. For instance, in *Application of True v.
Department of Health and Welfare,* 103 Idaho 151, 645 P.2d 891 (1982), the
court considered the constitutionality of a statute which permitted immediate revocation of conditional release status when (1) the "director of the
[mental health] department or his designated representative" believed that
the patient had failed to meet the conditions of his release and that
"conditions justifying hospitalization continue[d] to exist"; or when (2) the
director or his designate had reason to believe that the patient had
"relapsed" and was "again in need of hospitalization," based on the report
of two persons "who are either licensed physicians, health officers, designated examiners or peace officers, the prosecuting attorney or a judge of a
court". The court rejected the state's argument that the patient's ability to
appeal any hospitalization decision within 30 days and the additional right
to habeas relief adequately protected the patient's due process interests:

> [I]t cannot be said that [the appeal and habeas provisions] adequately
> protect the interests of a mental health patient whose conditional

release status has been revoked. Review under either provision is not mandatory. Neither provision requires that the patient be apprised of the reasons for his rehospitalization. Under these circumstances, there can be no assurances of meaningful review. But more importantly, both provisions are infirm because they place the burden on the patient to bring forth sufficient facts to justify relief from an order of rehospitalization. It is the state, in cases where it seeks to deprive an individual of a protectible liberty or property interest, which must bring forth sufficient facts justifying its summary action.

The court then went on to decide what process is due the patient who is the subject of a revocation proceeding:

In the instant situation, the conditionally released mental health patient's interest in insuring that the revocation of his right to remain at liberty be based on an accurate evaluation of the facts and diagnosis must be balanced against the Department's need to conduct its program of treatment of the mentally ill and mentally retarded with a minimum of judicially imposed interference. The court is of the opinion that although mental health patients are entitled to due process when the Department seeks to revoke their conditional release status, important differences between the conditional release program for mental health patients and the parole system are such that the procedures outlined in *Morrissey* for parole revocation, both in terms of timing and formality, are inappropriate in the instant case.

* * *

[T]iming becomes more critical in the instant case than it is in the parole setting. In the parole situation a delay in the revocation of an individual's parolee status, while highly undesirable in cases where revocation is found to be justified, does not present a serious threat to the degree of rehabilitation achieved prior to the violation. In contrast, in cases where a mental health patient is suspected of remission, the Department's interest in rehospitalization for immediate treatment is paramount, as the progress towards recovery which had been achieved is seriously jeopardized by a remission which is left untreated.

* * *

The great weight we accord the Department's need for immediate rehospitalization of a conditionally released mental health patient suspected of remission is such that the general rule that an individual be given an opportunity for a hearing before he is deprived of a protectible interest is inapplicable. The situation present when a decision is made to revoke the conditional release status of the patient is extraordinary: the patient because of a suspected remission in his mental condition possibly poses a danger to others and/or to himself.

Nonetheless, it would be wrong, and in certain instances tragic, to assume that all evaluations and reports that a conditionally released patient is in need of rehospitalization are accurate. In order to militate against the possibility of an erroneous decision that rehospitalization is warranted, the court is also of the opinion that a mental health patient whose conditional release status is subject to revocation is entitled to mandatory notice and a hearing to follow as soon as is reasonably possible after the patient's return to the hospital.

Specifically, the minimal due process requirements are: (1) prompt written notice to the patient of the reasons for and evidence relied on justifying rehospitalization as well as notice of the right to challenge the allegations and (2) a hearing before a neutral hearing body to be held as soon as is reasonably possible following the patient's rehospitalization, at which time the patient is to be afforded the right to counsel, the right to present evidence and examine witnesses, and upon a decision sustaining the order of rehospitalization, the right to a written statement by the fact-finding body as to the reasons for revocation of the patient's conditional release status. We stress that these are minimal requirements.

Most statutes are unclear as to whether revocation of conditional release begins an entirely new commitment period or instead only authorizes hospitalization for the remainder of the original commitment. Should this matter? Is it relevant to consider the effect that additional procedures will have on the state's willingness to engage in conditional release programs?

A second issue connected with conditional release that has yet to be extensively litigated concerns the types of limitations the constitution places on the conditions which may be imposed as part of such a program. For instance, in a jurisdiction which recognizes a right to refuse medication, may release be conditioned upon the patient's agreement to accept medication?

E. VOLUNTARY ADMISSION PROCEDURES

Since the end of the second World War, there has been a growing interest in avoiding involuntary commitment proceedings by encouraging "voluntary" admission of people with mental disorders; today every state but Alabama allows people to admit themselves for psychiatric treatment. Nationally, such admissions comprise just under 50% of the mental hospital population and about 85% of the population in psychiatric units of general hospitals. S. Brakel, J. Parry & B. Weiner, The Mentally Disabled and the Law 178–79 (1985). One early explanation of why voluntary status has been so favored asserted:

> [Voluntary admission] enjoys the unique position of being favored by all of the groups concerned with influencing legislation in this field. The medical profession endorses this procedure because of its simplicity and the complete lack of any court action. The patient who can recognize his illness and seek hospitalization on his own volition is the one who will actively participate in his treatment, cooperate with his doctor, and benefit the most from the treatment. As a result the voluntary patient will be discharged more rapidly, thereby alleviating the generally crowded conditions that exist in most mental facilities. Those who are concerned with civil liberties of mental patients are reassured, since the dangers of wrongful detention exist only in involuntary hospitalization procedures.

Comment, "Hospitalization of the Mentally Disabled in Pennsylvania: The Mental Health–Mental Retardation Act of 1966," 71 Dick.L.Rev. 307, 308–09 (1967). This section examines the procedures associated with hospitalizing a person whom the state is willing to admit as a "voluntary" patient.

GILBOY, SCHMIDT, "VOLUNTARY" HOSPITALIZATION OF THE MENTALLY ILL

66 N.W.L.Rev. 429.
(1971).

Both the medical and legal proponents of voluntary care share a conception of voluntary admission as an individual decision to accept mental treatment, made entirely apart from involuntary commitment procedures, thereby avoiding the therapeutic and legal problems of coercion. We have recently studied the use of voluntary admission procedures in Illinois, a state in which a substantial majority of persons hospitalized in mental institutions are now admitted under voluntary procedures. The results of our study indicate that the foregoing conception is wrong.

In a majority of cases voluntary admission is utilized to hospitalize persons who are already in some form of official custody. Voluntary admission avoids procedural complexity and the need for officials to assume responsibility, both inherent drawbacks to compulsory commitment from the officials' point of view. Individuals are therefore induced to voluntarily commit themselves with the threat of involuntary commitment as the principal means of persuasion, and with little concern for the adequacy of the information on which the individual's decision is based or whether it is "voluntary" at all.

* * *

Although our study was limited to analysis of relevant statistical data and direct personal observation of commitment procedures in Illinois, that state's procedures for commitment of the mentally ill are similar to those of many other states.

DEFINITION OF VOLUNTARY ADMISSION

Under Illinois law there are two different procedures for voluntary admission to mental hospitals. Under the first procedure, known as "informal admission," an individual is admitted to a mental hospital without formal application and is free to leave at any time during normal day-shift hours. Under the second procedure, known as "voluntary admission," an individual is admitted to a mental hospital upon formal application and is free to leave "within 5 days, excluding Saturdays, Sundays and holidays, after he gives any professional staff person notice of his desire to leave, . . ." However, during that 5–day notice period, the hospital officials may ask a court to hold an involuntary commitment hearing, which must be set within 5 days after such petition. The patient continues to be hospitalized pending a final order of the court at the hearing. Thus, informal admission may be described as an entirely voluntary process. Voluntary admission, in contrast, requires an initial voluntary decision on the part of the patient, but, once that decision is made, the patient is subject to restraint on his right to leave the hospital, and may be required to remain a week or more after he expresses a desire to leave.

A striking preliminary fact which our study disclosed is that informal admission is almost never utilized. In fact, in only about one percent of the cases admitted to mental institutions in Illinois is "informal admission" utilized. In contrast, voluntary admission is used in about 68% of all cases. The reason for the greater use of voluntary admission appears to be the additional restraining power the procedure gives the hospital over the patient. "With 'informal admission' the units just do not feel enough control over the patient," one hospital admissions officer remarked. Another hospital official described informal admission as an "inconvenience" to hospital staff personnel and an unnecessary "allowance" to patients. In one case described to us by an admissions officer, informal admission was used to house overnight an individual admittedly not in need of hospitalization, but for whom no other immediate shelter could be found.

The almost total refusal to use the entirely voluntary informal admission procedure is suggestive at the outset of the general attitude of officials toward voluntary admission procedures. The value of such procedures to officials, as will be more evident below, is not primarily in allowing individuals to remain in control of their own circumstances, but rather in hospitalizing individuals with a minimum of official responsibility and difficulty.

POLICE CUSTODY CASES

The case which proponents of voluntary admission almost always have in mind is that of an individual who arrives at a mental institution by himself, or accompanied by a physician, family, relatives or friends, and asks to be admitted for treatment. We call these "non-custody cases" to denote the absence of any official custody prior to the individual's decision to commit himself.

* * *

Our study disclosed that about 40% of all voluntarily admitted patients are brought to the mental hospital by the police and in about 55% of the cases where individuals are brought to the hospital by the police, voluntary admission results. While some studies of civil commitment have recognized that a significant number of persons are brought to mental institutions by the police, there has been little recognition that such cases often result in voluntary rather than involuntary commitment.

* * *

It is important to understand the difference between these police custody cases and the non-custody cases which proponents of voluntary care have usually assumed. In non-custody cases, the individual is making a choice between voluntarily committing himself or remaining outside the hospital, which is a fairly simple choice. The application form for voluntary admission discloses the restrictions on the right to leave the hospital which that status will impose.

In police custody cases, on the other hand, the alternatives as they appear to the individual are voluntary admission versus involuntary commitment. This is a much more difficult decision. In these cases, to make a reasonable choice, the individual must be informed about the nature of the involuntary commitment process since that is the major alternative before him. [M]ost persons unquestionably have only the vaguest idea, if any at all, about the nature of the involuntary commitment procedure. Indeed, most persons probably have only a vague idea of the substantive legal standard to be applied at such a hearing.

The typical practice in cases, however, is to explain voluntary admission to the patient in a very cursory manner, describing it as a desirable alternative to involuntary commitment. The explanation "If you sign a voluntary admission it will only be between you and the doctor and not the judge," is typical. To regard the uninformed decision to accept hospitalization as "voluntary" is highly artificial.

COURT CASES

Our study disclosed that approximately 10–11% of voluntary admissions to mental hospitals result from decisions made, or announced, in court at the time of an involuntary commitment hearing. Voluntary admission occurs in approximately 35% of the cases which come to court for involuntary commitment hearings. The court hearing may be the result of initial involuntary commitment on the basis of an emergency petition or physician's certificate as described earlier. However, in about 60% of cases the court hearing follows an initial criminal arrest.

* * *

A decision to accept voluntary admission by a defendant at a court hearing raises the same issue of adequate disclosure discussed earlier in connection with voluntary admission of persons brought by the police to the hospital admissions office. It might be expected that the involvement of the public defender and the judge at the time of a court hearing would insure that any decision on admission would be fully informed. However, the judges involved appear to give no consideration to the defendant's awareness of his situation. Any indication that the public defender and state's attorney are agreeable to voluntary admission and that the patient will agree is sufficient to dispose of the case. There is no inquiry to ascertain whether the defendant understands the choices before him and the decision he is making. The public defender, because of the time pressures to which he is subject and the non-adversary conception of his job, does not seek to advise patients of their rights so that they can make an informed judgment. Rather, the public defender makes his own judgment as to whether voluntary admission is appropriate and, if so, then urges the defendant to accept such hospitalization in a manner not unlike that of admissions officers in cases discussed earlier.

Where persons come to civil commitment hearings after having initially been arrested on criminal charges (a majority of the cases in Chicago), a further legal issue is raised. In these cases the individuals are under an added pressure: the threat of criminal prosecution if they should successfully resist civil commitment. If the individual is committed, voluntarily or involuntarily, the criminal charge against him is usually dropped.

* * *

Our study disclosed that in a majority of the cases in which voluntary admission procedures were used, the individuals were already under some form of official custody and were faced with the threat of involuntary commitment proceedings as the principal alternative to voluntary admission.

Questions and Comments

1. *The informed consent model of voluntary admission.* Gilboy and Schmidt suggest that many voluntary admissions in Illinois are not really voluntary because of the implicit and explicit pressures exerted on those who agree to such admissions and because of the failure to explain to them the nature and consequence of such admissions. Would their concerns be addressed by imposing an informed consent requirement on the voluntary admission process? As discussed in Chapter Three, the informed consent doctrine requires that, before treatment is administered, the potential patient must (1) be told of its risks and benefits; (2) be able to competently assess them; and (3) make a voluntary decision to undergo the treatment based on this assessment. The three aspects of the doctrine as they might apply in the voluntary admission context are discussed below.

Disclosure of Information. Gilboy and Schmidt's research indicates that persons who are admitted as voluntary patients rarely have their options fully explained to them and as a result have only vague notions about them. Presumably, all potential patients should be told about the alternatives open to them: the nature and consequences of involuntary commitment (and of the criminal process, if this is a disposition being considered) and the nature and consequences of voluntary commitment. Is this enough?

Competency. As developed in Chapter Nine, determining whether the information which is imparted is competently assessed is problematic, given the difficulty of defining competency. But it is worth noting that every study of the issue has concluded that most voluntary patients have significant difficulty understanding their situation. The best constructed study, which involved interviews of 50 voluntary patients within two days of their admission, found that "a large percentage of the patients who voluntarily entered [the] hospital were not competent to consent to their own admission." Appelbaum, Mirkin & Bateman, "Empirical Assessment of Competency to Consent to Psychiatric Hospitalization," 138 Am.J.Psych. 1170, 1174 (1981). This finding held "whether competency was defined on narrow clinical grounds, with a broader clinically oriented focus, in terms that measure understanding of legal rights, or by means of criteria that combined all of these definitions." Id. Interestingly, the study also found that "50% of the patients did not acknowledge their need to be in a psychiatric hospital; the vast majority of these denied it outright." Id. at 1173.

Another study reported interviews with 100 voluntary patients, each of whom had signed a form setting out their rights, as well as their obligation to remain for three days after giving notice of intent to leave. The interviews, conducted five days after admission, produced the following results:

1. Patient unable to make relevant answer to questions   13 patients
2. Patient responsive to questions but had no relevant information   18 patients
3. Patient responsive but had erroneous information   24 patients
4. Patient had incomplete information   37 patients
5. Patient had complete information   8 patients

Ten days after admission 33 of the patients were interviewed again. Fifteen showed a higher level of understanding at the second interview than they had at the first. Olin & Olin, "Informed Consent in Voluntary Mental Hospital Admissions," 132 Am.J.Psychiat. 938 (1975). See also, Grossman & Summers, "A Study of the Capacity of Schizophrenic Patients to Give Informed Consent," 31 J.Hosp. & Comm.Psychiat. 205 (1980); Palmer & Wohl, "Voluntary–Admission Forms: Does the Patient Know What He's Signing?", 23 J.Hosp. & Comm.Psychiat. 250 (1972).

Voluntariness. The claim that many voluntary admissions are not voluntary is made forthrightly by Szasz:

> What is called voluntary admission is really not voluntary. It is perhaps quasi-voluntary. What we call voluntary admission to a mental hospital doesn't resemble voluntary admission to a medical hospital, for example, for pneumonia. It is rather a kind of voluntary involuntary admission. This so-called voluntary admission to a mental hospital is a procedure, which, more often than not, could be paraphrased as follows. It is as if the patient were told: 'If you don't go to the hospital by signing this piece of paper, then we'll get you in by having someone else sign another piece of paper.'

Hearings on the Constitutional Rights of the Mentally Ill Before the Subcomm. on Constitutional Rights of the Senate Comm. on the Judiciary, 87th Cong., 1st Sess. 265 (1961).

Assume that the police have brought in to a receiving ward a person whom they believe to be mentally disabled. Assume further that this person has been fully informed of and understands the difference between voluntary and involuntary hospitalization and the fact that the government has the authority to institute involuntary commitment proceedings against him. In what sense would the implicit or explicit threat to exercise such authority render a decision by this person to be a voluntary patient "involuntary"?

Consider the law on plea bargaining, the process by which criminal defendants agree to plead guilty in exchange for a reduced charge or sentence. The Supreme Court has made clear that a guilty plea produced by this process may be rendered involuntary by "coercion, terror, inducements, [and] subtle or blatant threats." *Boykin v. Alabama*, 395 U.S. 238, 89 S.Ct. 1709, 23 L.Ed.2d 274 (1969). At the same time, the Court has refused to invalidate guilty pleas simply because the defendant's situation is an unpleasant one. So long as a guilty plea represents a reasoned choice from among alternatives that are legitimately offered by the prosecution, it is not "involuntary". *Bordenkircher v. Hayes*, 434 U.S. 357, 98 S.Ct. 663, 54 L.Ed.2d 604 (1978); *Brady v. United States*, 397 U.S. 742, 90 S.Ct. 1463, 25 L.Ed.2d 747 (1970). Would the decision to be a voluntary patient described above be "involuntary" under these cases? If not, is there still a reason for withholding the voluntary label from such a person?

2. *Alternatives to the informed consent model.* In light of the difficulties with the informed consent model of voluntary admission, particularly with respect to ensuring competent decisionmaking, various alternatives have been proposed. The first alternative is to allow voluntary admission of anyone who is "suitable" for such admission and fails to object to it. Several states appear to permit so-called "non-protesting" admissions. See, e.g., Mass Gen.Laws Ann. ch. 123, § 10(a); D.C.Code 1981, § 21–513.

> Although such [provisions] slight the value of individual autonomy that the informed consent is designed to foster, it would be no worse than the present system and would have the additional virtue of avoiding pretense. This system could, in addition, be augmented with the kind of internal review procedures (e.g. utilization review, staff conferences) that the Supreme Court indicated were adequate to protect the rights of minors admitted by their parents [in *Parham v. J.R.*]. Such a change would maximize therapeutic interests, while relegating more formal, legalistic proceedings to the background.

Appelbaum, Mirkin & Bateman, supra at 1175. Are provisions which permit admission of non-protesting persons an end-run around the procedural requirements of involuntary commitment? Or are they justified by the "need for a simple, non-traumatic admission process for those individuals who either do not recognize their need for hospitalization or are unwilling to seek admission, but nevertheless do not object when others initiate the admission process?" Note, "District of Columbia Hospitalization of the Mentally Ill Act," 65 Colum.L.Rev. 1062, 1065 (1965). In the past, many of the admissions under such statutes have been of senile persons who make no objection to psychiatric hospitalization. See Application for Certification of William R, 9 Misc.2d 1084, 172 N.Y.S.2d 869 (1958).

The second alternative to an informed consent model of voluntary admission is to appoint a guardian for all persons who assent to or do not protest hospitalization. The guardian's function would be to decide whether hospitalization is in the person's best interests, considering all relevant factors, including the person's wishes. This substituted judgement model is widely used as a method of institutionalizing minors and the developmentally disabled. Very often the guardian is one of the putative patient's relatives, but it could be a judge or a public guardian. Does this approach provide any better protection against the practices observed by Gilboy and Schmidt?

A third alternative, of course, is to prohibit admission into a public psychiatric facility unless the person meets the criteria for involuntary commitment. Presumably, this would bar some people who want or need treatment from obtaining it. Some commentators argue against *any* procedure which has this effect:

> In the vast majority of involuntary *and* voluntary cases, it is the family or relatives who move toward, pressure for, or insist on commitment. If state law enforcement personnel are involved, it is as often as not at the request of the family or relatives. In many instances where it orders commitment, the state's judicial machinery merely formalizes and sanctions a decision arrived at by the family and the family doctor. In admitting a mentally disabled person to one of its institutions, the state often does no more than facilitate the provision of wanted treatment that is difficult or too costly to obtain otherwise. With respect to the commitment process, the patient himself . . . may be confused or indifferent, generally agitated, unable to understand its necessity, or simply unable to comprehend. The phenomenon of a freely derived, fully conscious, voluntary decision to enter a mental facility (particularly a public facility) is as rare as knowing, overt resistance to involuntary commitment. In short, the voluntary-involuntary dichotomy of mental institutionalization, the traditional roles that are assigned to the participants in this dichotomized process, and many of the laws and procedures enacted to regulate it suffer from their irrelevance to practical situations.

S. Brakel, J. Parry and B. Weiner, The Mentally Disabled and the Law 32 (1985).

3. *The Supreme Court and voluntary commitment.* In *Zinermon v. Burch*, ___ U.S. ___, 110 S.Ct. 975, 108 L.Ed.2d 100 (1990), the plaintiff was asked to sign forms giving his consent to admission and treatment, even though staff evaluation showed that, upon his arrival at the evaluating facility, he was "hallucinating, confused, psychotic, and believed he was 'in heaven.'" Within the next three days, he signed voluntary admission forms on two other occasions. He subsequently brought a § 1983 action against the state of Florida, alleging that his due process rights were violated by the staff when they admitted him as a voluntary patient knowing he was incompetent, rather than affording him the procedural protections granted those subjected to involuntary commitment. Although the U.S. Supreme Court did not address the merits, it held that this claim was justiciable in federal court under § 1983. Portions of the Court's opinion may be of interest in deciding between the informed consent model or one of the alternative approaches:

> The Florida statutes, of course, do not allow incompetent persons to be admitted as "voluntary" patients. . . . A patient who is willing to sign forms but incapable of informed consent certainly cannot be relied on to protest his "voluntary" admission and demand that the involuntary placement procedure be followed. The staff are the only persons

in a position to take notice of any misuse of the voluntary admission process, and to ensure that the proper procedure is followed.

Florida chose to delegate to petitioners a broad power to admit patients to FSH, i.e., to effect what, in the absence of informed consent, is a substantial deprivation of liberty. Because petitioners had state authority to deprive persons of liberty, the Constitution imposed on them the State's concomitant duty to see that no deprivation occurs without adequate procedural protections.

It may be permissible constitutionally for a State to have a statutory scheme like Florida's, which gives state officials broad power and little guidance in admitting mental patients. But when those officials fail to provide constitutionally required procedural safeguards to a person whom they deprive of liberty, the state officials cannot then escape liability. . . . It is immaterial whether the due process violation Burch alleges is best described as arising from petitioners' failure to comply with state procedures for admitting involuntary patients, or from the absence of a specific requirement that petitioners determine whether a patient is competent to consent to voluntary admission.

(4.) *Release of voluntary patients.* The procedure for releasing voluntary patients under the Illinois statute described by Gilboy and Schmidt is similar to that found in most states. Typically, a voluntary patient who wants to leave the hospital may not do so immediately but must give notice, ranging from three to ten days, during which time the hospital may initiate commitment proceedings if it feels involuntary commitment is warranted. This restraint on release has been justified by Guttmacher and Weihofen, Psychiatry and the Law 306 (1952), as follows:

> With regard to provisions for release, two opposing considerations must be weighed. On the one hand, complete freedom to leave the hospital at any time will almost certainly lead a number of patients to leave a few days after being admitted, for restlessness and dissatisfaction with the restrains of hospitalization are common and natural, especially during the first period of adjustment. This makes the admission a complete waste of time and money. On the other hand, refusal to release a voluntary patient on demand would not only be difficult to justify legally but would be highly undesirable, because resort to voluntary admission will be discouraged unless it is made quite clear that a patient may change his mind and leave. Most voluntary admission statutes meet the problem by providing that a voluntary patient shall be released within a specified number of days after he gives written notice of his desire to leave, unless in the meanwhile the hospital authorities start proceedings to have his status changed to that of involuntary patient.

Some courts have struck down such advance notice provisions. *In Ex parte Romero,* 51 N.M. 210, 181 P.2d 811 (1947), for instance, the patient "was admitted to the sanitarium on his written application . . . and the certificate of a doctor of medicine." Four days after admission he verbally requested release but was denied, under authority of a statute which permitted detention of a voluntary patient for ten days after notice of an intent to leave. The court held that the statute violated the due process clause:

> The respondent urges that by the voluntary act of the petitioner in making the request for admission, he contracted with it to there remain and receive treatment until ten days after written notice of his desire or intention to terminate the same was given, unless sooner released. Obviously, it does not require citation of authority that one may not enforce such a contract made with a person he knows to be so disordered in mind as to require treatment in an institution for the treatment of mental diseases.

Consider also *Ex parte Lloyd*, 13 F.Supp. 1005 (E.D.Ky.1936) which construed a federal statute that authorized the Secretary of the Treasury to order treatment of those addicts who applied for it "for the maximum amount of time estimated by the Surgeon General . . . as necessary to effect a cure". The court rejected the contention of the government that the statute should be construed to authorize specific enforcement of an addict's agreement to undergo treatment. Such a construction, held the court, would violate the due process clause and the thirteenth amendment, which prohibits involuntary servitude except as a punishment for crime.

> The full intent of the[se] provisions could be defeated with obvious facility if citizens could be held to involuntary servitude or enforced imprisonment, through the guise of such contracts. The contract exposes the petitioner to liability for any damages suffered as the result of the breach but not to involuntary servitude in any form nor to the loss of his liberty or any of its essential attributes without due process of law.

In contrast to *Romero* and *Lloyd*, consider *Ortega v. Rasor*, 291 F.Supp. 748 (S.D.Fla.1968). There, pursuant to the Narcotic Rehabilitation Act of 1966, the successor to the statute construed in *Lloyd*, the petitioner "voluntarily requested the Court to order him civilly committed for treatment of a narcotic addiction." As part of standard procedure, he signed a form waiving his right to further hearing if a psychiatrist designated by the Surgeon General found, after a 30–day evaluation period in the hospital, that he was "an addict who is likely to be rehabilitated through treatment." The petitioner also agreed that if such a finding were made, the court could enter a order, in his absence and without further hearing, committing him to the care and custody of the Surgeon General for a treatment period not to exceed six months and such posthospitalization treatment as was authorized by the Act. After the 30–day evaluation period, the examining psychiatrist submitted a report making the requisite findings and the court ordered the petitioner committed.

In holding that the petitioner could not withdraw from the treatment, the district court (the same court that entered the commitment order) stated:

> . . . In the case at bar, the Court is not concerned with a situation of compulsory treatment as such. The petitioner . . . initially instituted the proceeding for his civil commitment with the filing of a petition on his own behalf. . . . The Court, having independently recollected the hearing held pursuant to Mr. Ortega's petition for commitment,

which hearing was brought before the Court by the government, and having reviewed the transcript of that hearing, is convinced that the petitioner acted of his own volition in requesting civil commitment and not because he was under the influence of narcotics and did not know what he was doing. The transcript of the hearing as well as the petition for voluntary civil commitment and Waiver of Further Court Appearance, both signed by Mr. Ortega established without a doubt that Mr. Ortega was fully apprised of his responsibilities under the Act and in fact understood those responsibilities. The Court will not permit the petitioner to terminate his treatment simply because the road to recovery is bumpy.

In *Romero* and *Lloyd* the admission process was non-judicial; in *Ortega,* a court was involved. Should this matter? Is there any other explanation for the difference in the results reached in these decisions? More generally, would invalidating the notice-and-detention provisions found in most state statutes make any practical difference? Couldn't the patient who demands release be discharged and then immediately detained and subjected to involuntary commitment proceedings?

5. *Review of voluntary patients; conversion to voluntary status.* Many patients who are admitted voluntarily never request release, especially those who are admitted under the non-protesting admissions statutes described earlier. Are voluntary patients entitled to periodic review, as is true with involuntary patients? As the next section indicates, there has been considerable litigation on this issue in connection with specific types of "voluntary" patients, i.e., the developmentally disabled and children. As a general matter, these cases mandate some type of review, although not necessarily judicial.

Some courts have considered the review issue in the context of conversion of involuntary patients to voluntary status. Many states authorize this conversion whenever the hospital staff believes the change is indicated, in the belief that a voluntary relationship enhances therapy. See, e.g., Ark.Stats. § 59–1412; N.Y.Code § 9.23. One court has found that the patient subject to such conversion in status is entitled to a judicial hearing reviewing the change as well as the same sort of periodic review provided involuntary patients. *Matter of Buttonow*, 23 N.Y.2d 385, 297 N.Y.S.2d 97, 244 N.E.2d 677 (1968). The dissenting opinion in *Buttonow* stated, in part: "[T]he salutary effect of voluntary status may be impaired by repeated judicial proceedings, or worse, remove the incentive of the institutions to arrange for conversions of status." Id. at 684 (Breitel, J., dissenting). Perhaps relevant here is recent literature indicating that voluntary patients are hospitalized twice as long as involuntary patients, and are less frequently considered to have received maximum benefits from their hospitalization. Nicholson, "Characteristics Associated with Change in the Legal Status of Involuntary Psychiatric Patients," 39 Hosp. & Comm. Psychiat. 424 (1988).

V. COMMITMENT OF OTHER POPULATIONS

As noted at the outset of this chapter, most states have enacted separate commitment statutes for certain groups of mentally disabled individuals. The most prominent such groups are insanity acquittees, prison and jail inmates requiring psychiatric treatment, substance abusers, the developmentally disabled, and children with mental disability. This section examines the special considerations involved in commitment of these groups, with frequent comparison to the preceding materials.

A. INSANITY ACQUITTEES

Every state permits immediate commitment of persons who have been found not guilty by reason of insanity. Some states require a hearing before such commitment, but most states allow the acquittee to be committed "automatically" for a short period of time, at which point a hearing is held to determine whether further commitment is proper. Almost all states also provide for later periodic judicial review, although in a few jurisdictions release is left up to the initiation of the hospital or the acquittee. One might argue that because insanity acquittees have by definition eluded conviction, they are similarly situated to persons subject to regular civil commitment and thus should be processed according to the same standards and procedures. But the Supreme Court has indicated that the constitution does not require such an equation.

JONES v. UNITED STATES
Supreme Court of the United States, 1983.
463 U.S. 354, 103 S.Ct. 3043, 77 L.Ed.2d 694.

JUSTICE POWELL delivered the opinion of the Court.

The question presented is whether petitioner, who was committed to a mental hospital upon being acquitted of a criminal offense by reason of insanity, must be released because he has been hospitalized for a period longer than he might have served in prison had he been convicted.

I

In the District of Columbia a criminal defendant may be acquitted by reason of insanity if his insanity is "affirmatively established by a preponderance of the evidence." D.C.Code § 24–301(j) (1981). If he successfully invokes the insanity defense, he is committed to a mental hospital. § 24–301(d)(1). The statute provides several ways of obtaining release. Within 50 days of commitment the acquittee is entitled to a judicial hearing to determine his eligibility for release, at which he has the burden of proving by a preponderance of the evidence that he is no longer mentally ill or dangerous. § 24–301(d)(2).[3] If he fails to meet this burden at the 50–day hearing, the committed acquittee subsequently may be released, with court approval, upon certification of his recovery by the hospital chief of service. § 24–301(e). Alternatively, the acquittee is entitled to a judicial hearing every six months at which he may establish by a preponderance of the evidence that he is entitled to release. § 24–301(k).

Independent of its provision for the commitment of insanity acquitees, the District of Columbia also has adopted a civil-commitment procedure, under which an individual may be committed upon clear and convincing proof by the Government that he is mentally ill and likely to injure himself or others. § 21–545(b). The individual may demand a jury in the civil-commitment proceeding. § 21–544. Once committed, a patient may be released at any time upon certification of recovery by the hospital chief of service. §§ 21–546, 21–548. Alternatively, the patient is entitled after the first 90 days, and subsequently at 6–month intervals, to request a judicial hearing at which he may gain his release by proving by a preponderance of the evidence that he is no longer mentally ill or dangerous. §§ 21–546, 21–547.

II

On September 19, 1975, petitioner was arrested for attempting to steal a jacket from a department store. The next day he was arraigned in the District of Columbia Superior Court on a charge of attempted petit larceny, a misdemeanor punishable by a maximum prison sentence of one year. The court ordered petitioner committed to St. Elizabeths, a public hospital for the mentally ill, for a determination of his competency to stand trial. On March 1, 1976, a hospital psychologist submitted a report to the court stating that petitioner was competent to stand trial, that petitioner suffered from "Schizophrenia, paranoid type," and that petitioner's alleged offense was "the product of his mental disease." The court ruled that petitioner was competent to stand trial. Petitioner subsequently decided to plead not guilty by reason of insanity. The Government did not contest the plea, and it entered into a stipulation of facts with petitioner. On March 12, 1976, the Superior Court found petitioner not guilty by reason of insanity and committed him to St. Elizabeths pursuant to § 24–301(d)(1).

On May 25, 1976, the court held the 50–day hearing required by § 24–301(d)(2)(A). A psychologist from St. Elizabeths testified on behalf of the Government that, in the opinion of the staff, petitioner continued to suffer from paranoid schizophrenia and that "because his illness is still quite active, he is still a danger to himself and to others." Petitioner's counsel conducted a brief cross-examination, and presented

---

3. The statute does not specify the standard for determining release, but the District of Columbia Court of Appeals held in this case that, as in release proceedings under § 24–301(e) and § 21–545(b), the confined person must show that he is either no longer mentally ill or no longer dangerous to himself or others. See 432 A.2d 364, 372, and n. 16 (1981) (en banc).

no evidence.[8] The court then found that "the defendant-patient is mentally ill and as a result of his mental illness, at this time, he constitutes a danger to himself or others." Petitioner was returned to St. Elizabeths. Petitioner obtained new counsel and, following some procedural confusion, a second release hearing was held on February 22, 1977. By that date petitioner had been hospitalized for more than one year, the maximum period he could have spent in prison if he had been convicted. On that basis he demanded that he be released unconditionally or recommitted pursuant to the civil-commitment standards in § 21–545(b), including a jury trial and proof by clear and convincing evidence of his mental illness and dangerousness.

III

It is clear that "commitment for any purpose constitutes a significant deprivation of liberty that requires due process protection." *Addington v. Texas,* 441 U.S. 418, 425, 99 S.Ct. 1804, 1809, 60 L.Ed.2d 323 (1979). Therefore, a State must have "a constitutionally adequate purpose for the confinement." *O'Connor v. Donaldson,* 422 U.S. 563, 574, 95 S.Ct. 2486, 2493, 45 L.Ed.2d 396 (1975). Congress has determined that a criminal defendant found not guilty by reason of insanity in the District of Columbia should be committed indefinitely to a mental institution for treatment and the protection of society. Petitioner does not contest the Government's authority to commit a mentally ill and dangerous person indefinitely to a mental institution, but rather contends that "the petitioner's trial was not a constitutionally adequate hearing to justify an indefinite commitment."

Petitioner's argument rests principally on *Addington v. Texas, supra,* in which the Court held that the Due Process Clause requires the Government in a civil-commitment proceeding to demonstrate by clear and convincing evidence that the individual is mentally ill and dangerous. Petitioner contends that these due process standards were not met in his case because the judgment of not guilty by reason of insanity did not constitute a finding of present mental illness and dangerousness and because it was established only by a preponderance of the evidence. Petitioner then concludes that the Government's only conceivably legitimate justification for automatic commitment is to ensure that insanity acquittees do not escape confinement entirely, and that this interest can justify commitment at most for a period equal to the maximum prison sentence the acquittee could have received if convicted. Because petitioner has been hospitalized for longer than the one year he might have served in prison, he asserts that he should be released unconditionally or recommitted under the District's civil-commitment procedures.

---

8. Petitioner's counsel seemed concerned primarily about obtaining a transfer for petitioner to a less restrictive wing of the hospital. See Tr. 11–12.

A

We turn first to the question whether the finding of insanity at the criminal trial is sufficiently probative of mental illness and dangerousness to justify commitment. A verdict of not guilty by reason of insanity establishes two facts: (i) the defendant committed an act that constitutes a criminal offense, and (ii) he committed the act because of mental illness. Congress has determined that these findings constitute an adequate basis for hospitalizing the acquittee as a dangerous and mentally ill person. See H.R.Rep. No. 91–907, *supra*, at 74 (expressing fear that "dangerous criminals, particularly psychopaths, [may] win acquittals of serious criminal charges on grounds of insanity" and yet "escape hospital commitment"); S.Rep. No. 1170, 84th Cong., 1st Sess., 13 (1955) ("Where [the] accused has pleaded insanity as a defense to a crime, and the jury has found that the defendant was, in fact, insane at the time the crime was committed, it is just and reasonable in the Committee's opinion that the insanity, once established, should be presumed to continue and that the accused should automatically be confined for treatment until it can be shown that he has recovered"). We cannot say that it was unreasonable and therefore unconstitutional for Congress to make this determination.

The fact that a person has been found, beyond a reasonable doubt, to have committed a criminal act certainly indicates dangerousness. Indeed, this concrete evidence generally may be at least as persuasive as any predictions about dangerousness that might be made in a civil-commitment proceeding.[13] We do not agree with petitioner's suggestion that the requisite dangerousness is not established by proof that a person committed a non-violent crime against property. This Court never has held that "violence," however that term might be defined, is a prerequisite for a constitutional commitment.[14]

Nor can we say that it was unreasonable for Congress to determine that the insanity acquittal supports an inference of continuing mental

---

13. In attacking the predictive value of the insanity acquittal, petitioner complains that "[w]hen Congress enacted the present statutory scheme, it did not cite any empirical evidence indicating that mentally ill persons who have committed a criminal act are likely to commit additional dangerous acts in the future." He further argues that the available research fails to support the predictive value of prior dangerous acts. We do not agree with the suggestion that Congress' power to legislate in this area depends on the research conducted by the psychiatric community. We have recognized repeatedly the "uncertainty of diagnosis in this field and the tentativeness of professional judgment. The only certain thing that can be said about the present state of knowledge and therapy regarding mental disease is that science has not reached finality of judgment. . . ." The lesson we have drawn is not that government may not act in the face of this uncertainty, but rather that courts should pay particular deference to reasonable legislative judgments.

14. See *Overholser v. O'Beirne,* 112 App. D.C. 267, 276, 302 F.2d 852, 861 (1961) (Burger, J.) ("[T]o describe the theft of watches and jewelry as 'non-dangerous' is to confuse danger with violence. Larceny is usually less violent than murder or assault, but in terms of public policy the purpose of the statute is the same as to both") (footnote omitted). It also may be noted that crimes of theft frequently may result in violence from the efforts of the criminal to escape or the victim to protect property or the police to apprehend the fleeing criminal.

illness. It comports with common sense to conclude that someone whose mental illness was sufficient to lead him to commit a criminal act is likely to remain ill and in need of treatment. The precise evidentiary force of the insanity acquittal, of course, may vary from case to case, but the Due Process Clause does not require Congress to make classifications that fit every individual with the same degree of relevance. Because a hearing is provided within 50 days of the commitment, there is assurance that every acquittee has prompt opportunity to obtain release if he has recovered.

Petitioner also argues that, whatever the evidentiary value of the insanity acquittal, the Government lacks a legitimate reason for committing insanity acquittees automatically because it can introduce the insanity acquittal as evidence in a subsequent civil proceeding. This argument fails to consider the Government's strong interest in avoiding the need to conduct a *de novo* commitment hearing following every insanity acquittal—a hearing at which a jury trial may be demanded, § 21–544, and at which the Government bears the burden of proof by clear and convincing evidence. Instead of focusing on the critical question whether the acquittee has recovered, the new proceeding likely would have to relitigate much of the criminal trial. These problems accent the Government's important interest in automatic commitment. See *Mathews v. Eldridge,* 424 U.S. 319, 348, 96 S.Ct. 893, 909, 47 L.Ed.2d 18 (1976). We therefore conclude that a finding of not guilty by reason of insanity is a sufficient foundation for commitment of an insanity acquittee for the purposes of treatment and the protection of society.

B

Petitioner next contends that his indefinite commitment is unconstitutional because the proof of his insanity was based only on a preponderance of the evidence, as compared to *Addington's* civil-commitment requirement of proof by clear and convincing evidence. In equating these situations, petitioner ignores important differences between the class of potential civil-commitment candidates and the class of insanity acquittees that justify differing standards of proof. The *Addington* Court expressed particular concern that members of the public could be confined on the basis of "some abnormal behavior which might be perceived by some as symptomatic of a mental or emotional disorder, but which is in fact within a range of conduct that is generally acceptable." In view of this concern, the Court deemed it inappropriate to ask the individual "to share equally with society the risk of error." But since automatic commitment under § 24–301(d)(1) follows only if the *acquittee himself* advances insanity as a defense and proves that his criminal act was a product of his mental illness, there is good reason for diminished concern as to the risk of error. More important, the proof that he committed a criminal act as a result of mental illness eliminates the risk that he is being committed for mere "idiosyncratic behavior." A criminal act by definition is not "within a range of conduct that is generally acceptable."

We therefore conclude that concerns critical to our decision in *Addington* are diminished or absent in the case of insanity acquittees. Accordingly, there is no reason for adopting the same standard of proof in both cases. "[D]ue process is flexible and calls for such procedural protections as the particular situation demands." The preponderance of the evidence standard comports with due process for commitment of insanity acquitees.[17]

C

The remaining question is whether petitioner nonetheless is entitled to his release because he has been hospitalized for a period longer than he could have been incarcerated if convicted. The Due Process Clause "requires that the nature and duration of commitment bear some reasonable relation to the purpose for which the individual is committed." *Jackson v. Indiana*, 406 U.S. 715, 738, 92 S.Ct. 1845, 1858, 32 L.Ed.2d 435 (1972). The purpose of commitment following an insanity acquittal, like that of civil commitment, is to treat the individual's mental illness and protect him and society from his potential dangerousness. The committed acquittee is entitled to release when he has recovered his sanity or is no longer dangerous. And because it is impossible to predict how long it will take for any given individual to recover—or indeed whether he ever will recover—Congress has chosen, as it has with respect to civil commitment, to leave the length of commitment indeterminate, subject to periodic review of the patient's suitability for release.

In light of the congressional purposes underlying commitment of insanity acquittees, we think petitioner clearly errs in contending that an acquittee's hypothetical maximum sentence provides the constitutional limit for his commitment. A particular sentence of incarceration is chosen to reflect society's view of the proper response to commission of a particular criminal offense, based on a variety of considerations such as retribution, deterrence, and rehabilitation. The State may punish a person convicted of a crime even if satisfied that he is unlikely to commit further crimes.

Different considerations underlie commitment of an insanity acquittee. As he was not convicted, he may not be punished. His confinement rests on his continuing illness and dangerousness. Thus, under the District of Columbia statute, no matter how serious the act committed by the acquittee, he may be released within 50 days of his acquittal if he has recovered. In contrast, one who committed a less

---

17. A defendant could be required to prove his insanity by a higher standard than a preponderance of the evidence. See *Leland v. Oregon*, 343 U.S. 790, 799, 72 S.Ct. 1002, 1007, 96 L.Ed. 1302 (1952). Such an additional requirement hardly would benefit a criminal defendant who wants to raise the insanity defense, yet imposition of a higher standard would be a likely legislative response to a holding that an insanity acquittal could support automatic commitment only if the verdict were supported by clear and convincing evidence.

serious act may be confined for a longer period if he remains ill and dangerous. There simply is no necessary correlation between severity of the offense and length of time necessary for recovery. The length of the acquittee's hypothetical criminal sentence therefore is irrelevant to the purposes of his commitment.

IV

We hold that when a criminal defendant establishes by a preponderance of the evidence that he is not guilty of a crime by reason of insanity, the Constitution permits the Government, on the basis of the insanity judgment, to confine him to a mental institution until such time as he has regained his sanity or is no longer a danger to himself or society. This holding accords with the widely and reasonably held view that insanity acquittees constitute a special class that should be treated differently from other candidates for commitment.

*   *   *

JUSTICE BRENNAN, with whom JUSTICE MARSHALL and JUSTICE BLACKMUN join, dissenting.

*   *   *

1. Our precedents in other commitment contexts are inconsistent with the argument that the mere facts of past criminal behavior and mental illness justify indefinite commitment without the benefits of the minimum due process standards associated with civil commitment, most importantly proof of present mental illness and dangerousness by clear and convincing evidence. In *Addington* itself, the petitioner did not dispute that he had engaged in a wide variety of assaultive conduct that could have been the basis for criminal charges had the State chosen to prosecute him. Similarly, the petitioner in *Jackson v. Indiana*, 406 U.S. 715, 92 S.Ct. 1845, 32 L.Ed.2d 435 (1972), had been charged with two robberies, yet we required the State to follow its civil commitment procedures if it wished to commit him for more than a strictly limited period. As the Court indicates, these cases are perhaps distinguishable on the ground that there was never proof that a *crime* had been committed, although in *Addington* the petitioner's violent acts were before the jury. That objection, however, cannot be leveled at *Baxstrom v. Herold*, 383 U.S. 107, 86 S.Ct. 760, 15 L.Ed.2d 620 (1966), or *Humphrey v. Cady, supra.*

The petitioner in *Baxstrom* had been convicted of assault and sentenced to a term in prison, during which he was certified as insane by a prison physician. At the expiration of his criminal sentence, he was committed involuntarily to a state mental hospital under procedures substantially less protective than those used for civil commitment. We held that, once he had served his sentence, Baxstrom could not be treated differently from other candidates for civil commitment. The principal difference between this case and *Baxstrom* is petitioner's admission, intrinsic to an insanity plea in the District of Columbia at the time of his trial, that his crime was "the product" of his mental illness. *Humphrey,* however, indicates the limited importance of that distinction.

In *Humphrey,* the petitioner had been convicted of contributing to the delinquency of a minor, the court had determined that his crime was "probably directly motivated by a desire for sexual excitement," and the State had established his "need" for psychiatric treatment by a preponderance of the evidence at a special hearing. He was committed for treatment for the maximum period for which he could have been incarcerated as punishment for his crime—as in this case, one year—and at the end of that period his commitment was renewed for five more years after a judicial hearing on his present mental illness and dangerousness. Thus, the situation was almost precisely identical to that in this case after petitioner's February 1977 hearing—the defendant had been found to have committed a criminal act beyond a reasonable doubt, a connection between that act and a mental disorder had been established by a preponderance of the evidence, and he had been confined for longer than the maximum sentence he could have received. If anything, Humphrey had received *more* protections than Michael Jones; the State had borne the burden of proof by a preponderance of the evidence at his "release hearing," *ibid.,* and his recommitment was for a strictly limited time. Nevertheless, we held that Humphrey's constitutional challenge to the renewal order had substantial merit, because Humphrey had not received the procedural protections given persons subject to civil commitment.

2. The Government's interests in committing petitioner are the same interests involved in *Addington, O'Connor, Baxstrom,* and *Humphrey* —isolation, protection, and treatment of a person who may, through no fault of his own, cause harm to others or to himself. Whenever involuntary commitment is a possibility, the Government has a strong interest in accurate, efficient commitment decisions. Nevertheless, *Addington* held both that the government's interest in accuracy was not impaired by a requirement that it bear the burden of persuasion by clear and convincing evidence, and that the individual's interests in liberty and autonomy required the government to bear at least that burden. An acquittal by reason of insanity of a single, nonviolent misdemeanor is not a constitutionally adequate substitute for the due process protections of *Addington* and *O'Connor, i.e.,* proof by clear and convincing evidence of present mental illness or dangerousness, with the government bearing the burden of persuasion.

* * *

Close reading of the Court's opinion reveals the utter emptiness of the legislative judgment it finds so unproblematic. Today's decision may overrule *Humphrey* by implication. It does not, however, purport to overrule *Baxstrom* or any of the cases which have followed *Baxstrom.* It is clear, therefore, that the separate facts of criminality and mental illness cannot support indefinite psychiatric commitment, for both were present in *Baxstrom.* The Court's careful phrasing indicates as much:

"someone *whose mental illness was sufficient to lead him to commit a criminal act* is likely to remain ill and in need of treatment." The Court relies on a *connection* between mental condition and criminal conduct that is unique to verdicts of "not guilty by reason of insanity." Yet the relevance of that connection, as opposed to each of its separate components, is far from a matter of obvious "common sense." None of the available evidence that criminal behavior by the mentally ill is likely to repeat itself distinguishes between behaviors that were "the product" of mental illness and those that were not. It is completely unlikely that persons acquitted by reason of insanity display a rate of future "dangerous" activity higher than civil committees with similar arrest records, or than persons convicted of crimes who are later found to be mentally ill. The causal connection between mental condition and criminal behavior that "not guilty by reason of insanity" formulations universally include is more a social judgment than a sound basis for determining dangerousness.

Given the close similarity of the governmental interests at issue in this case and those at issue in *Addington,* and the highly imperfect "fit" between the findings required for an insanity acquittal and those required under *O'Connor* to support an indefinite commitment, I cannot agree that the Government should be excused from the burden that *Addington* held was required by due process.[16]

Questions and Comments

1. *"Automatic" commitment.* In parts III(A) and III(B) of its opinion in *Jones,* the Supreme Court focused primarily on the constitutionality of "automatically" committing persons acquitted by reason of insanity. The Court sanctioned confinement without a hearing for at least 50 days when a criminal adjudication establishes beyond a reasonable doubt that the defendant has committed a criminal act and by a preponderance of the evidence that the defendant was insane at the time of the act. Does the Court's reasoning in Part III(B) of the opinion sanction automatic commitment in jurisdictions which allow an insanity verdict based on a reasonable doubt about sanity?[t] Even if it does not, could resort to automatic commitment in such jurisdictions be supported by analogizing to emergency

---

16. Note that extended institutionalization may effectively make it impossible for an individual to prove that he is no longer mentally ill and dangerous, both because it deprives him of the economic wherewithal to obtain independent medical judgments and because the treatment he receives may make it difficult to demonstrate recovery. The current emphasis on using psychotropic drugs to eliminate the characteristic signs and symptoms of mental illness, especially schizophrenia, may render mental patients docile and unlikely to engage in violent or bizarre behaviors while they are institutionalized, but it does not "cure" them or allow them to demonstrate that they would remain nonviolent if they were not drugged. See American Psychiatric Assn., Statement on the Insanity Defense 15–16 (1982). At petitioner's May 1976 hearing, the Government relied on testimony that petitioner was "not always responsive in a positive way to what goes on" and was "not a very active participant in the informal activities on the Ward" to support its contention that he had not recovered. The amount of medication he was receiving, however, made it unlikely he could be an active participant in anything.

t. About 15 states require the state to prove sanity beyond a reasonable doubt. See pp. 502–504.

commitment in the civil commitment context, which is normally permitted on a showing well below the preponderance level?

Of course, even if only minimal proof of mental disability and dangerousness is sufficient for automatic commitment, one might question the Court's conclusion that the evidence adduced at a criminal trial (or, as in *Jones,* pursuant to a plea bargain) meets this standard. At most, all that is proven at such proceedings is that, at some time in the past, the defendant committed an antisocial act while insane. Do you agree with the Court's reasoning in Part III(A) that this finding is sufficient to support an "automatic" finding of present mental illness and dangerousness?

2. *Timing of hearing.* In holding that automatic commitment is permissible, *Jones* stated: "Because a hearing is provided within 50 days of the commitment, there is assurance that every acquittee has prompt opportunity to obtain release if he has recovered." Does the opinion *require* a "prompt" hearing (within 50 days) for the acquittee who has been automatically committed?

3. *Burden and standard of proof at the commitment hearing.* While *Jones* can be construed to require a hearing at some point after automatic commitment, it probably also sanctions the type of hearing authorized by the District of Columbia, which places the burden of proof on the acquittee by a preponderance of the evidence. See Ellis, "The Consequences of the Insanity Defense: Proposals to Reform Post–Acquittal Commitment Law," 35 Cath.U.L.Rev. 961, 972 (1986). Whether or not *Jones* so holds, a large number of states, as well as the District of Columbia, continue to place the burden of proof on the acquittee at the commitment hearing; some even require the acquittee to produce *clear and convincing* proof of noncommittability.[u] Of those that place the burden on the state, many require merely a preponderance of the evidence showing. See S. Brakel, J. Parry & B. Weiner, The Mentally Disabled and the Law 786–795 (1985) (chart). Obviously, all of these statutes would be unconstitutional in the civil commitment context, given *Addington.* On what grounds might they be upheld in the post-insanity acquittal context? Several possibilities exist.

Risk of Error Analysis. First, consider again the reasoning in Part III(B) of *Jones* finding that such statutes are constitutional because there is "good reason for diminished concern as to the risk of error." By the time of the review hearing, is it still plausible to say that the risk of error on the issue of present mental disability and dangerousness is sufficiently diminished by proof at trial of insanity and a criminal act to differentiate this situation from civil commitment?

The Public Safety Rationale. Most courts justify placing more of an evidentiary burden on insanity acquittees than on others subject to commitment on a different ground—that insanity acquittees, as a class, are more dangerous than other groups. See, e.g., *People v. Chavez,* 629 P.2d 1040, 1047–8 (Colo.1981). There is no doubt that insanity acquittees are more likely to have committed serious antisocial behavior than persons who are subjected to civil commitment. But one study has suggested that this fact

---

u. The federal Insanity Defense Reform Act of 1984 requires those acquitted of "violent" crimes to prove noncommittability by clear and convincing evidence. 18 U.S.C. § 4243(d).

does not correlate with a greater likelihood of recidivism. See Note, "Commitment and Release of Persons Found Not Guilty by Reason of Insanity: A Georgia Perspective," 15 Ga.L.Rev. 1065, 1079 (1981). At the least, shouldn't those acquittees charged with "minor" crimes (akin to the type of act which might also trigger civil commitment) be treated the same as those subjected to civil commitment? See American Bar Association Criminal Justice Mental Health Standard 7–7.3(b). Or does the fact that acquittees have been charged with crime, albeit minor, make them different?

More fundamentally, even if one is willing to assume that insanity acquittees are more dangerous than others, is adjustment of the burden and standard of proof the proper response? If the legal system wants to recognize formally the perception that acquittees are a greater threat to public safety, an alternative might be to adopt a presumption to that effect. Such a presumption would require the acquittee to come forward with some evidence of nondangerousness (i.e. carry the burden of production), but leave the ultimate burden of proof (i.e., the burden of persuasion) on the government by whatever standard of proof is considered appropriate (e.g., by clear and convincing evidence or a preponderance of the evidence). The threshold for adopting a presumption is that it must rest on an established probability. In addition, in order to deter any tendency to rely on presumptions for proving *all* probable facts, some other reason for the presumption is usually required, such as the difficulty of proving the issue, the opponent's superior access to evidence relating to the issue, or the desire to promote a special policy. McCormick, Handbook of the Law of Evidence § 348, at 806–07 (3d. ed. 1982). Would a presumption of dangerousness for insanity acquittees be proper? A presumption of mental illness?

The Lack of Autonomy Rationale. Another argument against applying *Addington* to commitment of insanity acquittees, at least those charged with violent crime, is advanced by Ingber in "Rules for An Exceptional Class: The Commitment and Release of Persons Acquitted of Violent Offenses by Reason on Insanity," 57 N.Y.U.L.Rev. 281, 301–02, 309 (1982). Ingber notes that one reason for limiting exercise of the police power in the civil commitment context is the societal interest in fostering autonomy. But, he contends, the insanity acquittee, unlike the person subjected to civil commitment, has been found deficient as an autonomous human being. Therefore the acquittee charged with a violent crime may be committed under a lower standard of proof.

> In a civil hearing, the state's interest in the safety of its citizens is partly offset by its interest in promoting autonomy; not so in a violent acquittee's commitment hearing. Thus, the state has a greater net interest in favor of a lower standard of proof in the latter hearing. In a word, it has no reason to be concerned about the effects such a standard will have on the autonomy of persons at large in society. The greater net state interest in a lower standard supports a reduction of the standard to a preponderance of the evidence.

Is this reasoning persuasive? Would it support not only reducing the standard of proof but shifting the burden of proof to the defendant?

The Clean-up Doctrine. Finally, consider the strength of what has been called the "clean-up doctrine", see Note, "Commitment Following an Insanity Acquittal," 94 Harv.L.Rev. 605, 617 (1981), as support for placing a heavier burden on insanity acquittees than on those subjected to civil commitment.

> If an insanity acquittee is wrongly committed, so the argument goes, he was probably sane at trial and therefore wrongly acquitted of the crime in the first place. 'While the acquittee therefore may be deprived erroneously of his liberty in the *commitment* process, the liberty he loses is likely to be liberty which society mistakenly had permitted him to retain in the *criminal* process.'

Id. at 618 (emphasis in original).

4. *Commitment criteria.* How closely should the criteria for post-insanity acquittal commitment track the criteria for civil commitment? The same considerations that govern the choice of the burden and standard of proof are influential here as well. Generally, although the language of commitment statutes for insanity acquittees tends to be similar, if not identical, to that found in civil commitment statutes, it is often construed or applied so as to make release more difficult for the insanity acquittee.

The Supreme Court in *Jones* does not make definitive statements about the proper commitment criteria for insanity acquittees, but its position can be gleaned from the opinion. In summarizing its holding, the Court stated that an acquittee who is found insane by a preponderance of the evidence may be confined to a mental institution "until such time as he has regained his sanity or is no longer a danger to himself or society." Several aspects of the quoted portion of this statement are noteworthy (although they may be dicta given the facts of *Jones*).

First, the Court's language would appear to permit release of acquittees who show either that they are no longer "insane" *or* that they are no longer dangerous. This language is taken from judicial interpretation of the District of Columbia statute at issue in *Jones*. See *Jones*, n. 3. Other courts, however, have upheld release provisions that require the absence of *both* mental illness and dangerousness. For instance, finding that the legislature "did not intend to [apply] the civil-commitment standards," the Supreme Court of Wisconsin held that continued commitment of an acquittee is permissible upon proof of dangerousness alone; no proof of mental illness is necessary. *State v. Gebarski*, 90 Wis.2d 754, 280 N.W.2d 672 (1979). See also, *Harris v. Ballone*, 681 F.2d 225 (4th Cir.1982). As noted at the outset of this chapter, prolonged "pure" preventive detention (i.e., detention based solely on a finding of dangerousness) has traditionally been permitted only in the most extreme circumstances. Do insanity acquittees fit within this category?

Two other aspects of the Court's summary statement allude to the content of the commitment criteria. First, the statement, and indeed the entire opinion, refers to recovery and proof of "sanity" rather than mental illness or mental disability. Should this usage be read to mean that the definition of mental disability for purposes of post-insanity acquittal commitment must be tied to the mental disease or defect requirement of the insanity defense? Or should it be defined as it is under civil commitment statutes? Note that the former definition is narrower and thus would make it easier for the acquittee to win release.[v]

The Court also speaks of "danger to self" as a commitment criterion. Should an insanity acquittee be committable under the special commitment provisions discussed above solely on the ground that he or she is mentally disabled and suicidal or gravely disabled? In other words, should parens patriae commitment be permissible other than through normal commitment standards and procedures?

Finally, in other portions of *Jones* the Court gives some clues as to how it would define danger to others in the post-acquittal context. In note 14, for instance, it asserts that crimes against property should be included within the definition of dangerous acts. In some jurisdictions, danger to property is not a ground for civil commitment. Would adopting the Court's interpretation of the dangerousness for commitment of insanity acquittees be permissible in such jurisdictions? Lower courts have also held that a showing of imminence is not required in order to commit insanity acquittees. See, e.g., *Hill v. State,* 358 So.2d 190 (Fla.App.1978). Is this warranted?

5. *Procedures.* The only procedural aspect of the post-acquittal commitment hearing addressed by *Jones* was the right to jury trial. In a footnote, the Court stated:

> The District of Columbia provides for a jury at civil-commitment hearings, . . . and petitioner contends that equal protection requires that insanity acquittees also be permitted to demand a jury at the 50–day hearing. Because we determine that an acquittee's commitment is based on the judgment of insanity at the criminal trial, rather than solely on the findings at the 50–day hearing, . . . the relevant equal protection comparison concerns the procedures available at the criminal trial and at a civil-commitment hearing. We therefore agree with the Court of Appeals that the absence of a jury at the 50–day hearing 'is justified by the fact that the acquittee has had a right to a jury determination of his sanity at the time of the offense.'

463 U.S. at 362 n. 10, 103 S.Ct. at 3048 n. 10. Would the Court's analysis justify denying an acquittee counsel or other rights normally associated with civil commitment? Switching from equal protection analysis to a due process perspective, recall that two principal reasons given by the Supreme Court for relaxing procedures in the civil commitment context are the medical nature of the issues involved and the need to avoid procedures which will deter friends and families from seeking treatment. See *Addington,* supra; *Parham v. J.R.* Are these concerns present in the post-insanity acquittal context? What other state interests should be weighed in the balance in deciding how much process is due?

6. *Duration of commitment.* Despite the Supreme Court's holding in *Jones,* several commentators have argued, and several state statutes provide, that commitment of acquittees be limited to the maximum sentence the acquittee would have received had he or she been found responsible for the

---

v. See pp. 511–512 for a discussion of the mental disease or defect requirement in insanity cases.

crime charged. One rationale for such a rule is that commitment of insanity acquittees is, contrary to the Court's assertion, punitive and thus should be limited by the relevant criminal sentence. Three judges of the District of Columbia Court of Appeals panel in the *Jones* case reasoned as follows:

> [A]cquittees are not confined to mental institutions for medical reasons alone. They are confined there in part because society is unwilling to allow those who have committed crimes to escape without paying for their crimes. The intent of the statute is partially punitive, and thus the [stricter procedures governing commitment and release of acquittees] reflect this added burden on the defendant. Because of this punitive purpose, the maximum statutory period of confinement becomes relevant, for at that point society no longer has a valid interest in continued confinement on the basis of a shortcut procedure.

Consider also this alternative critique of this aspect of *Jones*, from Ellis, supra at 981–82:

> The majority's analysis attempts to answer the wrong question. The issue is not how long Jones could be lawfully committed, but rather how long he could be confined under procedures different from those employed for general commitment patients. The Court is correct in stating that treatment needs should be a determining factor in ascertaining the appropriate length of commitment. But the duration of the applicability of special commitment procedures should be set independently by principles of fairness and equality. Those principles require that special commitment be limited to the period of time during which the individual could have been confined had he been convicted.
>
> *   *   *
>
> . . . The state interest occasioned by attempted petit larceny is finite and measured by the maximum sentence; it does not increase when the offender proves to be mentally disabled. Any greater interest in confining the disabled offender must arise from his disability rather than his offense. Confining an acquittee for a longer period than the maximum sentence for his crime can only be justified by his continuing treatment or habilitation needs, and at that point, the fact of his offense becomes irrelevant. Therefore, there is no justification for treating him differently than general commitment patients who have a continuing treatment or habilitation need. Thus general commitment procedures should be the only means of extending such a commitment.

In practice, insanity acquittees tend to spend about the same amount of time in the hospital as do convicted persons charged with similar crimes, although the time periods vary from state to state. Once released, insanity acquittees are no less likely to recidivate than released felons who were charged with similar offenses. Indeed, most research indicates a lower rate of recidivism for insanity acquittees. See, e.g., Pasewark, Pantle & Steadman, "Detention and Rearrest Rates of People Found Not Guilty by Reason of Insanity," 139 Am.J.Psychiat. 893 (1982).

7. *The Oregon review board.* As with civil commitment, perhaps more important than the various standards and procedures accompanying post-acquittal commitment are the systemic measures established for handling

insanity acquittees who are determined to be mentally ill and dangerous. In 1977, the Oregon legislature enacted legislation setting up an innovative approach toward this problem. Or.Rev.Stat. §§ 161.327 to 161.336. Its most significant innovation was to shift responsibility for committed acquittees from the trial court to a Psychiatric Security Review Board (PSRB), on the theory that courts lack the staff, expertise and motivation to assure adequate treatment and monitoring of acquittees. The PSRB consists of five members, usually a psychiatrist, a psychologist, a person with expertise in parole and probation matters, a criminal trial lawyer, and a member of the general public. It has jurisdiction over all committed acquittees for the term of the maximum sentence they would have received had there been a conviction. It has authority to arrange treatment in many different types of programs, and leans heavily on conditional release arrangements. Any acquittee dissatisfied with the Board's disposition of his or her case may appeal to the courts. During the first five years of its operation, 6% of the 295 people conditionally released under the PSRB's authority were arrested for felony charges. Rogers, Bloom, & Mason, "After Oregon's Insanity Defense: A Comparison of Conditional Release and Hospitalization," 5 Int'l J.L. & Psychiat. 391, 398 (1982).

B. PRISON AND JAIL INMATES

Of those mentally disordered individuals who are processed through the criminal justice system, far fewer than one percent are acquitted by reason of insanity. Only a slightly larger proportion are sentenced under the types of special sentencing provisions discussed in Chapter Seven, such as those which establish indeterminate sentences and separate treatment facilities for persons found to be "mentally disordered sex offenders." The vast majority of mentally disordered persons who are charged with crime and not diverted out of the system prior to adjudication are convicted and sentenced to jail or prison. It has been estimated that roughly 14% of all convicted felons may be psychotic, that anywhere from 9.5% to 29% are mentally retarded, and that perhaps another 35% have character disorders. S. Brakel, J. Parry, B. Weiner, The Mentally Disabled and the Law 736–37 (1985). At some point during their sentence, many of these people need treatment that cannot be provided in jail or prison. Until 1980, in most states these people could be transferred to a mental health facility (either within the correctional system or within the mental health system) on the sayso of a mental health professional. That has now changed.

VITEK v. JONES

Supreme Court of the United States, 1980.
445 U.S. 480, 100 S.Ct. 1254, 63 L.Ed.2d 552.

MR. JUSTICE WHITE delivered the opinion of the Court, except as to Part IV–B.

The question in this case is whether the Due Process Clause of the Fourteenth Amendment entitles a prisoner convicted and incarcerated in the State of Nebraska to certain procedural protections, including notice, an adversary hearing, and provision of counsel, before he is transferred involuntarily to a state mental hospital for treatment of a mental disease or defect.

I

Nebraska Rev.Stat. § 83–176(2) (1976) authorizes the Director of Correctional Services to designate any available, suitable, and appropriate residence facility or institution as a place of confinement for any state prisoner and to transfer a prisoner from one place of confinement to another. Section 83–180(1), however, provides that when a designated physician or psychologist finds that a prisoner "suffers from a mental disease or defect" and "cannot be given proper treatment in that facility," the director may transfer him for examination, study, and treatment to another institution within or without the Department of Correctional Services. Any prisoner so transferred to a mental hospital is to be returned to the Department if, prior to the expiration of his sentence, treatment is no longer necessary. Upon expiration of sentence, if the State desires to retain the prisoner in a mental hospital, civil commitment proceedings must be promptly commenced. § 83–180(3).

On May 31, 1974, Jones was convicted of robbery and sentenced to a term of three to nine years in state prison. He was transferred to the penitentiary hospital in January 1975. Two days later he was placed in solitary confinement, where he set his mattress on fire, burning himself severely. He was treated in the burn unit of a private hospital. Upon his release and based on findings required by § 83–180 that he was suffering from a mental illness or defect and could not receive proper treatment in the penal complex, he was transferred to the security unit of the Lincoln Regional Center, a state mental hospital under the jurisdiction of the Department of Public Institutions.

Jones challeng[es] on procedural due process grounds the adequacy of the procedures by which the Nebraska statutes permit transfers from the prison complex to a mental hospital.

* * *

III

On the merits, the threshold question in this case is whether the involuntary transfer of a Nebraska state prisoner to a mental hospital implicates a liberty interest that is protected by the Due Process Clause.

* * *

Undoubtedly, a valid criminal conviction and prison sentence extinguish a defendant's right to freedom from confinement. Such a conviction and sentence sufficiently extinguish a defendant's liberty "to empower the State to confine him in any of its prisons." *Meachum v. Fano,* 427 U.S., at 224, 96 S.Ct., at 2538 (emphasis deleted). It is also true that changes in the conditions of confinement having a substantial adverse impact on the prisoner are not alone sufficient to invoke the protections of the Due Process Clause "[a]s long as the conditions or degree of confinement to which the prisoner is subjected is within the sentence imposed upon him."

Appellants maintain that the transfer of a prisoner to a mental hospital is within the range of confinement justified by imposition of a prison sentence, at least after certification by a qualified person that a prisoner suffers from a mental disease or defect. We cannot agree. None of our decisions holds that conviction for a crime entitles a State not only to confine the convicted person but also to determine that he has a mental illness and to subject him involuntarily to institutional care in a mental hospital. Such consequences visited on the prisoner are qualitatively different from the punishment characteristically suffered by a person convicted of crime. Our cases recognize as much and reflect an understanding that involuntary commitment to a mental hospital is not within the range of conditions of confinement to which a prison sentence subjects an individual. *Baxstrom v. Herold,* 383 U.S. 107, 86 S.Ct. 760, 15 L.Ed.2d 620 (1966); *Specht v. Patterson,* 386 U.S. 605, 87 S.Ct. 1209, 18 L.Ed.2d 326 (1967); *Humphrey v. Cady,* 405 U.S. 504, 92 S.Ct. 1048, 31 L.Ed.2d 394 (1972); *Jackson v. Indiana,* 406 U.S. 715, 724, 725, 92 S.Ct. 1845, 1851, 32 L.Ed.2d 435 (1972). A criminal conviction and sentence of imprisonment extinguish an individual's right to freedom from confinement for the term of his sentence, but they do not authorize the State to classify him as mentally ill and to subject him to involuntary psychiatric treatment without affording him additional due process protections.

In light of the findings made by the District Court, Jones' involuntary transfer to the Lincoln Regional Center pursuant to § 83–180, for the purpose of psychiatric treatment, implicated a liberty interest protected by the Due Process Clause. Many of the restrictions on the prisoner's freedom of action at the Lincoln Regional Center by themselves might not constitute the deprivation of a liberty interest retained by a prisoner. But here, the stigmatizing consequences of a transfer to a mental hospital for involuntary psychiatric treatment, coupled with the subjection of the prisoner to mandatory behavior modification as a treatment for mental illness, constitute the kind of deprivations of liberty that requires procedural protections.

IV

The District Court held that to afford sufficient protection to the liberty interest it had identified, the State was required to observe the following minimum procedures before transferring a prisoner to a mental hospital:

"A. Written notice to the prisoner that a transfer to a mental hospital is being considered;

"B. A hearing, sufficiently after the notice to permit the prisoner to prepare, at which disclosure to the prisoner is made of the evidence being relied upon for the transfer and at which an opportunity to be heard in person and to present documentary evidence is given;

"C. An opportunity at the hearing to present testimony of witnesses by the defense and to confront and cross-examine witnesses called by the state, except upon a finding, not arbitrarily made, of good cause for not permitting such presentation, confrontation, or cross-examination;

"D. An independent decisionmaker;

"E. A written statement by the fact-finder as to the evidence relied on and the reasons for transferring the inmate;

"F. Availability of legal counsel, furnished by the state, if the inmate is financially unable to furnish his own; and

"G. Effective and timely notice of all the foregoing rights."

A

We think the District Court properly identified and weighed the relevant factors in arriving at its judgment. Concededly the interest of the State in segregating and treating mentally ill patients is strong. The interest of the prisoner in not being arbitrarily classified as mentally ill and subjected to unwelcome treatment is also powerful, however; and as the District Court found, the risk of error in making the determinations required by § 83–180 is substantial enough to warrant appropriate procedural safeguards against error.

We recognize that the inquiry involved in determining whether or not to transfer an inmate to a mental hospital for treatment involves a question that is essentially medical. The question whether an individual is mentally ill and cannot be treated in prison "turns on the meaning of the facts which must be interpreted by expert psychiatrists and psychologists." *Addington v. Texas,* 441 U.S., at 429, 99 S.Ct., at 1811. The medical nature of the inquiry, however, does not justify dispensing with due process requirements. It is precisely "[t]he subtleties and nuances of psychiatric diagnoses" that justify the requirement of adversary hearings.

Because prisoners facing involuntary transfer to a mental hospital are threatened with immediate deprivation of liberty interests they are currently enjoying and because of the inherent risk of a mistaken transfer, the District Court properly determined that procedures similar to those required by the Court in *Morrissey v. Brewer,* 408 U.S. 471, 92 S.Ct. 2593, 33 L.Ed.2d 484 (1972), were appropriate in the circumstances present here.

The notice requirement imposed by the District Court no more than recognizes that notice is essential to afford the prisoner an opportunity to challenge the contemplated action and to understand the nature of what is happening to him. Furthermore, in view of the nature of the determinations that must accompany the transfer to a mental hospital, we think each of the elements of the hearing specified by the District Court was appropriate. The interests of the State in avoiding disruption was recognized by limiting in appropriate circumstances the prisoner's right to call witnesses, to confront and cross examine. The District Court also avoided unnecessary intrusion into either medical or correctional judgments by providing that the independent decisionmaker conducting the transfer hearing need not come from outside the prison or hospital administration.

B

The District Court did go beyond the requirements imposed by prior cases by holding that counsel must be made available to inmates facing transfer hearings if they are financially unable to furnish their own. We have not required the automatic appointment of counsel for indigent prisoners facing other deprivations of liberty, *Gagnon v. Scarpelli*, 411 U.S., at 790, 93 S.Ct., at 1763; but we have recognized that prisoners who are illiterate and uneducated have a greater need for assistance in exercising their rights. *Gagnon v. Scarpelli, supra*, at 786–787, 93 S.Ct., at 1761–1762. A prisoner thought to be suffering from a mental disease or defect requiring involuntary treatment probably has an even greater need for legal assistance, for such a prisoner is more likely to be unable to understand or exercise his rights. In these circumstances, it is appropriate that counsel be provided to indigent prisoners whom the State seeks to treat as mentally ill.

V

Because Mr. Justice Powell, while believing that Jones was entitled to competent help at the hearing, would not require the State to furnish a licensed attorney to aid him, the judgment below is affirmed as modified to conform with the separate opinion filed by Mr. Justice Powell.

So ordered.

[On the right to counsel issue, Mr. Justice Powell's concurring opinion, reprinted at pp. 724–725, found that due process requires only "a qualified and independent advisor" who "may be . . . a licensed psychiatrist or other mental health professional." The remaining four members of the Court dissented on the ground that the case was moot.]

Questions and Comments

1. *Comparison to civil commitment.* Although *Vitek* clearly held that something more than a diagnosis from a mental health professional is necessary before a prison-to-hospital transfer may take place, it just as clearly does not require as much process as most states provide those subject to civil commitment.[w] Prior to *Vitek* some lower courts held that the equal protection clause required civil commitment procedures prior to such transfers. In *United States ex rel. Schuster v. Herold*, 410 F.2d 1071 (2d Cir.), cert. denied 396 U.S. 847, 90 S.Ct. 81, 24 L.Ed.2d 96 (1969), for instance, the court held that the prison inmate subjected to a transfer should be accorded "substantially the same procedures . . . as are granted

---

w. Note that the Supreme Court has yet to indicate whether civil commitment requires anything more in the way of pro- cedural formality than it provides prisoners subject to hospital transfers.

to civilians when they are involuntarily committed to a mental hospital." Id. at 1084. Accord, *Matthews v. Hardy*, 420 F.2d 607 (D.C.Cir.1969), cert. denied 397 U.S. 1010, 90 S.Ct. 1231, 25 L.Ed.2d 423 (1970). The *Schuster* court based its decision primarily on the Supreme Court's decision in *Baxstrom v. Herold*, 383 U.S. 107, 86 S.Ct. 760, 15 L.Ed.2d 620 (1966). It will be recalled that *Baxstrom* held unconstitutional, under the equal protection clause, a New York law providing a relatively informal commitment process for prisoners who were on the verge of completing their prison term; the Court reasoned that prisoners who have served their terms are similarly situated to persons subjected to civil commitment and therefore may only be committed pursuant to normal civil commitment procedures. If raised by the petitioner in *Vitek*, should *Baxstrom* and equal protection analysis have governed the decision, as *Schuster* suggests?

Instead of equal protection analysis, the Court relied on *Morrissey v. Brewer* and *Gagnon v. Scarpelli*, which dealt with the procedures necessary to revoke probation and parole under the due process clause. Recall that traditional due process analysis, under *Mathews v. Eldridge*, 424 U.S. 319, 96 S.Ct. 893, 47 L.Ed.2d 18 (1976), requires balancing (1) the significance of the private interest to be adjudicated under the procedures at issue; (2) the risk of an erroneous deprivation under the procedures; and (3) the government's interest in maintaining them. In *Vitek*, the Court identified two private interests affected by transfer: the stigma associated with being labelled mentally disordered and the possibility of compelled treatment. There are at least two other possible drawbacks to transfer: the "strong likelihood that an inmate transferred to a mental health facility will be paroled later than a like inmate who remained in the correctional facility" (given "that most parole authorities would be wary of releasing a person from a mental health facility directly to the community"), and the possibility that transferees will be denied good-time credits for the time they are in the hospital. Churgin, The Transfer of Inmates to Mental Health Facilities," in Monahan & Steadman, eds., Mentally Disordered Offenders 220 (1983). Are these factors enough to make prison-to-hospital transfers equivalent to the deprivation of liberty associated with civil commitment? Are there any relevant differences between transfers and commitment with respect to the second and third prongs of the *Mathews v. Eldridge* analysis?

2. *Pre-trial detainees.* A separate transfer issue arises in the context of pretrial detention. Of the six million or so people who pass through the jails each year, "it is estimated that 600,000 of them are seriously mentally ill." S. Brakel, J. Parry, B. Weiner, The Mentally Disabled and the Law 736 (1985). Although some of these people have been convicted and sentenced to serve time in jail, most are there because they have been unable to make bail and thus are confined pending trial or some other proceeding. Of this latter group, many will eventually be evaluated for and found incompetent to stand trial, a procedure explored in Chapter Nine. But a large number are not found incompetent, yet need treatment that cannot be provided in jail. See Steadman, McCarty & Morrissey, The Mentally Ill in Jail: Planning for Essential Services (1989). Should *Vitek* apply to these people? Or is civil commitment the proper route? If the latter, should commitment *criteria* as well as procedures be applicable?

3. *Hospital-to-prison transfers.* Usually a person transferred to a mental health facility will eventually be returned to the prison.[x] Sometimes, this retransfer may be premature (if, for example, the hospital believes the person is a "troublemaker"). Is such a person entitled to a hearing to review the hospital's decision? At least two courts have considered this issue; they reached opposite results. *Burchett v. Bower,* 355 F.Supp. 1278 (D.Ariz.1973) (yes); *Cruz v. Ward,* 558 F.2d 658 (2d Cir.1977) (no).

If such a hearing is held, what criteria should apply? Perhaps of relevance here is *Bowring v. Godwin,* 551 F.2d 44 (4th Cir.1977), which found a right to psychiatric treatment for prisoners, but only when that treatment is a "medical necessity":

> [A prisoner] is entitled to psychological or psychiatric treatment if a physician or other health care provider, exercising ordinary skill and care at the time of observation, concludes with reasonable medical certainty (1) that the prisoner's symptoms evidence a serious disease or injury; (2) that such disease or injury is curable or may be substantially alleviated; and (3) that the potential for harm to the prisoner by reason of delay or the denial of care would be substantial.

Cf. *Estelle v. Gamble,* 429 U.S. 97, 97 S.Ct. 285, 50 L.Ed.2d 251 (1976) (holding that the eighth amendment obligates the government to provide medical care for prisoners, but only to the extent necessary to avoid "deliberate indifference to serious medical needs of prisoners.")

C. CHEMICALLY DEPENDENT PERSONS

SAMUEL BRAKEL, JOHN PARRY AND BARBARA WEINER, THE MENTALLY DISABLED AND THE LAW

(Chicago: American Bar Foundation, 1985).
pp. 41–43.

About two-thirds (32) of the states have special statutes for the commitment of alcoholic persons. Slightly fewer (29) have procedures for institutionalizing persons addicted to drugs. These are civil commitment statutes. A minority of states—9 in the case of alcoholics, 16 for drug addicts—also have separate statutes providing for the mental health processing of chemical substance addicts who have been charged with or convicted of a crime. . . . It should not be supposed that states without special provisions lack the power to commit persons with drug or alcohol dependency or that they do in fact refrain from institutionalizing such persons. The traditional interpretation of the mentally ill commitment laws is that they are broad enough to cover these groups. . . .

The statutory definitions of an alcoholic or drug-addicted person have undergone considerable modernization over the past 10 to 15 years, with substantial similarity in the language used in many states. Even among more varying formulations, one can often find at least the

---

x. No court has yet addressed whether transferees are entitled to periodic review. Presumably, at the least, hospitalization is limited by the length of the sentence.

traces of a common "standard" definition. The description of an alcoholic in the Colorado law contains most of the standard elements: "a person who habitually lacks self-control as to the use of alcoholic beverages or uses alcoholic beverages to the extent that his health is substantially impaired or endangered or his social or economic function is substantially disrupted." The reference to habit or chronicity of abuse is common to all formulations. The laws of a few states add or substitute language that emphasizes the threat of the individual's condition to others. In the Texas statute, for example, an alcoholic is someone who among other things "endangers public morals, health, safety or welfare." In Nevada, the perceived danger is to the "health, safety or welfare of [the alcoholic] himself or any other person or group of persons."

The definitions of committable drug addicts show more diversity. A few are phrased like the provisions covering alcoholics, substituting "narcotic drug" or "chemical substance" for "alcoholic beverages." Several states—Massachusetts is one—expressly exclude users of alcohol or tobacco from the definition of the drug addicted, but others are silent on this point. [A] state such as Hawaii employs one statutory definition for all "substance abuse." A person suffering from it is described as one who "uses narcotic, stimulant, depressant, or hallucinogenic drugs or alcohol to an extent which interferes with his personal, social, family, or economic life." The definitions in many states are quite lengthy, touching on the nature of the substance, the fact that its use is illegal or strictly circumscribed, the level and length of dependency, its psychic and behavioral effects, and the threat posed by the user to the community.

* * *

Nationally, in 1980–81, "alcohol disorders"—cases in which the primary diagnosis is alcoholism—accounted for 22% of the admissions to public (state and county) mental institutions, 9% of those to private mental hospitals, and 8% of those to general hospitals with psychiatric units. Combined, the proportion is 13%, some 136,000 out of the total of slightly more than one million mentally disordered persons admitted to the nation's inpatient facilities. One can only guess the number of cases in which alcoholism figures as a secondary or contributing factor toward institutionalization, though it is sure to be comparably high if not higher. The total number of persons with alcohol disorders admitted to public mental institutions in 1981 was 71,864, while the number of resident alcoholic patients stood at 6,708, a comparatively low figure only because the comparatively short periods of hospitalization for alcoholics (11 days was the median in 1975) keep the in-residence totals from accumulating higher.

In 1952, drug addicts constituted less than 1% of all first admissions to state mental institutions and 0.1% of the resident population. By 1967 these figures had more than doubled, to 2.1% and 0.4%, respectively. The most recent figures (which comprise readmissions as well as first-time entries for 1981) are 5.0% and 2.0% —that is, 19,370 admissions for "drug disorders" and 1,879 in residence. These numbers pale in the light of the full incidence of drug abuse in this country. In 1965, the United States Bureau of Narcotics reported over 57,000 known active addicts. Today, with broader definitions and more "liberal" diagnosis to match increased abuse, the figures are staggering: the National Institute of Mental Health reports estimates of half a million heroin addicts alone; 10 million Americans are reported to have "tried" cocaine; 42 million have tried marijuana, with 16 million identified as "current users," among whom many of the heaviest users are adolescents of high school age. In addition, there are untold numbers of adults and teenagers who abuse barbiturates and other sedatives, tranquilizers, amphetamines and other stimulants, and hallucinogenic drugs.

Questions and Comments

1. *Police power commitment.* In *Robinson v. California,* 370 U.S. 660, 82 S.Ct. 1417, 8 L.Ed.2d 758 (1962), the Supreme Court held that drug and alcohol addiction per se may not be punished criminally because, among other things, addiction is not a voluntary act. But in *Powell v. Texas,* 392 U.S. 514, 88 S.Ct. 2145, 20 L.Ed.2d 1254 (1968), it made clear that if an addict commits any type of crime, even if it is being drunk in public, then he or she may be punished. Thus criminal sanctions continue to be society's primary response to addicts who commit antisocial acts. Brakel, et al., supra at 43.

Nonetheless, as the excerpt suggests, most states also authorize commitment of such addicts. Wexler has argued that such commitment is inappropriate, at least as applied to those addicted to narcotics (in particular heroin). He first contends that drug addicts are much less likely to commit *violent* crime than the general population, given the sense of well being that accompanies drug taking. Second, he argues that the fact that some addicts are relatively more likely to commit *property* offenses in order to finance their habits should not authorize their commitment on police power grounds:

> In addition to the offensiveness of committing people partially because they are poor (we would not be willing to commit nonaddict poor people simply on a showing that they were likely to steal), we are faced with the argument that
>
> > the virtual certainty that addicts will break the law is in a direct sense the state's own fault. An addict's need for narcotics is by definition beyond his control. By denying him legal access to narcotics, the state makes him *ipso facto* an habitual criminal. By obliging him to obtain his drugs at exorbitant black market prices, the same legislative policy also drives poor addicts inexorably to theft. It flouts fundamental fairness for the state to force a man to commit crimes and at the same time to punish or confine him on grounds of his resultant criminality.

Fundamental fairness or not, current law and practice permits the state *both* to punish and to commit because of the resultant criminality. . . .

One response to this problem, Wexler notes, is to establish drug maintenance programs (such as methadone treatments). If such programs were properly implemented, then neither the criminal law or preventive detention would be necessary, since addicts would not need to steal. However, if maintenance programs are not thought feasible or wise, the state should still be forced to rely on the criminal law rather than commitment for handling addicts. He explains: "Only if we had a sure-fire cure for addiction by brief confinement or by some miracle drug might we, by analogy to a quarantine, preventively detain to avoid rather minor offenses such as property crimes."

Wexler then recommends a hybrid sanction-control approach to the problem:

> Instead of preventive detention . . . we could devise an acceptable alternative: the criminal law process could be used to detect those addicts who commit or attempt property offenses and, by enabling them to elect treatment in lieu of punishment, could be used to encourage them to seek treatment for their addiction. . . . Proper completion of treatment should result in vitiating the criminal proceedings, but an uncooperative attitude toward therapy could result in a transfer to the criminal system, with, however, credit toward the criminal sentence for all time spent in the therapeutic process. Interestingly and perhaps significantly for this peno-therapeutic paradigm, a study of the federal Narcotic Addict Rehabilitation Act, which has provision both for pure civil commitment and for the election of treatment while criminal charges remain pending, found the success rate under the latter provision to exceed the success rate under the former, which, according to the authors of the study, suggests that external legal pressure to comply with the program is a factor in success.[y]

D. Wexler, Mental Health Law 37–39 (1981).

Do you agree with Wexler's analysis? Recall that the standard justifications for police power commitment of the mentally ill are that the mentally ill are either more dangerous, more treatable or less deterrable than the general population. Do addicts fit into any of these categories? If property theft by poverty-stricken addicts is the state's "fault", should either civil commitment *or* criminal sanction be permissible? Finally, does any of this apply to alcoholics?

2. *Parens patriae commitment.* Wexler also has doubts about the propriety of committing narcotics addicts under the parens patriae power.

> Drug addicts . . . are seldom classified as psychotic, and they ordinarily retain contact with reality. If addicts are to be considered incompetent, then, it must be because their overpowering compulsion to consume drugs prevents them from reaching a rational decision regard-

---

y. The civil provisions of the Narcotic Addict Rehabilitation Act of 1966 are dis- cussed at pp. 754–755 in the context of "voluntary" commitment [footnote by eds].

ing treatment. . . . But it is true, of course, that some addicts *do* decide to enter treatment, and that cuts against a blanket notion equating addiction with incompetence. One commentator has argued rather persuasively that addiction should not in itself establish incompetency.

> But if addicts have lost their powers of self-control, so have all chain smokers and compulsive gamblers. They have all lost control over a partial and clearly limited area of conduct, but not over conduct or decision-making capacity generally. They are unable to decide not to smoke or gamble, but they are as competent to decide to attempt a cure of their habit as to decide whether to undergo an operation or to come in out of the rain. Addiction, as a shorthand expression for compulsive psychological dependence, makes no man a ward of the state unless his weakness has some additional effects on his mental processes generally.

Wexler points out that the benefit the addict receives from commitment is also unclear. First, the addict may prefer his addicted state to confinement and indefinite supervision or even to his or her previous life prior to addiction. Second, there is "virtually no empirical data to support the claim that institutionalization in a drug-free environment followed by an intensive aftercare supervision offers even a fair chance of cure for the average narcotic addict." [z] Thus, "so long as the addict may be physically committed and subjected to the traditional abstinence approaches, the validity of the paternalistic intervention will remain questionable . . ." However, Wexler suggests, a court might be able to order *outpatient* commitment, perhaps to a maintenance program, "if the conceptual and empirical questions regarding the competency of addicts were resolved in the negative." Id. at 42–44.

How do you respond to this analysis? Does it have relevance for those addicted to alcohol?

D. THE DEVELOPMENTALLY DISABLED

The term "developmental disability" was not widely used until the 1970's. It is meant to designate a large group of mentally disordered individuals who are distinguished from both the mentally ill and alcohol and drug addicts. Under the federal Developmentally Disabled Assistance and Bill of Rights Act, 42 U.S.C. §§ 6000, 6001(7), the term is defined to include:

> a severe, chronic disability of a person which (A) is attributable to a mental or physical impairment or combination of mental and physical impairments; (B) is manifested before the person attains age twenty-two; (C) is likely to continue indefinitely; (D) results in substantial functional limitations in three or more of the following areas of major life activity: (i) self-care, (ii) receptive and expressive language, (iii) learning, (iv) mobility, (v) capacity for independent living, and (vi)

---

z. This is a quote from the 1967 Task Force Report on Narcotics and Drug Abuse issued by the President's Commission on Law Enforcement and the Administration of Justice. More recent programs evidence only slightly better results. See, e.g., Beck, "We Can Stem Drug Abuse," 68 A.B.A.J. 691 (1982).

economic self-sufficiency; and (E) reflects the person's need for a combination and sequence of special, interdisciplinary, or generic care, treatment or other services which are of lifelong or extended duration and are individually planned and coordinated.

The group of mentally disordered individuals most commonly categorized as developmentally disabled are the mentally retarded. But also included are people who suffer from learning disabilities, epilepsy, cerebral palsy and autism.

About 35 states have special commitment statutes for the developmentally disabled; about 25 use this term specifically, while the rest focus on the mentally retarded. In many of these states, the differences between this special commitment statute and the commitment statute for the mentally ill are insignificant. However, in several states the commitment criteria for the developmentally disabled are both broader and more narrow: many permit commitment based on a finding of a need for treatment, at the same time dangerousness is removed as a criterion. Additionally, the latter statutes tend to be more vague in setting out the procedures to be followed in the commitment process. Some appear to contemplate only "voluntary" admissions, initiated either by the person or the person's relatives or guardian. S. Brakel, J. Parry, B. Weiner, The Mentally Disabled and the Law 37–39 (1985). As the following case makes clear, there have been other differences as well.

IN RE HOP

Supreme Court of California, 1981.
29 Cal.3d 82, 171 Cal.Rptr. 721, 623 P.2d 282.

RICHARDSON, JUSTICE.

We are presented with a habeas corpus petition filed on behalf of Irene Hop who is a developmentally disabled adult woman presently suffering from juvenile ceroid lipofunscinosis (Spielmeyer Vogt or Batten disease). The petition, verified by her counsel of record, recites that since 1975 she has been under the care of Inland Counties Regional Center (the Center), that she has neither guardian of her person or estate nor conservator, and that for several years she had been cared for at the Salem–Christian Home in Ontario, California but on February 15, 1979, on the petition of her mother, she was placed in respondent Lanterman State Hospital, a more confining facility, as a nonprotesting developmentally disabled person. It is further alleged that she lacked the ability to object to her transfer to respondent, and that through successive but unsuccessful petitions for habeas corpus she has been unable to obtain any judicial review of the propriety of her initial transfer and confinement at respondent hospital.

The central issue presented is whether the statutory scheme which permits the placement of "nonprotesting" developmentally disabled adults in state hospitals for an indefinite time meets the constitutional requirements of due process and equal protection of the laws. We will conclude that the present statutory procedures are constitutionally infirm.

* * *

THE STATUTORY COMMITMENT AND RELEASE PROCEDURES

Hop was placed in a state hospital under the provisions of Welfare and Institutions Code section 4825 which authorizes "the admission of an adult developmentally disabled person to a state hospital . . . upon the application of the person's parent or guardian or conservator in accordance with the provisions of Sections 4653 and 4803." Sections 4653 and 4803 permit placement in a state hospital if the regional center recommends such placement and "an employee or designee" of the regional center certifies that no objection has been made to the placement by either the person recommended or any person acting on his behalf. Section 6000.5 authorizes the state hospital to accept a person so recommended.

Respondent contends that Hop's placement was "voluntary," stressing that any person acting on her behalf and objecting to her placement could obtain her freedom pursuant to habeas corpus release authorized by section 4800 et seq. or pursuant to the administrative process described in the Release Procedures Manual used by the state hospitals for the developmentally disabled. We examine and summarize these suggested procedures.

Section 4800 et seq. provides that every person (who, for convenience, we hereafter describe as the ward) admitted or committed to a state hospital or other related facility "shall have a right to a hearing by writ of habeas corpus for his release . . . after he or any person acting on his behalf makes a request for release to any member of the staff. . . ." Judicial review occurs in the appropriate superior court which may either order the ward's release, or conduct an evidentiary hearing following which, if the court finds that the ward is not developmentally disabled or is disabled but "able to provide safely for his basic personal needs for food, shelter, and clothing, he shall be immediately released." If the ward needs care and there is a responsible person, regional center, or other agency willing and able to assume such care the court may release the ward to such responsible person or agency. If the ward is found to be developmentally disabled and without parent, and lacking but needing a conservator the court "shall order the appropriate regional center or the state department to initiate . . . proceedings for the appointment of a conservator. . . ." (§ 4801.)

The Release Procedures Manual provides the necessary steps to be taken when a voluntary or nonprotesting developmentally disabled resident, verbally or nonverbally, indicates that he or she wishes to leave the facility. Within 24 hours a "validity conference" must be held at which the staff evaluates the request. If staff concludes that harm may result from immediate release, the regional center must be notified and asked to determine within five days whether commitment procedures pursuant to section 6500 or community placement should be initiated. If a petition for commitment is filed at the regional center's request, the ward's status is changed to that of a "detainee" under section 6506 which authorizes detention in a state hospital pending a commitment hearing. If no commitment petition is filed and a community placement is not immediately available the ward is placed on "administrative hold," and detained in the hospital while a formal request for release is forwarded to the superior court.

* * *

The Nature of the Placement

Respondent argues that we need not examine the constitutionality of section 4825 placements because persons placed under the section are admittees, not committees, who are free either to leave or to object to their confinement. Respondent stresses the fact that admission of the ward is conditioned upon a lack of any objection and that requests for release by a parent, guardian, or conservator or by the ward herself will be honored (§ 4800 and the Release Procedures Manual). It is argued that "there is really no need for any hearing. Persons who are in any way capable of objecting may do so. . . . Persons who are so low functioning that they cannot in any way object could not assist in any hearing on their behalf anyway."

* * *

Respondent's argument contains an inherent analytical difficulty. Hop is presumed sufficiently *competent* to understand the need for her to object to her placement when it has been initiated by a third party, her mother. At the same time she is presumed *incompetent* to a degree which would prevent her from requesting admission or, once confined, obtaining unilaterally and without review her own release. In short, although they are incompetent on their own to get in or out, non-protesting developmentally disabled adults are statutorily presumed competent enough to be able to object to hospital placement initiated by others. The ward's dilemma is akin to that faced by the admittee described in a recent article, "If you try to leave, they go to court to make you stay; if you do not try to leave, you demonstrate that you want to stay." (Ferleger et al., *Anti–Institutionalization: The Promise of the Pennhurst Case* (1979) 31 Stan.L.Rev. 717, 737.)

It is difficult to accept the thesis that a lack of objection may be construed as an affirmative request for placement by those who otherwise are deemed incompetent to request hospital admission. Nor can a lack of objection before or after admission be construed as a waiver of constitutional rights to which a ward may otherwise be entitled. The failure to object to a commitment by a third party who is neither conservator nor legal representative is no waiver.

* * *

At this point, a complicating companion problem is presented, namely, a role conflict arising from the fact that the agency responsible for the care and therapy of the ward is the entity which is given the added duty of notice and explanation of the ward's constitutional rights. The regional centers and hospital staffs charged with care, treatment, and therapy, are simultaneously entrusted with notice and explanation of rights. This role conflict may be further aggravated by an additional subtle pressure favoring hospital treatment as opposed to community placement of the ward. Local community placement may be difficult to locate and also expensive, and its cost may be borne locally by a regional center's budget. Hospital placements are funded from statewide sources. The centers, charged with administering and paying for therapy and care, and also with recommending and finding suitable placement, must simultaneously determine whether an objection to the proposed hospital placement has been made. (§ 4620 et seq.). A subtle strain is thereby placed on the center's impartial neutrality and detachment which unconsciously in its administrative decision may thereby favor hospital placements at state expense.

From all of the foregoing considerations we conclude that a developmentally disabled adult placed in a state hospital at the request of one not so legally authorized (see, e.g., § 5358) may not be deemed a "voluntary" admittee because he or she neither requested nor knowingly agreed to the placement. It follows that the present statutory scheme which permits indefinite placement of such nonprotesting developmentally disabled adults in a state hospital without any hearing constitutes a denial of due process of law.

EQUAL PROTECTION

No other class of adults similarly situated and in need of protective custody may lawfully be placed in a state hospital without a knowing and intelligent waiver of rights, or a request, or a judicial determination that placement is appropriate. No rational basis has been suggested for denying to the incompetent developmentally disabled those procedural rights which are readily granted to other incompetent adults for whom state hospital placement is sought.

*　*　*

Neither the benevolent intent of the Legislature, nor of those involved in the care of the developmentally disabled, nor the force of the legislative directive mandating the least restrictive placements for the developmentally disabled renders constitutional the legislative scheme which denies them the procedural safeguards of a hearing which is uniformly extended to other potential wards.

From the foregoing we conclude that the placement of Irene Hop in a state hospital at the request of her mother, in the absence of either a judicial determination regarding her disability or a knowing and intelligent request for admission was unconstitutional. She is entitled to a judicial hearing on the question of whether, because of developmental disability she is gravely disabled or a danger to herself or others and whether placement in a state hospital is warranted. We analogize her situation to that of proposed conservatees under the Lanterman–Petris–Short Act. As such she is entitled to the same congeries of rights

including the right to a jury trial on demand * * * and to the
application of the standard of proof beyond a reasonable doubt.

* * *

DISPOSITION

Our holding does not require the immediate release either of Hop
or of those presently held in state hospitals under the authority of
section 4825. We reaffirm our cautionary observation in *Roger S.,*
supra, that "A precipitous release of these [adults] to families and
community facilities unprepared to care for them could be both disruptive to the treatment program and potentially harmful to the [patient]
and the community." Hop is, however, entitled to a prompt hearing
which complies with the requirements herein described. She will also
be entitled to the appointment of counsel, for, consistent with the views
expressed by us in *Roger S.,* "[i]nasmuch as a minor [or a developmentally disabled adult] may be presumed to lack the ability to marshal the
facts and evidence, to effectively speak for himself and to call and
examine witnesses, or to discover and propose alternative treatment
programs, due process also requires that counsel be provided. . . ."

* * *

Questions and Comments

1. *Equal protection and procedural formality.* The "non-protesting",
"voluntary" admission procedure found unconstitutional in *Hop* is a relatively common alternative to involuntary commitment in many states.[a] It
is used more frequently with the developmentally disabled than with the
mentally ill, apparently because those in the former group are much less
likely to voice objections. Although many mildly and moderately retarded
persons are capable of communicating, many are not. For these people, as
well as for the profoundly retarded, speaking of "involuntary" or "voluntary" commitment may be meaningless.

In *Matter of Harhut,* 385 N.W.2d 305 (Minn.1986), the court was
confronted with a statutory scheme for commitment of the mentally
retarded which, unlike the statute at issue in *Hop,* required an initial
judicial determination of committability but, like that statute, did not
establish periodic judicial review procedures. Lawyers for the petitioner, a
35–year–old man who was blind, mildly mentally retarded, and autistic "at
times", argued there was no rational or compelling basis for requiring
mentally retarded individuals to request judicial review when the state
mandated such review for the mentally ill and for chemically dependent
persons. The court rejected this argument, stating:

[T]he distinction between the commitment periods . . . is based on a
legislative judgment that mental retardation is, unlike chemical dependency or mental illness, a condition not usually susceptible of great or
rapid improvement. The legislature decided that indeterminate commitment subject to judicial review on the motion of the patient was the
more effective and efficient way to deal with the state's responsibility

a. See discussion of non-protesting admissions of the mentally ill, pp. 751–755.

to treat retarded persons. This is a legitimate public purpose, and it is not clear beyond a reasonable doubt that indeterminate commitment is an unreasonable means of assuring the state's interest.

Although the court found no equal protection violation, it did find that, under the due process clause, every mentally retarded person committed to an institution is entitled to have counsel receive the results of staff medical reviews; according to the statute, these reviews were to occur "as frequently as necessary but not less than annually." It further held that some type of judicial review—not necessarily rising to the level of a hearing—must occur once every three years (the review period for the mentally ill and chemically dependent was one year).

Perhaps worth noting is that between *Hop* and *Harhut* the United States Supreme Court decided *City of Cleburne v. Cleburne Living Center*, 473 U.S. 432, 105 S.Ct. 3249, 87 L.Ed.2d 313 (1985), which considered the constitutionality of a zoning ordinance that discriminated against the mentally retarded. As described by the *Harhut* court, in *Cleburne* "the Court declined to recognize mentally retarded persons as a suspect or quasi-suspect class since their situation is best addressed by legislative action, there has been a distinct legislative response showing that the mentally retarded are not politically powerless, and such a rule would open the door to creating a new series of quasi-suspect classifications." [b] Is *Cleburne* relevant here, given the classes being compared? More generally, is there a "rational basis" for permitting "non-protesting admission" and patient-initiated review for the developmentally disabled in those jurisdictions which do not permit either for the mentally ill?

2. *Commitment criteria.* As noted in the introduction to this subsection, many statutes governing commitment of the developmentally disabled allow confinement based merely on a finding of disability and a "need for treatment"—or, to use more modern terminology, "habilitation" or "training in survival skills." At least one court has found such statutes unconstitutional. See, e.g., *Kinner v. State*, 382 So.2d 756 (Fla.App.1980) (the statute must include "criteria limiting persons who may be involuntarily committed to those who lack the capacity to weigh for themselves the risks of freedom and the benefits of hospitalization and/or to those who are dangerous to themselves or others.). See also, *People v. Reliford*, 65 Ill. App.3d 177, 21 Ill.Dec. 778, 382 N.E.2d 72 (1978). In contrast, one court has upheld against a vagueness challenge a statute which permitted commitment if the court certifies simply that the person is "mentally deficient." *Matter of Vandenberg*, 48 Or.App. 609, 617 P.2d 675 (1980). The court found that, unlike the criteria for commitment of the mentally ill, "the standard for commitment [under this statute] is set by scientific tests monitoring levels of intellectual functioning and adaptive behavior." The statute and accompanying regulations permitted court certification only if the examining institution found (a) that the person met the definition of mental retardation found in the Manual of the American Association of Mental Deficiency and (b) that "admission to a state institution for the mentally retarded [is] the optimal available plan and is in the best

b. *Cleburne* is discussed in detail in Chapter Twelve.

interest of the person and the community." The definition of mental retardation in the Manual did not require consideration of the person's ability to understand or consent to treatment.

Is there a reasonable basis for establishing broader commitment criteria for the developmentally disabled? Does the "voluntary" label provide such a basis? How does the *Hop* court answer these questions?

3. *Alternatives to institutionalization.* Given the obvious disabilities of many of the developmentally disabled, the major problem connected with their commitment is not that it frequently coerces people who do not want or need state-provided habilitation but that it usually means long-term institutionalization in mega-facilities that are inadequate at providing training and even tend to accentuate dependency and deterioration. See Ferleger, "Anti–Institutionalization: The Promise of the *Pennhurst* Case," 31 Stanford L.Rev. 717, 720–724 (1979). The least restrictive alternative doctrine has particular applicability here. Dwybad and Herr have suggested that, once it is determined that a developmentally disabled person is incapable of giving meaningful consent and requires close supervision due to a lack of survival skills, the relevant placement criteria should be "whether any in-home supportive services or respite care services could be provided as an alternative to removal from home surroundings; factually-grounded expectations of effective treatment in other settings; and a realistic assessment of whether the benefits to the resident of removal from community surroundings outweigh the harms." Dwybad & Herr, "Unnecessary Coercion: An End to Involuntary Civil Commitment of Retarded Persons," 31 Stanford L.Rev. 753, 764 (1979). Unfortunately, many localities are lacking in either home or community services for the developmentally disabled. Indeed, most of the litigation which attempts to force states to create alternatives to institutions has been brought on behalf of this group. These efforts, and the legislation they have spawned, are discussed in Chapters Ten, Eleven and Twelve.

E. CHILDREN

Until the 1950's, the procedures for committing children were usually similar, if not identical, to those governing commitment of adults. But since that time, in conjunction with the general trend toward voluntary hospitalization, most states have enacted special statutes allowing "voluntary" admission of children on the petition of their parents or guardians. By the mid–1970's, three-quarters of the states had special statutory provisions allowing parents to commit their children to mental institutions without a court hearing or any lesser form of judicial oversight and leaving release up to the hospital and the parents. Toward the end of the 1970's, motivated by the reforms of adult commitment, some of these states had revised their statutes to require adult-type hearings, at least when the child objected to commitment or requested release. S. Brakel, J. Parry & B. Weiner, The Mentally Disabled and the Law 43–44 (1985). It was in this context that the Supreme Court decided *Parham v. J.R.*

PARHAM v. J.R. ET AL.

Supreme Court of the United States, 1979.
442 U.S. 584, 99 S.Ct. 2493, 61 L.Ed.2d 101.

[The plaintiffs in this class action were two minors who had been institutionalized in a psychiatric facility operated by the state of Georgia at the initiation of their guardians. One of the plaintiffs, J.L., was initially admitted into Central State Hospital at the age of six. At the time of his admission he had been expelled from school for "uncontrollable behavior" and had manifested "extremely aggressive" behavior at home. For a period of time J.L. was permitted to go home, but his behavior during these visits was "erratic," and the parents asked for discontinuance of the home visits. Two years later a new program was implemented that permitted J.L. to live at home and attend school in the hospital. However, when the parents found they were unable to control J.L.'s behavior, they requested his readmission into Central State Hospital.

The second plaintiff, J.R., was declared a neglected child and removed from his natural parents when he was three months old. He lived in a succession of foster homes until he reached the age of seven, when his disruptive and "incorrigible" behavior both at home and school led his seventh set of foster parents to request his removal. J.R. was thereafter institutionalized in Central State Hospital at the initiative of the Georgia Department of Family and Student Services. At the time of his admission, he was diagnosed as "borderline retarded" and suffering from "unsocialized aggressive reaction."]

MR. CHIEF JUSTICE BURGER delivered the opinion of the Court.

The question presented in this appeal is what process is constitutionally due a minor child whose parents or guardian seek state administered institutional mental health care for the child and specifically whether an adversary proceeding is required prior to or after the commitment.

* * *

A three-judge District Court was convened pursuant to 28 U.S.C. §§ 2281 and 2284. After considering expert and lay testimony and extensive exhibits and after visiting two of the State's regional mental health hospitals, the District Court held that Georgia's statutory scheme was unconstitutional because it failed to protect adequately the appellees' due process rights.

To remedy this violation the court enjoined future commitments based on the procedures in the Georgia statute. It also commanded Georgia to appropriate and expend whatever amount was "reasonably necessary" to provide nonhospital facilities deemed by the appellant state officials to be the most appropriate for the treatment of those members of plaintiffs' class, who could be treated in a less drastic, nonhospital environment.

Appellants challenged all aspects of the District Court's judgment.

* * *

Georgia Code, § 88–503.1 provides for the voluntary admission to a state regional hospital of children such as J.L. and J.R. Under that provision admission begins with an application for hospitalization signed by a "parent or guardian." Upon application the superintendent of each hospital is given the power to admit temporarily any child for "observation and diagnosis." If, after observation, the superintendent finds "evidence of mental illness" and that the child is "suitable for treatment" in the hospital, then the child may be admitted "for such period and under such conditions as may be authorized by law."

Georgia's mental health statute also provides for the discharge of voluntary patients. Any child who has been hospitalized for more than five days may be discharged at the request of a parent or guardian. Even without a request for discharge, however, the superintendent of each regional hospital has an affirmative duty to release any child "who has recovered from his mental illness or who has sufficiently improved that the superintendent determines that hospitalization of the patient is no longer desirable."

Georgia's Mental Health Director has not published any statewide regulations defining what specific procedures each superintendent must employ when admitting a child under 18. Instead, each regional hospital's superintendent is responsible for the procedures in his or her facility. There is substantial variation among the institutions with regard to their admission procedures and their procedures for review of patients after they have been admitted.

* * *

[At Southwestern Hospital, after] a child is admitted, the hospital has weekly reviews of his condition performed by its internal medical and professional staff. There also are monthly reviews of each child by a group composed of hospital staff not involved in the weekly reviews and by community clinic staff people. The average stay for each child who was being treated at Southwestern in 1975 was 100 days.

* * *

[At Atlanta Regional Hospital, after] admission the staff reviews the condition of each child every week. In addition, there are monthly utilization reviews by nonstaff mental health professionals; this review considers a random sample of children's cases. The average length of each child's stay in 1975 was 161 days.

* * *

[The Court described similar procedures at three other facilities].

* * *

III

* * *

The parties agree that our prior holdings have set out a general approach for testing challenged state procedures under a due process claim.   Assuming the existence of a protectible property or liberty interest, the Court has required a balancing of a number of factors:

> "First, the private interest that will be affected by the official action; second, the risk of an erroneous deprivation of such interest through the procedures used, and the probable value, if any, of additional or substitute procedural safeguards; and finally, the Government's interest, including the function involved and the fiscal and administrative burdens that the additional or substitute procedural requirement would entail."

Mathews v. Eldridge, 424 U.S. 319, 335, 96 S.Ct. 893, 903, 47 L.Ed.2d 18 (1976).

In applying these criteria, we must consider first the child's interest in not being committed.   Normally, however, since this interest is inextricably linked with the parents' interest in and obligation for the welfare and health of the child, the private interest at stake is a combination of the child's and parents' concerns.   Next we must examine the State's interest in the procedures it has adopted for commitment and treatment of children.   Finally, we must consider how well Georgia's procedures protect against arbitrariness in the decision to commit a child to a state mental hospital.

(a) It is not disputed that a child, in common with adults, has a substantial liberty interest in not being confined unnecessarily for medical treatment and that the State's involvement in the commitment decision constitutes state action under the Fourteenth Amendment.

We also recognize that commitment sometimes produces adverse social consequences for the child because of the reaction of some to the discovery that the child has received psychiatric care.   This reaction, however, need not be equated with the community response resulting from being labeled by the state as delinquent, criminal, or mentally ill and possibly dangerous.   The state through its voluntary commitment procedures does not "label" the child; it provides a diagnosis and treatment that medical specialists conclude the child requires.   In terms of public reaction, the child who exhibits abnormal behavior may be seriously injured by an erroneous decision not to commit.   Appellees overlook a significant source of the public reaction to the mentally ill, for what is truly "stigmatizing" is the symptomatology of a mental or emotional illness.   The pattern of untreated, abnormal behavior—even if nondangerous—arouses at least as much negative reaction as treatment that becomes public knowledge.   A person needing, but not receiving, appropriate medical care may well face even greater social ostracism resulting from the observable symptoms of an untreated disorder.

However, we need not decide what effect these factors might have in a different case.   For purposes of this decision, we assume that a child has a protectible interest not only in being free of unnecessary bodily restraints but also in not being labeled erroneously by some because of an improper decision by the state hospital superintendent.

(b) We next deal with the interests of the parents who have decided, on the basis of their observations and independent professional recommendations, that their child needs institutional care. Appellees argue that the constitutional rights of the child are of such magnitude and the likelihood of parental abuse is so great that the parents' traditional interests in and responsibility for the upbringing of their child must be subordinated at least to the extent of providing a formal adversary hearing prior to a voluntary commitment.

Our jurisprudence historically has reflected Western Civilization concepts of the family as a unit with broad parental authority over minor children. Our cases have consistently followed that course; our constitutional system long ago rejected any notion that a child is "the mere creature of the State" and, on the contrary, asserted that parents generally "have the right, coupled with the high duty, to recognize and prepare [their children] for additional obligations."

Surely, this includes a "high duty" to recognize symptoms of illness and to seek and follow medical advice. The law's concept of the family rests on a presumption that parents possess what a child lacks in maturity, experience, and capacity for judgment required for making life's difficult decisions. More important, historically it has recognized that natural bonds of affection lead parents to act in the best interests of their children.

As with so many other legal presumptions, experience and reality may rebut what the law accepts as a starting point; the incidence of child neglect and abuse cases attests to this. That some parents "may at times be acting against the interests of their child" creates a basis for caution, but is hardly a reason to discard wholesale those pages of human experience that teach that parents generally do act in the child's best interests. The statist notion that governmental power should supersede parental authority in *all* cases because *some* parents abuse and neglect children is repugnant to American tradition.

Nonetheless, we have recognized that a state is not without constitutional control over parental discretion in dealing with children when their physical or mental health is jeopardized. Moreover, the Court recently declared unconstitutional a state statute that granted parents an absolute veto over a minor child's decision to have an abortion. Planned Parenthood of Missouri v. Danforth, 428 U.S. 52, 96 S.Ct. 2831, 49 L.Ed.2d 788 (1976). Appellees urge that these precedents limiting the traditional rights of parents, if viewed in the context of the liberty interest of the child and the likelihood of parental abuse, require us to hold that the parents' decision to have a child admitted to a mental hospital must be subjected to an exacting constitutional scrutiny, including a formal, adversary preadmission hearing.

Appellees' argument, however, sweeps too broadly. Simply because the decision of a parent is not agreeable to a child or because it involves risks does not automatically transfer the power to make that decision from the parents to some agency or officer of the state. The same characterizations can be made for a tonsillectomy, appendectomy or other medical procedure. Most children, even in adolescence, simply are not able to make sound judgments concerning many decisions, including their need for medical care or treatment. Parents can and must make those judgments. * * * The fact that a child may balk at hospitalization or complain about a parental refusal to provide cosmetic surgery does not diminish the parents' authority to decide what is best for the child.

* * *

Appellees place particular reliance on *Planned Parenthood,* arguing that its holding indicates how little deference to parents is appropriate when the child is exercising a constitutional right. The basic situation in that case, however, was very different; *Planned Parenthood* involved an absolute parental veto over the child's ability to obtain an abortion. Parents in Georgia in no sense have an absolute right to commit their children to state mental hospitals; the statute requires the superintendent of each regional hospital to exercise independent judgment as to the child's need for confinement.

In defining the respective rights and prerogatives of the child and parent in the voluntary commitment setting, we conclude that our precedents permit the parents to retain a substantial, if not the dominant, role in the decision, absent a finding of neglect or abuse, and that the traditional presumption that the parents act in the best interests of their child should apply. We also conclude, however, that the child's rights and the nature of the commitment decision are such that parents cannot always have absolute and unreviewable discretion to decide whether to have a child institutionalized. They, of course, retain plenary authority to seek such care for their children, subject to a physician's independent examination and medical judgment.

(c) The State obviously has a significant interest in confining the use of its costly mental health facilities to cases of genuine need. The Georgia program seeks first to determine whether the patient seeking admission has an illness that calls for in-patient treatment. To accomplish this purpose, the State has charged the superintendents of each regional hospital with the responsibility for determining, before authorizing an admission, whether a prospective patient is mentally ill and whether the patient will likely benefit from hospital care. In addition, the State has imposed a continuing duty on hospital superintendents to release any patient who has recovered to the point where hospitalization is no longer needed.

* * *

The State also has a genuine interest in allocating priority to the diagnosis and treatment of patients as soon as they are admitted to a hospital rather than to time-consuming procedural minuets before the admission. One factor that must be considered is the utilization of the time of psychiatrists, psychologists and other behavioral specialists in preparing for and participating in hearings rather than performing the task for which their special training has fitted them. Behavioral experts in courtrooms and hearings are of little help to patients.

The *amicus* brief of the American Psychiatric Association points out at page 20 that the average staff psychiatrist in a hospital presently is able to devote only 47% of his time to direct patient care. One consequence of increasing the procedures the state must provide prior to a child's voluntary admission will be that mental health professionals will be diverted even more from the treatment of patients in order to travel to and participate in—and wait for—what could be hundreds—or even thousands—of hearings each year. Obviously the cost of these procedures would come from the public monies the legislature intended for mental health care.

(d) We now turn to consideration of what process protects adequately the child's constitutional rights by reducing risks of error without unduly trenching on traditional parental authority and without undercutting "efforts to further the legitimate interests of both the state and the patient that are served by" voluntary commitments. We conclude that the risk of error inherent in the parental decision to have a child institutionalized for mental health care is sufficiently great that some kind of inquiry should be made by a "neutral factfinder" to determine whether the statutory requirements for admission are satisfied. That inquiry must carefully probe the child's background using all available sources, including, but not limited to, parents, schools and other social agencies. Of course, the review must also include an interview with the child. It is necessary that the decisionmaker have the authority to refuse to admit any child who does not satisfy the medical standards for admission. Finally, it is necessary that the child's continuing need for commitment be reviewed periodically by a similarly independent procedure.[15]

We are satisfied that such procedures will protect the child from an erroneous admission decision in a way that neither unduly burdens the states nor inhibits parental decisions to seek state help.

Due process has never been thought to require that the neutral and detached trier of fact be law-trained or a judicial or administrative officer. Surely, this is the case as to medical decisions for "neither judges nor administrative hearing officers are better qualified than psychiatrists to render psychiatric judgments." Thus, a staff physician will suffice, so long as he or she is free to evaluate independently the child's mental and emotional condition and need for treatment.

It is not necessary that the deciding physician conduct a formal or quasi-formal hearing. A state is free to require such a hearing, but due process is not violated by use of informal traditional medical investiga-

---

15. As we discuss more fully later, the District Court did not decide and we therefore have no reason to consider at this time what procedures for review are independently necessary to justify continuing a child's confinement. We merely hold that a subsequent, independent review of the patient's condition provides a necessary check against possible arbitrariness in the *initial* admission decision.

tive techniques. Since well-established medical procedures already exist, we do not undertake to outline with specificity precisely what this investigation must involve. The mode and procedure of medical diagnostic procedures is not the business of judges. What is best for a child is an individual medical decision that must be left to the judgment of physicians in each case. We do no more than emphasize that the decision should represent an independent judgment of what the child requires and that all sources of information that are traditionally relied on by physicians and behavioral specialists should be consulted. * * * [One of the] problem(s) with requiring a formalized, factfinding hearing lies in the danger it poses for significant intrusion into the parent-child relationship. Pitting the parents and child as adversaries often will be at odds with the presumption that parents act in the best interests of their child. It is one thing to require a neutral physician to make a careful review of the parents' decision in order to make sure it is proper from a medical standpoint; it is a wholly different matter to employ an adversary contest to ascertain whether the parents' motivation is consistent with the child's interests.

Moreover, it is appropriate to inquire into how such a hearing would contribute to the long range successful treatment of the patient. Surely, there is a risk that it would exacerbate whatever tensions already existed between the child and the parents. Since the parents can and usually do play a significant role in the treatment while the child is hospitalized and even more so after release, there is a serious risk that an adversary confrontation will adversely affect the ability of the parents to assist the child while in the hospital. Moreover, it will make his subsequent return home more difficult. These unfortunate results are especially critical with an emotionally disturbed child; they seem likely to occur in the context of an adversary hearing in which the parents testify. A confrontation over such intimate family relationships would distress the normal adult parents and the impact on a disturbed child almost certainly would be significantly greater.

* * *

By expressing some confidence in the medical decisionmaking process, we are by no means suggesting it is error free. On occasion parents may initially mislead an admitting physician or a physician may erroneously diagnose the child as needing institutional care either because of negligence or an overabundance of caution. That there may be risks of error in the process affords no rational predicate for holding unconstitutional an entire statutory and administrative scheme that is generally followed in more than 30 states. "[P]rocedural due process rules are shaped by the risk of error inherent in the truthfinding process as applied to the generality of cases, not the rare exceptions." In general, we are satisfied that an independent medical decisionmaking process, which includes the thorough psychiatric investigation described earlier followed by additional periodic review of a child's condition, will protect children who should not be admitted; we do not believe the risks of error in that process would be significantly reduced by a more formal, judicial-type hearing.

* * *

IV

(a) Our discussion in Part III was directed at the situation where a child's natural parents request his admission to a state mental hospital. Some members of appellees' class, including J.R., were wards of the State of Georgia at the time of their admission. Obviously their situation differs from those members of the class who have natural parents. While the determination of what process is due varies somewhat when the state, rather than a natural parent, makes the request for commitment, we conclude that the differences in the two situations do not justify requiring different procedures at the time of the child's initial admission to the hospital.

For a ward of the State, there may well be no adult who knows him thoroughly and who cares for him deeply. * * * Contrary to the suggestion of the dissent, however, we cannot assume that when the State of Georgia has custody of a child it acts so differently from a natural parent in seeking medical assistance for the child. [T]here is no evidence that the State, acting as guardian, attempted to admit any child for reasons unrelated to the child's need for treatment. Indeed, neither the District Court nor the appellees have suggested that wards of the State should receive any constitutional treatment different from children with natural parents.

* * *

Once we accept that the State's application of a child for admission to a hospital is made in good faith, then the question is whether the medical decisionmaking approach of the admitting physician is adequate to satisfy due process. We have already recognized that an independent medical judgment made from the perspective of the best interests of the child after a careful investigation is an acceptable means of justifying a voluntary commitment. We do not believe that the soundness of this decisionmaking is any the less reasonable in this setting.

Indeed, if anything, the decision with regard to wards of the State may well be even more reasonable in light of the extensive written records that are compiled about each child while in the State's custody.

* * *

Since the state agency having custody and control of the child *in loco parentis* has a duty to consider the best interests of the child with respect to a decision on commitment to a mental hospital, the State may constitutionally allow that custodial agency to speak for the child, subject, of course, to the restrictions governing natural parents.

* * *

(b) It is possible that the procedures required in reviewing a ward's need for continuing care should be different from those used to review a child with natural parents. As we have suggested earlier, the issue of what process is due to justify continuing a voluntary commitment must be considered by the District Court on remand. In making that inquiry the District Court might well consider whether wards of the State should be treated with respect to continuing therapy differently from children with natural parents.

The absence of an adult who cares deeply for a child has little effect on the reliability of the initial admission decision, but it may have some effect on how long a child will remain in the hospital. We noted in *Addington v. Texas, supra,* —— U.S., at ——, 99 S.Ct., at 1811, "the concern of family and friends generally will provide continuous opportunities for an erroneous commitment to be corrected." For a child without natural parents, we must acknowledge the risk of being "lost in the shuffle."

* * *

Whether wards of the State generally have received less protection than children with natural parents, and, if so, what should be done about it, however, are matters that must be decided in the first instance by the District Court on remand, if the Court concludes the issue is still alive. * * * [W]e are satisfied that Georgia's medical factfinding processes are reasonable and consistent with constitutional guarantees. Accordingly, it was error to hold unconstitutional the State's procedures for admitting a child for treatment to a state mental hospital. The judgment is therefore reversed and the case is remanded to the District Court for further proceedings consistent with this opinion.

Reversed and remanded.

* * *

MR. JUSTICE BRENNAN, with whom MR. JUSTICE MARSHALL and MR. JUSTICE STEVENS join, concurring in part and dissenting in part.

* * *

I

RIGHTS OF CHILDREN COMMITTED TO MENTAL INSTITUTIONS

It may well be argued that children are entitled to more protection than are adults. The consequences of an erroneous commitment decision are more tragic where children are involved. Children, on the average, are confined for longer periods than are adults. Moreover, childhood is a particularly vulnerable time of life and children erroneously institutionalized during their formative years may bear the scars for the rest of their lives. Furthermore, the provision of satisfactory institutionalized mental care for children generally requires a substantial financial commitment that too often has not been forthcoming.

* * *

In addition, the chances of an erroneous commitment decision are particularly great where children are involved. Even under the best of circumstances psychiatric diagnosis and therapy decisions are fraught with uncertainties. These uncertainties are aggravated when, as under the Georgia practice, the psychiatrist interviews the child during a period of abnormal stress in connection with the commitment, and without adequate time or opportunity to become acquainted with the patient. These uncertainties may be further aggravated when economic and social class separate doctor and child, thereby frustrating the accurate diagnosis of pathology.

These compounded uncertainties often lead to erroneous commitments since psychiatrists tend to err on the side of medical caution and therefore hospitalize patients for whom other dispositions would be more beneficial. The National Institute of Mental Health recently found that only 36% of patients below age 20 who were confined at St. Elizabeths Hospital actually required such hospitalization. Of particular relevance to this case, a Georgia study Commission on Mental Health Services for Children and Youth concluded that more than half of the State's institutionalized children were not in need of confinement if other forms of care were made available or used.

* * *

II

RIGHTS OF CHILDREN COMMITTED BY THEIR PARENTS

* * *

I believe that States may legitimately postpone formal commitment proceedings when parents seek in-patient psychiatric treatment for their children. Such children may be admitted, for a limited period, without prior hearing, so long as the admitting psychiatrist first interviews parent and child and concludes that short term in-patient treatment would be appropriate.

I do not believe, however, that the present Georgia juvenile commitment scheme is constitutional in its entirety. Although Georgia may postpone formal commitment hearings, when parents seek to commit their children, the State cannot dispense with such hearings altogether.

* * *

The informal postadmission procedures that Georgia now follows are simply not enough to qualify as hearings—let alone reasonably prompt hearings. The procedures lack all the traditional due process safeguards. Commitment decisions are made *ex parte*. Georgia's institutionalized juveniles are not informed of the reasons for their commitment; nor do they enjoy the right to be present at the commitment determination, nor the right to representation, the right to be heard, the right to be confronted with adverse witnesses, the right to cross-examine, or the right to offer evidence of their own. By any standard of due process, these procedures are deficient.

The special considerations that militate against preadmission commitment hearings when parents seek to hospitalize their children do not militate against reasonably prompt postadmission commitment hearings. In the first place, postadmission hearings would not delay the commencement of needed treatment. Children could be cared for by the State pending the disposition decision.

Second, the interest in avoiding family discord would be less significant at this stage since the family autonomy already will have been fractured by the institutionalization of the child. In any event, postadmission hearings are unlikely to disrupt family relationships. At later hearings the case for and against commitment would be based upon the observations of the hospital staff and the judgments of the staff psychiatrists, rather than upon parental observations and recommendations. The doctors urging commitment, and not the parents, would stand as the child's adversaries. As a consequence, postadmission commitment hearings are unlikely to involve direct challenges to parental authority, judgment or veracity. To defend the child, the child's advocate need not dispute the parents' original decision to seek medical treatment for their child, or even, for that matter, their observations concerning the child's behavior. The advocate need only argue, for example, that the child had sufficiently improved during his hospital stay to warrant out-patient treatment or outright discharge. Conflict between doctor and advocate on this question is unlikely to lead to family discord.

As a consequence, the prospect of a postadmission hearing is unlikely to deter parents from seeking medical attention for their children and the hearing itself is unlikely to so traumatize parent and child as to make the child's eventual return to the family impracticable.

* * *

III

RIGHTS OF CHILDREN COMMITTED BY THEIR STATE GUARDIANS

Georgia does not accord prior hearings to juvenile wards of the State of Georgia committed by state social workers acting *in loco parentis*. The Court dismisses a challenge to this practice on the grounds that state social workers are obliged by statute to act in the children's best interest.

* * *

To my mind, there is no justification for denying children committed by their social workers the prior hearings that the Constitution typically requires. * * * [First, the] rule that parents speak for their children, even if it were applicable in the commitment context, cannot be transmuted into a rule that state social workers speak for their minor clients. The rule in favor of deference to parental authority is designed to shield parental control of childrearing from state interference. * * *(The social worker-child relationship is not deserving of the special protection and deference accorded to the parent-child relationship and state officials acting *in loco parentis* cannot be equated with parents.)

Second, the special considerations that justify postponement of formal commitment proceedings whenever parents seek to hospitalize their children are absent when the children are wards of the State and are being committed upon the recommendations of their social workers. The prospect of preadmission hearings is not likely to deter state social workers from discharging their duties and securing psychiatric attention for their disturbed clients. Moreover, since the children will already be in some form of state custody as wards of the State, prehospitalization hearings will not prevent needy children from receiving state care during the pendency of the commitment proceedings. Finally, hearings in which the decisions of state social workers are reviewed by other state officials are not likely to traumatize the children or to hinder their eventual recovery.

For these reasons I believe that, in the absence of exigent circumstances, juveniles committed upon the recommendation of their social workers are entitled to preadmission commitment hearings. As a consequence, I would hold Georgia's present practice of denying these juveniles prior hearings unconstitutional.

Questions and Comments

1. **Institutionalized Juveniles.** In a companion case to *Parham, Secretary of Public Welfare of Penn. v. Institutionalized Juveniles*, 442 U.S. 640, 99 S.Ct. 2523, 61 L.Ed.2d 142 (1979), the Court upheld Pennsylvania's system for committing mentally ill and mentally retarded children on the petition of their parents or guardian. As it had in *Parham*, the Court stressed the thoroughness of the preadmission procedure.

> No child is admitted without at least one and often more psychiatric examinations by an independent team of mental health professionals whose sole concern under the statute is whether the child needs and can benefit from institutional care. The treatment team not only interviews the child and parents but also compiles a full background history from all available sources. If the treatment team concludes that institutional care is not in the child's best interest, it must refuse the child's admission. Finally, every child's condition is reviewed at least every 30 days.

Also as in *Parham*, the Court declined to decide what, if any, judicial postadmission procedures are required.

2. *Children's competence.* The majority opinion in *Parham* states that "[m]ost children, even in adolescence, simply are not able to make sound judgments concerning many decisions, including their need for medical care or treatment." The available studies indicate, to the contrary, that by age 14 minors are typically as competent as adults in making treatment decisions and that some children under that age are equally competent. See, e.g., Weithorn & Campbell, "The Competency of Children and Adolescents to Make Informed Treatment Decisions," 53 Child Dev. 1589 (1982). Most of the research in this area has involved "nonclinical" populations, however. What impact, if any, should these findings have on the due process analysis of commitment of minors?

3. *Parental and governmental good faith.* In holding that children subject to commitment are not entitled to the procedural protections afforded adults, the Court's decisions in *Parham* and *Institutionalized Juveniles* rely in part on the assumption that most parents seeking such commitment act in the "best interest" of their children. There is significant research disputing this assumption. For instance, one review concluded: "[O]ne thing that is clear from a variety of statistical data is that both the decision to place a child in an institution and the selection of the type of institution for him are dependent to a great extent on factors other than the needs of the child." D. Pappenfort, ed., Child Caring, Social Policy and the Institution 112 (1973).

Rather than the child, it may be the parents who are disturbed. One study of Philadelphia admissions indicated that, in 25 percent of the cases in which complainants alleged someone was mentally ill, it was the complainant, not the prospective patient, who was mentally ill. T. Scheff, Being Mentally Ill: A Sociological Theory 171 (1966). Others have noted that a child may be made the scapegoat for conflicts, disabilities or emotional deficiencies of the parents or siblings. Vogel & Bell, "The Emotionally Disturbed Child as the Family Scapegoat," in A Modern Introduction to the Family 412 (N. Bell & E. Vogel rev. ed. 1968). Even if the parents are relatively "normal", they may decide to hospitalize their child for reasons that have little to do with his or her needs. For example, the district court in *Institutionalized Juveniles* found, based on extensive expert testimony, that the parents' decision to hospitalize a mentally retarded child may be the result of community pressure, emotional difficulties in dealing with the child, or financial problems connected with providing necessary care.[c]

On the other hand, the social worker who is in charge of a child who is a ward of the state is presumably not affected by such considerations when making placement decisions. Are there other reasons for suspecting the sincerity of a social worker's decision to seek institutionalization of such a child? Note that the guardianship statutes of several states bar state social service officials from serving as guardians out of a fear of conflict of interest. Legal Counsel for the Elderly, Decisionmaking, Incapacity and the Elderly 75 (1987).

4. *The independent decisionmaker.* The *Parham* Court placed considerable faith in the psychiatric interview as a means of ferreting out inappropriate petitions, whether they be by parents or state guardians. Ellis, in "Volunteering Children: Parental Commitment of Minors to Mental Institutions," 62 Cal.L.Rev. 840, 864 (1974) has questioned the efficacy of this type of review:

> Experience shows that in the most blatant cases of parental error psychiatrists do screen out admissions which are not warranted by apparent pathology in the child. In less obvious cases, however,

---

c. Financially strapped parents of mentally and physically handicapped children have received a significant boost with the Education for All Handicapped Children Act, 20 U.S.C. §§ 1400–1461 (1976), which provides federal and state funding for "mainstreaming" handicapped children in the public school system. This Act, which is discussed in detail in Chapter Eleven, may have taken some pressure off the commitment system.

psychiatrists may fail to perform an effective screening function. There are three reasons for this failure: (1) The performance of psychiatrists in precommitment interviews and examinations is often perfunctory and tends toward overdiagnosis; (2) Psychiatrists may be insensitive to legally important commitment issues; (3) The effectiveness of the psychiatrist in the admitting process is weakened by uncertainty over whose agent he or she is in such circumstances—the parent's or the child's.

On the latter point, Ellis notes: "While the goal of the psychiatrist will be expressed—and perceived—as the best welfare of the child-patient, it is the parent who has come to seek help, whose situation seems most desperate, who seems the most reliable source of information about what is wrong, who is closest to the psychiatrist in age and social outlook, and who is paying the psychiatrist's fee." Id. at 866.

There is little information bearing on the number of "inappropriate" admissions of children under procedures like those in use in Georgia. The figures provided by Justice Brennan in dissent suggesting that a large number of children are improperly hospitalized are probably as much a reflection on the unavailability of community resources as an indication of the accuracy of decisions made by admitting clinicians. However, it is worth noting that the amicus brief submitted by the American Psychiatric Association, upon which the majority heavily relies, questioned the wisdom of leaving the hospitalization decision to a psychiatrist in all circumstances.

> While Amici agree with appellant that psychiatric diagnosis—i.e., identification of specific mental illnesses—are medically reliable, we recognize that this fact is not dispositive of the issue of when a hearing is constitutionally required. Even if a child is properly diagnosed, it does not follow that hospitalization is necessary or desirable. Rather, Amici believe that in appropriate circumstances a due process hearing may provide a reasonable forum for deciding what care should be provided to a properly diagnosed child.

Amicus Brief for the American Psychiatric Association, et. al., at 24. Specifically, the APA advocated following the Georgia procedure only when (a) parents in an intact family wish to admit (b) a preadolescent child (c) to an accredited institution (d) for a short-term period (e.g., less than 45 days). In all other circumstances, concluded the APA, the danger of inappropriate placement merits affording the child due process protections.

5. *Postadmission review.* In *Parham* the Court required some sort of "independent review of the patient's condition" but then remanded to the district court for a determination as to the precise postadmission procedure mandated by the constitution. Several states provide for automatic judicial review procedures akin to those provided in adult commitment. Many, however, provide such review only at the child's request. In other states, because they are "voluntary" patients, children are not entitled to either periodic review or habeas review. At the same time, because they are children, they cannot give notice of an intention to leave, as can adult voluntary patients, unless they obtain approval of their parents or guardian. Ellis, supra at 847.

Although the postadmission issue is at least as important as the issues addressed by the Court, the only guidance the Court provided on remand was to indicate that children confined pursuant to a petition by the state may be entitled to more procedural oversight than children whose confinement was sought by their parents. This was because parents are more likely to make sure their children do not get "lost in the shuffle." Are parents any more likely to seek release of their children than the state is of its wards? Consider Shoenberger, " 'Voluntary' Commitment of Mentally Ill or Retarded Children: Child Abuse by the Supreme Court," 7 U.Dayton L.Rev. 1, 30 (1981):

> Once a family decides to institutionalize a mentally retarded child . . . reopening that emotionally charged decision is very difficult, even in the context of available supportive social services for in-home care that, if previously available, might have prevented institutionalization. Indeed, every time a family member visits the retarded individual, "all the old guilt feelings and indecisiveness surge up about whether or not they made the right decision."

6. *Criteria.* Do the differences between adults and children permit different *standards* of commitment as well as different procedures? As with some of the statutes governing commitment of the developmentally disabled, the Georgia statute at issue in *Parham* permits admission of the child solely upon a finding by the admitting psychiatrist that the child is mentally disordered and suitable for treatment. Had the Supreme Court been asked to address the constitutionality of these criteria, how should it have held? Would a decision upholding the statute be consistent with *O'Connor v. Donaldson?*

7. *Implications of* Parham. Should the reasoning found in *Parham* be extended to *adult* civil commitment, thus permitting commitment of adults under a need for treatment criterion as interpreted by a "neutral physician?" How much of the Court's rationale for its decision in *Parham* is dependent upon some special characteristic of children and their situation? At the least, could *Parham's* reasoning be applied to commitment of the adult developmentally disabled, given the fact that they are often wards of their relatives or the state?

Chapter Nine

COMPETENCY DETERMINATIONS

I. INTRODUCTION

The issue of competency—the capacity to decide or to perform certain functions—permeates both the criminal and civil justice systems, although the precise decisions to be made and functions to be carried out vary from context to context. In civil cases, for instance, competency may refer to a capacity to understand and approve the terms of a contract or a will, manage financial affairs, or make treatment decisions. In criminal cases, it may designate the capacity to comprehend legal proceedings and communicate with an attorney, or to understand and waive certain rights, such as the right to remain silent.

In all of these situations, the state may intervene to ensure that a person is capable of performing the required tasks. More significantly, if the state determines the person is incompetent, it may deprive him or her of liberty, property or the option to act. In the illustrative civil situations noted above, the incompetent person may be prohibited from making a contract or will or unable to have it implemented, required to surrender control of financial or personal affairs to a guardian, or subjected to civil commitment. In the noted criminal-law situations, the person found incompetent may be forcibly treated, in a hospital or elsewhere, for the purpose of "restoring" competency to undergo legal proceedings and make waiver decisions; in the meantime he or she will be prevented from obtaining adjudication of the pending charges.

The primary justification for these types of interventions stems from this society's preference for autonomy—the freedom to make and act upon one's decisions. We value autonomy because we assume people are ordinarily the best judges of their own interests and because, even if they are not, taking away their opportunity to decide would show insufficient respect for the person. Because of this preference for autonomy, we generally allow individuals considerable latitude when engaging in behavior that is not directly harmful to others. But when a person appears to lack autonomy, either because of externally imposed coercion or—more relevant to this book—"internal" causes, we are less likely to respect his or her choices, even if they affect no one else. Because these people are not deemed to be able to function or to make decisions in their own best interests, we are more willing to override their decisions even if doing so will make them feel degraded or minimized. At the least, many would argue, the state's parens patriae power—its power to act as parent for disabled citizens—authorizes interfering with an incompetent person when harm to self would otherwise result and the intervention will not itself cause harm.[a] Beyond this, there may even be an affirmative *duty* to intervene under such circumstances.

To take an extreme example, suppose a man is unable to control his bodily movements and is unable to speak. When asked a question, his head might nod "yes" or "no" completely randomly. Most would agree that taking some important action—say, giving or withholding experimental but potentially life-saving treatment—based on such a nod would be improper. There is no necessary correlation between the nod and the person's "true" desires. Indeed, the nod is not really a "choice" in any sense of the word; acting on it could be viewed as an insult to him. Therefore, consistent with the autonomy preference, the state is justified in attempting to enable him to respond in a meaningful fashion and, if that fails, in making the decision for him if a decision is necessary.

a. See discussion of the parens patriae power at pp. 651–669.

A second possible justification for refusing to honor the man's "decision" and allowing government intervention under these circumstances is more general in nature. Not only would acting on a random nod be insulting to the individual; it would also make a mockery of the concept of autonomy itself. It would suggest that society sanctions random decisionmaking. Thus, ensuring competency of the individual protects not only his or her interests but those of society at large.

The central issue addressed in this chapter is the extent to which the state may intervene to further these interests when a person who is allegedly mentally disabled wants to, is asked to, or is required to perform a particular task. Although it will allude to a number of such tasks, this chapter will focus on management of essential survival chores, making treatment decisions, assisting counsel at trial, and waiving constitutional rights. Before looking at these issues, we will look more closely at the competency notion.

II.   GENERAL CONSIDERATIONS

TEST CASES

In the following four cases, the subjects were found incompetent. Reflect on whether you agree as you read the following materials.

Case 1.   Mr. B, a 43 year-old man, has long-standing glaucoma in both eyes. In one eye, vision remains only for motion. In the other eye, vision is better, though poorly controlled by medication. Mr. B's ophthalmologist has proposed a drainage procedure for the second eye which has a high chance of improving his vision for several months (at which time it could be undertaken again) and a negligible chance of damaging the eye. Although Mr. B expresses concern about the pressure in his eye and is fearful of going blind, he refuses the drainage procedure, explaining that his "voices" would be "angry with him" if he underwent the procedure. When his reasons for refusal are explored further, he notes that his mother had a similar drainage procedure which had not been helpful. He then discusses his attachment to his mother, stating that he feels that whatever happened to his mother will also happen to him.[b]

Case 2.   Ms. N. is 72 years old and is presently in the intensive care unit of General Hospital in Nashville, Tenn., because of gangrenous condition in her two feet. Doctors estimate that the probability of her surviving without amputation of the feet is 5 to 10% and the probability of survival after amputation is about 50%, with possible severe psychotic results. Ms. N. refuses to consent to the amputation or consider the possibility that it is necessary to

---

b. This case is adapted from Appelbaum & Roth, "Clinical Issues in the Assessment of Competency," 138 Am.J. Psychiat. 1462, 1464 (1981). The authors conclude that the patient was "apparently incompetent", thus permitting doctors to override the refusal.

save her life. She feels very strongly that her physical condition is improving and that she will recover without the necessity of surgery. When asked if she would prefer to die rather than lose her feet, she answered "possibly." The flesh on her feet is black, shriveled, rotting, and stinking; she believes their appearance is a result of soot or dirt.[c]

Case 3. Ms. K. dies, leaving only $1.00 of a sizeable estate to her only child, Ms. R., with the rest going to a church. Testimony at a will contest proceeding reveals that, when asked why she wanted to distribute her estate in this way, Ms. K. stated that she had not gotten along well with R., that while living with the R.s she had been required to do things which she did not want to do, that Mr. R. had made a derogatory remark concerning Germans (K. was of German descent), that the R.s were lacking in religious spirit, and that Ms. R. had tried to kill her by putting glass in her pudding. She also stated that she (Ms. K.) had failed to contribute enough in support of the church. Independent evidence disclosed that the daughter had prepared the pudding with the glass in it but that the glass was there accidentally. Furthermore, Ms. K. had been assured by many people that such was the case, but she persisted in believing that her daughter had wanted to harm her.[d]

Case 4. Mr. F., diagnosed as suffering from manic-depressive psychosis, began to emerge from the depressed phase in August. Previously frugal and cautious, he began driving at high speeds, to be sexually more active with his wife and to discuss the purchase of land for development. In September, against the advice of his lawyer, he contracted for land in the Catskills and talked about erecting a 400 room hotel with a marina and golf course. On September 23, he signed another contract—after his lawyer counseled against it and withdrew from negotiations—to buy more property, on which he planned to erect a drug store and merchandise mart. Under this contract, title was not to change hands until October 20. Within two weeks of signing the contract, he arranged for a title search, giving correct details concerning the property and price, and asked that the search be completed within a week. He also persuaded a former employee to join in the enterprise, promising him a salary and a Lincoln Continental when the project was complete, had a sign erected on the premises stating that F. Drug Company and merchandise mart were coming soon, hired an architect, initiated a mortgage application, hired laborers to begin digging, filed plans with city officials, and went to Albany to obtain

c. These facts are taken from State Dept. Human Services v. Northern, 563 S.W.2d 197 (Tenn.App.1978), where the court authorized amputation of Ms. Northern's foot if her condition "has developed to such a critical stage as to demand immediate amputation to save her life." Ms. Northern died in 1978 as a result of a clot from gangrenous tissue; the surgery was never performed because of complications rendering it more dangerous.

d. The case is based on In re Klein's Estate, 28 Wash.2d 456, 183 P.2d 518 (1947), in which the court declared Ms. Klein's will void.

the necessary approval for building. He also went to a psychiatrist to get help for his wife, who he stated was trying to stop his activities. This psychiatrist saw him on three subsequent occasions. On October 8th Mr. F. was hospitalized after purchasing a hunting gun, with all doctors agreeing on a diagnosis of manic-depressive psychosis.[e]

DUNCAN KENNEDY, DISTRIBUTIVE AND PATERNALISTIC MOTIVES IN CONTRACT AND TORT LAW, WITH SPECIAL REFERENCE TO COMPULSORY TERMS AND UNEQUAL BARGAINING POWER

41 Md.L.Rev., 563, 642–646.
(1982).

The principled anti-paternalist admits readily that one sometimes has to overrule another's choice in his best interest, but argues that those cases are explained by incapacity, or perhaps by another similar principled exception to the general idea that people are autonomous. (Likewise, the principled paternalist will argue that there are some cases in which people should be allowed to choose on their own—the two positions are indistinguishable for the purposes of my argument here.) . . .

The idea of incapacity will *sometimes* help in explaining the actor's decision to intervene. Sometimes one feels that the other has really and truly lost selfhood, become a walking automaton or disintegrated, so that someone has simply to take care of them, make decisions for them, control their lives. As the actor, you have to worry that you will make bad custodial decisions, but not that you will be criticized for intervening at all. But those are extreme cases, and the difficulties with paternalism arise in situations where you have occasion to act without being able to appeal to any such blanket permission as is afforded by the other being just crazy.

* * *

The problem with the notion of capacity in [the more typical] setting is not that it's positively wrong—just that it doesn't help. The strategy is to divide the decision into two parts, hoping that will make it easier than if the question whether to act is treated as a single whole. First, we try to decide whether the other possesses a trait or quality called "ability to determine her own best interests." If she does, we accede to her wishes even if in that particular case we are convinced that her action is not in her best interests. If it were truly easier to decide the presence or absence of the quality of capacity than to decide on balance whether we should intervene, treating that question all together, then capacity would be useful. But the question of capacity is

e. This case is based on Faber v. Sweet Style Mfg. Corp., 40 Misc.2d 212, 242 N.Y.S.2d 763 (1963), in which the court voided Faber's second contract on the ground of incompetency.

hopelessly intertwined with the question of what the other wants to do in this particular case.

First, there is no such "thing" as capacity, and there can be no such thing as its "absence" either. We ask the question of capacity already oriented to the further question whether we will have to let the person do something injurious to herself. There is no other reason to ask the question. Now if you ask me to *answer* the question without knowing what the potentially injurious thing is, it seems to me I should refuse. I don't believe that capacity exists except as capacity-to-make-this-decision. But as soon as I am deciding the issue of capacity-to-make-this decision, I find myself considering all the factors, testing my intuition of the other's false consciousness, the severity of the consequences, the possibility that I want to render the other dependent through paternalism, just as I would if I frankly admitted at the beginning that it's just a big mess, with no principled way to find your way through.

I come back to ad hoc paternalism, by which I mean that in fear and trembling you approach each case determined to act if that's the best thing to do, recognizing that influencing another's choice—another's life—in the wrong direction, or so as to reinforce their condition of dependence, is a crime against them. Of course, I haven't proved the impossibility of a principled anti-paternalist stance. I think I've undermined the idea that we can decide when to act and when not to act through a notion like: "Do not overrule the choice of a person who has the capacity to choose on their own". . . .

* * *

. . . Principled anti-paternalism is a defense mechanism. One way to deal with the pain and fear of having to make an ad hoc paternalist decision—one way to deny the pain and fear—is to claim that you "had" to do what you did because principle (say, the principle of incapacity) required it. That the principle doesn't really work is less important than that it anesthetizes. . . .

The following selections are more optimistic about our ability to define competency independently of the decision to be made. Although they focus on competency to make treatment decisions, they may well be relevant to competency in other contexts as well.

PAUL APPELBAUM & LOREN ROTH, COMPETENCY
TO CONSENT TO RESEARCH: A PSYCHIATRIC
OVERVIEW

39 Arch.Gen.Psychiat. 951, 952–56.
(1982).

* * *

EVIDENCING A CHOICE

The least rigorous standard for competency . . . is the subject's actual communication of a decision as to his participation in the proposed project. This requirement has been phrased as demanding that the subject "manifest his consent" or "express a positive interest in taking part".

* * *

To the uninitiated, operationalizing the requirement that the subject evidence a choice may seem a trivial exercise; in most instances one need only ask the subject whether or not he desires to participate. There are occasions, however, in which the communication from the subject will be so ambiguous as to raise serious questions about whether or not consent has occurred. These include cases in which the subject's verbal and behavioral responses diverge (for example, when a subject declines to participate in a study requiring venipuncture, then rolls up his sleeve and holds out his arm to the experimenter).

* * *

FACTUAL UNDERSTANDING OF THE ISSUES

The subject's understanding of the issues relevant to participation is the single factor that has been most widely accepted as a standard for competency. A typical formulation requires that the subject have "the cognitive capacity to consider the relevant issues". Those areas that have been considered to be crucial for the subject to understand include "the nature of the procedure, its risks, and other relevant information," "the nature and likelihood of success of the proposed treatment and . . . of its risks and side-effects," "the available options, their advantages and disadvantages," "the knowledge that he has a choice to make," "who he is, where he is, what he is reading and what he is doing in signing the paper," and "the consequences of participation or non-participation."

* * *

The rigor of the requirement of understanding obviously increases with the amount and complexity of material that is required to be understood. Some writers make understanding the sine qua non of their standard of competency, and it has long been the primary element of legal tests of contractual and testamentary capacity.

"Factual understanding" actually encompasses two different standards: one can require, as many writers do, that the subject have the "ability to understand," or more strictly, one can insist that the subject manifest "actual understanding" of the material.

* * *

Means of demonstrating a subject's actual understanding of issues related to his decision include, in increasing order of difficulty, asking him to repeat the information provided, asking him to paraphrase it in his own words, and requiring that he display an ability to put some or all of the information to practical use. One difficulty in testing understanding of the consequences of a decision (often conceptualized as the risks and benefits) is the possibility of divergence between what the investigator perceives as a benefit or a risk and the subject's view of the matter. Consequences of participation, such as prolonged hospitalization, which are often thought of as a disadvantage, might seem quite desirable to a socially isolated or otherwise impoverished subject.

RATIONAL MANIPULATION OF INFORMATION

One step beyond measuring factual understanding is determining how the information that the subject assimilates is utilized in the decision-making process. The rubrics by which this standard is discussed include judgment, rationality, rational weighing of risks and benefits, reality testing, and decision-making capacity. Legal rules concerning contractual and testimonial capacity traditionally have recognized at least one defect of rationality, the presence of "insane delusions," as grounds for invalidating a person's acts.

* * *

The subjective nature of any assessment of rationality frequently has been pointed to as a major obstacle to the successful use of such a test. But an even greater problem may lie in the consensus of most experts today that an impairment of rationality does not necessarily affect global decision-making ability, that is, that the impact of delusions, for example, may be limited to a discrete area of mental functioning. Although this belief awaits definitive empirical verification, it indicates the possible utility of a test of rationality directed to the specific decision at hand rather than to the person's general functioning.

* * *

APPRECIATION OF THE NATURE OF THE SITUATION

The strictest standard for competency requires that, once understanding has been attained, the rational manipulation of information take place in the context of the subject's appreciation of the nature of his situation.

Appreciation is distinct from factual understanding in that it requires the subject to consider the relevance to his immediate situation of those facts he has understood previously in the abstract. It differs from the rational manipulation of information by requiring that the subject take certain crucial data into consideration, rather than merely asking him to manipulate rationally whatever information is already at hand. This has been phrased in a variety of ways, asking that the subject "appreciate the consequences of giving or withholding consent," have "a sense of who he is and why he is agreeing," recognize, "in a mature fashion, the implications of alternative courses of action and appreciate both cognitively and affectively the nature of the thing to be decided," or "appreciate what is relevant to forming a judgment of the issue in question—i.e., ... consider relevant evidence."

* * *

Whether the extent of the subject's appreciation needs to coincide precisely with the investigator's is a controversial topic. Some commentators have suggested that, in a therapeutic setting, the patient need only "understand the nature of the mental condition which the psychiatrist believes him to have," without necessarily agreeing with that judgment. Such a standard, however, more closely resembles a factual-understanding test than a genuine test of appreciation. Although some people may be uncomfortable with such a criterion, of necessity the subject's views (e.g., on the presence or absence of illness or the results of accepting or refusing participation) ultimately must be measured by their correspondence with the consensus of knowledgeable (usually professional) opinion on those issues.

Choosing the Standard

Despite wide variation in the wording of many attempts to define the standards for competency, they appear, as was just shown, to be classifiable into four general categories. Rather than deriving a single standard for competency from this discussion of the relevant mental functions and the psychopathologic states that may impair them, one is left with a range of testable functions that, depending on where the line is drawn, can yield multiple standards for competency of varying stringency. Furthermore, it is clear from this approach that any of the four resulting standards, or some combination of them, are "legitimate" as long as they can be justified from some reasonable policy perspective.

ELYN SAKS, COMPETENCY TO MAKE PSYCHIATRIC TREATMENT DECISIONS
(Forthcoming).

[There are] three criteria that any adequate competency standard must meet. First, the standard must faithfully identify those abilities that are intuitively necessary to making decisions (I shall call this criterion the "abilities" criterion). For instance, an ability to understand what one is deciding is probably necessary to making competent decisions. Is an ability to reason also necessary? And what about the ability to know one's true needs and values? Of course the standard will not require all of the abilities that the ideal decisionmaker exercises, for the case *is* ideal. Yet *some* of these abilities are necessary to making any decision, and it is part of the job of a competency standard to help us decide which ones are necessary, and which are not.

The second criterion (the "unconventionality" criterion) requires that a competency standard protect the expression of personal values and beliefs, however unconventional, since one important purpose of competency doctrine is to allow people to pursue their interests according to their own lights. This criterion limits the range and level of abilities we can require under the "abilities" criterion, warning us that even "ideal" decisionmaking may simply be a product of convention. Indeed, we cannot require even the beliefs (still less the desires) of the ideal decisionmaker unless we can show them to be knowably correct. Freedom to decide, in other words, includes freedom to decide what is true no less than what is good.

The third criterion (the "irrationality" criterion) requires that a competency standard designate a reasonably small class of individuals as incompetent in the face of the pervasive influence of the irrational and the unconscious. Indeed, if any person in whose decisionmaking irrational processes were shown to be present were deemed incompetent, then there would be virtually *no* competent decisionmakers to be found; psychiatrists and psychologists have convincingly demonstrated the ever-present influence of primitive hopes, wishes, and fears on the mental lives of us all. Thus, irrational processes may hopelessly compromise certain types of mental function that we posit in the ideal case. An apparently intact reasoner, for example, may choose a treatment because of fantasies of merger with the doctor/parent, or, less fancifully perhaps, because he overvalues a vivid memory. Like the "unconventionality" criterion, the "irrationality" criterion limits the reach of the "abilities" criterion because many abilities inextricably implicate irrationality.

* * *

. . . [These criteria] enable us to replace our vague, inchoate notion of competency with a more rigorously-formulated standard—a standard that is nonetheless true to our pre-reflective convictions. Two very simple competency standards will show us the criteria at work.

According to the first standard, a person is competent if her decision merely "evidences a choice." This standard does not require particular beliefs and values on the part of the patient, and so it avoids trenching on the expression of unconventional beliefs and values. Similarly, the standard does not require rationality, so that the pervasive irrationality of decisionmaking is unproblematic. While the standard thus meets the "unconventionality" and "irrationality" criteria, it squarely violates the "abilities" criterion. Two-year-olds, after all, can say "yes" and "no," yet we need not honor their choices. What further abilities competency requires—and why—will concern us below, but the simple capacity to evince some choice is clearly not enough.

A second proposed competency standard suffers from precisely the opposite problem. This standard deems a person competent only if he makes a reasonable decision. A "reasonable result" standard selects people who are quite likely to have adequate decisionmaking abilities. At least they have shown themselves able to make this particular decision—by definition their choice is good. But while the standard may effectively meet the "abilities" criterion, it plainly violates the "unconventionality" and "irrationality" criteria. To require a reasonable outcome is to bar the expression of idiosyncratic preference and goals, and to require an integrity of the reasoning process that many may lack. Thus the second standard must fail: requiring people to live according to someone else's conception of the good completely frustrates the purposes of competency doctrine.

For very different reasons, then, these two preliminary standards fail to meet the three criteria for an adequate standard of competency. We would do better to focus on the kinds of abilities that, on the face of it, are necessary to adequate decisionmaking—e.g. understanding and reasoning. . . .

A. The "Pure Understanding" View

The first standard—the "pure understanding" standard—deems a person competent if he can assimilate the information that the caregiver provides. "Understanding" in this sense is nothing more than comprehension; the patient need neither accept nor believe the information in order to be competent. . . . The "pure understanding" view finds patients incompetent who have organic deficits that prevent them from grasping the meaning of what is said, who are too disorganized or agitated to attend to information or to communicate understanding, or who are unable to retain information for even a short period of time.

The "pure understanding" view has the clear advantage of meeting the "unconventionality" and "irrationality" criteria without qualification. It gives full scope to unconventionality. Indeed, it allows patients to express not only unconventional desires, but also unconventional beliefs: it makes no inquiry into the truth of their beliefs. Moreover, the "pure understanding" view incapacitates only a relatively small group of patients. Because it in no way requires rationality, defending its cutoff point in the face of pervasive irrationality is unproblematic.

Although the "pure understanding" view meets the "unconventionality" and "irrationality" criteria, it fails to meet the "abilities" criterion. While *comprehending* information is clearly necessary to decisionmaking—imagine being asked to make a decision described in a foreign language—comprehension alone is not enough. Unless one credits the theory to some degree, the comprehension is pointless. . . . We want decisionmakers at least to *consider* the information provided—requiring actual belief may unnecessarily infringe on the "abilities" criterion— because making a decision in one's best interests requires knowing how those interests are likely to be affected, and the information may well supply that knowledge.

B. The "Modified Understanding" View

The second competency standard, the "modified understanding" view, attempts to remedy the shortcomings of the "pure understanding" view, while largely retaining its advantages. In its most prevalent form, the "modified understanding" view says that, to be competent, the patient must comprehend the information that the doctor provides, and must also believe that the *doctor* believes it. This theory does seem to put the patient in an adequate position to make a decision, and thus to meet the challenge of the "abilities" criterion. To recognize that the doctor believes the information is at least to have an incentive to *consider* it; our society regards doctors as possessing some knowledge about health. The "modified understanding" view also seems to satisfy the "unconventionality" and "irrationality" criteria. Because it requires only one, fairly uncontroversial belief, it infringes on the decisionmaker's freedom to believe to only a small degree. In addition, it requires little in the way of rationality.

The "modified understanding" view, however, is finally untenable. . . . [W]hile belief that information is worth considering is necessary for and prior to belief that it is true, it does not go far enough; one must also be able to come to acceptable beliefs about its truth. Decisions, after all, are made on the basis of beliefs and values, so that it is what one *believes,* not what one *considers* believing, that essentially determines one's decisions. . . .

C. The "Understanding and Belief" Views

Unlike the "modified understanding" view, "understanding and belief" theories require that the decisionmaker have the ability to assess all evidence relevant to her decision. These theories exist in more naive and less naive forms. According to the more naive version, a person is competent if she not only comprehends the information that the caregiver provides, but also *believes* the information. This theory is naive to the extent that it assumes that caregivers can discern the truth—truth, especially medical truth, is most elusive. It is also naive to reason that the doctor's version of the truth is the best we have, and so must be believed. Absent clear criteria for truth, it is for each person to determine whose "truth" is real: that is one of the points of the "unconventionality" criterion. The naive theory also conflicts with the "irrationality" criterion insofar as it identifies a large class as incompetent because their beliefs deviate in a minor way from the "received" position—perhaps, indeed, because they are subject to the influence of the irrational.

Sophisticated "understanding and belief" theories are more skeptical about authoritative versions of the truth, requiring a decisionmaker only to comprehend the caregiver's information and to form no patently false beliefs about the material elements of the information. For example, while a naive "understanding and belief" view requires the patient to believe that a treatment will help when her doctor holds the same belief, a sophisticated "understanding and belief" view requires only that the patient avoid patently false beliefs about the treatment— that, for example, it will cause a nuclear explosion. The law's predominant competency test is a sophisticated "understanding and belief" theory of this kind, which characterizes as "delusional" those beliefs that are so patently false that those who hold them must have suffered a severe breakdown of their ability to assess evidence. The concept of a delusion is the law's answer to the concerns of the "unconventionality" and "irrationality" criteria; because only patently false beliefs vitiate capacity, the conflict with the "unconventionality" criterion is minimal; because only patent irrationality disqualifies the patient, the conflict with the "irrationality" criterion is minimal as well.

Some conflict remains, however. The "understanding and belief" view does limit what one may believe (in a way it does not limit what one may desire), and so threatens to trench on merely unconventional behavior. The limitation makes sense, however: unless one's belief in some way conforms to the world, it represents a failed attempt to describe the world. By contrast, one is entitled to choose values and desires without constraint because values and desires are neither objectively right nor objectively wrong in a straightforward way; to value something unpopular is not to hold a false value, whereas to believe that the moon is made of green cheese is to hold a false belief. Placing limits on what one can believe is also reasonable because medical treatment decisions take effect in the world. Since the point of a treatment decision is to achieve the best adaptation of one's desires and values to the world, the decisionmaker must have some *grasp* of the world. Thus, some tension between the "abilities" criterion and the "unconventionality" criterion is inevitable.

D. The "Full Reasoning" View

Another competency standard, the "full reasoning" view, demands a level of reasoning ability greater than the capacity to assess evidence that the "understanding and belief" view requires. . . .

The "full reasoning" view is untenable because it inevitably produces "unconventionality" and "irrationality" problems, and is not clearly warranted by the "abilities" criterion. . . .

First, fully intact reasoning may not be necessary for adequate decisionmaking, just as, for example, speaking with a good accent is not necessary for basic communication in a foreign language (compare knowing rudimentary vocabulary and syntax). Second, what qualities of reasoning are "good" may be open to dispute (just as linguists disagree over the appropriate accent for a dead language). In short, the "abilities criterion" does not clearly require good reasoning. And if the nature of good reasoning is controversial, to require some particular form of reasoning is to discriminate against deviancy, and so to violate the "unconventionality" criterion.

The "full reasoning" view also raises acute "irrationality" problems. Even generally effective decisionmakers accord undue weight to vivid examples, misuse statistics, and misunderstand probabilities. They may also be profoundly affected by irrational and unconscious factors. If, as under the "full reasoning" view, less than patent irrationality makes one incompetent, then most, if not all, people are incompetent, because people's reasoning is invaded to some degree by irrational processes. This result is clearly untenable, and so we must reject the "full reasoning" view.

Our investigations have revealed that the "pure" and "modified understanding" views fail to equip the patient adequately to make decisions, while the "full reasoning" view requires a facility in reasoning that few, if any, achieve. Of "understanding and belief" views, sophisticated versions . . . are the most satisfactory. It seems reasonable to focus on a severe inability to assess evidence . . . because decisions take effect in the world: Gross misconceptions about the world are likely to impair the quality of decisionmaking.

* * *

[Thus, a] concept of treatment competency that is consistent with settled law and adequate to the philosophical problems posed by the "unconventionality" and "irrationality" criteria will make use of the concept of a delusion to remedy that gap. Put simply, treatment competency will require comprehension of the treatment information, along with an absence of delusions, or patently unsupported beliefs, about the matters covered by that information.

Questions and Comments

1. *Levels of competency.* Appelbaum and Roth contend that competency tests can be divided into four categories. Saks, on the other hand, discerns at least six. Between the two excerpts, how many distinct competency tests are put forward? Can you rank them in ascending order of "competency"? Or are they not comparable?

2. *Varying competency with the choice to be made.* Many commentators have argued that differing levels of competency should be required depending upon the decision being made. For instance, Appelbaum and Roth, in the above excerpt, state that "any of the four categories of [standards], or some combination of them, are 'legitimate' as long as they can be justified from some reasonable policy perspective." This idea is expanded upon in Roth, Meisel & Lidz, "Tests of Competency to Consent to Treatment," 134 Am.J. Psychiat. 279, 283 (1977):

> When there is a favorable risk/benefit ratio to the proposed treatment in the opinion of the person determining competency and the patient consents to the treatment, there does not seem to be any reason to stand in the way of administering treatment. To accomplish this, a test employing a low threshold of competency may be applied to find even a marginal patient competent so that his or her decision may be honored. This is what happens daily when uncomprehending patients are permitted to sign themselves into the hospital. Similarly, when the risk/benefit ratio is favorable and the patient refuses treatment, a test employing a higher threshold of competency may be applied. Under such a test even a somewhat knowledgeable patient may be found incompetent so that consent may be sought from a substitute decision maker and treatment administered despite the patient's refusal. An example would be the patient withdrawing from alcohol who,

although intermittently resistive, is nevertheless administered sedative medication. In both of these cases, in which the risk/benefit ratio is favorable, the bias of physicians, other health professionals, and judges is usually skewed toward providing treatment. Therefore, a test of competency is applied that will permit the treatment to be administered irrespective of the patient's actual or potential understanding.

However, there is a growing reluctance on the part of our society to permit patients to undergo treatments that are extremely risky or for which the benefits are highly speculative. Thus if the risk/benefit ratio is unfavorable or questionable and the patient refuses treatment, a test employing a low threshold of competency may be selected so that the patient will be found competent and his or her refusal honored. This is what happens in the area of sterilization of mentally retarded people, in which at least from the perspective of the retarded individual, the risk/benefit ratio is questionable. On the other hand, when the risk/benefit ratio is unfavorable or questionable and the patient consents to treatment, a test using a higher threshold of competency may be applied preventing even some fairly knowledgeable patients from undergoing treatment. The judicial opinion in the well-known Kaimowitz psychosurgery case delineated a high test of competency to be employed in that experimental setting.

Drane offers a similar proposal. He states that for "medical decisions that are not dangerous and are objectively in the patient's best interests" all that is required is awareness "in the sense of being in contact with one's situation" and assent. A higher level of competency should be required for situations in which "the diagnosis is doubtful, or the condition chronic", where "diagnosis is certain but the treatment is more dangerous or not quite so effective" or where "there are alternative treatments, or no treatment at all is an alternative". Here the person "must be able to understand the risks and outcomes of the different options and then be able to make a decision based on this understanding." Finally, "for those treatment decisions that are very dangerous" (that is, where "the decision involves not a balancing of what are widely recognized as reasonable alternatives or a reasonable response to a doubtful diagnosis, but a choice that seems to violate reasonableness"), the person must "appreciate what he or she is doing" and "the implications of the medical information for his or her life," a standard which contemplates "an understanding that is both technical and personal, intellectual and emotional." Drane, "The Many Faces of Competency," 15 The Hastings Cent. Rep. No. 2, 17, 18–19 (April, 1985). See also, Schwartz & Blank, "Shifting Competency During Hospitalization: A Model for Informed Consent Decisions," 37 Hosp. & Comm. Psychiat. 1256 (1986).

While these comments pertain to competency to make treatment decisions, similar contentions have been made about other contexts. For instance, it is often said that the level of competency necessary to enter into a contract is greater than the level needed to make a will, see, e.g., *McPheters v. Hapke*, 94 Idaho 744, 497 P.2d 1045 (1972), and that pleading guilty requires more capacity than does going to trial. See, e.g., *Sieling v. Eyman*, 478 F.2d 211 (9th Cir.1973). These statements could be interpreted to mean merely that making a contract or pleading guilty requires understanding more facts, or facts that are more complicated, than does making a will or going to trial (where most decisions will be made by a lawyer). But in context the courts that make these statements appear to be recognizing different *levels* of competency for different types of decisions. Thus, if one followed the courts' suggestion, factual understanding might be sufficient to be competent to stand trial or write a valid will, while full "appreciation" of the situation might be required to plead guilty or make a contract.

Saks disagrees with the "different levels" thesis. She argues that one standard—the understanding and belief standard—should apply to all situations.

> All competency areas encompass decisions ranging from very important to trivial, so that ranking competency areas as generally more or less consequential is extremely difficult. For example, a medical decision may prevent the immediate death of a young, otherwise healthy person, or it may provide relief from a minor headache. A will may dispose of the vast estate of a person whose family is in dire need, or the small estate of a person who has one wealthy, remote relative. And a trial decision may lead to either the death penalty or a day in jail. Because of this, to say that will-making as an area is less important than other competency areas—in particular, than the area of treatment choice—is impermissible, even though will-making involves interests of people other than the testator (he may care for them more than for himself, as it were), and even though it involves only property. The plain fact is that we cannot decide whether liberty, health, or property is more important without knowing how much of each, and with what further consequences: an abstract ranking is simply not possible.

> * * *

> Indeed, if varying the level of competency based on the importance of decisions made sense, a competency theorist might urge us to *lower* the level of competency for potentially consequential decisions. Because people care more about more consequential decisions, we should arguably permit them to choose what they will have to live with. Moreover, taking away consequential decisions may entail a greater assault on individual dignity. For example, telling a person that he can decide what kind of ice cream to have, but not where to live, may more seriously injure his self-esteem. Such a theory, indeed, seems already to inform some areas of the law. For example, some states permit minors to accept or to reject psychiatric treatment without regard to their competency, presumably because the decision is so important. In short, if varying levels of competency is acceptable at all, *lowering* the level of competency for crucial decisions would be most in the spirit of competency doctrine.

With whom do you agree? Under Saks' approach, could we allow voluntary admissions of non-protesting persons (discussed at pp. 751–755)? Should a person be able to consent to extremely experimental and life-threatening treatment if he or she is only able to meet Saks' understanding and belief test? Under the approach advocated by Roth, Meisel and Lidz, who should make the decision as to whether a treatment is "favorable", "questionable" or "dangerous"? Once that decision is made, do you agree with Drane's proposal as to the competency level that should be required for the treatment in question? Should there be differing levels of competency with respect to the *same* treatment, depending upon whether the person is refusing or consenting, as Roth, Meisel and Lidz suggest?

3. *Other possible competency tests.* All of the tests discussed above are essentially cognitive in orientation. Traditionally, competency has been conceptualized as a matter of awareness, understanding, and reasoning ability. But competency can be viewed from other perspectives as well. Two other approaches are worth mentioning.

Volitional Test. Analogous to some versions of the insanity defense, one could require not only a minimal level of cognitive functioning but also a demonstration that the choice being made is "voluntary." Although assessing whether a choice is or is not an exercise of "free will" is problematic conceptually,[f] the rationale for requiring a volitional inquiry is straightforward: a person is not acting autonomously if his or her choices are "compelled." For instance, a severely depressed, suicidal person confronted with various treatment options may understand all of them but find it very difficult to resist choosing the most dangerous treatment, even though the remaining treatments are just as effective. Roth, Meisel and Lidz report the following case: "A 49 year-old woman whose understanding of treatment was otherwise intact, when informed that there was a 1 in 3,000 chance of dying from ECT, replied, " 'I hope I am the one.' " Roth, Meisel & Lidz, supra at 282. Should such a person be considered competent to make this treatment decision?

Different Person Test. A second approach is described and critiqued by Saks, supra.

> The "different person" theory rationalizes our intuition that mentally ill choices are incompetent by focusing on the change in personality that mental illness brings about, and the effects of that change on decisional capacity. The theory holds that a person is incompetent, not if what appear to be her values and beliefs are unacceptable according to some external standard, but rather if they are not *her* values and beliefs, because she has been transformed by mental illness into a "different person." The idea is that the person has lost touch with her own values and ways of looking at the world: she is simply not *herself.* The testamentary capacity cases, with their symbolic notion of testation as representative of the testator's psychic will, at times use language suggestive of this theory, as when they say that a will is not truly the "testator's." The "different person" theory deftly sidesteps the "irrationality" and "unconventionality" criteria; the decisionmaker's irrationality is irrelevant, and her thinking and feeling are not forced into a conventional mold. All that the "different person" theory requires is that the decisionmaker be true to herself.

f. See pp. 516–527 for a discussion of this issue in the context of the insanity defense.

* * *

[The different person theory also finesses the abilities criterion]. . . . [O]n the face of it, the "different person" can himself be quite capable. But the "different person," because he is not the true self, does not know the true self's values and needs, and to that extent *is* incapable of making a decision that expresses those values and needs. Similarly, the "different person" theory responds to the concern that the evaluator may choose among the decisionmaker's competing values when they conflict, thus undermining the purpose of competency doctrine. In truth it is the real self who makes the value choice, which the evaluator simply reflects in his decision. . . .

Mental illness is often described in a way that lends itself to the "different person" theory. For example, a mentally ill person is said to suffer "ego alien" impulses and thoughts, and, on recovery, to return to his "premorbid personality." Sometimes he does not even remember his experiences and, when he does, he may not recognize himself in them: he *feels* as if he was then a different person. The "different person" theory predicts that the recovered psychiatric patient will repudiate the choices and actions of his mentally ill self, and will thank the treatment provider for overriding his refusal and requiring treatment.

On examination, however, this theory is not as compelling as it seems. The problem is that the classic model does not fit all, or even most, mental illness—still less the choices made by its sufferers. Most obviously, some patients never return to their "premorbid" personalities, and so their mentally ill choices *become* authentic. Yet even when their illness is temporary, recovered patients may well not repudiate their past choices and thank their caregivers. Of course, all such patients might be unduly grudging. But it seems far more plausible to suppose that many of their choices are *misidentified* as "mentally ill" choices, or—even though truly "mentally ill"—are not experienced as the choices of a different person.

The essential problem is that determining reliably which choices are "mentally ill" and will later be repudiated is very difficult. . . .

See also, Faden & Beauchamp, A History of Informed Consent 262–269 (1986).

4. *The* Katz *Case.* A case that might help flesh out some of the concepts discussed above is *Katz v. Superior Court,* 73 Cal.App.3d 952, 141 Cal.Rptr. 234 (1977), which involved a guardianship proceeding. The proposed wards were young adults (over the age of majority) who had become members of the Unification Church, headed by Reverend Moon. The parents of these individuals claimed that psychological pressure exerted by the church had impaired the physical and mental health of their children; specifically, it was alleged that the children had experienced "abrupt personality changes," and were the victims "of mind control through hypnosis, mesmerism, and/or brainwashing." 141 Cal.Rptr. at 239 n. 7. The father of one of the children testified that while his daughter was in the church "she became somewhat child-like in her belief and acceptance of this unitary system of beliefs, and her interests were almost totally

devoted to that system of beliefs, to the exclusion of virtually all else." He noted that her voice had changed from being hoarse to high-pitched. He also believed she was being "imposed upon" because she received no compensation outside of minimal food and a place to sleep for her constant work for the church. On cross-examination, he acknowledged that she had looked healthy. Id. at 246.

One of the experts for the parents testified as follows:

It is my opinion that all five of these well-meaning, well-intentioned young people—Jan Kaplan, Leslie Brown, John Hovard, Jacqueline Katz and Barbara Underwood—have several symptoms which are not present in the average individual of their ages and background.

During my interviews with them, it was as though these individuals responded to a pre-set (i.e., there was an effort made to answer all questions out of a limited set of answers). This limited set of answers appeared to be alien or inconsistent with those of their non-cult peers.

They all suffered from gross lack of information regarding current events; they all seemed to be preoccupied with a concern about their selfishness, but all reported that they worked as much as twenty hours a day.

They all showed a moderate degree of memory impairment, especially about their childhoods; their functional vocabulary in terms of the words that they used during the interview was limited and constricted.

Their affects were blunted, emotionality frozen in a child-like inappropriate smile to all input, whether it be hostile or otherwise.

They were all wide-eyed, had short attention spans and a decreased ability towards abstractions; they were full of inconsistencies, contradictions and confabulations when pressured.

They uniformly held that the Unification Church was not responsible for anything unless it was positive.

They had very little concern for previous and future personal goals; they were paranoid about previous relationships, and had defensive attitudes toward id urges.

Their inner sense of authority was lost, and all responded as if they were influenced by an outside authority.

They all showed various degrees of regression and child-like attitudes, especially when stressed.

In general, they did not respond as one would expect from their background and personality types.

The expert did not diagnose any of them psychotic nor did he give them any other standard psychiatric diagnosis, but he did predict that staying in the church environment for the next six months would not be in the best interests of their health. Id. at 248–49.

The children testified at trial, and described their beliefs. They stated that their mode of living was one they had chosen to follow. They denied any coercive persuasion and pointed out that there was no physical restraint involved. One member of the group had left the church, but returned after four days of reflection. They "insisted on their competency". Id. at 250. They also introduced expert testimony which asserted that "the experiences relied upon by the parents' experts were no more than usually accompany devotion to a religious belief." Id. at 250.

Assume the issue is whether the children's decision to stay with the Unification Church was a competent one.[g] What if Saks' "understanding and belief" test were applied to the *Katz* facts? The different person theory? A competency test which recognized a volitional component? One of the standards described by Roth, et al.? Should the fact that religious preferences are involved raise the level of incompetency required before state intervention may take place? Should the fact that the parents only wanted the children to go through a "deprogramming" session after which they would be free to return to the church lower the level of incompetency required for intervention?

III. GUARDIANSHIP

A. HISTORY AND DEVELOPMENT

SAMUEL BRAKEL, JOHN PARRY AND BARBARA WEINER, THE MENTALLY DISABLED AND THE LAW

Chicago, American Bar Foundation, 3d ed. pp. 369–370.
(1985).

Incompetency proceedings are of a much earlier origin than hospitalization proceedings. For example, in Rome in the first century B.C., elaborate provisions were made for the protection of the property of the mentally disabled, while none at all existed for their person. This pattern was followed in England and also in colonial America, where several of the colonies passed legislation designed to protect the estates of "insane persons" long before the colonial governments became concerned with the personal welfare of the mentally disabled.

No institution for the care of the mentally disabled existed in England until long after the Norman Conquest. Guardianship of the mentally disabled in medieval England was the function of the lord of the manor, who was charged with protecting their proprietary and personal interests. This guardianship actually applied to both the person and the property of the insane, but the chief reason for its existence was apparently proprietary, stemming from the desire to prevent the mentally disabled from becoming a public burden or dissipating their assets to the detriment of their heirs.

It would seem that originally this guardianship, or *tutorship* as it was called, was applicable only to mentally deficient persons. By the beginning of the fourteenth century, however, guardianship was ex-

---

g. The court did not frame the issue this way, but rather held that guardianship could be imposed only if the children were "gravely disabled", as defined by California's commitment law. Since there was "no real showing . . . that the [proposed wards] are physically unhealthy, or actually deprived of, or unable to secure food, clothing and shelter," the court denied the petition for guardianship. *Katz* and the standards for guardianship are discussed further in the next section of this chapter.

panded to include mentally ill persons and was formally recognized as a duty of the Crown.

The king's guardianship was exercised through the Lord Chancellor, by virtue of a special commission issued to him by the Crown rather than by the general authority of the chancery court. In exercising the power, the Chancellor held an inquisition to determine the condition of the mentally disabled person and to appoint a committee for his person and property if he was adjudged an "idiot" or a "lunatic." It was the further duty of the chancery court to supervise and control the conduct of such a committee.

In the United States responsibility for incompetents was deemed to be vested in the people. Either by inheritance from the common law or by expressed constitutional and statutory provisions, jurisdiction over the person and property of incompetents was assumed by the courts of equity.

The doctrine of *parens patriae*, which obligates the state to care for the vulnerable and the less fortunate, provides both the primary philosophical justification and the legal basis for our guardianship laws. More recently, the principle that the state should exercise its power against the individual only so far as is absolutely necessary has made the individual circumstances of the ward an important basis for state action. Thus, incompetency and guardianship are often viewed in gradations that attempt to approximate the range of capacities enjoyed by mentally disabled persons.

GARY MELTON, JOHN PETRILA, NORMAN POYTHRESS & CHRISTOPHER SLOBOGIN, PSYCHOLOGICAL EVALUATIONS FOR THE COURTS: A HANDBOOK FOR MENTAL HEALTH PROFESSIONALS AND LAWYERS

(New York: Guilfford Press, 1987).
pp. 246–247.

In some jurisdictions, there are separate provisions for appointment of a guardian of one's person (e.g., with authority over health care decisions, decisions about housing and food) and a guardian of one's estate (e.g., with authority over the making of contracts to sell one's property, management of bank accounts and trusts, and payments of debts). The latter type of guardian is often called a *conservator* or *committee*, although this nomenclature is not consistent across jurisdictions.

In addition to, or instead of this distinction, some jurisdictions also distinguish between *general* (plenary) and *specific* guardianship. As the name implies, in the latter form of guardianship, the guardian's powers are restricted to particular types of decisions. Thus, with respect to guardianship of the person, the guardian may have authority only to make a specific treatment decision (e.g., consent to a specific course of treatment that has been proposed) or "nonroutine" treatment decisions (e.g., consent to any major surgery); the disabled person would remain free to make other health care decisions. Similarly, a disabled person under limited guardianship of the estate might be able to make decisions about the property, except with respect to a particular complicated business deal that has been proposed, or any purchase over $100. On the other hand, under general guardianship, the guardian has total control of the individual's person, estate, or both. Obviously, limited guardianship schemes are more respectful of disabled persons' autonomy. . . .

Beyond these distinctions about the *scope* of guardianship, it is also important to recognize disparate *bases* of guardianship. In most instances, individuals are found, on the basis of particularized evidence, to lack specific or general capacities. They are actually (or *de facto*) incompetent and in need of a guardian to make decisions for them. On the other hand, some people are *presumed* to require a guardian. Regardless of their *de facto* level of competency, they are incompetent in law (*de jure*). For example, even though older minors are often as competent as adults to make decisions of various types, they are *de jure* incompetent for most purposes and, as a result, lack legal authority to act on their own behalf. Even in those instances in which the law permits some minors to make decisions independently, they generally are presumed incompetent until they are able to rebut this presumption. Because there is such a strong legal presumption of minors' incompetency, there usually is no need to adjudicate their need for guardianship. In most cases, there also is no need to determine who the guardian will be. Children are generally subject to the wishes of their "natural" guardians—their parents—who are presumed, in the absence of strong evidence to the contrary, to act in their best interests.

Civilly committed adults may also find themselves presumed incompetent to make many decisions. Civil commitment sometimes carries collateral loss of rights to marry, possess a driver's license, refuse intrusive treatments, manage one's property, and so forth. In such instances, there often is no need to appoint a guardian, in that state statutes provide authority to particular officials to make decisions on behalf of the committed person. . . .

B. THE BASIS FOR INTERVENTION

QUINN ESTATE

54 Pa.D. & C.2d 405 (Phila. County Orphans' Ct. 1971).

SILVERSTEIN, J., December 8, 1971.—By decree dated July 15, 1971, pursuant to petition filed by Manuel Kaufman, Deputy Welfare Commissioner of the City of Philadelphia, a citation issued directed to Kathryn M. Quinn to show cause why she should not be adjudged an incompetent and a guardian of her estate appointed. At the hearing on August 19, 1971, Francis I. Farley, Esquire, appeared on behalf of Kathryn M. Quinn. Kathryn M. Quinn was not present although Mr.

Farley advised the court that he had written Miss Quinn two letters advising her to be present.

Sara Downey, a social worker in the Adult Services Department of Public Welfare, testified that she has visited Miss Quinn, who is 56 years old, once a week since February 1971. That from her observation, there was no heat in the house. The interior of the house is in poor condition. Miss Quinn keeps two dogs and two cats whose leavings cover the floors. Apparently, Miss Quinn makes no attempt to clean up the house. There are roaches and flies in abundance in the house. The plumbing is not operative and Miss Quinn uses a drain in the backyard as a toilet. Trash accumulates in the house and yard. An abatement crew from License and Inspection spent two days cleaning out the house and yard but trash is accumulating again.

Miss Quinn receives a welfare check of $101.60 each month. Frequently, Miss Quinn denies that the check has arrived. Miss Downey has been in touch with the Philadelphia Electric Company which has threatened to terminate service for nonpayment of its bills. The gas company has also threatened to terminate service and advises Miss Downey that Miss Quinn refuses entrance to their meter reader. There are outstanding bills from the telephone, gas and electric companies, as well as Graduate Hospital ($29.00), Wanamaker's ($330.72), water and sewer taxes ($37.28) and real estate taxes ($168.35). Miss Downey testified that from her observation Miss Quinn is incapable of making decisions concerning her day-to-day life. Sometimes she is lucid and at other times she has told Miss Downey that she feels she is living in a nightmare.

Miss Downey stated she had explained the nature of the guardianship proceedings to Miss Quinn, who had only laughed. It was Miss Downey's opinion that Miss Quinn did not understand the nature of the proceedings.

Mrs. John Lannutti, a niece of the alleged incompetent, confirmed Miss Downey's testimony concerning the conditions in which Miss Quinn is living. She stated that when she had visited the house years past, it was always neat and clean. She had not been to the house for two years before her visit in March 1971. That in the intervening period Kathryn Quinn's physical condition had deteriorated markedly.

Dr. Alfred Duncan, a psychiatrist with the Mental Health and Retardation Unit of the City of Philadelphia, testified that he examined Kathryn Quinn at the request of Miss Downey on April 28, 1971. He found no organic deficit and found her general health to be unremarkable. He did, however, reach a diagnosis of residual schizophrenia. He stated that " * * * as one of the characteristics of residual schizophrenia, the likelihood of her being inclined to manage affairs to any degree is small." Dr. Duncan stated that the prognosis was that Miss Quinn's condition was likely to remain static. That she might improve if she would attend a mental health center and take medication, but she refused to do so.

* * *

In considering the evidence and the motion to dismiss, I am aware that the Incompetents' Estates Act of February 28, 1956, P.L. (1955) 1154, 50 P.S. § 3101, et seq., which empowers a court to declare a person mentally incompetent and to place such individual's business affairs in the hands of another for management is "a dangerous statute easily capable of abuse".

The Incompetents' Estates Act, as amended, provides under "Definitions": "(3) 'Incompetent' means a person who, because of mental infirmities of old age, mental illness, mental deficiency, drug addiction or inebriety, is unable to manage his property, or is liable to dissipate it or become the victim of designing persons": 50 P.S. § 3102.

The standard of proof in incompetency proceedings has been repeatedly set forth by the Supreme Court: "Mental capacity and competency are to be presumed and before any person shall be deprived of the right to handle his or her own property and manage his or her own affairs there must be *clear* and *convincing* proof of mental incompetency and such proof must be *preponderating*".

I am satisfied from the testimony that Kathryn Quinn is incompetent as defined in the act.

* * *

The uncontradicted testimony of the wretched conditions in which the alleged incompetent apparently willingly lives and of her personal habits is clear evidence of her inability to manage her own affairs.

For the above reasons, I enter the attached decree.

SUR EXCEPTIONS TO DECREE

KLEIN, ADM. J., March 13, 1972.—It is crystal clear that Kathryn Quinn is an elderly woman, suffering from schizophrenia, who without supervision might soon die of malnutrition and neglect. Judge Silverstein, after a most careful study of the matter, wrote a comprehensive adjudication, in which he reviewed the factual situations and the applicable law and adjudged the respondent incompetent and appointed John L. Steward, Director of the Adult Services Division of the Department of Public Welfare of the City of Philadelphia, guardian of her estate.

Judge Silverstein's order was obviously correct and serves the best interests of this unfortunate woman.

ESTATE OF GALVIN v. GALVIN

112 Ill.App.3d 677, 68 Ill.Dec. 370, 445 N.E.2d 1223.

Appellate Court of Illinois, First District, First Division, 1983.

* * *

GOLDBERG, JUSTICE:

After a hearing, the trial court denied the petition of Mildred Tobias (petitioner) to be appointed guardian of the estate and person of Harold Galvin (respondent). Petitioner appeals.

Petitioner called Dr. William Reotutar, a qualified physician, to testify. The doctor testified he first treated respondent in October of 1980, after respondent had been admitted to St. Anne's Hospital. Respondent was suffering from "advanced multiple arthritis." Also, the respondent had a "cerebral vascular accident" or stroke.

* * *

Respondent was readmitted to the hospital in the fall of 1981 for treatment of his heart, cerebral, and arthritic conditions. The witness diagnosed another stroke and noted that respondent was "a little bit confused at times and was a little bit agitated at times." A psychiatric consultant observed that respondent experienced "some delusions" and "hallucinations." Dr. Reotutar diagnosed the respondent as having "organic brain syndrome" which describes "behavioral disorder due to some degeneration or atrophy of the brain cells." Respondent remained in the hospital for about two months. Respondent is currently under medication for his heart condition. Failure to take the medication as prescribed could endanger his life. While his heart condition is currently stable, the condition is irreversible. Similarly organic brain syndrome is irreversible and progressive. Although the doctor did not know how respondent handled his financial affairs, he believed respondent was disabled and unable to manage his affairs. On cross-examination the doctor testified that the respondent had made some recent improvement. He stated the respondent was "more oriented and more realistic."

Under questioning by the trial judge, respondent testified he owns the three-flat building in which he lives. He occupies the basement apartment with two men, John and Mike. They do not pay rent but respondent does collect rent from the other two apartments. Respondent handles his own financial affairs and has a checking account which currently has a balance of $350. Respondent receives social security of about $550 per month. Respondent did not believe he had a heart condition but he continues to take the medication prescribed by the doctor.

Under adverse examination by counsel for petitioner, the respondent testified he never had a checking account, he invented the snowmobile, at one time he had a pet black widow spider, and he could produce fire by pointing his finger. He also testified that John and Mike sometimes prepare his meals but he can and sometimes does prepare his own meals. He stated he could shop by himself and go to the laundromat with use of his walker and pulling a shopping cart. He testified he was able to take care of himself and did not want a guardian.

During the examination of respondent, the trial judge interrupted the proceedings and stated, "There is no way in God's world that I am going to adjudicate him a disabled person. He is physically suffering from some disability. . . . He is eccentric . . . but there is no way I am going to adjudicate him in need of a guardian. . . . He lives a bizarre, strange life. I might not want to do it, but unless you can make an offer of proof that is going to show me that he does not understand the things he's doing—. He understands."

Thereafter, counsel for petitioner made an oral offer of proof that John and Mike would testify respondent had no concept of time relationship, believed he had been a co-worker with the Shah of Iran, and the men plan to move out of respondent's apartment so that respondent would be left alone. In addition, petitioner's attorney offered to call Lorraine Polinski, cousin of the respondent, for examination. . . . The attorney stated this witness would testify that she had hired an attorney and that "She insisted a will be drawn, naming her as executor of this estate." The witness has recommended to respondent that he go to Oak Forest [Hospital]. Also, the respondent is "constantly" at petitioner's home where she and her mother "take care of" the respondent. In addition . . . the respondent [went] outside without shoes or stockings and wearing only slippers during sub-zero weather. Also, "another neighbor" would testify that when respondent went to the hospital his shopping and other needs were provided by the petitioner. The trial judge refused the offer of proof and denied the petition.

In this court, petitioner contends the decision of the trial court was against the manifest weight of the evidence and petitioner was denied due process because the trial judge abused his discretion and did not allow her to a full opportunity to present her case. We disagree.

A trial court is mandated to adjudicate a person incompetent and appoint a guardian only when the alleged incompetent is "not fully able to manage his person or estate . . .." (Ill.Rev.Stat.1981, ch. 110½, pars. 11a–2, 11a–3.) The pertinent statute applicable to the case before us was amended effective as of September 16, 1979.

* * *

" 'Disabled person' defined. 'Disabled person' means a person 18 years or older who (a) because of mental deterioration or physical incapacity is not fully able to manage his person or estate, or (b) is mentally ill or developmentally disabled and who because of his mental illness or developmental disability is not fully able to manage his person or estate, or (c) because of gambling, idleness, debauchery or excessive use of intoxicants or drugs, so spends or wastes his estate as to expose himself or his family to want or suffering.

"Adjudication of disability—Power to appoint guardian. (a) Upon
the filing of a petition by a reputable person or by the alleged disabled
person himself or on its own motion, the court may adjudge a person to
be a disabled person and may appoint (1) a guardian of his person, if
because of his disability he lacks sufficient understanding or capacity
to make or communicate responsible decisions concerning the care of
his person, or (2) a guardian of his estate, if because of his disability he
is unable to manage his estate or financial affairs or (3) a guardian of
his person and of his estate.

"Guardianship shall be utilized only as is necessary to promote the
well-being of the disabled person, to protect him from neglect, exploitation, or abuse, and to encourage development of his maximum self-
reliance and independence. Guardianship shall be ordered only to the
extent necessitated by the individual's actual mental, physical and
adaptive limitations."

In commenting specifically upon these portions of the pertinent
statute, this court stated that the legislature made these amendments
"an express part of the statutory scheme for appointed guardians for
disabled adults."

* * *

"Under the new sections, the legislature has made it clear that
although a person may be a disabled person, in the statutory sense of
not being fully able to manage his person, a guardian is not therefore
permissible or appropriate, if that person is capable of making and
communicating responsible decisions concerning the care of his person.
Thus, a person who was physically unable to care for himself, but who
could direct others in such activity, would not necessarily need a
guardian over his person. Similarly, a person might be a 'disabled
person' but nevertheless not be in need of a guardian over his estate,
because with help from others he is able to direct and manage his
affairs and estate."

* * *

In the case at bar, it is clear the respondent suffers from some
physical disability and has some mental peculiarities. Nevertheless,
with particular reference to the above citation, we cannot say the
determination of the trial judge that respondent was not unable to
manage his person and estate is contrary to the manifest weight of the
evidence.

* * *

Questions and Comments

1. *Typical criteria for guardianship.* The statute involved in
Quinn —focusing on the effect of various types of conditions on a person's
ability to manage property and resist the manipulation of others—was
typical of guardianship statutes until the early 1970's. The Illinois statute
at issue in *Galvin* reflects the modern trend, which has been described as a
movement toward "criteria that minimize the importance of the results of
an individual's decision and instead examine the ability of the individual to
go through the cognitive process of making rational decisions." S. Brakel,

J. Parry and B. Weiner, The Mentally Disabled and the Law 371 (1985). Almost all statutes in this latter grouping (including Illinois') adopt some version of the Uniform Probate Code, which defines an incapacitated person as "any person who is impaired by reason of mental illness, mental deficiency, physical illness or disability, advanced age . . . or other cause (except minority) to the extent that he lacks sufficient understanding or capacity to make or communicate responsible decisions concerning his person." National Conference of Commissioners on Uniform State Law, Uniform Probate Code § 5 (4th ed. 1975). Another "modern" formulation is provided by the American Bar Association's model statute, which authorizes general guardianship only for "adults whose ability to receive and evaluate information effectively and/or to communicate decisions is impaired to such an extent that they lack the capacity to manage their financial resources and/or meet essential requirements for their physical health or safety." Ch. 1, § 3.

With reference to the materials in the previous section, what level of competency do these various formulations imply? Are they significantly different from one another? What type of competency standard *should* apply in this context? The following three notes explore this last issue further.

2. *Vagueness doctrine and guardianship.* One way in which the courts have attempted to refine the criteria for guardianship has been through vagueness analysis. In *Katz v. Superior Court*, 73 Cal.App.3d 952, 141 Cal.Rptr. 234 (1st Dist.1977), the court analyzed the constitutionality of a statute which provided that the court "shall appoint a conservator of the . . . person . . . [first] of any adult person who by reason of advanced age, illness, injury, mental weakness, intemperance, addiction to drugs or other disability, or other cause is unable to properly care for himself or his property, or [second] who for said causes or for any other cause is likely to be deceived or imposed upon by artful or designing persons." The court found the second ground unconstitutionally vague, at least when applied to guardianships of the person, stating in part: "In an age of subliminal advertising, television exposure and psychological salesmanships, everyone is exposed to artful and designing persons at every turn. It is impossible to measure the degree of likelihood that some will succumb." Id. at 244. The first ground survived constitutional challenge, but only after the court construed it as equivalent to the definition of grave disability in California's commitment law. The court justified this interpretation by stating: "If an adult person is less than gravely disabled we find no warrant for depriving him or her of liberty and freedom of action under either [the guardianship statute] or [the civil commitment statute]." Id. at 252–53. Thus, according to *Katz*, a person may not be subjected to guardianship of the person unless he or she is "unable to provide for his basic personal needs for food, clothing or shelter." See Cal.Code § 5008(h).

In a similar vein is *In re Boyer*, 636 P.2d 1085 (Utah 1981). There the Utah Supreme Court construed a statute which adopted verbatim the language of the Uniform Probate Code, quoted in note 1. Utah Code Ann. 1953, § 75–1–201(18). The statute was challenged on the ground that the words "capacity to make or communicate responsible decisions concerning his person" would allow appointment of a guardian for a person "who makes decisions regarded by some as irresponsible, even though he has sufficient capacity to make personal management decisions which allow him to function in a manner acceptable to himself and without any threat of injury to himself." The court agreed, but avoided declaring the statute unconstitutionally vague by construing it to require an impairment which renders the individual "unable to care for his personal safety or unable to attend to and provide for such necessities as food, shelter, clothing, and medical care, without which physical injury of illness may occur." Id. at 1089.

Recall the comment in note 1 that modern guardianship statutes try to focus the inquiry more on the quality of the person's thought process than on the "results of the individual's decision." Do the *Katz* and *Boyer* decisions return the law of guardianship to a consideration of the "results of the individual's decision" rather than an examination "of the ability of the individual to go through the cognitive process of making rational decisions?" If so, is there a way out of this circle? Is the material in section II of this chapter any help?

3. *Civil commitment criteria and guardianship.* In developing guardianship criteria, *Katz* explicitly and *Boyer* implicitly adopt language found in statutes authorizing parens patriae commitment (discussed at pp. 674–677). The Uniform Probate Code and the ABA statute, although more oriented toward the quality of the person's cognitive processes, also focus on the types of impairment that the inability to care commitment criterion does.

This relationship is worth noting in light of modern attempts to differentiate incompetency determinations from commitment decisions. Until the 1970's, most states equated the two, a correlation which was symbolized by the practice in many states of delegating commitment authority to probate courts. In these states, institutionalized persons were presumed incompetent at least until release and perhaps until a court "restored" them to competency. Thus, these people not only lost the authority to make their own treatment decisions but also were automatically deprived, with no further judicial proceeding necessary, of the right to vote, possess a driver's license, manage property or marry. Today most states specifically eliminate the presumption of incompetency for institutionalized persons and require a separate incompetency adjudication. S. Brakel, J. Parry, B. Weiner, The Mentally Disabled and the Law 258 (1985). Although a number of states still grant hospital administrators some authority over patients' financial affairs (e.g., disposition of social security benefits) and a few allow other restrictions "necessary for the patient's medical welfare," see, e.g., Utah Code Ann.1953, § 64–7–45(1), no state allows the mere fact of commitment to substitute for a general incompetency determination. Given the close relation between current incompetency criteria and parens patriae commitment criteria noted above, is this modern development an efficient use of judicial resources?

4. *Guardianship and the least restrictive alternative doctrine.* If a person is incompetent to make everyday decisions, and as a result is eligible for both commitment or guardianship, what criteria should govern

the selection of an option? In answering this question one might need to take into account the different types of guardianship available. First, as noted previously, while guardians traditionally exerted complete power over the ward, in more recent times a distinction has developed between guardianships of the estate and guardianships of the person. *Quinn* involved the former, *Galvin* involved both. Making the distinction between the two can often be difficult. For instance, in *Quinn* is the guardianship sought really a guardianship of the estate? Put another way, does the court have statutory authority to do what it did?

Also noted in the introductory materials is the movement away from "general" guardianship toward "specific" or "limited" guardianship, whether the guardianship is of the person or of the estate. Ideally, perhaps, general guardianships should be rare. That is, the court should be careful to give control to the guardian only in those areas where the ward has demonstrated incompetence. Thus, a court should gauge a person's ability to vote, handle varying levels of financial transactions, make decisions about food and shelter, choose from among various types of treatment and so on, and shape the guardianship accordingly. A number of states attempt to implement this idea statutorily. See, e.g., Idaho Code § 56–239(d); Me.Rev.Stat.Ann., tit. 18, § 3512. One commentator has even called for abolition of general guardianship, in order to encourage narrower grants of power to the guardian. Frolik, "Plenary Guardianship: An Analysis, A Critique and a Proposal for Reform," 23 Ariz.L.Rev. 599, 653 (1981). Could the guardianship in *Quinn* have been further limited? A 1978 ABA study of limited guardianship provisions in six states found that they were rarely used. Id. A 1985 Illinois study produced similar results. See Legal Counsel for the Elderly, Decisionmaking, Incapacity and the Elderly 77 (1987).

A third way in which the least restrictive means idea might be implemented is through provision for temporary guardianships, ranging from 15 days to 6 months. Normally used as a stopgap measure after a guardian dies or is removed or in emergency situations, the procedures associated with such guardianships are usually very informal. 44 C.J.S. Insane Persons § 38 (1982). The Uniform Guardianship and Protective Proceeding Act does not even provide for a hearing prior to establishment of a temporary arrangement (although the duration of the guardianship is limited to 15 days). § 2–208.

Finally, there may be circumstances where even a clear finding of incompetency does not merit imposition of a guardianship. There are a number of other possibly "less restrictive" protective arrangements. These include "protective services" (in which case workers are appointed to supervise the person and ensure that he or she receives community services, voluntarily or involuntarily), powers of attorney, "living wills" (by which a person authorizes certain actions contingent upon certain conditions developing), court authorizations of single transactions (e.g., kidney transplants), representative payee arrangements (used for receipt of welfare entitlements), trusts, joint tenancies, and transfers of property. See Schmidt & Peters, "Legal Incompetents' Need for Guardians in Florida," 15 Bull.Am.Acad.Psychiat. & L. 69, 82 (1987). If a less restrictive alternative is available, would it be justifiable, for reasons analogous to those used to justify relaxed criteria for outpatient commitment,[h] to intervene at a level of competency higher than the level required to establish a guardianship?

5. *Procedures.* Every state provides for a hearing to determine the need for guardianship. Concerns connected with notice, the right to be present, the right to a public jury trial, application of the rules of evidence and most other aspects of the hearing are similar to those that arise in the civil commitment context, discussed in Chapter Eight. As a result, the procedures tend to be similar.

In some jurisdictions, however, fewer procedural protections are provided at guardianship proceedings, based on the perception that the intervention occasioned by guardianship is less substantial. For instance, in *Rud v. Dahl,* 578 F.2d 674, 679 (7th Cir.1978), the court held that counsel for the prospective ward is not "an essential element of due process" at guardianship proceedings:

> First of all, the nature of the intrusion on liberty interests from an adjudication of incompetency is far less than the intrusion resulting from other types of proceedings in which the presence of counsel has been mandated. Involuntary incarceration, for example, does not result from an incompetency proceeding. Moreover, the technical skills of an attorney are less important, as the procedural and evidentiary rules of an incompetency proceeding are considerably less strict than those applicable in other types of civil and criminal proceedings. Finally, the costs associated with the mandatory appointment of counsel will undermine one of the essential purposes of the proceeding itself—protection of the limited resources of the incompetent's estate from dissipation—for few alleged incompetents will be able to effect a 'knowing and intelligent' waiver of undesired counsel.

In many jurisdictions, representation of the ward is required but only by a guardian ad litem, who functions not as an advocate for the client's views but rather acts according to what he or she feels is in the best interests of the proposed ward. Sherman, "Guardianship: Time for a Reassessment," 49 Fordham L.Rev. 350, 354 (1980).

For similar reasons, many courts have upheld application of the preponderance of the evidence standard at guardianship proceedings despite the Supreme Court's ruling in *Addington v. Texas,* 441 U.S. 418, 99 S.Ct. 1804, 60 L.Ed.2d 323 (1979), requiring the clear and convincing standard at civil commitment proceedings. As explained by one court:

> We do not feel that more harm will befall an individual who is erroneously subjected to guardianship than to an individual who is in need of a guardian but is erroneously denied one. If an individual is erroneously subjected to a guardianship, then [state law] allows such a ward to file a petition for the removal of his guardian.

Guardianship of Roe, 383 Mass. 415, 421 N.E.2d 40 (1981).

6. *Who may serve as guardian.* The filing of a petition for guardianship is generally considered "jurisdictional"; that is, the court may appoint anyone guardian, not just the petitioner. See *Brown v. Storz,* 710 S.W.2d

h. See pp. 687–689.

402 (Mo.App.1986). Most state statutes establish priorities for deciding who should be guardian, with family members and relatives occupying the foremost positions. See, e.g., Uniform Guardian and Protective Proceeding Act §§ 2–205, 2–309. However, nonfamily members have been appointed in lieu of available and willing family members when "(1) the family member has an adverse interest to that of the ward; (2) there is dissension within the family; (3) the family member lacks business ability; or (4) some other substantial reason for disqualification exists." Legal Counsel for the Elderly, supra at 75. An increasing number of states are also requiring that guardians meet certain qualifications and even undergo training programs. See, e.g., West's Fla.Stat.Ann. § 744.344 et seq.

At least 29 states provide for public guardians. Legal Counsel for the Elderly, supra at 76, n. 90. Intended primarily for those with no relatives or relatives who are unsuitable as guardians, the public guardian device appears to fill a significant need. A study of institutionalized individuals in Florida found that over 11,000 people were probably legally incompetent and in need of either a guardianship of the person, guardianship of the estate, or both. Schmidt & Peters, supra at 78. The identity of the public guardian varies widely among jurisdictions. For instance, some states specifically authorize departments of mental health or social services to serve as public guardians. Others specifically prohibit these entities from serving, because they often provide the treatment or services about which the guardian must decide, thus creating a possible conflict of interest. Legal Counsel for the Elderly, supra at 76. Evidence of such a conflict is provided by a study of the Minnesota system, which found that some social service agencies refused to provide services unless the individual consented to become a ward of the agency. Levy, "Protecting the Mentally Retarded: An Empirical Survey and Evaluation of the Establishment of State Guardianship in Minnesota," 49 Minn.L.Rev. 821, 857 (1965).

Other studies of public guardianship have found that, even if the conflict of interest problem is solved, the responsible agencies are often overburdened and impersonal in nature, thus resulting in a tendency to institutionalize their wards. Frolik, supra at 648. At the same time, in theory at least, public guardians should offer greater sophistication and expertise and should be more in tune with available services than are private guardians. Id. at 646. One possible method of reducing the negative and accentuating the positive aspects of public guardianship is to create a nonprofit corporation using concerned citizens as guardians, as New York has done with the Association for Retarded Citizens. Id. at 648–49. Based on the available information, who would have been the best guardian in *Quinn* and *Galvin*?

7. *Restoration of competency.* The general practice with respect to terminating a guardianship is described by S. Brakel, J. Parry and B. Weiner, supra at 392–93:

Restoration is a legal determination that individuals who have been adjudged incompetent are now able to manage their business and personal affairs adequately. The law presumes that persons who are adjudicated incompetent remain so. In order for wards to regain their competent status they normally must vindicate themselves in a separate judicial proceeding or, in a few states, be discharged from a mental institution. This second method is a holdover from the time when it was common to merge commitment and competency hearings. It avoids the need to prevail in a hearing that may be even more difficult than challenging an assertion of incompetency in the first instance.

* * *

. . . Thirty-nine jurisdictions permit wards to apply for restoration themselves. Forty jurisdictions state essentially that anyone with an interest in the matter may initiate proceedings on behalf of the ward. California is unique because the legislature enacted a statute that provides for automatic restoration unless the conservator applies for reappointment. A number of other states require periodic review of guardianships, while Illinois and Virginia specify that the court of proper jurisdiction may initiate the proceedings on its own. . . .

As noted, not all states require periodic judicial review of an incompetency finding. Is this constitutional, in light of the Supreme Court's decision in *Parham v. J.R.,* discussed at pp. 787–802? Would it matter if, as is true in most states, the guardian is required to file periodic reports with the court on the status of the ward?

C. POWERS AND DUTIES OF THE GUARDIAN

Within the scope of whatever kind of guardianship is established (i.e. of the person or of the estate, general or limited), the guardian has authority to make decisions concerning the ward. However, there are two further types of limitations on this authority. First, the guardian is supposed to take only those actions which will be in the "best interests" of the ward; that is, the guardian is in a fiduciary relationship with the ward. In some jurisdictions, the best interest test has been modified to require the guardian to make the decision that the ward would have made had he or she been competent. Both the best interest and substituted judgment standards are discussed further below.

The second type of limitation on the guardian's authority bars unmonitored surrogate decisions in certain instances. For instance, a guardian of the estate, even one with general powers, is often prohibited by statute from executing a will for the ward, and usually must obtain a court order before selling real property or revoking certain types of trusts. Similarly, a guardian of the person, although authorized to make most medical decisions for the ward, must usually seek court approval before consenting to certain types of procedures viewed as "extraordinary", such as abortion, psychosurgery, organ transplants, or sterilization. The following materials focus on sterilization as paradigmatic of the situations in which guardians must make difficult choices, although several other situations are discussed as well.

MATTER OF GUARDIANSHIP OF HAYES

Supreme Court of Washington, 1980.
93 Wash.2d 228, 608 P.2d 635.

*   *   *

HOROWITZ, JUSTICE.

*   *   *

Petitioner Sharon Hayes is the mother of Edith Melissa Maria Hayes, who was born severely mentally retarded on December 17, 1963. She petitioned the Superior Court for an order appointing her as the guardian of Edith's person and specifically authorizing a sterilization procedure on Edith. The court dismissed the petition on a motion for summary judgment on the ground it had no authority to issue an order for sterilization of a retarded person.

*   *   *

Edith Hayes is severely mentally retarded as a result of a birth defect. Now 16 years old, she functions at the level of a four to five year old. Her physical development, though, has been commensurate with her age. She is thus capable of conceiving and bearing children, while being unable at present to understand her own reproductive functions or exercise independent judgment in her relationship with males. Her mother and doctors believe she is sexually active and quite likely to become pregnant. Her parents are understandably concerned that Edith is engaging in these sexual activities. Furthermore, her parents and doctors feel the long term effects of conventional birth control methods are potentially harmful, and that sterilization is the most desirable method to ensure that Edith does not conceive an unwanted child.

Edith's parents are sensitive to her special needs and concerned about her physical and emotional health, both now and in the future. They have sought appropriate medical care and education for her, and provided her with responsible and adequate supervision. During the year or so that Edith has been capable of becoming pregnant, though, they have become frustrated, depressed and emotionally drained by the stress of seeking an effective and safe method of contraception. They believe it is impossible to supervise her activities closely enough to prevent her from becoming involved in sexual relations. Thus, with the consent of Edith's father, Sharon Hayes petitioned for an order appointing her guardian and authorizing a sterilization procedure for Edith.

I

JURISDICTION

Edith's court appointed guardian ad litem contended below, and now maintains on appeal, that a superior court has no power to authorize a sterilization absent specific statutory authority. He cites in support of that view cases from other jurisdictions in which courts have concurred that specific statutory authority is required.

* * *

The courts of this state have long recognized the inherent power of the superior court "to hear *and determine* all matters legal and equitable in all proceedings known to the common law." Original jurisdiction is granted to superior courts over all cases and proceedings in which jurisdiction is not vested exclusively in some other court by Washington Const. art. 4, § 6.

* * *

We therefore hold that Washington Const. art. 4, § 6 gives the superior courts of this state the jurisdiction to entertain and act upon a request for an order authorizing sterilization of a mentally incompetent person.

II

STANDARDS FOR STERILIZATION

Our conclusion that superior courts have the power to grant a petition for sterilization does not mean that power must be exercised. Sterilization touches upon the individual's right of privacy and the fundamental right to procreate. It is an unalterable procedure with serious effects on the lives of the mentally retarded person and those upon whom he or she may depend. Therefore, it should be undertaken only after careful consideration of all relevant factors. We conclude this opinion with a set of guidelines setting out of the questions which must be asked and answered before an order authorizing sterilization of a mentally incompetent person could be issued. First, however, the consideration which are important to this determination can be best illuminated by discussing briefly the historical context from which they arise.

Sterilization of the mentally ill, mentally retarded, criminals, and sufferers from certain debilitating diseases became popular in this country in the early 20th century. The theory of "eugenic sterilization" was that the above-named traits and diseases, widely believed at that time to be hereditary, could be eliminated to the benefit of all society by simply preventing procreation.

More than 20 states passed statutes authorizing eugenic sterilizations. Washington passed a punitive sterilization law aimed at habitual criminals and certain sex offenders in 1909. The law exists today as RCW 9.92.100. Another statute, also enacted early in the century, denied certain persons, including the mentally retarded, the right to marry unless it is established that procreation by the couple is impossible. RCW 26.04.030, repealed by Laws of 1979, 1st Ex.Sess., ch. 128, § 4. While this statute did not authorize sterilizations, it was clearly based on eugenic principles.

In 1921 the Washington legislature enacted a law providing for sterilization of certain mentally retarded, mentally ill and habitually criminal persons restrained in a state institution. Laws of 1921, ch. 53, p. 162. This statute was held unconstitutional because of its failure to provide adequate procedural safeguards in *In re Hendrickson,* 12 Wash. 2d 600, 123 P.2d 322 (1942).

The United States Supreme Court upheld the constitutionality of a eugenic sterilization law which provided adequate procedural safeguards, however, in *Buck v. Bell,* 274 U.S. 200, 47 S.Ct. 584, 71 L.Ed. 1000 (1927). Since that time it has generally been believed that eugenic sterilization statutes are constitutional although, as noted above, more recent Supreme Court decisions suggest the importance of respecting the individual's constitutional rights of privacy and procreation.

More recently scientific evidence has demonstrated little or no relationship between genetic inheritance and such conditions as mental retardation, criminal behavior, and diseases such as epilepsy. Geneticists have discovered, for example, that some forms of mental retardation appear to have no hereditary component at all, while in some others the element of heredity is only one of a number of factors which may contribute to the condition. In short the theoretical foundation for eugenic sterilization as a method of improving society has been disproved.

At the same time other previously unchallenged assumptions about mentally retarded persons have been shown to be unreliable. It has been found, for example, that far from being an insignificant event for the retarded person, sterilization can have longlasting detrimental emotional effects. Furthermore, while retarded persons, especially children, are often highly suggestible, there is evidence they are also capable of learning and adhering to strict rules of social behavior. Many retarded persons are capable of having normal children and being good parents.

Of great significance for the problem faced here is the fact that, unlike the situation of a normal and necessary medical procedure, in the question of sterilization the interests of the parents of a retarded person cannot be presumed to be identical to those of the child. The problem of parental consent to sterilization is of great concern to professionals in the field of mental health, and the overwhelming weight of opinion of those who have studied the problem appears to be that consent of a parent or guardian is a questionable or inadequate basis for sterilization. It is thus clear that in any proceedings to determine whether an order for sterilization should issue, the retarded person must be represented, as here, by a disinterested guardian ad litem.

Despite all that has been said thus far, in the rare case sterilization may indeed be in the best interests of the retarded person. However, the court must exercise care to protect the individual's right of privacy, and thereby not unnecessarily invade that right. Substantial medical evidence must be adduced, and the burden on the proponent of sterilization will be to show by clear, cogent and convincing evidence that such a procedure is in the best interest of the retarded person.

Among the factors to be considered are the age and educability of the individual. For example, a child in her early teens may be incapable at present of understanding the consequences of sexual activity, or exercising judgment in relations with the opposite sex, but may also have the potential to develop the required understanding and judgment through continued education and developmental programs.

A related consideration is the potential of the individual as a parent. As noted above, many retarded persons are capable of becoming good parents, and in only a fraction of cases is it likely that offspring would inherit a genetic form of mental retardation that would make parenting more difficult.

Another group of relevant factors involve the degree to which sterilization is medically indicated as the last and best resort for the individual. Can it be shown by clear, cogent and convincing evidence, for example, that other methods of birth control are inapplicable or unworkable?

In considering these factors, several courts have developed sterilization guidelines. With the assistance of the brief of Amicus Mental Health Law Project, a careful review of these considerations allows us to provide the superior court with standards to be followed in exercising its jurisdiction to issue an order authorizing sterilization of a mentally incompetent individual.

The decision can only be made in a superior court proceeding in which (1) the incompetent individual is represented by a disinterested guardian ad litem, (2) the court has received independent advice based upon a comprehensive medical, psychological, and social evaluation of the individual, and (3) to the greatest extent possible, the court has elicited and taken into account the view of the incompetent individual.

Within this framework, the judge must first find by clear, cogent and convincing evidence that the individual is (1) incapable of making his or her own decision about sterilization, and (2) unlikely to develop sufficiently to make an informed judgment about sterilization in the foreseeable future.

Next, it must be proved by clear, cogent and convincing evidence that there is a need for contraception. The judge must find that the individual is (1) physically capable of procreation, and (2) likely to engage in sexual activity at the present or in the near future under circumstances likely to result in pregnancy, and must find in addition that (3) the nature and extent of the individual's disability, as determined by empirical evidence and not solely on the basis of standardized tests, renders him or her permanently incapable of caring for a child, even with reasonable assistance.

Finally, there must be no alternatives to sterilization. The judge must find that by clear, cogent and convincing evidence (1) all less drastic contraceptive methods, including supervision, education and training, have been proved unworkable or inapplicable, and (2) the proposed method of sterilization entails the least invasion of the body of the individual. In addition, it must be shown by clear, cogent and convincing evidence that (3) the current state of scientific and medical knowledge does not suggest either (a) that a reversible sterilization procedure or other less drastic contraceptive method will shortly be available, or (b) that science is on the threshold of an advance in the treatment of the individual's disability.

There is a heavy presumption against sterilization of an individual incapable of informed consent that must be overcome by the person or entity requesting sterilization. This burden will be even harder to overcome in the case of a minor incompetent, whose youth may make it difficult or impossible to prove by clear, cogent and convincing evidence that he or she will never be capable of making an informed judgment about sterilization or of caring for a child.

Review of the facts in this case in light of these standards make it clear that the burden has not yet been met. It cannot be said that Edith Hayes will be unable to understand sexual activity or control her behavior in the future. The medical testimony and report of the mental health board are not detailed enough to provide clear, cogent and convincing evidence in this regard. Edith's youth is of particular concern, since she has many years of education before her. Furthermore, although there is evidence that some methods of birth control have already been tried, there is insufficient proof that no conventional form of contraception is a reasonable and medically acceptable alternative to sterilization. Nor is there any evidence such a procedure would not have detrimental effects on Edith's future emotional or physical health. Finally, there is no evidence that a pregnancy would be physically or emotionally hazardous to Edith, and insufficient evidence that she would never be capable of being a good parent.

Additional factfinding at the trial level will help the superior court judge answer the questions set out in this opinion. Therefore, the case is reversed and remanded for further proceedings consistent with this opinion.

* * *

Questions and Comments

1. *The competency standard for sterilization.* Assuming there is the requisite statutory or judicial authority, when may a court authorize or undertake a surrogate decision concerning sterilization? The formulation found in *Hayes* is widely followed. Looking closely at the guidelines of that case, it would appear that if a person is competent to understand the sterilization process and its consequences and refuses the procedure, the state may take no further action. Conversely, if the person is incapable of understanding the procedure and its consequences, *Hayes* appears to hold that he or she is incompetent for purposes of making the sterilization

decision and that a surrogate decision (taking into account such factors as the likelihood of sexual activity and the person's parenting ability) is permitted.

Is this the correct competency test? Consider this excerpt from Scott, "Sterilization of Mentally Retarded Persons: Reproductive Rights and Family Privacy," 1986 Duke L.J. 806, 837–38 (1986):

> The autonomy interest of the mentally retarded person in deciding whether to have a child is obscured under laws based on the paternalism model because of the requirement of a threshold inquiry into whether the person is competent to make an informed medical decision about sterilization. If she is not, the law presumes that she is incapable of making the reproductive decision and that a surrogate (the court) must weigh her interests and make the decision for her. The ability to make an informed medical decision involves a level of cognitive functioning that many mentally retarded persons lack. However, a person who is unable to make this implementing decision might nonetheless be capable of making the underlying decision to have or to forgo having a child. This decision is fundamentally different from the medical sterilization decision and requires different capabilities. By specifying competency to make the medical decision as the threshold requirement, laws based on the paternalism model distort and even foreclose the inquiry into the individual's ability to make the decision whether to have a child.
>
> Under the autonomy model, competency to make a meaningful choice to procreate rests on the individual's ability to fulfill the basic responsibilities of parenthood. A mildly impaired person may have this ability regardless of whether she is legally competent to make medical decisions regarding sterilization. Her interest in making her own reproductive decisions should be legally protected. On the other hand, a severely disabled person's childlike wish for a baby does not signify a meaningful choice. A decision to have a child is, most importantly, a decision to become a parent—to assume a role that requires a minimal level of competency. If the individual lacks this capability and the state would predictably intervene to remove any child produced in order to protect it, then the choice to have a child is not a legally protectable exercise in personal autonomy. Thus, the interest in autonomy is derivative of the underlying interest in having children. If the retarded individual lacks the ability to exercise the substantive interest, she lacks the interest in making the choice.

Under Scott's approach, what should be the competency standard for decisionmaking about abortion?

2. *Best interests analysis.* Assuming a person is found incompetent to make the sterilization decision under the appropriate standard, what factors will justify making a surrogate decision in favor of the procedure? In other words, when is sterilization in an incompetent person's best interests? *Hayes* lists several factors. Note that the court seems to consider sterilization the option of last resort, by requiring a showing that there are no "less drastic" contraceptives that "have been proved unworkable". Other courts are even more restrictive. For instance, one court

allowed sterilization of an incompetent person only upon a finding that the procedure is medically essential "to preserve the life or physical or mental health of the incompetent person." In the *Matter of A.W.,* 637 P.2d 366, 375 (Colo.1981).

Are these types of "least restrictive alternative" rules sensible? If the person is not competent to make a decision about having children, should we prefer a nonpermanent procedure such as contraceptive pills or an intrauterine device? If sterilization is not performed, but because of the increased risks of pregnancy and increased burden on the family, the person is eventually institutionalized, has the "least drastic" method been pursued?

3. *The substituted judgment standard.* Some courts eschew best interests analysis in favor of a substituted judgment test. This approach was described in *Matter of Moe,* 385 Mass. 555, 432 N.E.2d 712 (1982), which also involved a sterilization decision:

> In utilizing the doctrine of substituted judgment, this court seeks to maintain the integrity of the incompetent person by giving the individual a forum in which his or her rights may be exercised. The court dons 'the mental mantle of the incompetent' and substitutes itself as nearly as possible for the individual in the decision making process. In utilizing the doctrine the court does not decide what is necessarily the best decision but rather what decision would be made by the incompetent person if he or she were competent.

The factors the court then listed as considerations in making the substituted judgment decision are virtually identical to those listed in *Hayes,* except that the court added that the individual's religious beliefs, if any, must be ascertained. Would a substituted judgment analysis be any different than a best interests analysis on the *Hayes* facts? Does application of the substituted judgment test make sense in such a situation?

4. *Relevance of the ward's desires.* Under both the best interest and substituted judgment tests, at least as described by *Hayes* and *Moe,* the decisionmaker is to inquire into and take into account the ward's desires. Does this requirement make sense when the individual has been found incompetent?

Should any weight be given to a previous statement made while the person is *competent*? Suppose, for instance, that a woman of 20 suffers an incapacitating head injury which leaves her sexually active but at the mental age of 5, unable either to understand the sterilization procedure or to make a decision concerning having a child. One year before the accident, she had indicated that she would never want to be sterilized or otherwise give up her capacity to have children. Should this fact bar a court under either test from authorizing sterilization? Would it make any difference if the reason given for not wanting sterilization was based on religious preferences? In the alternative, what if, a year before the accident, she had indicated she never wanted to have children?

Consider *Cruzan v. Harmon,* 760 S.W.2d 408 (Mo.1988), a case in front of the U.S. Supreme Court at the time this book went to press. There, the parents and co-guardians of Nancy Cruzan requested the termination of procedures which were sustaining the life of their daughter, a twenty-six year old woman who as a result of an automobile accident was in a permanent vegetative state, but not legally dead under state law. The trial court found that, before the accident, Nancy had been a "vivacious, active, outgoing, independent person who preferred to do for herself." It also found that about a year prior to her accident, she had "discussions with her then housemate, friend and co-worker," during which "she expressed the feeling that she would not wish to continue living if she couldn't be at least halfway normal." The court characterized these conversations as "somewhat serious." The finding that Nancy's "lifestyle and other statements to family and friends suggest that she would not wish to continue her present existence without hope as it is," heavily influenced the trial court in ordering the state of Missouri to honor the co-guardians' request.

The Missouri Supreme Court reversed, calling the evidence about Nancy's wishes "inherently unreliable and thus insufficient to support the co-guardians' claim to exercise substituted judgment on Nancy's behalf." The court concluded: "The State's interest is in preservation of life, not only Nancy's life, but also the lives of persons similarly situated yet without the support of a loving family. This interest outweighs any rights invoked on Nancy's behalf to terminate treatment in the face of the uncertainty of Nancy's wishes and her own right to life." Id. at 426. What is the state's interest in the sterilization context? The individual's interest?

5. *Intervention for the benefit of third parties.* Many courts which have sanctioned surrogate decisionmaking in the sterilization context have emphasized that the decision should take into account only the interests of the ward. For instance, in *Moe* supra, the court stated: "No sterilization is to be compelled on the basis of any State or parental interest." 432 N.E.2d at 721. Does the *Hayes* court take a position on this issue? *Should* third party interests be taken into account?

In answering this last question, it might be useful to consider a case involving a decision other than sterilization. *In re Guardianship of Pescinski*, 67 Wis.2d 4, 226 N.W.2d 180 (1975) addressed whether a court may order an operation to remove the kidney of an incompetent person in order to save the life of a relative. The court described the facts as follows:

. . . The appellant, Janice Pescinski Lausier, on her own petition, was appointed guardian of the person of her brother, the respondent, Richard Pescinski. In 1958, Richard was declared incompetent and was committed to Winnebago State Hospital. He has been a committed mental patient since that date, classified as a schizophrenic, chronic, catatonic type.

On January 31, 1974, Janice Pescinski Lausier petitioned for permission to Dr. H.M. Kauffman to conduct tests to determine whether Richard Pescinski was a suitable donor for a kidney transplant for the benefit of his sister, Elaine Jeske. Elaine had both kidneys surgically removed in 1970 because she was suffering from kidney failure diagnosed as chronic glomerulonephritis. In order to sustain her life, she was put on a dialysis machine, which functions as an artificial kidney. Because of the deterioration of Elaine, the petition contended that a kidney transplant was needed. Subsequent tests were completed establishing that Richard was a suitable donor, and a hearing was then held on the subject of whether permission should be granted to perform the transplant. The guardian ad litem would not give consent to the transplant and the county court held that it did not have the power to give consent for the operation.

At the time of the hearing Elaine was thirty-eight and her brother Richard was thirty-nine. Evidence was produced at the hearing that the other members of the Pescinski family had been ruled out as possible donors on the basis of either age or health. The father, aged seventy, and the mother, aged sixty-seven, were eliminated as possible donors by Dr. Kauffman because, as a matter of principle, he would not perform the operation on a donor over sixty. A similar rationale was applied by Dr. Kauffman as to all of the six minor children of Elaine, the doctor concluding that he "would not personally use their kidneys" as a matter of his "own moral conviction." Mrs. Jeske's sister, Mrs. Lausier, was excluded as a donor because she has diabetes. Another brother, Ralph Pescinski, testified that he was forty-three years old, had been married twenty years and had ten children, nine of whom remained at home. He is a dairy farmer and did not care to be a donor because there would be nobody to take over his farm and he felt he had a duty to his family to refuse. He further testified that he had a stomach disorder which required a special diet and had a rupture on his left side. He had been to see Dr. Capati at the Neillsville Clinic, who told him he should not get involved and that his family should come first.

The testimony showed that Richard was suffering from schizophrenia—catatonic type, and that while he was in contact with his environment there was marked indifference in his behavior. Dr. Hoffman, the medical director at the Good Samaritan Home, West Bend, Wisconsin, testified that in layman's terms Richard's mental disease was a flight from reality. He estimated Richard's mental capacity to be age twelve. No evidence in the record indicates that Richard consented to the transplant.

The court then upheld the trial court's decision prohibiting the operation.

"A guardian of the person has the care of the ward's person and must look to the latter's health, education, and support." The guardian must act, if at all, "loyally in the best interests of his ward." There is absolutely no evidence here that any interests of the ward will be served by the transplant.

. . . We decline to adopt the concept of "substituted judgment" which was specifically approved by the Kentucky Court of Appeals in Strunk v. Strunk, 445 S.W.2d 145 (Ky.1969). In that case, the Kentucky court held a court of equity had the power to permit the removal of a kidney from an incompetent ward of the state upon the petition of his committee who was also his mother. . . .

. . . Historically, the substituted judgment doctrine was used to allow gifts of the property of an incompetent. If applied literally, it would allow a trial court, or this court, to change the designation on a life insurance policy or make an election for an incompetent widow, without the requirement of a statute authorizing these acts and contrary to prior decisions of this court.

We conclude that the doctrine should not be adopted in this state.

We, therefore, must affirm the lower court's decision that it was without power to approve the operation, and we further decide that there is no such power in this court. An incompetent particularly should have his own interests protected. Certainly no advantage should be taken of him. In the absence of real consent on his part, and in a situation where no benefit to him has been established, we fail to find any authority for the county court, or this court, to approve this operation.

In his dissent, Justice Day argued in favor of the substituted judgment test:

I think the court as a court of equity does have authority to permit the kidney transplant operation requested in the petition of the guardian of Richard Pescinski. I agree with the reasoning of the Court of Appeals of the state of Kentucky [in *Strunk*] . . . That case involved the authorization of a transplant from a 27–year–old incompetent to his 28–year–old brother. The court in that case did find, based on the testimony of a psychiatrist, that while the incompetent had the mental age of six, it would be of benefit to him to keep his brother alive so that his brother could visit him on occasion[.] . . . In the case before us, if the incompetent brother should happily recover from his mental illness, he would undoubtedly be happy to learn that the transplant of one of his kidneys to his sister saved her life. This at least would be a normal response and hence the transplant is not without benefit to him.

The majority opinion would forever condemn the incompetent to be always a receiver, a taker, but never a giver. For in holding that only those things which financially or physically benefit the incompetent may be done by the court, he is forever excluded from doing the decent thing, the charitable thing. The British courts have not so held. Two British cases cited in Strunk permitted the estate of an incompetent to provide a pension for a faithful servant in one instance and in another to help an indigent brother—this by the device known as "substituted judgment" where the court in effect does for the incompetent what it is sure he would do himself if he had the power to act. This approach gives the incompetent the benefit of the doubt, endows him with the finest qualities of his humanity, assumes the goodness of his nature instead of assuming the opposite.

6. *Procedure. Hayes* is typical in its requirement that a court be involved in the sterilization decision. For instance, in *Moe*, 432 N.E.2d at 716–17, the court stated:

Since sterilization is an extraordinary and highly intrusive form of medical treatment that irreversibly extinguishes the ward's fundamental right of procreative choice, we conclude that a guardian must obtain a proper judicial order for the procedure before he or she can validly consent to it. Guardians and parents, therefore, absent statutory or judicial authorization, cannot consent to the sterilization of a ward in their care or custody.

What makes sterilization "extraordinary" and "intrusive", compared for instance to a decision regarding financial affairs? In another Massachusetts case, the court identified several factors to be considered in determining whether there must be a court order before medical intervention may take place:

> [T]he extent of impairment of the patient's mental faculties, whether the patient is in custody of a State institution, the prognosis without the proposed treatment, the prognosis with the proposed treatment, the complexity, risk and novelty of the proposed treatment, its possible side effects, the patient's level of understanding and probable reaction, the urgency of decision, the consent of the patient, spouse or guardian, the good faith of those who participate in the decision, the clarity of professional opinion as to what is good medical practice, the interests of third persons, and the administrative requirements of any institution involved.

Matter of Spring, 380 Mass. 629, 405 N.E.2d 115 (1980).

Scott, supra at 859–863, disagrees with the requirement that a judicial hearing be held in all sterilization cases, relying in part on *Parham v. J.R.* (*Parham,* reprinted at pp. 787–799, permitted parents to commit their children if an independent assessment by a mental health professional concurs.) Scott argues that in some cases a *Parham*-type arrangement is sufficient to authorize the sterilization decision, at least when the ward's parents are the surrogate decisionmakers:

> [If a "reliable clinical evaluation" finds that] the child is not potentially capable of reproductive choice, she is less at risk than the child for whom hospitalization is sought. Parents seeking sterilization are not trying to "dump" their retarded child. Their initiative may well be an effort to facilitate her continued care at home. Thus, potential conflicts of interest would seem less probable in this situation than when psychiatric hospitalization is proposed.

> * * *

> Mentally disabled persons who will require lifelong care clearly lack the capacity to care for a child. They also have a greater interest in family continuity and stability than do those who are less disabled. Thus, only minimal procedural requirements are desirable. If a reliable clinical evaluation shows that the person lacks the capacity to care for herself, little risk is created by avoiding a judicial proceeding altogether and permitting the sterilization to be performed upon parental request and authorization.

> In the case of a less disabled person who is potentially capable of caring for herself, but who clearly lacks an interest in reproduction, judicial review is desirable if the procedural costs to the individual and her family are outweighed by the potential for reducing error. Alternatively, procedural costs might be reduced without unduly sacrificing

accuracy by using a less formal review forum similar to a hospital ethics committee. Such a committee could undertake nonadversarial review of the expert's evaluation to ensure that it is competent, independent and based on all relevant information. The committee could consult with other experts or with the parents. Such a nonjudicial review mechanism would protect family privacy and stability to a greater degree than would a judicial proceeding.

If the disability is less severe, the possibility of underestimating the interest in reproductive choice becomes greater, and the costs of procedural protection become more acceptable. Thus, if the findings of the expert raise any ambiguity about the individual's potential interest in reproductive choice, judicial review is warranted.

Mandatory judicial review may also be indicated if the person protests the sterilization in any meaningful way, regardless of her level of disability. The incompetent person's protest should not be a bar to her parent's decision. Nonetheless, it would justify mandatory judicial scrutiny of her lack of competency.

7. *Hospitalizing the ward.* Similar issues arise in the context of making decisions about psychiatric treatment. Is a decision to hospitalize the ward in a mental institution "extraordinary", so that hospitalization may not take place unless procedures for involuntary commitment are followed? Or may a guardian avoid court disposition by admitting the ward as a "voluntary" patient? In most states today, a guardian may not follow the latter course, at least if the ward objects to hospitalization. In the words of one court:

> If we were not to require at least substantial compliance with the [involuntary commitment] law to fully protect the rights of incompetents it would be possible for an unscrupulous person to have himself appointed guardian and then lock his ward in a mental institution and proceed to waste the ward's estate. If a state and the judiciary are not vigilant in the protection of the rights of incompetents it is likely to lead to the abuse of the person and estate of such incompetents. The mentally ill are unable to think and care for themselves in a normal manner and of necessity depend upon the state and the courts for protection. . . . We . . . must hold in this case that the ward was not afforded either procedural or substantive due process. . . .

Von Luce v. Rankin, 267 Ark. 34, 588 S.W.2d 445 (1979). In *Von Luce* the ward protested the hospitalization. Should involuntary proceedings be required if the ward does not protest? To what extent does *Parham* undercut *Von Luce* and permit a guardian to "voluntary in" his or her ward if a mental health professional employed by the hospital sanctions the decision?

An even more controversial issue has been the guardian's authority to consent to various types of psychiatric treatments, ranging from drug therapy to psychosurgery. That issue is addressed in the next section, as part of a discussion on the larger issue of when persons with mental disability have the right to refuse or consent to psychiatric treatment.

IV. THE RIGHT TO REFUSE AND CONSENT TO PSYCHIATRIC TREATMENT

In Chapter Three, we discussed the informed consent doctrine, which is normally thought to require professionals who are engaged in treating patients to honor an informed, voluntary decision by a competent individual. This common law doctrine regulates the relationship between doctor and patient by imposing liability on doctors who do not obtain informed consent for nonemergency treatment. However, when the treatment at issue is psychiatric in nature and the patient is thought to be seriously mentally ill (as opposed to anguished or neurotic), the informed consent doctrine has not found uniform acceptance. For instance, until the 1970's people who were civilly committed or hospitalized as incompetent to stand trial or criminally insane could be forcibly medicated regardless of their competency to make treatment decisions. Apparently, the assumption was that since these people were subject to involuntary institutionalization, they were not competent to veto a particular treatment decision. At the same time, they were not competent to insist on certain types of treatment. Similarly, uninstitutionalized persons who were supervised by guardians (of the person) had little or no control over their treatment.

These practices continue today in a number of jurisdictions. However, several courts have now recognized a "right to refuse" psychotropic medication for institutionalized populations, in the process constitutionalizing a version of the informed consent doctrine in that context. The precise scope of this right is still being fleshed out; its application to other types of treatment is also unclear. This section first examines the right to refuse antipsychotic medication; it then addresses consent and refusal with respect to three other psychiatric treatment techniques: electro-convulsive therapy, psychosurgery, and behavior modification.

A. PSYCHOACTIVE MEDICATION

WASHINGTON v. HARPER
Supreme Court of the United States, 1990.
___ U.S. ___, 110 S.Ct. 1028, ___ L.Ed.2d ___.

JUSTICE KENNEDY delivered the opinion of the Court.

The central question before us is whether a judicial hearing is required before the State may treat a mentally ill prisoner with antipsychotic drugs against his will. Resolution of the case requires us to discuss the protections afforded the prisoner under the Due Process Clause of the Fourteenth Amendment.

I

Respondent Walter Harper was sentenced to prison in 1976 for robbery. From 1976 to 1980, he was incarcerated at the Washington's

State Penitentiary. Most of that time, respondent was housed in the prison's mental health unit, where he consented to the administration of antipsychotic drugs. Antipsychotic drugs, sometimes called "neuroleptic" or "psychotropic drugs," are medications commonly used in treating mental disorders such as schizophrenia. As found by the trial court, the effect of these and similar drugs is to alter the chemical balance in the brain, the desired result being that the medication will assist the patient in organizing his or her thought processes and regaining a rational state of mind.

Respondent was paroled in 1980 on the condition that he participate in psychiatric treatment. While on parole, he continued to receive treatment at the psychiatric ward at Harborview Medical Center in Seattle, and was later sent to Western State hospital pursuant to a civil commitment order. In December 1981, the State revoked respondent's parole after he assaulted two nurses at a hospital in Seattle.

Upon his return to prison, respondent was sent to the Special Offender Center (SOC or Center), a 144-bed correctional institute established by the Washington Department of Corrections to diagnose and treat convicted felons with serious mental disorders. At the Center, psychiatrists first diagnosed respondent as suffering from a manic-depressive disorder. At first, respondent gave voluntary consent to treatment, including the administration of antipsychotic medications. In November 1982, he refused to continue taking the prescribed medications. The treating physician then sought to medicate respondent over his objections, pursuant to SOC Policy 600.30.

Policy 600.30 was developed in partial response to this Court's decision in *Vitek v. Jones*, 445 U.S. 480, 100 S.Ct. 1254, 63 L.Ed.2d 552 (1980).[i] The Policy has several substantive and procedural components. First, if a psychiatrist determines that an inmate should be treated with antipsychotic drugs but the inmate does not consent, the inmate may be subjected to involuntary treatment with the drugs only if he (1) suffers from a "mental disorder" and (2) is "gravely disabled" or poses a "likelihood of serious harm" to himself, others, or their property.[3]

---

i. *Vitek* is reprinted at pp. 770–774.

3. The Policy's definitions of the terms "mental disorder," "gravely disabled," and "likelihood of serious harm" are identical to the definitions of the terms as they are used in the state involuntary commitment statute. "Mental disorder" means "any organic, mental, or emotional impairment which has substantial adverse effects on an individual's cognitive or volitional functions." Wash.Rev.Code § 71.05.020(2) (1987). "Gravely disabled" means "a condition in which a person, as a result of a mental disorder: (a) [i]s in danger of serious physical harm resulting from a failure to provide for his essential human needs of health or safety, or (b) manifests severe deterioration in routine functioning evi-

denced by repeated and escalating loss of cognitive or volitional control over his or her actions and is not receiving such care as is essential for his or her health or safety." § 71.05.020(1). "Likelihood of serious harm" means "either: (a) [a] substantial risk that physical harm will be inflicted by an individual upon his own person, as evidenced by threats or attempts to commit suicide or inflict physical harm on one's self, (b) a substantial risk that physical harm will be inflicted by an individual upon another, as evidenced by behavior which has caused such harm or which places another person or persons in reasonable fear of sustaining such harm, or (c) a substantial risk that physical harm will be inflicted by an individual upon the proper-

Only a psychiatrist may order or approve the medication. Second, an inmate who refuses to take the medication voluntarily is entitled to a hearing before a special committee consisting of a psychiatrist, psychologist, and the Associate Superintendent of the Center, none of whom may be, at the time of the hearing, involved in the inmate's treatment or diagnosis. If the committee determines by a majority vote that the inmate suffers from a mental disorder and is gravely disabled or dangerous, the inmate may be medicated against his will, provided the psychiatrist is in the majority.

Third, the inmate has certain procedural rights before, during, and after the hearing. He must be given at least 24 hours' notice of the Center's intent to convene an involuntary medication hearing, during which time he may not be medicated. In addition, he must receive notice of the tentative diagnosis, the factual basis for the diagnosis, and why the staff believes medication is necessary. At the hearing, the inmate has the right to attend; to present evidence, including witnesses; to cross-examine staff witnesses; and to the assistance of a lay advisor who has not been involved in his case and who understands the psychiatric issues involved. Minutes of the hearing must be kept, and a copy provided to the inmate. The inmate has the right to appeal the committee's decision to the Superintendent of the Center within 24 hours, and the Superintendent must decide the appeal within 24 hours after its receipt. The inmate may seek judicial review of a committee decision in state court by means of a personal restraint petition or extraordinary writ.

Fourth, after the initial hearing, involuntary medication can continue only with periodic review. When respondent first refused medication, a committee, again composed of a non-treating psychiatrist, a psychologist, and the Center's Associate Superintendent was required to review an inmate's case after the first seven days of treatment. If the committee reapproved the treatment, the treating psychiatrist was required to review the case and prepare a report for the Department of Corrections medical director every 14 days while treatment continued.

In this case, respondent was absent when members of the Center staff met with the committee before the hearing. The committee then conducted the hearing in accordance with the Policy, with respondent being present and assisted by a nurse practitioner from another institution. The committee found that respondent was a danger to others as a result of a mental disease or disorder, and approved the involuntary administration of antipsychotic drugs. On appeal, the Superintendent upheld the committee's findings. Beginning on November 23, 1982, respondent was involuntarily medicated for about one year. Periodic review occurred in accordance with the Policy.

In November 1983, respondent was transferred from the Center to the Washington State Reformatory. While there, he took no medica-

ty of others, as evidenced by behavior which has caused substantial loss or dam- age to the property of others." § 71.05.020(3).

tion, and as a result, his condition deteriorated. He was retransferred to the Center after only one month. Respondent was the subject of another committee hearing in accordance with Policy 600.30, and the committee again approved medication against his will. Respondent continued to receive antipsychotic drugs, subject to the required periodic reviews, until he was transferred to the Washington State Penitentiary in June 1986.

In February 1985, respondent filed suit in state court under 42 U.S.C. § 1983 against various individual defendants and the State, claiming that the failure to provide a judicial hearing before the involuntary administration of antipsychotic medication violated the Due Process, Equal Protection, and Free Speech clauses of both the federal and state constitutions, as well as state tort law. He sought both damages and declaratory and injunctive relief. After a bench trial in March 1987, the court held that, although respondent had a liberty interest in not being subjected to the involuntary administration of antipsychotic medication, the procedures contained in the Policy met the requirements of due process as stated in *Vitek*.

On appeal, the Washington Supreme Court reversed and remanded the case to the trial court. Agreeing with the trial court that respondent had a liberty interest in refusing antipsychotic medications, the Court concluded that the "highly intrusive nature" of treatment with antipsychotic medications warranted greater procedural protections than those necessary to protect the liberty interest at stake in *Vitek*. It held that, under the Due Process Clause, the State could administer antipsychotic medication to a competent, nonconsenting inmate only if, in a judicial hearing at which the inmate had the full panoply of adversarial procedural protections, the State proved by "clear, cogent, and convincing" evidence that the administration of antipsychotic medication was both necessary and effective for furthering a compelling state interest.

We granted certiorari, and we reverse.

*   *   *

III

*   *   *

Restated in the terms of this case, the substantive issue is what factual circumstances must exist before the State may administer antipsychotic drugs to the prisoner against his will; the procedural issue is whether the State's nonjudicial mechanisms used to determine the facts in a particular case are sufficient. The Washington Supreme Court in effect ruled upon the substance of the inmate's right, as well as the procedural guarantees, and both are encompassed by our grant of certiorari. We address these questions beginning with the substantive one.

*   *   *

We have no doubt that respondent possesses a significant liberty interest in avoiding the unwanted administration of antipsychotic drugs under the Due Process Clause of the Fourteenth Amendment. *Vitek.* Upon full consideration of the state administrative scheme, however, we find that the Due Process Clause confers upon respondent no greater right than that recognized under state law.

Respondent contends that the State, under the mandate of the Due Process Clause, may not override his choice to refuse antipsychotic drugs unless he has been found to be incompetent, and then only if the factfinder makes a substituted judgment that he, if competent, would consent to drug treatment. We disagree. The extent of a prisoner's right under the Clause to avoid the unwanted administration of antipsychotic drugs must be defined in the context of the inmate's confinement. The Policy under review requires the State to establish, by a medical finding, that a mental disorder exists which is likely to cause harm if not treated. Moreover, the fact that the medication must first be prescribed by a psychiatrist, and then approved by a reviewing psychiatrist, ensures that the treatment in question will be ordered only if it is in the prisoner's medical interests, given the legitimate needs of his institutional confinement.[8] These standards, which recognize both the prisoner's medical interests and the State's interests, meet the demands of the Due Process Clause.

* * *

There can be little doubt as to both the legitimacy and the importance of the governmental interest presented here. There are few cases in which the State's interest in combating the danger posed by a person to both himself and others is greater than in a prison environment, which, "by definition," is made up of persons with "a demonstrated proclivity for antisocial criminal, and often violent, conduct." We confront here the State's obligations, not just its interests. The State has undertaken the obligation to provide prisoners with medical treatment consistent not only with their own medical interests, but also with the needs of the institution. Prison administrators have not only an interest in ensuring the safety of prison staffs and administrative

8. The dissent contends that the SOC Policy permits respondent's doctors to treat him with antipsychotic medications against his will without reference to whether the treatment is medically appropriate. For various reasons, we disagree. That an inmate is mentally ill and dangerous is a necessary condition to medication, but not a sufficient condition; before the hearing committee determines whether these requirements are met, the inmate's treating physician must first make the decision that medication is appropriate. The SOC is a facility whose purpose is not to warehouse the mentally ill, but to diagnose and treat convicted felons, with the desired goal being that they will recover to the point where they can function in a normal prison environment. In keeping with this purpose, an SOC psychiatrist must first prescribe the antipsychotic medication for the inmate, and the inmate must refuse it, before the Policy is invoked. Unlike the dissent, we will not assume that physicians will prescribe these drugs for reasons unrelated to the medical needs of the patients; indeed, the ethics of the medical profession are to the contrary. See Hippocratic Oath; American Psychiatric Association, Principles of Medical Ethics With Annotations Especially Applicable to Psychiatry, in Codes of Professional Responsibility 129–135 (R. Gorlin ed. 1986). . . .

personnel, but the duty to take reasonable measures for the prisoners' own safety. These concerns have added weight when a penal institution, like the Special Offender Center, is restricted to inmates with mental illnesses. Where an inmate's mental disability is the root cause of the threat he poses to the inmate population, the State's interest in decreasing the danger to others necessarily encompasses an interest in providing him with medical treatment for his illness.

Special Offender Center Policy 600.30 is a rational means of furthering the State's legitimate objectives. Its exclusive application is to inmates who are mentally ill and who, as a result of their illness, are gravely disabled or represent a significant danger to themselves or others. The drugs may be administered for no purpose other than treatment, and only under the direction of a licensed psychiatrist. There is considerable debate over the potential side effects of antipsychotic medications, but there is little dispute in the psychiatric profession that proper use of the drugs is one of the most effective means of treating and controlling a mental illness likely to cause violent behavior.

The alternative means proffered by respondent for accommodating his interest in rejecting the forced administration of antipsychotic drugs do not demonstrate the invalidity of the State's policy. Respondent's main contention is that, as a precondition to antipsychotic drug treatment, the State must find him incompetent, and then obtain court approval of the treatment using a "substituted judgment" standard. The suggested rule takes no account of the legitimate governmental interest in treating him where medically appropriate for the purpose of reducing the danger he poses. A rule that is in no way responsive to the State's legitimate interests is not a proper accommodation, and can be rejected out of hand. Nor are physical restraints or seclusion "alternative[s] that fully accommodat[e] the prisoner's rights at de minimis cost to valid penological interests." Physical restraints are effective only in the short term, and can have serious physical side effects when used on a resisting inmate, as well as leaving the staff at risk of injury while putting the restraints on or tending to the inmate who is in them. Furthermore, respondent has failed to demonstrate that physical restraints or seclusion are acceptable substitutes for antipsychotic drugs, in terms of either their medical effectiveness or their toll on limited prison resources.

We hold that, given the requirements of the prison environment, the Due Process Clause permits the State to treat a prison inmate who has a serious mental illness with antipsychotic drugs against his will, if the inmate is dangerous to himself or others and the treatment is in the inmate's medical interest. Policy 600.30 comports with these requirements; we therefore reject respondent's contention that its substantive standards are deficient under the Constitution.

IV

Having determined that state law recognizes a liberty interest . . . protected by the Due Process Clause, which permits refusal of antipsychotic drugs unless certain preconditions are met, we address next what procedural protections are necessary to ensure that the decision to medicate an inmate against his will is neither arbitrary nor erroneous under the standards we have discussed above. The Washington Supreme Court held that a full judicial hearing, with the inmate being represented by counsel, was required by the Due Process Clause before the State could administer antipsychotic drugs to him against his will. In addition, the court held that the State must justify the authorization of involuntary administration of antipsychotic drugs by "clear, cogent, and convincing" evidence. We hold that the administrative hearing procedures set by the SOC Policy do comport with procedural due process, and conclude that the Washington Supreme Court erred in requiring a judicial hearing as a prerequisite for the involuntary treatment of prison inmates.

A

The primary point of disagreement between the parties is whether due process requires a judicial decisionmaker. As written, the Policy requires that the decision whether to medicate an inmate against his will be made by a hearing committee composed of a psychiatrist, psychologist, and the Center's Associate Superintendent. None of the committee members may be involved, at the time of the hearing, in the inmate's treatment or diagnosis; members are not disqualified from sitting on the committee, however, if they have treated or diagnosed the inmate in the past. The committee's decision is subject to review by the Superintendent; if the inmate so desires, he may seek judicial review of the decision in a state court. Respondent contends that only a court should make the decision to medicate an inmate against his will.

Respondent's interest in avoiding the unwarranted administration of antipsychotic drugs is not insubstantial. The forcible injection of medication into a nonconsenting person's body represents a substantial interference with that person's liberty. The purpose of the drugs is to alter the chemical balance in a patient's brain, leading to changes, intended to be beneficial, in his or her cognitive processes. While the therapeutic benefits of antipsychotic drugs are well documented, it is also true that the drugs can have serious, even fatal, side effects. One such side effect identified by the trial court is acute dystonia, a severe involuntary spasm of the upper body, tongue, throat, or eyes. The trial court found that it may be treated and reversed within a few minutes through use of the medication Cogentin. Other side effects include akathesia (motor restlessness, often characterized by an inability to sit still); neuroleptic malignant syndrome (a relatively rare condition which can lead to death from cardiac dysfunction); and tardive dyskinesia, perhaps the most discussed side effect of antipsychotic drugs.

Tardive dyskinesia is a neurological disorder, irreversible in some cases, that is characterized by involuntary, uncontrollable movements of various muscles, especially around the face. The State, respondent, and amici sharply disagree about the frequency with which tardive dyskinesia occurs, its severity, and the medical profession's ability to treat, arrest, or reverse the condition. A fair reading of the evidence, however, suggests that the proportion of patients treated with antipsychotic drugs who exhibit the symptoms of tardive dyskinesia ranges from 10% to 25%. According to the American Psychiatric Association, studies of the condition indicate that 60% of tardive dyskinesia is mild or minimal in effect, and about 10% may be characterized as severe.

Notwithstanding the risks that are involved, we conclude that an inmate's interests are adequately protected, and perhaps better served, by allowing the decision to medicate to be made by medical professionals rather than a judge. The Due Process Clause "has never been thought to require that the neutral and detached trier of fact be law trained or a judicial or administrative officer." *Parham v. J.R.* Though it cannot be doubted that the decision to medicate has societal and legal implications, the Constitution does not prohibit the State from permitting medical personnel to make the decision under fair procedural mechanisms. Particularly where the patient is mentally disturbed, his own intentions will be difficult to assess, and will be changeable in any event. Respondent's own history of accepting and then refusing drug treatment illustrates the point. We cannot make the facile assumption that the patient's intentions, or a substituted judgment approximating those intentions, can be determined in a single judicial hearing apart from the realities of frequent and ongoing clinical observation by medical professionals. Our holding in *Parham* that a judicial hearing was not required prior to the voluntary commitment of a child to a mental hospital was based on similar observations:

> ". . . [D]ue process is not violated by use of informal, traditional medical investigative techniques. . . . The mode and procedure of medical diagnostic procedures is not the business of judges. . . .
> Although we acknowledge the fallibility of medical and psychiatric diagnosis, we do not accept the notion that the shortcomings of specialists can always be avoided by shifting the decision from a trained specialist using the traditional tools of medical science to an untrained judge or administrative hearing officer after a judicial-type hearing. Even after a hearing, the nonspecialist decisionmaker must make a medical-psychiatric decision. Common human experience and scholarly opinions suggest that the supposed protections of an adversary proceeding to determine the appropriateness of medical decisions for the commitment and treatment of mental and emotional illness may well be more illusory than real."

Nor can we ignore the fact that requiring judicial hearings will divert scarce prison resources, both money and the staff's time, from the care and treatment of mentally ill inmates.

* * *

[A]dequate procedures exist here. In particular, independence of the decisionmaker is addressed to our satisfaction by these procedures. None of the hearing committee members may be involved in the inmate's current treatment or diagnosis. . . . In the absence of record evidence to the contrary, we are not willing to presume that members of the staff lack the necessary independence to provide an inmate with a full and fair hearing in accordance with the Policy. In previous cases involving medical decisions implicating similar liberty interests, we have approved use of similar internal decisionmakers. See *Vitek*; *Parham*.[13] As we reasoned in *Vitek*, it is only by permitting persons connected with the institution to make these decisions that courts are able to avoid "unnecessary intrusion into either medical or correctional judgments." *Vitek*.

B

The procedures established by the Center are sufficient to meet the requirements of due process in all other respects, and we reject respondent's arguments to the contrary. The Policy provides for notice, the right to be present at an adversary hearing, and the right to present and cross-examine witnesses. See *Vitek*. The procedural protections are not vitiated by meetings between the committee members and staff before the hearing. Absent evidence of resulting bias, or evidence that

---

13. In an attempt to prove that internal decisionmakers lack the independence necessary to render imparital decisions, respondent and various amici refer us to other cases in which it is alleged that antipsychotic drugs were prescribed not for medical purposes, but to control or discipline mentally ill patients. We rejected a similar claim in *Parham*, and do so again here, using much the same reasoning. "That such a practice may take place in some institutions in some places affords no basis for a finding as to [Washington's] program," *Parham*, particularly in light of the trial court's finding here that the administration of antipsychotic drugs to respondent was consistent with good medical practice. Moreover, the practical effect of mandating an outside decisionmaker such as an "independent psychiatrist" or judge in these circumstances may be chimerical. Review of the literature indicates that outside decisionmakers concur with the treating physician's decision to treat a patient involuntarily in most, if not all, cases. See Bloom, Faulkner, Holm, & Rawlinson, "An Empirical View of Patients Exercising Their Right to Refuse Treatment", 7 Int'l J. Law & Psychiatry 315, 325 (1984) (independent examining physician used in Oregon psychiatric hospital concurred in decision to involuntarily medicate patients in 95% of cases); Hickman, Resnick, & Olson, "Right to Refuse Psychotropic Medication:

An Interdisciplinary Proposal", 6 Mental Disability Law Reporter 122, 130 (1982) (independent reviewing psychiatrist used in Ohio affirmed the recommendation of internal reviewer in 100% of cases). Review by judges of decisions to override a patient's objections to medication yields similar results. Appelbaum, "The Right to Refuse Treatment With Antipsychotic Medications: Retrospect and Prospect", 145 Am. J. Psychiatry 413, 417–418 (1988). In comparison, other studies reveal that review by internal decisionmakers is hardly as lackluster as the dissent suggests. See Hickman, Resnick, & Olson, supra, at 130 (internal reviewer approved of involuntary treatment in 75% of cases); Zito, Lentz, Routt, & Olson, "The Treatment Review Panel: A Solution to Treatment Refusal?", 12 Bull.Am.Acad.Psychiatry Law 349 (1984) (internal review panel used in Minnesota mental hospital approved of involuntary medication in 67% of cases). See generally Appelbaum & Hoge, "The Right to Refuse Treatment: What the Research Reveals", 4 Behavioral Sciences & the Law 279, 288–290 (1986) (summarizing results of studies on how various institutions review patients' decisions to refuse antipsychotic medications and noting "the infrequency with which refusals are allowed, regardless of the system or the decisionmaker").

the actual decision is made before the hearing, allowing respondent to contest the staff's position at the hearing satisfies the requirement that the opportunity to be heard "must be granted at a meaningful time and in a meaningful manner." We reject also respondent's contention that the hearing must be conducted in accordance with the rules of evidence or that a "clear, cogent, and convincing" standard of proof is necessary. This standard is neither required nor helpful when medical personnel are making the judgment required by the regulations here. See *Vitek.* Finally, we note that under state law an inmate may obtain judicial review of the hearing committee's decision by way of a personal restraint petition or petition for an extraordinary writ, and that the trial court found that the record compiled under the Policy was adequate to allow such review.

Respondent contends that the Policy is nonetheless deficient because it does not allow him to be represented by counsel. We disagree. "[I]t is less than crystal clear why lawyers must be available to identify possible errors in medical judgment." Given the nature of the decision to be made, we conclude that the provision of an independent lay advisor who understands the psychiatric issues involved is sufficient protection. See *Vitek* (Powell, J., concurring).

V

In sum, we hold that the regulation before us is permissible under the Constitution. It is an accommodation between an inmate's liberty interest in avoiding the forced administration of antipsychotic drugs and the State's interests in providing appropriate medical treatment to reduce the danger that an inmate suffering from a serious mental disorder represents to himself or others. The Due Process Clause does require certain essential procedural protections, all of which are provided by the regulation before us. The judgment of the Washington Supreme Court is reversed and the case remanded for further proceedings.

It is so ordered.

JUSTICE STEVENS, with whom JUSTICE BRENNAN and JUSTICE MAR-SHALL join, concurring in part and dissenting in part.

* * *

I

The Court acknowledges that under the Fourteenth Amendment "respondent possesses a significant liberty interest in avoiding the unwanted administration of antipsychotic drugs," but then virtually ignores the several dimensions of that liberty. They are both physical and intellectual. Every violation of a person's bodily integrity is an invasion of his or her liberty. The invasion is particularly intrusive if it creates a substantial risk of permanent injury and premature death. Moreover, any such action is degrading if it overrides a competent person's choice to reject a specific form of medical treatment. And when the purpose or effect of forced drugging is to alter the will and the mind of the subject, it constitutes a deprivation of liberty in the most literal and fundamental sense.

> "The makers of our Constitution undertook to secure conditions favorable to the pursuit of happiness. They recognized the significance of man's spiritual nature, of his feelings and of his intellect. They knew that only a part of the pain, pleasure and satisfactions of life are to be found in material things. They sought to protect Americans in their beliefs, their thoughts, their emotions and their sensations. They conferred, as against the Government, the right to be let alone—the most comprehensive of rights and the right most valued by civilized men." Olmstead v. United States, 277 U.S. 438, 478, 48 S.Ct. 564, 572, 72 L.Ed. 944 (1928) (Brandeis, J., dissenting).

The liberty of citizens to resist the administration of mind altering drugs arises from our Nation's most basic values.

The record of one of Walter Harper's involuntary medication hearings at the Special Offense Center (SOC) notes: "Inmate Harper stated he would rather die th[a]n take medication." That Harper would be so opposed to taking psychotropic drugs is not surprising: as the Court acknowledges, these drugs both "alter the chemical balance in a patient's brain" and can cause irreversible and fatal side effects.[5] The prolixin injections that Harper was receiving at the time of his statement exemplify the intrusiveness of psychotropic drugs on a person's body and mind. Prolixin acts "at all levels of the central nervous system as well as on multiple organ systems." It can induce catatonic-like states, alter electroencephalographic tracings, and cause swelling of the brain. Adverse reactions include drowsiness, excitement, restlessness, bizarre dreams, hypertension, nausea, vomiting, loss of appetite, salivation, dry mouth, perspiration, headache, constipation, blurred vision, impotency, eczema, jaundice, tremors, and muscle spasms. As with all psychotropic drugs, prolixin may cause tardive dyskinesia, an often irreversible syndrome of uncontrollable movements that can prevent a person from exercising basic functions such as driving an automobile, and neuroleptic malignant syndrome, which is

---

5. The Court relies heavily on the brief filed by the American Psychiatric Association and the Washington State Psychiatric Association as Amici Curiae (Psychiatrists' Brief), to discount the severity of these drugs. However, medical findings discussed in other briefs support the conclusions of the Washington Supreme Court and challenge the reliability of the Psychiatrists' Brief. For example, the Brief for American Psychological Association as Amicus Curiae (Psychologists' Brief) points out that the observation of tardive dyskinesia has been increasing "at an alarming rate" since the 1950–1970 data relied on by the Psychiatrists' Brief, and that "the chance of suffering this potentially devas-tating disorder is greater than one in four." See also Brief for Coalition for the Fundamental Rights and Equality of Ex-Patients as Amicus Curiae 16–18 (court findings and recent literature on side effects); Brief for National Association of Protection and Advocacy Systems et al. Amici Curiae 7–16 (same). Psychiatrists also may not be entirely disinterested experts. The psychologists charge: "As a psychiatrist has written, '[l]itigation from patients suffering from TD [tardive dyskinesia] is expected to explode within the next five years. Some psychiatrists and other physicians continue to minimize the seriousness of TD . . . [despite] continual warnings.'"

30% fatal for those who suffer from it. The risk of side effects increases over time.

The Washington Supreme Court properly equated the intrusiveness of this mind altering drug treatment with electroconvulsive therapy or psychosurgery. It agreed with the Supreme Judicial Court of Massachusetts' determination that the drugs have a " 'profound effect' " on a person's " 'thought processes' " and a " 'well-established likelihood of severe and irreversible adverse side effects,' " and that they therefore should be treated " 'in the same manner we would treat psychosurgery or electroconvulsive therapy.' " There is no doubt, as the State Supreme Court and other courts that have analyzed the issue have concluded, that a competent individual's right to refuse such medication is a fundamental liberty interest deserving the highest order of protection.

II

Arguably, any of three quite different state interests might be advanced to justify a deprivation of this liberty interest. The State might seek to compel Harper to submit to a mind altering drug treatment program as punishment for the crime he committed in 1976, as a "cure" for his mental illness, or as a mechanism to maintain order in the prison. The Court today recognizes Harper's liberty interest only as against the first justification.

Forced administration of antipsychotic medication may not be used as a form of punishment. This conclusion follows inexorably from our holding in *Vitek v. Jones* that the Constitution provides convicted felon the protection of due process against an involuntary transfer from the prison population to a mental hospital for psychiatric treatment.

*   *   *

The Court does not suggest that psychotropic drugs, any more than transfer for medical treatment, may be forced on prisoners as a necessary condition of their incarceration or as a disciplinary measure. Rather, it holds:

> "[G]iven the requirements of the prison environment, the Due Process Clause permits the State to treat a prison inmate who has a serious mental illness with antipsychotic drugs against his will, if the inmate is dangerous to himself or others and the treatment is in the inmate's medical interest. Policy 600.30 comports with these requirements; we therefore reject respondent's contention that its substantive standards are deficient under the Constitution."

Crucial to the Court's exposition of this substantive due process standard is the condition that these drugs "may be administered for no purpose other than treatment," and that "the treatment in question will be ordered only if it is in the prisoner's medical interests, given the legitimate needs of his institutional confinement." Thus, although the

Court does not find, as Harper urges, an absolute liberty interest of a competent person to refuse psychotropic drugs, it does recognize that the substantive protections of the Due Process Clause limit the forced administration of psychotropic drugs to all but those inmates whose medical interests would be advanced by such treatment.

[W]hether or not the State's alleged interest in providing medically beneficial treatment to those in its custody who are mentally ill may alone override the refusal of psychotropic drugs by a presumptively competent person, a plain reading of Policy 600.30 reveals that it does not meet the substantive standard set forth by the Court. Even on the Court's terms, the Policy is constitutionally insufficient.

Policy 600.30 permits forced administration of psychotropic drugs on a mentally ill inmate based purely on the impact that his disorder has on the security of the prison environment. The provisions of the Policy make no reference to any expected benefit to the inmate's medical condition. . . . Although any application of Policy 600.30 requires a medical judgment as to a prisoner's mental condition and the cause of his behavior, the Policy does not require a determination that forced medication would advance his medical interest. Use of psychotropic drugs, the State readily admits, serves to ease the institutional and administrative burdens of maintaining prison security and provides a means of managing an unruly prison population and preventing property damage. By focusing on the risk that the inmate's mental condition poses to other people and property, the Policy allows the State to exercise either parens patriae authority or police authority to override a prisoner's liberty interest in refusing psychotropic drugs. Thus, most unfortunately, there is simply no basis for the Court's assertion that medication under the Policy must be to advance the prisoner's medical interest.

* * *

The State advances security concerns as a justification for forced medication in two distinct circumstances. A SOC Policy provision not at issue in this case permits 72 hours of involuntary medication on an emergency basis when "an inmate is suffering from a mental disorder and as a result of that disorder presents an imminent likelihood of serious harm to himself or others." In contrast to the imminent danger of injury that triggers the emergency medication provisions, a general risk of illness-induced injury or property damage—evidenced by no more than past behavior—allows long-term, involuntary medication of an inmate with psychotropic drugs under Policy 600.30. This ongoing interest in security and management is a penological concern of a constitutionally distinct magnitude from the necessity of responding to emergencies. It is difficult to imagine what, if any, limits would restrain such a general concern of prison adminstrators who believe that prison environments are, " 'by definition,' . . . made up of persons with 'a demonstrated proclivity for antisocial criminal, and often violent, conduct.' " A rule that allows prison administrators to address potential security risks by forcing psychotropic drugs on mentally ill inmates for prolonged periods is unquestionably an "exaggerated response" to that concern.

[T]he record before us does not establish that a more narrowly drawn policy withdrawing psychotropics from only those inmates who actually refuse consent[15] and who do not pose an imminent threat of serious harm[16] would increase the marginal costs of SOC administration. Harper's own record reveals that administrative segregation and standard disciplinary sanctions were frequently imposed on him over and above forced medication and thus would add no new costs. Similarly, intramuscular injections of psychotropics, such as those frequently forced on Harper, entail no greater risk than administration of less dangerous drugs such as tranquilizers. Use of psychotropic drugs simply to suppress an inmate's potential violence, rather than to achieve therapeutic results, may also undermine the efficacy of other available treatment programs that would better address his illness.

[T]he flaw in Washington's Policy 600.30—and the basic error in the Court's opinion today—is the failure to divorce from each other the two justifications for forced medication [i.e., security and rehabilitation] and to consider the extent to which the Policy is reasonably related to

15. There is no evidence that more than a small fraction of inmates would refuse drugs under a voluntary policy. Harper himself voluntarily took psychotropics for six years, and intermittently consented to them after 1982. See e.g., *Rogers v. Okin*, 478 F.Supp. 1342, 1369 (Mass. 1979) (only 12 of 1,000 institutionalized patients refused psychotropic drugs for prolonged periods during the two years that judicial restraining order was in effect), modified, 634 F.2d 650 (CA1 1980), vacated and remanded, sub nom. *Mills v. Rogers*, 457 U.S. 291, 102 S.Ct. 2442, 73 L.Ed.2d 16 (1982). The efficacy of forced drugging is also marginal; involuntary patients have a poorer prognosis than cooperative patients. See Rogers & Webster, "Assessing Treatability in Mentally Disordered Offenders", 13 Law and Human Behavior 19, 20–21 (1989).

16. As the Court notes, properly used, these drugs are "one of the most effective means of treating and controlling" certain incurable mental illnesses, but they are not a panacea for long-term care of all patients.

"[T]he maintenance treatment literature . . . shows that many patients (approximately 30%) relapse despite receiving neuroleptic medication, while neuroleptics can be withdrawn from other patients for many months and in some cases for years without relapse. Standard maintenance medication treatment strategies, though they are indisputably effective in group comparisons, may be quite inefficient in addressing the treatment requirements of the individual patient." Lieberman et al., "Reply to Ethics of Drug Discontinuation Studies in Schizophrenia," 46 Archives of General Psychiatry 387, 387 (1989) (footnotes omitted).

Indeed, the drugs appear to have produced at most minor "savings" in Harper's case. Dr. Petrich reported that "medications are not satisfactory in containing the worst excesses of his labile and irritable behavior. He is uncooperative when on medication." [A] therapy supervisor reported before Harper's involuntary medication began: "during the time in which he assaulted the nurse at Cabrini he was on neuroleptic medication yet there is indication that he was psychotic. However, during his stay at SOC he has been off of all neuroleptic medications and at times has shown some preoccupation and appearance of psychosis but has not become assaultive. His problems on medication, such as the paradoxical effect from the neuroleptic medications, may be precipitated by increased doses of neuroleptic medications and may cause an exacerbation of his psychosis. Though Mr. Harper is focused on psychosomatic problems from neuroleptic medications as per the side effects, the real problem may be that the psychosis is exacerbated by neuroleptic medications."

either interest. The State, and arguably the Court, allows the SOC to blend the state interests in responding to emergencies and in convenient prison administration with the individual's interest in receiving beneficial medical treatment. The result is a muddled rationale that allows the "exaggerated response" of forced psychotropic medication on the basis of purely institutional concerns. So serving institutional convenience eviscerates the inmate's substantive liberty interest in the integrity of his body and mind.

III

The procedures of Policy 600.30 are also constitutionally deficient. Whether or not the State ever may order involuntary administration of psychotropic drugs to a mentally ill person who has been committed to its custody but has not been declared incompetent, it is at least clear that any decision approving such drugs must be made by an impartial professional concerned not with institutional interests, but only with the individual's best interests. The critical defect in Policy 600.30 is the failure to have the treatment decision made or reviewed by an impartial person or tribunal.[20]

* * *

The decisionmakers [under Policy 600.30] have two disqualifying conflicts of interest. First, the panel members must review the work of treating physicians who are their colleagues and who, in turn, regularly review their decisions. Such an in-house system pits the interests of an inmate who objects to forced medication against the judgment not only of his doctor, but often his doctor's colleagues.[22] Furthermore, the Court's conclusion that "[n]one of the hearing committee members may be involved in the inmate's current treatment or diagnosis" overlooks the fact that Policy 600.30 allows a treating psychiatrist to participate in all but the initial seven-day medication approval. This revolving door operated in Harper's case. Dr. Petrich treated Harper through

---

20. It is not necessary to reach the question whether the decision to force psychotropic drugs on a competent person against his will must be approved by a judge, or by an administrative tribunal of professionals who are not members of the prison staff, in order to conclude that the mechanism of Policy 600.30 violates procedural due process. The choice is not between medical experts on the one hand and judges on the other; the choice is between decisionmakers who are biased and those who are not.

22. As regular SOC staff, 600.30 committee members are: "susceptible to implicit or explicit pressure for cooperation ('If you support my orders, I'll support yours'). It is instructive that month after month, year after year, this 'review' panel always voted for more medication—despite the scientific literature showing that periodic respites from drugs are advisable and

that prolonged use of antipsychotic drugs is proper only when the medical need is clear and compelling." Psychologists' Brief 26–27 (footnote omitted).

Rates of approval by different review bodies are of limited value, of course, because institutions will presumably adjust their medication practices over time to obtain approval under different standards or by different reviewing bodies. However, New Jersey's review of involuntary psychotropic medication in mental institutions is instructive. In 1980 external review by an "independent psychiatrist" who was not otherwise employed by the Department of Human Services resulted in discontinuation or reduction of 59% of dosages. After the Department moved to an internal peer review system, that percentage dropped to 2.5% of cases. Brief for New Jersey Department of Public Advocate as Amicus Curiae 38–54.

1982 and recommended involuntary medication on October 27, 1982. Dr. Loeken, staff psychologist Giles, and Assistant Superintendent Stark authorized medication for seven days after a 600.30 hearing on November 23, 1982. Dr. Petrich then replaced Dr. Loeken on the committee, and with Giles and Stark approved long-term involuntary medication on December 8, 1982. Solely under this authority, Dr. Petrich prescribed more psychotropic medication for Harper on December 8, 1982 and throughout the following year.

Second, the panel members, as regular staff of the Center, must be concerned not only with the inmate's best medical interests, but also with the most convenient means of controlling the mentally disturbed inmate. The mere fact that a decision is made by a doctor does not make it "certain that professional judgment in fact was exercised." The structure of the SOC committee virtually insures that it will not be. While the initial inquiry into the mental bases for an inmate's behavior is medical, the ultimate medication decision under Policy 600.30 turns on an assessment of the risk that an inmate's condition imposes on the institution. The prescribing physician and each member of the review committee must therefore wear two hats. This hybrid function disables the independent exercise of each decisionmaker's professional judgment. The structure of the review committee further confuses the objective of the inquiry; two of the committee members are not trained or licensed to prescribe psychotropic drugs, and one has no medical expertise at all. The trump by institutional interests is dramatized by the fact that appeals of committee decisions under the Policy are made solely to the SOC Superintendent.

* * *

The institutional bias that is inherent in the identity of the decisionmakers is unchecked by other aspects of Policy 600.30. The committee need not consider whether less intrusive procedures would be effective, or even if the prescribed medication would be beneficial to the prisoner, before approving involuntary medication. Findings regarding the severity or the probability of potential side effects of drugs and dosages are not required. And, although the Policy does not prescribe a standard of proof necessary for any factual determination upon which a medication decision rests, the Court gratuitously advises that the "clear, cogent, and convincing" standard adopted by the State Supreme Court would be unnecessary.

Nor is the 600.30 hearing likely to raise these issues fairly and completely. An inmate recommended for involuntary medication is no more capable of " 'speaking effectively for himself' " on these "issues which are 'complex or otherwise difficult to develop or present' " than an inmate recommended for transfer to a mental hospital. *Vitek* (Powell, J., concurring in part). Although single doses of some psychotropic drugs are designed to be effective for a full month, the inmate may not refuse the very medication he is contesting until 24 hours before his hearing. Policy 600.30 also does not allow the inmate to be represented by counsel at hearings, but only to have present an advisor, who is appointed by the SOC. These advisors, of questionable loyalties and efficacy, cannot provide the "independent assistance" required for an inmate fairly to understand and participate in the hearing process.[30] In addition, although the Policy gives the inmate a "limitable right to present testimony through his own witnesses and to confront and cross-examine witnesses," in the next paragraph it takes that right away for reasons that "include, but are not limited to such things as irrelevance, lack of necessity, redundancy, possible reprisals, or other reasons relating to institutional interests of security, order, and rehabilitation." Finally, because Policy 600.30 provides a hearing only for the seven-day committee, and just a paper record for the long-term committee, the inmate has no opportunity at all to present his objections to the more crucial decision to medicate him on a long-term basis.

In sum, it is difficult to imagine how a committee convened under Policy 600.30 could conceivably discover, much less be persuaded to overrule, an erroneous or arbitrary decision to medicate or to maintain a specific dosage or type of drug. Institutional control infects the decisionmakers and the entire procedure. . . .

I continue to believe that "even the inmate retains an unalienable interest in liberty—at the very minimum the right to be treated with dignity—which the Constitution may never ignore." A competent individual's right to refuse psychotropic medication is an aspect of liberty requiring the highest order of protection under the Fourteenth Amendment. Accordingly, . . . I respectfully dissent from the Court's opinion and judgment.

Questions and Comments

1. *The rationale for a right to refuse.* The majority opinion in *Harper* relies on the due process clause in holding that a prisoner has a "right" to refuse unwanted antipsychotic drugs. Other possible bases for a right to refuse which have been advanced by various courts and commentators include: (1) the first amendment's protection of thought and expression; (2) the eighth amendment's prohibition against cruel and unusual punishment; (3) the equal protection clause's requirement that like classes be treated alike (here the comparable class is the non-mentally ill, who are protected by the informed consent doctrine); and (4) the "penumbral" right to privacy's protection of bodily integrity. See 2 Men.Dis.L.Rep. 43, 46 (1977) (discussing these and other bases for the right). Among the lower court decisions which have found a constitutional right to refuse medication, most have relied on the latter theory. See, e.g., *United States v.*

---

30. The prisoner is introduced to, and may consult with, his appointed advisor at the commencement of the hearing. Harper's advisor on November 23, 1982, a nurse practitioner from Washington State Reformatory, asked Harper three questions in the hearing. The other five advisors appointed for Harper never spoke in the hearings. All five were apparently staff at the SOC: SOC Psychiatric Social Worker Hyden (who sat for the SOC Assistant Superintendent on the next 180–day committee that reapproved Harper's medication), a prison chaplain, two registered nurses, and a correctional officer.

Charters, 863 F.2d 302 (4th Cir. 1988) (dealing with patients found incompetent to stand trial); *Rogers v. Okin*, 634 F.2d 650 (1st Cir. 1980) (civilly committed patients); *Rennie v. Klein*, 653 F.2d 836 (3d Cir. 1981) (civilly committed patients). Is the right to privacy approach significantly different from the Supreme Court's approach in *Harper*? Of the various approaches, which is the most persuasive? How would the choice of a particular constitutional basis affect the scope of the right?

2. *The substantive scope of the right.* Focusing solely on the scope of the right, rather than the procedures for implementing it, what are the implications of *Harper* for persons who are civilly committed? For those who are committed after acquittal by reason of insanity? If prison confinement is indistinguishable from commitment in this regard, does *any* involuntarily committed person have a federal constitutional right to refuse medication after *Harper*?

In the civil committment context, other courts have arrived at standards different both from each other and from the policy at issue in *Harper*. In *Rogers v. Commissioner*, 390 Mass. 489, 458 N.E.2d 308 (1983), the Supreme Judicial Court of Massachusetts developed standards under Massachusetts law similar to those adopted by the Washington Supreme Court in *Harper*. The holding can be summarized as follows:

(1) Administration of antipsychotic medication over a competent patient's objection is permissible if the patient "poses an imminent threat of harm to himself or others, and . . . if there is no less intrusive alternative to antipsychotic drugs." Id. at 321.

(2) Otherwise, forcible medication is permissible only if the patient is incompetent to made a treatment decision. A *doctor's* determination of incompetency will justify forcible medication only if the medication is necessary "to prevent the 'immediate, substantial, and irreversible deterioration of a serious mental illness,' in cases in which 'even the smallest of avoidable delays would be intolerable.'" Id. at 322.

(3) If medication is necessary beyond this emergency period, and in all other circumstances, incompetence must be determined by a judge, at a hearing with notice and a guardian ad litem appointed to assist the court in the treatment decision. Id. at 322–23.

(4) If the judge finds the patient incompetent, he or she must make a substituted judgment decision and approve a treatment plan. Either the judge or a court-appointed guardian must monitor the subsequent treatment process. Id. at 318.

Similar to *Rogers*, *Rennie v. Klein*, 653 F.2d 836 (3d Cir. 1981), permitted forcible medication of those who are imminently dangerous to self or others, and of those for whom "there is a significant possibility" of harm to self, provided medication is the least intrusive means of accomplishing the state's goals of treatment and security. But *Rennie* also denied a right to refuse to competent, nondangerous patients, if the medication "would probably improve the patient's condition within a significantly shorter time period" than alternative treatment plans. Id. at 852. Other courts have reduced the right even further, holding that the patient's competency "is properly treated as simply another factor in the ultimate medical decision to administer the medication involuntarily." *United States v. Charters*, 863 F.2d 302 (4th Cir. 1988).

3. *Procedures.* What are the procedural implications of *Harper* for civilly committed patients? The majority relies heavily not only on *Vitek v. Jones*, which involved the due process rights of prisoners transferred to mental hospitals, but also on *Parham v. J.R.*, which involved the civil commitment of children. Are the citations to either *Vitek* or *Parham* apposite in deciding upon the proper procedures for implementing the right to refuse?

Consider the following methods of implementing the right in non-emergency situations: (1) judicial determination and monitoring (see *Rogers*, described in note 2); (2) judicial appointment of a guardian who makes all treatment decisions (an option permitted by *Rogers* after the initial judicial intervention, see note 2); (3) review by professionals from outside the institution (required by the trial court in *Rennie*, 462 F.Supp. 1131, 1147 (D.N.J. 1978)); (4) review by professionals from the same institution (as permitted in *Harper*); (5) a judicial determination at the commitment hearing, with no further review (see Stromberg & Stone, "A Model State Law on Civil Commitment of the Mentally Ill," 20 Harv.J.Legis. 265, 356–57 (1983)); (6) no review of the professional's decision (see e.g., *Dautremont v. Broadlawns Hosp.*, 827 F.2d 291 (8th Cir.1987)). In light of the realities described in *Harper*, which option do you prefer? If some type of hearing is appropriate, what standard of proof should apply? Should the patient be entitled to an advocate?

4. *Uninstitutionalized persons' right to refuse.* The caselaw described above concerns the right of institutionalized persons to refuse medication. In contrast to the narrowed right accorded this population, the non-mentally ill individual, as noted at the beginning of this section, is normally entitled to the protections of the informed consent doctrine, which provides a relatively robust right to refuse. What is the scope of the right for the non-institutionalized person who is mentally ill?

In re Guardianship of Roe, 383 Mass. 415, 421 N.E.2d 40 (1981), involved the right of a 21 year-old ward to refuse medication after his release from the hospital. The Massachusetts Supreme Court held that the ward's guardian, his father, could not unilaterally make the treatment decision for the ward unless there was an "emergency". Otherwise, a court must make the treatment decision. Further the court could authorize forcible medication only if one of two circumstances were met:

> (1) where a judicial substituted judgment determination indicates that the incompetent individual would, if competent, accept antipsychotic drugs, or (2) where there exists a State interest of sufficient magnitude to override the individual's right to refuse. If the asserted State interest is the prevention of violent conduct by non-institutionalized mentally ill individuals, then, upon a showing equivalent to that necessary to commit an individual against his will, the State is entitled to force the individual to choose, by way of substituted judgment,

either involuntary commitment or medication with antipsychotic drugs.

Id. at 61.

Two issues are raised by *Roe*. The first has to do with the role of the court vis-a-vis the role of the guardian. Do you agree with *Roe's* requirement that a court order be obtained prior to forcibly medicating a ward whose validly appointed guardian has consented to the treatment?[j] The second issue concerns the consequences of a refusal by an uninstitutionalized person. As indicated above, under *Roe,* if a dangerous person chooses hospitalization over medication, then the state must acquiesce in that choice. May the person continue to refuse medication once in the hospital? In a footnote, the *Roe* court stated: "We do not address the question of whether and to what extent the State interest in *institutional* order and safety may be capable of overwhelming the right of an involuntarily committed individual to refuse medical treatment . . .." Id. at 61 n. 23 (emphasis in original).

5. *Benefits and costs of the right to refuse.* Some research on the impact of the right to refuse litigation is reported in the following excerpt from Brooks, "The Right to Refuse Antipsychotic Medication: Law and Policy," 39 Rutgers L.Rev. 339, 367–374 (1987).

Benefits

* * *

Decreasing the amount of medication used was an objective of refusal litigation. . . . Studies show that there has been a substantial lowering of individual dosages in a number of hospitals. . . .

Another aspect of "too much drugs" is "too many different drugs." The practice of polypharmacy, though widely disapproved, was widespread in pre-litigation years. Current data from Napa State indicate that polypharmacy has been virtually eliminated. In 1974 a mean of 2.3 drugs were used for a single patient in the first eight weeks of confinement, with a range up to five different drugs. In 1983 [after a consent decree required review of refusals by outside psychiatrists] the mean during the same period of time was only 1.1. . . .

A third benefit would result from changing types of medications to see whether patients respond less dysphorically and with fewer side effects to a medication different from one originally prescribed. There is no hard data on this important change, so we can only speculate about it, but there is anecdotal data that this now occurs more frequently than before.

A fourth benefit would be reducing the incidence of inappropriate delegation by physicians to other staff prescribing medication. This was once a major problem. . . . In Davis v. Hubbard, the court found that, at Lima State Hospital in Ohio, PRN orders were being written that permitted attendants to decide when medication should be administered. These PRN orders often had no termination or review

j. The answer to this question may depend upon whether one views antipsychotic medication as an "extraordinary treatment" (see pp. 845–847).

date. It was further reported that attendants could obtain medication from the pharmacy by submitting appropriate forms "without a physician's signature." In Ohio hospitals such PRN orders have been eliminated. Inappropriate delegations have been terminated.

A fifth benefit has been the encouragement of processes of negotiation and participation by patients in their own treatment programs, a process that is initiated when a patient refuses medication. . . . The process of negotiation is not only responsive to patient needs, but also encourages patient autonomy and enhances patient dignity. [Moreover], research has indicated that negative reaction to medication is a powerful predictor of noncompliance and poor outcome.

* * *

Patient Costs

What are the costs to the patient? One is delay in treatment. In states like Massachusetts, the procedure requires a judicial hearing to determine whether the patient is competent to refuse. Veliz and James show that there are long delays between the refusal, the petition to compel medication, and the hearing, on average four and one-half months, and ranging from two to seven months. But . . . [i]t is not obvious that patients actually suffer from such delays, nor do Veliz and James present any data to that effect. Put otherwise, there is no evidence that the delays cause patients to "rot."

It has been argued that a significant cost to refusing patients would be longer stays in the hospital. Do refusers, in fact, spend more time in the hospital than consenters? Evidence suggests that refusers are discharged at approximately the same rate as consenters. Refusal seems not to prolong hospitalization.

Do refusers deteriorate, remain the same, or improve? . . . Hargreaves and associates studied forty-seven cases (out of 2,700 reviews) in which refusals were upheld. Deterioration occurred in twenty-five patients of whom twenty were remedicated. No adverse consequences were seen in eight patients. The outcome was "unclear" for the rest. There was thus no harm to the patient in approximately 50 percent of these refusals, and presumably little harm to the twenty who were remedicated.

Have a larger number of antisocial incidents occurred because refusing patients went untreated? Psychiatrists had predicted outbreaks of violence and disruption by non-medicated refusers. Have there been transfers to locked wards, self-injurious behaviors, property destruction, suicide attempts, verbal threats, assaults, AWOLs, escapes, or displays of non-cooperation? Were seclusion and restraint used more extensively? A Minnesota study shows no statistical difference in these areas between refusers and consenters.

Costs to Staff and State

* * *

It is to be expected that many staff members, though not all, would find refusals a burden. . . . Hargreaves and associates asked doctors and nurses for their views about refusal at Napa State. Eighty-five percent of the doctors thought the refusal consent decree made their work more difficult. Nurses were more negative than doctors, saying that the decree went "too far." Twenty-five percent of nurses thought that the consent decree was "absurd." Ninety percent of nurses said that the consent decree made their jobs more difficult. Many felt that the decree was a waste of money, that it impaired treatment quality and made their work more dangerous. . . . It is difficult to evaluate such reactions since they are subjective and unsupported by specific illustrations of ways in which work has been made "more difficult." Some increases in difficulty surely result from an increase in the complexity of the caring task in response to legitimate patient needs. But are there inappropriate burdens unrelated to providing care? . . . A crucial aspect of the problem is that there is a long history of neglect of public sector patients. Any legal requirement that strikes at this neglect increases a burden. It is not clear how this particular "cost" should be weighed as against the benefits described.

Finally, we reach a twofold cost to the state. The first is the cost of hearings, which requires paying outside reviewers, lawyers, and others. The second is the cost involved in diverting personnel from other functions to the job of preparing for and appearing at hearings.

Hargreaves and associates have calculated that salary costs for outside psychiatric reviewers, patient advocates, hospital support staff, departmental staff, and the like, came to over $300,000 in the first year of the consent decree at Napa State Hospital. A "hidden" cost included the diversion of clinicians from other duties to the preparation of paper work for reviews. Since there were 2,800 reviews, each single review cost approximately $100. Hargreaves estimates that at this rate it would cost approximately $1–$1.5 million per year for reviews in all five major mental hospitals in California.

* * *

[I]s the cost too high because relatively few patients refuse and even fewer refusals are upheld? . . . The first data available from the Boston State Hospital, involved in the *Rogers* case, showed an incidence of about 9 percent refusals for 1,400 patients. Later data shows a proportion of refusals in a variety of hospitals ranging from 2.4 and 5 percent to 15 percent.

The data on refusal overrides shows proportions ranging from 100 percent of overrides in a study of nine patients to only 67 percent of overrides in a study of 19 Minnesota patients. In other words, in Minnesota, one-third of refusals were upheld, a much larger proportion than anywhere else. It has been suggested that the greater deference in Minnesota to refusals is a result of the fact that only one member of the five-member Anoka Treatment Review Panel was a physician.

It has been argued that the significance to the patient of a right to refuse has been exaggerated and should be abandoned. It has also been argued that even such a small incidence as 5% refusals interferes with the treatment of more than 15,000 patients a year, assuming an annual commitment rate of 300,000.

B. ELECTROCONVULSIVE THERAPY AND PSYCHOSURGERY

ELECTROCONVULSIVE THERAPY CONSENSUS DEVELOPMENT CONFERENCE STATEMENT

Vol. 5, No. 11, 1985.
U.S.Dept. of Health and Human Services, Public Health Service, National Institutes of Health, Office of Medical Applications of Research.

Electroconvulsive therapy (ECT) is a treatment for severe mental illness in which a brief application of electric stimulus is used to produce a generalized seizure. In the United States in the 1940's and 1950's, the treatment was often administered to the most severely disturbed patients residing in large mental institutions. As often occurs with new therapies, ECT was used for a variety of disorders, frequently in high doses and for long periods. Many of these efforts proved ineffective, and some even harmful. Moreover, its use as a means of managing unruly patients, for whom other treatments were not then available, contributed to the perception of ECT as an abusive instrument of behavioral control for patients in mental institutions for the chronically ill. With the introduction of effective psychopharmacologic medications and the development of judicial and regulatory restrictions, the use of ECT has waned.

The treatment is now used primarily in general hospital psychiatric units and in psychiatric hospitals. A National Institute of Mental Health hospital survey estimated that 33,384 patients admitted to hospital psychiatric services during 1980 were treated with ECT, representing approximately 2.4% of all psychiatric admissions.

* * *

The efficacy of ECT has been established most convincingly in the treatment of delusional and severe endogenous depressions, which make up a clinically important minority of depressive disorders. Some studies find ECT to be of at least equal efficacy to medication treatments, and others find ECT to be superior to medication. Not a single controlled study has shown another form of treatment to be superior to ECT in short-term management of severe depressions. It must be noted, however, that those studies that found ECT to be superior to medication were not designed to study the persistence of this advantage of ECT beyond the short term. Moreover, the available evidence suggests that relapse rates in the year following ECT are likely to be high unless maintenance antidepressant medications are subsequently prescribed.

* * *

Electroconvulsive therapy and lithium appear to be equally effective for acute mania, and either is superior to hospitalization without somatic therapy. A treatment regimen in which ECT is used for the acute episode, followed by lithium maintenance, does not appear to be associated with an increased risk of early relapse compared with lithium treatment alone.

*   *   *

Neuroleptics are the first line of treatment of schizophrenia. The evidence for the efficacy of ECT in schizophrenia is not compelling but is strongest for those schizophrenic patients with a shorter duration of illness, a more acute onset, and more intense affective symptoms. It has not been useful in chronically ill schizophrenic patients.

*   *   *

In early days of ECT, mortality was a significant problem. The commonly quoted overall mortality rate in the first few decades was 0.1%, or one per 1,000. Over the years, safer methods of administration have been developed, including the use of short-acting anesthetics, muscle relaxants, and adequate oxygenation. Present mortality is very low. In the least favorable recent series reported, there were 2.9 deaths per 10,000 patients. In another series, 4.5 deaths per 100,000 patients were reported. Overall, the risk is not different from that associated with the use of short-acting barbiturate anesthetics. The risk of death from anesthesia, although very small, is present and should be considered when evaluating the setting for performing ECT.

In the past, up to 40% of patients suffered from various complications, the most common being vertebral compression fractures. With present techniques, these risks have been virtually eliminated. In one recent study of almost 25,000 treatments, a complication rate of one per 1,300 to 1,400 treatments was found. These included laryngospasm, circulatory insufficiency, tooth damage, vertebral compression fractures, . . . peripheral nerve palsy, skin burns, ...

NOTE, REGULATION OF ELECTROCONVULSIVE THERAPY

75 Mich.L.Rev. 363, 367–369.
(1976).

Of far greater concern are the mental complications of ECT—particularly disorientation and loss of memory. Disorientation may be so complete that the patient will not remember the names of people around him and, in rare cases, his occupation. Such confusion has been reported to persist for as long as six months after treatment. This effect may actually be a necessary part of the therapy, for some clinicians believe that the extent of the treatment's eventual success is directly proportional to the amount of temporary disorientation. That loss of memory is also a frequent result of ECT is not seriously questioned. However, the scope and length of the loss is a subject of vigorous debate within the psychiatric profession. Total amnesia typically occurs throughout the entire course of a series of treatments. Some authorities state that memory usually returns within a few weeks of the final treatment; however, there are also reports of permanent memory impairment. Memory loss may extend to events occurring before or after the treatment. Although other serious mental complications of ECT are not thoroughly documented, there is some evidence indicating that ECT may cause brain damage and impairment of learning ability.

PLOTKIN, LIMITING THE THERAPEUTIC ORGY: MENTAL PATIENTS' RIGHT TO REFUSE TREATMENT
72 Nw.L.Rev. 461, 466–71.
(1978).

The earliest example of psychosurgery dates back to the Inca civilization where the perforation of the skull was used to "cure" mental illness by supposedly releasing evil spirits from the brain. Now, as then, psychosurgery is simply "[b]rain surgery performed for the relief of mental and psychic symptoms." The difference between psychosurgery and routine brain surgery is that psychosurgery is used to alter behavior.

After early research by Fulton and Jacobsen catalogued the disappearance of frustration, temper tantrums, and anxiety toward learning tasks following frontal cortex ablation in two chimpanzees, modern surgeons began to contemplate psychosurgery as a viable treatment technique. The Portuguese team of Moniz and Lima introduced bilateral prefrontal lobotomy on humans in 1936. They hypothesized that "by interrupting some of the connections between the prefrontal lobes and other parts of the brain, some modifications might be brought about in the mental processes of psychotic individuals."

In 1936, on the strength of Moniz's results, Freeman and Watts, the American "pioneers" of psychosurgery, performed the first "standard" lobotomy in the United States. They were able to achieve a bleaching of emotional tone and a quieting of anxiety in psychotic patients. They reported that:

> [patients] are not apathetic, lacking all emotion, after lobotomy; rather, the emotion attaches itself to external happenings rather than to inner experiences. Patients * * * are usually cheerful, responsive, affectionate and unreserved. They are outspoken, often critical of others and lacking in embarrassment. * * * Some patients are distractible, others have single track minds; some are indolent, others are human dynamos. The most striking and constant change from the pre-operative personality lies in a certain unselfconsciousness.

> * * * The patient emerges from operation with an immature personality that is at first poorly equipped for maintaining him in a competitive society; but with the passage of time there is progressive improvement, so that in about one-half of the cases earning a living again becomes possible.

* * *

As a result of both the frequency of psychosurgery's negative effects and the increasing availability of psychotropic drugs, a significant decline in the use of psychosurgery occurred during the 1950's, especially in state hospitals. Nevertheless, psychosurgery, while dormant, did not disappear; in fact, it has rallied in the last decade. A small group of neurosurgeons are struggling to devise methods for increasing the specificity of therapeutic results, while diminishing the unfavorable personality effects associated with classical lobotomies.

Current procedures, allegedly aiming only at specific sites in the brain, emphasize extremely precise localization and limitation of the operation to achieve therapeutic benefit without use of extensive cutting techniques. Generally, more favorable results have been reported with these localized procedures. The severe emotional blunting, impaired intellectual functioning, and extensive somatic side effects which accompanied the older techniques are today reported to occur with less frequency.

* * *

R. CULLITON, PSYCHOSURGERY: NATIONAL COMMISSION ISSUES SURPRISINGLY FAVORABLE REPORT
194 Science 299.
(1976).

[I]t came as something of a surprise when the [National Commission for the Protection of Human Subjects of Biomedical and Behavioral Research] adopted its report that "encourages" the Secretary of Health, Education, and Welfare to support research on psychosurgery and that, in general, treats psychosurgery benignly. Asked by *Science* what it was that influenced the commission favorably, its chairman, J. Kenneth Ryan of Harvard Medical School, replied, "We looked at the data and saw they did not support our prejudices. I, for one, did not expect to come out in favor of psychosurgery. But we saw that some very sick people had been helped by it, and that it did not destroy their intelligence or rob them of feelings. Their marriages were intact. They were able to work. The operation shouldn't be banned."

In saying this, Ryan and the other commissioners are by no means endorsing the clearly destructive prefrontal lobotomies that were performed on an estimated 40,000 to 50,000 mental patients 25 years ago. . . . What they are approving is study of the newer forms of contemporary surgery [stereotactic surgery] in which only small, selective areas of brain tissue are destroyed.

The data that so impressed the commission were gathered by scientists who were asked to undertake special investigations of psychosurgery. One man surveyed the world literature of the past 5 years and two teams of researchers personally evaluated the psychological and neurological status of patients who had psychosurgery between 1965 and 1975. Between them, they interviewed and administered a battery of tests to 61 psychosurgery patients. Most of the patients were middle-aged, all were white, and all suffered from long-standing and very debilitating mental illness.

One of the studies was conducted by Hans–Lukas Teuber and his colleagues, Suzanne Corkin and Thomas E. Twitchell, at the Massachusetts Institute of Technology. Teuber, a neurophysiologist, was chosen by the commission for two reasons. For nearly 30 years, Teuber has been studying the side effects of brain injury, dealing with previously healthy individuals who suffered brain damage in an accident or in combat. The commission thought him particularly well qualified to examine patients whose brains had been selectively damaged by psychosurgery. In addition, it was no secret that Teuber did not think much of psychosurgery. . . .

Teuber studied 34 men and women who had been operated on by the same surgeon. Each had a cingulotomy, an operation in which a bundle of nerve fibers connecting the frontal lobes with the limbic system (thought to be the seat of emotions) is interrupted by precise, well-placed lesions. The amount of tissue that is destroyed is very small.

The 34 cingulotomy patients were operated on for a variety of problems including persistent pain and depression, depression alone, obsessive-compulsive illness, anxiety neurosis, and borderline schizophrenia. In terms of success, Teuber reports that the patients with pain accompanied by depression "stand out." Nine of 11 such patients were cured of long-standing illness that had been refractory to drugs, psychotherapy, and electroshock. Five of seven patients with depression alone were markedly better after psychosurgery. The rest did not do so well. Four patients who had obsessive-compulsive disorders, for example, were as resistant to psychosurgery as they were to everything else. The reactions of the other patients were mixed and no clear pattern could be found; the investigators were left with the preliminary conclusion that cingulotomy appears to be the most effective for patients with depression alone or accompanied with pain.

Teuber's observations are remarkably similar to those of Allan F. Mirsky of Boston University School of Medicine, who, with Maressa Hecht Orzack, also did a study for the commission. Mirsky is well known for his research on brain functioning in primates and human beings. If they had any prejudice against psychosurgery before they undertook this study, they kept it to themselves. In a recent telephone interview with *Science,* Orzack said they were "neutral" or, perhaps, a little "skeptical." However, she says, "when we began seeing the patients, we were just amazed."

Mirsky, Orzack, and their colleagues, evaluated 27 patients who had psychosurgery performed by one of three surgeons. One of them practices in the Northeast, the other two on the West Coast. None of the three performs the same kind of operation. Therefore, the type and the amount of brain tissue that is targeted for destruction varies from surgeon to surgeon. On the basis of their examinations, the researchers concluded that 14 of the 27 patients "derived considerable benefit" from psychosurgery; most of them had been treated for depression. Several others showed "slight" or "moderate" improvement. There was no evidence of serious side effects.

ADEN v. YOUNGER

Court of Appeal, Fourth District, Division 1, 1976.
57 Cal.App.3d 662, 129 Cal.Rptr. 535.

GERALD BROWN, PRESIDING JUSTICE.

Petitioners Jane Doe and Betty Roe are mentally ill. Doe has had electroconvulsive therapy (ECT) and may need further voluntary treatments. Roe wants a surgical "Multiple target procedure," or psychosurgery. . . .

* * *

The Attorney General, the Director of Health, and the Board of Medical Examiners are respondents.

The law involved in this petition is part of the Lanterman–Petris–Short Act (Welf. & Inst.Code §§ 5000–5404.1). The law changes conditions under which psychosurgery and shock treatment can be performed. The changes applicable to persons involuntarily detained and persons voluntarily admitted to state hospitals, private mental institutions, county psychiatric hospitals and certain mentally retarded persons, are:

Psychosurgery: (§§ 5325, 5326, 5326.3.)

Patients have the right to refuse psychosurgery and the professional person in charge of the facility may not deny them that right. If a patient refuses consent, it must be entered on the record.

If a patient wants psychosurgery, then the conditions for performing such surgery include:

(a) The patient must give written informed consent, dated, witnessed and entered in his record. The consent may be withdrawn at any time. An oral explanation by the doctor is necessary.

(b) The patient must have capacity to consent.

(c) An oral explanation must be given to a responsible relative, guardian or conservator.

(d) The reasons for surgery must be in the patient's treatment record, other treatments must be exhausted and surgery must be critically needed.

(e) Three appointed physicians (two board-certified psychiatrists or neurosurgeons), must examine the patient and unanimously agree with the treating physician's determinations and that the patient has capacity to consent. There must be a 72–hour wait after the patient's written consent before surgery.

Shock Treatment: (§ 5326.4.)

If the treating physician feels shock treatments are necessary, he must give an extensive oral explanation to the patient and his relative, guardian, or conservator.

Shock treatments shall be performed only after:

(a) The patient gives written informed consent.

(b) The patient has capacity to consent.

(c) A relative, guardian or conservator has been given a thorough oral explanation.

(d) "Adequate documentation" has been entered in the patient's record. All other treatments have been exhausted and the treatment is critically needed.

(e) There has been a review by three appointed physicians (two board-certified) who agree with the treating physician that the patient has capacity to consent.

If the patient does not have the capacity to consent, shock treatments can be given if conditions (c), (d) and (e) are met.

No shock treatments may be given if the patient is able to give informed consent and refuses.

* * *

The petitioners, and amici curiae in support of the petition for writ of mandate, rest their attack on the amended and added Welfare & Institutions Code sections on several asserted constitutional infirmities:

* * *

A. EQUAL PROTECTION

Petitioners' equal protection arguments [i.e., that they should be able to obtain psychosurgery or ECT treatment as easily as non-mental patients] are without merit.

* * *

Mental patients are distinct from other ill patients in two special circumstances. First, their competence to accede to treatment is more questionable than that of other patients. Mental patients' incompetence may not be presumed solely by their hospitalization (§ 5331), but it is common knowledge mentally-ill persons are more likely to lack the ability to understand the nature of a medical procedure and appreciate its risks. Second, their ability to voluntarily accept treatment is questionable. The impossibility of an involuntarily detained person voluntarily giving informed consent to these medical procedures is fully treated in *Kaimowitz v. Department of Mental Health for the State of Michigan.* "Voluntary" patients, newly included within the protection of the "Patients' Bill of Rights" (§ 5325) are susceptible to many of the pressures placed on involuntary patients. The Legislature's inclusion of these "voluntary" patients recognizes the fact the "voluntary" label is a creation of the Legislature, and often only means the patient did not formally protest hospitalization. These circumstances make the separate treatment of mental patients clearly rationally related to the objective of insuring their rights to refuse treatment. The special regulation of psychosurgery and ECT is also a reasonable classification because these procedures, associated with *mental* illness, present a great danger of violating the patient's rights.

B. VAGUENESS

[The court found that the provisions in both the psychosurgery and ECT statute requiring that the treatment be "critically needed" were unconstitutionally vague because they provided "no guide to the degree of need required".]

* * *

A patient with acute depression and suicidal tendencies would come within the standard if the form of treatment were essential to protect his life. But what of the patient who does not have self-destructive tendencies and is completely dysfunctional psychologically? Does an inability to remain employed or married qualify as a "critical" condition? Must there be a danger of deterioration, or is a stable condition of severe psychosis critical? If all other forms of appropriate therapies have been attempted, has a "critical" need for ECT or psychosurgery been established?

It seems probable the legislative intent was to require a compelling need for these forms of treatment beyond the mere existence of a behavioral or mental disorder. There seems to be a tacit assumption by the Legislature the cure is sometimes more harmful than the disease, and only the most dangerous and harmful conditions should be so treated. Some persons of "common intelligence" may agree an assessment of impending injury, absent prompt treatment, gives rise to a critical need. Others of like intelligence may demand considerably more, or somewhat less. We conclude on its face the "critically needed" criterion is impermissibly vague.

C. DUE PROCESS

The regulation of ECT and psychosurgery is a legitimate exercise of the state's inherent police power. The state has an interest in seeing that these procedures, like other medical procedures, are performed under circumstances insuring maximum safety for the patient. Arrayed against these legitimate state interests are equally valid considerations of rights of privacy, freedom of speech and thought, and the right to medical treatment.

[The court found that the first two rights—the right to privacy and the right to freedom of speech and thought—could be treated together as aspects of the right to "privacy of the mind" or "freedom of thought".]

* * *

Freedom of thought is intimately touched upon by any regulation of procedures affecting thought and feelings. In an effort to protect freedom of thought, the state has put procedural and substantive obstacles in the path of those who both need and desire certain forms of treatment, and in that way their freedom of thought remains impaired because they cannot get treatment. Psychosurgery and ECT are viewed, rightly or wrongly, as drastic, radical forms of treatment compared to psychotherapy or drug therapy, and indicative of more severe illness. Public exposure, or even disclosure to limited numbers of government representatives, may have a chilling effect on patients' efforts to undergo these treatments, thereby restricting their freedom of thought. Some patients will be denied treatment as a natural and intended result of this legislation. Although the reasons for such denials may be the patients' own best interests, such regulation must be justified by a compelling state interest.

* * *

[T]he state's interests, as expressed in the challenged law, may be summarized as the protection of the right to refuse treatment and the prevention of unnecessary administration of hazardous and intrusive treatments. The test of the constitutionality of these provisions will be whether each of them furthers a compelling state interest and is necessary to accomplish the purpose.

* * *

[A]n analysis of the review procedures involved in each form of treatment will be considered separately.

Consent to psychosurgery is regulated and applied differently to three groups of patients: incompetent, involuntary, and all others. The state's interest in protecting patients from unconsented-to and unnecessary administrations of psychosurgery clearly justifies a review procedure which insures the competence of the patient and the truly voluntary nature of his consent. The incompetent patient is incapable of consenting to such a procedure, and the state's interest in protecting him from such procedures fully justifies the attendant invasion of privacy. Although there are substantial problems of procedural due process involved, a review of a patient's competence by a review committee is constitutional where, as here, there is reason to suspect incompetence.

The involuntary patient presents the dilemma of either prohibiting the administration of psychosurgery to such patients (see *Kaimowitz v. Department of Mental Health for the State of Michigan, supra,* 2 Prison L.Rptr. 433), or providing for a substitute decision-making process. Because the voluntariness of such a patient's consent can never be adequately confirmed, the establishment of a review committee to make the treatment decision for the patient is justified by the state's compelling interest in preventing involuntary administration of psychosurgery.

The substantive review of proposed treatments for competent and voluntary patients is a different problem. Once the competency of the patient and voluntariness of the consent is confirmed, what interest of the state can justify the substitution of the review committee's decision for that of the patient and his physician?

The hazardous, experimental nature of psychosurgery is a legitimate reason for the state to regulate its use as a treatment of last resort. Requiring unanimity by the review committee insures each approved treatment is an appropriate use of an experimental procedure. The importance of assuring that consents to psychosurgery be voluntarily given by informed, competent mental patients, plus the need to regulate an experimental procedure, justify the Legislature's decision to remove these considerations from the sole discretion of the treating physician. There are sound reasons why the treating physician's assessment of his patient's competency and voluntariness may not always be objective, and he may not necessarily be the best or most objective judge of how appropriate an experimental procedure would be. Because the consequences to the patient of such a procedure are so serious, and the effects he may suffer are so intrusive and irreversible, tort damages are totally inadequate. The need for some form of restraint is a sufficiently compelling state interest to justify the attendant invasion of the patient's right to privacy. That right to privacy is not absolute and must give way to appropriate regulation.

The new regulatory scheme as it applies to "shock treatment" is almost identical to the regulatory system for psychosurgery. The review procedures of section 5326.3, as applied to involuntary or incompetent patients, function the same as those under section 5326.4, and the review is also constitutional. These procedures for involuntary patients provide for a substitute decision-making process because of the difficulty of acquiring a truly voluntary consent to such a procedure. In the case of incompetent patients, the substitute decision-making process permits the use of this form of treatment for patients who cannot consent for themselves. These applications of section 5326.4 are constitutional for the reasons previously discussed.

The thorny question in section 5326.4 concerns the application of the review system to voluntary competent patients. As already noted, the state has a compelling interest in assuring the competency and voluntariness of patients who undergo this form of treatment. To this end, the review system is compatible with due process. However, once the competency of a voluntary patient has been confirmed, and the truly voluntary nature of his consent is determined, the state has little excuse to invoke the substitute decision-making process. "Shock treatment", or more precisely ECT, is not an experimental procedure, nor are its hazards as serious as those of psychosurgery. . . . Where informed consent is adequately insured, there is no justification for infringing upon the patient's right to privacy in selecting and consenting to the treatment. The state has varied interests which are served by the regulation of ECT, but these interests are not served where the patient and his physician are the best judges of the patient's health, safety and welfare.

Therefore, insofar as section 5326.4 applies to competent and voluntary patients who have given competent, voluntary and informed consent, it is unconstitutional. Substantive review is proper for involuntary or incompetent patients because there is a need for a substitute decision-maker. Any possible need which exists for the voluntary and competent patient cannot prevail in the face of the serious infringement to the patient's right to privacy as guaranteed by *Roe v. Wade*, 410 U.S. 113, 93 S.Ct. 705, 35 L.Ed.2d 147.

* * *

Relying upon *Jacobson v. Massachusetts*, 197 U.S. 11, 25 S.Ct. 358, 49 L.Ed. 643, petitioners also assert a constitutional right to care for one's own health is unconstitutionally invaded by the new procedure. We reject the notion the case recognizes any such fundamental right. The court deciding *Jacobson* held the vaccination of citizens against smallpox is a valid exercise of the state's police power. Petitioners also unmeritoriously assert a constitutional right to medical treatment. Where this right is concerned, due process requires only that the state, once it has institutionalized a person for the purpose of treatment, provide reasonable treatment or release the person. In the present case, any denial of treatment is tantamount to a finding that that particular form of treatment is not reasonable. It is not a denial of any or all treatment.

Questions and Comments

1. *Consent to treatment.* *Aden* represents a case in which patients sought treatment rather than refused it. The extent to which persons with mental disability have a right to *some* type of therapy is addressed in subsequent chapters. Here the issue is not whether there is a general entitlement to psychiatric treatment but whether a person who wants a particular treatment (or at least does not refuse it) may be forced to undergo scrutiny and jump procedural hurdles that are not ordinarily required when treatment is sought.

Assume that a person (1) wants psychosurgery or ECT; (2) asserts he or she is competent to consent to such treatment; and (3) is considered competent by the treating physician. May the state require this person to show that the treatment is "critically needed" (as defined in *Aden*) and to convince a review board that he or she is competent before the treatment may occur? *Aden* holds that if the patient is "voluntary" and wants ECT, the answer to this question is no. But if the patient wants psychosurgery, or is an involuntary patient and wants ECT, the answer is yes. Is *Aden's* differentiation between ECT and psychosurgery, involuntary and voluntary patients defensible? How should persons who are not hospitalized and who want psychosurgery or ECT be handled?

2. *Kaimowitz.* Other courts have also stressed differences between hospitalized patients and other patients in determining the scope of the "right to consent" to intrusive psychiatric treatment. *Aden* relies on *Kaimowitz v. Department of Mental Health*, No. 73–19434–AW (Cir.Ct. of Wayne Cty., Mich., July 10, 1973), *abstracted* in 13 Crim.L.Rep. 2452 (1974), the best-known case addressing the implications of allowing institutionalized individuals to consent to psychosurgery. *Kaimowitz* is reprinted at pp.

206–215, but is briefly summarized here. The case arose when one "John Doe", who was in a state hospital after being committed under Michigan's sex psychopath statute, signed an "informed consent" form and obtained signatures from his parents authorizing doctors to implant depth electrodes in him. The treatment was part of an experimental program designed to determine whether psychosurgery would reduce aggression. Attorney Kaimowitz became aware of the planned operation and petitioned the court for a restraining order. The court granted relief, concluding that, when the person who consents is involuntarily detained by the state, "the three basic elements of informed consent—competency, knowledge, and voluntariness—cannot be ascertained with a degree of reliability warranting resort to use of such an invasive procedure."

With respect to competency, the court found that

> [i]nstitutionalization tends to strip the individual of the support which permits him to maintain his sense of self-worth and the value of his own physical and mental integrity. An involuntarily confined mental patient clearly has diminished capacity for making a decision about irreversible experimental psychosurgery.

On the knowledge prong, the court held that, from the record developed in the case, "the facts surrounding experimental brain surgery are profoundly uncertain, and the lack of knowledge on the subject makes a knowledgeable consent to psychosurgery literally impossible." Finally, concerning the voluntariness issue, the court stated:

> Involuntarily confined mental patients live in an inherently coercive institutional environment. Indirect and subtle psychological coercion has profound effect upon the patient population. Involuntarily confined patients cannot reason as equals with the doctors and administrators over whether they should undergo psychosurgery. They are not able to voluntarily give informed consent because of the inherent inequality in their position.[23]

What are the implications of the court's reasoning for involuntarily committed patients who consent to *other* types of treatment? For nonhospitalized persons who want to consent to psychosurgery? At the end of its opinion, the court stated: "When the state of medical knowledge develops to the extent that the type of psychosurgical intervention proposed here becomes an accepted neurosurgical procedure and is no longer experimen-

---

23. It should be emphasized that once John Doe was released in this case and returned to the community he withdrew all consent to the performance of the proposed experiment. His withdrawal of consent under these circumstances should be compared with his response . . . to questions placed to him [while he was] waiting the implantation of depth electrodes. The significant questions and answers are as follows:

"1. Would you seek psychosurgery if you were not confined to an institution?

A. Yes, if after testing this showed it would be of help.

2. Do you believe that psychosurgery is a way to obtain your release from the institution?

A. No, but it would be a step in obtaining my release. It is like any other therapy or program to help persons to function again.

3. Would you seek psychosurgery if there were other ways to obtain your release?

A. Yes. If psychosurgery were the only means of helping my physical problem after a period of testing."

tal, it is possible, with appropriate review mechanisms, that involuntarily detained mental patients could consent to such an operation." Doesn't this language undercut the reasoning in the rest of the opinion?

3. *Ranking treatments.* Assuming the state may make it more difficult procedurally to consent to certain types of treatment, how does one decide which treatments to put in this category? This question is of course related to the previous discussion concerning when a guardian's or clinician's decision about treatment for a refusing or nonprotesting patient must be subject to further monitoring, judicial or otherwise. But the issues are not necessarily identical. In addition to reviewing the previous materials on the subject, consider Professor Shapiro's attempt, in "Legislating the Control of Behavior Control: Autonomy and the Coercive Use of Organic Therapies," 47 S.Cal.L.Rev. 237, 256 n. 51 (1974), to identify factors relevant to determining when judicial or administrative oversight of a treatment decision might be most useful:

> (1) the extent to which the effects of the therapy upon mentation are reversible;

> (2) the extent to which the resulting psychic state is "foreign," "abnormal," or "unnatural" for the person in question, rather than simply a restoration of his prior psychic state (this is closely related to the "magnitude" or "intensity" of the change);

> (3) the rapidity with which the effects occur;

> (4) the scope of the change in the total "ecology" of the mind's functions;

> (5) the extent to which one can resist acting in ways impelled by the psychic effects of the therapy; and

> (6) the duration of the change.

Is this list comprehensive enough? Should the extent to which the treatment is considered "experimental" be added as a criterion?

It may also be useful at this point to revisit an issue alluded to at the beginning of this chapter (see pp. 816–819). If a treatment is considered so extraordinary that special procedural precautions are mandated before a consenting person is permitted to undergo the treatment, should we, for the same reason, raise the level of competency required to make the decision (perhaps requiring "full appreciation" of the treatment and its consequences)? Should we also make it particularly easy to refuse the treatment (perhaps by honoring any indication of refusal, regardless of the person's mental capacity)? Conversely, if a treatment is not extraordinary, should we facilitate consent (perhaps by allowing it upon mere assent of the patient) and make refusal more difficult?

C. BEHAVIOR MODIFICATION TECHNIQUES

PLOTKIN, LIMITING THE THERAPEUTIC ORGY: MENTAL PATIENTS' RIGHT TO REFUSE TREATMENT

72 Nw.L.Rev. 461, 479–81.
(1978).

Behavior therapy is the application of systematically-obtained empirical data and theoretical concepts to describe and remedy abnormal patterns of behavior. It is, in other words, a systematic means of controlling human behavior based on the assumption, drawn from research upon animal and human subjects, that a person's maladaptive behavior is an effort to reduce or avoid problems by escape.

Pavlov's classical animal conditioning experiments stirred other behavioralists to apply his experimental procedures to the study of human behavior. Although there has yet to evolve a single, universally accepted technique, most practitioners subscribe to one of three common methods of behavior therapy: desensitization, aversion therapy, and operant conditioning.

Desensitization is a counterconditioning technique in which a person is exposed to an unpleasant or feared experience in gradual steps. During this gradual exposure, the therapist attempts to elicit responses from the person that are antagonistic to the anxiety usually provoked by the unpleasant stimulus. It is hoped that this will desensitize the patient by weakening his or her association between the anxiety and the stress-inducing situation.

Aversion therapy is used to eliminate various forms of undesirable behavior by punishing the person each time the specified behavior occurs. The punishment, or aversive stimulus, may occur at the same time as the undesired behavior, or it may closely follow after exhibition of the behavior.

Operant conditioning attempts to control behavior by reinforcing only desired behaviors. The principle "is that behavior is primarily influenced by what follows it—its consequences—and that in order to change behavior the consequences of that behavior should be altered." Rather than punishing, or negatively reinforcing maladaptive behavior, the principle of operant conditioning is to withhold approval for such actions so that the unwanted behavior will ultimately become "extinct."

Behavior therapies, in one form or another, have been extensively used in institutions. One estimator suggested that "half the nation's public mental hospitals have projects based on behavior therapy concepts." On the basis of such experience, behaviorists claim that they now have reliable scientific data proving that their techniques are effective.

KNECHT v. GILLMAN

United States Court of Appeals, Eighth Circuit, 1973.
488 F.2d 1136.

ROSS, CIRCUIT JUDGE.

This is an action by Gary Knecht and Ronald Stevenson, both in the custody of the State of Iowa, against officials of that state, under 42 U.S.C. § 1983. Their complaint alleged that they had been subjected to injections of the drug apomorphine at the Iowa Security Medical Facility (ISMF) without their consent and that the use of said drug by the defendants constituted cruel and unusual punishment in violation of the eighth amendment. The trial court dismissed their complaint for injunctive relief. We reverse with directions to enjoin the defendants from further use of the drug except pursuant to specific guidelines hereinafter set forth.

* * * [T]he evidence contained in the report of the magistrate showed that apomorphine had been administered at ISMF for some time prior to the hearing as "aversive stimuli" in the treatment of inmates with behavior problems. The drug was administered by intramuscular injection by a nurse after an inmate had violated the behavior protocol established for him by the staff. Dr. Loeffelholz testified that the drug could be injected for such pieces of behavior as not getting up, for giving cigarettes against orders, for talking, for swearing, or for lying. Other inmates or members of the staff would report on these violations of the protocol and the injection would be given by the nurse without the nurse or any doctor having personally observed the violation and without specific authorization of the doctor.

When it was determined to administer the drug, the inmate was taken to a room near the nurses' station which contained only a water closet and there given the injection. He was then exercised and within about fifteen minutes he began vomiting. The vomiting lasted from fifteen minutes to an hour. There is also a temporary cardiovascular effect which involves some change in blood pressure and "in the heart." This aversion type "therapy" is based on "Pavlovian conditioning."

The record is not clear as to whether or not the drug was always used with the initial consent of the inmate. It has apparently been administered in a few instances in the past without obtaining written consent of the inmate and once the consent is given, withdrawal thereof was not permitted. Apparently, at the time of trial apomorphine was not being used unless the inmate signed an initial consent, but there is no indication that the authorities now permit an inmate to withdraw his consent once it is given. Neither is there any indication in the record that the procedure has been changed to require the prior approval of a physician each time the drug is administered. Likewise there is no indication that there has been any change in the procedure which permits the administration of the drug upon reports of fellow inmates despite a recommendation by the magistrate that this practice should be avoided.

The testimony relating to the medical acceptability of this treatment is not conclusive. Dr. Steven Fox of the University of Iowa testified that behavior modification by aversive stimuli is a "highly questionable technique" and that only a 20% to 50% success is claimed. He stated that it is not being used elsewhere to his knowledge and that its use is really punishment worse than a controlled beating since the one administering the drug can't control it after it is administered.

On the other hand, Dr. Loeffelholz of the ISMF staff testified that there had been a 50% to 60% effect in modifying behavior by the use of apomorphine at ISMF. There is no evidence that the drug is used at any other inmate medical facility in any other state.

The Iowa Security Medical Facility is established by Section 223.1, Code of Iowa, 1973. It is an institution for persons displaying evidence of mental illness or psychological disorders and requiring diagnostic services and treatment in a security setting.

* * *

* * * [T]he purpose of confinement at ISMF is not penal in nature, but rather one of examination, diagnosis and treatment. Naturally, examination and diagnosis, by their very definition, do not encompass the administration of drugs. Thus, when that course of conduct is taken with respect to any particular patient, he is the recipient of treatment.

The use of apomorphine, then, can be justified only if it can be said to be treatment. Based upon the testimony adduced at the hearing and the findings made by the magistrate and adopted by the trial court, it is not possible to say that the use of apomorphine is a recognized and acceptable medical practice in institutions such as ISMF. Neither can we say, however, that its use on inmates who knowingly and intelligently consent to the treatment, should be prohibited on a medical or a legal basis. The authorities who testified at the evidentiary hearing indicate that some form of consent is now obtained prior to this treatment. The only question then is whether, under the eighth amendment, its use should be prohibited absent such consent; and if so what procedure must be followed to prevent abuses in the treatment procedures and to make certain the consent is knowingly and intelligently made.

At the outset we note that the mere characterization of an act as "treatment" does not insulate it from eighth amendment scrutiny.

* * *

Here we have a situation in which an inmate may be subjected to a morphine base drug which induces vomiting for an extended period of time. Whether it is called "aversive stimuli" or punishment, the act of forcing someone to vomit for a fifteen minute period for committing some minor breach of the rules can only be regarded as cruel and unusual unless the treatment is being administered to a patient who knowingly and intelligently has consented to it. To hold otherwise would be to ignore what each of us has learned from sad experience—that vomiting (especially in the presence of others) is a painful and debilitating experience. The use of this unproven drug for this purpose on an involuntary basis, is, in our opinion, cruel and unusual punishment prohibited by the eighth amendment.

We turn then to the question of how best to prevent abuse in the treatment procedures of consenting participants and how to make certain that the consent is knowingly and intelligently given.

* * *

In this case the trial court should enjoin the use of apomorphine in the treatment of inmates at the ISMF except when the following conditions are complied with:

1.   A written consent must be obtained from the inmate specifying the nature of the treatment, a written description of the purpose, risks and effects of treatment, and advising the inmate of his right to terminate the consent at any time. This consent must include a certification by a physician that the patient has read and understands all of the terms of the consent and that the inmate is mentally competent to understand fully all of the provisions thereof and give his consent thereto.

2.   The consent may be revoked at any time after it is given and if an inmate orally expresses an intention to revoke it to any member of the staff, a revocation form shall be provided for his signature at once.

3.   Each apomorphine injection shall be individually authorized by a doctor and be administered by a doctor, or by a nurse. It shall be authorized in each instance only upon information based on the personal observation of a member of the professional staff. Information from inmates or inmate aides of the observation of behavior in violation of an inmate's protocol shall not be sufficient to warrant such authorization.

The judgment of the district court is reversed with directions to grant the injunction under the terms hereinbefore set forth.

* * *

Questions and Comments

1.   *The definition of punishment.* Although the regimen followed in *Knecht* may seem particularly prone to abuse, conceivably any psychiatric treatment—ranging from psychotherapy to psychosurgery—could be used as punishment, depending upon how that concept is defined. Eighth amendment cases hold that the prohibition against cruel and unusual punishment "must draw its meaning from the evolving standards of decency that mark the progress of a maturing society." *Trop v. Dulles*, 356 U.S. 86, 101, 78 S.Ct. 590, 598, 2 L.Ed.2d 630 (1958). Prisoners have successfully used the clause to obtain court censure of corporal punishment, inadequate medical care, solitary confinement, assaults by guards, and generally abysmal conditions. But in reaching these results, the courts have usually

required demonstration of "barbarous" conditions that "shock the conscience". See Friedman, "Legal Regulation of Applied Behavior Analysis in Mental Institutions and Prisons," 17 Ariz.L.Rev. 39, 61–62 (1975). The Supreme Court has also been called upon to define punishment in *due process* cases alleging that certain conditions imposed on pretrial detainees constitute punishment prior to a determination of guilt. In *Bell v. Wolfish*, 441 U.S. 520, 99 S.Ct. 1861, 60 L.Ed.2d 447 (1979), the Court stated:

> If a particular condition or restriction of pretrial detention is reasonably related to a legitimate governmental objective, it does not, without more, amount to "punishment." Conversely, if a restriction or condition is not reasonably related to a legitimate goal—if it is arbitrary or purposeless—a court permissibly may infer that the purpose of the governmental action is punishment that may not constitutionally be inflicted upon detainees qua detainees.

The Court went on to permit a number of practices—such as limits on mail privileges, unannounced searches of detainees' living areas, and visual body cavity inspections—that it felt were related to legitimate security needs. See also, *United States v. Salerno,* reprinted at pp. 615–620.

There are a number of other factors that might be relevant to determining whether a particular treatment is punishment. Consider this excerpt from Friedman, supra at 70–71 n. 159:

> . . . The intent of the person applying the procedure is certainly one factor [in determining whether the procedure is punishment], though probably not a sufficient factor. Physical offensiveness or deprivation of things desired would probably be a second criterion. Even a combination of an actual intent to punish and an offensive procedure, however, would not necessarily define the procedure as punishment. Consider, for example, a normal appendectomy performed in the case of acute appendicitis by a sadistic surgeon who actually intends to punish his patient. In this case, the law would probably deem the procedure treatment rather than punishment despite the painful impact of the procedures and the surgeon's punitive intent. Thus the recognized therapeutic nature of a procedure would be another criterion. On the other hand, where a hazardous or intrusive procedure of recognized therapeutic value is utilized against a patient's will, it might be deemed punishment, despite its recognized therapeutic value, depending on the surgeon's punitive intent. Thus, the lack of consent of the patient to a procedure would be another criterion of punishment.

> The upshot of this discussion is that for a procedure to be considered punishment for eighth amendment purposes, it must first be physically offensive or depriving of things desired and imposed with an intent to punish. In addition, it must be either without recognized therapeutic value or with recognized therapeutic value but imposed without the patient's consent. In this latter instance, the patient's consent would remove the procedure from the category of punishment, making it unnecessary to say that he has waived his protection against cruel and unusual punishment. In the former instance, consent would not be permitted for the same reason one would not be permitted to consent to

mayhem; consent would not serve any legitimate interest of either the subject or society.

What procedures should be considered "physically offensive" or "depriving of things desired"? Should antipsychotic medication be included in the first category? Freedom to leave the hospital ward in the second? With respect to the therapeutic value of a procedure, could not any procedure be characterized as "therapeutic" in the abstract? For instance, in *Knecht* cannot one make a reasonable argument for the therapeutic value of apomorphine? Perhaps therapeutic value also should depend upon the type of symptom or event which is meant to be extinguished by use of the procedure? (Consider, for instance, the reasons clinicians gave for using apomorphine in *Knecht*.)

2. *The role of consent.* Finally, what role should the patient's consent play in deciding whether a procedure is punishment? In *Knecht* Dr. Fox testified that the use of apomorphine was "punishment worse than a controlled beating." Would an inmate's consent to a beating make it treatment? Do the considerations discussed in the materials on consent to psychosurgery apply to the *Knecht* facts as well?

3. *Operant conditioning.* Unlike the aversive conditioning at issue in *Knecht,* a number of "behavior modification" programs rely on positive reinforcement. As Plotkin points out, such operant conditioning procedures may rely upon "withholding approval" when unwanted behavior occurs. More frequently, at least in hospital settings, things such as private lockers or beds, visits with the ward psychiatrist, personal chairs, writing materials, movies, television programs, or grounds privileges are used as reinforcers. See Wexler, Mental Health Law 215–16 (1981). Is it possible to characterize these "token economy" programs as punishment? If so, would the patient's informed consent convert the program into treatment?

Assuming consent of the patient is required before a token economy program may be instituted, should such consent be revocable, as *Knecht* holds? Can "behavior modification" techniques work if consent is revocable?

V. COMPETENCY IN THE CRIMINAL PROCESS

At several points in the criminal process, the law requires that the criminal accused be "competent". For instance, the Supreme Court has held that, under the fifth amendment, a person may not be subjected to custodial interrogation unless he or she understands and voluntarily waives the right to remain silent and the right to have an attorney present during interrogation. *Miranda v. Arizona,* 384 U.S. 436, 86 S.Ct. 1602, 16 L.Ed.2d 694 (1966). It has also held, under the due process clause, that a guilty plea is not valid unless the accused understands the nature and consequences of the plea and enters the plea voluntarily. *Boykin v. Alabama,* 395 U.S. 238, 89 S.Ct. 1709, 23 L.Ed.2d 274 (1969). Similarly, an accused may not undergo trial unless he or she understands the trial process and can communicate with the attorney. *Drope v. Missouri,* 420 U.S. 162, 95 S.Ct. 896, 43 L.Ed.2d 103 (1975). After conviction, most states require that the defendant be competent to participate in the sentencing proceeding, a rule the Court is likely to constitutionalize when given the opportunity to do so. Cf. *Green v. United States,* 365 U.S. 301, 304, 81 S.Ct. 653, 655, 5 L.Ed.2d 670 (1961) ("The most persuasive counsel may not be able to speak for a defendant [at sentencing] as the defendant might, with halting eloquence, speak for himself."). Finally, the Court has held that persons convicted of capital murder and sentenced to death may not be executed unless competent to understand what is happening to them. *Ford v. Wainwright,* 477 U.S. 399, 106 S.Ct. 2595, 91 L.Ed.2d 335 (1986).

Thus, a finding of incompetency could stall the criminal process at a number of different points. One can imagine a quite different system. Analogous to the plenary power given a guardian of the person, the lawyer for a criminal defendant found incompetent could be empowered to act and make decisions for the defendant. But, in contrast to most areas of the civil law, the criminal law has made incompetency an absolute bar to action under a wide variety of circumstances. The wisdom of this distinction should be considered throughout this section.

The first topic discussed is "competency to proceed" with a given proceeding, which includes competency to stand trial and competency to be sentenced. Then "decisional competency" is examined, in particular competency to plead guilty and competency to waive rights associated with interrogation. As developed below, these competencies differ from the first type in that they require the defendant to make a particular decision. Finally, the chapter closes with materials concerning competency to be executed, which fits neither of the first two categories. Indeed, this last subject has only a minimal connection to the autonomy interests that underlie the competency notion.

A. COMPETENCY TO PROCEED

1. *Criteria*

GARY MELTON, JOHN PETRILA, NORMAN
POYTHRESS AND CHRIS SLOBOGIN,
PSYCHOLOGICAL EVALUATIONS FOR THE COURTS
(New York: Guilford Press) 66–69.
(1987).

(A) HISTORIC ANTECEDENTS

The requirement that an individual must be competent in order to undergo the criminal process originated in the common law, and has been traced at least to the 17th century. The English system of criminal justice incorporated, as does the American system today, a requirement that the defendant plead to the charge prior to trial.

Some commentators believe that the concept of "competency" first arose as a reaction by the English courts to defendants who, rather than making the required plea, stood mute. The court in such a case then sought to ascertain whether the defendant was "mute of malice" or "mute by visitation of God." If the individual fell into the first category, the court sought to force a plea by use of a process in which increasingly heavier weights were placed upon the individual's chest. If the individual fell in the latter category, he or she was spared this ordeal. The category "mute by visitation from God" initially included the literally deaf and mute, but over time was expanded to include the "lunatic."

While the requirement that the defendant be competent may have developed as a practical response to a practical problem, it also seems to have its roots in a more general concern that it was simply unfair to subject certain types of individuals to trial. Thus, Blackstone observed that a defendant who before arraignment for an offense "becomes mad, he ought not to be arraigned for it; because he is not able to plead to it with that advice and caution that he ought. And if, after he has pleaded, the prisoner becomes mad, he shall not be tried: for how can he make his defense?" As judicial decisions began formalizing the competency doctrine, the idea that it was unfair to try an individual who lacked the ability to defend himself was maintained. For example, in *Frith's Case,* the court found that trial must be postponed until the defendant "by collecting together his intellects, and having them entire, he shall be able so to model his defense and to ward off the punishment of the law."

American courts, which relied heavily upon English common law both substantively and procedurally, also utilized the competency doctrine. In 1835, for instance, the man who attempted to assassinate President Andrew Jackson was declared unfit to stand trial. In 1899, a federal court of appeals gave the doctrine constitutional status, observing that "it is fundamental that an insane person can neither plead to an arraignment, be subjected to a trial, or, after trial, receive judgment, or, after judgment, undergo punishment; . . . to the same effect are all the common-law authorities. . . . It is not 'due process of law' to subject an insane person to trial upon an indictment involving liberty or life." Over the years, the doctrine has retained this constitutional status, with the United States Supreme Court only recently finding the principle that an incompetent defendant may not be tried "fundamental to an adversary system of justice." [*Drope v. Missouri,* 420 U.S. 162, 172, 95 S.Ct. 162, 43 L.Ed.2d 103 (1975)].

As competency law has developed, the underlying value at stake has remained constant: The doctrine is necessary to preserve the essential fairness of the criminal justice system. As one commentator has observed, the defendant must be competent so that (1) the trial or plea hearing will arrive at accurate results ("one who cannot comprehend the proceedings may not appreciate what information is relevant to the proof of his innocence"); (2) the criminal process will be dignified ("the adversary form of the criminal proceeding necessarily rests on the assumption that defendant will be a conscious and intelligent participant; the trial of a defendant who cannot fulfill this expectation appears inappropriate and irrational"); and (3) the imposition of any punishment will be morally justified ("in part there is the notion that the state is justified in imposing sanctions only where there is a possibility that the person convicted will realize the moral reprehensibility of his conduct").

[I]deally, the criminal process should provide a trial between adversaries as evenly matched as possible. It was in recognition of the fact that this was often not the case that the Supreme Court handed down its well-known criminal law decisions of the 1960s, which guaranteed defendants the rights to be represented by counsel, to confront their accusers, and to present witnesses on their own behalf. However, this entire process posits a defendant able to *participate* in his or her own defense. Without the competency doctrine, the rights afforded would be useless for at least some individuals, and the process itself would be a sham.

(B) Current Formulation of the Competency Test

The United States Supreme Court, in the case of *Dusky v. United States* [362 U.S. 402, 80 S.Ct. 788, 4 L.Ed.2d 824 (1960)], established the modern legal definition of competency to stand trial. The Court held that "the test must be whether he [the defendant] has sufficient present ability to consult with his attorney with a reasonable degree of rational understanding and a rational as well as factual understanding of proceedings against him." . . . While the Court did not amplify the meaning of this language, the test enunciated suggests that competency to stand trial has several core elements.

First, competency assesses the defendant's *present* ability to consult with counsel and to understand the proceedings. It therefore differs fundamentally from the test for criminal responsibility, which is a *retrospective* inquiry focusing on the defendant's state of mind at the time of the offense.

Second, the test focuses on the defendant's *capacity*, not willingness, to relate to the attorney and understand the proceedings. The defendant who refuses to talk to the attorney even though capable of doing so is making a rational choice knowing the consequences. Unless the lack of motivation is based on irrational factors, thereby calling into question one's capacity to assist in one's defense, it is not ground for an incompetency finding.

Third, the requirement that the defendant possess a "reasonable" degree of understanding suggests that the test as applied to a particular case is a flexible one. "Perfect" or complete understanding on the part of the defendant will not be required—in fact, most observers agree that the threshold for a finding of competency is not particularly high.

Fourth, the emphasis on the presence or absence of "rational" and "factual" understanding suggests an emphasis on cognitive functioning. It is important to note that the test equates neither mental illness nor the defendant's need for treatment with lack of competency. Indeed, the presence of mental illness is relevant only insofar as that illness affects one's "rational understanding" as one consults with counsel and undergoes criminal trial. Thus, the mere fact that a defendant is psychotic does not mean that he or she is incompetent to stand trial; only if the illness impairs the defendant's ability to participate in the defense is the legal test met.

There have been a number of efforts by the courts, by legislative draftsmen, and by clinicians to add content to the rather sparsely worded standard enunciated by the Supreme Court. These efforts typically focus on two generic issues: the defendant's capacity to *understand* the criminal process, including the role of the participants in that process; and the defendant's ability to *function* in that process, primarily through consulting with counsel in the preparation of a defense. For example, one federal court concluded that a defendant will be found competent if the following hold true:

1. The defendant has "the mental capacity to appreciate his presence in relation to time, place, and things."

2. The defendant has "sufficient elementary mental processes to apprehend (i.e., to seize and grasp with what mind he has) that he is in a court of justice, charged with a criminal offense."

3. The defendant understands that there is a judge on the bench.

4. The defendant "understands that a prosecutor is present who will try to convict him of a criminal charge."

5. The defendant "understands that a lawyer will undertake to defend him against that charge."

6. The defendant understands that "he is expected to tell his lawyer the circumstances, to the best of his mental ability (whether colored or not by mental aberration) the facts surrounding him at the time and place where the law violation is alleged to have been committed."

7. The defendant understands that there will be a jury present to determine guilt or innocence.

8. The defendant "has memory sufficient to relate those things in his own personal manner."

* * *

Most state statutes simply adopt or provide variations on the test announced in *Dusky*. For instance, the Michigan statute directs that "the court shall determine the capacity of one to assist in his own defense by his ability to perform in the preparation of his defense." The New Jersey statute, on the other hand, is very explicit. It is nearly identical to the judicially articulated test noted above. . . .

* * *

In addition to the efforts of judges and legislators, clinicians have developed a number of checklists and tests designed to assist the clinician in the actual evaluation of competency. For instance, the Group for the Advancement of Psychiatry, composed primarily of psychiatrists, has derived a 21–item list from existing test instruments [see Table 4–1]. It has cautioned, however, that the list is meant only to identify areas of inquiry and should not leave the impression that "enormous legal sophistication is required of both psychiatrist and defendant."

Table 4–1
List of Items Relevant to Competency to Stand Trial   ⚹

Competency to Stand Trial may involve the ability of a defendant:
1. To understand his current legal situation.
2. To understand the charges against him.
3. To understand the facts relevant to his case.
4. To understand the legal issues and procedures in his case.
5. To understand legal defenses available in his behalf.
6. To understand the dispositions, pleas, and penalties possible.
7. To appraise the likely outcomes.
8. To appraise the roles of defense counsel, the prosecuting attorney, the judge, the jury, the witnesses, and the defendant.
9. To identify and locate witnesses.
10. To relate to defense counsel.
11. To trust and to communicate relevantly with his counsel.
12. To comprehend instructions and advice.
13. To make decisions after receiving advice.
14. To maintain a collaborative relationship with his attorney and to help plan legal strategy.
15. To follow testimony for contradictions or errors.
16. To testify relevantly and be cross-examined if necessary.
17. To challenge prosecution witnesses.
18. To tolerate stress at the trial and while awaiting trial.
19. To refrain from irrational and unmanageable behavior during the trial.
20. To disclose pertinent facts surrounding the alleged offense.
21. To protect himself and to utilize the legal safeguards available to him.

* * *

Questions and Comments

1. *Competency to be sentenced.* Another competency to proceed issue that arises with increasing frequency concerns the convicted offender's capacity to participate in the sentencing process. Although to get to the sentencing stage a defendant will have been found either competent to stand trial or competent to plead guilty, decompensation between adjudication and sentence can occur. In *Saddler v. United States,* 531 F.2d 83 (2d Cir.1976), the Second Circuit held that sentencing must be postponed in

such situations if the judge has "reasonable grounds to believe that the defendant may not have a level of awareness sufficient to understand the nature of the proceeding or to exercise the right of allocution." (The right of allocution—which exists in the federal courts and most state courts but is not constitutionally required—provides the defendant with an opportunity to speak in his or her behalf and offer information in mitigation of punishment prior to its imposition.) The American Bar Association recommends simply adopting the *Dusky* test as the proper standard for determining competency to be sentenced. ABA, Criminal Justice Mental Health Standards, 7–5.2(a)(i).

Unlike the Second Circuit and most other courts, the ABA would also allow provisional sentencing of the offender found incompetent, so long as the offender is accorded an opportunity, once restored to competency, to exercise the right of allocution. 7–5.2(b). The ABA justifies this approach as follows:

> A logical corollary of the rule requiring defendant allocution at sentencing is that incompetent defendants may not be sentenced during the period of their incompetency, particularly if they are unable personally to address the sentencing court. If, however, the right is not recognized as absolute, there is no need to suspend sentencing proceedings for a convicted defendant represented by counsel, particularly if a thorough presentence report has been prepared and presented to the sentencing court. . . . If defense counsel is afforded an opportunity to contest the contents of the presentence report and to advance data omitted from it, the chances are relatively slight that a defendant's incompetence will frustrate the submission and consideration of information useful to a sentencing decision. Moreover, deferred sentencing may be significantly more oppressive to a defendant, particularly if coupled with commitment for treatment or rehabilitation to restore or attain competence, than imposition of a sentence during the enforcement of which the defendant may receive appropriate treatment or habilitation.

Id. at 271–72. Do you agree? What if the offender is not restorable to competency? Assuming the validity of the ABA's position, could much the same argument be made in favor of *trying* defendants while incompetent?

Note that "competency to proceed" issues can arise any time the defendant is subject to a proceeding. Thus, for instance, Florida requires a determination of competency prior to probation revocation hearings and revocation of conditional release for insanity acquittees. Fla.R.Crim.Pro. Rule 3.210(a)(1).

2. *Understanding the proceedings.* Under any competency to proceed standard, the criminal defendant must have some understanding of the proceedings to which he or she will be subjected. Typically, as the above material suggests, it is thought the defendant should grasp the roles of the judge, prosecutor and defense attorney and the general nature of the adversary process. One issue that has arisen in this regard is the extent to which cynical, but perhaps plausible, views of the process suggest incompetency. For instance, one competency interview "protocol" gives a high score (meaning a score suggesting competency) to a statement that the

judge is "fair", and a low score to a statement that the judge is "unjust", "too harsh", or "wrong."   The same protocol gives low scores for the statement that a defendant's biggest concern with his lawyer is "tardiness" and for a statement that, in disagreeing with his attorney, the defendant might feel there is "no sense arguing."   See description of the Competency Screening Test, in Roesch & Golding, Competency to Stand Trial 60–61 (1980).   Are these ratings "fair"?

The defendant should also be able to understand the *specific* case against him or her.   As the above material suggests, this is generally thought to include the charges or issues to be resolved, the consequences of an adverse decision, and the crucial arguments for and against the defense.

✗ 3. *Providing information; amnesia.*   Whether seen as a due process or effective assistance of counsel concern, a key reason underlying the competency to proceed requirement is the belief that defendants must be able to provide the defense attorney with a coherent account of their side of the story.   Thus, it is important that the defendant be able to recall and describe the time period surrounding the alleged offense.   Yet many defendants have or claim to have amnesia for this time period.   Such amnesia could be "organic" (i.e., caused by a blow to the head suffered at the time of the offense, or by excessive ingestion of intoxicants prior to the offense), "psychogenic" (the result of a psychological defense mechanism such as "repression," which allows a person to "forget" a traumatic event), or an aspect of malingering.

When, if ever, should amnesia require a finding of incompetency? Most courts hold that amnesia per se is not a bar to a finding of competency.   Probably the leading case in this area is *Wilson v. United States,* 391 F.2d 460 (D.C.Cir.1968).   The facts of the case were as follows:

> Appellant was tried and convicted on five counts of assault with a pistol and robbery.   The evidence presented at trial was certainly sufficient to sustain the conviction. . . .   The testimony revealed that on October 2, 1964, at about 9:00 P.M., Gerald Fells, who had just parked his car and begun walking down the street, was robbed at gunpoint by two men who took his car keys and stole his car.   The robbers held handkerchiefs to their faces and consequently Mr. Fells could not make a positive identification.   Nevertheless he testified at trial that appellant "closely resembled" one of his two assailants.

> A short time later, at about 9:20 P.M., two men held up a pharmacy on Connecticut Avenue and escaped with over $400 in cash and three bottles of the drug Desadrine.   At trial an employee of the pharmacy positively identified appellant as one of the robbers.   Soon after the robbery a police lookout was broadcast for two Negroes driving Mr. Fells' yellow Mustang and believed to have committed the pharmacy holdup.   Two officers in a police cruiser spotted the stolen car heading south on Connecticut Avenue and began to pursue it.   During the ensuing high-speed chase the suspects' stolen car missed a curve, ran off the road, and crashed into a tree.   One of the two men found in the demolished car was dead; the other, the appellant here, was unconscious.   Money, a gun, a bottle of Desadrine, some of Mr. Fells' effects,

and a stocking mask and hat resembling those worn by the robbers were found scattered about the wreckage.

In the accident appellant fractured his skull and ruptured several blood vessels in his brain. He remained unconscious for three weeks. He still suffers from a partial paralysis and a slight speech defect. He cannot now, and almost certainly never will, remember anything that happened from the afternoon of the robberies until he regained consciousness three weeks later. Except for this memory loss appellant's mental condition is normal. He suffers from no mental disease or defect, and apparently never has.

* * *

The Government's witness, Doctor Economou, testified that appellant had permanent retrograde amnesia and would not be able to aid in his own defense in terms of remembering any of the acts alleged in the indictment. He had "no doubt" that appellant was not feigning. However, the doctor also testified that the appellant did have a rational understanding of the charges against him, that he suffered from no mental disorder, and that, but for the amnesia and slight physical sequelae of the accident, he was in good health . . .

The probate judge held that "amnesia per se in a case where recollection was present during the time of the alleged offenses and where defendant has the ability to construct a knowledge of what happened from other sources and where he has the present ability to follow the course of the proceedings against him and discuss them rationally with his attorney does not constitute incompetency per se. . . ." The judge left open to defense counsel the option of renewing the incompetence claim if formal discovery and other sources of information did not disclose sufficient facts to enable Wilson to receive a fair trial. Wilson renewed his claim of incompetency before trial, but the trial judge found him competent as well. He was then tried without a jury and convicted.

The D.C. Circuit agreed with the thrust of the probate judge's opinion, but modified the test he applied in the following manner:

. . . The accused must be able to perform the functions which "are essential to the fairness and accuracy of a criminal proceeding."

A prediction of the amnesic defendant's ability to perform these functions must, of course, be made before trial at the competency hearing. But where the case is allowed to go to trial, at its conclusion the trial judge should determine whether the defendant has in fact been able to perform these functions. He should, before imposing sentence, make detailed written findings, after taking any additional evidence deemed necessary, concerning the effect of the amnesia on the fairness of the trial. In making these findings the court should consider the following factors:

(1) The extent to which the amnesia affected the defendant's ability to consult with and assist his lawyer.

(2) The extent to which the amnesia affected the defendant's ability to testify in his own behalf.

(3) The extent to which the evidence in suit could be extrinsically reconstructed in view of the defendant's amnesia. Such evidence would include evidence relating to the crime itself as well as any reasonably possible alibi.

(4) The extent to which the Government assisted the defendant and his counsel in that reconstruction.

(5) The strength of the prosecution's case. Most important here will be whether the Government's case is such as to negate all reasonable hypothesis of innocence. If there is any substantial possibility that the accused could, but for his amnesia, establish an alibi or other defense, it should be presumed that he would have been able to do so.

(6) Any other facts and circumstances which would indicate whether or not the defendant had a fair trial. After finding all the facts relevant to the fairness of the trial, considering the amnesia, the court will then make a judgment whether, under applicable principles of due process, the conviction should stand.[4]

If the court determines that the conviction may not stand because of the unfairness of the trial caused by the defendant's amnesia, the court will vacate the conviction and give the Government an opportunity to retry the case. If on retrial the Government is unable to overcome the unfairness which would have thus voided the first conviction, the indictment will be dismissed.

Judge Fahy argued in dissent that the indictment against the defendant should have been dismissed:

Appellant by reason of physical brain injury has not simply been completely and permanently deprived of all knowledge of the robbery itself but of all knowledge of anything covering the entire period surrounding it. To try him for crimes which occurred during this period is thus to try him for something about which he is mentally absent altogether, and this for a cause not attributable to his voluntary conduct. The effect is very much as though he were tried in absentia notwithstanding his physical presence at the time of trial.

* * *

The remand proceedings required by the court cannot solve the problem presented by this case. Appellant will no more be able to assist his counsel, and his counsel will no more be able effectively to assist him, at the remand hearing than at the trial itself. The terms of the

---

4. It would of course be desirable that defendants not only be competent to stand trial, but also have present awareness of their whereabouts and activities at the time of the crime of which they are accused. But courts have not considered such awareness as an essential ingredient of competence itself. As Judge Leventhal [in concurrence] points out, the man accused of committing a crime while drunk may have no recollection concerning the alleged events. And in the so-called "delayed arrest" narcotics cases, while the guilty man may remember his crime, the innocent accused may remember nothing at all about his activities at the critical time. Yet this court, while acknowledging that a delayed arrest may entail loss of memory, has never considered such lack of memory as going directly to competence to stand trial. Instead, it has required that where there has been substantial delay in arrest there can be a conviction only if the Government's case has strong corroboration. This approach . . . makes the probability of prejudice, not lack of memory per se, controlling.

remand in substance required a hearing on the issue of prejudice. To try separately this issue would leave us where we are now, with the added difficulty that at the remand hearing it appears appellant would be required to testify whether or not he wished to do so, raising another Fifth Amendment problem. If the case is to turn on the issue of prejudice we should determine now that prejudice is inherent in the situation. . . .

Is the majority's approach fair? What possible defenses might Wilson have been able to raise based on memory of the time period surrounding the alleged offense? Are the intoxication and delayed arrest cases referred to by the majority good precedent? Under Judge Fahy's approach, would it matter whether the amnesia was organic, psychogenic or feigned? In terms of providing assistance to counsel, isn't the result the same, regardless of the reason for the amnesia?

4. *Relationship with attorney.* As a final consideration, every competency to proceed standard requires some ability to communicate with the attorney. If the above requirements are met, this usually will not be a problem. But occasionally a person who is otherwise competent may, as a result of paranoia, develop an irrational distrust of the attorney. Perhaps relevant to this situation is *Morris v. Slappy,* 461 U.S. 1, 103 S.Ct. 1610, 75 L.Ed.2d 610 (1983), in which the defendant claimed ineffective assistance of counsel because his initial counsel became ill and was replaced with an attorney with whom he did not feel comfortable. The Ninth Circuit upheld this claim, finding that, while a defendant does not have an unqualified right to appointment of counsel of choice, the sixth amendment right to counsel would "be without substance if it did not include the right to a meaningful attorney-client relationship." The Supreme Court reversed, stating: "No court could possibly guarantee that a defendant will develop the kind of rapport with his attorney—privately retained or provided by the public—that the Court of Appeals thought part of the Sixth Amendment guarantee to counsel."

5. *The importance of context.* Several commentators have argued that the competency to proceed determination should be context-dependent; in other words, the complexity of the case is a relevant consideration in making the competency determination. See, e.g., Robey, "Criteria for Competency to Stand Trial: A Checklist for Psychiatrists," 122 Am. J.Psychiat. 616, 620 (1965); Roesch & Golding, supra at 82. On this view, for instance, a person may be competent to proceed when charged with a vagrancy violation because he understands the relatively simple charge and because the evidence to be challenged consists entirely of testimony by one police officer, but may be incompetent to proceed on a homicide charge based on circumstantial evidence that will take two weeks to introduce.

COMPETENCY PROBLEM

With these considerations in mind, decide whether the individual interviewed below, whose psychological tests indicate an intelligence quotient of 52, is competent to proceed on a charge of attempted rape. The interview is transcribed verbatim to give the flavor of a typical competency examination.

Q: Hello. This is Dr. Smith and I'm Dr. Falkin. Are you Phil Jones?

A: Yeah.

Q: We would like to talk to you briefly about the criminal case against you. Do you know where you are?

A: Some hospital.

Q: Do you know the name of the hospital?

A: Uh-uh [meaning no].

Q: Do you know what time it is?

A: I really don't know. I can't tell time too good.

Q: Do you have a watch?

A: Uh-uh.

Q: You talked to someone here last week didn't you?

A: Yes sir.

Q: Do you remember the name of that person?

A: I think her name was Sally [real name was Shelley].

Q: Sally?

A: Yeah.

Q: Do you remember what she told you about what was going to happen today?

A: No.

Q: Do you have any idea what is happening today? What we're here for? Why we're asking you questions?

A: Uh-uh.

Q: Can you guess?

A: Something 'bout going to court.

Q: Can you go any further than that?

A: That's all I know.

Q: Did your lawyer talk to you about this at all?

A: Uh-uh.

Q: He didn't say anything about it?

A: He didn't say nothing.

Q: Okay. Can you tell me your attorney's name? Your lawyer's name?

A: I don't know his name neither.

Q: Do you get along with your attorney?

A: He don't care about the case.

Q: How do you know?

A: I just know.

Q: Can you talk to him?

A: He don't talk much.

Q: How many times have you seen him?

A: One time [this turns out to be true].

Q: Just one?

A: Uh-huh [meaning yes].

Q: Do you ever talk to him on the phone?

A: No.

Q: Do you know what he looks like?

A: He's tall and uh, uh, tall and skinny [this is accurate].

Q: The one time you saw him where did you see him?

A: Uh—the courthouse. And he's supposed to let me know when I'm supposed to go back to court, but I ain't heard nothing yet.

Q: Why were you at the courthouse?

A: Uh—something about, something about a girl.

Q: Did you see a judge there?

A: Yeah—the only thing he told me, to stay out of trouble and don't go over there where she's at and he told me to stay out of Greenbrier [the area where the alleged incident occurred].

Q: Did he say anything else?

A: That's all.

Q: You're sure?

A: Yeah, that's all he said.

Q: Did he say anything about why you were in court?

A: Yeah, uh, he asked me that and he said something like—uh you know it's a—uh bad charge against me.

Q: A what?

A: That it's a bad charge against me.

Q: What was it?

A: 'Tempted rape, that's all. The only thing I done—I didn't try to rape her or nothing like that—the only thing I done was pushed her down in the bushes and that's all I did. I don't 'member doing anything else.

Q: The police report says you waited for her and tried to take off her clothes. Is that right?

A: I don't know 'bout that.

Q: After you pushed her in the bushes what happened?

A: She said she was taking medicine, so I jumped on my bike and went to the Seven-Day Junior [a convenience store next to his brother's gas station].

Q: You don't remember anything else?

A: Nope. [The victim claimed that Jones had pushed her and tried to take off her belt. When she screamed, he got on his bike and left. She mentioned nothing about medicine.]

Q: Do you know what an insanity defense is?

A: No.

Q: An insanity defense is—your lawyer might tell the judge or the jury that you were having emotional or mental problems when you pushed the girl.

A: I didn't do nothing wrong.

Q: Would you let your lawyer argue that—the insanity defense?

A: All I done was pushed her in the bushes.

Q: So you are saying you would not be willing to plead guilty to your charges? You would not want to tell the judge that you did something bad?

A: I never done nothing bad.

Q: Let's assume that you had done something bad. Would you be willing to tell the judge that if you could get a good deal?

A: I never done nothing bad.

* * *

Q: What is it—what does the word attempt mean to you?

A: Umm—taking something that belongs to somebody else.

Q: Attempt means that?

A: Yeah.

Q: Do you know the difference between rape and attempted rape?

A: No.

Q: Will you try to think about it and tell me? The difference between rape and attempted rape?

A: (Long pause). That's all I know.

Q: Do you think you're going to go to court?

A: Huh?

Q: Is this, are you going to—are you going to have a trial?

A: Yeah, I hope so.

Q: You hope so. What happens in a trial in a courtroom?

A: I really don't know.

Q: What's your idea of what happens in a trial?

A: Sometimes they throw it out of court.

Q: Throw it out of court. Throw what out of court?

A: Uh, if you, if you, if ah, if ah, if you done it or didn't do it.

Q: And what happens if you throw it out of court—which way does it go?

A: (Pause). I don't know which way it goes.

Q: If you go to court will you see a prosecutor?

A: The prosecutor, yeah.

Q: What does he do?

A: He's . . . ah, I don't know.

Q: He brings the case against you for the state. He tries to convict you.

A: Yeah, he's wants to, uh, get me (laughs).

Q: What could he do to you if he got you?

A: Uh, he'd send me to the state farm [apparently referring to a mental hospital, where Mr. Jones had been briefly confined once before ten years earlier].

Q: The state farm?

A: Yeah, I'd have to stay at the state farm for a long time.

Q: What if the judge said you had to go to jail instead of the state farm?

A: Jail.

Q: Do you understand what a jail is?

A: It's got bars.

Q: If you had to choose between jail and the state farm, where would you like to go?

A: I don't know.

Q: Can you think about it and tell me?

A: Uh . . . The people at the state farm make fun.

Q: They make fun of you?

A: Yeah.

* * *

Q: What temperature do you think it is outside?

A: (Pause). Four o'clock.

Q: No, temperature.

A: (Pause). I don't know.

Q: Do you know what temperature means?

A: No.

Q: How hot or cold do you think it is?

A: I don't know.

Q: Weren't you outside today?

A: Yeah. I never did get cold much.

Q: You were outside today, right?

A: Uh-huh.

Q: I thought it was pretty cold, I thought it was really cold, I thought it was almost freezing. It was like almost about to snow [in fact the day was quite warm].

A: Felt like it.

Q: Do you know the month and the day and the year?

A: I don't know the date.

Q: Do you have any idea what month it is?

A: Um . . . no.

Q: What season of the year is it?

A: I don't know that either.

Q: You don't?

A: No.

Q: How about the year. Do you keep up with the years at all?

A: No.

Q: Okay, if I'd say it's either March or November or August, which month seems most right [it was November]?

A: August.

Q: Seems like August to you?

A: Yeah.

Q: What is August like? When we talk about the month of August what do you think about? Or what makes right now seem like August?

A: Cold weather.

Q: Cold weather?

A: Cold weather.

Q: Okay, what months make you think about warm weather? Can you name some months?

A: I don't know the months. I ain't gone through school.

Q: Do you know how many months there are in a year?

A: (Pause). Seven.

Q: Seven? Can you count to seven?

A: No.

Q: How far can you count?

A: Um, not too far.

*   *   *

Q: You say you got a divorce. What happens when you get a divorce and what is a divorce?

A: Just me and her just separated. She got her divorce and I got mine.

Q: If you found a stamped letter laying on the walk somewhere and you were walking along and it was just laying there like somebody just dropped it, what would you do with it?

A: Um, turn it into the postman.

Q: You'd turn it into the postman? Can you count money?

A: Um, not too good.

Q: If I gave you a ten dollar bill and asked for half of it back how much of it would you give me back?

A: (Pause). Five.

Q: Okay. Then you gave me the five dollars back and I said you can have half of that back, I'll give half of it back to you. Then how much would I be giving you back?

(R. & S.) Mental Health, 2d Ed. ACB—31

A: (Long pause). Four.

Q: Four? If your little girl would start crying what would you think would be wrong with her, what would be the—just crying—what would be some of the things that that could mean?

A: She be crying for something.

Q: Like what maybe?

A: Um, like uh, candy bar or something.

Q: Could there be other reasons?

A: Sometimes she cries and she gets a high fever and she gets sick sometimes.

Q: So she cries sometimes when she's sick? And any other things that you can think about that would make a little child that age cry?

A: Uh uh.

Q: A couple more questions and then we're going to stop I think. But I'm gonna list several things and you try to pick out the thing in the list of three or four things that I say that might be different. Okay? Orange, apple, a pear, baby rattle.

A: Um, baby rattle.

Q: Baby rattle. You picked that out because of what?

A: I don't know why I picked it out, it was a baby rattle.

Q: Okay, let's try it again. Hammer, saw, a square, and an ice cream cone.

A: (Pause). Ice cream cone.

Q: Okay, why did you say an ice cream cone?

A: You can eat an ice cream cone.

Mr. Jones chopped wood for a living. In order to make the competency to proceed decision, what additional information would you want?[k] If you think that the defendant is not at present competent to proceed, do you think he is "restorable" to competency? If so, should he be hospitalized for this purpose? Or can steps short of that be taken?

2. Procedures for Assessing Competency to Proceed

In *Pate v. Robinson,* 383 U.S. 375, 86 S.Ct. 836, 15 L.Ed.2d 815 (1966), the Supreme Court held that the due process clause requires the trial court to order an inquiry into competency to stand trial any time there is a "bona fide doubt" on the issue. The one case in which it has applied the standard was *Drope v. Missouri,* 420 U.S. 162, 95 S.Ct. 896, 43 L.Ed.2d 103 (1975), in which Drope was charged, along with two others, with the forcible rape of his wife. At the time of trial, Drope had been found competent, based largely on a report submitted by a psychiatrist. The report stated that the defendant had no "delusions,

k. When shown the videotape from which this interview was transcribed, approximately half of a group of state court judges stated they would have found the defendant competent to stand trial; the other half found him incompetent. Before his case was resolved, Mr. Jones died from exposure.

illusions, hallucinations," was "well-oriented in all spheres," and "was able, without trouble to answer questions testing judgement." The report also noted, however, that the defendant "had difficulty in participating well," "had a difficult time relating," and was "markedly circumstantial and irrelevant in his speech." Furthermore, the defendant's wife testified at trial that the defendant was sick, that he would roll down the stairs when he did not "get his way or [was] worried about something," and that he had choked her the Sunday evening before trial (an event which removed her initial reluctance about pursuing the prosecution). On the second day of trial, the defendant shot himself, apparently in a suicide attempt. The Missouri Court of Appeals found that neither the psychiatric report nor the suicide attempt created a reasonable doubt as to the defendant's competence. The Supreme Court reversed. While the Court noted that neither the report nor the defense attorney's motion for a continuance after the suicide attempt provided facts "bearing specifically on the issue of petitioner's competence to stand trial," it found that "the record reveals a failure to give proper weight to the information suggesting incompetence which came to light during trial." Thus, a competency evaluation should have been ordered on the second day of the trial. In the course of its opinion, the Court stated:

> [E]vidence of defendant's irrational behavior, his demeanor at trial, and any prior medical opinion on competence to stand trial are all relevant in determining whether further inquiry is required, but even one of these factors standing alone may, in some circumstances, be sufficient. There are, of course, no fixed or immutable signs which invariably indicate the need for further inquiry to determine fitness to proceed; the question is often a difficult one in which a wide range of manifestations and subtle nuances are implicated. That they are difficult to evaluate is suggested by the varying opinions trained psychiatrists can entertain on the same facts.

Id. at 180, 95 S.Ct. at 908.

In most jurisdictions, any party—the defense attorney, the prosecutor, or the trial judge sua sponte—may raise the competency issue. If the court finds that a bona fide doubt about competency exists, and if the incompetency appears related to mental disability (which is usually the case), the court orders one or more mental health professionals to perform an evaluation. Typically, this assessment is performed in a hospital, where the defendant may be "evaluated" for several weeks or even months. See Burt & Morris, "A Proposal for Abolition of the Incompetency Plea," 40 U.Chi.L.Rev. 66, 88 (1972). Since the 1970's many states have tried to shorten the duration of hospital evaluations; many have also moved toward providing outpatient evaluations either in the jail or, if the defendant has obtained pretrial release, in a local clinic. S. Brakel, J. Parry & B. Weiner, The Mentally Disabled and the Law 697 (1985).

Very often, the report which results from the evaluation is the only information available to the court.   Twenty-four states explicitly allow the competency decision to be based solely on the expert's report, unless one of the parties disagrees with its conclusions.   Id. at 703.   In North Carolina, a survey of 55 North Carolina judges disclosed that 59% of them virtually never hold a formal hearing to assess evidence of the defendant's competency.   R. Roesch & S. Golding, Competency to Stand Trial 193 (1980).   If a hearing does take place, it is usually informal and perfunctory.   In the survey noted above, 35% of the judges said they never disagreed with the clinical report and the remaining 65% stated that disagreement was rare.   Id.   See also, H. Steadman, Beating a Rap?: Defendants Found Incompetent to Stand Trial 54 (1979) (roughly 90% agreement between report and judicial decision).   States vary as to which party bears the burden of proof, with the tendency being to put the burden on the party alleging incompetency.   Only one state requires proof of incompetency by clear and convincing evidence.   The rest adopt the preponderance of the evidence standard.   Brakel, Parry & Weiner, supra at 703.

If the defendant is found competent to stand proceed, then, of course, the proceedings resume.   If the defendant is found incompetent, he or she is almost always required to undergo treatment for the purpose of restoring competency.   This treatment usually takes place in a hospital, although again there is some movement toward outpatient treatment.   In *Jackson v. Indiana,* 406 U.S. 715, 92 S.Ct. 1845, 32 L.Ed.2d 435 (1972), the Supreme Court imposed limitations on the duration of treatment to restore competency:

> A person charged by a State with a criminal offense who is committed solely on account of his incapacity to proceed to trial cannot be held more than a reasonable period of time necessary to determine whether there is a substantial probability that he will attain the capacity in the foreseeable future.   If it is determined that this is not the case, then the State must either institute the customary civil commitment proceedings that would be required to commit indefinitely another citizen or release the defendant.

Id. at 737–38, 92 S.Ct. at 1858.   *Jackson* is discussed in more detail after the following notes on procedural issues.

Questions and Comments

1.   *The bona fide doubt standard.*   In *Drope* the Supreme Court listed three factors—evidence of defendant's irrational behavior, his demeanor at trial and any prior medical opinion on competence to stand trial—and then stated that "even one of these factors standing alone may, in some circumstances, be sufficient."   Is this standard too low?   Consider the following description of how the evaluation system works in practice, from Melton, et al., Psychological Evaluations for the Courts, at 70–71:

> Unfortunately, the low threshold for seeking competency, while perhaps necessary from a constitutional perspective, has encouraged mis-

use of the system. Data on attorney's rationales for referral suggest
that the evaluation is often precipitated by concerns that are in some
sense illegitimate.

One prominent reason for evaluation is simply attorney ignorance.
Rosenberg and McGarry found that only 10 of 28 trial attorneys they
interviewed had any knowledge at all of the legal standards for
incompetency. Similarly, attorneys (and clinicians) may frequently
confuse incompetency with mental disorder per se or with insanity,
and may request evaluation of the former when in fact they want an
evaluation on the latter issues.

Even when there is no such conceptual confusion, competency evaluation referrals are sometimes used to obtain information relevant to a
defense based on the defendant's mental state at the time of the offense
or to a dispositional plan. For example, in a questionnaire study of
defense attorneys who had referred their clients to Dorothea Dix
Hospital in North Carolina for an evaluation of competency to stand
trial, almost half indicated that they were actually seeking an opinion
as to the defendant's criminal responsibility. They also indicated that
they hoped to obtain information relating to disposition. Why do
attorneys who understand the law misuse it in this way? In fairness,
some states have no procedures for obtaining evaluation of an indigent
defendant's mental state at the time of the offense or treatment needs.
In other states, however, the procedures for obtaining such evaluations
do exist; they appear to be neglected because they are more cumbersome than those associated with obtaining an evaluation of competency
to stand trial.

Of more concern than these abuses is evidence suggesting that incompetency referrals are used as a ruse to force treatment of bizarre
persons who do not meet dangerousness requirements for civil commitment. Stone has suggested that, when police learn the strictures of
"imminent dangerousness" in the context of civil commitment, they
are more likely to rely on the criminal justice system to force entry of
"crazy" people "disturbing the peace" into the mental health system.
When a defendant acts bizarrely or presents management problems in
jail, he or she is most readily placed in the mental health system
through a request for an evaluation of competency, particularly since
the court itself or the prosecution may raise the question. Thus, the
sheriff can call the prosecutor or the judge and—with a court order,
perfunctorily obtained—can have the defendant transferred from the
jail to the mental health system, ostensibly for an evaluation of
competency. This circumvents the need to establish that the defendant meets civil commitment standards through a procedure affording
due process rights. Such a shortcut through system boundaries is
spurious not only because of the insult to defendants' rights. It may
also fail on pragmatic grounds. Forensic units may lack clear authority to provide involuntary treatment to defendants admitted for evaluation. Moreover, hospitals may—and should—limit their intervention
to the scope of orders for admission. Consequently, defendants should

be returned to the jail quickly, immediately after competency is evaluated.

Finally, and perhaps most objectionable, competency referrals may be for purely strategic reasons unrelated to any concern with defendants' mental status. Perhaps foremost among these purposes is simply delay. In a case where the alleged offense has created public uproar, defense counsel may succeed in bringing about the defendant's removal from the community until public emotions have calmed by having him or her hospitalized for a competency evaluation. Similarly, if the evidence is weak but the public sentiment for prosecution is strong, prosecutors may have the defendant "put away" for a period through a competency evaluation. The result may be pretrial detention without the opportunity for bail.

The abuses for strategic purposes unrelated to mental status extend beyond delay. In particular, prosecutors may use competency evaluations as a means of discovery. Even if the defendant's statements during a competency evaluation are inadmissible at trial on the issue of guilt, they may provide the prosecution with leads in its investigation if information from the evaluation is available to all parties. Regardless of whether this is the primary intention, prosecutors may use competency evaluations effectively to interrogate and investigate defendants in derogation of Fifth and Sixth Amendment protections.[1]

Interestingly, in a survey of North Carolina judges, Roesch and Golding found that judges suspect abuses of the competency referral process, especially by defense attorneys who misunderstand the concept or who merely seek delay. Nonetheless, the majority of judges reported that they routinely grant motions for competency evaluations without requiring evidence that there is cause to raise the issue.

Additional evidence suggesting that the system is misused comes from Roesch and Golding, supra at 47–49. In a review of ten studies of the evaluation process, they found that the percentage of defendants referred for evaluation who were subsequently found incompetent varied from 1.2% to 77%, with the proportion of defendants found incompetent across the studies averaging 30%. Moreover, this latter figure probably overstates the number of defendants who were actually incompetent, since mental health professionals tend to err on the side of an incompetency finding, id. at 49, yet, as noted above, judges usually rubberstamp their conclusions. Thus, it is probable that a significant number of those referred for evaluation should not have been. Is there any way to modify the bona fide doubt standard to discourage these abuses?

2. *Community evaluations.* An indirect way to discourage abuse of the competency system is the development of a community evaluation system. If an order authorizing a competency evaluation results only in a brief evaluation either in jail or in the local clinic, attorneys who seek a competency evaluation to delay trial or remove the defendant from the community will have nothing to gain from an illegitimate referral. Roesch

1. See pp. 471–476 for a discussion of the application of the fifth amendment to competency evaluations.

and Golding have demonstrated that a relatively brief interview in the community can arrive at results on the competency issue that are at least as reliable as those reached by hospital clinicians after prolonged observation of the defendant in the hospital. Roesch & Golding, supra at 188–191. Given this finding, one could argue that outpatient evaluations are required under least restrictive alternative analysis. The right to pretrial release and the right to speedy trial may also be infringed by prolonged pretrial hospitalization.[m]

In light of these considerations, should hospitalization for the purpose of evaluating the competency of an individual be prohibited? Alternatively, in addition to a showing that there is a bona fide doubt about competency, should there be a showing that the criteria for civil commitment are met? If the latter route is appropriate, and the defense attorney is the one who raises the competency issue, what role should he or she play at the commitment hearing, if any? Might a conflict of interest arise in this situation?

3. *Parties who may raise the issue.* Another means of limiting abuse of the competency evaluation process is to prohibit the judge or the prosecution, or both, from raising the issue. See, e.g., Eizenstadt, "Mental Competency to Stand Trial," 4 Harv.Civ.Rts.Civ.Lib.L.Rev. 379, 384–85 (1969). Is such a prohibition justifiable?

Given the possibly adverse consequences of a competency evaluation, should the *defense attorney* be barred from raising the issue if the client does not want it raised? The American Bar Association Criminal Justice Mental Health Standards require the defense attorney to move for an evaluation of competency whenever he or she "has a good faith doubt as to the defendant's competence," even over the client's objection. Standard 7–4.2. The commentary to the standard justifies this approach as follows:

> Because the trial of an incompetent defendant necessarily is invalid as a violation of due process, a defense lawyer's duty to maintain the integrity of judicial proceedings requires that the trial court be advised of the defendant's possible incompetence.[16] Ultimately, this requirement provides protections for criminal defendants. In addition, to permit defense counsel to proceed to trial with incompetent clients deprives defendants of their personal right to participate in and to control the thrust of their defense. It further assumes that defense attorneys properly determine the best interests of their clients. Criminal defendants, even though represented by trial counsel, have the exclusive right to make certain critical decisions, e.g., to waive or demand jury trial, to decide whether or not to testify in personal defense, and to decide the plea to be entered. Obviously, incompetent

---

m. Note, however, that the state may deny pretrial release for a legitimate "regulatory" reason, United States v. Salerno, reprinted at pp. 615–620, and that statutes which implement the speedy trial right usually exempt time spent performing a competency evaluation or undergoing treatment to restore competency from the time period relevant to determining whether the right is violated. See, e.g., 18 U.S.C. § 3161(h)(4).

16. See Model Rules of Professional Conduct 3.3(a)(1) ("A lawyer shall not knowingly . . . make a false statement of material fact or law to a tribunal").

defendants cannot make these decisions and they may not be made by their attorneys.

Standard 7–4.2(c) recommends a clear requirement that defense counsel raise the issue of a defendant's present mental incompetence whenever counsel has a good faith doubt about competence. It resolves the difficult conflict of concerns inherent in such circumstances . . . in favor of counsel's obligation to the court. The conflict, if it exists, arises from a perceived pragmatic failure of the criminal justice system to live up to its promise, in that the deficiencies in the system of incompetence evaluation and treatment implicitly threaten excessive or inappropriate sanctions against defendants. The standard takes the position that, if such problems exist, the thrust should be to correct the problems, not to permit a pragmatic but philosophically unsound mechanism to avoid them. If elements of unfairness are eliminated from the system, defendants will have little reason to prefer a pragmatic avoidance of the competence issue in favor of trial on the merits.

Uphoff, in "The Role of the Criminal Defense Lawyer in Representing the Mentally Impaired Defendant: Zealous Advocate or Officer of the Court?", 1988 Wisc.L.Rev. 65, 89–96, criticizes the ABA approach:

Although truth, and efficient, fair results are important systemic goals, the lawyer's role in the adversary system generally permits her to represent her client zealously even at the expense of these systemic goals. It is not enough to state in conclusory fashion that requiring defense counsel to assume an officer-of-the-court role serves these systemic goals. Rather, if defense counsel for a mentally impaired defendant is to play a different, lesser role than zealous advocate, it should be incumbent on those who wish to change counsel's role to provide the authority or to explain the policy warranting such a change.

The commentary to ABA Standard 7–4.2, however, offers little authority for its restricted view of defense counsel's role. It suggests that defense counsel's failure to disclose a doubt about her client's competency constitutes a false statement of material fact. Certainly counsel, as an officer of the court, has a duty to avoid perpetrating a fraud on the court. Yet, the ethics codes, acclaiming the virtues of the adversary system and the principle of zealous partisanship, generally permit a criminal defense lawyer to withhold information or even create a misleading impression. The controversy surrounding the lawyer's duty to divulge a client's perjury reflects the limited scope of the criminal defense lawyer's obligation to disclose a client's fraud and the importance of the value of confidentiality. While the Model Rules now require disclosure of a client's intention to commit perjury, it is a major leap to equate nondisclosure of defense counsel's doubts about a client's competence with fraud. . . .

. . . A number of courts have held that a lawyer can be compelled to testify regarding counsel's opinion of a client's competency even though the lawyer's observations would involve privileged client communications, but the better reasoned position is that a lawyer's opinion about a client's competence or state of mind is inextricably mixed with the client's private communications. Accordingly, the lawyer should not be forced to raise competency and thereby disclose privileged matters unless that disclosure is consistent with the client's interests or wishes.

* * *

. . . If a lawyer does not adequately investigate the [competency] issue or fails to raise competency without a legitimate reason, that lawyer's representation should be deemed inadequate. Yet it is neither unduly burdensome nor difficult to scrutinize trial counsel's reasons for not acting.

Appellate review of the limited instances in which counsel decides for strategic reasons not to raise competency is less costly overall to the criminal justice system than obligating defense counsel to act whenever she has a reasonable doubt. If defense lawyers strictly adhere to this duty, they will be raising competency in many cases in which the client ultimately will be found competent. This will mean additional court hearings, unnecessary hospitalization, and increased costs for all of the major participants in the criminal justice system.

Moreover, even if counsel raises competency, the defendant still has a right to challenge the doctor's opinion. At this hearing, the defense lawyer, whose request triggered the evaluation in the first place, will be representing the defendant. The defendant may be understandably reluctant to trust defense counsel in view of counsel's previous actions. Furthermore, defense counsel's role at this hearing will be impossibly complicated. She cannot act as an advocate while at the same time offering testimony, based in part on confidential communications, that is adverse to her client.

* * *

. . . If the prosecutor or the trial court feels that the judicial process is being demeaned by proceeding against an incompetent defendant, either can raise competency. Similarly, either can raise the issue if defense counsel appears to be inadequately protecting a mentally ill client.

Which stance is more persuasive? We will revisit this issue in the subsection on decisional competency.

4. *Hearing procedures.* A final method of discouraging abuse of the system is to formalize the competency determination process. If the parties know that the results of an evaluation (and thus its necessity) will be closely scrutinized by a court, they may be less willing to initiate the process in the first place. Independent of this practical concern is whether the constitution *requires* more formal proceedings than presently occur. In particular: (1) is the present tendency to allow the competency decision to be made by stipulation of the parties proper? and (2) is the preponderance of the evidence standard high enough?

Might the answers to these questions depend upon whether the evaluator(s) find the defendant competent or incompetent? One could argue that the consequence of a determination of *in*competency is analogous to civil commitment. But one court has refused to equate the competency and commitment situations—at least when the issue is whether a jury trial is required in the former context—on the ground a finding of incompetency results only in temporary confinement, while commitment may result in permanent hospitalization. *State ex rel. Matalik v. Schubert,* 57 Wis.2d 315, 204 N.W.2d 13 (1973). Consider this reasoning in light of the next case.

3. Disposition

JACKSON v. INDIANA
Supreme Court of the United States, 1972.
406 U.S. 715, 92 S.Ct. 1845, 32 L.Ed.2d 435.

* * *

MR. JUSTICE BLACKMUN delivered the opinion of the Court.

We are here concerned with the constitutionality of certain aspects of Indiana's system for pretrial commitment of one accused of crime.

Petitioner, Theon Jackson, is a mentally defective deaf mute with a mental level of a pre-school child. He cannot read, write, or otherwise communicate except through limited sign language. In May 1968, at age 27, he was charged in the Criminal Court of Marion County, Indiana, with separate robberies of two women. The offenses were alleged to have occurred the preceding July. The first involved property (a purse and its contents) of the value of four dollars. The second concerned five dollars in money. The record sheds no light on these charges since, upon receipt of not-guilty pleas from Jackson, the trial court set in motion the Indiana procedures for determining his competency to stand trial. Ind.Ann.Stat. § 9–1706a (Supp.1971), now Ind. Code 35–5–3–2 (1971).

As the statute requires, the court appointed two psychiatrists to examine Jackson. A competency hearing was subsequently held at which petitioner was represented by counsel. The court received the examining doctors' joint written report and oral testimony from them and from a deaf-school interpreter through whom they had attempted to communicate with petitioner. The report concluded that Jackson's almost non-existent communication skill, together with his lack of hearing and his mental deficiency, left him unable to understand the nature of the charges against him or to participate in his defense. One doctor testified that it was extremely unlikely that petitioner could ever learn to read or write and questioned whether petitioner even had the ability to develop any proficiency in sign language. He believed that the interpreter had not been able to communicate with petitioner to any great extent and testified that petitioner's "prognosis appears rather dim." The other doctor testified that even if Jackson were not a deaf mute, he would be incompetent to stand trial, and doubted whether petitioner had sufficient intelligence ever to develop the necessary communication skills. The interpreter testified that Indiana had no facilities that could help someone as badly off as Jackson to learn minimal communication skills.

On this evidence, the trial court found that Jackson "lack[ed] comprehension sufficient to make his defense," § 9–1706a, and ordered him committed to the Indiana Department of Mental Health until such time as that Department should certify to the court that "the defendant is sane."

Petitioner's counsel then filed a motion for a new trial, contending that there was no evidence that Jackson was "insane," or that he would ever attain a status which the court might regard as "sane" in the sense of competency to stand trial. Counsel argued that Jackson's commitment under these circumstances amounted to a "life sentence" without his ever having been convicted of a crime, and that the commitment therefore deprived Jackson of his Fourteenth Amendment rights to due process and equal protection, and constituted cruel and unusual punishment under the Eighth Amendment made applicable to the States through the Fourteenth. The trial court denied the motion. On appeal the Supreme Court of Indiana affirmed, with one judge dissenting, 253 Ind. 487, 255 N.E.2d 515 (1970). Rehearing was denied with two judges dissenting. We granted certiorari[.] . . .

For the reasons set forth below, we conclude that, on the record before us, Indiana cannot constitutionally commit the petitioner for an indefinite period simply on account of his incompetency to stand trial on the charges filed against him. Accordingly, we reverse.

I

INDIANA COMMITMENT PROCEDURES

Section 9–1706a contains both the procedural and substantive requirements for pretrial commitment of incompetent criminal defendants in Indiana. If at any time before submission of the case to the court or jury the trial judge has "reasonable ground" to believe the defendant "to be insane," he must appoint two examining physicians and schedule a competency hearing. The hearing is to the court alone, without a jury. The examining physicians' testimony and "other evidence" may be adduced on the issue of incompetency. If the court finds the defendant "has not comprehension sufficient to understand the proceedings and make his defense," trial is delayed or continued and the defendant is remanded to the state department of mental health to be confined in an "appropriate psychiatric institution." The section further provides that "[w]henever the defendant shall become sane" the superintendent of the institution shall certify that fact to the court, and the court shall order him brought on to trial. The court may also make such an order *sua sponte.* There is no statutory provision for periodic review of the defendant's condition by either the court or mental health authorities. Section 9–1706a by its terms does not accord the defendant any right to counsel at the competency hearing or otherwise describe the nature of the hearing; but Jackson was represented by counsel who cross-examined the testifying doctors carefully and called witnesses on behalf of the petitioner-defendant.

Petitioner's central contention is that the State, in seeking in effect to commit him to a mental institution indefinitely, should have been required to invoke the standards and procedures of Ind.Ann.Stat. § 22–1907, now Ind.Code 16–15–1–3 (1971), governing commitment of "feeble-minded" persons. That section provides that upon application of a "reputable citizen of the county" and accompanying certificate of a reputable physician that a person is "feeble-minded and is *not insane* or epileptic" (emphasis supplied), a circuit court judge shall appoint two physicians to examine such person. After notice, a hearing is held at which the patient is entitled to be represented by counsel. If the judge determines that the individual is indeed "feeble-minded," he enters an order of commitment and directs the clerk of the court to apply for the person's admission "to the superintendent of the institution for feeble-minded persons located in the district in which said county is situated." A person committed under this section may be released "at any time," provided that "in the judgment of the superintendent, the mental and physical condition of the patient justifies it." The statutes do not define either "feeble-mindedness" or "insanity" as used in § 22–1907. But a statute establishing a special institution for care of such persons, § 22–1801, IC 1971, 16–15–4–1, refers to the duty of the State to provide care for its citizens who are "feeble-minded, and are therefore unable properly to care for themselves." These provisions evidently afford the State a vehicle for commitment of persons in need of custodial care who are "not insane" and therefore do not qualify as "mentally ill" under the State's general involuntary civil commitment scheme. . . .

[The Court then described the standards and procedures under the "general involuntary commitment" statute, which was similar to the statute for commitment of mentally retarded persons, except that it only allows commitment "in the interest of the welfare of such person or the welfare of others of the community in which such person resides."]

* * *

II

EQUAL PROTECTION

Because the evidence established little likelihood of improvement in petitioner's condition, he argues that commitment under § 9–1706a in his case amounted to a commitment for life. This deprived him of equal protection, he contends, because, absent the criminal charges pending against him, the State would have had to proceed under other statutes generally applicable to all other citizens: either the commitment procedures for feeble-minded persons, or those for mentally ill persons. He argues that under these other statutes (1) the decision whether to commit would have been made according to a different standard, (2) if commitment were warranted, applicable standards for release would have been more lenient, (3) if committed under § 22–1907, he could have been assigned to a special institution affording appropriate care, and (4) he would then have been entitled to certain privileges not now available to him.

In Baxstrom v. Herold, 383 U.S. 107, 86 S.Ct. 760, 15 L.Ed.2d 620 (1966), the Court held that a state prisoner civilly committed at the end of his prison sentence on the finding of a surrogate was denied equal protection when he was deprived of a jury trial that the State made generally available to all other persons civilly committed. Rejecting the State's argument that Baxstrom's conviction and sentence constituted adequate justification for the difference in procedures, the Court said that "there is no conceivable basis for distinguishing the commitment of a person who is nearing the end of a penal term from all other civil commitments." . . . The Court also held that Baxstrom was denied equal protection by commitment to an institution maintained by the state corrections department for "dangerously mentally ill" persons, without a judicial determination of his "dangerous propensities" afforded all others so committed.

If criminal conviction and imposition of sentence are insufficient to justify less procedural and substantive protection against indefinite commitment than that generally available to all others, the mere filing of criminal charges surely cannot suffice. . . .

Respondent argues, however, that because the record fails to establish affirmatively that Jackson will never improve, his commitment "until sane" is not really an indeterminate one. It is only temporary, pending possible change in his condition. Thus, presumably, it cannot be judged against commitments under other state statutes that are truly indeterminate. The State relies on the lack of "exactitude" with which psychiatry can predict the future course of mental illness. . . .

Were the State's factual premise that Jackson's commitment is only temporary a valid one, this might well be a different case. But the record does not support that premise. . . . [In addition to the evidence already described] the court . . . heard petitioner's mother testify that Jackson already had undergone rudimentary out-patient training communications skills from the deaf and dumb school in Indianapolis over a period of three years without noticeable success. There is nothing in the record that even points to any possibility that Jackson's present condition can be remedied at any future time.

* * *

We therefore must turn to the question whether, because of the pendency of the criminal charges that triggered the State's invocation of § 9–1706a, Jackson was deprived of substantial rights to which he would have been entitled under either of the other two state commitment statutes. *Baxstrom* held that the State cannot withhold from a few the procedural protections or the substantive requirements for commitment that are available to all others. In this case commitment procedures under all three statutes appear substantially similar: notice, examination by two doctors, and a full judicial hearing at which the individual is represented by counsel and can cross-examine witnesses and introduce evidence. Under each of the three statutes, the commitment determination is made by the court alone, and appellate review is available.

In contrast, however, what the State must show to commit a defendant under § 9–1706a, and the circumstances under which an individual so committed may be released, are substantially different from the standards under the other two statutes. [With respect to the criteria for commitment, the Court reiterated its earlier comparison of the statutes.]

More important, an individual committed as feeble-minded is eligible for release when his condition "justifies it," § 22–1814, and an individual civilly committed as mentally ill when the "superintendent or administrator shall discharge such person *or* [when] cured of such illness." § 22–1223 (emphasis supplied). Thus, in either case release is appropriate when the individual no longer requires the custodial care or treatment or detention that occasioned the commitment, or when the department of mental health believes release would be in his best interests. The evidence available concerning Jackson's past employment and home care strongly suggests that under these standards he might be eligible for release at almost any time, even if he did not improve. On the other hand, by the terms of his present § 9–1706a commitment, he will not be entitled to release at all, absent an unlikely substantial change for the better in his condition.

Baxstrom did not deal with the standard for release, but its rationale is applicable here. The harm to the individual is just as great if the State, without reasonable justification, can apply standards making his commitment a permanent one when standards generally applicable to all others afford him a substantial opportunity for early release.

As we noted above, we cannot conclude that pending criminal charges provide a greater justification for different treatment than conviction and sentence. Consequently, we hold that by subjecting Jackson to a more lenient commitment standard and to a more stringent standard of release than those generally applicable to all others not charged with offenses, and by thus condemning him in effect to permanent institutionalization without the showing required for commitment or the opportunity for release afforded by § 22–1209 or § 22–1907, Indiana deprived petitioner of equal protection of the laws under the Fourteenth Amendment.

III

DUE PROCESS

For reasons closely related to those discussed in Part II above, we also hold that Indiana's indefinite commitment of a criminal defendant solely on account of his incompetency to stand trial does not square with the Fourteenth Amendment's guarantee of due process.

* * *

The States have traditionally exercised broad power to commit persons found to be mentally ill. The substantive limitations on the exercise of this power and the procedures for invoking it vary drastically among the States. The particular fashion in which the power is exercised—for instance, through various forms of civil commitment, defective delinquency laws, sexual psychopath laws, commitment of persons acquitted by reason of insanity—reflects different combinations of distinct bases for commitment sought to be vindicated. The bases that have been articulated include dangerousness to self, dangerousness to others, and the need for care or treatment or training. Considering the number of persons affected, it is perhaps remarkable that the substantive constitutional limitations on this power have not been more frequently litigated.

We need not address these broad questions here. It is clear that Jackson's commitment rests on proceedings that did not purport to bring into play, indeed did not even consider relevant, *any* of the articulated bases for exercise of Indiana's power of indefinite commitment. The state statutes contain at least two alternative methods for invoking this power. But Jackson was not afforded any "formal commitment proceedings addressed to [his] ability to function in society," or to society's interest in his restraint, or to the State's ability to aid him in attaining competency through custodial care or compulsory treatment, the ostensible purpose of the commitment. At the least, due process requires that the nature and duration of commitment bear some reasonable relation to the purpose for which the individual is committed.

We hold, consequently, that a person charged by a State with a criminal offense who is committed solely on account of his incapacity to proceed to trial cannot be held more than the reasonable period of time necessary to determine whether there is a substantial probability that he will attain that capacity in the foreseeable future. If it is determined that this is not the case, then the State must either institute the customary civil commitment proceeding that would be required to commit indefinitely any other citizen, or release the defendant. Furthermore, even if it is determined that the defendant probably soon will be able to stand trial, his continued commitment must be justified by progress toward that goal. In light of differing state facilities and procedures and a lack of evidence in this record, we do not think it appropriate for us to attempt to prescribe arbitrary time limits. We note, however, that petitioner Jackson has now been confined for three and one-half years on a record that sufficiently establishes the lack of a substantial probability that he will ever be able to participate fully in a trial.

These conclusions make it unnecessary for us to reach petitioner's Eighth–Fourteenth Amendment claim.

IV

DISPOSITION OF THE CHARGES

Petitioner also urges that fundamental fairness requires that the charges against him now be dismissed. The thrust of his argument is that the record amply establishes his lack of criminal responsibility at the time the crimes are alleged to have been committed. The Indiana court did not discuss this question. Apparently it believed that by reason of Jackson's incompetency commitment the State was entitled to hold the charges pending indefinitely. On this record, Jackson's claim is a substantial one. For a number of reasons, however, we believe the issue is not sufficiently ripe for ultimate decision by us at this time.

A. Petitioner argues that he has already made out a complete insanity defense. Jackson's criminal responsibility at the time of the alleged offenses, however, is a distinct issue from his competency to stand trial. The competency hearing below was not directed to criminal responsibility, and evidence relevant to it was presented only incidentally. Thus, in any event, we would have to remand for further consideration of Jackson's condition in the light of Indiana's law of criminal responsibility.

B. Dismissal of charges against an incompetent accused has usually been thought to be justified on grounds not squarely presented here: particularly, the Sixth–Fourteenth Amendment right to a speedy trial, or the denial of due process inherent in holding pending criminal charges indefinitely over the head of one who will never have a chance to prove his innocence. Jackson did not present the Sixth–Fourteenth Amendment issue to the state courts. Nor did the highest state court rule on the due process issue, if indeed it was presented to that court in precisely the above-described form. We think, in light of our holdings in Parts II and III, that the Indiana courts should have the first opportunity to determine these issues.

C. Both courts and commentators have noted the desirability of permitting some proceedings to go forward despite the defendant's incompetency. For instance, § 4.06(3) of the Model Penal Code would permit an incompetent accused's attorney to contest any issue "susceptible of fair determination prior to trial and without the personal participation of the defendant." An alternative draft of § 4.06(4) of the Model Penal Code would also permit an evidentiary hearing at which certain defenses, not including lack of criminal responsibility, could be raised by defense counsel on the basis of which the court might quash the indictment. Some States have statutory provisions permitting pretrial motions to be made or even allowing the incompetent defendant a trial at which to establish his innocence, without permitting a conviction. We do not read this Court's previous decisions to preclude the States from allowing, at a minimum, an incompetent defendant to raise certain defenses such as insufficiency of the indictment, or make certain pretrial motions through counsel. Of course, if the Indiana courts conclude that Jackson was almost certainly not capable of criminal responsibility when the offenses were committed, dismissal of the charges might be warranted. But even if this is not the case, Jackson may have other good defenses that could sustain dismissal or acquittal and that might now be asserted. We do not know if Indiana would approve procedures such as those mentioned here, but these possibilities will be open on remand.

Reversed and remanded.

Questions and Comments

1. *Analyzing* Jackson. With respect to the equal protection basis for *Jackson,* is the Court correct when it concludes that those found incompetent to stand trial are similarly situated to civil committees or to prisoners who have served their sentences? Is the Court's finding in this regard consistent with its decision in *Jones v. United States,* reprinted at pp. 756–762, which held that those acquitted by reason of insanity are not similarly situated to civil committees? With respect to the due process basis of *Jackson,* would the Court's holding authorize hospitalization of an incompetent individual beyond the maximum sentence permitted for the alleged crime?

2. *State implementation of* Jackson. Reaction to *Jackson* has been diverse. As of 1986, eighteen states limit hospitalization of those found incompetent to stand trial to 18 months or less, at which time they must either be released or civilly committed. Fifteen states and the District of Columbia set the limit with reference to the maximum potential sentence for the crime charged. Most of these jurisdictions provide that the limit shall be the lesser of the length of the potential sentence (or some proportion thereof) and a given period of time (ranging from 15 months to 10 years). The remaining states either explicitly place no limits on commitment of defendants found incompetent or rely upon the courts to rule in individual cases. Golding & Roesch, "Competency for Adjudication: An International Analysis," in D. Weisstub (ed.), 4 Law and Mental Health: International Perspectives (1988).

A separate but analogous concern is when the charge against an incompetent defendant must be dismissed. The Supreme Court in *Jackson* avoided deciding this issue. As a result, even if the state is required to release or civilly commit an incompetent person under *Jackson,* it is not required to dismiss the charge. Many states link dismissal with the end of the "*Jackson* treatment period", others do not provide for dismissal until after release from civil commitment, and several make no explicit provision for dismissal. Golding & Roesch, supra at 130. Possibly relevant here is *Klopfer v. North Carolina,* 386 U.S. 213, 87 S.Ct. 988, 18 L.Ed.2d 1 (1967), decided before *Jackson.* There, the Court found unconstitutional a prosecutor's use of a "nolle prosequi with leave", a procedural device discharging the accused from custody but permitting prosecution in the future. The Court ruled that by postponing (indefinitely) prosecution, the state denied the defendant the right to speedy trial guaranteed under the sixth amendment. The Court stated: "The petitioner is not relieved of the limitations placed upon his liberty by the prosecution merely because its suspension permits him to go. The pendency of the indictment may subject him to public scorn and deprive him of employment."

3. *The clinical perspective.* How sensible are the various approaches adopted by the states in response to *Jackson?* According to Stone, in Mental Health and Law: A System in Transition 212–13 (1975), six months should be the outer limit for hospitalization of incompetent individuals in most cases:

> Six months is a period much longer than that shown to be necessary to treat most civilly committed patients, particularly since the advent of drug therapy. It is my belief that after 6 months, the vast majority of the alleged incompetents will be in one of two categories: those who are competent to stand trial, and those who are suffering from mental disabilities, such as mental retardation, brain damage, or chronic deteriorated states such that restoration to competency, ever, is unlikely. The first group should be brought to trial, and charges against the second group should be dropped. A small residual category of persons not clearly in either group could, under carefully reviewed procedures, be confined for another 6 months and then disposed of as previously indicated. In the case of those charged with minor offenses, the time should be even shorter and the reviewing court should promptly consider alternatives to prolonged incarceration such as probation, outpatient care, or dismissal of the charges. Courts should, of course, be attentive to any tendency to subvert the previously discussed limits by periodic recommitments on dubious minor charges.

4. *Incompetent defendants' right to refuse.* As is true in the civil commitment context, the predominant treatment of those found incompetent is antipsychotic medication. In light of *Harper v. Washington*, reprinted at pp. 848–864, and *Jackson,* what are the arguments that the latter group should have no right to refuse such medication? In response, consider this analysis of the facts in *United States v. Charters*, 829 F.2d 479, 493–94 (1987), rev'd, 863 F.2d 302 (4th Cir.1988):

> First, there is no certainty that Charters would become competent if medicated. The district court acknowledged that "there is no way of knowing" whether the medication would render Charters competent. In view of the significant risk that antipsychotic drugs will cause serious injury to Charters, including a risk of permanent injury, the mere possibility (not even the "probability") that the government might realize its desire to try Charters can be given little weight against the countervailing considerations.
>
> Second, it is questionable that the government's interest in having a fair trial would be realized by trying a heavily medicated defendant. Fentiman, Whose Right is it Anyway?: Rethinking Competency to Stand Trial in Light of the Synthetically Sane Insanity Defendant, 40 U.Miami L.Rev. 1109 (1986); Note, Antipsychotic Drugs and Fitness to Stand Trial: The Right of the Unfit Accused to Refuse Treatment, 52 U.Chi.L.Rev. 773 (1985). As the commentators have argued, the real government interest at issue here is not simply an interest in trying an accused; rather, the government's interest is in a fair trial in which

the accused's guilt or innocence is correctly determined. Even if we were to assume that forcibly medicating Charters would make him competent to stand trial, there is good reason to question whether the government's interest in a fair trial will be well served by placing a heavily medicated defendant before a jury. The sanity of the defendant at the time he committed the crime is usually the primary issue in the trial of an "incompetent" defendant made "competent" through the administration of drugs. However, if the defendant is heavily medicated during the trial, the jury may get a false impression of the defendant's mental state at the time of the crime. See Fentiman, supra; Note, Antipsychotic Drugs and Fitness to Stand Trial, supra.

Just as medication can create misimpressions about the defendant's sanity at the time of the crime, its effects can cause other important misimpressions about the defendant's mental state. For example, two common side effects of antipsychotic medication are akinesia and akathisia. The first makes the defendant apathetic and unemotional. The second makes him agitated and restless. As a result, the jury may be misled by the demeanor of a defendant who appears not to care about the crime (or the victim) or who appears overly anxious at particular moments. Furthermore, as the result of akinesia, the defendant may become so apathetic that he is unwilling (if not unable) to assist his attorney in the defense.

Finally, even were it clear that the medication would render Charters competent and there were no threat that the jury would be misled by his demeanor, we do not think that the government's interest in trying Charters would justify administering antipsychotic drugs against his will. Although we do not intend to downplay the importance of the government's obvious interest in resolving the guilt or innocence of a particular defendant, the interest does not permit such a draconian invasion of the individual's freedom and the risk of permanent physical injury.

The *Charters* court also rejected the state's argument that forcible medication should be permitted on parens patriae grounds. The court stated: "The parens patriae interest cannot justify compelled medication until the need for an individual guardian or custodian has been determined, the guardian or custodian appointed, and the guardian or custodian has recommended that the medication be administered."

At one time, a number of courts adhered to an "automatic bar" rule, prohibiting trial of those defendants who were restored to competency solely through medication. Winick, "Psychotropic Medication and Competence to Stand Trial," 3 Am.Bar Found. Research J. 769, 775 (1968). The automatic bar rule prohibited trial of medicated defendants whether or not they refused the medication. The result was a revolving door effect: defendants who were rendered competent through medication and sent back for trial were returned to the hospital untried because the trial judge ordered them taken off medication, thus allowing deterioration into incompetency. Id. at 773.

Today most states permit forcible medication, as well as trial of medicated defendants, and attempt to handle the "demeanor problem" identified by the *Charters* court in one of two ways. The first, exemplified by the ABA Criminal Justice Mental Health Standard 7–4.14(b), is to allow "either party . . . to introduce evidence regarding the treatment or habilitation and its effects" and to require the court to give appropriate instructions. The second approach was outlined by the court in *State v. Hayes*, 118 N.H. 458, 389 A.2d 1379 (1978). *Hayes* permits the state to compel medication of an incompetent defendant initially, but

> [i]f the defendant by his own voluntary choice, made while competent, becomes incompetent to stand trial because he withdraws from the medication, he may be deemed to have waived his right to be tried while competent. The trial court should however carefully examine the defendant on the record, while competent, to establish the following: that the defendant understands that if he is taken off the psychotropic medication he may become legally incompetent to stand trial; that he understands that he has a constitutional right not to be tried while legally incompetent; that the defendant voluntarily gives up this right by requesting that he be taken off the psychotropic medication; and that he understands that the trial will continue whatever his condition may be.

The court also held that, in the event an effective waiver is made, the defendant may still be kept on medication until the point prior to trial when withdrawing medication would reproduce most nearly the defendant's mental state at the time of the offense. Thus, for instance, if a defendant had previously been on medication, but stopped taking it two weeks prior to the offense, the state should be able to forcibly medicate until two weeks prior to trial.

In some states the "treatment" provided those committed on incompetency grounds consists not only of the usual modalities but also of classes meant to provide information about plea bargaining, the roles of courtroom personnel, courtroom procedure and appropriate courtroom behavior. Pendleton, "Treatment of Persons Found Incompetent to Stand Trial," 137 Am. J.Psychiat. 1098 (1980). May a defendant be forced to take these classes?

5. *Reform proposals. Jackson's* ruling that a person charged with a criminal offense who is not restorable to competency must either be released or civilly committed has been attacked from two directions. From the state's point of view, *Jackson* is problematic because it results in release (or relatively insecure civil confinement) of dangerous, mentally unstable individuals. From the defendant's perspective, *Jackson* as implemented results in prolonged confinement of those who have not been found guilty of any crime; indeed, as noted above, many states still permit periods of hospitalization ranging well beyond six months. These two strains of thought have coalesced into a suggestion that, after reasonable attempts at restoration have been made, defendants who remain incompetent should be tried.

The proposal that unrestorably incompetent defendants be tried comes in several forms: (1) At the end of trial but before a verdict is reached, the court determines—along the lines suggested by *Wilson* when dealing with amnesic defendants (see pp. 895–898)—whether the defendant's participation was necessary and lacking. If so, no verdict is reached; if not, the factfinder reaches a verdict and it stands; (2) The defendant is tried through to verdict at an "innocent only" trial, which results in release of the defendant if there is acquittal, and a vacation of the verdict and a "*Jackson* disposition" if there is conviction. Paull, "S.B. 133: The Near Resolution of a Major Problem: Fitness in the Criminal Law," 56 Chi–Kent L.Rev. 1107, 1118–19 (1980); (3) The defendant is tried through to verdict at a "super-fair" trial (at which a particularly high burden is placed on the prosecution and restrictions on discovery are loosened) whose verdict— whether acquittal or conviction—is final. See Burt & Morris, "A Proposal for the Abolition of the Incompetency Plea" 40 U.Chi.L.Rev. 66, 77 (1972). Combining various aspects of these proposals, the American Bar Association has recommended still another approach for handling those it calls the "permanently incompetent" (i.e., those who are still incompetent after 12 to 18 months of treatment). Under the ABA proposal, permanently incompetent individuals who are charged with minor crimes are released or civilly committed. Those charged with serious felonies are tried; however, if conviction results the defendant is *committed* under the procedures and criteria applicable to those found not guilty by reason of insanity.

Which of these procedures, if any, is constitutional under current law? Does the last paragraph of *Jackson* sanction any of these approaches? Several commentators have argued that language in *Pate* to the effect that convicting an incompetent person violates due process is dictum, since that case (as well as *Drope*) focused on the procedural issue of when a hearing to determine competency must be held, rather than on the substantive issue of when if ever a person may be tried despite incompetency. See, e.g., Burt & Morris, supra at 75–76. Moreover, in *Drope* the Court stated that deferring the competency hearing until after trial "may have advantages." 420 U.S. at 182, 95 S.Ct. at 909. If all of these options are constitutional, are any preferable to *Jackson's* approach?

B. DECISIONAL COMPETENCY

SIELING v. EYMAN
United States Court of Appeals, Ninth Circuit, 1973.
478 F.2d 211.

* * *

Sieling bases his right to relief on the ground that his guilty pleas were invalid. He contends that he was mentally incompetent to enter them. In substance, his argument is that neither the finding of competency to stand trial nor the guilty plea proceedings, held in the trial court, adequately resolved the question of his competency to waive his constitutional right to trial. He points out that his competency to make such a waiver was not at issue at the competency hearing, and accordingly, the trial court never made a finding on that issue; further, he argues that the colloquy immediately preceding his guilty plea cannot suffice to resolve the question, because it consisted of no more than the usual inquiry concerning voluntariness, lack of coercion, and understanding of the consequences, and therefore did not extend into the area of his mental competency at all.

Support for Sieling's argument is found in Westbrook v. Arizona, 384 U.S. 150, 86 S.Ct. 1320, 16 L.Ed.2d 429 (1966). In that decision, the Supreme Court gave recognition to a distinction between a defendant's mental competency to stand trial, and his competency to waive his right to counsel at trial. The Court held that a trial court finding, under Arizona Criminal Rule 250, that the defendant was competent to assist counsel in his defense, did not suffice as a finding that he was also competent to waive such a fundamental constitutional right as the right to the assistance of counsel.

A plea of guilty "is itself a conviction. Like a verdict of a jury it is conclusive. More is not required; the court has nothing to do but give judgment and sentence." Several federal constitutional rights are involved in a waiver that takes place when a plea of guilty is entered in a state criminal trial. First, is the privilege against compulsory self-incrimination guaranteed by the Fifth Amendment and applicable to the States by reason of the Fourteenth. Second, is the right to trial by jury. Third, is the right to confront one's accusers. Consequently, the courts must exercise the "utmost solicitude of which [they] are capable in canvassing the matter with the accused to make sure he has a full understanding of what the plea connotes and of its consequence." Boykin v. Alabama, 395 U.S. at 243–244, 89 S.Ct. at 1712.

It is of course well settled that a defendant in a criminal trial cannot be deemed to abandon any fundamental constitutional protection unless there is both "an intelligent and competent waiver by the accused." Johnson v. Zerbst, 304 U.S. 458, 465, 58 S.Ct. 1019, 1023, 82 L.Ed. 1461 (1938); Westbrook v. Arizona, *supra*. In the typical case— that is, when the defendant's sanity or mental capacity has not been put in issue—the determination of the validity of the waiver by the defendant can be assessed with an assumption that he is mentally capable of making the weighty decisions involved in giving up his right to counsel, cross-examination, trial by jury, or his privilege against self-incrimination. However, where a substantial question of a defendant's mental capacity has arisen in a criminal proceeding, it is logically inconsistent to suggest that his waiver can be examined by mere reference to those criteria we examine in cases where the defendant is presumed competent, since in the latter cases no inquiry into the defendant's mental capacity to make the waiver is made. Cf. Pate v. Robinson, 383 U.S. 375, 384, 86 S.Ct. 836, 15 L.Ed.2d 815 (1966). If a defendant who can be presumed competent pleads guilty, a court can assess the adequacy of his waiver by examination of the objective evidence in the record, such as the advice given him by the court as to the nature of the charge, the waivers resulting from the plea and the sentencing prospects, as well as the defendant's statements or responses made in open court. Where the question of a defendant's lack of mental capacity lurks in the background, however, the same inquiry, while still necessary, fails to completely resolve the question of whether the defendant can properly be said to have had a "rational, as well as a factual, understanding" that he is giving up a constitutional right.

We think *Westbrook* makes it plain that, where a defendant's competency has been put in issue, the trial court must look further than to the usual "objective" criteria in determining the adequacy of a constitutional waiver. In *Westbrook,* although the state court had, after hearing, concluded that the defendant was mentally competent to stand trial, the Supreme Court deemed it essential that a further "inquiry into the issue of his competence to waive his constitutional right to the assistance of counsel . . ." was required. It was not suggested there, nor has it been in this case, that the state court's determination that the accused was competent to stand trial was incorrect. The clear implication, then, is that such a determination is inadequate because it does not measure the defendant's capacity by a high enough standard. While the Court did not suggest a standard, it is reasonable to conclude from the Court's language that the degree of competency required to waive a constitutional right is that degree which enables him to make decisions of very serious import. Judge Hufstedler, in Schoeller v. Dunbar, 423 F.2d 1183, 1194 (9th Cir.1970) has suggested the following standard: "A defendant is not competent to plead guilty if a mental illness has substantially impaired his ability to make a reasoned choice among the alternatives presented to him and to understand the nature of the consequences of his plea." We think this formulation is the appropriate one, for it requires a court to assess a defendant's competency with specific reference to the gravity of the decisions with which the defendant is faced.

The examination and inquiry into Sieling's competency, made by the state court here, was not directed at such a level of competency. Under Rule 250, Arizona Rules of Criminal Procedure, the trial court's inquiry is directed to whether a defendant is ". . . able to understand the proceedings and to assist in his defense." In *Westbrook,* that same Arizona determination was held insufficient for waiver of counsel purposes. If such a determination is deficient on the facts of *Westbrook,* we think *a fortiori* it is a deficient basis for upholding a plea of guilty.

* * *

Questions and Comments

1. *Competency to plead guilty.* Roughly 90% of all criminal cases are resolved through pleas of guilty. Thus it would seem—contrary to the impression one gets from caselaw and commentary—that a criminal defendant's competency to plead guilty and participate in plea negotiations, rather than his or her competency to stand trial, should be the primary focus of the parties in most cases (as it was in earlier times—see pp. 889–890). Many authorities suggest that, in practical terms, this oversight is of little import. For instance, the American Bar Association has stated: "Ordinarily, absent additional information bearing on defendant's competence, a finding made that the defendant is competent to stand trial should be sufficient to establish the defendant's competence to plead guilty." Criminal Justice Mental Health Standard 7–5.1(a)(i). Most federal courts

have also found, contrary to *Sieling*, that *Dusky's* language suffices in this context. See, e.g., *Allard v. Helgemoe*, 572 F.2d 1 (1st Cir.1978) and cases cited therein.

However, some differences between the two situations are worth noting. On the one hand, the person pleading guilty will not have to undergo the stress of trial. On the other, as *Sieling* points out, unlike the person going to trial, the person who pleads guilty necessarily waives the rights to jury trial and trial counsel, the right to confront one's accusers, and the privilege against self-incrimination. Moreover, the defendant's suggestibility (i.e., likelihood of going along unthinkingly with the suggestions of others) may be more relevant in the latter context, since the Supreme Court has held that a guilty plea must not only be "intelligent" and "knowing" but also "voluntary." *Boykin v. Alabama*, 395 U.S. 238, 89 S.Ct. 1709, 23 L.Ed.2d 274 (1969).

In practice, is the *Sieling* standard likely to "create a class of semi-competent defendants who are not protected from prosecution because they have been found competent to stand trial, but who are denied the leniency of the plea bargaining process because they are not competent to plead guilty?" Note, "Competence to Plead Guilty: A New Standard," 1974 Duke Law Journal 149, 170. On the other hand, does equation of the standards lead to inappropriate guilty pleas?

2. *Distinguishing competency to proceed and decisional competency.* Bonnie has suggested a different way of looking at these issues which may help explain why most courts have not followed *Sieling*.[n] He argues that because competency to stand trial (and other competency to proceed standards) require only generalized capacities—a capacity to understand the proceedings and an ability to relate to an attorney—they are not "decisional" competencies like competency to plead guilty or competency to waive an attorney, which require making a specified decision. He analogizes pleading guilty to treatment decisionmaking, which also involves making a specific decision. He then points to the notion, developed by those who have analyzed treatment decisionmaking, that the level of competency required to *consent* to a recommended treatment should be lower than the level of competency required for a refusal (discussed at pp. 816–819). Assuming this idea is valid, can you see how courts might feel justified in equating competency to plead guilty with competency to stand trial despite the differences between the two identified above? Does the same analogy explain why competency to waive one's attorney is uniformly regarded to be much "higher" than either competency to stand trial or competency to plead guilty?

3. *Waiving the right to be tried while competent.* Although the competency to proceed notion may not encompass any specific decisional capacity, the decision to *waive* the right to be tried while competent raises a decisional competency issue. These materials have alluded to at least three points in the criminal process where such a waiver may occur. First, the issue arises when the defense attorney is confronted by a client who

n. The following ideas were suggested by a paper written by Professor Bonnie for the MacArthur Program of Research on Mental Health and the Law, entitled "Competency in the Criminal Process," dated 2/6/89.

objects to undergoing the competency evaluation process despite objective indicia raising a bona fide doubt about competency. It also arises when the client insists on going to trial in an unmedicated state despite evidence that foregoing medication will make it unlikely he or she will be competent during trial. Finally, it may arise when a defendant has been found "permanently incompetent" but insists on a trial, perhaps to obtain vindication, avoid civil commitment, or avoid having charges pending indefinitely.

When should a defendant be allowed to waive the right to be tried while competent? In *Pate v. Robinson,* the Supreme Court stated "it is contradictory to argue that a defendant may be incompetent and yet knowingly or intelligently 'waive' his right to have the court determine his capacity to stand trial." Winick, in "Incompetency to Stand Trial: An Assessment of Costs and Benefits, and a Proposal for Reform," 39 Rutgers L.Rev. 243, 265–66 (1987), disagrees, at least when the defense attorney is in agreement with the client who wants to waive the right:

> In a variety of contexts, defense attorneys acting alone are permitted to waive the rights of their clients without consulting with them. The failure of defense counsel to raise a timely objection to the admissibility of a confession, even though this may go to the accuracy of the guilt determination process, is deemed sufficient to waive the issue without any necessity for the defendant's concurrence. Similarly, the failure of defense counsel to challenge the composition of the grand or petit jury constitutes waiver without any necessity of the defendant's participation in the decision. Furthermore, counsel's failure without consulting the defendant to cross-examine a witness or to raise and preserve a point may waive important constitutional rights of his client. If such consultation is not a prerequisite to the waiver of at least certain of the defendant's fundamental constitutional rights, why should such significance be placed on ascertaining the defendant's capacity to engage in the very consultation that is itself unnecessary, or to possess an understanding of the proceedings that would make such consultation meaningful? If the waiver of certain fundamental trial rights can be accomplished without the necessity of the defendant even being consulted, why isn't the judgment of the defendant and his attorney that trial is in the defendant's best interests honored, even if there may be serious reason to question his competency?

> In fact, even in the criminal process, incompetent defendants are permitted to waive certain rights. For example, the defendant is permitted to waive his due process right to a hearing to contest whether he is competent to stand trial. Where defense counsel agrees to stipulate to the evaluators' reports and the prosecutor agrees, absent objection by the defendant, no hearing is held. The Supreme Court has also allowed a defendant whose competency was questionable to waive his constitutional right to be present at the trial itself by conducting himself in a disorderly and disruptive manner.[o]

o. Here Winick is referring to *Allen v. Illinois,* 397 U.S. 337, 90 S.Ct. 1057, 25 L.Ed.2d 353 (1970), in which the Court held that a disruptive defendant may be re- moved from the courtroom, bound and gagged, or held in contempt, at the judge's discretion. [Footnote by eds.]

When the client and the defense attorney are in agreement that the right to be tried while competent should be waived, Winick suggests that the client's choice should be honored whenever it is "clearly articulated." Although this level of competency is at the low end of the spectrum, Winick justifies his approach as follows:

> . . . Because an individual able to express a choice is exercising at least some autonomy, respect for the principle of autonomy makes it appropriate to utilize a presumption of competency to guide the decisionmaker in such cases. The presumption is not an irrebutable presumption; it does not decide the case. Rather, the presumption guides decision by reminding the decisionmaker of the importance of autonomy values in resolving the competency question. It functions as a weight on the scales, a weight that can be outweighed by other values (e.g., principles of beneficence or justice), but which will predominate in their absence and sometimes even in their presence. When the competing values at stake are respect for autonomy and a desire to act in the individual's best interests or to protect him from harm, the competency question should turn on an assessment of the degree of autonomy present and the risk/benefit ratio of the activity in question. . . .

> . . . A presumption in favor of accepting the defendant's choice, if clearly expressed, to stand trial or plead guilty notwithstanding his mental impairment should be applied, particularly where defense counsel concurs in his choice. Counsel's concurrence will presumably eliminate instances in which the defendant's choice is based on irrelevant reasons ("I will plead guilty because I am an insect"), or irrational beliefs ("I will stand trial and thereby become a movie star"), or on outright delusions ("I am an extraterrestrial and will return to my planet"). Moreover, the concurrence of the defendant's attorney in his decision to stand trial or plead is strong evidence that the risk/benefit ratio of his choice is acceptable compared to an adjudication of incompetency; in short, that the defendant's decision is not an unreasonable one. At a minimum, a relatively low standard of competency and minimal scrutiny should be applied where the defendant, with the concurrence of his attorney, expresses the wish to stand trial, and a higher standard and more intense scrutiny where the state asserts that the defendant should be tried over his objection that he is incompetent.

Id. at 271–72.

Winick's argument implies that if the attorney and the client *disagree* on whether to waive the right to be tried while competent a higher level of competency is required in order for there to be a valid waiver. Such disagreement is perhaps most likely to occur at the initial stages of the process, when the attorney, for ethical or strategic reasons, believes the client should undergo a competency evaluation but the client objects. Recall the American Bar Association recommendation that the attorney override the client's wishes in this regard, and Uphoff's rejection of this view (see pp. 909–911). In light of the above materials, with whom do you agree? If you were the attorney for Phil Jones, subject of the interview at pp. 898–904, would you press for a competency evaluation if he insisted he did not want to go to the "state farm" (hospital) again?

4. *Other client waivers.* As *Seiling* suggests, there are a number of other situations in which "decisional" competency could be implicated. According to the American Bar Association's Model Rules of Professional Conduct, for instance, the client, not the lawyer, should be the ultimate authority for all "fundamental decisions" in the criminal process. In addition to deciding whether or not to plead guilty, the rule lists as "fundamental" decisions to waive the right to jury trial, testify, and forego an appeal. Proposed Rule 1.2(a) (Final Draft 1982). Should Winick's approach be followed in assessing a defendant's decision in these circumstances? That is, if the defendant and the attorney are in agreement, should the client's articulation of a choice be sufficient?

Left unclear by the ABA Rule is how much control the defendant should have over the legal strategy of the case (outside of the decision to testify). One issue that arises occasionally in this regard is whether an insanity defense may be raised over the defendant's objection. Several courts have required a separate hearing to determine whether an objecting defendant is voluntarily and intelligently waiving the defense; if so, the defendant's wishes are honored. See, e.g., *Frendak v. United States*, 408 A.2d 364 (D.C.App.1979). At least one prominent court, however, has permitted assertion of the defense over the defendant's objection, even if the defendant is *competent* to make such a decision, on the ground that it would be morally repugnant to convict a person who was insane at the time of the offense. *Whalem v. United States*, 346 F.2d 812 (D.C.Cir.1965).

Under the *Frendak* approach, note that a finding of competency to stand trial does not necessarily mean the person is competent to make a decision about the insanity defense; a separate hearing is required in *all* cases. How does this result comport with Winick's and Bonnie's analysis of decisional competency? Under the *Whalem* approach, the defendant's wishes are to be taken into account but are not dispositive. Is this justifiable? Judge Bazelon, who wrote *Whalem*, undoubtedly would support a competent nondangerous person's right to refuse psychiatric treatment. Cf. Bazelon, "Implementing the Right to Treatment," 36 Chicago L.Rev. 742 (1969). How, if at all, is compelling the assertion of an insanity defense different from compelling treatment over a competent person's objection?

5. *Voluntariness.* Under the constitution, most waiver decisions in the criminal context must not only be "knowing and intelligent" but also "voluntary." [p] For instance, as noted earlier, the Supreme Court has held that guilty pleas must be knowing, intelligent and voluntary. Similarly, waiver of the right to counsel and of the insanity defense must be voluntary.

The law of confessions has provided the most comprehensive definition of voluntariness, in part because it is governed by two separate constitutional provisions. As with guilty pleas, a confession is invalid under the

---

p. Note the analogy here to the informed consent doctrine, which requires not only a competent decision based on full disclosure of relevant information, but also that the decision be voluntary. See Chapter Three.

due process clause if, in the totality of the circumstances, it is involuntarily made. *Brown v. Mississippi,* 297 U.S. 278, 56 S.Ct. 461, 80 L.Ed. 682 (1936). Additionally, a confession may be considered inadmissible by virtue of the fifth amendment's privilege against self-incrimination, as interpreted by *Miranda v. Arizona,* 384 U.S. 436, 86 S.Ct. 1602, 16 L.Ed.2d 694 (1966). *Miranda* requires that, before every "custodial interrogation", the police must inform the defendant of the right to remain silent and the right to an attorney during the interrogation; if these warnings are not given, any admissions obtained during the interrogation are not admissible (even though, in fact, the admissions may not be "coerced"; thus, this part of *Miranda* devised a prophylactic rule designed to provide defendants with information concerning their right to remain silent). If the warnings are given, subsequent admissions may still be inadmissible if the state is unable to show by a preponderance of the evidence that they were given after a knowing, intelligent and voluntary waiver of the right to remain silent. On the other hand, if the admissions are made before custodial interrogation begins or are the product of a valid post-warning waiver, then they are admissible. The following materials further explore, in the interrogation context, the problematic "voluntariness" issue.

COLORADO v. CONNELLY

Supreme Court of the United States, 1986.
479 U.S. 157, 107 S.Ct. 515, 93 L.Ed.2d 473.

* * *

CHIEF JUSTICE REHNQUIST delivered the opinion of the Court.

* * *

I

On August 18, 1983, Officer Patrick Anderson of the Denver Police Department was in uniform, working in an off-duty capacity in downtown Denver. Respondent Francis Connelly approached Officer Anderson and, without any prompting, stated that he had murdered someone and wanted to talk about it. Anderson immediately advised respondent that he had the right to remain silent, that anything he said could be used against him in court, and that he had the right to an attorney prior to any police questioning. See *Miranda v. Arizona,* 384 U.S. 436, 86 S.Ct. 1602, 16 L.Ed.2d 694 (1966). Respondent stated that he understood these rights but he still wanted to talk about the murder. Understandably bewildered by this confession, Officer Anderson asked respondent several questions. Connelly denied that he had been drinking, denied that he had been taking any drugs, and stated that, in the past, he had been a patient in several mental hospitals. Officer Anderson again told Connelly that he was under no obligation to say anything. Connelly replied that it was "all right," and that he would talk to Officer Anderson because his conscience had been bothering him. To Officer Anderson, respondent appeared to understand fully the nature of his acts.

Shortly thereafter, Homicide Detective Stephen Antuna arrived. Respondent was again advised of his rights, and Detective Antuna asked him "what he had on his mind." Respondent answered that he had come all the way from Boston to confess to the murder of Mary Ann Junta, a young girl whom he had killed in Denver sometime during November 1982. Respondent was taken to police headquarters, and a search of police records revealed that the body of an unidentified female had been found in April 1983. Respondent openly detailed his story to Detective Antuna and Sergeant Thomas Haney, and readily agreed to take the officers to the scene of the killing. Under Connelly's sole direction, the two officers and respondent proceeded in a police vehicle to the location of the crime. Respondent pointed out the exact location of the murder. Throughout this episode, Detective Antuna perceived no indication whatsoever that respondent was suffering from any kind of mental illness.

Respondent was held overnight. During an interview with the public defender's office the following morning, he became visibly disoriented. He began giving confused answers to questions, and for the first time, stated that "voices" had told him to come to Denver and that he had followed the directions of these voices in confessing. Respondent was sent to a state hospital for evaluation. He was initially found incompetent to assist in his own defense. By March 1984, however, the doctors evaluating respondent determined that he was competent to proceed to trial.

At a preliminary hearing, respondent moved to suppress all of his statements. Doctor Jeffrey Metzner, a psychiatrist employed by the state hospital, testified that respondent was suffering from chronic schizophrenia and was in a psychotic state at least as of August 17, 1983, the day before he confessed. Metzner's interviews with respondent revealed that respondent was following the "voice of God." This voice instructed respondent to withdraw money from the bank, to buy an airplane ticket, and to fly from Boston to Denver. When respondent arrived from Boston, God's voice became stronger and told respondent either to confess to the killing or to commit suicide. Reluctantly following the command of the voices, respondent approached Officer Anderson and confessed.

Dr. Metzner testified that, in his expert opinion, respondent was experiencing "command hallucinations." This condition interfered with respondent's "volitional abilities; that is, his ability to make free and rational choices." Dr. Metzner further testified that Connelly's illness did not significantly impair his cognitive abilities. Thus, respondent understood the rights he had when Officer Anderson and Detective Antuna advised him that he need not speak. Dr. Metzner admitted that the "voices" could in reality be Connelly's interpretation of his own guilt, but explained that in his opinion, Connelly's psychosis motivated his confession.

On the basis of this evidence the Colorado trial court decided that respondent's statements must be suppressed because they were "involuntary." [T]he court ruled that a confession is admissible only if it is a product of the defendant's rational intellect and "free will." Although the court found that the police had done nothing wrong or coercive in securing respondent's confession, Connelly's illness destroyed his volition and compelled him to confess. The trial court also found that Connelly's mental state vitiated his attempted waiver of the right to counsel and the privilege against compulsory self-incrimination. Accordingly, respondent's initial statements and his custodial confession were suppressed.

The Colorado Supreme Court affirmed. In that court's view, the proper test for admissibility is whether the statements are "the product of a rational intellect and a free will." Indeed, "the absence of police coercion or duress does not foreclose a finding of involuntariness. One's capacity for rational judgment and free choice may be overborne as much by certain forms of severe mental illness as by external pressure." The court found that the very admission of the evidence in a court of law was sufficient state action to implicate the Due Process Clause of the Fourteenth Amendment to the United States Constitution. The evidence fully supported the conclusion that respondent's initial statement was not the product of a rational intellect and a free will. The court then considered respondent's attempted waiver of his constitutional rights and found that respondent's mental condition precluded his ability to make a valid waiver. The Colorado Supreme Court thus affirmed the trial court's decision to suppress all of Connelly's statements.

II

The Due Process Clause of the Fourteenth Amendment provides that no State shall "deprive any person of life, liberty, or property, without due process of law." Just last Term, in *Miller v. Fenton,* we held that by virtue of the Due Process Clause "certain interrogation techniques, either in isolation or as applied to the unique characteristics of a particular suspect, are so offensive to a civilized system of justice that they must be condemned."

Indeed, coercive government misconduct was the catalyst for this Court's seminal confession case, *Brown v. Mississippi,* 297 U.S. 278, 56 S.Ct. 461, 80 L.Ed. 682 (1936). In that case, police officers extracted confessions from the accused through brutal torture. The Court had little difficulty concluding that even though the Fifth Amendment did not at that time apply to the States, the actions of the police were "revolting to the sense of justice." The Court has retained this due process focus, even after holding, in *Malloy v. Hogan,* 378 U.S. 1, 84 S.Ct. 1489, 12 L.Ed.2d 653 (1964), that the Fifth Amendment privilege against compulsory self-incrimination applies to the States.

Thus the cases considered by this Court over the 50 years since *Brown v. Mississippi* have focused upon the crucial element of police overreaching. While each confession case has turned on its own set of factors justifying the conclusion that police conduct was oppressive, all have contained a substantial element of coercive police conduct. Absent police conduct causally related to the confession, there is simply no basis for concluding that any state actor has deprived a criminal defendant of due process of law. Respondent correctly notes that as interrogators have turned to more subtle forms of psychological persuasion, courts have found the mental condition of the defendant a more significant factor in the "voluntariness" calculus. But this fact does not justify a conclusion that a defendant's mental condition, by itself and apart from its relation to official coercion, should ever dispose of the inquiry into constitutional "voluntariness."

Respondent relies on *Blackburn v. Alabama,* 361 U.S. 199, 80 S.Ct. 274, 4 L.Ed.2d 242 (1960), and *Townsend v. Sain,* 372 U.S. 293, 83 S.Ct. 745, 9 L.Ed.2d 770 (1963), for the proposition that the "deficient mental condition of the defendants in those cases was sufficient to render their confessions involuntary." But respondent's reading of *Blackburn* and *Townsend* ignores the integral element of police overreaching present in both cases. In *Blackburn,* the Court found that the petitioner was probably insane at the time of his confession and the police learned during the interrogation that Blackburn had a history of mental problems. The police exploited this weakness with coercive tactics: "The eight- to nine-hour sustained interrogation in a tiny room which was upon occasion literally filled with police officers; the absence of Blackburn's friends, relatives, or legal counsel; [and] the composition of the confession by the Deputy Sheriff rather than by Blackburn." These tactics supported a finding that the confession was involuntary. Indeed, the Court specifically condemned police activity that "wrings a confession out of an accused against his will." *Townsend* presented a similar instance of police wrongdoing. In that case, a police physician had given Townsend a drug with truth-serum properties. The subsequent confession, obtained by officers who knew that Townsend had been given drugs, was held involuntary. These two cases demonstrate that while mental condition is surely relevant to an individual's susceptibility to police coercion, mere examination of the confessant's state of mind can never conclude the due process inquiry.

* * *

"[T]he central purpose of a criminal trial is to decide the factual question of the defendant's guilt or innocence" and while we have previously held that exclusion of evidence may be necessary to protect constitutional guarantees, both the necessity for the collateral inquiry and the exclusion of evidence deflect a criminal trial from its basic purpose. Respondent would now have us require sweeping inquiries into the state of mind of a criminal defendant who has confessed, inquiries quite divorced from any coercion brought to bear on the defendant by the State. We think the Constitution rightly leaves this sort of inquiry to be resolved by state laws governing the admission of evidence and erects no standard of its own in this area. A statement rendered by one in the condition of respondent might be proved to be quite unreliable, but this is a matter to be governed by the evidentiary laws of the forum, see, *e.g.,* Fed.Rule Evid. 601, and not by the Due

Process Clause of the Fourteenth Amendment. "The aim of the requirement of due process is not to exclude presumptively false evidence, but to prevent fundamental unfairness in the use of evidence, whether true or false.". . .

We hold that coercive police activity is a necessary predicate to the finding that a confession is not "voluntary" within the meaning of the Due Process Clause of the Fourteenth Amendment. We also conclude that the taking of respondent's statements, and their admission into evidence, constitute no violation of that Clause.

III

* * *

We also think that the Supreme Court of Colorado was mistaken in its analysis of the question of whether respondent had waived his *Miranda* rights in this case.[3] Of course, a waiver must at a minimum be "voluntary" to be effective against an accused. The Supreme Court of Colorado in addressing this question relied on the testimony of the court-appointed psychiatrist to the effect that respondent was not capable of making a "free decision with respect to his constitutional right of silence . . . and his constitutional right to confer with a lawyer before talking to the police."

We think that the Supreme Court of Colorado erred in importing into this area of constitutional law notions of "free will" that have no place there. There is obviously no reason to require more in the way of a "voluntariness" inquiry in the *Miranda* waiver context than in the Fourteenth Amendment confession context. The sole concern of the Fifth Amendment, on which *Miranda* was based, is governmental coercion.

* * *

IV

The judgment of the Supreme Court of Colorado is accordingly reversed, and the cause remanded for further proceedings not inconsistent with this opinion.

* * *

JUSTICE STEVENS, concurring in the judgment in part and dissenting in part.

* * *

When the officer whom respondent approached elected to handcuff him and to take him into custody, the police assumed a fundamentally different relationship with him. Prior to that moment, the police had no duty to give respondent *Miranda* warnings and had every right to continue their exploratory conversation with him. Once the custodial relationship was established, however, the questioning assumed a presumptively coercive character. In my opinion the questioning could

---

3. Petitioner conceded at oral argument that when Officer Anderson handcuffed respondent, the custody requirement of *Miranda* was satisfied. For purposes of our decision we accept that concession, and we similarly assume that the police officers "interrogated" respondent within the meaning of *Miranda*.

not thereafter go forward in the absence of a valid waiver of respondent's constitutional rights unless he was provided with counsel. Since it is undisputed that respondent was not then competent to stand trial, I would also conclude that he was not competent to waive his constitutional right to remain silent.

The Court seems to believe that a waiver can be voluntary even if it is not the product of an exercise of the defendant's " 'free will.' " The Court's position is not only incomprehensible to me; it is also foreclosed by the Court's recent pronouncement in *Moran v. Burbine* that "the relinquishment of the right must have been voluntary in the sense that it was the product of a free and deliberate choice . . .". Because respondent's waiver was not voluntary in that sense, his custodial interrogation was presumptively coercive. The Colorado Supreme Court was unquestionably correct in concluding that his post-custodial incriminatory statements were inadmissible.

Accordingly, I concur in the judgment insofar as it applies to respondent's precustodial statements but respectfully dissent from the Court's disposition of the question that was not presented by the certiorari petition.

JUSTICE BRENNAN, with whom JUSTICE MARSHALL joins, dissenting.

* * *

I

The respondent's seriously impaired mental condition is clear on the record of this case. At the time of his confession, Mr. Connelly suffered from a "longstanding severe mental disorder," diagnosed as chronic paranoid schizophrenia. He had been hospitalized for psychiatric reasons five times prior to his confession; his longest hospitalization lasted for seven months. Mr. Connelly heard imaginary voices and saw nonexistent objects. He believed that his father was God, and that he was a reincarnation of Jesus.

At the time of his confession, Mr. Connelly's mental problems included "grandiose and delusional thinking." He had a known history of "thought withdrawal and insertion." Although physicians had treated Mr. Connelly "with a wide variety of medications in the past including antipsychotic medications," he had not taken any antipsychotic medications for at least six months prior to his confession. Following his arrest, Mr. Connelly initially was found incompetent to stand trial because the court-appointed psychiatrist, Dr. Metzner, "wasn't very confident that he could consistently relate accurate information." Dr. Metzner testified that Mr. Connelly was unable "to make free and rational choices" due to auditory hallucinations: "[W]hen he was read his *Miranda* rights, he probably had the capacity to know that he was being read his *Miranda* rights [but] he wasn't able to use that information because of the command hallucinations that he had experienced." He achieved competency to stand trial only after six months of hospitalization and treatment with antipsychotic and sedative medications.

* * *

II

* * *

A

* * *

While it is true that police overreaching has been an element of every confession case to date, it is also true that in every case the Court has made clear that ensuring that a confession is a product of free will is an independent concern. The fact that involuntary confessions have always been excluded in part because of police overreaching signifies only that this is a case of first impression. Until today, we have never upheld the admission of a confession that does not reflect the exercise of free will.

* * *

B

Since the Court redefines voluntary confessions to include confessions by mentally ill individuals, the reliability of these confessions becomes a central concern. [W]e have to date not required a finding of reliability for involuntary confessions only because *all* such confessions have been excluded upon a finding of involuntariness, regardless of reliability. The Court's adoption today of a restrictive definition of an "involuntary" confession will require heightened scrutiny of a confession's reliability.

The instant case starkly highlights the danger of admitting a confession by a person with a severe mental illness. The trial court made no findings concerning the reliability of Mr. Connelly's involuntary confession, since it believed that the confession was excludable on the basis of involuntariness. However, the overwhelming evidence in the record points to the unreliability of Mr. Connelly's delusional mind. Mr. Connelly was found incompetent to stand trial because he was unable to relate accurate information, and the court-appointed psychiatrist indicated that Mr. Connelly was actively hallucinating and exhibited delusional thinking at the time of his confession. The Court, in fact, concedes that "[a] statement rendered by one in the condition of respondent might be proved to be quite unreliable. . . ."

Moreover, the record is barren of any corroboration of the mentally ill defendant's confession. No physical evidence links the defendant to the alleged crime. Police did not identify the alleged victim's body as the woman named by the defendant. Mr. Connelly identified the alleged scene of the crime, but it has not been verified that the unidentified body was found there or that a crime actually occurred there. There is not a shred of competent evidence in this record linking the defendant to the charged homicide. There is only Mr. Connelly's confession.

Minimum standards of due process should require that the trial court find substantial indicia of reliability, on the basis of evidence extrinsic to the confession itself, before admitting the confession of a mentally ill person into evidence. I would require the trial court to make such a finding on remand. To hold otherwise allows the State to imprison and possibly to execute a mentally ill defendant based solely upon an inherently unreliable confession.

III

* * *

B

The Court imports its voluntariness analysis, which makes police coercion a requirement for a finding of involuntariness, into its evaluation of the waiver of *Miranda* rights. My reasoning in Part II, applies *a fortiori* to involuntary confessions made in custody involving the waiver of constitutional rights. I will not repeat here what I said there.

I turn then to the second requirement, apart from the voluntariness requirement, that the State must satisfy to establish a waiver of *Miranda* rights. Besides being voluntary, the waiver must be knowing and intelligent. We recently noted that "the waiver must have been made with a full awareness both of the nature of the right being abandoned and the consequences of the decision to abandon it." The two requirements are independent: "Only if the 'totality of the circumstances surrounding the interrogation' reveal *both* an uncoerced choice *and* the requisite level of comprehension may a court properly conclude that the *Miranda* rights have been waived."

* * *

Since the Colorado Supreme Court found that Mr. Connelly was "clearly" unable to make an "intelligent" decision, clearly its judgment should be affirmed. The Court reverses the entire judgment, however, without explaining how a "mistaken view of voluntariness" could "taint" this independent justification for suppressing the custodial confession, but leaving the Supreme Court of Colorado free on remand to reconsider other issues, not inconsistent with the Court's opinion. Such would include, in my view, whether the requirement of a knowing and intelligent waiver was satisfied.

I dissent.

Questions and Comments

1. *Evaluating the voluntariness of confessions.* The majority in *Connelly* holds that "absent police conduct causally related to the confession", a confession is "voluntary" under the due process clause. When is a statement "caused" by police? Consider this comment from Grano, "Voluntariness, Free Will, and the Law of Confessions," 65 Va.L.Rev. 859, 886–87 (1979):

> Causal language . . . is not helpful in solving concrete cases. Philosophical attempts to explain causation usually focus on the realm of

physical impacts and motion, as the example of one billiard ball striking another classicially illustrates. When one billiard ball strikes another, it may be appropriate to view the first ball as both a necessary and sufficient cause of the second ball's motion. To say, however, that one individual "caused" another to do something is to use the notion of causation in quite a different sense. With respect to confessions, the conduct of the police, proper or improper, never can be considered a sufficient cause of a resulting confession; the defendant's choice to confess always will be a necessary cause, except in those few cases where hypnosis, a drug, or some other procedure negates the defendant's consciousness. [On the other hand, l]ike the billiard ball, the police conduct can [always] be considered a necessary cause of a resulting confession, except perhaps when a suspect comes to the station desiring to confess. Were admissibility of confessions thus to turn on the sufficiency of the police interrogation process as a cause, few confessions would be suppressed; were it to turn on the necessity of the process as a causal factor, few confessions would be admitted. Neither extreme, of course, describes the law of confessions.

Even if the statements that Connelly made in response to police questions were "caused" by the police, neither a due process or *Miranda* violation necessarily occurred. The majority in *Connelly* requires not only police "causation" but also police "coercion" for there to be a constitutional violation. What are the differences between the majority's and Justice Stevens's definition of "coercion"? More generally, assuming police causation, how much additional pressure by the police is necessary before a confession becomes "coerced" and "involuntary"? Again, an excerpt from Grano, discussing "the extent to which the state may impair the mental freedom of suspects to secure confessions," might be useful:

> A subjective standard of voluntariness, taking into account all the defendant's weakness and infirmities, would make it exceedingly difficult to procure admissible confessions. The vast majority of defendants, weak or strong, initially are disinclined to provide the police self-incriminating statements. The objective of the interrogation session is to overcome this initial unwillingness without creating a risk that an innocent person will falsely confess. To take into account the peculiar weaknesses of each defendant would frustrate this objective, for the permissible level of police pressure would then decrease in direct proportion to the weakness of the suspect, thus leaving room for little more than volunteered statements.

*   *   *

Nevertheless, we cannot ignore the Court's numerous references to defendants' subjective characteristics. In Haley v. Ohio, for example, a fifteen-year-old boy arrested for murder confessed after continuous interrogation between midnight and five o'clock in the morning. In finding the confession involuntary, the Court reasoned that a fifteen-year-old cannot be judged by the more exacting standards of maturity. Similarly, the Court consistently has held that a defendant's physical or mental condition is a relevant factor [citing, inter alia, *Blackburn*]. The Court thus recently held involuntary a confession obtained from a wounded defendant in a hospital intensive care unit.

Cases such as these reflect society's basic sense of justice. Indeed, it would seem inconceivable to hold a child or a gravely ill person to the same powers of resistance as the normal adult. Thus, the mental freedom test cannot remain true to our fundamental normative judgments unless we incorporate some of the defendant's individual characteristics. . . .

. . . Characteristics that are feigned easily and difficult to verify properly may be excluded, much as they are in everyday discourse and in the substantive criminal law. We generally do not excuse conduct because of social adversity, peculiar personality traits, abnormal temperament, or low intelligence; rather, we expect an individual to overcome these conditions or characteristics. We do, however, morally empathize with the physically or mentally ill, the feeble, the very young, and the very old. These, moreover, are stark characteristics that an interrogating officer can be expected to recognize.

* * *

Thus, the mental freedom component of the due process voluntariness test should ask whether a person of ordinary firmness, innocent or guilty, having the defendant's age, physical condition, and relevant mental abnormalities (but not otherwise having the defendant's personality traits, temperament, intelligence, or social background), and strongly preferring not to confess, would find the interrogation pressures overbearing. Although primarily objective, this test takes sufficient account of the defendant's individual capacities to satisfy our fundamental moral concerns about impairment of mental freedom.

Id. at 900–906.

2. *The cognitive aspect of voluntariness.* In addition to considering a person's capacity to withstand police pressure, should we evaluate the person's cognitive capacity when determining voluntariness? Assuming that the police action is insufficient for "coercion", is the resulting confession always "voluntary", even if the confessor does not grasp its significance for the prosecution's case? How does the majority answer this question? Justice Stevens and Justice Brennan? Is it relevant, as both Stevens and Brennan seem to think, that Connelly may have been incompetent to stand trial when he made the statements?

Finally, note the majority's holding that, even if the statements were voluntarily obtained, state evidentiary law might bar their admission on remand. How do you evaluate Connelly's chances for success on this score?

3. *Voluntariness in other contexts.* In other areas involving decisional competency and waiver—e.g., pleading guilty, deciding whether to raise an insanity defense, deciding whether to forego an appeal—the defendant is represented by an attorney, thus diminishing if not removing altogether pressure from the police and the prosecutor. Does *Connelly* thus eliminate voluntariness as a due process or fifth amendment issue in these contexts? Or is its threshold requirement of state coercion relevant only to the interrogation context? If the latter, does *Connelly* mean that a person's confession might be accepted and his guilty plea rejected, despite no change in mental condition?

If you were the judge in the Phil Jones case, supra at pp. 898–904, would you accept a plea of guilty from him, knowing that his attorney had suggested that he do so?

C. DIGNITARIAN COMPETENCY

FORD v. WAINWRIGHT

Supreme Court of the United States, 1986.
477 U.S. 399, 106 S.Ct. 2595, 91 L.Ed.2d 335.

* * *

JUSTICE MARSHALL announced the judgment of the Court and delivered the opinion of the Court with respect to Parts I and II . . .

For centuries no jurisdiction has countenanced the execution of the insane, yet this Court has never decided whether the Constitution forbids the practice. Today we keep faith with our common-law heritage in holding that it does.

I

Alvin Bernard Ford was convicted of murder in 1974 and sentenced to death. There is no suggestion that he was incompetent at the time of his offense, at trial, or at sentencing. In early 1982, however, Ford began to manifest gradual changes in behavior. They began as an occasional peculiar idea or confused perception, but became more serious over time. After reading in the newspaper that the Ku Klux Klan had held a rally in nearby Jacksonville, Florida, Ford developed an obsession focused upon the Klan. His letters to various people reveal endless brooding about his "Klan work," and an increasingly pervasive delusion that he had become the target of a complex conspiracy, involving the Klan and assorted others, designed to force him to commit suicide. He believed that the prison guards, part of the conspiracy, had been killing people and putting the bodies in the concrete enclosures used for beds. Later, he began to believe that his women relatives were being tortured and sexually abused somewhere in the prison. This notion developed into a delusion that the people who were tormenting him at the prison had taken members of Ford's family hostage. The hostage delusion took firm hold and expanded, until Ford was reporting that 135 of his friends and family were being held hostage in the prison, and that only he could help them. By "day 287" of the "hostage crisis," the list of hostages had expanded to include "senators, Senator Kennedy, and many other leaders." In a letter to the Attorney General of Florida, written in 1983, Ford appeared to assume authority for ending the "crisis," claiming to have fired a number of prison officials. He began to refer to himself as "Pope John Paul, III," and reported having appointed nine new justices to the Florida Supreme Court.

Counsel for Ford asked a psychiatrist who had examined Ford earlier, Dr. Jamal Amin, to continue seeing him and to recommend appropriate treatment. On the basis of roughly 14 months of evaluation, taped conversations between Ford and his attorneys, letters written by Ford, interviews with Ford's acquaintances, and various medical records, Dr. Amin concluded in 1983 that Ford suffered from "a severe, uncontrollable, mental disease which closely resembles 'Paranoid Schizophrenia With Suicide Potential' "—a "major mental disorder . . . severe enough to substantially affect Mr. Ford's present ability to assist in the defense of his life."

Ford subsequently refused to see Dr. Amin again, believing him to have joined the conspiracy against him, and Ford's counsel sought assistance from Dr. Harold Kaufman, who interviewed Ford in November 1983. Ford told Dr. Kaufman that "I know there is some sort of death penalty, but I'm free to go whenever I want because it would be illegal and the executioner would be executed." When asked if he would be executed, Ford replied: "I can't be executed because of the landmark case. I won. Ford v. State will prevent executions all over." These statements appeared amidst long streams of seemingly unrelated thoughts in rapid succession. Dr. Kaufman concluded that Ford had no understanding of why he was being executed, made no connection between the homicide of which he had been convicted and the death penalty, and indeed sincerely believed that he would not be executed because he owned the prisons and could control the Governor through mind waves. Dr. Kaufman found that there was "no reasonable possibility that Mr. Ford was dissembling, malingering or otherwise putting on a performance. . . ." The following month, in an interview with his attorneys, Ford regressed further into nearly complete incomprehensibility, speaking only in a code characterized by intermittent use of the word "one," making statements such as "Hands one, face one. Mafia one. God one, father one, Pope one. Pope one. Leader one."

Counsel for Ford invoked the procedures of Florida law governing the determination of competency of a condemned inmate, Fla.Stat. § 922.07 (1985). Following the procedures set forth in the statute, the Governor of Florida appointed a panel of three psychiatrists to evaluate whether, under § 922.07(2), Ford had "the mental capacity to understand the nature of the death penalty and the reasons why it was imposed upon him." At a single meeting, the three psychiatrists together interviewed Ford for approximately 30 minutes. Each doctor then filed a separate two- or three-page report with the Governor, to whom the statute delegates the final decision. One doctor concluded that Ford suffered from "psychosis with paranoia" but had "enough cognitive functioning to understand the nature and the effects of the death penalty, and why it is to be imposed on him." Another found that, although Ford was "psychotic," he did "know fully what can happen to him." The third concluded that Ford had a "severe adaptational disorder," but did "comprehend his total situation including being sentenced to death, and all of the implications of that penalty." He believed that Ford's disorder, "although severe, seem[ed] contrived and recently learned." Thus, the interview produced three different diagnoses, but accord on the question of sanity as defined by state law.

The Governor's decision was announced on April 30, 1984, when, without explanation or statement, he signed a death warrant for Ford's execution.

II

* * *

There is now little room for doubt that the Eighth Amendment's ban on cruel and unusual punishment embraces, at a minimum, those modes or acts of punishment that had been considered cruel and unusual at the time that the Bill of Rights was adopted. "Although the Framers may have intended the Eighth Amendment to go beyond the scope of its English counterpart, their use of the language of the English Bill of Rights is convincing proof that they intended to provide at least the same protection. . . ."

Moreover, the Eighth Amendment's proscriptions are not limited to those practices condemned by the common law in 1789. Not bound by the sparing humanitarian concessions of our forebears, the Amendment also recognizes the "evolving standards of decency that mark the progress of a maturing society." *Trop v. Dulles,* 356 U.S. 86, 101, 78 S.Ct. 590, 598, 2 L.Ed.2d 630 (1958) (plurality opinion). In addition to considering the barbarous methods generally outlawed in the 18th century, therefore, this Court takes into account objective evidence of contemporary values before determining whether a particular punishment comports with the fundamental human dignity that the Amendment protects.

A

We begin, then, with the common law. The bar against executing a prisoner who has lost his sanity bears impressive historical credentials; the practice consistently has been branded "savage and inhuman." 4 W. Blackstone, Commentaries * 24–* 25 (hereinafter Blackstone). Blackstone explained:

> "[I]diots and lunatics are not chargeable for their own acts, if committed when under these incapacities: no, not even for treason itself. Also, if a man in his sound memory commits a capital offence, and before arraignment for it, he becomes mad, he ought not to be arraigned for it: because he is not able to plead to it with that advice and caution that he ought. And if, after he has pleaded, the prisoner becomes mad, he shall not be tried: for how can he make his defence? If, after he be tried and found guilty, he loses his senses before judgment, judgment shall not be pronounced; and if, after judgment, he becomes of nonsane memory, execution shall be stayed: for peradventure, says the humanity of the English law, had the prisoner been of sound memory, he might have alleged something in stay of judgment or execution." *Ibid.* (footnotes omitted).

Sir Edward Coke had earlier expressed the same view of the common law of England: "[B]y intendment of Law the execution of the offender is for example, . . . but so it is not when a mad man is executed, but should be a miserable spectacle, both against Law, and of extream inhumanity and cruelty, and can be no example to others."

As is often true of common-law principles, the reasons for the rule are less sure and less uniform than the rule itself. One explanation is that the execution of an insane person simply offends humanity, another, that it provides no example to others and thus contributes nothing to whatever deterrence value is intended to be served by capital punishment. Other commentators postulate religious underpinnings: that it is uncharitable to dispatch an offender "into another world, when he is not of a capacity to fit himself for it." It is also said that execution serves no purpose in these cases because madness is its own punishment: *furiosus solo furore punitur.* More recent commentators opine that the community's quest for "retribution"—the need to offset a criminal act by a punishment of equivalent "moral quality"—is not served by execution of an insane person, which has a "lesser value" than that of the crime for which he is to be punished. Unanimity of rationale, therefore, we do not find. "But whatever the reason of the law is, it is plain the law is so." We know of virtually no authority condoning the execution of the insane at English common law.

Further indications suggest that this solid proscription was carried to America, where it was early observed that "the judge is bound" to stay the execution upon insanity of the prisoner. . . .

B

This ancestral legacy has not outlived its time. Today, no State in the Union permits the execution of the insane. It is clear that the ancient and humane limitation upon the State's ability to execute its sentences has a firm a hold upon the jurisprudence of today as it had centuries ago in England. The various reasons put forth in support of the common-law restriction have no less logical, moral, and practical force than they did when first voiced. For today, no less than before, we may seriously question the retributive value of executing a person who has no comprehension of why he has been singled out and stripped of his fundamental right to life. Similarly, the natural abhorrence civilized societies feel at killing one who has no capacity to come to grips with his own conscience or deity is still vivid today. And the intuition that such an execution simply offends humanity is evidently shared across this Nation. Faced with such widespread evidence of a restriction upon sovereign power, this Court is compelled to conclude that the Eighth Amendment prohibits a State from carrying out a sentence of death upon a prisoner who is insane. Whether its aim be to protect the condemned from fear and pain without comfort of understanding, or to protect the dignity of society itself from the barbarity of exacting mindless vengeance, the restriction finds enforcement in the Eighth Amendment.

* * *

JUSTICE POWELL, concurring in part and concurring in the judgment.

* * *

A

As the Court recognizes, the ancient prohibition on execution of the insane rested on differing theories. . . .

[The contention that prohibiting execution of the insane is justified as a way of preserving the defendant's ability to make arguments on his own behalf] has slight merit today. Modern practice provides far more extensive review of convictions and sentences than did the common law, including not only direct appeal but ordinarily both state and federal collateral review. Throughout this process, the defendant has access to counsel, by constitutional right at trial, and by employment or appointment at other stages of the process whenever the defendant raises substantial claims. Nor does the defendant merely have the right to counsel's assistance; he also has the right to the *effective* assistance of counsel at trial and on appeal. These guarantees are far broader than those enjoyed by criminal defendants at common law. It is thus unlikely indeed that a defendant today could go to his death with knowledge of undiscovered trial error that might set him free.

In addition, in cases tried at common law execution often followed fairly quickly after trial, so that incompetence at the time of execution was linked as a practical matter with incompetence at the trial itself. Our decisions already recognize, however, that a defendant must be competent to stand trial, and thus the notion that a defendant must be able to assist in his defense is largely provided for. . . .

B

The more general concern of the common law—that executions of the insane are simply cruel—retains its vitality. It is as true today as when Coke lived that most men and women value the opportunity to prepare, mentally and spiritually, for their death. Moreover, today as at common law, one of the death penalty's critical justifications, its retributive force, depends on the defendant's awareness of the penalty's existence and purpose. Thus, it remains true that executions of the insane both impose a uniquely cruel penalty and are inconsistent with one of the chief purposes of executions generally. For precisely these reasons, Florida requires the Governor to stay executions of those who "d[o] not have the mental capacity to understand the nature of the death penalty and why it was imposed" on them. A number of States have more rigorous standards, but none disputes the need to require that those who are executed know the fact of their impending execution and the reason for it.

Such a standard appropriately defines the kind of mental deficiency that should trigger the Eighth Amendment prohibition. If the defendant perceives the connection between his crime and his punishment, the retributive goal of the criminal law is satisfied. And only if the defendant is aware that his death is approaching can he prepare himself for his passing. Accordingly, I would hold that the Eighth Amendment forbids the execution only of those who are unaware of the punishment they are about to suffer and why they are to suffer it.

Petitioner's claim of insanity plainly fits within this standard. According to petitioner's proffered psychiatric examination, petitioner does not know that he is to be executed, but rather believes that the death penalty has been invalidated. If this assessment is correct, petitioner cannot connect his execution to the crime for which he was convicted.

* * *

[The opinion of JUSTICE O'CONNOR, concurring in part and dissenting in part, in which JUSTICE WHITE joined, and the dissenting opinion of JUSTICE REHNQUIST, in which CHIEF JUSTICE BURGER joined, are deleted.]

Questions and Comments

1. *The rationale for the competency requirement in death penalty cases.* The Court in *Ford* notes at least six rationales that might justify its rule that a person be competent prior to execution: (1) an incompetent person might be unable to provide counsel with last minute information leading to vacation of the sentence; (2) madness is punishment enough in itself; (3) an incompetent person cannot make peace with God; (4) execution of an incompetent person has no deterrent effect on the population; (5) such execution "is a miserable spectacle . . . of extreme inhumanity and cruelty"; (6) the retribution or vengeance meant to be realized by execution cannot be exacted from an incompetent person. Do any of these rationales distinguish the incompetent from the competent sufficiently to justify a prohibition against execution only of the incompetent? Might it not be more "cruel" to execute a fully aware individual than one who is not? Research indicates that, for some individuals, psychosis is a defense mechanism against the horrors of the death penalty. Bluestone & McGahee, "Reaction to Extreme Stress: Impending Death by Execution," 119 Am.J. Psychiat. 392 (1962).

For a view that, of the rationales advanced by the Court, only the retributive one is supportable, see Ward, "Competency for Execution: Problems in Law and Psychiatry," 14 Fla.St.U.L.Rev. 35, 49–56 (1986).q As described by Ward:

> The retributive theory of competency for execution is predicated upon an assumption that every wrong act must be avenged by a punitive act of equal quality. Presumably, killing an insane person does not satisfy the societal interest in reprisal for the previous wrong as well as does killing a sane person. Therefore, imposing the death penalty on

q. Ward also argues, however, that the rule could be supported on the additional ground that society is ambivalent about the death penalty and thus "the number of death penalties imposed should be decreased in various ways," including the incompetency bar. Id. at 56.

incompetent prisoners exacts a punishment less valuable than the crime itself.

Id. at 54. See also, Hazard & Louisell, "Death, the State, and the Insane: Stay of Execution," 9 UCLA L.Rev. 381 (1962).

The competency requirements discussed previously in this chapter have derived primarily from a concern for individual autonomy, and only secondarily from a desire to achieve societal goals. Can the same be said for the requirement imposed by the Court in *Ford*?

2. *The competency standard.* The criteria for determining competency to be executed presumably vary depending upon the rationale chosen. Is Florida's statutory definition of competency—representative of the rule followed by a majority of states—sufficient, as Justice Powell suggests? An alternative standard—a version of which is followed by most of the remaining states—was quoted by Justice Frankfurter in his dissenting opinion in *Solesbee v. Balkcom,* 339 U.S. 9, 20 n. 3, 70 S.Ct. 457, 462 n. 3, 94 L.Ed. 604 (1950):

> After sentence of death, the test of insanity is whether the prisoner has not 'from the defects of his faculties, sufficient intelligence to understand the nature of the proceedings against him, what he was tried for, the purpose of his punishment, the impending fate which awaits him, a sufficient understanding to know any fact which might exist which would make his punishment unjust or unlawful, and the intelligence requisite to convey such information to his attorneys or the court.'

(Quoting *In re Smith,* 176 P. at 823). This language reads like a competency to proceed standard. Is it better than the Florida language?

Under either standard, how should the word "understand" be defined? In *Johnson v. Cabana,* 818 F.2d 333 (5th Cir.1987), the court dismissed as irrelevant expert testimony that the prisoner "appeared too calm and too much in control to appreciate the gravity of his situation." In contrast, in *Musselwhite v. State,* 215 Miss. 363, 60 So.2d 807 (1952), the court found the prisoner incompetent because the testimony revealed "that if he were taken to the electric chair, he would not quail or take account of its significance." Does not this latter language, which suggests that the prisoner must have an "emotional appreciation" of the situation, better reflect the retributive rationale? On the other hand, would a sociopath ever meet this standard?

3. *Procedures.* The second issue the Court addressed in *Ford* was the proper procedure for determining competency to be executed. As recounted above, Florida allowed the governor to make the final decision on competency, based on reports from three psychiatrists. Three members of the Court joined Justice Marshall in deciding that the due process clause required more: specifically, a hearing on the competency issue, presided over by a judicial officer, at which the prisoner would have the right to be present with counsel and confront the experts. Justice O'Connor, joined by Justice White, also concluded that due process was violated by the Florida procedure, but indicated that all the state was constitutionally required to provide was some procedure for receiving the written submissions of the

prisoner. Justice Rehnquist, joined by Chief Justice Burger, voted to uphold the Florida procedure.

As a result of this lineup, Justice Powell's opinion was controlling on the procedural issue. He agreed with Marshall that the Florida procedures were inadequate, but stated: "I would not require the kind of full-scale 'sanity trial' that Justice Marshall appears to find necessary." In explaining this stance, he stated:

First, the Eighth Amendment claim at issue can arise only after the prisoner has been validly convicted of a capital crime and sentenced to death. Thus, in this case the State has a substantial and legitimate interest in taking petitioner's life as punishment for his crime. That interest is not called into question by petitioner's claim. Rather, the only question raised is not whether, but when, his execution may take place. This question is important, but it is not comparable to the antecedent question whether petitioner should be executed at all. It follows that this Court's decisions imposing heightened procedural requirements on capital trials and sentencing proceedings do not apply in this context.

Second, petitioner does not make his claim of insanity against a neutral background. On the contrary, in order to have been convicted and sentenced, petitioner must have been judged competent to stand trial, or his competency must have been sufficiently clear as not to raise a serious question for the trial court. The State therefore may properly presume that petitioner remains sane at the time sentence is to be carried out, and may require a substantial threshold showing of insanity merely to trigger the hearing process.

Finally, the sanity issue in this type of case does not resemble the basic issues at trial or sentencing. Unlike issues of historical fact, the question of petitioner's sanity calls for a basically subjective judgment. And unlike the determination of whether the death penalty is appropriate in a particular case, the competency determination depends substantially on expert analysis in a discipline fraught with "subtleties and nuances." This combination of factors means that ordinary adversarial procedures—complete with live testimony, cross-examination, and oral argument by counsel—are not necessarily the best means of arriving at sound, consistent judgments as to a defendant's sanity. Cf. *Parham v. J.R.*

477 U.S. at 425–26, 106 S.Ct. at 2609–10. In light of this reasoning, Justice Powell concluded that the state needed only to provide an "impartial officer or board that can receive evidence and argument from the prisoner's counsel, including psychiatric evidence that may differ from the State's own psychiatric examination." Id. at 427, 100 S.Ct. at 2610.

If the rationale for the prohibition on executing incompetent prisoners is retributive, as defined by Ward (see note 1), does the individual have *any* interest in making sure the conclusion about competency is accurate? Should the individual even have "standing" to raise the issue?

4. *Treating the incompetent.* If a person is found incompetent to be executed, should he or she have the right to refuse treatment that will

restore and maintain competency to be executed? Are the reasons given by Justice Powell in justifying minimal procedures at the competency determination relevant here as well? In *State v. Perry*, 545 So.2d 1049 (La.1989), the Louisiana Supreme Court held that a death row inmate with a severe psychosis may be forcibly medicated in an attempt to make him competent to be executed. The U.S. Supreme Court has decided to review the case. ____ U.S. ____, 110 S.Ct. 1317, 108 L.Ed.2d 492 (1989).

A separate problem is ethical rather than legal. It involves the role of the mental health professional in restoring competency. As noted in Note, "Medical Ethics and Competency to be Executed," 96 Yale L.J. 167, 178–79 (1986),

> the express purpose of competency treatment is to guarantee that the patient will be killed. Each treatment strategy to heal the inmate is in fact another strategy to ensure his death. No intervening acts save the minuscule likelihood that, once sane, the inmate will articulate a heretofore unknown reason for a stay of execution, will prevent the execution that the physician has made possible.

In response to this dilemma, the American Medical Association has adopted the following position: "The physician, as a member of a profession dedicated to the preserving of life when there is hope of doing so, should not be a participant in a legally authorized execution." Is this rigid stance ethical in view of the suffering an untreated person might experience? Consider also the fact that many persons on death row decide they would rather be executed than continue living in prison. See White, "Defendants Who Elect Execution," 48 U.Pitt.L.Rev. 853, 854–55 (1987).

5. *Decisional competency and the death penalty.* In this regard, how competent must a person on death row be before he or she can abort collateral proceedings and demand that the state carry out the death sentence? Cf. *Gilmore v. Utah,* 429 U.S. 1012, 1013, 97 S.Ct. 436, 437, 50 L.Ed.2d 632 (1976) (in which the Supreme Court held that Gilmore could waive further judicial review of his case and proceed to execution because he "made a knowing and intelligent waiver of any and all federal rights he might have asserted . . .".). At least one court has required a relatively high level of competency in this situation (i.e., higher than what is required for competency to proceed), given the irreversibility of the decision. *Franz v. State,* 296 Ark. 181, 188–89, 754 S.W.2d 839, 843 (1988).

Chapter Ten

POST-COMMITMENT ISSUES

Table of Sections

I. INTRODUCTION

The Supreme Court has made clear that "a state is under no constitutional duty to provide substantive services for those within its borders." Youngberg v. Romeo, 457 U.S. 307, 316, 102 S.Ct. 2452, 2458, 73 L.Ed.2d 28 (1982). But after the state intervenes in a person's life, it must obey constitutional dictates. This chapter focuses on the states' constitutional obligations toward those it has involuntarily committed through civil or criminal process. It also examines the constitutional prerogatives of "voluntary" patients who are voluntary in name only (e.g., nonprotesting admittees, children committed by their parents, individuals committed by their guardians). The various *statutory* enactments which may require the state to provide services for certain populations (e.g., the Education for All Handicapped Children Act) are discussed in Part III of this book.

The extent to which the state is obligated under the constitution to provide for the needs and demands of those whom it has deprived of liberty is a matter of considerable complexity. For instance, can one justifiably conclude that the state has met its constitutional duty if it provides decent living quarters for those it involuntarily hospitalizes? If it must provide more, is mere prevention of deterioration enough? Or must the state afford committed individuals treatment or habilitation [a] that will improve their condition? Assuming a duty to provide something more than food and shelter for those it deprives of liberty, is the state also obligated to create community resources when community treatment or habilitation is deemed more effective than traditional hospital treatment? Within an institutional environment (whether or not it is in the "community") to what extent may the state limit access to mail and phone service, contact with the opposite sex, exercise and so on? When, if ever, must the state pay a patient for work performed at the institution?

Additionally, assessing the scope of the constitutional right to treatment and habilitation raises systemic concerns more dramatically than other issues addressed in this book. Do courts have the expertise to assess the effectiveness of treatment? Do they have the authority to force states to create new treatment facilities and programs? If so, how is this authority to be enforced?

These are the primary issues examined in this chapter. To provide a realistic backdrop to this discussion, the following excerpt, describing the experiences of several patients in the Texas mental health system, is offered.

JOSEPH NOCERA, THE LONG, LONESOME ROAD
Texas Monthly 43–53.
(1986).

* * *

A real mental health system does not exist in Texas. Instead, a group of independent fiefdoms and power bases all operate under the loose rubric of the Texas Department of Mental Health and Mental Retardation (MHMR). State hospitals are one power base, and local mental health authorities are another. Probate judges try to get mentally ill people into state hospitals, while hospital social workers try just as hard to get them out. There is even a federal judge involved in running the state hospital. As a result of a class-action suit brought a dozen years ago on the behalf of patients, federal district judge Barefoot Sanders is immersed in every aspect of hospital life, and although his intimidating presence has made the hospitals marginally better, the improvements have come at the expense of the local authorities. Part of the reason that everyone seems to be working at cross-purposes is that there is honest disagreement about how best to treat the mentally ill. But the chaos that reigns in the Texas mental health system also results from some of the worst reasons imaginable: bureaucratic infighting and turf battles, and a preference for the status quo over innovation or change.

Fred Thomas is in many ways typical of the people who populate that system. He is black. He is poor. He is unquestionably a tough

a. Habilitation is the term used to refer to treatment and education of the developmentally disabled.

case, partly because of the severity of his illness, but also because, as I discovered in the five months I spent with him a year ago, he lacks the motivation to try to make something of his life. Though instilling such motivation is perhaps the most fundamental goal of the modern mental health movement, the Texas system has seemed utterly helpless to change Fred. Instead, the system has been content to process him into the state hospital and process him out—always sending him back to his mother's house, where inevitably and tragically he would revert to his old ways. Although Texas' mental health hospitals are no longer hellholes, they are still little more than benign jails. One former social worker used to tell patients about to be released: "If you can survive in this place, you can survive anything." When I first met Fred Thomas, he had learned to survive in the hospital. The question confronting him was whether he could survive beyond its walls.

* * *

On a bright April day, in a large outdoor area of the Austin State Hospital, Fred Thomas sat down across from me at a picnic table. In hospital jargon, he was in the Harris K patio—the Harris K unit being the drab, one-story, pentagon shaped building that surrounds the patio. The men on Fred's ward were outdoors for an hour of "exercise"—thus satisfying one of Judge Sanders' requirements for structured daily activities. As far as I could see, only two men were actually exercising: a member of the ward staff and a patient were shooting baskets through a worn, bent rim. A few other patients were walking, somewhat frantically, along a cement pathway. The rest were either sitting in chairs or sprawling out under one of the pecan trees, fast asleep. At least half of them were smoking—and constantly fending off requests for a nearly finished cigarette. Almost all the patients wore dirty, ill-fitting clothes. Most of them looked harmless enough, except for one, a black, middle-aged schizophrenic with a Fu Manchu moustache who was standing in the center of the patio screaming about the CIA and the KGB. I would later learn that he was Donald Peterson.

Before coming over to the table, Fred had been among those trying to get someone to give him a cigarette. He was wearing a grimy sweatshirt, slightly tattered green jogging pants, and old-fashioned high-top sneakers without socks. Upon reaching the table, Fred sat down across from me, but at first he ignored me, concentrating instead on the cigarette he had scored. He lighted the cigarette and inhaled with excruciating slowness, savoring each puff as if it might be his last. Before his first admission, Fred had never smoked. But because cigarettes are so integral to life in a state hospital—even to the extent that they are used as carrots in Austin's behavior modification program—he now smoked so much that his fingers had permanent tobacco stains. When his cigarette was finished, he looked up and began talking.

Fred's speech was characterized by what psychiatrists call "loose association" or "tangential thought"—that is, skipping rapidly from one topic to the next, usually with a tenuous thread linking each new thought to the one before it. When I introduced myself, he said, "Joe. Where you gonna go, Joe? Joe Willie Namath." And that led him to a brief discussion of Namath's bad knees, and on to trees and bees, and then to the birds and the bees, and then to honey, which led to girls, and finally to a recently released patient whom he claimed had been his girlfriend.

[T]hat April marked the beginning of Fred's fifth stay at the Austin State Hospital. After his initial admission in 1979, he had managed to stay out of the hospital for four years. But between March 1984 and March 1985, he had been in three times.

* * *

It's 8 a.m. on a Thursday in early May: time for the "morning meds" in Ward B, one of the four male wards in the Harris K unit (there are two female wards). Ward B has been Fred Thomas' home for more than a month.

The heart of an Austin State Hospital ward is the central dayroom, no larger than a bank president's office; it is filled with beat-up chairs, a few card tables, and a television set that is constantly on. Plexiglass windows and locked doors separate the dayroom and a nurse's station, from which the ward staff keeps watch over its charges. There are some 25 men in the Ward B dayroom this morning, at least 7 more than the ward was intended to hold. During the time I spent at Harris K, the dayroom was constantly overcrowded, which greatly increased the level of agitation and even danger. Fred, however, does not seem agitated. He is wearing a clean pair of short pants, a new T-shirt, and his ever-present basketball sneakers, unlaced. He is standing in front of a full-length mirror, mumbling to himself. No one seems to notice.

[T]he two mental health workers sitting in the nurse's station don't notice Fred because, by their lights, he is being good. To such non-professionals, who make less than a good grocery clerk, a patient's goodness is measured entirely on the basis of how little trouble he causes. Fred may be incoherent, but at least he's not starting a fight. Besides, they are busy with their morning ration of paperwork, which is voluminous, as usual.

The other patients don't take any special note of Fred because most of them are equally absorbed in their own private worlds. . . . Three or four men are sitting stonily in chairs, grumbling angrily at the walls. Another man erupts into loud, incomprehensible laughter. A new patient tries to flick something off his shoulder, a motion he repeats again and again; there is nothing there. In the bathroom an extremely delusional, muscular man stuffs magazines down a toilet. The man's parents conceived him (so the story goes) while both were patients at Rusk State Hospital. He has been flushing magazines down the toilet every morning for over a week, ever since someone sent dozens of old copies of the New Yorker to Ward B.

Although all the patients were roused out of bed two hours ago, the only things they have been required to do so far are brush their teeth, comb their hair, and make their beds, activities that exhaust no more than five minutes apiece. Thus the rest of their time has been spent doing what they're doing now—milling about. When you're confined to a state hospital ward, you're forced to spend a lot of time with your thoughts, however terrifying they might be. This cruel fact cannot possibly help anyone get better, but that's the way it is. Other than the television, there are very few distractions. Milling about is the basic activity in the ward.

In the middle of the low-level chaos, a nurse holding a carton containing the morning medication walks into the nurse's station. Her name is Sue Dennison. "Okay," she announces in a tone that is both firm and pleasant, "get in line for your morning meds." The two mental health workers go into the dayroom to help the patients form a scraggly line. One by one the patients step up to the nurse's station to receive their medication. The psychotropic drugs they take—with names like Thorazine, Navane, Prolixin, Mellaril, and Haldol—are the primary, indeed, the only, form of real treatment they will receive in the hospital. And while there is no doubt that most of the people in this dayroom need the drugs desperately, there is considerable doubt as to whether some of them might not also benefit from other forms of help—from therapy, for instance. The issue of alternative treatments, which is the subject of a fierce national debate, does not get addressed in Austin. It is drugs that can prop people up the fastest, and get them out the quickest, and soak up the least amount of money. So drugs are what is used.

The first person Sue Dennison sees on this Thursday morning is a short, shy, soft-spoken man who looks about fifty years old. He is a murderer. In June 1980, six weeks after being released from the state hospital, he shot his next-door neighbor. He had heard voices telling him the neighbor was about to shoot him. Every time the doctors think he is well enough to stand trial, he is sent to prison. But as soon as he gets to prison, he regresses and has to be returned to the state hospital.

"How are you feeling today?" Dennison asks him. A few days before, the man had asked a ward staffer if the attendant was going to kill him soon. "Oh, just fine," he says meekly.

Next, a young black man steps up to the window. He has a little goatee and wears a baseball cap turned backward. When he sees Dennison, he puts his chin on the window ledge and stares at her salaciously. "Come on Michael," she says. "I can't give you your medicine if you're doing that." He keeps staring.

Michael is retarded. He was committed by a probate judge in Harris County, thus making him Austin's problem instead of Houston's. Harris County washed its hands of him not long after he arrived by sending a letter to the hospital stating that Michael could not be returned to Houston because the city lacked an "appropriate placement." But Austin doesn't have any place for him either. He belongs in a state school for the mentally retarded, but he can't get into one; the waiting period is about two years. Judge Sanders' monitors have raised the issue of retarded people languishing in the state hospitals. But what can the staff on Ward B do? All they can do is wait.

[B]ringing up the end of the line is Donald Peterson (not his real name). He is the toughest patient on the ward; he has lived at least half of his adult life in an institution—either a mental hospital or Huntsville State Prison (for armed robbery). The other patients are afraid of him. The staff prefers to keeps its distance too. Peterson, who looks old beyond his 44 years, hasn't shaved or bathed in days. He smells of stale cigarettes and rancid sweat, and the other patients have been complaining about him. Eventually, staff will have to force Peterson to take a shower, but they're not in any hurry. The last time they tried to make Peterson clean up—it happened about a week ago—one of the mental health workers wound up with torn ligaments in his thumb.

Don Peterson seems quite comfortable living in Ward B. And why not? His life on the outside is unrelievedly sad. His elderly father refuses to have anything to do with him. The mental health system barely knows he exists. He sleeps in a sickeningly ramshackle house in a Houston ghetto with a dozen other mentally ill people. For human companionship, he hangs out at the Star of Hope Mission in downtown Houston, where he is prey for thugs.

In the hospital, on the other hand, his living conditions are dramatically improved, he knows the ropes, and he can play the hunter instead of the prey. Soon after [one patient] arrived, for instance, Peterson sidled up to him on a bench with a can of Coke in his hand and asked with a smirk, "Do you think I can kill you with this?" Peterson also, from time to time, initiates sex with other men in the ward. This is not uncommon among the patients; even Fred was once caught trading a sexual act for cigarettes.

. . . After Sue Dennison gives Peterson his medicine, he quickly walks away—a little too quickly, in Dennison's opinion. She believes Peterson has been "cheeking his meds" lately—that is, only pretending to take his medication until he can get to the bathroom and spit it out. She thinks this because he has begun talking about how John Kennedy and Martin Luther King have deputized him "to be with white women." The mental health workers stop Peterson before he can get to the bathroom. He glares at them for a few seconds, but finally he swallows.

After Fred takes his morning medication and has breakfast in the ward cafeteria, he gets his two-cigarette allotment from the ward's "point store" (patients trade "points" they have earned in return for cigarettes or candy or coffee).

* * *

What happened to Fred in the past month offers a short course in the vagaries of patient care at the state hospital. His commitment began on March 26, when he was admitted to Ward B as an "acute" patient, a status that legally limits his stay to a maximum of ninety days. He told the admissions staff glumly, "This is where I belong."

The doctor for Wards A and B (A is one of the female wards) was a kindly, Egyptian-born psychiatrist whose command of English was tentative at best, and who had a reputation for being cautious—too cautious, in fact, for the bureaucracy, which felt that he was gumming up the works by not releasing patients quickly enough. After about twenty minutes with Fred, the doctor diagnosed his illness as "Schizophrenia undifferentiated chronic"—very much in line with previous diagnoses—and prescribed Prolixin, a safe choice that also reflected Fred's history.

A month later Fred's first doctor left the hospital; he was replaced by a Cuban-born psychiatrist named Heriberto Cabada. Brusque and garrulous, Cabada was almost the complete opposite in temperament from his predecessor, with whom he shares only one apparent trait: heavily accented English. (Like most state hospitals, Austin is full of foreign-born and trained psychiatrists.) A large man with a pronounced girth who favored guayabera shirts and a three-day growth of beard, Cabada was the shortest of the short-timers. In little more than a month he would finish and move to Miami to begin what he hoped to be a lucrative private practice. Wards A and B were about the last place on earth he wanted to be. "This is a first-year resident's rotation," he groused to anyone within earshot. But he knew why he had been brought in.

In his three years at the hospital, Cabada had learned how to play the game, and he had become fairly cynical about it. He knew how to keep his head down whenever there was trouble; he had learned that lesson when one of his patients committed suicide while he was on vacation, and he nearly lost his residency as a result. Although he bridled at the paperwork ("It's a wonder we have time to see any patients at all"), he knew the importance of leaving a paper trail to keep the court and the bureaucracy satisfied. He knew he was there to prescribe drugs and not to administer psychotherapy. "This is a place to stabilize people and to get them out," he said bluntly. And when he got to Wards A and B, he immediately understood what was expected of him. Within a week, Cabada has released enough patients that the census on Ward B had dropped from 24 to 18. "I love that Cabada," said one of the workers on the ward.

And when Cabada saw Fred Thomas for the first time—fifteen minutes on the morning of May 2—he knew what was expected of him there too. Prolixin, which the previous doctor had prescribed, was popular in community outpatient clinics because it was the only drug at the time that could be given by injection with long-lasting (up to two weeks) effect. But the imperative at the state hospital makes Prolixin much less ideal because it is so slow-acting compared with most other psychotropic drugs. As Cabada noted in Fred's chart, the patient "is progressing slowly, although he is not at the point where he should be." To speed things along, Cabada decided to switch Fred to Haldol, a potent, fast-acting, highly sedative drug. Haldol is as popular inside the hospital as Prolixin is outside. At an initial dose of thirty milligrams a day, Fred was more drugged, and more sedated, and feeling more side effects than he had in his life.

Late one afternoon, a few days after the change, I got an inkling of how Haldol was affecting Fred. The patients were out on the patio; Fred was sitting in a chair he had pulled out from the ward. He was in a bad way. His lips were tight and trembled slightly, and he constantly touched them. He scratched his legs until they were white with scratch marks, and he was very groggy. Peterson came up to Fred and started screaming at him; Fred barely noticed. Instead he began talking to himself softly; "Rolling bowling green."

* * *

[While Dr. Cabada was on vacation, Fred was seen by a Dr. Kerr. According to Kerr, "When I was in medical school, we were always taught that a psychotic person was schizophrenic until proven otherwise." But after working in state hospitals, Kerr came to believe that many of the delusional patients he saw were not afflicted solely with schizophrenia or solely with manic depression, but rather with some combination of the two. Kerr rediagnosed Fred as suffering from a "schizoaffective disorder" and put him on Tegretol, 200 milligram three times a day, stating "There is nothing empirical about this. All you can do is bring your experience and your training." On this drug, Fred improved to the point where the hospital staff considered releasing him to a community facility].

* * *

No one can doubt that deinstitutionalization has done a lot of good. Many who didn't need to be there were languishing in mental hospitals; their lives have been immeasurably improved. In 1970 alone, the Austin State Hospital's population dropped from 3400 to 1800, and almost all releases were easy cases. But if deinstitutionalization has done some unquestioned good, it has also had its share of unintended consequences. Look around downtown Houston, where as many as 2000 mentally ill people, "freed" from the state hospital, wander the streets like modern-day paupers, and you quickly realize how far the promise of deinstitutionalization is from the reality. The miracle drugs that were going to "cure" the mentally ill have turned out to be not so miraculous after all—helpful, yes, but not miraculous. The extensive network of community programs and halfway houses that were expected to absorb the thousands of mentally ill streaming out of state hospitals never developed—especially not in Texas, where the state hospitals still pull in nearly 80 per cent of all the mental health money even as their populations have been reduced by more than two thirds. A patient's right under the law to be released from a state hospital commitment after ninety days has been largely responsible for the so-called revolving door syndrome, in which patients spend their lives shuttling back and forth from the hospital to the community. The right to live in the least restrictive environment has meant that thousands of mentally ill people, not sick enough to be confined to a hospital ward but still desperately in need of care, live in the least restrictive environment imaginable: the streets.

And yet the pressure on the state hospitals to "get the census down" remains as inexorable as ever. It comes from state and federal law and from a society still unwilling to admit that deinstitutionalization has not worked the way it was supposed to. And it also comes from Judge Sanders. The judge's mental health monitors—the people overseeing the hospital system on his behalf—deny that depopulation is their intent, but they cannot deny the result. Their goal is purely to improve conditions at the state hospital, with little thought given to how the judge's orders will affect the rest of the system. Several years ago, when Judge Sanders, acting on the masters' recommendations, ordered that the staff-to-patient ratio be significantly lowered, his aim was to make each ward a less dangerous place. But since the hospitals didn't have the money to hire the hundreds of staff members needed to comply with the order, they reacted—predictably—not by adding staff but by increasing medication dosages for the patients, to get them out more quickly. The hospitals can say—and do say, all the time—that they are only doing their job while complying with a court order. The judge can say that he is doing his job. (The population in Austin today is around 550.) And meanwhile, a few thousand more mentally ill people are released to the streets, where they find . . . nothing.

Well, not exactly nothing. Houston, for example, does have some outpatient clinics, some apartments for mentally ill people, and one small halfway house to serve the thousands of mentally ill people who live in the city. The halfway house is Tarry Hall, on a residential street in Montrose. It has 27 beds. It is the reality of deinstitutionalization in Houston. . . .

* * *

"Hygiene and room check are now beginning."

It was 9:15 a.m. . . ., and the voice booming over the intercom belonged to Dennis Milam, a bearded, sandaled social worker who is third in command at Tarry Hall. By this time, the residents (as Tarry Hall calls its clientele) had been awake for nearly three hours, and theoretically they should have finished their hygiene and room chores. Instead, most were in the same position as Fred. They hadn't even started.

Tarry Hall is a deceptively large house built in the shape of a square doughnut. Its central feature is an outdoor courtyard surrounded by four wide corridors. In the front of the building is a pool room, and in the back, a den. Because it has a TV and a stereo, the den serves much the same function as the dayroom in Austin; it is where the residents can usually be found when they have nothing else to do. It was where Talvin Paul—a 25–year–old graduate of Grambling who was Fred's caseworker—now found his new charge.

"Have you taken a shower yet, Fred?" asked Talvin.

"Too early for that, man." Fred stared straight ahead while Talvin spoke. "One of the expectations around here is that everybody takes a shower," Talvin said. Still, Fred didn't move. It was 9:25. Over the intercom Dennis said, "Fred Thomas, you are needed in your room." Fred crushed his cigarette butt into the floor—ignoring Talvin's admonition to put it in an ashtray—and shuffled off to his room.

The purpose of the hygiene and room chores is to instill a sense of responsibility in the residents, and those who accomplish their daily tasks are rewarded with access to their money and cigarettes and with the accumulation of free time—time they can spend away from the halfway house. Fred and his new roommate, another recent arrival from Austin, listened impassively as Dennis explained what was expected of them each morning: besides making their beds and putting their clothes away, they were supposed to sweep, mop, and dust their rooms. In addition, each would soon be given a household chore (Fred was eventually assigned a bathroom to keep clean). "Do you understand?" asked Dennis. Fred nodded and began picking up his sheets. But as soon as Dennis left, Fred dropped the sheets, wandered back into the den, and turned on the stereo. It was 9:35.

Fifteen minutes later, Dennis found him. "In the morning," he said, "we don't have the stereo or TV on." He flicked the music off. "Your roommate is sweeping the room right now, so why don't you get the mop?" Annoyed by that, Fred nonetheless got a mop and dragged it behind him toward his bedroom. When he got there he gave the floor a few halfhearted passes. But as soon as the coast was clear, Fred started to walk back to the den. Talvin spotted him. "Fred," he shouted, "you need to be in your room!"

That was more than Fred could bear. He stalked past Talvin into the den and again turned on the stereo. When Talvin caught up with him, Fred glared. "Why are you trying to punish me, man?" he asked. It was 10:15.

Today hygiene and room check took nearly two hours. Up until a few months ago, it had taken a half-hour. Back then, the staff had encouraged residents to look for work, and the residents themselves had run a meeting every Friday to decide how much free time each person had earned. Now the staff was spending its time encouraging residents to comb their hair, and the Friday meeting was run by staff members, who had already decided how much time each resident had earned. Things were different because the residents were different; the mentally ill people whom Tarry Hall once treated had been much less sick than the ones it treated now.

That era had only recently ended, yet it was already viewed nostalgically by the Tarry Hall staff. It had been more fun to work with higher functioning residents: they were more motivated to succeed and easier to reach, and the psychic rewards for the staff were much more immediate. Tarry Hall had enjoyed a great deal of independence in the old days. Stripped of that independence, Tarry Hall was bitter.

For most of its eight-year existence, the halfway house had successfully resisted efforts to make it a port of entry for released state hospital patients. Never mind that Tarry Hall was the only county-funded halfway house in the city and that there were mentally ill people in the streets of Houston who needed the kind of help Tarry Hall could offer. For years Tarry Hall administrators refused to admit that those two facts were connected.

Early in 1985, however, in its never-ending effort to reduce hospital populations, MHMR began dangling money in front of local mental health agencies as an inducement to treat more mentally ill people. Each agency would receive $35.50 per patient per day that the census was reduced in Austin. Gradually, the Harris County mental health authorities began making changes aimed at keeping more people out of the hospital. For instance, they assigned caseworkers to monitor the progress of recently released state hospital patients. They also began scrambling for more placement possibilities: inevitably, they saw Tarry Hall as a luxury they could no longer afford. In late March 1985 Tarry Hall had begun accepting its first handful of residents from Austin.

The change from without imposed on Tarry Hall also brought changes from within. Tarry Hall used to have a library: now the library was being converted to a point store. The former clientele had attended current-events classes; the new clientele took walks in the neighborhood. In general sights were lowered. Among the staff members, who had agreed to the changes only because they had no other choice, morale was very weak.

The question that remained unanswered was whether the new Tarry Hall was equipped to help its new residents. For years the staff had done a good job with the people it chose to work with. Now, though the residents were different, the staff was the same. Could the staff teach residents to comb their hair and take a shower as well as they had once taught current events? Could Tarry Hall motivate the truly unmotivated? As Fred had shown, it would be no easy trick.

* * *

One morning in early July I decided to see how the other half lived—the mentally ill people in Houston who do not have one of the 27 beds in Tarry Hall or access to the other facilities available to the lucky few. I went looking for Don Peterson [who had been released unconditionally at about the same time Fred was released].

I started at the [Reverend] Armstrong house where Peterson lived and talked my way inside for a quick glance around. I didn't find

Peterson, but what I did find left me reeling. Peterson's tiny bedroom, which he shared with two other people, was particularly gruesome. A spoon on his bureau had been there for so long that whatever food it once held had turned moldy and black and so hard that it appeared glued to the surface. I saw a black woman walking around naked. I tried to talk to her, but two young white "attendants" shooed me away. The attendants would be fired a few weeks later when Armstrong found them "misusing one of the girls," as he phrased it, though not sexually, he quickly added. Before I left, one of the tenants told me that Peterson usually hung out at the Star of Hope Mission during the day.

That's where I found Peterson, sitting in a lower downtown parking lot across the street from the mission, a large, two-story building that can accommodate as many as five hundred homeless every night. Next to him was a white teenager, a runaway. Despite the heat, Peterson wore his usual four shirts, a vest, a jacket, and a pair of new tan cowboy boots. Sweat was dripping from the end of his moustache, and a dirty winger coat lay on the sidewalk next to him. He held a Burger King bag that contained a bottle of Thunderbird wine, which he had bought from someone at the mission for 13 cents.

Every day Peterson got up before dawn and took a bus downtown in order to be at the mission in time for breakfast, which began at 5 a.m. He usually stayed through the dinner hour. I thought at first that he came because the food was better, but he quickly disabused me. "Rev's [Reverend Armstrong's] food's about the same." So why did he do it? "Dunno," he said. "Guess it's cause this is where all my friends are." He pointed in the direction of the runaway. I asked him what his friend's name was. He didn't know.

The real reason for Peterson's routine was that the Star of Hope Mission came the closest to approximating life in an institution. He was used to the barter economy of the state hospital; that also existed among the transient population. He was even used to the danger. The runaway told me, somewhat nervously, that in the last week there had been four stabbings outside the mission. From reading the newspaper you can get the impression that mentally ill people commit an inordinate number of violent crimes. At a place like the Star of Hope Mission, you quickly see that the opposite is true: their sickness makes them easy targets.

* * *

You didn't have to spend much time in Houston mental health circles to hear the allegations about the Reverend Alvin Armstrong. They were rampant. There were allegations of sexual abuse at his house, of serious untreated illness, and more. From time to time, someone in the bureaucracy would poke around, but the investigations were always halfhearted at best. The system's dirty little secret is that it needs Armstrong, desperately, to provide his wretched shelter. However many mentally ill people are wandering the streets of Houston, there would be hundreds more without the Alvin Armstrongs of the world. Mentally ill street people shame the society that lets them live as they do. In Armstrong's house, tucked away in the ghetto, they are out of sight and out of mind.

Everyone in the system knew how bad this house was; everyone felt helpless to do anything. The existence of places like Armstrong's was seen as a fact of life in the mental health business—one of the awful, unintended consequences of deinstitutionalization. A social worker who refers patients to Armstrong told me that she couldn't bring herself to visit the house. "I don't want to see it," she said. "I don't want to know where I'm sending them."

*   *   *

II. THEORETICAL UNDERPINNINGS OF THE RIGHT TO TREATMENT AND HABILITATION

DONALDSON v. O'CONNOR

United States Court of Appeals, Fifth Circuit, 1974.
493 F.2d 507, 519–531.

*   *   *

The question for decision, whether patients involuntarily civilly committed in state mental hospitals have a constitutional right to treatment, has never been addressed by any of the federal courts of appeals. Four district courts, however, have decided the question within the last three years, three of which held that there is a constitutional right to treatment. The Court of Appeals for the District of Columbia Circuit, in a landmark case decided eight years ago, took note in dictum of the existence and seriousness of the question, although in the same case the court held that the Hospitalization of the Mentally Ill Act of 1964 creates a *statutory* right to treatment on the part of mental patients in the District of Columbia.[11] The idea of a constitutional right to treatment has received an unusual amount of scholarly discussion and support, and there is now an enormous range of precedent relevant to, although not squarely in point with, the issue. The idea has been current at least since 1960, since the publication in the May 1960 issue of the American Bar Association Journal of an article by Dr. Morton Birnbaum, a forensic medical doctor now generally credited with being the father of the idea of a right to treatment. The A.B.A. Journal editorially endorsed the idea shortly after the publication of Dr. Birnbaum's article.

We hold that a person involuntarily civilly committed to a state mental hospital has a constitutional right to receive such individual treatment as will give him a reasonable opportunity to be cured or to improve his mental condition.

11. Rouse v. Cameron, 1966, 125 U.S. App.D.C. 366, 373 F.2d 451.

In reaching this result, we begin by noting the indisputable fact that civil commitment entails a "massive curtailment of liberty" in the constitutional sense. [B]eyond this, the conclusion that the due process clause guarantees a right to treatment rests upon a two-part theory. The first part begins with the fundamental, and all but universally accepted, proposition that "any nontrivial governmental abridgement of [any] freedom [which is part of the 'liberty' the Fourteenth Amendment says shall not be denied without due process of law] must be justified in terms of some 'permissible governmental goal.'" Once this "fairly sweeping concept of substantive due process" is assumed, the next step is to ask precisely what government interests justify the massive abridgement of liberty civil commitment entails.

* * *

The key point of the first part of the theory of a due process right to treatment is that where, as in Donaldson's case, the rationale for confinement is the *"parens patriae"* rationale that the patient is in need of treatment, the due process clause requires that minimally adequate treatment be in fact provided. This in turn requires that, at least for the nondangerous patient, constitutionally minimum standards of treatment be established and enforced. As Judge Johnson expressed it in the *Wyatt* case: "To deprive any citizen of his or her liberty upon the altruistic theory that the confinement is for humane therapeutic reasons and then fail to provide adequate treatment violates the very fundamentals of due process." Wyatt v. Stickney, 325 F.Supp. at 785. This key step in the theory also draws considerable support from, if indeed it is not compelled by, the Supreme Court's recent decision in Jackson v. Indiana, 1972, 406 U.S. 715, 92 S.Ct. 1845, 32 L.Ed.2d 435. In *Jackson,* the Supreme Court established the rule that "[a]t the least, due process requires that the nature and duration of commitment bear some reasonable relation to the purposes for which the individual is committed". If the "purpose" of commitment is treatment, and treatment is not provided, then the "nature" of the commitment bears no "reasonable relation" to its "purpose", and the constitutional rule of *Jackson* is violated.

This much represents the first part of the theory of a due process right to treatment; persons committed under what we have termed a *parens patriae* ground for commitment must be given treatment lest the involuntary commitment amount to an arbitrary exercise of government power proscribed by the due process clause. The second part of the theory draws no distinctions between persons committed under *"parens patriae"* rationales and those committed under "police power" rationales. This part begins with the recognition that, under our system of justice, long-term detention is, as a matter of due process, generally permitted only when an individual is (1) proved, in a proceeding subject to the rigorous constitutional limitations of the due process clause of the fourteenth amendment and the Bill of Rights, (2) to have committed a *specific act* defined as an offense against the state. Moreover, detention, under the criminal process, is usually allowed only for a period of time explicitly fixed by the prisoner's sentence. The second part of the theory of a due process right to treatment is based on the principle that when the three central limitations on the government's power to detain—that detention be in retribution for a specific offense; that it be limited to a fixed term; and that it be permitted after a proceeding where fundamental procedural safeguards are observed— are absent, there must be a *quid pro quo* extended by the government to justify confinement.[21] And the *quid pro quo* most commonly recognized is the provision of rehabilitative treatment, or, where rehabilitation is impossible, minimally adequate habilitation and care, beyond the subsistence level custodial care that would be provided in a penitentiary.

* * *

The appellants argue strenuously that a right to constitutionally adequate treatment should not be recognized, because such a right cannot be governed by judicially manageable or ascertainable standards. In making the argument, they rely heavily upon the Northern District of Georgia's decision in Burnham v. Department of Public Health, 1972, 349 F.Supp. 1335, 1341–1343. In *Burnham,* the district judge held that a class action seeking declaratory and injunctive relief requiring the Georgia Department of Public Health to provide treatment at Georgia mental hospitals presented a nonjusticiable controversy. He quoted Baker v. Carr, 1962, 369 U.S. 186, 198, 82 S.Ct. 691, 700, 7 L.Ed.2d 663, for the proposition that determining whether a suit was justiciable requires determining whether "the duty asserted can be judicially identified and its breach judicially determined, and whether protection for the right asserted can be judicially molded". He then cited the ambiguity of the dictionary definition of treatment, a passage from a law review article noting the fact that there are as many as forty different methods of psychotherapy, and a passage from the Supreme Court's decision in Greenwood v. United States, 1956, 350 U.S. 366, 76 S.Ct. 410, 100 L.Ed. 412, concerning the "tentativeness" and "uncertainty" of "professional judgment" in the mental health field. He concluded: "[T]he claimed duty (i.e. to 'adequately' or 'constitutionally treat') defies judicial identity and therefore prohibits its breach from being judicially defined."

The defendants' argument can be answered on two levels. First, we doubt whether, even if we were to concede that courts are incapable of formulating standards of adequate treatment in the abstract, we could or should for that reason alone hold that no right to treatment

---

21. In Welsch v. Likins, 1974, 373 F.Supp. 487, the District of Minnesota described, and rejected, a different *quid pro quo* rationale for a right to treatment. We also reject the rationale described by the *Welsch* court, and the rationale we embrace should be carefully contrasted with it:

One theory is that commitment pursuant to civil statutes generally lacks the procedural safeguards afforded those charged with criminal offense. The constitutional justification for this abridgment of *procedural rights* is that the purpose of commitment is treatment. (Emphasis supplied).

Welsch v. Likins, 373 F.Supp. at 496.

can be recognized or enforced. There will be cases—and the case at bar is one—where it will be possible to make determination whether a given individual has been denied his right to treatment without formulating in the abstract what constitutes "adequate" treatment.

* * *

We do not, however, concede that determining what constitutes adequate treatment is beyond the competence of the judiciary. In deciding in individual cases whether treatment is adequate, there are a number of devices open to the courts, as Judge Bazelon noted in discussing the implementation of the statutory right to treatment in the landmark case of Rouse v. Cameron:

> But lack of finality [of professional judgment] cannot relieve the court of its duty to render an informed decision. Counsel for the patient and the government can be helpful in presenting pertinent data concerning standards for mental care, and, particularly when the patient is indigent and cannot present experts of his own, the court may appoint independent experts. Assistance might be obtained from such sources as the American Psychiatric Association, which has published standards and is continually engaged in studying the problems of mental care. The court could also consider inviting the psychiatric and legal communities to establish procedures by which expert assistance can be best provided.

There are by now many cases where courts have undertaken to determine whether treatment in an individual case is adequate or have ordered that determination to be made by a trial court. Even in cases like *Wyatt* and *Burnham,* when courts are asked to undertake the more difficult task of fashioning institution-wide standards of adequacy, the task should not be beyond them. The experience of the *Wyatt* case bears this out. In *Wyatt,* agreement was reached among the parties on almost all of the minimum standards for adequate treatment ordered by the district court, and the defendants joined in submitting the standards to the district court. These stipulated standards were supported and supplemented by testimony from numerous expert witnesses. Moreover, there was a striking degree of consensus among the experts, including the experts presented by the defendants, as to the minimum standards for adequate treatment. The standards developed have not been challenged by the defendants in the appeal now pending before this Court.

In summary, we hold that where a nondangerous patient is involuntarily civilly committed to a state mental hospital, the only constitutionally permissible purpose of confinement is to provide treatment, and that such a patient has a constitutional right to such treatment as will help him to be cured or to improve his mental condition. . . .

O'CONNOR v. DONALDSON

Supreme Court of the United States, 1975.
422 U.S. 563, 95 S.Ct. 2486, 45 L.Ed.2d 396.

JUSTICE BURGER, concurring.

[The Supreme Court's majority opinion in this case, reprinted at pp. 649–654, avoided the right to treatment issue. However, Chief Justice Burger, in a concurring opinion, directly addressed it, arguing that no such right should be recognized. In the first part of his concurrence, also reprinted at pp. 654–656, he responded to the Fifth Circuit's "first theory" justifying the right to treatment by disputing that court's apparent conclusion that "with respect to persons who are not physically dangerous, a State has no power to confine the mentally ill except for the purpose of providing them with treatment." Burger contended that, historically, parens patriae commitment had been primarily for custodial care, not treatment. Even today, "it remains a stubborn fact that there are many forms of mental illness which are not understood, some of which are untreatable in the sense that no effective therapy has yet been discovered for them, and that rates of 'cure' are generally low." Burger also noted the uncertainty of psychiatric diagnosis and the difficulty of treating mentally ill individuals who are unwilling to recognize they are ill. He concluded: "It may be that some persons in . . . these categories, and there may be others, are unable to function in society and will suffer real harm to themselves unless provided with care in a sheltered environment." Burger then addressed the Fifth Circuit's "second theory" justifying a constitutional right to treatment.]

B

Alternatively, it has been argued that a Fourteenth Amendment right to treatment for involuntarily confined mental patients derives from the fact that many of the safeguards of the criminal process are not present in civil commitment. The Court of Appeals described this theory as follows:

"[A] due process right to treatment is based on the principle that when the three central limitations on the government's power to detain—that detention be in retribution for a specific offense; that it be limited to a fixed term; and that it be permitted after a proceeding where the fundamental procedural safeguards are observed—are absent, there must be a *quid pro quo* extended by the government to justify confinement. And the *quid pro quo* most commonly recognized is the provision of rehabilitative treatment." 493 F.2d, at 522.

To the extent that this theory may be read to permit a State to confine an individual simply because it is willing to provide treatment, regardless of the subject's ability to function in society, it raises the gravest of constitutional problems, and I have no doubt the Court of Appeals would agree on this score. As a justification for a constitutional right to such treatment, the *quid pro quo* theory suffers from equally serious defects.

It is too well established to require extended discussion that due process is not an inflexible concept. Rather, its requirements are determined in particular instances by identifying and accommodating the interests of the individual and society. Where claims that the State is acting in the best interests of an individual are said to justify reduced procedural and substantive safeguards, this Court's decisions require that they be "candidly appraised." However, in so doing judges are not free to read their private notions of public policy or public health into the Constitution.

The *quid pro quo* theory is a sharp departure from, and cannot coexist with, due process principles. As an initial matter, the theory presupposes that essentially the same interests are involved in every situation where a State seeks to confine an individual; that assumption, however, is incorrect. It is elementary that the justification for the criminal process and the unique deprivation of liberty which it can impose requires that it be invoked only for commission of a specific offense prohibited by legislative enactment.[7] But it would be incongruous, for example, to apply the same limitation when quarantine is imposed by the State to protect the public from a highly communicable disease.

A more troublesome feature of the *quid pro quo* theory is that it would elevate a concern for essentially procedural safeguards into a new substantive constitutional right. Rather than inquiring whether strict standards of proof or periodic redetermination of a patient's condition are required in civil confinement, the theory accepts the absence of such safeguards but insists that the State provide benefits which, in the view of a court, are adequate "compensation" for confinement. In light of the wide divergence of medical opinion regarding the diagnosis of and proper therapy for mental abnormalities, that prospect is especially troubling in this area and cannot be squared with the principle that "courts may not substitute for the judgments of legislators their own understanding of the public welfare, but must instead concern themselves with the validity under the Constitution of the methods which the legislature has selected." Of course, questions regarding the adequacy of procedure and the power of a State to continue particular confinements are ultimately for the courts, aided by expert opinion to the extent that is found helpful. But I am not persuaded that we should abandon the traditional limitations on the scope of judicial review.

---

7. This is not to imply that I accept all of the Court of Appeals' conclusions regarding the limitations upon the States' power to detain persons who commit crimes. For example, the notion that confinement must be "for a fixed term" is difficult to square with the widespread practice of indeterminate sentencing, at least where the upper limit is a life sentence.

YOUNGBERG v. ROMEO

Supreme Court of the United States, 1982.
457 U.S. 307, 102 S.Ct. 2452, 73 L.Ed.2d 28.

JUSTICE POWELL delivered the opinion of the Court.

The question presented is whether respondent, involuntarily committed to a state institution for the mentally retarded, has substantive rights under the Due Process Clause of the Fourteenth Amendment to (i) safe conditions of confinement; (ii) freedom from bodily restraints; and (iii) training or "habilitation." Respondent sued under 42 U.S.C. § 1983 three administrators of the institution, claiming damages for the alleged breach of his constitutional rights.

I

Respondent Nicholas Romeo is profoundly retarded. Although 33 years old, he has the mental capacity of an 18–month–old child, with an I.Q. between 8 and 10. He cannot talk and lacks the most basic self-care skills. Until he was 26, respondent lived with his parents in Philadelphia. But after the death of his father in May 1974, his mother was unable to care for him. Within two weeks of the father's death, respondent's mother sought his temporary admission to a nearby Pennsylvania hospital.

Shortly thereafter, she asked the Philadelphia County Court of Common Pleas to admit Romeo to a state facility on a permanent basis. Her petition to the court explained that she was unable to care for Romeo or control his violence.[2] As part of the commitment process, Romeo was examined by a physician and a psychologist. They both certified that respondent was severely retarded and unable to care for himself. On June 11, 1974, the Court of Common Pleas committed respondent to the Pennhurst State School and Hospital, pursuant to the applicable involuntary commitment provision of the Pennsylvania Mental Health and Mental Retardation Act.

At Pennhurst, Romeo was injured on numerous occasions, both by his own violence and by the reactions of other residents to him. Respondent's mother became concerned about these injuries. After objecting to respondent's treatment several times, she filed this complaint on November 4, 1976, in the United States District Court for the Eastern District of Pennsylvania as his next friend. The complaint alleged that "[d]uring the period July, 1974 to the present, plaintiff has suffered injuries on at least sixty-three occasions." The complaint originally sought damages and injunctive relief from Pennhurst's director and two supervisors; it alleged that these officials knew, or should have known, that Romeo was suffering injuries and that they failed to

2. Mrs. Romeo's petition to the Court of Common Pleas stated: "Since my husband's death I am unable to handle him. He becomes violent—kicks, punches, breaks glass; He can't speak—wants to express himself but can't. He is [a] constant 24 hr. care. [W]ithout my husband I am unable to care for him."

institute appropriate preventive procedures, thus violating his rights under the Eighth and Fourteenth Amendments.

Thereafter, in late 1976, Romeo was transferred from his ward to the hospital for treatment of a broken arm. While in the infirmary, and by order of a doctor, he was physically restrained during portions of each day. These restraints were ordered by Dr. Gabroy, not a defendant here, to protect Romeo and others in the hospital, some of whom were in traction or were being treated intravenously. Although respondent normally would have returned to his ward when his arm healed, the parties to this litigation agreed that he should remain in the hospital due to the pending lawsuit. Nevertheless, in December 1977, a second amended complaint was filed alleging that the defendants were restraining respondent for prolonged periods on a routine basis. The second amended complaint also added a claim for damages to compensate Romeo for the defendants' failure to provide him with appropriate "treatment or programs for his mental retardation." All claims for injunctive relief were dropped prior to trial because respondent is a member of the class seeking such relief in another action.[6]

An 8–day jury trial was held in April 1978. Petitioners introduced evidence that respondent participated in several programs teaching basic self-care skills.[7] A comprehensive behavior-modification program was designed by staff members to reduce Romeo's aggressive behavior,[8] but that program was never implemented because of his mother's objections. Respondent introduced evidence of his injuries and of conditions in his unit.

At the close of the trial, the court instructed the jury that "if any or all of the defendants were aware of and failed to take all reasonable steps to prevent repeated attacks upon Nicholas Romeo," such failure deprived him of constitutional rights. The jury also was instructed that if the defendants shackled Romeo or denied him treatment "as a punishment for filing this lawsuit," his constitutional rights were violated under the Eighth Amendment. Finally, the jury was instructed that only if they found the defendants "deliberate[ly] indifferen[t] to the serious medical [and psychological] needs" of Romeo could they find that his Eighth and Fourteenth Amendment rights had been violated. The jury returned a verdict for the defendants, on which judgment was entered.

The Court of Appeals for the Third Circuit, sitting en banc, reversed and remanded for a new trial. The court held that the Eighth

6. *Pennhurst State School and Hospital v. Halderman,* 451 U.S. 1, 101 S.Ct. 1531, 67 L.Ed.2d 694 (1981) (remanded for further proceedings).

7. Prior to his transfer to Pennhurst's hospital ward, Romeo participated in programs dealing with feeding, showering, drying, dressing, self-control, and toilet training, as well as a program providing interaction with staff members.

Some programs continued while respondent was in the hospital, and they reduced respondent's aggressive behavior to some extent.

8. The program called for short periods of separation from other residents and for use of "muffs" on plaintiff's hands for short periods of time, *i.e.,* five minutes, to prevent him from harming himself or others.

Amendment, prohibiting cruel and unusual punishment of those convicted of crimes, was not an appropriate source for determining the rights of the involuntarily committed. Rather, the Fourteenth Amendment and the liberty interest protected by that Amendment provided the proper constitutional basis for these rights. In applying the Fourteenth Amendment, the court found that the involuntarily committed retain liberty interests in freedom of movement and in personal security. These were "fundamental liberties" that can be limited only by an "overriding, non-punitive" state interest. It further found that the involuntarily committed have a liberty interest in habilitation designed to "treat" their mental retardation.

The en banc court did not, however, agree on the relevant standard to be used in determining whether Romeo's rights had been violated. Because physical restraint "raises a presumption of a punitive sanction," the majority of the Court of Appeals concluded that it can be justified only by "compelling necessity." A somewhat different standard was appropriate for the failure to provide for a resident's safety. The majority considered that such a failure must be justified by a showing of "substantial necessity." Finally, the majority held that when treatment has been administered, those responsible are liable only if the treatment is not "acceptable in the light of present medical or other scientific knowledge." [14]

Chief Judge Seitz, concurring in the judgment, considered the standards articulated by the majority as indistinguishable from those applicable to medical malpractice claims. In Chief Judge Seitz' view, the Constitution "only requires that the courts make certain that professional judgment in fact was exercised." He concluded that the appropriate standard was whether the defendants' conduct was "such a substantial departure from accepted professional judgment, practice, or standards in the care and treatment of this plaintiff as to demonstrate that the defendants did not base their conduct on a professional judgment."

We granted the petition for certiorari because of the importance of the question presented to the administration of state institutions for the mentally retarded.

II

We consider here for the first time the substantive rights of involuntarily committed mentally retarded persons under the Four-

---

14. Actually, the court divided the right-to-treatment claim into three categories and adopted three standards, but only the standard described in text is at issue before this Court. The Court of Appeals also stated that if a jury finds that *no* treatment has been administered, it may hold the institution's administrators liable unless they can provide a compelling explanation for the lack of treatment, but respondent does not discuss this precise standard in his brief and it does not appear to be relevant to the facts of this case. In addition, the court considered "least intrusive" analysis appropriate to justify severe intrusions on individual dignity such as permanent physical alteration or surgical intervention, but respondent concedes that this issue is not present in this case.

teenth Amendment to the Constitution. In this case, respondent has been committed under the laws of Pennsylvania, and he does not challenge the commitment. Rather, he argues that he has a constitutionally protected liberty interest in safety, freedom of movement, and training within the institution; and that petitioners infringed these rights by failing to provide constitutionally required conditions of confinement.

The mere fact that Romeo has been committed under proper procedures does not deprive him of all substantive liberty interests under the Fourteenth Amendment. See, *e.g., Vitek v. Jones,* 445 U.S. 480, 491–494, 100 S.Ct. 1254, 1262–1264, 63 L.Ed.2d 552 (1980). Indeed, the state concedes that respondent has a right to adequate food, shelter, clothing, and medical care. We must decide whether liberty interests also exist in safety, freedom of movement, and training. If such interests do exist, we must further decide whether they have been infringed in this case.

A

Respondent's first two claims involve liberty interests recognized by prior decisions of this Court, interests that involuntary commitment proceedings do not extinguish. The first is a claim to safe conditions. In the past, this Court has noted that the right to personal security constitutes a "historic liberty interest" protected substantively by the Due Process Clause. And that right is not extinguished by lawful confinement, even for penal purposes. If it is cruel and unusual punishment to hold convicted criminals in unsafe conditions, it must be unconstitutional to confine the involuntarily committed—who may not be punished at all—in unsafe conditions.

Next, respondent claims a right to freedom from bodily restraint. In other contexts, the existence of such an interest is clear in the prior decisions of this Court. Indeed, "[l]iberty from bodily restraint always has been recognized as the core of the liberty protected by the Due Process Clause from arbitrary governmental action." This interest survives criminal conviction and incarceration. Similarly, it must also survive involuntary commitment.

B

Respondent's remaining claim is more troubling. In his words, he asserts a "constitutional right to minimally adequate habilitation." This is a substantive due process claim that is said to be grounded in the liberty component of the Due Process Clause of the Fourteenth Amendment.[19] The term "habilitation," used in psychiatry, is not

---

19. Respondent also argues that because he was committed for care and treatment under state law he has a state substantive right to habilitation, which is entitled to substantive, not procedural, protection under the Due Process Clause of the Fourteenth Amendment. But this argument is made for the first time in respondent's brief to this Court. It was not advanced in the courts below, and was not argued to the Court of Appeals as a ground for reversing the trial court. Given the uncertainty of Pennsylvania law and the lack of any guidance on this issue from the

defined precisely or consistently in the opinions below or in the briefs of the parties or the *amici*.[20] [T]he term refers to "training and development of needed skills." Respondent emphasizes that the right he asserts is for "minimal" training, and he would leave the type and extent of training to be determined on a case-by-case basis "in light of present medical or other scientific knowledge."

In addressing the asserted right to training, we start from established principles. As a general matter, a State is under no constitutional duty to provide substantive services for those within its border. See *Harris v. McRae*, 448 U.S. 297, 318, 100 S.Ct. 2671, 2689, 65 L.Ed.2d 784 (1980) (publicly funded abortions); *Maher v. Roe*, 432 U.S. 464, 469, 97 S.Ct. 2376, 2380, 53 L.Ed.2d 484 (1977) (medical treatment). When a person is institutionalized—and wholly dependent on the State—it is conceded by petitioners that a duty to provide certain services and care does exist, although even then a State necessarily has considerable discretion in determining the nature and scope of its responsibilities. Nor must a State "choose between attacking every aspect of a problem or not attacking the problem at all."

Respondent, in light of the severe character of his retardation, concedes that no amount of training will make possible his release. And he does not argue that if he were still at home, the State would have an obligation to provide training at its expense. The record reveals that respondent's primary needs are bodily safety and a minimum of physical restraint, and respondent clearly claims training related to these needs. As we have recognized that there is a constitutionally protected liberty interest in safety and freedom from restraint, training may be necessary to avoid unconstitutional infringement of those rights. On the basis of the record before us, it is quite uncertain whether respondent seeks any "habilitation" or training unrelated to safety and freedom from bodily restraints. In his brief to this Court, Romeo indicates that even the self-care programs he seeks are needed to reduce his aggressive behavior. And in his offer of proof to the trial court, respondent repeatedly indicated that, if allowed to testify, his experts would show that additional training programs, including self-care programs, were needed to reduce his aggressive behavior. If, as seems the case, respondent seeks only training related to safety and freedom from restraints, this case does not present the difficult question whether a mentally retarded person, involuntarily committed to a state institution, has some general constitutional right to training *per se*, even when no type or amount of training would lead to freedom.[23]

lower federal courts, we decline to consider it now.

20. Professionals in the habilitation of the mentally retarded disagree strongly on the question whether effective training of all severely or profoundly retarded individuals is even possible.

23. In the trial court, respondent asserted that "state officials at a state mental hospital have a duty to provide residents . . . with such treatment as will afford them a reasonable opportunity to acquire and maintain those life skills necessary to cope as effectively as their capacities permit." But this claim to a sweeping *per se* right was dropped thereafter. In his brief to this Court, respondent does not repeat it and, at oral argument, respon-

Chief Judge Seitz, in language apparently adopted by respondent, observed:

> "I believe that the plaintiff has a constitutional right to minimally adequate care and treatment. The existence of a constitutional right to care and treatment is no longer a novel legal proposition."

Chief Judge Seitz did not identify or otherwise define—beyond the right to reasonable safety and freedom from physical restraint—the "minimally adequate care and treatment" that appropriately may be required for this respondent. In the circumstances presented by this case, and on the basis of the record developed to date, we agree with his view and conclude that respondent's liberty interests require the State to provide minimally adequate or reasonable training to ensure safety and freedom from undue restraint. In view of the kinds of treatment sought by respondent and the evidence of record, we need go no further in this case.

III

A

We have established that Romeo retains liberty interests in safety and freedom from bodily restraint. Yet these interests are not absolute; indeed to some extent they are in conflict. In operating an institution such as Pennhurst, there are occasions in which it is necessary for the State to restrain the movement of residents—for example, to protect them as well as others from violence. Similar restraints may also be appropriate in a training program. And an institution cannot protect its residents from all danger of violence if it is to permit them to have any freedom of movement. The question then is not simply whether a liberty interest has been infringed but whether the extent or nature of the restraint or lack of absolute safety is such as to violate due process.

Accordingly, whether respondent's constitutional rights have been violated must be determined by balancing his liberty interests against the relevant state interests. If there is to be any uniformity in protecting these interests, this balancing cannot be left to the unguided discretion of a judge or jury. We therefore turn to consider the proper standard for determining whether a State adequately has protected the rights of the involuntarily committed mentally retarded.

B

We think the standard articulated by Chief Judge Seitz affords the necessary guidance and reflects the proper balance between the legitimate interests of the State and the rights of the involuntarily committed to reasonable conditions of safety and freedom from unreasonable restraints. He would have held that "the Constitution only requires that the courts make certain that professional judgment in fact was

dent's counsel explicitly disavowed any claim that respondent is constitutionally entitled to such treatment as would enable him "to achieve his maximum potential."

exercised. It is not appropriate for the courts to specify which of several professionally acceptable choices should have been made." Persons who have been involuntarily committed are entitled to more considerate treatment and conditions of confinement than criminals whose conditions of confinement are designed to punish. At the same time, this standard is lower than the "compelling" or "substantial" necessity tests the Court of Appeals would require a State to meet to justify use of restraints or conditions of less than absolute safety. We think this requirement would place an undue burden on the administration of institutions such as Pennhurst and also would restrict unnecessarily the exercise of professional judgment as to the needs of residents.

Moreover, we agree that respondent is entitled to minimally adequate training. In this case, the minimally adequate training required by the Constitution is such training as may be reasonable in light of respondent's liberty interests in safety and freedom from unreasonable restraints. In determining what is "reasonable"—in this and in any case presenting a claim for training by a State—we emphasize that courts must show deference to the judgment exercised by a qualified professional. By so limiting judicial review of challenges to conditions in state institutions, interference by the federal judiciary with the internal operations of these institutions should be minimized. Moreover, there certainly is no reason to think judges or juries are better qualified than appropriate professionals in making such decisions. For these reasons, the decision, if made by a professional,[30] is presumptively valid; liability may be imposed only when the decision by the professional is such a substantial departure from accepted professional judgment, practice, or standards as to demonstrate that the person responsible actually did not base the decision on such a judgment. In an action for damages against a professional in his individual capacity, however, the professional will not be liable if he was unable to satisfy his normal professional standards because of budgetary constraints; in such a situation, good-faith immunity would bar liability.

IV

In deciding this case, we have weighed those postcommitment interests cognizable as liberty interests under the Due Process Clause of the Fourteenth Amendment against legitimate state interests and in light of the constraints under which most state institutions necessarily operate. We repeat that the State concedes a duty to provide adequate food, shelter, clothing, and medical care. These are the essentials of

---

30. By "professional" decisionmaker, we mean a person competent, whether by education, training or experience, to make the particular decision at issue. Long-term treatment decisions normally should be made by persons with degrees in medicine or nursing, or with appropriate training in areas such as psychology, physi-cal therapy, or the care and training of the retarded. Of course, day-to-day decisions regarding care—including decisions that must be made without delay—necessarily will be made in many instances by employees without formal training but who are subject to the supervision of qualified persons.

the care that the State must provide. The State also has the unquestioned duty to provide reasonable safety for all residents and personnel
within the institution. And it may not restrain residents except when
and to the extent professional judgment deems this necessary to assure
such safety or to provide needed training. In this case, therefore, the
State is under a duty to provide respondent with such training as an
appropriate professional would consider reasonable to ensure his safety
and to facilitate his ability to function free from bodily restraints. It
may well be unreasonable not to provide training when training could
significantly reduce the need for restraints or the likelihood of violence.

Respondent thus enjoys constitutionally protected interests in conditions of reasonable care and safety, reasonably nonrestrictive confinement conditions, and such training as may be required by these interests. Such conditions of confinement would comport fully with the
purpose of respondent's commitment. Cf. *Jackson v. Indiana*, 406 U.S.
715, 738, 92 S.Ct. 1845, 1858, 32 L.Ed.2d 435 (1972). In determining
whether the State has met its obligations in these respects, decisions
made by the appropriate professional are entitled to a presumption of
correctness. Such a presumption is necessary to enable institutions of
this type—often, unfortunately, overcrowded and understaffed—to continue to function. A single professional may have to make decisions
with respect to a number of residents with widely varying needs and
problems in the course of a normal day. The administrators, and
particularly professional personnel, should not be required to make
each decision in the shadow of an action for damages.

In this case, we conclude that the jury was erroneously instructed
on the assumption that the proper standard of liability was that of the
Eighth Amendment. We vacate the decision of the Court of Appeals
and remand for further proceedings consistent with this decision.

So ordered.

JUSTICE BLACKMUN, with whom JUSTICE BRENNAN and JUSTICE
O'CONNOR join, concurring.

I join the Court's opinion. I write separately, however, to make
clear why I believe that opinion properly leaves unresolved two difficult
and important issues.

The first is whether the Commonwealth of Pennsylvania could
accept respondent for "care and treatment," as it did under the Pennsylvania Mental Health and Mental Retardation Act of 1966, and then
constitutionally refuse to provide him any "treatment," as that term is
defined by state law. Were that question properly before us, in my
view there would be a serious issue whether, as a matter of due process,
the State could so refuse. I therefore do not find that issue to be a
"frivolous" one, as the Chief Justice does.

In *Jackson v. Indiana*, 406 U.S. 715, 92 S.Ct. 1845, 32 L.Ed.2d 435
(1972), this Court, by a unanimous vote of all participating Justices,
suggested a constitutional standard for evaluating the conditions of a

civilly committed person's confinement: "At the least, due process requires that the nature and duration of commitment bear some reasonable relation to the purpose for which the individual is committed."

* * *

In respondent's case, the majority and principal concurring opinions in the Court of Appeals agreed that "[b]y basing [respondent's] deprivation of liberty at least partially upon a promise of treatment, the state ineluctably has committed the community's resources to providing minimal treatment." Neither opinion clarified, however, whether respondent in fact had been totally denied "treatment," as that term is defined under Pennsylvania law. To the extent that the majority addressed the question, it found that "the evidence in the record, although somewhat contradictory, suggests not so much a total failure to treat as an inadequacy of treatment."

This Court's reading of the record, supports that conclusion. Moreover, the Court today finds that respondent's entitlement to "treatment" under Pennsylvania law was not properly raised below. Given this uncertainty in the record, I am in accord with the Court's decision not to address the constitutionality of a State's total failure to provide "treatment" to an individual committed under state law for "care and treatment."

The second difficult question left open today is whether respondent has an independent constitutional claim, grounded in the Due Process Clause of the Fourteenth Amendment, to that "habilitation" or training necessary to *preserve* those basic self-care skills he possessed when he first entered Pennhurst—for example, the ability to dress himself and care for his personal hygiene. In my view, it would be consistent with the Court's reasoning today to include within the "minimally adequate training required by the Constitution," such training as is reasonably necessary to prevent a person's pre-existing self-care skills from *deteriorating* because of his commitment.

The Court makes clear that even after a person is committed to a state institution, he is entitled to such training as is necessary to prevent unreasonable losses of additional liberty as a result of his confinement—for example, unreasonable bodily restraints or unsafe institutional conditions. If a person could demonstrate that he entered a state institution with minimal self-care skills, but lost those skills after commitment because of the State's unreasonable refusal to provide him training, then, it seems to me, he has alleged a loss of liberty quite distinct from—and as serious as—the loss of safety and freedom from unreasonable restraints. For many mentally retarded people, the difference between the capacity to do things for themselves within an institution and total dependence on the institution for all of their needs is as much liberty as they ever will know.

Although respondent asserts a claim of this kind, I agree with the Court that "[o]n the basis of the record before us, it is quite uncertain whether respondent [in fact] seeks any 'habilitation' or training unrelated to safety and freedom from bodily restraints." Since the Court finds respondent constitutionally entitled at least to "such training as may be reasonable in light of [his] liberty interests in safety and freedom from unreasonable restraints," I accept its decision not to address respondent's additional claim.

If respondent actually seeks habilitation in self-care skills not merely to reduce his aggressive tendencies, but also to maintain those basic self-care skills necessary to his personal autonomy within Pennhurst, I believe he is free on remand to assert that claim.

* * *

The Court finds it premature to resolve this constitutional question on this less than fully developed record. Because I agree with that conclusion, I concur in the Court's opinion.

CHIEF JUSTICE BURGER, concurring in the judgment.

I agree with much of the Court's opinion. However, I would hold flatly that respondent has no constitutional right to training, or "habilitation," *per se.* The parties, and the Court, acknowledge that respondent cannot function outside the state institution, even with the assistance of relatives. Indeed, even now neither respondent nor his family seeks his discharge from state care. Under these circumstances, the State's provision of food, shelter, medical care, and living conditions as safe as the inherent nature of the institutional environment reasonably allows, serves to justify the State's custody of respondent. The State did not seek custody of respondent; his family understandably sought the State's aid to meet a serious need.

I agree with the Court that some amount of self-care instruction may be necessary to avoid unreasonable infringement of a mentally retarded person's interests in safety and freedom from restraint; but it seems clear to me that the Constitution does not otherwise place an affirmative duty on the State to provide any particular kind of training or habilitation—even such as might be encompassed under the essentially standardless rubric "minimally adequate training," to which the Court refers. Since respondent asserts a right to "minimally adequate" habilitation "[q]uite apart from its relationship to decent care," unlike the Court I see no way to avoid the issue.*

I also point out that, under the Court's own standards, it is largely irrelevant whether respondent's experts were of the opinion that "additional training programs, including self-care programs, were needed to

---

* Indeed, in the trial court respondent asserted a broad claim to such "treatment as [would] afford [him] a reasonable opportunity to acquire and maintain those life skills necessary to cope as effectively as [his] capacities permit."

Respondent also maintains that, because state law purportedly creates a right to "care and treatment," he has a *federal substantive* right under the Due Process Clause to enforcement of this state right. This contention is obviously frivolous; were every substantive right created by state law enforceable under the Due Process Clause, the distinction between state and federal law would quickly be obliterated.

reduce [respondent's] aggressive behavior,"—a prescription far easier for "spectators" to give than for an institution to implement. The training program devised for respondent by petitioners and other professionals at Pennhurst was, according to the Court's opinion, "presumptively valid"; and "liability may be imposed only when the decision by the professional is such a substantial departure from accepted professional judgment, practice, or standards as to demonstrate that the person responsible actually did not base the decision on such a judgment." Thus, even if respondent could demonstrate that the training programs at Pennhurst were inconsistent with generally accepted or prevailing professional practice—if indeed there be such—this would not avail him so long as his training regimen was actually prescribed by the institution's professional staff.

* * *

Questions and Comments

1. *Choosing a rationale.* Of the various constitutional theories described in the preceding opinions, which is the most convincing? The first rationale advanced by the Fifth Circuit (discussed also by Justice Blackmun in *Youngberg*) is premised on *Jackson v. Indiana's* notion that the nature of confinement must bear a reasonable relationship to its purpose. Does a right to treatment for civilly committed patients necessarily flow from this premise, in light of the points made by Chief Justice Burger in his concurring opinion in *Donaldson?* Recall that, in *Jackson* itself, the Court required that all persons committed for restoration of competency to stand trial receive treatment to effect that restoration unless they are unrestorable, in which case they should be released *or* civilly committed. Does this holding support Burger's assertions about the possible purposes of civil commitment?

In response, consider this excerpt from *Wyatt v. Aderholt,* 503 F.2d 1305, 1313 (5th Cir.1974), in which the Fifth Circuit addressed a contention similar to Burger's.

> [W]e find it impossible to accept the [state's] underlying premise that the 'need for care' for the mentally ill—and to relieve their families, friends, or guardians of the burden of doing so—can supply a constitutional justification for civil commitment . . . The state interest thus asserted may be, strictly speaking, a 'rational' state interest. But we find it so trivial beside the major personal interests against which it is to be weighed that we cannot possibly accept it as a justification for the deprivations of liberty involved.

Note also that a majority of states today recognize by statute a right to treatment for every committed patient, whether committed under parens patriae or police power authority (although some states make the provision of treatment contingent on funding). S. Brakel, J. Parry & B. Weiner, The Mentally Disabled and the Law 337 (1985). Of what significance is this fact in evaluating the importance of *Jackson* in establishing a constitutional right to treatment? In his *Youngberg* concurrence, how does Burger amend his *Donaldson* argument to take into account this modern statutory development? Does Justice Powell's *Youngberg* opinion foreclose a right to treatment based on the "*Jackson*" rationale?

With respect to the Fifth Circuit's second rationale for a constitutional right to treatment (the "quid pro quo" theory), does not the court's reasoning imply that provision of treatment is the only justification for affording civil committees fewer procedural and substantive protections than criminal defendants? To what extent *are* the differences between civil commitment and the criminal process justified by an assumed treatment orientation of the former (cf. *Addington, Parham, Allen v. Illinois*)?

Turning to the Supreme Court's reasoning in *Youngberg*, note that it avoided reliance on the eighth amendment's cruel and unusual punishment clause. Some lower courts have based a right to treatment on this provision in light of the Supreme Court's opinion in *Robinson v. California*, 370 U.S. 660, 82 S.Ct. 1417, 8 L.Ed.2d 758 (1962), which held that the clause prohibits criminal punishment of a person for the status of being an addict. In *Welsch v. Likins*, 373 F.Supp. 487, 496–7 (D.Minn.1974), for instance, the court held that confining someone who is mentally ill and dangerous without treatment is like punishing someone for being an addict, and thus is a violation of the eighth amendment. One reason for rejecting this approach to the right to treatment is that the cruel and unusual punishment clause has normally been applied only to criminal punishment. See *Bell v. Wolfish*, 441 U.S. 520, 99 S.Ct. 1861, 60 L.Ed.2d 447 (1979) (claims brought by pretrial detainees about conditions imposed on them prior to trial not actionable under the eighth amendment). Assuming this problem is overcome, is *Robinson* good precedent for establishing a right to treatment?

In *Youngberg*, the Court focused instead on the liberty interests of committed patients under the due process clause. Relying on this clause, the majority clearly established a right to "minimally adequate treatment" which, "in this case," consisted of a right to safe conditions and freedom from bodily restraint. At first glance, this formulation may seem narrow. But consider the following excerpt from Note, "The Supreme Court: 1981 Term," 96 Harv.L.Rev. 62, 82–84 (1982):

> Although the Court [in *Youngberg*] sidestepped a direct affirmation of broad rights to habilitation, Justice Powell's liberty-based rationale for a constitutional right to training may lead to a comparable result by any of three avenues. First, although Justice Powell failed to define the scope of "training related to safety and freedom from restraints," he explicitly included training necessary to prevent the violence of self-destructive behavior that creates both a more dangerous institutional environment and a heightened need for bodily restraint. Moreover, the right must encompass training based upon individualized evaluations of patients; only such training can reasonably ensure effective protection of a given patient's liberty interest. Most significantly, Justice Powell's formulation may itself imply a right to habilitative treatment. Training in basic self-care skills—such as dressing oneself and reading—fits within his formulation, because substantial psychiatric study shows that such training reduces violent and self-destructive behavior.

Second, if logically extended, Justice Powell's liberty-based rationale would justify even broad constitutional rights to treatment. As Justice Blackmum observed in his concurrence, a constitutional right to 'such training as is reasonably necessary to prevent a person's pre-existing self-care skills from deteriorating' is 'consistent' with the majority's opinion. The deterioration of basic skills, Justice Blackmum noted, presents 'a loss of liberty quite distinct from—and as serious as—the loss of safety and freedom from unreasonable restraints.'

Third, the Court's reasoning implies the existence of expansive rights that protect the patient's principal liberty interest—the interest in release from involuntary confinement. Psychiatrists have observed that the absence of the training necessary to improve a person's basic skills can unduly prolong confinement. Thus, the majority's liberty-based rationale suggests that mental patients have a constitutional right to habilitative rather than merely protective treatment.

A variant of this last possible interpretation of *Youngberg* was proposed in Spece, "Preserving the Right to Treatment: A Critical Assessment and Constructive Development of Constitutional Right to Treatment Theories," 20 Ariz.L.Rev. 1, 33–46 (1978). Relying on least restrictive alternative theory, Spece argued that "virtually all patients are entitled to superior, individual treatment . . . unless the state can meet the heavy burden of demonstrating either that treatment would neither hasten release nor enhance freedom within the institution or that confinement with treatment would be less effective than confinement simpliciter in achieving the state's commitment goals." Id. at 34–35. According to Spece, this theory "comfortably accommodates the confinement of those who are untreatable but otherwise committable." Id. at 44. At the same time, Spece asserts, it requires the state to provide treatment for virtually every patient who is treatable. To what extent does *Youngberg* endorse this theory? In the majority opinion, look at both the penultimate paragraph and footnote 14.

2. *The professional judgment standard.* Note that whatever the ultimate scope of the right to treatment, the question as to whether that right has been infringed may well depend upon how courts construe *Youngberg's* professional judgment standard. For instance, even if patients have a right to treatment or habilitation that will enable them to leave the hospital as soon as possible, deciding whether a particular treatment program implements that right may depend solely upon whether "professional judgment was exercised" in deciding upon the program. Note also that *Youngberg* stated that if the reason professional judgment is not exercised or implemented is budgetary, then damages cannot be awarded against an individual professional (the "good faith" defense). However, the Court made no comment on the viability of a "budgetary defense" in an individual or class action suit seeking to enjoin the state to provide treatment.

3. *Aftermath of* Youngberg. Since *Youngberg,* no federal court has subscribed to the Fifth Circuit's version of the right to treatment as the right "to such treatment as will help [the patient] be cured or to improve his mental condition." Some courts hearing individual and class actions claiming a right to habilitation or treatment have read *Youngberg* very

narrowly. For instance, one court held that because members of the plaintiff class were relatively high functioning mildly or moderately retarded individuals they did not need training "to enhance . . . their right to liberty of movement" and thus were not guaranteed treatment under the constitution. *Phillips v. Thompson,* 715 F.2d 365 (7th Cir.1983). However, most courts seem willing to interpret *Youngberg* to mandate something more than just the treatment necessary to ensure safety and the ability to function free of bodily restraints. Representative of this trend is the Second Circuit's decision in *Society for Good Will to Retarded Children, Inc. v. Cuomo,* 737 F.2d 1239 (2d Cir.1984). Although it held that after *Youngberg* the constitution does not require the state to provide treatment designed to improve a mentally retarded individual's condition, the Second Circuit endorsed Justice Blackmun's right-to-avoid-deterioration standard. See also, *Assoc. for Retarded Citizens of North Dakota v. Olson,* 561 F.Supp. 473, 487 (D.N.D.1982), affirmed 713 F.2d 1384 (8th Cir.1983).

Courts have expanded upon *Youngberg* in other ways as well. Some courts have broadly defined the professional judgment rule. One court stated in dictum that a psychiatric decision should not be characterized as "professional" where "it is not based on a view as to how best to operate a mental health facility." *Johnson v. Brelje,* 701 F.2d 1201, 1209 n. 9 (7th Cir.1983). Another held that professional judgment is not exercised when "the professional's stated judgment was modified to conform to the *available* treatment, rather than the *appropriate* treatment, for the plaintiff's condition." *Thomas S. v. Morrow,* 601 F.Supp. 1055, 1059 (W.D.N.C.1984) (emphasis in original). Many courts have also rejected the "budgetary defense" in injunction suits. For instance, in *Clark v. Cohen,* 613 F.Supp. 684, 704 (E.D.Pa.1985), the court compelled placement of a mildly retarded patient in the community over financially-based objections by the state, emphasizing that professional judgment, to be entitled to judicial deference, "has to be based on medical or psychological criteria and not on exigency, administrative convenience, or other non-medical criteria." See also, *Thomas S. v. Morrow,* supra at 375. Third, although *Youngberg* obviously involved an involuntarily committed individual, most courts have refused to distinguish between involuntary and voluntary patients in applying its ruling. See, e.g., *Society for Good Will to Retarded Children, Inc. v. Cuomo,* supra at 1245–46 ("[O]nce [the state] chose to house . . . voluntary patients, thus making them dependent on the state, it was required to do so in a manner that would not deprive them of constitutional rights").

Finally, it should be noted that some state courts have relied on state statutory language rather than the federal constitution in imposing wide-ranging treatment obligations on the government. See, e.g., *Arnold v. Sarn,* No. C–432355 (Ariz.Super.Ct., Maricopa Cty., May 29, 1985). This development is discussed further in Section IV of this chapter.

III. IMPLEMENTING THE RIGHT: *WYATT v. STICKNEY*

The following section examines various aspects of one "right to treatment" case, originally styled as *Wyatt v. Stickney*. Although filed over a decade before *Youngberg* and based on a theory of the right to treatment that was not endorsed by that decision, the *Wyatt* litigation is a useful focal point for further study of post-commitment treatment issues for a number of reasons. First, as the first major class action brought to enforce a systemwide right to treatment and habilitation, the case has had a significant impact on judicial and legislative decisions around the country that are still in force today. Second, *Wyatt's* long procedural history provides a particularly good illustration of the vagaries of attempting to implement judicially the right to treatment and habilitation. Third, even assuming *Youngberg* effectively narrows the scope of the right to treatment, *Wyatt* has many lessons to offer future litigators. As the previous notes indicate, *Youngberg* has not deterred courts from using constitutional or statutory language as a basis for reviewing decisions by state hospital employees and administrators. Moreover, most of these more recent cases are, like *Wyatt* (and unlike *Youngberg*), class action suits which involve requests for injunctive relief. In *Wyatt v. Aderholt,* 503 F.2d 1305, 1316 (5th Cir.1974), the court explained why this kind of suit is likely to be preferred over individual actions:

> . . . In the first place, habeas corpus relief and tort damages are available only after the fact of a failure to provide individual treatment. Here the plaintiffs seek preventive relief, to assure in advance that mental patients will at least have the *chance* to receive adequate treatment by proscribing the maintenance of conditions that foredoom *all* mental patients *inevitably* to inadequate mental treatment. Moreover, there are special reasons why reliance upon individual suits by mental patients would be especially inappropriate. Mental patients are particularly unlikely to be aware of their legal rights. They are likely to have especially limited access to legal assistance. Individual suits may be protracted and expensive, and individual mental patients may therefore be deterred from bringing them. And individual suits may produce distortive therapeutic effects within an institution, since a staff may tend to give especially good—or especially harsh—treatment to patients the staff expects or knows to be litigious.

(Emphasis in original). Given the likelihood of injunctive actions, the tactical lessons derived from the *Wyatt* litigation will continue to be useful, regardless of the theoretical underpinnings of the right to treatment ultimately settled upon.

Ironically, as initially conceived *Wyatt v. Stickney* was not a right to treatment suit. Filed in October, 1970, the original action was brought on behalf of patients at Bryce Hospital in Tuscaloosa, Alabama asking for an injunction prohibiting anticipated layoffs of hospital personnel (which were to occur because a cut in the Alabama cigarette tax reduced the money available to the state hospital system). Although Ricky Wyatt, a patient, was the named plaintiff, in fact "a fairly small number of staff, not a group of indignant patients or their relatives" was the "motivating power behind the suit." Stickney, "*Wyatt v. Stickney:* The Right to Treatment," in Bonnie, ed., Psychiatrists and the Legal Process: Diagnosis and Debate 274, 278 (1977). Under the auspices of federal district court judge Frank Johnson, however, the suit triggered a wide-ranging investigation of the deplorable conditions at Bryce and other institutions in Alabama [b] and resulted in substantial changes in the system. In the original *Wyatt* decision, Judge Johnson, relying on a "*Jackson*" theory of the right to treatment, held that every civilly committed patient possesses "a constitutional right to receive such individual treatment as will give them a realistic opportunity to be cured or to improve his or her mental condition." 325 F.Supp. 781, 784 (M.D.Ala.1981). The decision set out below is his enforcement decree. Note that it contains standards for virtually every aspect of hospital operation, ranging from the proper temperature of hot water, to the number of social workers and clerk typists per unit, to the types of documents which must be included in each patient's files. The materials following the decision use *Wyatt* and its progeny to provide a flavor of right to treatment litigation and its consequences.

WYATT v. STICKNEY

United States District Court, Middle District Alabama, 1972.
344 F.Supp. 373.

ORDER AND DECREE

JOHNSON, CHIEF JUDGE.

This class action originally was filed on October 23, 1970, in behalf of patients involuntarily confined for mental treatment purposes at Bryce Hospital, Tuscaloosa, Alabama. On March 12, 1971, in a formal opinion and decree, this Court held that these involuntarily committed patients "unquestionably have a constitutional right to receive such individual treatment as will give each of them a realistic opportunity to be cured or to improve his or her mental condition." The Court further held that patients at Bryce were being denied their right to treatment and that defendants, per their request, would be allowed six months in which to raise the level of care at Bryce to the constitutionally required minimum. Wyatt v. Stickney, 325 F.Supp. 781 (M.D.Ala.1971). In this decree, the Court ordered defendants to file reports defining the mission and functions of Bryce Hospital, specifying the objective and subjective standards required to furnish adequate care to the treatable mentally

---

b. The *Wyatt* record is replete with accounts of patients who died or were seriously harmed as a result of inattention by staff, as well descriptions of patient abuse, of filthy conditions, and of general neglect. For instance, the record disclosed that, at one of the institutions involved in the *Wyatt* litigation, four patients had died "due to understaffing, lack of supervision, and brutality."

One of the four died after a garden hose had been inserted into his rectum for

five minutes by a working patient who was cleaning him; one died when a fellow patient hosed him with scalding water; another died when soapy water was forced into his mouth; and a fourth died from a self-administered overdose of drugs which had been inadequately secured.

Wyatt v. Aderholt, 503 F.2d 1305, 1311 n. 6. (5th Cir. 1974).

ill and detailing the hospital's progress toward the implementation of minimum constitutional standards. Subsequent to this order, plaintiffs, by motion to amend granted August 12, 1971, enlarged their class to include patients involuntarily confined for mental treatment at Searcy Hospital and at Partlow State School and Hospital for the mentally retarded.

On September 23, 1971, defendants filed their final report, from which this Court concluded on December 10, 1971, that defendants had failed to promulgate and implement a treatment program satisfying minimum medical and constitutional requisites. Generally, the Court found that defendants' treatment program was deficient in three fundamental areas. It failed to provide: (1) a humane psychological and physical environment, (2) qualified staff in numbers sufficient to administer adequate treatment and (3) individualized treatment plans. More specifically, the Court found that many conditions, such as nontherapeutic, uncompensated work assignments, and the absence of any semblance of privacy, constituted dehumanizing factors contributing to the degeneration of the patients' self-esteem. The physical facilities at Bryce were overcrowded and plagued by fire and other emergency hazards. The Court found also that most staff members were poorly trained and that staffing ratios were so inadequate as to render the administration of effective treatment impossible. The Court concluded, therefore, that whatever treatment was provided at Bryce was grossly deficient and failed to satisfy minimum medical and constitutional standards. Based upon this conclusion, the Court ordered that a formal hearing be held at which the parties and amici [3] would have the opportunity to submit proposed standards for constitutionally adequate treatment and to present expert testimony in support of their proposals.

Pursuant to this order, a hearing was held at which the foremost authorities on mental health in the United States appeared and testified as to the minimum medical and constitutional requisites for public institutions, such as Bryce and Searcy, designed to treat the mentally ill. At this hearing, the parties and amici submitted their proposed standards, and now have filed briefs in support of them. Moreover, the parties and amici have stipulated to a broad spectrum of conditions they feel are mandatory for a constitutionally acceptable minimum treatment program. This Court, having considered the evidence in the case, as well as the briefs, proposed standards and stipulations of the parties, has concluded that the standards set out in Appendix A to this decree are medical and constitutional minimums. Consequently, the Court will order their implementation. In so ordering, however, the

---

3. The amici in this case, including the United States of America, the American Orthopsychiatric Association, the American Psychological Association, the American Civil Liberties Union, and the American Association on Mental Deficiency, have performed exemplary service for which this Court is indeed grateful.

[Note the absence of the American Psychiatric Association, which declined Judge Johnson's offer to participate. Eds.]

Court emphasizes that these standards are, indeed, both medical and constitutional minimums and should be viewed as such. The Court urges that once this order is effectuated, defendants not become complacent and self-satisfied. Rather, they should dedicate themselves to providing physical conditions and treatment programs at Alabama's mental institutions that substantially exceed medical and constitutional minimums.

In addition to asking that their proposed standards be effectuated, plaintiffs and amici have requested other relief designed to guarantee the provision of constitutional and humane treatment. Pursuant to one such request for relief, this Court has determined that it is appropriate to order the initiation of human rights committees to function as standing committees of the Bryce and Searcy facilities. The Court will appoint the members of these committees who shall have review of all research proposals and all rehabilitation programs, to ensure that the dignity and the human rights of patients are preserved. The committees also shall advise and assist patients who allege that their legal rights have been infringed or that the Mental Health Board has failed to comply with judicially ordered guidelines. At their discretion, the committees may consult appropriate, independent specialists who shall be compensated by the defendant Board. Seven members shall comprise the human rights committee for each institution. . . .

This Court will reserve ruling upon other forms of relief advocated by plaintiffs and amici, including their prayer for the appointment of a master and a professional advisory committee to oversee the implementation of the court-ordered minimum constitutional standards.[6] Federal courts are reluctant to assume control of any organization, but especially one operated by a state. This reluctance, combined with defendants' expressed intent that this order will be implemented forthwith and in good faith, causes the Court to withhold its decision on these appointments. Nevertheless, defendants, as well as the other parties and amici in this case, are placed on notice that unless defendants do comply satisfactorily with this order, the Court will be obligated to appoint a master.

Because the availability of financing may bear upon the implementation of this order, the Court is constrained to emphasize at this juncture that a failure by defendants to comply with this decree cannot be justified by a lack of operating funds. As previously established by this Court:

6. The Court's decision to reserve its ruling on the appointment of a master necessitates the reservation also of the Court's appointing a professional advisory committee to aid the master. Nevertheless, the Court notes that the professional mental health community in the United States has responded with enthusiasm to the proposed initiation of such a committee to assist in the upgrading of Alabama's mental health facilities. Consequently, this Court strongly recommends to defendants that they develop a professional advisory committee comprised of amenable professionals from throughout the country who are able to provide the expertise the evidence reflects is important to the successful implementation of this order.

"There can be no legal (or moral) justification for the State of Alabama's failing to afford treatment—and adequate treatment from a medical standpoint—to the several thousand patients who have been civilly committed to Bryce's for treatment purposes. To deprive any citizen of his or her liberty upon the altruistic theory that the confinement is for humane therapeutic reasons and then fail to provide adequate treatment violates the very fundamentals of due process."

From the above, it follows consistently, of course, that the unavailability of neither funds, nor staff and facilities, will justify a default by defendants in the provision of suitable treatment for the mentally ill.

Despite the possibility that defendants will encounter financial difficulties in the implementation of this order, this Court has decided to reserve ruling also upon plaintiffs' motion that defendant Mental Health Board be directed to sell or encumber portions of its land holdings in order to raise funds. Similarly, this Court will reserve ruling on plaintiffs' motion seeking an injunction against the treasurer and the comptroller of the State authorizing expenditures for nonessential State functions, and on other aspects of plaintiffs' requested relief designed to ameliorate the financial problems incident to the implementation of this order. The Court stresses, however, the extreme importance and the grave immediacy of the need for proper funding of the State's public mental health facilities. The responsibility for appropriate funding ultimately must fall, of course, upon the State Legislature and, to a lesser degree, upon the defendant Mental Health Board of Alabama. For the present time, the Court will defer to those bodies in hopes that they will proceed with the realization and understanding that what is involved in this case is not representative of ordinary governmental functions such as paving roads and maintaining buildings. Rather, what is so inextricably intertwined with how the Legislature and Mental Health Board respond to the revelations of this litigation is the very preservation of human life and dignity. Not only are the lives of the patients currently confined at Bryce and Searcy at stake, but also at issue are the well-being and security of every citizen of Alabama. As is true in the case of any disease, no one is immune from the peril of mental illness. The problem, therefore, cannot be overemphasized and a prompt response from the Legislature, the Mental Health Board and other responsible State officials, is imperative.

In the event, though, that the Legislature fails to satisfy its well-defined constitutional obligation, and the Mental Health Board, because of lack of funding or any other legally insufficient reason, fails to implement fully the standards herein ordered, it will be necessary for the Court to take affirmative steps, including appointing a master, to ensure that proper funding is realized [8] and that adequate treatment is

8. The Court understands and appreciates that the Legislature is not due back in regular session until May, 1973. Nevertheless, special sessions of the Legislature are frequent occurrences in Alabama, and there has never been a time when such a session was more urgently required. If the Legislature does not act promptly to appro-

available for the mentally ill of Alabama.

This Court now must consider that aspect of plaintiffs' motion of March 15, 1972, seeking an injunction against further commitments to Bryce and Searcy until such time as adequate treatment is supplied in those hospitals. Indisputably, the evidence in this case reflects that no treatment program at the Bryce–Searcy facilities approaches constitutional standards. Nevertheless, because of the alternatives to commitment commonly utilized in Alabama, as well as in other states, the Court is fearful that granting plaintiffs' request at the present time would serve only to punish and further deprive Alabama's mentally ill.

* * *

Appendix A

MINIMUM Constitutional STANDARDS for Adequate Treatment of The Mentally Ill

I. *Definitions:*

    a. "Hospital"—Bryce and Searcy Hospitals.

    b. "Patients"—all persons who are now confined and all persons who may in the future be confined at Bryce and Searcy Hospitals pursuant to an involuntary civil commitment procedure.

    c. "Qualified Mental Health Professional"—

      (1) a psychiatrist with three years of residency training in psychiatry;

      (2) a psychologist with a doctoral degree from an accredited program;

      (3) a social worker with a master's degree from an accredited program and two years of clinical experience under the supervision of a Qualified Mental Health Professional;

      (4) a registered nurse with a graduate degree in psychiatric nursing and two years of clinical experience under the supervision of a Qualified Mental Health Professional.

    d. "Non–Professional Staff Member"—an employee of the hospital, other than a Qualified Mental Health Professional, whose duties require contact with or supervision of patients.

II. *Humane Psychological and Physical Environment*

    1. Patients have a right to privacy and dignity.

    2. Patients have a right to the least restrictive conditions necessary to achieve the purposes of commitment.

    3. No person shall be deemed incompetent to manage his affairs, to contract, to hold professional or occupational or vehicle operator's

priate the necessary funding for mental health, the Court will be compelled to grant plaintiffs' motion to add various State officials and agencies as additional parties to this litigation, and to utilize other avenues of fund raising.

licenses, to marry and obtain a divorce, to register and vote, or to make a will *solely* by reason of his admission or commitment to the hospital.

4. Patients shall have the same rights to visitation and telephone communications as patients at other public hospitals, except to the extent that the Qualified Mental Health Professional responsible for formulation of a particular patient's treatment plan writes an order imposing special restrictions. The written order must be renewed after each periodic review of the treatment plan if any restrictions are to be continued. Patients shall have an unrestricted right to visitation with attorneys and with private physicians and other health professionals.

5. Patients shall have an unrestricted right to send sealed mail. Patients shall have an unrestricted right to receive sealed mail from their attorneys, private physicians, and other mental health professionals, from courts, and government officials. Patients shall have a right to receive sealed mail from others, except to the extent that the Qualified Mental Health Professional responsible for formulation of a particular patient's treatment plan writes an order imposing special restrictions on receipt of sealed mail. The written order must be renewed after each periodic review of the treatment plan if any restrictions are to be continued.

6. Patients have a right to be free from unnecessary or excessive medication. No medication shall be administered unless at the written order of a physician. The superintendent of the hospital and the attending physician shall be responsible for all medication given or administered to a patient. The use of medication shall not exceed standards of use that are advocated by the United States Food and Drug Administration. Notation of each individual's medication shall be kept in his medical records. At least weekly the attending physician shall review the drug regimen of each patient under his care. All prescriptions shall be written with a termination date, which shall not exceed 30 days. Medication shall not be used as punishment, for the convenience of staff, as a substitute for program, or in quantities that interfere with the patient's treatment program.

7. Patients have a right to be free from physical restraint and isolation. Except for emergency situations, in which it is likely that patients could harm themselves or others and in which less restrictive means of restraint are not feasible, patients may be physically restrained or placed in isolation only on a Qualified Mental Health Professional's written order which explains the rationale for such action. The written order may be entered only after the Qualified Mental Health Professional has personally seen the patient concerned and evaluated whatever episode or situation is said to call for restraint or isolation. Emergency use of restraints or isolation shall be for no more than one hour, by which time a Qualified Mental Health Professional shall have been consulted and shall have entered an appropriate order in writing. Such written order shall be effective for no more than 24 hours and must be renewed if restraint and isolation are to be

continued. While in restraint or isolation the patient must be seen by qualified ward personnel who will chart the patient's physical condition (if it is compromised) and psychiatric condition every hour. The patient must have bathroom privileges every hour and must be bathed every 12 hours.

8. Patients shall have a right not to be subjected to experimental research without the express and informed consent of the patient, if the patient is able to give such consent, and of his guardian or next of kin, after opportunities for consultation with independent specialists and with legal counsel. Such proposed research shall first have been reviewed and approved by the institution's Human Rights Committee before such consent shall be sought. Prior to such approval the Committee shall determine that such research complies with the principles of the Statement on the Use of Human Subjects for Research of the American Association on Mental Deficiency and with the principles for research involving human subjects required by the United States Department of Health, Education and Welfare for projects supported by that agency.

9. Patients have a right not to be subjected to treatment procedures such as lobotomy, electro-convulsive treatment, adversive reinforcement conditioning or other unusual or hazardous treatment procedures without their express and informed consent after consultation with counsel or interested party of the patient's choice.

10. Patients have a right to receive prompt and adequate medical treatment for any physical ailments.

11. Patients have a right to wear their own clothes and to keep and use their own personal possessions except insofar as such clothes or personal possessions may be determined by a Qualified Mental Health Professional to be dangerous or otherwise inappropriate to the treatment regimen.

12. The hospital has an obligation to supply an adequate allowance of clothing to any patients who do not have suitable clothing of their own. Patients shall have the opportunity to select from various types of neat, clean, and seasonable clothing. Such clothing shall be considered the patient's throughout his stay in the hospital.

13. The hospital shall make provision for the laundering of patient clothing.

14. Patients have a right to regular physical exercise several times a week. Moreover, it shall be the duty of the hospital to provide facilities and equipment for such exercise.

15. Patients have a right to be outdoors at regular and frequent intervals, in the absence of medical considerations.

16. The right to religious worship shall be accorded to each patient who desires such opportunities. Provisions for such worship shall be made available to all patients on a nondiscriminatory basis. No individual shall be coerced into engaging in any religious activities.

17. The institution shall provide, with adequate supervision, suitable opportunities for the patient's interaction with members of the opposite sex.

18. The following rules shall govern patient labor:

A. *Hospital Maintenance* No patient shall be required to perform labor which involves the operation and maintenance of the hospital or for which the hospital is under contract with an outside organization. Privileges or release from the hospital shall not be conditioned upon the performance of labor covered by this provision. Patients may voluntarily engage in such labor if the labor is compensated in accordance with the minimum wage laws of the Fair Labor Standards Act, 29 U.S.C. § 206 as amended, 1966.

B. *Therapeutic Tasks and Therapeutic Labor*

(1) Patients may be required to perform therapeutic tasks which do not involve the operation and maintenance of the hospital, provided the specific task or any change in assignment is:

    a. An integrated part of the patient's treatment plan and approved as a therapeutic activity by a Qualified Mental Health Professional responsible for supervising the patient's treatment; and

    b. Supervised by a staff member to oversee the therapeutic aspects of the activity.

(2) Patients may voluntarily engage in therapeutic labor for which the hospital would otherwise have to pay an employee, provided the specific labor or any change in labor assignment is:

    a. An integrated part of the patient's treatment plan and approved as a therapeutic activity by a Qualified Mental Health Professional responsible for supervising the patient's treatment; and

    b. Supervised by a staff member to oversee the therapeutic aspects of the activity; and

    c. Compensated in accordance with the minimum wage laws of the Fair Labor Standards Act, 29 U.S.C. § 206 as amended, 1966.

C. *Personal Housekeeping* Patients may be required to perform tasks of a personal housekeeping nature such as the making of one's own bed.

D. Payment to patients pursuant to these paragraphs shall not be applied to the costs of hospitalization.

19. *Physical Facilities*

A patient has a right to a humane psychological and physical environment within the hospital facilities. These facilities shall be designed to afford patients with comfort and safety, promote dignity, and ensure privacy. The facilities shall be designed to make a positive contribution to the efficient attainment of the treatment goals of the hospital.

A. *Resident Unit*

The number of patients in a multi-patient room shall not exceed six persons. There shall be allocated a minimum of 80 square feet of floor space per patient in a multi-patient room. Screens or curtains shall be provided to ensure privacy within the resident unit. Single rooms shall have a minimum of 100 square feet of floor space. Each patient will be furnished with a comfortable bed with adequate changes of linen, a closet or locker for his personal belongings, a chair, and a bedside table.

B. *Toilets and Lavatories*

There will be one toilet provided for each eight patients and one lavatory for each six patients. A lavatory will be provided with each toilet facility. The toilets will be installed in separate stalls to ensure privacy, will be clean and free of odor, and will be equipped with appropriate safety devices for the physically handicapped.

C. *Showers*

There will be one tub or shower for each 15 patients. If a central bathing area is provided, each shower area will be divided by curtains to ensure privacy. Showers and tubs will be equipped with adequate safety accessories.

D. *Day Room*

The minimum day room area shall be 40 square feet per patient. Day rooms will be attractive and adequately furnished with reading lamps, tables, chairs, television and other recreational facilities. They will be conveniently located to patients' bedrooms and shall have outside windows. There shall be at least one day room area on each bedroom floor in a multi-story hospital. Areas used for corridor traffic cannot be counted as day room space; nor can a chapel with fixed pews be counted as a day room area.

E. *Dining Facilities*

The minimum dining room area shall be ten square feet per patient. The dining room shall be separate from the kitchen and will be furnished with comfortable chairs and tables with hard, washable surfaces.

F. *Linen Servicing and Handling*

The hospital shall provide adequate facilities and equipment for handling clean and soiled bedding and other linen. There must be frequent changes of bedding and other linen, no less than every seven days to assure patient comfort.

G. *Housekeeping*

Regular housekeeping and maintenance procedures which will en-sure that the hospital is maintained in a safe, clean, and attractive condition will be developed and implemented.

H. *Geriatric and Other Nonambulatory Mental Patients*

There must be special facilities for geriatric and other nonambu-latory patients to assure their safety and comfort, including special fittings on toilets and wheelchairs. Appropriate provision shall be made to permit nonambulatory patients to communicate their needs to staff.

I. *Physical Plant*

(1) Pursuant to an established routine maintenance and repair program, the physical plant shall be kept in a continuous state of good repair and operation in accordance with the needs of the health, comfort, safety and well-being of the patients.

(2) Adequate heating, air conditioning and ventilation systems and equipment shall be afforded to maintain temperatures and air changes which are required for the comfort of patients at all times and the removal of undesired heat, steam and offensive odors. Such facilities shall ensure that the temperature in the hospital shall not exceed 83° F nor fall below 68°F.

(3) Thermostatically controlled hot water shall be provided in adequate quantities and maintained at the required temperature for patient or resident use (110°F at the fixture) and for mechanical dishwashing and laundry use (180°F at the equipment).

(4) Adequate refuse facilities will be provided so that solid waste, rubbish and other refuse will be collected and disposed of in a manner which will prohibit transmission of disease and not create a nuisance or fire hazard or provide a breeding place for rodents and insects.

(5) The physical facilities must meet all fire and safety standards established by the state and locality. In addition, the hospital shall meet such provisions of the Life Safety Code of the National Fire Protection Association (21st edition, 1967) as are applicable to hospitals.

19A. The hospital shall meet all standards established by the state for general hospitals, insofar as they are relevant to psychiatric facilities.

20. *Nutritional Standards*

Patients, except for the non-mobile, shall eat or be fed in dining rooms. The diet for patients will provide at a minimum the Recom-mended Daily Dietary Allowances as developed by the National Acade-my of Sciences. Menus shall be satisfying and nutritionally adequate to provide the Recommended Daily Dietary Allowances. In developing such menus, the hospital will utilize the Low Cost Food Plan of the

Department of Agriculture. The hospital will not spend less per patient for raw food, including the value of donated food, than the most recent per person costs of the Low Cost Food Plan for the Southern Region of the United States, as compiled by the United States Department of Agriculture, for appropriate groupings of patients, discounted for any savings which might result from institutional procurement of such food. Provisions shall be made for special therapeutic diets and for substitutes at the request of the patient, or his guardian or next of kin, in accordance with the religious requirements of any patient's faith. Denial of a nutritionally adequate diet shall not be used as punishment.

III. *Qualified Staff in Numbers Sufficient to Administer Adequate Treatment*

21. Each Qualified Mental Health Professional shall meet all licensing and certification requirements promulgated by the State of Alabama for persons engaged in private practice of the same profession elsewhere in Alabama. Other staff members shall meet the same licensing and certification requirements as persons who engage in private practice of their speciality elsewhere in Alabama.

22. a. All Non–Professional Staff Members who have not had prior clinical experience in a mental institution shall have a substantial orientation training.

b. Staff members on all levels shall have regularly scheduled in-service training.

23. Each Non–Professional Staff Member shall be under the direct supervision of a Qualified Mental Health Professional.

24. *Staffing Ratios*

The hospital shall have the following minimum numbers of treatment personnel per 250 patients. Qualified Mental Health Professionals trained in particular disciplines may in appropriate situations perform services or functions traditionally performed by members of other disciplines. Changes in staff deployment may be made with prior approval of this Court upon a clear and convincing demonstration that the proposed deviation from this staffing structure will enhance the treatment of the patients.

Classification	Number of Employees
Unit Director	1
Psychiatrist (3 years' residency training in psychiatry)	2
MD (Registered physicians)	4
Nurses (RN)	12
Licensed Practical Nurses	6
Aide III	6
Aide II	16
Aide I	70

Classification	Number of Employees
Hospital Orderly	10
Clerk Stenographer II	3
Clerk Typist II	3
Unit Administrator	1
Administrative Clerk	1
Psychologist (Ph.D.) (doctoral degree from accredited program)	1
Psychologist (M.A.)	1
Psychologist (B.S.)	2
Social Worker (MSW) (from accredited program)	2
Social Worker (B.A.)	5
Patient Activity Therapist (M.S.)	1
Patient Activity Aide	10
Mental Health Technician	10
Dental Hygienist	1
Chaplain	5
Vocational Rehabilitation Counselor	1
Volunteer Services Worker	1
Mental Health Field Representative	1
Dietitian	1
Food Service Supervisor	1
Cook II	2
Cook I	3
Food Service Worker	15
Vehicle Driver	1
Housekeeper	10
Messenger	1
Maintenance Repairman	2

IV. *Individualized Treatment Plans*

25. Each patient shall have a comprehensive physical and mental examination and review of behavioral status within 48 hours after admission to the hospital.

26. Each patient shall have an individualized treatment plan. This plan shall be developed by appropriate Qualified Mental Health Professionals, including a psychiatrist, and implemented as soon as possible—in any event no later than five days after the patient's admission. Each individualized treatment plan shall contain:

a. a statement of the nature of the specific problems and specific needs of the patient;

b. a statement of the least restrictive treatment conditions necessary to achieve the purposes of commitment;

c. a description of intermediate and long-range treatment goals, with a projected timetable for their attainment;

d.   a statement and rationale for the plan of treatment for achieving these intermediate and long-range goals;

e.   a specification of staff responsibility and a description of proposed staff involvement with the patient in order to attain these treatment goals;

f.   criteria for release to less restrictive treatment conditions, and criteria for discharge;

g.   a notation of any therapeutic tasks and labor to be performed by the patient in accordance with Standard 18.

27.   As part of his treatment plan, each patient shall have an individualized post-hospitalization plan. This plan shall be developed by a Qualified Mental Health Professional as soon as practicable after the patient's admission to the hospital.

28.   In the interests of continuity of care, whenever possible, one Qualified Mental Health Professional (who need not have been involved with the development of the treatment plan) shall be responsible for supervising the implementation of the treatment plan, integrating the various aspects of the treatment program and recording the patient's progress. This Qualified Mental Health Professional shall also be responsible for ensuring that the patient is released, where appropriate, into a less restrictive form of treatment.

29.   The treatment plan shall be continuously reviewed by the Qualified Mental Health Professional responsible for supervising the implementation of the plan and shall be modified if necessary. Moreover, at least every 90 days, each patient shall receive a mental examination from, and his treatment plan shall be reviewed by, a Qualified Mental Health Professional other than the professional responsible for supervising the implementation of the plan.

30.   In addition to treatment for mental disorders, patients confined at mental health institutions also are entitled to and shall receive appropriate treatment for physical illnesses such as tuberculosis. In providing medical care, the State Board of Mental Health shall take advantage of whatever community-based facilities are appropriate and available and shall coordinate the patient's treatment for mental illness with his medical treatment.

31.   Complete patient records shall be kept on the ward in which the patient is placed and shall be available to anyone properly authorized in writing by the patient. These records shall include:

a.   Identification data, including the patient's legal status;

b.   A patient history, including but not limited to:

(1) family data, educational background, and employment record;

(2) prior medical history, both physical and mental, including prior hospitalization;

c. The chief complaints of the patient and the chief complaints of others regarding the patient;

d. An evaluation which notes the onset of illness, the circumstances leading to admission, attitudes, behavior, estimate of intellectual functioning, memory functioning, orientation, and an inventory of the patient's assets in descriptive, not interpretative, fashion;

e. A summary of each physical examination which describes the results of the examination;

f. A copy of the individual treatment plan and any modifications thereto;

g. A detailed summary of the findings made by the reviewing Qualified Mental Health Professional after each periodic review of the treatment plan which analyzes the successes and failures of the treatment program and directs whatever modifications are necessary;

h. A copy of the individualized post-hospitalization plan and any modifications thereto, and a summary of the steps that have been taken to implement that plan;

i. A medication history and status, which includes the signed orders of the prescribing physician. Nurses shall indicate by signature that orders have been carried out;

j. A detailed summary of each significant contact by a Qualified Mental Health Professional with the patient;

k. A detailed summary on at least a weekly basis by a Qualified Mental Health Professional involved in the patient's treatment of the patient's progress along the treatment plan;

l. A weekly summary of the extent and nature of the patient's work activities described in Standard 18, *supra*, and the effect of such activity upon the patient's progress along the treatment plan;

m. A signed order by a Qualified Mental Health Professional for any restrictions on visitations and communication, as provided in Standards 4 and 5, *supra*;

n. A signed order by a Qualified Mental Health Professional for any physical restraints and isolation, as provided in Standard 7, *supra*;

o. A detailed summary of any extraordinary incident in the hospital involving the patient to be entered by a staff member noting that he has personal knowledge of the incident or specifying his other source of information, and initialed within 24 hours by a Qualified Mental Health Professional;

p. A summary by the superintendent of the hospital or his appointed agent of his findings after the 15–day review provided for in Standard 33 *infra*.

32. In addition to complying with all the other standards herein, a hospital shall make special provisions for the treatment of patients who are children and young adults. These provisions shall include but are not limited to:

    a. Opportunities for publicly supported education suitable to the educational needs of the patient. This program of education must, in the opinion of the attending Qualified Mental Health Professional, be compatible with the patient's mental condition and his treatment program, and otherwise be in the patient's best interest.

    b. A treatment plan which considers the chronological, maturational, and developmental level of the patient;

    c. Sufficient Qualified Mental Health Professionals, teachers, and staff members with specialized skills in the care and treatment of children and young adults;

    d. Recreation and play opportunities in the open air where possible and appropriate residential facilities;

    e. Arrangements for contact between the hospital and the family of the patient.

33. No later than 15 days after a patient is committed to the hospital, the superintendent of the hospital or his appointed, professionally qualified agent shall examine the committed patient and shall determine whether the patient continues to require hospitalization and whether a treatment plan complying with Standard 26 has been implemented. If the patient no longer requires hospitalization in accordance with the standards for commitment, or if a treatment plan has not been implemented, he must be released immediately unless he agrees to continue with treatment on a voluntary basis.

34. The Mental Health Board and its agents have an affirmative duty to provide adequate transitional treatment and care for all patients released after a period of involuntary confinement. Transitional care and treatment possibilities include, but are not limited to, psychiatric day care, treatment in the home by a visiting therapist, nursing home or extended care, out-patient treatment, and treatment in the psychiatric ward of a general hospital.

V. *Miscellaneous*

35. Each patient and his family, guardian, or next friend shall promptly upon the patient's admission receive written notice, in language he understands, of all the above standards for adequate treatment. In addition a copy of all the above standards shall be posted in each ward.

Questions and Comments

1. *The Partlow order.* As noted by the court, a second filing in the *Wyatt* case dealt with conditions in Partlow State School and Hospital, an

institution for the mentally retarded. Judge Johnson's order concerning Partlow was similar to the order governing Bryce and Searcy, except that it was even more extensive. See *Wyatt v. Stickney,* 344 F.Supp. 387 (M.D.Ala. 1972). For instance, in the course of defining the meaning of "adequate habilitation" for residents of Partlow, the order specified the class size, length of school year and minimum length of school day. The guidelines for the first two areas varied depending upon the patient's degree of retardation, while the length of the school day was fixed at 6 hours for all groups. Id. at 397.

2. *Subsequent history of* Wyatt *litigation.* Both of Judge Johnson's orders were substantially affirmed in *Wyatt v. Aderholt,* 503 F.2d 1305 (5th Cir.1974). In 1977, claiming that Alabama had not complied with the 1972 orders, plaintiffs asked the court to appoint a receiver who would supervise the functions of the Alabama mental health bureaucracy. Judge Johnson agreed that there had been "substantial noncompliance" in a number of areas. He granted the plaintiffs' motion, giving them three weeks to nominate a receiver. However, because the governor had also asked to be appointed as receiver, the court gave the governor ten weeks to file "specific proposals as to the remedial steps [he] will take if appointed receiver." *Wyatt v. Ireland,* 515 F.Supp. 888 (M.D.Ala.1981). The governor was eventually appointed as the receiver.

In the same suit, the defendants asked for a modification of the 1972 orders, which they claimed were too rigid. They charged that the court's overall approach "seriously detracted from resident care, treatment and training" because its inordinate recordkeeping requirements, its imposition of "ritualistic and meaningless" procedures, and its failure to stop the "harassment" of the human rights committees demoralized the staff. Id. at 838–39. The court refused to modify the original decree in any of these respects. Id. at 854–56. The defendants also asked for certain specific relief. They contended, for example, that requiring 6 hours of training per day, as the Partlow order did, was not always in the best interests of the residents, especially those who were profoundly or severely retarded. Id. at 816–17. Continuing a routine training regimen for patients who did not show substantial improvement could be "perjorative and demeaning" and might even constitute "cruel and inhuman treatment." Id. at 837. Instead, the defendants argued, residents who failed to improve with extensive education and training should be switched to "a full program of enriching activities, work activities, sheltered employment, physical exercise and therapies, and such other programs that tend to give meaning and dignity to their lives." Id. at 821. The court rejected this request, stating that, if granted, it would "threaten [the] constitutional right [of each resident] . . . to a habilitation program which will maximize his human abilities and enhance his ability to cope with his environment." Id. at 854. How does this holding compare to *Youngberg's?* See footnote 23 of that opinion.

In September, 1986, sixteen years after the initial complaint was filed, the *Wyatt* suit was officially settled. As part of the settlement agreement, the state of Alabama agreed to make "reasonable efforts" to achieve full accreditation by the relevant accrediting authorities. The agreement also required the state to make "substantial progress" toward establishing needed community facilities. Further, the agreement established patient advocacy and quality assurance programs. An advisory committee, on which the plaintiffs' attorney sits, also informally monitors hospital compliance. Finally, despite the end of the suit, both parties agreed that the original standards set out in *Wyatt v. Stickney* still apply. *Wyatt v. Wallis,* Civil Action No. 3195–N Sept. 22, 1986. Thus, although the suit is officially ended, in a sense it is still ongoing.

3. *The impact of* Wyatt. Between 1970 and 1975, the population at Bryce Hospital was reduced by 61.3%. Although this reduction was due to a number of factors (e.g., the creation of community mental health centers and the initiation of federal welfare programs subsidizing nursing home care), it was,

> in significant part, . . . attributable to specific aspects of the *Wyatt* litigation. The ban on nontherapeutic patient labor 'made it undesirable to have a large number of productive individuals in the hospital'; pressure to comply with patient-staff ratios 'tended to create a climate in which discharge of patients was seen as beneficial;' and the publicity spawned by the suit 'probably created more favorable public attitudes toward return of patients to the community than had existed previously.'

2 M. Perlin, Mental Disability Law: Civil and Criminal 71. Between 1970 and 1975, expenditures of the Alabama Department of Health increased by over 327%. During this time, the state significantly improved its psychologist-patient and social worker-patient ratios. However, it hired only a small number of additional psychiatrists, which meant that the few who were on staff did not have the time to oversee some of the activities the court had ordered them to monitor (such as development and implementation of individualized treatment and post-hospitalization plans). As a "direct result" of the suit, the state installed air conditioning, shower and toilet partitions and pay phones, and allowed the patients to receive uncensured mail. Patient abuse declined significantly, primarily due to the reduction in patients, the increased number of supervisory personnel and the presence of human rights committees brought about by *Wyatt.* At the same time, staff became fearful of giving patients any "negative feedback" lest it be construed as abuse. Id. at 71–73. Although the overall effect of these changes was probably to improve the quality of care, there is no direct data concerning therapeutic success on an individual basis. L.R. Jones & R. Parlour, *Wyatt v. Stickney:* Retrospect and Prospect xi, xii (1981).

Wyatt was also influential at the national level. One commentator concluded that, because of *Wyatt,* thirty-five departments of mental health instituted changes in regulations governing treatment of patients. Schnibbe, "Changes in State Mental Health Service Systems Since *Wyatt,*" in Jones & Parlour, supra at 173, 174. Many states passed "Patients Bill of Rights" legislation which replicated to a greater or lesser extent the *Wyatt* order. "The *Wyatt* Standards: An Influential Force in State and Federal Rules," 28 Hosp. & Comm. Psychiat. 374 (1977). *Wyatt* also influenced the Task Force Panel on Legal and Ethical Issues of the President's Commission on Mental Health, which in turn motivated Congress' passage of the Bill of Rights section of the Mental Health Systems Act. 2 Perlin, supra at 73. This Act, passed in 1983, requested the states to revise their laws taking into account the recommendations of the President's Commission. 42 U.S.C. § 9501.

Finally, *Wyatt* influenced several courts, which issued *Wyatt*-type orders. See, e.g., *Welsch v. Likins*, 373 F.Supp. 487 (D.Minn.1974); *Gary W. v. Louisiana*, 437 F.Supp. 1209 (E.D.La.1976). Most of these decisions were narrower in scope than *Wyatt* but, in the areas they dealt with, the relief they granted was at least as extensive as that granted in *Wyatt*. The following notes examine more closely some of the issues addressed by the *Wyatt* litigation and subsequent cases, and the extent to which *Youngberg* has changed the legal landscape.

4. *Individualized treatment plans.* A widely copied aspect of the *Wyatt* order is the detailed blueprint it established for preparation of an individualized treatment plan for each patient. See Appendix, paras. 25–29. The individualized plan has become a standard feature of hospital administration in virtually every state. How "individualized" do these plans have to be? If they are not prepared or adhered to, what should the patient's remedy be? See Appendix, para. 33. May the patient force a change in the plan by refusing the treatment indicated?[c] Perhaps most importantly, after *Youngberg,* to what extent is a patient entitled, under the federal constitution, to internal or judicial review of the adequacy of the treatment plan and its implementation? See Appendix, paras. 28, 29, 33. Consider also this excerpt from *United States v. Charters*, 863 F.2d 302, 312–13 (4th Cir.1988), construing *Youngberg's* professional judgment rule.

> Making an acceptable professional judgment [in the treatment context] does not require any internal adversarial hearing. The decision may be based upon accepted medical practices in diagnosis, treatment and prognosis, with the aid of such technical tools and consultative techniques as are appropriate in the profession. . . . [T]he basis for the decision should be supported by adequate documentation, not only because of normal professional requirements, but as a potential aid to judicial review. One could of course imagine any number of special internal review and consultative practices specifically designed to ensure confidence in the professional basis of specific medical decisions, and medical professionals, aware of the constitutional standard under which they are operating, are of course free to employ any that seem appropriate.

5. *Treatment in the least restrictive conditions.* Another innovation in *Wyatt* was its application of the least restrictive alternative idea to treatment *within* the institution. See Appendix, para. 2. Although the language in the Bryce order is quite general, the Partlow order provided more detail as to how this aspect of the right to treatment was to be implemented.

c. As developed at pp. 848–870, civilly committed patients may not have a right to refuse medication. But if such a right exists, it may be in tension with the right to treatment.

> [T]he institution shall make every attempt to move residents from (1) more to less structured living; (2) larger to smaller facilities; (3) larger to smaller living units; (4) group to individual residences; (5) segregated from the community to integrated into the community living; (6) dependent to independent living.

344 F.Supp. 373, 396 (M.D.Ala.1972).

Some courts have been even more precise. In *Goodwin v. Shapiro,* 545 F.Supp. 826 (D.N.J.1982), the court created three levels of supervision designed to enforce the "presumption" that "all patients shall be restricted only to the extent which shall be clinically necessary or necessary to the Hospital's internal order and security, but not for administrative convenience." Id. at 847. Supervisory Level A, which allows the patient "maximum institutional flexibility subject only to curfews and the patient's individual responsibility for meeting treatment or obligations" applies to all patients who do not meet Level B or Level C criteria. Level B applies when "[t]here is a reasonable basis to believe that the patient could be a danger to him/herself, or to others, or might cause significant damage to the property of others" or when "[t]here is a reasonable basis to believe that the patient is an elopement risk." This level of restriction allows grounds privileges "for a reasonable period of time every day without supervision" and "additional on-ground activity, off-ground activity, weekend passes and other such unsupervised activities as the treatment team deems appropriate." Level C, which applies to those who are *clearly* dangerous to self, others or property, or who are clearly an elopement risk, contemplates "complete and constant" supervision.

The Third Circuit's decision in *Youngberg* held that the plaintiff had a right to treatment in the least intrusive manner, and devised a three-tier framework for review similar to that set out in *Goodwin. Romeo v. Youngberg,* 644 F.2d 147, 164–170 (3d Cir.1980). Although the Supreme Court's decision in *Youngberg* did not explicitly address the least intrusive means issue, in its conclusion it included in the list of rights the plaintiff enjoyed the right to "reasonably nonrestrictive confinement conditions." 457 U.S. at 324. However, the Court also rejected the contention that physical restrictions on liberty should only be imposed in the face of a "compelling" or "substantial necessity;" instead the professional judgment rule applies. Can *Youngberg* be construed to require a system similar to that ordered in *Goodwin?* Is such a system a good idea? Recall Hoffman and Foust's argument that effectiveness of treatment must be taken into account if the least restrictive idea is to make sense (see pp. 683–686).

6. *Restraints and seclusion.* One concrete application of the least restrictive idea arises when hospital staff decide to use physical restraints or seclusion. As indicated in *Youngberg,* restraints are any means of restricting a patient's ability to react physically, usually involving the use of devices such as cuffs, straps, mittens, or braces. "Seclusion . . . involves placing the patient in one of the individual sleeping rooms in the ward, usually furnished with only a bed, and locking the door." *Eckerhart v. Hensley,* 475 F.Supp. 908, 926 (W.D.Mo.1979). Although restraint and seclusion are considered necessary devices for protection of the patient or others and may even be useful treatment mechanisms when the patient is

experiencing "sensory overload," they can also be used to punish problem patients or as a substitute for adequate supervision in an understaffed facility. Schwitzgebel & Schwitzgebel, Law and Psychological Practice 47 (1980).

Note *Wyatt's* regulation of these two modalities. Appendix, para. 7. A number of states have enacted such provisions legislatively. Some courts provide even more protections. One court, for instance, imposed an absolute prohibition on the use of seclusion for the mentally retarded. *New York State Assoc. for Retarded Children v. Rockefeller,* 357 F.Supp. 752, 768 (E.D.N.Y.1973). In *Davis v. Balson,* 461 F.Supp. 842, 876 (N.D.Ohio 1978), the court required that, before restraints or seclusion can be used, a hearing preceded by 24 hour notice and presided over by an impartial decisionmaker must occur. At the hearing, the patient is to have the opportunity to call witnesses, the assistance of another resident or staff member if the patient is illiterate or the issues complex, and the right to a written statement of the findings of fact and the evidence relied upon. Another court allowed emergency restraint or seclusion without a hearing, but required a physician to write an order if the intervention goes beyond four hours. *Negron v. Ward,* 458 F.Supp. 748 (S.D.N.Y.1976). *Negron* also required that the patient be released every two hours, and barred continued restraint or seclusion after this release unless further overt violent gestures are made. If restraint for more than 48 hours occurs, a qualified psychiatrist not employed by the hospital must examine the patient and make a written report indicating whether continued intervention is justified. How viable are these decisions after *Youngberg?* Recall that the plaintiff in that case was subjected to "soft restraints", allegedly as part of a training regimen.

An analogous issue arises when the state wants to transfer a patient to a more secure unit, usually after the patient is alleged to have committed a crime. In *Jones v. Robinson,* 440 F.2d 249 (D.C.Cir.1971), the court required a procedure akin to that described in *Davis v. Balson,* supra, before transfer of an alleged rapist to a maximum security unit could take place. Is there justification for requiring more procedural formality here than when seclusion or restraints are contemplated?

7. *Privacy and communication.* The *Wyatt* order provided that patients "shall have an unrestricted right to send sealed mail" and conditioned access to the phone. See Appendix, paras. 5, 4. Two years later in *Procunier v. Martinez,* 416 U.S. 396, 94 S.Ct. 1800, 40 L.Ed.2d 224 (1974), the Supreme Court articulated the following test to be applied to regulation of prison inmate correspondence:

> First the regulation or practice in question must further an important or substantial government interest unrelated to the suppression of expression. Prison officials may not censor inmate correspondence simply to eliminate unflattering or unwelcome opinions or factually inaccurate statements. Rather they must show that a regulation authorizing mail censorship furthers one or more of the substantial governmental interests of security, order and habilitation. Second, the limitation on First Amendment freedoms must be no greater than is necessary or essential to the protection of the particular governmental

interest involved. Thus a restriction on inmate correspondence that furthers an important or substantial interest in penal administration will nevertheless be invalid if its sweep is unnecessarily broad.

In *Davis v. Balson,* 461 S.Supp. 842 (N.D.Ohio 1978), the court relied on *Martinez* in holding that interdicting letters from mental patients addressed to the Pope and the Queen of England was not permissible.

In light of this caselaw, consider the examples of actual or contemplated censorship provided in Davidson, "Mental Hospitals and the Civil Liberties Dilemma," 31 Mental Hygiene 371, 374–76 (1967):

A letter from a patient, addressed to a 12–year–old child, was in an envelope that was bordered by a bizarre design. The child's mother opened it and found a letter containing imaginative sexual proposals, all profusely illustrated by the patient with fine artistic skill. The father called the hospital in understandable indignation.

A high school team played baseball on the grounds of our hospital. A male patient fell in love with one of the boys—from a distance—and sent him a homosexual love letter.

A 70–year–old patient, whose 40–year–old daughter had applied for her commitment, sent a letter to her 10–year–old granddaughter, addressing it to her at school. She wrote: "Your mother is a whore. She sent me away to get rid of me so she could entertain men at home. She will do the same to you unless you send her away." The child read this letter, and was brutally shocked. The mother felt that the child was entitled to some protection from communications like this.

* * *

. . . In the last three years we have had to impose restrictions on the outgoing mail of 11 patients. Since we have 3,800 patients, that is not a bad ratio. ·. . .   The telephone has been a more troublesome instrument and, in three years we have had to put some restrictions on use of the phone by 26 patients, because the recipients of obscene, threatening, or other painful calls made protests to us.

* * *

Most acutely mental ill patients recover; and they would then be embarrassed by the delusional ideas expressed in their own handwriting. It may sound sanctimonious to say that we are censoring mail for the patient's own good; but, in truth, that *does* happen. I recall a lawyer who came to us in a manic attack. He sent out some very silly letters to his valued clients, overflowing with reckless and grandiose ideas. When he recovered, he found that they would never trust him again. He upbraided us for not stopping those foolish letters.

Statutes protect the privacy of patients by restricting any general revelation of their identities. Thus, we may not permit "pen pals" to fish for names of patients, no matter how worthy their project may be. Sometimes we get into trouble because a patient has written home identifying another patient as being in the same ward, thus violating that other patient's right of privacy. The only way we could plug that leak would be to censor the first patient's mail—but this is where we came in in the first place. As you see, it is not as simple as it sounds.

How should a hospital handle such situations? Is it permissible to indicate on the outside of the envelope that the sender is a mental patient?

Other censorship issues arose in connection with John Hinckley, who was hospitalized after his acquittal by reason of insanity on charges of shooting President Reagan and three others. Hospital officials routinely intercepted his outgoing mail. One letter they found requested aid in killing actress Jodie Foster, the actress about whom Hinckley apparently fantasized in his plotting to assassinate President Reagan. The letter was turned over to the F.B.I. Hinckley was also denied interviews with the media pursuant to the following policy:

> The purpose of this policy is to prohibit personal interviews of patients on the maximum security wards . . . by representatives of the media. This policy is being enacted based upon a concern that such interviews and publicity could adversely affect the clinical well-being and treatment progress of such patients. These maximum security patients . . . may be unable to understand the implications of their own statements to the media. It is felt that this policy is necessary in order to preserve the integrity of patients' treatment and to prevent a disruption of the therapeutic milieu of these wards.

The policy applied to all personal interviews, face-to-face and over the phone, but not to communication with the media by mail. In a suit brought in federal court, Hinckley alleged the policy violated his first amendment right. The court rejected Hinckley's claim, finding that the policy, as applied to Hinckley "is reasonably related to legitimate therapeutic and institutional interests." *U.S. v. Hinckley,* Criminal No. 81–0306, Nov. 28, 1989.

Note that *Wyatt* allowed restrictions on incoming mail, if a "Qualified Mental Health Professional" so orders (see Appendix, para. 5). Is this permissible under *Martinez?* Why was the *Wyatt* court willing to allow restrictions on incoming but not outgoing mail? If incoming mail is opened by staff, should the patient have the right to be present?

8. *Payment for maintenance labor.* *Wyatt* included relatively detailed rules concerning patient labor. See Appendix, para. 18. Particularly important are its provisions governing labor involving the operation and maintenance of the hospital or for which the hospital would otherwise have to pay an employee. See Appendix, paras. 18A and 18B(2). These provisions were thought necessary to prevent exploitation of patients. Through the mid–1970's hospitals routinely required patients to perform, without pay, housekeeping in the wards, grounds maintenance, laundry duty, cooking and farming. For instance, in *Weidenfeller v. Kidulis,* 380 F.Supp. 445 (E.D.Wis.1974) the court described a 44 year-old mentally retarded man who "mowed the grass, cleaned patients' rooms, and washed dishes in the kitchen," and a 31 year-old mentally retarded male whose "tasks included such endeavors as unloading various materials, cleaning toilets and sinks, and scrubbing the kitchen floor," neither of whom were paid. In a study of 154 institutions conducted in 1972, approximately 30% of the patient workers (out of a total of 32,180) were not paid at all, and 50% received less than $10.00 a week. Friedman, "The Mentally Handicapped Citizen and Institutional Labor," 87 Harv.L.Rev. 567, 568 (1974). Another study indi-

cated that patient labor saved the state of Pennsylvania roughly $10 million a year. See S. Brakel, J. Parry & B. Weiner, The Mentally Disabled and the Law 280 (1985).

In some hospitals, privileges were denied if a patient refused to perform hospital maintenance work. Moreover, there was some evidence that institutions were reluctant to release people whose work skills had become "valuable" to the institution. Friedman, supra at 361. One commentator even concluded that work programs exacerbated the "institutionalization" process: "formerly skilled persons can become satisfied dishwashers [while] patients on the wards who are not working and who could benefit from learning to wash dishes are denied this opportunity," thus "repeat[ing the patients'] pre-institutional role of failure, this time in the still more destructive role of public charge." Bartlett, "Institutional Peonage," Atlantic Monthly, July 1964 at 116.

Properly administered, however, hospital work programs have been defended "as a fair and equitable pact mutually beneficial to both parties and as an opportunity for secure work with limited demands not readily found in the society at large." Brakel, Parry & Weiner, supra at 281. Uncompensated maintenance labor has been viewed as "therapeutic" for the patient to the extent it develops "new skills to help economic self-sufficiency . . . [and] a sense of routine." It may also be "a means for the resident to contribute to the costs of his care," thus promoting a feeling of self-worth, and provide "relief from the boredom of doing nothing." Id. Contrary to the suggestion above that work may lead to dependency on the institution, others have argued that a meaningful work role "modifies the tendency for a 'person' to erode into a 'patient';" for the long-term or chronically ill, "it can serve as a pivotal force in rehabilitation." Schwartz, "Expanding a Sheltered Workshop to Replace Nonpaying Patients Jobs," 27 Hosp. & Comm. Psychiat. 98, 99 (1976).

To some extent, Judge Johnson seemed to have been persuaded by the latter arguments. Six months after the *Wyatt* decree was issued, he modified paragraph 18A requiring compensation for institution-maintaining labor, for reasons described in Note, "The *Wyatt* Case: Implementation of a Judicial Decree Ordering Institutional Change," 84 Yale L.J. 1338, 1376 (1975):

> Shortly after the decree was entered, the Partlow Human Rights committee began to note numerous complaints from patients who had been working without compensation before the issuance of the decree but who, after the issuance of the decree, were no longer allowed to work because the administration allegedly lacked the resources to pay them. 'These residents are now bored and anxious to be doing something,' the PHRC noted. This problem had not been foreseen by the court. It was eventually corrected by clarifying the decree to allow patients to perform uncompensated labor for therapeutic purposes.

Nonetheless, the courts have generally held that, with the exception of personal chores, maintenance labor must be compensated. Most commonly, these decisions rely on the provisions of the Fair Labor Standards Act. Plaintiffs have also argued, however, that the thirteenth amendment and the right to treatment require the same result. These three legal avenues are examined below.

The Thirteenth Amendment. The thirteenth amendment prohibits "slavery" and "involuntary servitude." Courts have held that a valid thirteenth amendment claim requires proof (1) that the work was done involuntarily and (2) that there is no compelling governmental interest justifying the involuntary labor. *Butler v. Perry,* 240 U.S. 328, 36 S.Ct. 258, 60 L.Ed. 672 (1916). With respect to the involuntariness requirement, the Supreme Court has held, in the context of a criminal action against state officials based on an alleged violation of the thirteenth amendment, that unpaid labor is not involuntary unless it is produced by "the use or threat of physical restraint or physical injury" or "the use or threat of coercion through law or the legal process." *United States v. Kozminski,* 487 U.S. 931, 108 S.Ct. 2751, 101 L.Ed.2d 788 (1988). The Court went on to state:

> Our holding does not imply that evidence of other means of coercion, or of poor working conditions, or of the victim's special vulnerabilities is irrelevant in a prosecution under these statutes. [T]he vulnerabilities of the victim are relevant in determining whether the physical or legal coercion or threat thereof could plausibly have compelled the victim to serve. In addition, a trial court could properly find that evidence of other means of coercion or of extremely poor working conditions is relevant to corroborate disputed evidence regarding the use or threatened use of physical or legal coercion, the defendant's intention in using such means, or the causal effect of such conduct. We hold only that the jury must be instructed that compulsion of services by the use or threatened use of physical or legal coercion is a necessary incident of a condition of involuntary servitude.

One earlier case dealing with the application of the thirteenth amendment to patient labor stated that the "source of coercion" could be "said to be the boredom of institutional life and the belief of patients that it will be advantageous to them to appear to cooperate with the institution." Moreover, "coercion results from deprivation of the right to leave the ward on 'grounds' privileges or being otherwise restricted." *Downs v. Department of Public Welfare,* 368 F.Supp. 454, 458–59 (E.D.Pa.1973). Would any of these "sources of coercion" be found to implicate the thirteenth amendment today? Are there any other sources of coercion?

With respect to the second aspect of thirteenth amendment analysis, all courts agree that the government interest in requiring uncompensated patient labor is "compelling" if the labor can be characterized as "therapeutic." Most courts have placed a "heavy burden" on the plaintiff to demonstrate that a particular task is not therapeutic. *Weidenfuller v. Kidulis,* supra at 451. Thus, one court found that over 6,000 hours of work "at several different jobs, varying from food preparation and service to . . . cleaning and maintenance of the physical plant of the hospital" were "related to a therapeutic program of rehabilitation." *Estate of Buzzelle v. Colorado State Hospital,* 176 Colo. 554, 556, 491 P.2d 1369, 1370–71 (1971). Moreover, many courts have held that, under some circumstances, involuntary work that is admittedly *non*therapeutic fails to implicate the thirteenth amendment. In *Jobson v. Henne,* 355 F.2d 129 (2d Cir.1966), the

leading case in this regard, the court held that "the states are not . . .
foreclosed [by the thirteenth amendment] from requiring that a lawfully
committed inmate perform without compensation certain chores designed
to reduce the financial burden placed on a state by its program of treatment for the mentally retarded, if the chores are reasonably related to a
therapeutic program, or if not directly so related, chores of a normal house
keeping type and kind." Id. at 132. In *Krieger v. New York*, 54 Misc.2d
583, 283 N.Y.S.2d 86 (1966), the court found that a resident required to mop
floors, clean toilet bowls and other similar work "had no cause of action
[under the thirteenth amendment] because the work was 'of a normal
housekeeping type and kind.'" Id. at 89.

 Fair Labor Standards Act. Patient claims for compensation have been
much more successful when brought under the Fair Labor Standards Act,
which establishes minimum wage and maximum hour levels. 29 U.S.C.
§§ 201–219. In 1966, the Act was amended to apply to state hospitals and
institutions for the mentally disabled, with provision for payment below the
minimum wage to workers unable to work at a normal level because of
mental or physical handicap. In *Wyatt*, Judge Johnson ordered that, in
those circumstances when payment was due (recall the modification to the
order discussed earlier), it had to be in accordance with the FLSA. See
Appendix, paras. 18A, 18B(2)(c). Other courts went further. In *Souder v.
Brennan*, 367 F.Supp. 808 (D.D.C.1973), the court held that the Act applied
to virtually all work performed by patients at state institutions.

> Economic reality is the test of employment and the reality is that
> many patient-workers perform work for which they are in no way
> handicapped and from which the institution derives full economic
> benefit. So long as the institution derives any consequential economic
> benefit the economic reality test would indicate an employment rela-
> tionship rather than mere therapeutic exercise. To hold otherwise
> would make therapy the sole justification for thousands of positions as
> dishwashers, kitchen helpers, messengers, and the like.

Id. at 813. Obviously, *Souder's* definition of therapeutic work under the
FLSA, which is widely followed, is quite different from the typical definition of therapeutic work under the thirteenth amendment. Are there
reasons for this distinction? In any event, is it correct to assume, as the
Souder court seems to, that a particular job's economic benefit to the state
is inversely related to its "therapeutic value"? Is there a better way to
define the term?

 Souder has had a dampening effect on patient work programs. Even
with the provision for sub-minimum wage compensation for handicapped
individuals, most states discontinued such programs because of the financial burden imposed by decisions following the *Souder* rationale. Lebar,
"Worker–Patients: Receiving Therapy or Suffering Peonage?" 62 A.B.A.J.
219 (1976).

 The Right to Treatment. In response to this latter development,
plaintiffs have argued that the constitutional right to treatment *requires*
the state to provide such programs. Such an argument was made, for
instance, in *Schindenwolf v. Klein,* reported in 5 MDLR 60 (N.J.Super.Ct.,
Mercer Cty.1980); the result was a consent decree in which New Jersey

agreed to employ or provide vocational rehabilitation for 25% of the patients in five state facilities. Under the decree, this group of patients would be given institutional work assignments which do "not impede the residents' movement towards discharge" and which are neither "created nor maintained for the sole purpose of providing residents with activity." Id. at 63. The decree required that this work be compensated; personal housekeeping chores required of the patients need not be.

Of the arguments that can be advanced in support of the result in *Schindenwolf* the strongest derives from the least restrictive alternative rationale for the right to treatment. As described by Perlin, the plaintiffs' attorney in *Schindenwolf* litigation, the least restrictive alternative doctrine "mandates that infringement of individual interests and liberties go no further than that which is absolutely necessary for the achievement of the state's interest. Since the state's interest in confinement is treatment coupled with security, the right to work, especially in light of the demonstrated viability and success of therapeutic work programs, must be preserved." Perlin, "The Right to Voluntary, Compensated, Therapeutic Work as Part of the Right to Treatment: A New Theory in the Aftermath of *Souder,*" 7 Seton Hall L.Rev. 298, 332–33 (1976). Does the right to treatment rationale for patient work programs necessarily require that such programs be either voluntary or compensated? Consider the conclusion of Scoles & Fine, in "Aftercare and Rehabilitation in a Community Mental Health Center," Social Work 75, 78 (July, 1971), that "[n]othing appears to be a greater stimulus to engage in activities that reflect health instead of illness than to be paid for the product of those activities."

In light of the foregoing, reread the description of the work required of Fred Thomas by the staff at Tarry Hall (pp. 957–959). What is your analysis of the work arrangement? Should basic privileges such as access to one's own money be contingent on the performance of routine chores?

9. *Enforcing the right to treatment and habilitation.* Throughout the *Wyatt* litigation, Judge Johnson attempted to avoid dramatic confrontation with the state. His handling of the state's "budgetary defense" is one example. In *Wyatt v. Stickney,* he clearly stated that the state of Alabama would not be able to avoid constitutional dictates through pleading insolvency. As the decision indicates, he even contemplated ordering the state to sell land in order to provide funding for the hospital system. But the order was never issued. The Fifth Circuit was equally circumspect in this regard. In *Wyatt v. Aderholt,* 503 F.2d 1305, 1318 (5th Cir.1974), it stated that "[t]he serious constitutional questions presented by federal judicial action ordering the sale of state land, or altering the state budget, or which may otherwise arise in the problem of financing, in the event the governing authorities fail to move in good faith to ensure what all parties agree are minimal requirements, should not be adjudicated unnecessarily and prematurely." As this passage indicates, the court's caution resulted both from concern over the scope of federal judicial authority over state legislatures and from a perception that the state had been relatively cooperative up to that point.

When the state is *not* cooperative, what options short of the rather dubious step of ordering the state legislature to appropriate money are available to a federal court? One option is to close down the institutions. This approach has been taken in prison cases. See, e.g., *Ramos v. Lamm*, 485 F.Supp. 122, 169–70 (D.Colo.1979). A second option for the court is use of its contempt authority to force the relevant officials to act in accordance with the court order. On one occasion, for instance, the *Wyatt* plaintiffs moved to cite several Bryce staff members for violating paragraph 9 of the order concerning electroshock therapy. Although the citation was not granted, no further violations of this part of the order occurred. See Drake, "Judicial Implementation and *Wyatt v. Stickney*," 32 Ala.L.Rev. 299, 308 (1981).

Also illustrated by *Wyatt* is the use of masters and receivers. The receiver appointed in *Wyatt v. Ireland* was responsible for overseeing the operation of the Alabama hospitals and reporting to the court. Court-appointed officials can also perform more limited functions. As an example of the latter role, in *Lynch v. Baxley*, 386 F.Supp. 378 (M.D.Ala.1974), the court ordered special judges to preside over discharge hearings at Bryce and Searcy; over 3,100 patients were evaluated, and of that number 1,287 were discharged, 888 were committed, 777 were held pending placement, and 167 were voluntarily committed. Drake, supra at 309. Another potentially powerful enforcement mechanism is economic sanction. The court can assess damages for constitutional violations on a per patient, per day basis. Id. at 309–310.

A final enforcement mechanism, perhaps the most important, is a reliable information-gathering and advocacy system. Judge Johnson appointed human rights committees and monitors who were charged with reporting to the court about compliance with the order. His order also provided that "[p]atients shall have an unrestricted right to visitation with attorneys." Appendix, para. 4. Other approaches are legion. The Developmentally Disabled Assistance and Bill of Rights Act of 1975, 42 U.S.C. § 6012, provided funding for advocates for the developmentally disabled. Although supporting appropriations have since been drastically reduced, the model provided by the Act has encouraged state-funded advocacy services, usually relying on hospital employees. Many hospitals also have legal aid services, funded by a number of different mechanisms, which provide legal representation on discharge, "institutional" and civil legal issues. See Brakel, "Legal Aid in Mental Hospitals," 1981 Am.Bar. Found.Res.Journ. 23. One of the best known hospital operations, combining aspects of the advocacy services and legal aid, is the Mental Hygiene Legal Service (formerly the Mental Health Information Service) in New York. Composed of lawyers and mental health professionals, MHLS acts as an intermediary between hospital personnel and patients and between patients and the courts, informs patients of their rights, and investigates patients' claims. See Gupta, "New York's Mental Health Information Service: An Experiment in Due Process," 25 Rutgers L.Rev. 405 (1971).

An even more elaborate arrangement is suggested by Hoffman and Dunn, in "Guaranteeing the Right to Treatment," reprinted in Bonnie, ed., Psychiatrists and the Legal Process: Diagnosis and Debate 298 (1977). They propose that an administrative law model be used to implement the right to treatment. They suggest (1) the creation of a rule-making board, whose primary function would be to "promulgat[e] regulations to ensure the preservation of statutory and constitutional rights of mental patients;" (2) the designation of "treatment evaluators," psychiatrists who would be "authorized, if appropriate, to conduct informal but adversarial proceedings following alleged violations of patients' rights;" (3) the installation of a legal-aid services, which like New York's Mental Hygiene Legal Service would consist of full-time attorneys who would inform patients of their rights, investigate alleged violations and represent patients in proceedings before treatment evaluators, mental health judges, and other legal tribunals; and (4) the creation of a panel of mental health judges, who would develop an expertise in the mental health area and "preside over commitment proceedings and . . . appeals from some of the decisions made by treatment evaluators." Id. at 308–310, 317.

If a lawyer is involved in monitoring the rights of institutionalized persons, what should his or her role be? At least one commentator has suggested that the traditional adversarial stance is not appropriate in most situations:

> For the in-hospital lawyer to act in [an adversarial] fashion routinely, for him to take seriously and pursue uncompromisingly the bulk of patient complaints and grievances or to generally set himself up as a force hostile to the institution only spells disaster. It bogs the lawyer down in controversies of little merit whose ultimate outcome is often not in the best interests of either the individual patient or the general patient population. It causes him to lose the cooperation of the institutional staff without which—given the knowledge of and control over patients possessed by the staff—it is difficult to do the patients' interests justice. Carried far enough, this approach could also seriously hamper the institution's capacity to work to the benefit of the patients. The achievement of success in institutionally treating mental patients is already difficult enough—the illnesses may not be curable, the staff may be overworked and insufficiently expert, and the prospects upon discharge, even after improvement, may be dismal because the underlying or contributing conditions (problems of family, money, employment) remain unchanged. For a legal project to further reduce the chances of success by creating needless antagonisms between patients and staff and by intimidating medical or supervisory personnel and inhibiting them in carrying out their functions is irresponsible.

Brakel, supra at 90.

10. *The right to treatment in private institutions.* A number of states are now encouraging private operators to establish facilities for treatment and habilitation of the mentally disabled. For instance, Illinois is offering private interests long term contracts which provide state reimbursement for services rendered to patients, including institutional treatment. Are such facilities governed by the constitutional rulings described above? In other words, is there "state action" in such situations?

In *Blum v. Yaretsky,* 457 U.S. 991, 102 S.Ct. 2777, 73 L.Ed.2d 534 (1982), the Supreme Court held that medical residents of a private nursing home had failed to establish that a decision by the home to transfer them to a lower-level facility had a sufficient nexus with the state. Neither the fact that state funds paid for more than 90 percent of the cost of the patients' care nor the fact that the facility was extensively regulated by state agencies was deemed sufficient to establish state action. However, the court also noted that the home was not performing "a function that has traditionally been the exclusive prerogative of the State."

In *West v. Atkins,* 487 U.S. 42, 108 S.Ct. 2250, 101 L.Ed.2d 40 (1988), the Court indicated that this latter caveat may cover state-retained private caretakers. In *Atkins,* the Court held that Dr. Atkins, a private doctor hired by the state prison to operate two clinics each week at the prison, was a "state official acting under color of state law" for purposes of a civil rights action against the state:

> . . . It is the physician's function within the state system, not the precise terms of his employment, that determines whether his actions can fairly be attributed to the State. Whether a physician is on the state payroll or is paid by contract, the dispositive issue concerns the relationship among the State, the physician, and the prisoner. Contracting out prison medical care does not relieve the State of its constitutional duty to provide adequate medical treatment to those in its custody[.] . . . The State bore an affirmative obligation to provide adequate medical care to West; the State delegated that function to respondent Atkins; and respondent voluntarily assumed that obligation by contract.

Under the Court's decisions, would a halfway house such as Tarry Hall in Houston, described at pp. 957–959, be governed by the constitution?

11. *Reimbursement for treatment.* Every state has enacted legislation making voluntary *and* involuntary patients liable for the cost of their treatment. Forty-seven states extend this liability to the patient's relatives, usually including at least the patient's spouse, parents and adult children. S. Brakel, J. Parry & B. Weiner, The Mentally Disabled and the Law 168–170, Table 2.17. At least one court has held that since prisoners do not have to pay for the cost of their imprisonment, such statutes are unconstitutional. In *Department of Mental Hygiene v. Kirchner,* 60 Cal.2d 716, 36 Cal.Rptr. 488, 388 P.2d 720 (1964), the California Supreme Court declared:

> Whether the commitment is incidental to an alleged violation of a penal statute . . . or is essentially a civil commitment as in the instant case, the purposes of confinement and treatment or care in either case encompass the protection of society from the confined person, and his own protection and possible reclamation as a productive member of the body politic. Hence the cost of maintaining the state institution, including provision of adequate care for its inmates, cannot be arbitrarily charged to one class in the society; such assessment violates the equal protection clause.[d]

d. On remand from the U.S. Supreme Court, the California Supreme Court held that *Kirchner* was based on an interpreta-tion of the equal protection clause in the California constitution. 43 Cal.Rptr. 329, 400 P.2d 321 (1965). *Kirchner's* reach has

Most courts, contrary to *Kirchner*, have upheld state reimbursement statutes against such equal protection challenges. See, e.g., *In re Guardianship of Nelson*, 98 Wis.2d 261, 296 N.W.2d 736 (1980). Is there a rational basis for distinguishing between prisoners and patients in this regard? Might the state have to show *more* than a rational basis?

Consider in this regard *Chill v. Mississippi Hospital Reimbursement Commission*, 429 So.2d 574 (Miss.1983), in which the court held that, given a state statute which prohibited the state from seeking reimbursement "beyond ability to pay," "the legitimate needs and comforts of the patient and his or her dependents or surviving relatives" had an "absolute priority" over state claims. Id. 586–87. In *Nelson*, by contrast, the trial court's order granting the state all but $1,500 of the patient's $27,000 estate was affirmed. Might not the *Nelson* holding deter mentally disabled persons and their relatives from seeking treatment?

Assuming the state is entitled to reimbursement from the patient and relatives, how is the amount owed to be computed? Should every patient pay the same per diem amount or are those committed for treatment purposes liable for a greater amount than those committed primarily for incapacitative reasons?

A final question is whether the state may levy on funds the patients earn at the hospital. At the end of its provisions concerning patient labor, the *Wyatt* order states that "[p]ayment to patients pursuant to these paragraphs shall not be applied to the costs of hospitalization." See Appendix, para. 18D. What is the rationale for this rule? Consider the arguments in favor of allowing patient wages to setoff part of the costs of hospitalization in Kapp, "Residents of State Mental Institutions and Their Money (or, the State Giveth and the State Taketh Away)," 6 J.Psychiat. & Law 287, 304–05 (1979):

> [S]et-offs could provide a fair way to balance the resident's fundamental need to work (and to do so without exploitation), against the legitimate interest of the state mental health official in averting bankruptcy. The resident could be protected by a regulation limiting the percentage of his wages that could be set-off against his institutional charges, so that he would be assured of actually pocketing some of his earnings. Payment of wages, even if immediately recouped by the state, would give the resident knowledge that he or she is earning his or her room and board, and is not a mere ward of the state, knowledge which carries a sense of accomplishment, self-respect, and dignity of considerable therapeutic worth. Finally, permitting a resident to work and earn wages, even if they are subject to a set-off, could potentially provide him or her with certain tangible benefits including social security, state retirement payments, and workmen's compensation.

since been significantly curtailed. See, e.g., *Swoap v. Superior Court*, 10 Cal.3d 490, 111 Cal.Rptr. 136, 516 P.2d 840 (1973).

IV. THE RIGHT TO COMMUNITY SERVICES

In paragraph 34 of the order in *Wyatt v. Stickney,* the court decreed that the Alabama Mental Health Board and its agents "have an affirmative duty to provide adequate transitional treatment and care for all patients released after a period of involuntary confinement." A similar provision appeared in the Partlow order. 344 F.Supp. at 397, 407. Yet subsequently the court substantially undercut these provisions, as described in Note, "The *Wyatt* Case: Implementation of a Judicial Decree Ordering Institutional Change," 84 Yale L.J. 1339, 1374–75 (1975):

> Because some . . . members [of the Partlow Human Rights Committee] became concerned that certain former residents had not been properly placed outside the institution but instead were "dumped" into the community, [the Committee] raised the question of whether the decree and the committee's responsibility extended to residents who had been discharged from the institution. In response to a PHRC request for clarification of its responsibility, the district court explicitly restricted the committee to the institution.

> Because the PHRC was the only method the court had to supervise the decree, this restriction effectively limited the scope of the decree to the institution's walls. Yet it was clear that problems existed with residents released from the institution. Storekeepers in local communities complained of former residents engaging in such conduct as urinating on the floors, opening up and using packages of make-up, and bouncing on beds in furniture stores. Discharged residents allegedly engaged in improper sexual behavior, leading to complaints and criminal charges. Citizens of one town in Alabama applied for and were granted a state court injunction to close a halfway house for residents discharged from one of the *Wyatt* institutions, alleging that the house was so badly supervised that it constituted a nuisance which devalued local property. The lack of adequate post-institutional placement and followup was also evidenced by complaints received by the Alabama Mental Health Board from local mental health organizations, which stated that Partlow residents had been inappropriately placed under their care in facilities that were not suited to meet those persons' needs.

> The district court's decision to limit the PHRC's jurisdiction to the institution was probably founded on well-intentioned beliefs that the problems should be attacked one at a time. However, the court apparently failed to anticipate that the decree itself would create problems outside the institution, through the discharge of residents, and thus did not take sufficient measures to minimize these effects.

* * *

As this passage illustrates, for most patients a right to treatment is not particularly effective unless it also applies outside the institution. The following materials explore the right to treatment in the community.

LELSZ v. KAVANAGH

United States Court of Appeals, Fifth Circuit, 1987.
807 F.2d 1243.

EDITH H. JONES, CIRCUIT JUDGE:

This saga began in 1974 when a class action was filed against officials of the Texas Department of Mental Health and Mental Retardation (MHMR) alleging widespread abuses of mentally retarded patients and advocating their habilitation in the "least restrictive alternative" setting as a minimum standard of care. Simultaneously, a class represented by the same counsel were pursuing the same relief in Pennsylvania. In this appeal, we VACATE the district court's order dated June 5, 1985, which purports to enforce a consent decree between the class and the State by requiring the State to furlough no less than 279 class members from institutional to "community care" centers by September 1, 1986. For reasons elaborated upon below, the district court was without jurisdiction to award such state-law-based relief.

I. PROCEDURAL HISTORY

The class certified by the district court comprised approximately 2,400 residents of the Austin, Denton and Fort Worth state schools for the mentally retarded, representing approximately 26% of the "clients" of the State's thirteen institutional centers which care for the mentally retarded. In May, 1983, following at least two years of negotiations, a consent decree (the "Resolution and Settlement" or "R & S") was worked out between the parties. After giving appropriate notice and conducting an extensive hearing, the trial court approved the R & S. The court issued a lengthy opinion outlining the background of and legal basis for the consent decree. Order of July 21, 1983. The R & S is 21 pages long, consisting of 45 paragraphs of both specific and general guidelines and directives for the improvement of treatment of the mentally retarded.

The R & S set no timetable for developing community treatment centers, nor did it require the State to do more than exert its "best efforts" to provide such centers. Despite the lack of a timetable, the class representatives determined to press state officials for creation of community care centers by filing a "Motion for Community Placement" in February, 1985, less than two years after the R & S was entered. The motion requested that 779 class members, nearly one-third of those housed in the three state schools, be transferred immediately into the community. According to the class representatives, such a measure was necessary to fulfill the R & S. Further, the class contended that individualized habilitation profiles prepared for the class members by an interdisciplinary team of experts selected pursuant to the R & S reflected that 279 members of the class would be best served by transfer to community facilities. The State responded that it was in good faith complying with the R & S. Specifically, it had developed a comprehensive plan whereby 900 individuals from the thirteen state schools would be placed into community facilities during the 1985–87 biennium. . . . Obviously, a certain percentage of these statewide placements would be of class members, but the State was unable to estimate the number.

Following a hearing on the plaintiffs' motion, the district court ordered 279 class members to be transferred to community centers on or before September 1, 1986. Order of June 5, 1985. Because the . . . State had at the time of the hearing neither so placed those individuals nor guaranteed their transfer, the court found the State in breach of the R & S. The court chastised the State for foot-dragging and delay in implementing community placement, and the court insisted that the "feasible" plan for such furloughs developed by an expert retained in consequence of the class action was more "convincing" than the rationale adduced by the State. In response to the State's argument that it could not discriminatorily favor class members over residents of other institutions when making community placements, the court concluded that "if defendants wish to see in the court's obligation to enforce the Resolution and Settlement as to class members the creation of a 'two-tier' system in Texas, they may so name it. . . ." [4] The court also by its own account "overrode" state law procedures detailing the rights of parents in the determination of community placement, and replaced that law with a complex scheme designed by a court-appointed attorney. The Order of June 5 is the principal subject of this appeal. The State also appeals the denial of its motion to modify the June 5 Order to obtain similar relief.

II. JURISDICTION TO ENTER THE JUNE 5, 1985 ORDER

* * *

[Here the court noted that in *Pennhurst v. Halderman*, 465 U.S. 89, 104 S.Ct. 900, 79 L.Ed.2d 67 (1984) (*Pennhurst II*), the Supreme Court had held that the Eleventh Amendment prohibits federal courts from enforcing claims based on state law, unless the state consents to such suits. The court then proceeded to analyze the extent to which the district court's order rested on state law.]

III. THE STATE LAW BASIS FOR PROVISIONS OF THE RESOLUTION AND SETTLEMENT

Juxtaposing paragraphs 7 and 8 of the Resolution and Settlement, on which the district court rested its Order of June 5, 1985, with applicable state law reflects the congruence between them.

---

4. By its order, the district court re-allocated the $12.1 million appropriated by the Texas Legislature to create community placements for the clients of all thirteen state schools. The district court recognized that this sum was allocated to minimize the staff-to-patient ratios within all the state schools and was sufficient to make approximately 300 placements, per year, state wide. One must conclude that the district court knew that its order requiring such re-allocation of funds would disadvantage non-class residents of state schools.

II. Obligations of Defendants

7. The defendants will provide to each member of the plaintiff class habilitation tailored to the person's individual needs. In meeting the habilitation needs of members of the plaintiff class, the individual's particular circumstances, including age, degree of retardation and handicapping conditions, will be taken into account. Habilitation is that education, training and care required by each plaintiff class member to improve and develop the person's level of social and intellectual functioning, designed to maximize skills and development and to enhance ability to cope with the environment, and provided in the setting which is least restrictive of the person's liberty. Defendants will provide habilitation services necessary to meet the needs of plaintiff class members until such time as they no longer require services under this Resolution and Settlement.

8. Defendants will provide each member of the plaintiff class with the least restrictive alternative living conditions possible consistent with the person's particular circumstances, including age, degree of retardation and handicapping conditions. Consistent with the person's capacities, each member of the plaintiff class will be taught adequate skills to help the person progress within the environment and to live as independently as possible. Services will be offered with utmost regard for the class member's dignity and personal autonomy.

Tex.Rev.Civ.Stat.Ann. art. 5547–203 § 3.01A (Vernon Supp.1986) provides:

Community centers created pursuant to this Act are intended to be vital components in a continuum of services for the mentally ill and mentally retarded individuals of this state. It is the policy of this state that community centers strive to develop services for the mentally ill and mentally retarded that are effective alternatives to treatment in large residential facilities.

Tex.Rev.Civ.Stat.Ann. art. 5547–300 § 15 (Vernon Supp.1986) provides:

Each client shall have the right to live in the least restrictive habilitation setting appropriate to the individual's needs and be treated and served in the least intrusive manner appropriate to the individual's needs.

Recognizing the decisive impact of the foregoing state law, the July 21, 1983 district court Order approving the Resolution and Settlement states more than once that paragraphs 7 and 8 are governed by state law. The district court observed that "each of these provisions [of the R & S] effectuates rights explicitly protected by Texas law (if not implicitly by federal law), including those provisions concerning individual service plans and 'least restrictive alternative' living arrangements. . . ." The court noted that, "[a]lthough more detailed and far-reaching rights—including the right to habilitation in the least restrictive alternative living arrangement—have been located by district courts in the federal constitution and federal law, in this case it is likely that all such relief could and would have been predicated upon the more explicit Texas statutes. Tex.Rev.Civ.Stat.Ann. art. 5547–300 *et seq.*" As the district court recognized, state law confers on the class members, and on all other residents of state institutions for the mentally retarded, the right to live in the least restrictive setting. Because this is the right recognized in the Resolution and Settlement and enforced in the court's Order of June 5, 1985, that order plainly contravenes *Pennhurst II* unless some constitutional or federal right requires similar relief.

IV. THE CONSTITUTIONAL STANDARD OF CARE FOR THE MENTALLY RETARDED

The district court's uncertainty about the scope of federal support for a least restrictive environment was not misplaced. Appellees suggest, as a threshold matter, that the existence of a generalized "constitutional right" to community services for institutionalized mentally retarded people is not at issue before this Court. On the other hand, they contend that the constitutionally-based rights to enjoy safe conditions and to be free from harm, the right to be free from unnecessary institutionalization, and to have commitment bear some reasonable relation to its purpose are coextensive with the rights conferred in paragraphs 7 and 8 of the Resolution and Settlement. The distinction appellees seek to draw eludes us. Appellees are aware that the Supreme Court cases they cite do not cut such a swath.[8] In fact, the lower court cases on which appellees rely for their due process argument are precisely those which have considered, and uniformly rejected, a constitutionally-founded right to receive treatment in the least restrictive alternative setting.[9]

---

8. The Supreme Court cases relied upon by the appellees do not support the alleged relationship between community placements and the class members' rights to safety, freedom from bodily restraint, and minimally adequate habilitation. For example, the appellees have relied upon the landmark case of *Youngberg v. Romeo*, 457 U.S. 307, 102 S.Ct. 2452, 73 L.Ed.2d 28 (1982) in an attempt to transform the state right of a least restrictive environment into a federal right. The Supreme Court, however, refused to adopt the "least intrusive means" approach which had been relied upon by the Court of Appeals in its opinion in *Youngberg (Romeo v. Youngberg,* 644 F.2d 147 (3d Cir.1980) (en banc) (*See also Rennie v. Klein,* 720 F.2d 266, 268 (3d Cir. 1983)).

Another case, *Parham v. J.R.,* 442 U.S. 584, 99 S.Ct. 2493, 61 L.Ed.2d 101 (1979), is cited by appellees for the proposition that the mentally ill have a right to be free from unnecessary institutionalization. In *Parham* the issue under consideration involved possible *procedural* due process violations resulting from a state's procedures

for the commitment of minors. *Parham* had nothing to do with an individual's right to be confined in the least restrictive environment.

* * *

Finally, the appellees look to another Supreme Court case that addresses unacceptable commitment and review procedures for incompetent *criminal defendants. Jackson v. Indiana,* 406 U.S. 715, 92 S.Ct. 1845, 32 L.Ed.2d 435 (1972). Again, we find nothing in the case which would sway us toward appellees' view that the case supports a "least intrusive means" analysis. It merely holds that the nature and duration of a civil commitment must bear some reasonable relationship to the purpose for the confinement.

9. The appellees look to two cases, in particular, to support their argument favoring a constitutionally-founded right to receive treatment in the least restrictive alternative setting. In the first case, *Clark v. Cohen,* 794 F.2d 79 (3d Cir.1986), the Third Circuit entered an order directing the state to develop a program of commu-

In *Society for Good Will to Retarded Children v. Cuomo,* 737 F.2d 1239 (2d Cir.1984), the court stated, "we may consider only whether there is an entitlement to community placement or a 'least restrictive environment' under the federal Constitution. We hold that there is no such entitlement." The Second Circuit based its decision on the holding of *Youngberg v. Romeo,* 457 U.S. 307, 102 S.Ct. 2452, 73 L.Ed.2d 28 (1982), which confirmed the state's duty under the Fourteenth Amendment to provide adequate food, shelter, clothing, reasonable safety, and such training as "an appropriate professional would consider reasonable to ensure [a person's] safety and to facilitate his ability to function free from bodily restraints." *Youngberg* also held that in determining whether the state has met its obligations in these respects, decisions made by the appropriate professional are entitled to a presumption of correctness. "[L]iability may be imposed only when the decision by the professional is such a substantial departure from accepted professional judgment, practice, or standards as to demonstrate that the person responsible actually did not base the decision on such a judgment." The constitutional minimum standard of habilitation thus relates, not to the qualitative betterment of a retarded person's life, but only to the training necessary to afford him safety and freedom from bodily restraint. Whether that training is adequate must be determined in light of expert testimony; no constitutional violation exists unless the level of training is such a substantial departure from accepted professional judgment or standards as to demonstrate that the person responsible actually did not base the decision on such a judgment.

Reinforcing this view of *Youngberg* is *Society for Good Will, supra,* which further stated that "we may not look to whether the trial testimony established the superiority of a 'least restrictive environment' in general or of community placement in particular. Instead, we

nity services for a mildly retarded individual who had been confined to an institution for 28 years without the benefit of procedural due process. This case differs from the facts now under consideration since the Third Circuit was "dealing with a plaintiff who was committed without notice or hearing as a result of a petition containing an incorrect diagnosis, and who was retained against her will without a hearing for over 28 years." *Id.* at 86.

Clark was an *individual* case where the *only* method to remedy the effects of the unconstitutional confinement was community placement. In other words, community placement was not merely the *best* remedy for the plaintiff but the *only* remedy. The Third Circuit did *not* grant carte blanche, a constitutional right to community placement. Judge Becker in his concurrence noted that the Third Circuit had previously held in *Rennie v. Klein,* 720 F.2d 266 (3d Cir.1983) (en banc) that a right to habilitation did not include the

least restrictive alternative theory. *Clark,* 494 F.2d at 93 n. 9 (Becker, J. concurring).

As in *Clark, Thomas S. v. Morrow,* 781 F.2d 367 (4th Cir.1986) dealt with an *individual* situation where the plaintiff was found to be on the borderline between average intelligence and mild mental retardation. Thomas S. had the *potential* to live independently of the state's care, but was unable to live independently without *minimal* habilitation which involved a community setting. This community habilitation was not "better" care but the *only* way in which the state could remedy its past transgressions against Thomas S. At one point, he had been lodged in a night care unit operated in conjunction with a drug detoxification center (Thomas S. had no drug problems) which was incompatible with the treatment prescribed for him. At other points, he had been placed in a rest home that housed elderly and emotionally ill adults. Thomas S. was the only young person residing at this rest home.

may rule only on whether a decision to keep residents at SDC [Suffolk Developmental Center] is a rational decision based on professional judgment." *Society for Good Will,* 737 F.2d at 1249. The court in *Society for Good Will* therefore concluded that while experts disagreed on the appropriateness of institutionalization, retaining residents at the institution did not violate the professional judgment standard enunciated in *Youngberg.*

Appellees would distinguish *Society for Good Will* with the suggestion that the district court there ordered wholesale transfer of patients from an institution to community facilities, irrespective of individualized professional treatment recommendations. This observation is only partially correct. The Second Circuit noted that the number of placements ordered by the district court was virtually irreconcilable with the profound retardation of the majority of the institution's patients. On the other hand, the Second Circuit criticized the district court's willingness to substitute the judgment of plaintiffs' experts for that of the state's experts, in contravention of *Youngberg.* Critically, appellees' focus on the individual optimum habilitation plans misperceives the real issue, which was articulated by *Society for Good Will,* following *Youngberg.* The real issue is whether the existing level of habilitation represents a gross and unwarranted departure from the minimum standard necessary to preserve an individual's safety and freedom from physical restraint. Appellees' evidence in support of community placement in the district court concerned the optimum habilitation of each class member rather than the constitutional minimum standard. There is no evidence in the record concerning whether the State, at the time of the hearing leading to the June 5, 1985 Order, was denying class members the constitutional minimum standard. Moreover, the appellees never requested enforcement of the R & S to correct alleged failures to adequately protect clients from abuse or neglect or to remedy alleged inadequacies in adaptive equipment for physical therapy. The court never ordered any remedial action to improve these areas of care. No effort was made by any party to the Joint Motion for Community Placement, the expert consultant, or the district court to affect a substantive level of care, only its locale.

It is also worthwhile to observe that should the optimum standard of habilitation afforded class members by state law become coextensive with federal constitutional requirements, the emphasis of *Youngberg* on the judgment of the State's professionals will be thoroughly undermined. The constitutional standard in that instance would be determined by the views of expert witnesses, and outside consultants could effectively overrule state programs, contrary to *Youngberg.* While *Youngberg* may eventually have to be squared with the duty of a state to prevent deterioration of skills of the retarded committed to its institutions (*see Youngberg,* 457 U.S. at 327–29, 102 S.Ct. at 2464–65 (Blackmun, J. concurring)) this is by no means the same as requiring the State to provide the best care possible or the optimum location to improve the client's physical, mental and emotional conditions. As the

Second Circuit aptly noted in *Society for Good Will,* the due process clause only forbids *deprivations* of liberty without due process of law. "Where the state does not provide treatment designed to improve a mentally retarded individual's condition, it deprives the individual of nothing guaranteed by the Constitution; it simply fails to grant a benefit of optimal treatment that it is under no constitutional obligation to grant."

It is therefore our conclusion that the federal constitution does not confer on these class members a right to habilitation in the least restrictive environment. There being no constitutional scope to paragraphs 7 and 8 of the R & S, the district court's decree purporting to enforce them may not rest on that authority and is unauthorized.

V.   ENFORCEMENT OF THE R & S AS A CONSENT DECREE

*   *   *

[Here the court rejected the appellee's argument that by entering into the consent decree the state waived its Eleventh Amendment protection.]

The judgment of the district court is VACATED and the case REMANDED for further proceedings not inconsistent herewith.

WISDOM, CIRCUIT JUDGE, dissenting:

I agree with the majority's vacating the order of the district court. I would remand the case, however, for a hearing to determine whether the defendants have satisfied the Fourteenth Amendment criteria established in *Youngberg* as the minimum standards for the care of the mentally retarded.

I disagree with the majority's expansive view of the Eleventh Amendment and of *Pennhurst II.* The coexistence of similar federal and state rights and remedies does not deprive a federal court of jurisdiction. The plaintiffs brought the action in the federal court, alleging deprivation of their Fourteenth Amendment rights. As early as its order of May 13, 1983, the district court stated:

> The central focus of this case is the right of plaintiffs to safe conditions and to be free from harm, and the right to be free from unnecessary institutionalization. Also, the nature and duration of commitment must bear some reasonable relation to its purpose. The court recognizes the existence of these rights under the Fourteenth Amendment of the United States Constitution.

Order of May 13, 1983 (filed May 19, 1983), at 2–3. In its order of October 3, 1984, the district court again said:

> *Lelsz v. Kavanagh* was brought under the Fourteenth Amendment to the Constitution, and the court's primary obligation in this case is to enforce the Constitution.

The Eleventh Amendment enjoys no exalted position over the Fourteenth. If the plaintiffs have not had a full and fair hearing on their federal rights, they are entitled to one. The decision of the majority deprives them of a hearing on their federal claim.

Questions and Comments

1. *Community treatment for institutionalized patients.* *Lelsz* represents the predominant judicial response to the claim that the constitution requires the state to transfer institutionalized patients who can be treated outside the hospital to community facilities and to create such facilities if they don't exist. In line with *Lelsz* and *Society for Good Will,* cited in *Lelsz,* most courts hold that *Youngberg's* professional judgment rule is the dispositive test in this context: so long as such judgment is exercised, the resulting placement, whether it is an institution or a community facility, is constitutional. See e.g., *Rennie v. Klein,* 720 F.2d 266 (3d Cir.1983); *Phillips v. Thompson,* 715 F.2d 365, 368 (7th Cir.1983).

A few courts appear to reject this narrow view of *Youngberg,* however, at least under certain circumstances. In *Association of Retarded Children v. Olson,* 561 F.Supp. 473, 486 (D.N.D.1982), affirmed 713 F.2d 1384 (8th Cir.1983), the court construed *Youngberg* to mean "that a constitutional right to the least restrictive method of care or treatment exists . . . insofar as professional judgment determines that such alternatives would measurably enhance the resident's enjoyment of basic liberty interests." In *Thomas S. v. Morrow,* 601 F.Supp. 1055 (W.D.N.C.1984), affirmed 781 F.2d 367 (4th Cir.1986), the court applied this reasoning in finding that the plaintiff was entitled to a "a non-institutional specialized adult foster care situation" or "a group home with adults of average intelligence." The state had presented affidavits by state officials contending that the plaintiff's past treatment (which had consisted of placement in over 40 facilities, including mental hospitals) had been "minimally adequate". But the district court rejected this evidence as immaterial "because the professional's stated judgment was modified to conform to the *available* treatment, rather than to the *appropriate* treatment, for the plaintiff's condition." 601 F.Supp. at 1059. Instead the court relied on evidence the plaintiff presented, as well as evidence presented by other state-employed mental health professionals, in finding a "professional consensus" in favor of the ordered placement. Given the existence of the consent decree, how would this reasoning affect the outcome in *Lelsz?* See note 9 of the opinion.

2. *Community treatment for non-institutionalized patients.* Another important aspect of *Thomas S.* was the way in which both the district court and the circuit court of appeals in that case dealt with the fact that, at the time of the district court's final order, the plaintiff had been out of the hospital for about five months and was residing in a "detoxification and night care facility." The defendants argued that under such conditions—not involving commitment to an institution—the state is not infringing any liberty interests, and thus *Youngberg* did not apply. But both the district court and the Fourth Circuit held that the plaintiff's interest in liberty was implicated in this situation. As the Fourth Circuit put it:

Although during the course of this litigation Thomas's lodging has changed from a state hospital to a night care unit at a detoxification center, his status has not changed. He remains a legally incompetent adult who is a ward of a guardian appointed by the state. He did not choose to live at the detoxification center, and he is neither an alcoholic nor a drug addict. *Youngberg* does not suggest that an incompetent person sheds the basic liberty interests that the Court identified when state officials and his guardian move him from one facility to another.

See also, *Clark v. Cohen*, 794 F.2d 79 (3d Cir.), cert. denied 479 U.S. 962, 107 S.Ct. 459, 93 L.Ed.2d 404 (1986). Can this analysis be reconciled with *Youngberg's* statement that "a State is under no constitutional duty to provide substantive services for those within its borders"? What if Thomas had not been a ward of the state?

In "Beyond Least Restrictive Alternative Doctrine: A Constitutional Right to Treatment for Mentally Disabled Persons in the Community," 20 Loyola L.A.L.Rev. 1527 (1987), Costello and Preis conclude that when professional consensus indicates that a particular institutionalized individual or group of institutionalized individuals is "capable of functioning outside an institution with assistance, institutional care *cannot be* 'minimally adequate' treatment." Id. at 1552 (emphasis in original). They go on to argue that this reasoning should apply *whenever* a person or group of people can show that they require community treatment to avoid institutionalization, even if they are not hospitalized at the time they make the claim.

The risk of future involuntary hospitalization is a different kind of restriction on liberty from present institutional confinement. Nevertheless, for many mentally disabled persons caught in the "revolving door," it is a very real one. The crucial element of the revolving door is that it is a closed system: the mentally disabled person, once drawn into the mental health system, is thereafter constantly at risk of rehospitalization. This is not a hypothetical or far-fetched concern; the recidivism rate for persons identified as chronically mentally ill demonstrates the seriousness of the risk. For a person caught in the revolving door, just as for Nicholas Romeo, appropriate treatment and services are required to enable him or her to preserve and exercise liberty.

* * *

For mentally disabled individuals not part of the revolving door, institutionalization may still pose a very real threat. Too often, if the state perceives a mentally disabled person as a legitimate object of concern, under either the parens patriae or police power, the result will be a deprivation of liberty. Historically, institutional confinement has been the price exacted by the state from mentally disabled persons, in return for custodial care. As Governor Wallace of Alabama acknowledged as a defendant in *Wyatt v. Aderholt*, the "real clients" of the mental health system are the police, parents, and members of the community who do not want the responsibility of caring for—or learning to live with—disabled individuals.

Because of this demand, the state will probably not "just leave alone" mentally disabled persons perceived as non-dangerous but in need of protection and treatment. Under parens patriae, either the state will provide treatment services to enable them to function in the community, or it will place them in an institution.

A mentally disabled person who comes to the attention of the state through the criminal justice system, triggering the police power, is also likely to suffer a loss of liberty. If perceived as mentally disabled, he or she may be charged with a crime "for his or her own good" to make possible transfer from the jail to the state hospital. A misdemeanor charge may enable the court to order in-patient evaluation of competency to stand trial; such a commitment may extend to the maximum possible sentence for the charged offense. An acquittal on insanity grounds may yield the same result: confinement in a mental hospital for a fixed or open-ended term, depending upon the law of the jurisdiction.

* * *

A "minimally adequate" system of community-based programs and services, by increasing mentally disabled persons' ability to function in the community, will reduce the risk of state restriction on their liberty through the criminal justice or the civil mental health systems. Thus, the right to "minimally adequate" treatment in the community may be asserted for mentally disabled persons who are now inappropriately hospitalized, who have been institutionalized and are trapped in the "revolving door," or for those who, although never hospitalized, are dependent upon the state for assistance and thus subject to state restrictions on their liberty.

Do you agree? If the courts adopted the stance advocated by Costello and Preis, how would they enforce it?

3. *State law bases for the right to community treatment.* In light of the trend in the cases described above, it is important to consider alternatives to a federal constitution-based right to community services. Like *Lelsz, Dixon v. Weinberger,* 405 F.Supp. 974 (D.D.C.1975), was a class action brought in federal court alleging that hospitalized patients should be transferred to the community. More specifically, it alleged that, due to a deficiency in outpatient facilities, 43 percent of the patients in St. Elizabeths Hospital in Washington, D.C. were improperly institutionalized (based on an assessment by the hospital staff itself). However, the district court in *Dixon,* unlike the district court in *Lelsz,* relied exclusively on *state statutory* grounds in ordering the federal and District of Columbia governments to reallocate funds to create community facilities. The court found that the purpose of the District of Columbia's Hospitalization of the Mentally Ill Act was to return patients to a full and productive life in the community through care and treatment. It held further that patients were entitled to placement in the most appropriate setting, including non-hospital settings, and that the government had the primary responsibility for creating alternative settings.

To implement these findings, the court ordered the defendants to submit a plan for the creation of alternative facilities (including nursing homes, personal care homes, foster homes, and halfway houses). The plan was to specify how many patients qualified and how many would probably qualify for less restrictive treatment; why the remainder did not qualify; standards, procedures and personnel that would be used for care in alternative facilities; a timetable for implementation of the order; and the division of responsibility for implementation between the federal and District governments. The defendants submitted an "outline" of this plan in April, 1976, setting out the problems and tentative solutions. The District also indicated that it planned to construct two 400–bed nursing homes and to divert half of the hospital's budget for community care. The court subsequently ordered the defendants to implement the plan within six months. But the deadline passed, St. Elizabeth's lost its accreditation, and the plaintiff class remained in the hospital. As of 1989, many patients who had been identified as treatable in the community remained in the hospital, despite continued pressure by the court-appointed "*Dixon* committee".

A federal court ruling finding a right to community treatment based on local law, like the one in *Dixon,* is probably no longer possible, given the Supreme Court's decision in *Pennhurst II* (described in *Lelsz*). Partly as a result, *state* courts are beginning to flex their muscle in this area. For instance, in *Arnold v. Sarn,* No. C 432455 (Ariz.Super.Ct. Maricopa Cty. Mar. 15, 1985), the court found a right to community-based treatment for the chronically mentally ill based on statutory provisions which required the state mental health director to undertake "unified" mental health programs (including "the functions of state hospital and community mental health"), and to take "appropriate steps to provide health care services to the medically dependent citizens of this state." See Santiago, et al., "Changing a State Mental Health System Through Litigation: The Arizona Experiment," 143 Am.J.Psychiat. 1575 (1986). However, a California court rejected a similar claim, finding that the relevant statutory scheme merely expressed a preference for community-based treatment rather than a right; further, it held that even if such a right existed a court would lack authority to enforce it. *Mental Health Ass'n v. Deukmejian,* 186 Cal.App. 3d 1531, 233 Cal.Rptr. 130 (1986). Had *Lelsz* been brought in state court and relied on state law, should the plaintiff class have prevailed?

Another state law source for a right to community-based treatment is the state constitution, which usually contains provisions protecting liberty and privacy rights, as well as a provision guaranteeing due process of law. In some jurisdictions, these provisions have been construed to provide more protection to the mentally disabled than analogous provisions in the federal constitution. However, as of 1987, no jurisdiction had used these provisions to find a right to community-based treatment. Perlin, "State Constitutions and Statutes as Sources of Rights for the Mentally Disabled: The Last Frontier?" 20 Loyola L.A.L.Rev. 1249, 1292–3 (1987).

4. *Federal statutory grounds for a right to community treatment.* A final possible basis for a right to community-based treatment is federal statutory law. For instance, the Education for All Handicapped Children Act, 20 U.S.C. §§ 1411–1420, establishes an entitlement to education in the public school system for disabled children who qualify. Section 504 of the Rehabilitation Act of 1973, 29 U.S.C. § 794, which prohibits discrimination "solely by reason of . . . handicap," might also form the basis for a right to community treatment claim. Finally, the Developmentally Disabled Assistance and Bill of Rights Act, 42 U.S.C. §§ 6000–6081, which provides federal funds to those states willing to develop habilitation programs for

the developmentally disabled, provides that this group has "a right to appropriate treatment, services, and habilitation" in the "setting that is least restrictive of . . . personal liberty." Id. § 6010.

However, each of these statutes is limited in scope. The Education Act's provisions apply only to children, and have not been construed to require creation of programs beyond what can be accommodated by the public school system. See generally, Bartlett, "The Role of Cost in Educational Decisionmaking for the Handicapped Child," 48 Law & Contemp. Probs. 7 (1985). The Rehabilitation Act likewise has not been a particularly useful tool in efforts to obtain funding for community programs. For instance, one court held that even if institutionalized plaintiffs are able to show that similarly disabled persons have been placed in community facilities, the Act has not been violated. *Clark v. Cohen,* 794 F.2d 79, 84 n. 3 (3d Cir.1986). On the facts of *Lelsz,* might not § 504 have an *adverse* impact on the plaintiff's claim?

The DD Act is, on its face, potentially the most useful federal statute for those seeking a right to treatment in the community, since it clearly announces a right to treatment in a less restrictive setting, at least for all developmentally disabled individuals. However, in *Pennhurst State School & Hospital v. Halderman,* 451 U.S. 1, 101 S.Ct. 1531, 67 L.Ed.2d 694 (1981) (*Pennhurst I*), the Supreme Court destroyed any hope that this provision could be used to pressure states into creating community facilities. *Pennhurst* was the culmination of lengthy *Wyatt*-like litigation challenging the conditions of confinement at the Pennhurst institution for the mentally retarded in Pennsylvania. The Third Circuit had held that § 6010 of the DD Act created a substantive right in favor of the retarded, and that the conditions at Pennhurst violated those rights. 612 F.2d 84 (3d Cir.1979). The Supreme Court held, however, that § 6010 merely expresses a preference for treatment services in the least restrictive setting. The Court emphasized that courts should be cautious in attributing to Congress an intent to create rights when those rights impose affirmative obligations on the states to fund certain services. According to the Court, unless Congress unambiguously states its intent in such situations, no substantive right exists. The Court found "nothing" in the Act or its legislative history "to suggest that Congress intended to require the States to assume the high cost of providing 'appropriate treatment' in the 'least restrictive environment' to their mentally retarded citizens."

The extent to which federal and state statutes create treatment entitlements for the mentally disabled, independent of any deprivation of liberty by the state, is explored more fully in Part III of this book.

Part III

BENEFITS ELIGIBILITY AND LEGAL PROTECTION AGAINST DISCRIMINATION

Chapter Eleven

BENEFITS AND ENTITLEMENTS OF THE MENTALLY HANDICAPPED

Table of Sections

I. SPECIAL EDUCATIONAL BENEFITS

A. SCOPE OF GUARANTEED BENEFITS

BOARD OF EDUCATION v. ROWLEY

Supreme Court of the United States, 1982.
458 U.S. 176, 102 S.Ct. 3034, 73 L.Ed.2d 690.

JUSTICE REHNQUIST delivered the opinion of the Court.

This case presents a question of statutory interpretation. Petitioners contend that the Court of Appeals and the District Court misconstrued the requirements imposed by Congress upon States which receive federal funds under the Education of the Handicapped Act. We agree and reverse the judgment of the Court of Appeals.

I

The Education of the Handicapped Act (Act), 84 Stat. 175, as amended, 20 U.S.C. § 1401 *et seq.* (1976 ed. and Supp. IV), provides federal money to assist state and local agencies in educating handicapped children, and conditions such funding upon a State's compliance with extensive goals and procedures. The Act represents an ambitious

1026

federal effort to promote the education of handicapped children, and was passed in response to Congress' perception that a majority of handicapped children in the United States "were either totally excluded from schools or [were] sitting idly in regular classrooms awaiting the time when they were old enough to 'drop out.' " H.R.Rep. No. 94–332, p. 2 (1975) (H.R.Rep.).

* * *

In order to qualify for federal financial assistance under the Act, a State must demonstrate that it "has in effect a policy that assures all handicapped children the right to a free appropriate public education." 20 U.S.C. § 1412(1). That policy must be reflected in a state plan submitted to and approved by the Secretary of Education, § 1413, which describes in detail the goals, programs, and timetables under which the State intends to educate handicapped children within its borders. §§ 1412, 1413. States receiving money under the Act must provide education to the handicapped by priority, first "to handicapped children who are not receiving an education" and second "to handicapped children . . . with the most severe handicaps who are receiving an inadequate education," § 1412(3), and "to the maximum extent appropriate" must educate handicapped children "with children who are not handicapped." § 1412(5).[4] The Act broadly defines "handicapped children" to include "mentally retarded, hard of hearing, deaf, speech impaired, visually handicapped, seriously emotionally disturbed, orthopedically impaired, [and] other health impaired children, [and] children with specific learning disabilities." § 1401(1).

The "free appropriate public education" required by the Act is tailored to the unique needs of the handicapped child by means of an "individualized educational program" (IEP). § 1401(18). The IEP, which is prepared at a meeting between a qualified representative of the local educational agency, the child's teacher, the child's parents or guardian, and, where appropriate, the child, consists of a written document containing

> "(A) a statement of the present levels of educational performance of such child, (B) a statement of annual goals, including short-term instructional objectives, (C) a statement of the specific educational services to be provided to such child, and the extent to which such child will be able to participate in regular educational programs, (D) the projected date for initiation and anticipated duration of such services, and (E) appropriate objective criteria and evaluation procedures and schedules for determining, on at least an annual basis, whether instructional objectives are being achieved." § 1401(19).

4. Despite this preference for "mainstreaming" handicapped children—educating them with nonhandicapped children—Congress recognized that regular classrooms simply would not be a suitable setting for the education of many handicapped children. The Act expressly acknowledges that "the nature or severity of the handicap [may be] such that education in regular classes with the use of supplementary aids and services cannot be achieved satisfactorily." § 1412(5). The Act thus provides for the education of some handicapped children in separate classes or institutional settings. See *ibid.;* § 1413(a)(4).

Local or regional educational agencies must review, and where appropriate revise, each child's IEP at least annually. § 1414(a)(5). See also § 1413(a)(11).

In addition to the state plan and the IEP already described, the Act imposes extensive procedural requirements upon States receiving federal funds under its provisions. Parents or guardians of handicapped children must be notified of any proposed change in "the identification, evaluation, or educational placement of the child or the provision of a free appropriate public education to such child," and must be permitted to bring a complaint about "any matter relating to" such evaluation and education. §§ 1415(b)(1)(D) and (E).

Complaints brought by parents or guardians must be resolved at "an impartial due process hearing," and appeal to the state educational agency must be provided if the initial hearing is held at the local or regional level. §§ 1415(b)(2) and (c). Thereafter, "[a]ny party aggrieved by the findings and decision" of the state administrative hearing has "the right to bring a civil action with respect to the complaint . . . in any State court of competent jurisdiction or in a district court of the United States without regard to the amount in controversy." § 1415(e)(2).

Thus, although the Act leaves to the States the primary responsibility for developing and executing educational programs for handicapped children, it imposes significant requirements to be followed in the discharge of that responsibility. Compliance is assured by provisions permitting the withholding of federal funds upon determination that a participating state or local agency has failed to satisfy the requirements of the Act, §§ 1414(b)(2)(A), 1416, and by the provision for judicial review. At present, all States except New Mexico receive federal funds under the portions of the Act at issue today.

II

This case arose in connection with the education of Amy Rowley, a deaf student at the Furnace Woods School in the Hendrick Hudson Central School District, Peekskill, N.Y. Amy has minimal residual hearing and is an excellent lipreader. During the year before she began attending Furnace Woods, a meeting between her parents and school administrators resulted in a decision to place her in a regular kindergarten class in order to determine what supplemental services would be necessary to her education. Several members of the school administration prepared for Amy's arrival by attending a course in sign-language interpretation, and a teletype machine was installed in the principal's office to facilitate communication with her parents who are also deaf. At the end of the trial period it was determined that Amy should remain in the kindergarten class, but that she should be provided with an FM hearing aid which would amplify words spoken into a wireless receiver by the teacher or fellow students during certain classroom activities. Amy successfully completed her kindergarten year.

As required by the Act, an IEP was prepared for Amy during the fall of her first-grade year. The IEP provided that Amy should be educated in a regular classroom at Furnace Woods, should continue to use the FM hearing aid, and should receive instruction from a tutor for the deaf for one hour each day and from a speech therapist for three hours each week. The Rowleys agreed with parts of the IEP, but insisted that Amy also be provided a qualified sign-language interpreter in all her academic classes in lieu of the assistance proposed in other parts of the IEP. Such an interpreter had been placed in Amy's kindergarten class for a 2-week experimental period, but the interpreter had reported that Amy did not need his services at that time. The school administrators likewise concluded that Amy did not need such an interpreter in her first-grade classroom. They reached this conclusion after consulting the school district's Committee on the Handicapped, which had received expert evidence from Amy's parents on the importance of a sign-language interpreter, received testimony from Amy's teacher and other persons familiar with her academic and social progress, and visited a class for the deaf.

When their request for an interpreter was denied, the Rowleys demanded and received a hearing before an independent examiner. After receiving evidence from both sides, the examiner agreed with the administrators' determination that an interpreter was not necessary because "Amy was achieving educationally, academically, and socially" without such assistance. The examiner's decision was affirmed on appeal by the New York Commissioner of Education on the basis of substantial evidence in the record. Pursuant to the Act's provision for judicial review, the Rowleys then brought an action in the United States District Court for the Southern District of New York, claiming that the administrators' denial of the sign-language interpreter constituted a denial of the "free appropriate public education" guaranteed by the Act.

The District Court found that Amy "is a remarkably well-adjusted child" who interacts and communicates well with her classmates and has "developed an extraordinary rapport" with her teachers. It also found that "she performs better than the average child in her class and is advancing easily from grade to grade," but "that she understands considerably less of what goes on in class than she could if she were not deaf" and thus "is not learning as much, or performing as well academically, as she would without her handicap,". This disparity between Amy's achievement and her potential led the court to decide that she was not receiving a "free appropriate public education," which the court defined as "an opportunity to achieve [her] full potential commensurate with the opportunity provided to other children." According to the District Court, such a standard "requires that the potential of the handicapped child be measured and compared to his or her performance, and that the resulting differential or 'shortfall' be compared to the shortfall experienced by nonhandicapped children." The District Court's definition arose from its assumption that the responsibility for "giv[ing] content to the requirement of an 'appropriate education'" had "been left entirely to the [federal] courts and the hearing officers."

A divided panel of the United States Court of Appeals for the Second Circuit affirmed. The Court of Appeals "agree[d] with the [D]istrict [C]ourt's conclusions of law," and held that its "findings of fact [were] not clearly erroneous." 632 F.2d 945, 947 (1980).

We granted certiorari to review the lower courts' interpretation of the Act. Such review requires us to consider two questions: What is meant by the Act's requirement of a "free appropriate public education"? And what is the role of state and federal courts in exercising the review granted by 20 U.S.C. § 1415? We consider these questions separately.

III

A

This is the first case in which this Court has been called upon to interpret any provision of the Act. As noted previously, the District Court and the Court of Appeals concluded that "[t]he Act itself does not define 'appropriate education,'" 483 F.Supp., at 533, but leaves "to the courts and the hearing officers" the responsibility of "giv[ing] content to the requirement of an 'appropriate education.'" See also 632 F.2d, at 947. Petitioners contend that the definition of the phrase "free appropriate public education" used by the courts below overlooks the definition of that phrase actually found in the Act. Respondents agree that the Act defines "free appropriate public education," but contend that the statutory definition is not "functional" and thus "offers judges no guidance in their consideration of controversies involving 'the identification, evaluation, or educational placement of the child or the provision of a free appropriate public education.'" The United States, appearing as *amicus curiae* on behalf of respondents, states that "[a]lthough the Act includes definitions of a 'free appropriate public education' and other related terms, the statutory definitions do not adequately explain what is meant by 'appropriate.'"

We are loath to conclude that Congress failed to offer any assistance in defining the meaning of the principal substantive phrase used in the Act. It is beyond dispute that, contrary to the conclusions of the courts below, the Act does expressly define "free appropriate public education":

> "The term 'free appropriate public education' means *special education* and *related services* which (A) have been provided at public expense, under public supervision and direction, and without charge, (B) meet the standards of the State educational agency, (C) include an appropriate preschool, elementary, or secondary school education in the State involved, and (D) are provided in conformity with the individualized education program required under section 1414(a)(5) of this title." § 1401(18) (emphasis added).

"Special education," as referred to in this definition, means "specially designed instruction, at no cost to parents or guardians, to meet the unique needs of a handicapped child, including classroom instruction, instruction in physical education, home instruction, and instruction in hospitals and institutions." § 1401(16). "Related services" are defined as "transportation, and such developmental, corrective, and other supportive services . . . as may be required to assist a handicapped child to benefit from special education." § 1401(17).

Like many statutory definitions, this one tends toward the cryptic rather than the comprehensive, but that is scarcely a reason for abandoning the quest for legislative intent.

* * *

According to the definitions contained in the Act, a "free appropriate public education" consists of educational instruction specially designed to meet the unique needs of the handicapped child, supported by such services as are necessary to permit the child "to benefit" from the instruction. Almost as a checklist for adequacy under the Act, the definition also requires that such instruction and services be provided at public expense and under public supervision, meet the State's educational standards, approximate the grade levels used in the State's regular education, and comport with the child's IEP. Thus, if personalized instruction is being provided with sufficient supportive services to permit the child to benefit from the instruction, and the other items on the definitional checklist are satisfied, the child is receiving a "free appropriate public education" as defined by the Act.

* * *

Noticeably absent from the language of the statute is any substantive standard prescribing the level of education to be accorded handicapped children. Certainly the language of the statute contains no requirement like the one imposed by the lower courts—that States maximize the potential of handicapped children "commensurate with the opportunity provided to other children." That standard was expounded by the District Court without reference to the statutory definitions or even to the legislative history of the Act.

* * *

B

* * *

(ii)

Respondents contend that "the goal of the Act is to provide each handicapped child with an equal educational opportunity." We think, however, that the requirement that a State provide specialized educational services to handicapped children generates no additional requirement that the services so provided be sufficient to maximize each child's potential "commensurate with the opportunity provided other children."

* * *

(iii)

Implicit in the congressional purpose of providing access to a "free appropriate public education" is the requirement that the education to which access is provided be sufficient to confer some educational benefit upon the handicapped child. It would do little good for Congress to spend millions of dollars in providing access to a public education only to have the handicapped child receive no benefit from that education. The statutory definition of "free appropriate public education," in addition to requiring that States provide each child with "specially designed instruction," expressly requires the provision of "such . . . supportive services . . . as may be required to assist a handicapped child *to benefit* from special education." § 1401(17) (emphasis added). We therefore conclude that the "basic floor of opportunity" provided by the Act consists of access to specialized instruction and related services which are individually designed to provide educational benefit to the handicapped child.

The determination of when handicapped children are receiving sufficient educational benefits to satisfy the requirements of the Act presents a more difficult problem. The Act requires participating States to educate a wide spectrum of handicapped children, from the marginally hearing-impaired to the profoundly retarded and palsied. It is clear that the benefits obtainable by children at one end of the spectrum will differ dramatically from those obtainable by children at the other end, with infinite variations in between. One child may have little difficulty competing successfully in an academic setting with non-handicapped children while another child may encounter great difficulty in acquiring even the most basic of self-maintenance skills. We do not attempt today to establish any one test for determining the adequacy of educational benefits conferred upon all children covered by the Act. Because in this case we are presented with a handicapped child who is receiving substantial specialized instruction and related services, and who is performing above average in the regular classrooms of a public school system, we confine our analysis to that situation.

* * *

C

When the language of the Act and its legislative history are considered together, the requirements imposed by Congress become tolerably clear. Insofar as a State is required to provide a handicapped child with a "free appropriate public education," we hold that it satisfies this requirement by providing personalized instruction with sufficient support services to permit the child to benefit educationally from that instruction.

* * *

IV

A

As mentioned in Part I, the Act permits "[a]ny party aggrieved by the findings and decision" of the state administrative hearings "to bring a civil action" in "any State court of competent jurisdiction or in a district court of the United States without regard to the amount in controversy." § 1415(e)(2). The complaint, and therefore the civil action, may concern "any matter relating to the identification, evaluation, or educational placement of the child, or the provision of a free appropriate public education to such child." § 1415(b)(1)(E). In reviewing the complaint, the Act provides that a court "shall receive the record of the [state] administrative proceedings, shall hear additional evidence at the request of a party, and, basing its decision on the preponderance of the evidence, shall grant such relief as the court determines is appropriate." § 1415(e)(2).

The parties disagree sharply over the meaning of these provisions, petitioners contending that courts are given only limited authority to review for state compliance with the Act's procedural requirements and no power to review the substance of the state program, and respondents contending that the Act requires courts to exercise *de novo* review over state educational decisions and policies. We find petitioners' contention unpersuasive, for Congress expressly rejected provisions that would have so severely restricted the role of reviewing courts. In substituting the current language of the statute for language that would have made state administrative findings conclusive if supported by substantial evidence, the Conference Committee explained that courts were to make "independent decision[s] based on a preponderance of the evidence."

But although we find that this grant of authority is broader than claimed by petitioners, we think the fact that it is found in § 1415, which is entitled "Procedural safeguards," is not without significance. When the elaborate and highly specific procedural safeguards embodied in § 1415 are contrasted with the general and somewhat imprecise substantive admonitions contained in the Act, we think that the importance Congress attached to these procedural safeguards cannot be gainsaid. It seems to us no exaggeration to say that Congress placed every bit as much emphasis upon compliance with procedures giving parents and guardians a large measure of participation at every stage of the administrative process, see, *e.g.*, §§ 1415(a)–(d), as it did upon the measurement of the resulting IEP against a substantive standard. We think that the congressional emphasis upon full participation of concerned parties throughout the development of the IEP, as well as the requirements that state and local plans be submitted to the Secretary for approval, demonstrates the legislative conviction that adequate compliance with the procedures prescribed would in most cases assure much if not all of what Congress wished in the way of substantive content in an IEP.

Thus the provision that a reviewing court base its decision on the "preponderance of the evidence" is by no means an invitation to the courts to substitute their own notions of sound educational policy for those of the school authorities which they review. The very importance which Congress has attached to compliance with certain procedures in the preparation of an IEP would be frustrated if a court were permitted simply to set state decisions at nought. The fact that § 1415(e) requires that the reviewing court "receive the records of the [state] administrative proceedings" carries with it the implied requirement that due weight shall be given to these proceedings.

* * *

Therefore, a court's inquiry in suits brought under § 1415(e)(2) is twofold. First, has the State complied with the procedures set forth in the Act? And second, is the individualized educational program developed through the Act's procedures reasonably calculated to enable the child to receive educational benefits? If these requirements are met, the State has complied with the obligations imposed by Congress and the courts can require no more.

B

In assuring that the requirements of the Act have been met, courts must be careful to avoid imposing their view of preferable educational methods upon the States. The primary responsibility for formulating the education to be accorded a handicapped child, and for choosing the educational method most suitable to the child's needs, was left by the Act to state and local educational agencies in cooperation with the parents or guardian of the child.

We previously have cautioned that courts lack the "specialized knowledge and experience" necessary to resolve "persistent and difficult questions of educational policy." *San Antonio Independent School Dist. v. Rodriguez,* 411 U.S., at 42, 93 S.Ct., at 1301. We think that Congress shared that view when it passed the Act. As already demonstrated, Congress' intention was not that the Act displace the primacy of States in the field of education, but that States receive funds to assist them in extending their educational systems to the handicapped. Therefore, once a court determines that the requirements of the Act have been met, questions of methodology are for resolution by the States.

* * *

VI

Applying these principles to the facts of this case, we conclude that the Court of Appeals erred in affirming the decision of the District Court. Neither the District Court nor the Court of Appeals found that petitioners had failed to comply with the procedures of the Act, and the findings of neither court would support a conclusion that Amy's educational program failed to comply with the substantive requirements of the Act. On the contrary, the District Court found that the "evidence firmly establishes that Amy is receiving an 'adequate' education, since she performs better than the average child in her class and is advancing easily from grade to grade." 483 F.Supp., at 534. In light of this finding, and of the fact that Amy was receiving personalized instruction and related services calculated by the Furnace Woods school administrators to meet her educational needs, the lower courts should not have concluded that the Act requires the provision of a sign-language interpreter. Accordingly, the decision of the Court of Appeals is reversed, and the case is remanded for further proceedings consistent with this opinion.

So ordered.

*   *   *

[The concurring opinion of Mr. Justice Blackmun is omitted].

JUSTICE WHITE, with whom JUSTICE BRENNAN and JUSTICE MARSHALL join, dissenting.

In order to reach its result in this case, the majority opinion contradicts itself, the language of the statute, and the legislative history. Both the majority's standard for a "free appropriate education" and its standard for judicial review disregard congressional intent.

*   *   *

I

I agree that the language of the Act does not contain a substantive standard beyond requiring that the education offered must be "appropriate." However, if there are limits not evident from the face of the statute on what may be considered an "appropriate education," they must be found in the purpose of the statute or its legislative history.

*   *   *

The majority opinion announces a different substantive standard, that "Congress did not impose upon the States any greater substantive educational standard than would be necessary to make such access meaningful." *Ante,* at 3043. While "meaningful" is no more enlightening than "appropriate," the Court purports to clarify itself. Because Amy was provided with *some* specialized instruction from which she obtained *some* benefit and because she passed from grade to grade, she was receiving a meaningful and therefore appropriate education.

This falls far short of what the Act intended. *   *   * The basic floor of opportunity is as the courts below recognized, intended to eliminate the effects of the handicap, at least to the extent that the child will be given an equal opportunity to learn if that is reasonably possible. Amy Rowley, without a sign-language interpreter, comprehends less than half of what is said in the classroom—less than half of what normal children comprehend. This is hardly an equal opportunity to learn, even if Amy makes passing grades.

*   *   *

The issue before us is what standard the word "appropriate" incorporates when it is used to modify "education." The answer given by the Court is not a satisfactory one.

II

The Court's discussion of the standard for judicial review is as flawed as its discussion of a "free appropriate public education." According to the Court, a court can ask only whether the State has "complied with the procedures set forth in the Act" and whether the individualized education program is "reasonably calculated to enable the child to receive educational benefits." *Ante,* at 3051. Both the language of the Act and the legislative history, however, demonstrate that Congress intended the courts to conduct a far more searching inquiry.

* * *

There is no doubt that the state agency itself must make substantive decisions. The legislative history reveals that the courts are to consider, *de novo,* the same issues.

* * *

Thus, the Court's limitations on judicial review have no support in either the language of the Act or the legislative history. * * * I respectfully dissent.

Questions and Comments

1. *"Mainstreaming."* In enacting the EHA Congress signaled a clear preference for the educational "mainstreaming" of handicapped children. In fact, the statute specifically permits a placement in a special class or school only when the nature or severity of the handicap is such that regular classroom education cannot be achieved satisfactorily. 20 U.S.C. § 1412(5)(B). The preference for "mainstreaming" was a response to the past tendency of school districts to warehouse handicapped children in ill-equipped special classrooms or schools.

The notion of mainstreaming, whatever its educational benefits in a given case, will frequently coincide with the financial interests of the state in minimizing program costs. Parents, on the other hand, may prefer a special *residential* placement either because of their belief that such facilities may maximize the educational opportunities for their child or because it is more convenient or less disruptive to have the mentally disabled child reside outside the home. Moreover, in some instances, the choice to which the parent is responding is between a publicly operated day school facility and a privately operated residential facility particularly geared to deal with a specific disability.

To what extent does *Rowley,* which requires courts to accept programs devised by the school authorities so long as they provide some educational benefit, tacitly recognize that the schools must, in view of the budgetary limitations under which they operate, be free to take financial considerations into account in devising IEP's? Consider in this connection *Kerkam v. McKenzie,* 862 F.2d 884 (D.C.Cir.1988). There the Court of Appeals found that the district court wrongly applied the *Rowley* standard when it failed to find that a public day school placement for a severely mentally retarded child met the "same educational benefit" test.

2. *Parent's contribution.* May the parents of a handicapped child be called upon by the state to contribute to the cost of the education program required by the Act? In *Parks v. Pavkovic,* 557 F.Supp. 1280 (N.D.Ill.1983), affirmed 753 F.2d 1397 (7th Cir.1985), the state of Illinois was enjoined from requiring parents to pay a portion of their mentally disabled child's institutional living expenses. Illinois law sought to assess "responsible relative liability" against the parents of children receiving services from the Illinois Department of Mental Health and Developmental Disabilities. The court held that such an assessment, as to children placed in residential facilities for educational reasons, violates the EHA's mandate to states to provide a *free* appropriate public education.

POLK v. CENTRAL SUSQUEHANNA INTERMEDIATE UNIT 16

United States Court of Appeals, Third Circuit, 1988.
853 F.2d 171.

BECKER, CIRCUIT JUDGE.

This appeal requires that we examine the contours of the "free appropriate public education" requirement of the Education of the Handicapped Act, as amended, 20 U.S.C. §§ 1401–1461, (1982) (EHA), as it touches on the delivery of physical therapy, which is a "related service" under the EHA. Ronald and Cindy Polk are parents of Christopher Polk, a child with severe mental and physical impairments. They claim that defendants, the local school district and the larger administrative Intermediate Unit (which oversees special education for students in a five-county area) violated the EHA because they failed to provide Christopher with an adequate program of special education. Specifically, plaintiffs contend that defendants' failure to provide direct "hands-on" physical therapy from a licensed physical therapist once a week has hindered Christopher's progress in meeting his educational goals.

The district court granted summary judgment in favor of defendants. The court held that because Christopher derived "*some* educational benefit" from his educational program, the requirements of the EHA, as interpreted by the Supreme Court in *Board of Education v. Rowley* have been met.

We will reverse the district court's grant of summary judgment for two reasons. First, we discern a genuine issue of material fact as to whether the defendants, in violation of the EHA procedural requirement for *individualized* educational programs, have refused, as a blanket rule, to consider providing handicapped students with direct physical therapy from a licensed physical therapist. Second, we conclude that the district court applied the wrong standard in evaluating the appropriateness of the child's education. Although the district

court relied upon language from a recent Supreme Court case, it took
that language out of context and applied it beyond the narrow holding
of the Supreme Court's opinion. More specifically, we believe that the
district court erred in evaluating this severely handicapped child's
educational program by a standard under which even trivial advancement satisfied the substantive provisions of the EHA's guarantee of a
free and appropriate education. There is evidence in the record that
would support a finding that the program prescribed for Christopher
afforded no more than trivial progress. We will therefore reverse and
remand for further proceedings consistent with this opinion.

* * *

II. FACTS & PROCEDURAL HISTORY

Christopher Polk is severely developmentally disabled. At the age
of seven months he contracted encephalopathy, a disease of the brain
similar to cerebral palsy. He is also mentally retarded. Although
Christopher is fourteen years old, he has the functional and mental
capacity of a toddler. All parties agree that he requires "related
services" in order to learn. He receives special education from defendants, the Central Susquehanna Intermediate Unit # 16 (the IU) and
Central Columbia Area School District (the school district). Placed in a
class for the mentally handicapped, Christopher has a full-time personal classroom aide. His education consists of learning basic life skills
such as feeding himself, dressing himself, and using the toilet. He has
mastered sitting and kneeling, is learning to stand independently, and
is showing some potential for ambulation. Christopher is working on
basic concepts such as "behind," "in," "on," and "under," and the
identification of shapes, coins, and colors. Although he is cooperative,
Christopher finds such learning difficult because he has a short attention span.

Although the record is not clear on this point, until 1980, the
defendants apparently provided Christopher with direct physical therapy from a licensed physical therapist. Since that time, however,
under a newer, so-called consultative model, Christopher no longer
receives direct physical therapy from a physical therapist. Instead, a
physical therapist (one of two hired by the IU) comes once a month to
train Christopher's teacher in how to integrate physical therapy with
Christopher's education. Although the therapist may lay hands on
Christopher in demonstrating to the teacher the correct approach, he or
she does not provide any therapy to Christopher directly, but uses such
interaction to teach the teacher. Plaintiffs do not object to the consultative method per se, but argue that, to meet Christopher's individual
needs, the consultative method must be supplemented by direct ("hands
on") physical therapy.

In support of this position, plaintiffs adduced evidence that direct
physical therapy from a licensed physical therapist has significantly
expanded Christopher's physical capacities. In the summer of 1985,
Christopher received two weeks of intensive physical therapy from a

licensed physical therapist at Shriner's Hospital in Philadelphia. According to Christopher's parents, this brief treatment produced dramatic improvements in Christopher's physical capabilities. A doctor at Shriner's prescribed that Christopher receive at least one hour a week of direct physical therapy. Because the defendants were unwilling to provide direct physical therapy as part of Christopher's special education program, the Polks hired a licensed physical therapist, Nancy Brown, to work with Christopher at home. At the time of the hearing, she was seeing Christopher twice a week.

Plaintiffs acknowledge that the school program has benefited Christopher to some degree, but argue that his educational program is not appropriate because it is not individually tailored to his specific needs, as the EHA requires. Moreover, throughout all of the administrative and judicial proceedings that we now describe, plaintiffs have maintained that to comply with the EHA the defendants must provide, as part of Christopher's "free appropriate public education," one session a week with a licensed physical therapist.

Plaintiffs first challenged Christopher's IEP before a Commonwealth of Pennsylvania Department of Education Hearing Officer. At that hearing and in later depositions, the administrator of the IU, Christopher's teachers, the IU's physical therapy consultant, Christopher's current private physical therapist and his therapist from Shriner's all testified concerning Christopher's capabilities and educational needs. The Hearing Officer found that Christopher was benefiting from his education, and that his education was appropriate.

After exhausting administrative remedies to their dissatisfaction, the Polks brought suit in the district court for the Middle District of Pennsylvania.

*   *   *

[T]he district court granted summary judgment for the defendants. Relying on the Supreme Court's decision in *Rowley*, 458 U.S. at 206–07, 102 S.Ct. at 3050–51, the court held that the provisions of EHA had been met because Christopher had received *some* benefit from his education. This appeal followed.

Plaintiffs present two arguments on appeal. First, they submit that the defendants violated EHA's procedural requirements because Christopher's program is not truly individualized. Plaintiffs rely, in this regard, on the defendants' failure to provide direct ("hands on") physical therapy from a licensed physical therapist to *any* of the children in the intermediate unit (a fact they learned during Christopher's due process hearing before the state examiner). This failure, they contend, is evidence that the defendants have an inflexible rule prohibiting direct therapy and that such a rigid rule conflicts with the EHA's mandate of providing *individualized* education. Plaintiffs argue that genuine questions of material fact exist as to the defendants' willingness to provide direct physical therapy under any circumstances, and that such disputes preclude summary judgment.

Second, plaintiffs assert that Christopher's education is inadequate to meet his unique needs. They claim that the district court found Christopher's education appropriate only because it applied an erroneous legal standard in judging the educational benefit of Christopher's program.

III. ROLE OF PHYSICAL THERAPY IN PROVIDING A FREE APPROPRIATE PUBLIC EDUCATION UNDER THE EHA

For some handicapped children, the related services provided by the EHA serve as important facilitators of classroom learning.

*   *   *

For children like Christopher with severe disabilities, related services serve a dual purpose. First, because these children have extensive physical difficulties that often interfere with development in other areas, physical therapy is an essential prerequisite to education. For example, development of motor abilities is often the first step in overall educational development.[8]

As we explained in *Battle v. Pennsylvania*, 629 F.2d 269, 275 (3d Cir.1980), *cert. denied*, 452 U.S. 968, 101 S.Ct. 3123, 69 L.Ed.2d 981 (1981), in discussing children with severe emotional disturbances:

> Where basic self-help and social skills such as toilet training, dressing, feeding and communication are lacking, formal education begins at that point. If the child masters these fundamentals, the education moves on to more difficult but still very basic language, social and arithmetic skills, such as counting, making change, and identifying simple words.

Id. at 275.

Second, the physical therapy itself may form the core of a severely disabled child's special education. This court has recognized that "[t]he educational program of a handicapped child, particularly a severely and profoundly handicapped child . . . is very different from that of a non-handicapped child. The program may consist largely of 'related services' such as physical, occupational, or speech therapy." In Christopher's case, physical therapy is not merely a conduit to his education but constitutes, in and of itself, a major portion of his special education, teaching him basic skills such as toileting, feeding, ambulation, etc.

IV. THE PLAINTIFFS' PROCEDURAL CLAIM (THAT CHRISTOPHER'S EDUCATIONAL PLAN WAS NOT INDIVIDUALIZED)

As we noted above, the plaintiffs have offered to prove that the defendants never genuinely considered Christopher's unique needs because of a rigid policy of providing only consultative physical therapy. They adduced evidence during cross examination at the state administrative hearing that none of the 65 children in defendants' intermediate unit whose IEPs call for physical therapy actually receive direct physi-

---

8. Physical therapy is essential for a child like Christopher because, in order to learn basic skills, he must learn to use his muscles properly. A key function of physical therapy is to normalize tonic reflex patterns. *   *   *

cal therapy. The plaintiffs also contend that, since the adoption of the consultative model, this rigid policy has precluded the defendants from recognizing Christopher's individual needs in violation of the EHA. Plaintiffs submit that the district court did not recognize the force of this procedural argument, and hence erred in granting summary judgment when a genuine issue of material fact existed as to the willingness of the defendants to provide direct physical therapy to any child.

The defendants respond that it is, and always has been, their position that direct therapy would be provided, if needed. The therapist who consults monthly with Christopher's teacher testified before the Department of Education hearing examiner that she would provide therapy treatment directly if she determined that such therapy were appropriate. The previous physical therapy consultant and the administrator of the IU similarly claimed in testimony before the hearing examiner that direct physical therapy would be provided, if needed, but that such a case has never arisen for Christopher nor for any other student in the Unit.

Critical to resolution of this question are the Act's procedural protections. To repeat, the centerpiece of the procedural scheme is the IEP.

* * *

This system of procedural protection only works if the state devises an *individualized* program and is willing to address the handicapped child's "unique needs."

* * *

In our view, a rigid rule under which defendants refuse even to consider providing physical therapy, as did the rule struck down in *Battle*, would conflict with Christopher's procedural right to an individualized program. Drawing all reasonable inferences in favor of the non-moving party, we believe that a genuine dispute exists over whether the defendants would consider, under any circumstances, offering direct physical therapy, and that this dispute is over material facts, precluding summary judgment. Concomitantly, we believe that plaintiffs should be given an opportunity to continue their discovery into this question because the existence of a rigid rule prohibiting such therapy would violate the EHA. Therefore, we will reverse and remand the district court's decision for inquiry into whether defendants possess a rigid policy prohibiting the provision of direct physical therapy to children in the IU.

V. PLAINTIFFS' SUBSTANTIVE CLAIM (THAT THE COURT MISAPPLIED THE LEGAL STANDARD FOR EVALUATING APPROPRIATE EDUCATION)

A. *The Supreme Court's Opinion in Rowley*

We begin our discussion of the substantive protections of the EHA with the Supreme Court's opinion in *Board of Education v. Rowley,* 458 U.S. 176, 102 S.Ct. 3034, 73 L.Ed.2d 690 (1982), because the parties' arguments are so closely tied to that case; only in the context of *Rowley* can we intelligently present the parties' contentions and the district court's opinion.

* * *

Although the tenor of the *Rowley* opinion reflects the Court's reluctance to involve the courts in substantive determinations of appropriate education and its emphasis on the *procedural* protection of the IEP process, it is clear that the Court was not espousing an entirely toothless standard of substantive review. Rather, the *Rowley* Court described the level of benefit conferred by the Act as "meaningful." 458 U.S. at 192, 102 S.Ct. at 3043. As the Court explained:

> By passing the Act, Congress sought primarily to make public education available to handicapped children. But in seeking to provide such access to public education, Congress did not impose upon the States any greater substantive educational standard than would be necessary to make such access *meaningful*.

Id. (emphasis added). After noting the deference due to states on questions of education and the theme of *access* rather than a guarantee of any particular standard of benefit, the Court acknowledged that:

> Implicit in the congressional purpose of providing access to a "free appropriate public education" is the requirement that the education to which access is provided be sufficient to confer some educational benefit upon the handicapped child.

* * *

The preceding quotation demonstrates that the Supreme Court in *Rowley* did not abdicate responsibility for monitoring the substantive quality of education under the EHA. Instead, it held that the education must "provide educational benefit." The Court thus recognized that the substantive, independent judicial review envisioned by the EHA was not a hollow gesture. Instead, courts must ensure "a basic floor of opportunity" that is defined by an *individualized* program that confers benefit.

Finally, it is important to note that, notwithstanding *Rowley*'s broad language, the Court indicated that its holding might not cover every case brought under the EHA. Indeed, *Rowley* was an avowedly narrow opinion that relied significantly on the fact that Amy Rowley progressed successfully from grade to grade in a "mainstreamed" classroom.

* * *

Although we do not argue that *Rowley* "contradicts itself," *id.* at 212, 102 S.Ct. at 3053 (White, J., dissenting), we nevertheless note the tension in the *Rowley* majority opinion between its emphasis on procedural protection (almost to the exclusion of substantive inquiry) and its substantive component quoted and discussed *supra*. This tension is unresolved in the *Rowley* case itself because the facts of the case (including Amy Rowley's quite substantial benefit from her education) did not force the Court to confront squarely the fact that Congress cared about the quality of special education. In the case *sub judice*, however, the question of how much benefit is sufficient to be "meaningful" is inescapable. Therefore we must examine the Act's notion of "benefit" and apply a standard that is faithful to congressional intent and consistent with *Rowley.*

B. EHA Requires More than a De Minimis Benefit

We hold that the EHA calls for more than a trivial educational benefit. That holding rests on the Act and its legislative history as well as interpretation of *Rowley.*

1.

The opinion of the district court, anchored to the "some benefit" language of *Rowley,* 458 U.S. at 200, 102 S.Ct. at 3047, explained its holding as follows:

> The fact that Christopher would advance more quickly with intensive therapy rather than the therapy he now receives does not make the School District's program for Christopher defective. Programs need only render some benefit;—they need not maximize potential. . . .
>
> The Supreme Court has determined that the Act is primarily a procedural statute and does not impose a substantive duty on the state to provide a student with other than *some* educational benefits. Increased muscle tone may well fall outside of the scope of the requirement that Christopher receive some educational benefits from the program in which he is enrolled.

Plaintiffs argue on appeal that the district court applied the wrong standard in measuring the educational benefit of Christopher's program and that the case should be remanded for further proceedings consistent with the correct standard, one that requires more than a *de minimis* benefit. Defendants rejoin that *Rowley*'s announcement of a "some benefit" test precludes judicial inquiry into the substantive education conferred by the Act, so long as the handicapped child receives any benefit at all. Noting that Christopher's parents acknowledge that he derives some benefit from his education, defendants submit that the inquiry is over and that the district court's summary judgment must be affirmed.

* * *

This court recently has had occasion to interpret and apply the *Rowley* standard in the context of a severely impaired child. In *Board of Education v. Diamond,* 808 F.2d 987, 991 (3d Cir.1986), we expressly rejected the argument that when the Supreme Court in *Rowley* referred to "some benefit," it meant any benefit at all, even if the child nevertheless regressed. The case involved a child, Andrew Diamond, with severe physical, neurological, and emotional handicaps. Despite evidence that Andrew's learning skills were deteriorating and his behavior was becoming counterproductive, the state resisted transferring Andrew from his placement in a day program to a placement in a residential program. As a result, Andrew's parents put him in a residential program and paid for it themselves.

After a due process hearing, the school board was ordered to place Andrew in an appropriate residential setting. The school board filed an action in federal court seeking a day placement for Andrew. The district court, however, endorsed the residential placement and ordered the school district to reimburse Andrew's parents for the expenses incurred when paying for his residential placement themselves.

In *Diamond*, we thus confronted and rejected the very argument that the defendants make here:

> The School District's legal argument is that it is obliged by governing law to provide no more for Andrew Diamond than will be "of benefit" to him. The governing law, however, clearly imposes a higher standard.

Id. at 991. After observing that "the *Rowley* standard of enabling one to achieve passing marks and advance from grade to grade probably is not achievable for Andrew," *id.*, the court observed:

> But *Rowley* makes it perfectly clear that the Act requires a plan of instruction under which educational *progress* is likely. The School District's "of benefit" test is offered in defense of an educational plan under which educational regression actually occurred. Literally the School Board's plan might be conceived as conferring some benefit to Andrew in that less regression might occur under it than if Andrew Diamond had simply been left to vegetate. The Act, however, requires a plan likely to produce progress, not regression or trivial educational advancement.

Id. (emphasis in original). The teaching of *Diamond* is that, when the Supreme Court said "some benefit" in *Rowley*, it did not mean "some" as opposed to "none." Rather, "some" connotes an amount of benefit greater than mere trivial advancement.

Defendants seek to distinguish *Diamond*, arguing that *Diamond* was a more egregious case, whereby regression had occurred under the state's educational plan (there has been no regression here). Although we acknowledge that this distinction has some force, and that *Diamond* does indeed stand for the proposition that a child who is regressing (and whose regression can be reversed by reasonable means) is not receiving sufficient "benefit" under the Act, we believe that *Diamond* can and should be read more expansively.

Indeed, defendants' distinction of *Diamond*, if carried to its logical conclusion, would arguably render that case more expansive because progress for some severely handicapped children may require optimal benefit. As we noted in *Battle*, 629 F.2d at 269, severely handicapped children (unlike normal children) have a strong tendency to regress. A program calculated to lead to non-regression might actually, in the case of severely handicapped children, impose a greater burden on the state than one that requires a program designed to lead to more than trivial progress. The educational progress of a handicapped child (whether in life skills or in a more sophisticated program) can be understood as a continuum where the point of regression versus progress is less relevant than the conferral of benefit. We note that it is therefore possible to construe *Diamond*'s holding not solely as an issue of progress or regression but also as requiring that any educational benefit be more than *de minimis*.

* * *

Obviously, this court is in no position to determine the factual question whether the treatment the defendants currently provide for Christopher is appropriate. We are, however, obligated to correct errors of law on appeal, and we hold that the district court applied the wrong standard in granting summary judgment for defendants when it allowed for the possibility of only *de minimis* benefit.

* * *

We recognize the difficulty of measuring levels of benefit in severely handicapped children. Obviously, the question whether benefit is *de minimis* must be gauged in relation to the child's potential. However, we believe that the extent of the factual dispute concerning the level of benefit Christopher received from his educational program precludes summary judgment under the standard that we announce today. The judgment of the district court will therefore be reversed and the case remanded for further proceedings consistent with this opinion.

Questions and Comments

1. *The "some benefit" standard.* One of the grounds relied upon by the court in *Polk* to reverse the holding of the district court was an error in the lower court's failure to apply the correct substantive standard. What actually was the "test" employed by the District Court? Is the Court of Appeals' articulation of the governing standard consistent with the standard announced by the Supreme Court in *Rowley*? Does the excerpt from the District Court's opinion discussing the applicable standard set out in the *Polk* opinion support the Appellate Court's conclusion that the lower court applied a "de minimus" benefits standard?

In *Polk,* the parents of the child in question had conceded that the child was deriving "some benefit from his education." Why wasn't this concession dispositive? On what basis did the court find that the level of services required by the Act had perhaps not been met? Did the result turn on the fact that the services were deemed to be "de minimus", which is less than "some", or was the result based on some other ground?

2. *Related services.* Can the Act be construed to permit school boards to avoid the costs of residential placement because such placement can be characterized as "therapeutic" rather than educational? In *T.G. v. Board of Education of Piscataway,* 576 F.Supp. 420 (D.N.J.1983), an emotionally disturbed child was placed in a residential facility "to provide him with the controls and attention necessary for social and environmental development." In response to the parents' request for reimbursement for the cost of such placement, the school board denied the claim on the grounds that " 'psychotherapy' other than that necessary for diagnostic or evaluative purposes was not a 'related service' for which a local school district would

be responsible under the mandate of the Act." Id. at 422. In granting summary judgment for the parent-claimant the Court held that psychotherapy provided to an emotionally disturbed child is a related service under the Act since "the therapy was designed as an essential service to allow [the child] to simply benefit from the educational program planned for him." Id. at 424. See also, *Kruelle v. New Castle County School District*, 642 F.2d 687 (3d Cir.1981) (holding that 24–hour care in a residential setting was necessary to allow a profoundly mentally retarded child to learn).

3. *Related service requirements.* What other types of services might be considered related services necessary to assist a mentally handicapped child to benefit from his special education? Would the administering of psychotropic medication under medical supervision or the provision of psychotherapy during school hours be required by the Act?

4. *State educational benefits.* In administering the EHA, states may impose a higher substantive standard than those required by the Act itself. For instance, in *B.G. v. Cranford Board of Education*, 702 F.Supp. 1140 (D.N.J.1988), the court noted that the state of New Jersey by law requires school boards "to provide educational services according to how the student can *best* achieve success in learning." Id. at 1148. The court found that this standard required a residential placement of an emotionally disturbed child. The school district's day school placement of the child "though perhaps sufficient to satisfy the minimum federal standards under *Rowley*, is insufficient and inconsistent with New Jersey's requirements that B.G. be afforded a program that assures him the fullest opportunity to develop his intellectual capacities." Id. at 1157.

B. JUDICIAL REMEDIES TO SECURE BENEFITS

Section 615(e)(2) of the EHA (20 U.S.C. § 1415(e)(2)) provides: "Any party aggrieved by the findings and decision made [by the local or state educational agency] shall have the right to bring a civil action . . . in any State court of competent jurisdiction or in a district court of the United States without regard to the amount in controversy. In any action brought under this paragraph the court . . . *shall grant such relief as the court determines is appropriate.*" (Emphasis added.)

The Supreme Court has held that this section confers broad discretion upon the reviewing court to grant "appropriate" relief in light of the purposes of the EHA. At a minimum, this section allows injunctive relief. Under some circumstances, it also allows a court to award money damages. While the scope and circumstances of such awards have not been directly decided by the Supreme Court, the Court by way of dictum has tacitly acknowledged that the EHA permits the award of damages in exceptional circumstances. See, *Smith v. Robinson*, 468 U.S. 992, 1020 n. 24, 104 S.Ct. 3457, 3472 n. 24, 82 L.Ed.2d 746 (1984). A number of lower courts have found special circumstances justifying award of money damages to include instances where the school's offered program would constitute a risk to the child's physical health or where the school acts in bad faith by failing to comply with the EHA's procedural provisions in an egregious manner. See, e.g., *Miener v. Missouri*, 673 F.2d 969, 979–980 (8th Cir.1982); *Anderson v. Thompson*, 658 F.2d 1205, 1213–1214 (7th Cir.1981). In addition the Supreme Court has upheld the award of tuition reimbursement to parents who had unilaterally placed their child in private school contrary to the child's proposed IEP, after the district court determined that the private placement was appropriate. *Town of Burlington v. Department of Education*, 471 U.S. 359, 105 S.Ct. 1996, 85 L.Ed.2d 385 (1985).

Questions and Comments

1. *The "special circumstance" limitation.* What policy reasons might support the court's construction of section 615(e)(2) as limiting the award of money damages to special circumstances? Would the fact that such awards might deplete resources that would otherwise be available for special education programs and services be such a reason?

2. *Attorney fees.* The EHA as originally enacted contained no provision for award of attorney fees to prevailing parents. The effect of this provision was not clear until the Supreme Court holding in *Smith v. Robinson*, supra, that courts are without power to award attorney fees. Congress subsequently enacted the Handicapped Children's Protection Act of 1986 (P.L. 99–372), which amended the EHA to allow courts the discretion to award reasonable attorney fees to prevailing parents.

3. *States' immunity from suit in federal court.* Suppose a child's special education is provided by a state agency together with one or more local agencies acting in cooperation. Can parents sue the state itself on the grounds that it has failed to provide a free appropriate public education?

A number of earlier cases permitted suits against the state on the grounds that in enacting the EHA, Congress intended to invoke its power under the Fourteenth Amendment to abrogate states' immunity from suit under the 11th Amendment. See, e.g., *Parks v. Pavkovic*, 536 F.Supp. 296, 307 (N.D.Ill.1982) (on motion for preliminary injunction).

However, in *Dellmuth v. Muth*, ___ U.S. ___, 109 S.Ct. 2397, 105 L.Ed. 2d 181 (1989) the Supreme Court held that the language of the EHA does not evince an unmistakably clear intention to abrogate the states' constitutionally secured immunity from suit. Thus parents may be barred from collecting money damages (i.e., tuition reimbursement) from the state in a federal suit.

4. *Injunctive relief.* The Supreme Court recently considered a case in which a school district attempted to expel an emotionally disturbed child for violent conduct related to his disability. *Honig v. Doe*, 484 U.S. 305, 108 S.Ct. 592, 98 L.Ed.2d 686 (1988). After the child, responding to taunts, choked a classmate, the school district initially suspended the student, then proposed to exclude him permanently and extended the suspension pending expulsion proceedings. The Court held that these actions violated the EHA, which requires the school district to keep the child in his current placement pending review of its decisions as to changes in placement. 20 U.S.C. § 1415(e)(3) (the "stay put" provision).

The Court held that, pursuant to Department of Education policy, the school could suspend a student posing an immediate threat to the safety of others for 10 days, but that any suspension beyond that period constituted a change of placement which violated sec. 1415(e)(3) unless made with parental consent. In the absence of parental consent, school officials may seek judicial intervention. However, the "stay put" provision "effectively creates a presumption in favor of the child's current placement which school officials can overcome only by showing that maintaining the child in his or her current placement is substantially likely to result in injury either to himself or herself, or to others." 484 U.S. at 327, 108 S.Ct. at 606. The Supreme Court found that, in enjoining the school district from indefinitely suspending the child, the District Court properly balanced the child's educational interests against the school district's interest in maintaining a safe learning environment.

5. *Exhaustion of remedies.* Congress devised a multi-layered administrative procedural scheme intended to assure handicapped children access to special education. The Supreme Court has recognized that administrative remedies need not be exhausted if such would be "futile or inadequate." *Smith v. Robinson,* 468 U.S. 992, 1014 n. 17, 104 S.Ct. 3457, 3469 n. 17, 82 L.Ed.2d 746 (1984). Exhaustion by parents would be futile where the threatened discharge of the student from his private placement would prevent preservation of the status quo pending administrative review as required by 20 U.S.C. § 1415(e)(3), or where there exists no true administrative remedy due to state adherence to a policy which operates to deny a child a free appropriate public education in violation of the EHA. *Parks v. Pavkovic,* 536 F.Supp. 296, 302–303 (N.D.Ill.1982). The school may, in extraordinary circumstances, bypass administrative procedures if it can demonstrate an immediate need to temporarily enjoin a dangerous child from school attendance. *Honig v. Doe,* 484 U.S. 305, 327, 108 S.Ct. 592, 606, 98 L.Ed.2d 686 (1988). What circumstances will render exhaustion of remedies "futile and inadequate" necessarily will vary greatly from case to case.

II. SOCIAL SECURITY DISABILITY BENEFITS

A number of public programs and many private insurance plans provide compensation to persons who become disabled. Eligibility for the benefits provided by these programs is likely to turn on a determination of the existence of a disabling physical or mental impairment. The determination process can be complex to administer, especially in cases of psychiatric disabilities. In these cases, the determination of disability will in large part rest on the evaluator's interpretations of sometimes subtle symptoms. This section focuses on the disability benefits program created by the federal Social Security Act, the principal national program that awards benefits for disability. While the issues discussed in this section involve the application of a specific program, many of these problems will be encountered in the administration of any program that awards benefits to those whose disability is grounded on a psychiatric impairment. The case that follows is illustrative of the evidentiary issues that must be resolved in the adminis-tration of the Social Security Act.

A. PSYCHIATRIC DISORDERS AND THE DECISIONMAKING PROCESS

CHRISTENSEN v. BOWEN

United States District Court, Northern District of California, (1986).
633 F.Supp. 1214.

ORDER

CONTI, DISTRICT JUDGE.

Plaintiff brings this action pursuant to section 205(g) of the Social Security Act ("Act"), 42 U.S.C. section 405(g), to obtain judicial review of a "final decision" of the Secretary of Health and Human Services ("Secretary"), denying his claim for disability insurance benefits ("DIB").

In order to be affirmed on appeal, the Secretary's findings must be supported by substantial evidence and the Secretary must have applied the proper legal standards in denying plaintiff's claims. If the Secretary's findings are not supported by substantial evidence *or* are based upon a legal error, the Secretary's denial of benefits must be set aside. Substantial evidence is defined as "such relevant evidence as a reasonable mind might accept as adequate to support a conclusion," and it must be based on the record as a whole.

An individual is disabled under the Act if he is unable to,

> "engage in any substantial gainful activity by reason of any medically determinable physical or mental impairment which can be expected to result in death or which has lasted or can be expected to last for a continuous period of not less than twelve months."

42 U.S.C. section 423(d)(1)(A). The impairment must be "of such severity that the claimant is not only unable to do his previous work but cannot, considering his age, education, and work experience, engage in any other kind of substantial gainful work which exists in the national economy." 42 U.S.C. section 423(d)(2)(A). The claimant has the initial burden of establishing that he is unable to do his previous work, but once the claimant has made such a showing the burden shifts to the Secretary to come forward with specific findings showing that there is other substantial gainful activity that the claimant can per-form. *Bonilla v. Secretary of HEW*, 671 F.2d 1245, 1246 (9th Cir.1982); *Hall v. Secretary of HEW*, 602 F.2d 1372, 1375 (9th Cir.1979). Under the "medical-vocational guidelines" ("grids") promulgated by the Secretary, *see* Appendix 2 of Subpart P, 20 C.F.R. section 404.1501 *et seq.*, a claimant will be found capable of "other substantial gainful employment" if he meets certain age, educational, skill and exertional requirements.

While the medical-vocational guidelines provide some evidence of a claimant's ability to engage in substantial gainful work, however, it is well established that they are not of themselves sufficient to meet the Secretary's burden of proving nondisability. In *Lightfoot v. Mathews,* for example, this court held that a disability claimant's capacity to work "must be assessed in terms of age, education, work experience and impairments," and that "[t]his requires a finding of capacity to work which is expressed in specific kinds of jobs . . . not simply in terms of catch-all categories." 430 F.Supp. 620, 621 (N.D.Cal.1977). Similarly, in *Hall v. Secretary of HEW,* the Ninth Circuit Court of Appeals stated that the Secretary must "come forward with specific findings showing that the claimant has the physical and mental capacity to perform specified jobs," and that "the better method to demonstrate this is through the testimony of a vocational expert," although such testimony "would not be required when the availability of work is established by other reliable evidence." 602 F.2d 1372, 1377 (9th Cir.1979). * * *

I. Background.

Plaintiff in this case filed an application for DIB on November 17, 1983, alleging inability to work since May 6, 1983. The application was denied initially and on reconsideration by the Social Security Administration ("SSA"). Accordingly, plaintiff filed for a hearing before an administrative law judge ("ALJ") pursuant to 42 U.S.C. § 405(b). On March 7, 1985, the ALJ determined that plaintiff retained the residual functional capacity to perform work that did not involve high levels of stress, and therefore was not disabled. The Appeals Council affirmed the ALJ's findings on April 23, 1985, whereupon plaintiff filed the present action with this court.

Plaintiff is a 56–year old male who has a Bachelor's degree from Sacramento State College. His work history consists of 36 years of uninterrupted employment with Sears Roebuck Company as an operating superintendent and operating manager. When he last worked, he was responsible for the hiring, firing and discipline of 380 employees, in addition to the implementation of budgetary guidelines from Sears headquarters in Chicago. He worked a minimum of 10 hours per day and sometimes worked as many as 12 to 16 hours per day.

Plaintiff's alleged disability began in May 1983. At that time he consulted Dr. Thomas Ball for symptoms of significant work-induced stress, including severe depression, crying spells, suicidal tendencies, chronic fatigue, loss of appetite and a decreased sexual drive. Pursuant to the recommendations of Dr. Ball and plaintiff's work supervisor, plaintiff took a leave of absence from his job for a five-week period. Plaintiff returned to work on July 5, 1983. He continued to experience serious mental problems, including illegible handwriting, speaking with hesitation, difficulty in composing his thoughts, and a fear of leaving his office. Consequently, plaintiff again left work at Sears on August 7, 1983, and has not worked since.

Dr. Ball continued to treat plaintiff throughout 1983 and 1984. Dr. Ball prescribed Adapin, Xanax, and Halcion. In a report dated June 25, 1984, Dr. Ball indicated that plaintiff's "domestic activities" were unaffected by his mental condition, with the exception of sleeping difficulties, and that plaintiff's capacity to cope with the pressures of ordinary work seemed to be average. He noted, however, that plaintiff had no inclination to return to the stressful circumstances of his previous managerial position, but felt himself more capable of functioning in a work situation that was primarily physical. In a subsequent report dated September 11, 1984, Dr. Ball prescribed plaintiff's psychiatric symptoms as few, mild, and "not incapacitating."

In a consultative psychiatric evaluation dated August 14, 1984, Kathryn H. Knutsson, M.D. gave the following impression:

> This patient could benefit from appropriate anti-depressant medication and talking type of psychotherapy. He is bottled up within himself; is very self-critical. If he is able to learn new skills he would be able to work on for many years. When I saw him on 12/20/83 he was obviously not ready to return to work.

In a report dated September 17, 1984, Robert C. Burr, M.D., stated:

> He seems to have many of the anal-compulsive character traits often seen in people who are predisposed to depression. At present he *seems to be able to function adequately as long as he is placed in a sheltered environment in which very little is actually required of him. The idea of returning to the competitive work world seems to produce instant anxiety.*
>
> Mr. Christensen is obviously doing better than he did when he was still working at Sears in the summer of 1983. He does not appear to have recovered to the point where he could return to work.

Tr. at 189 (emphasis added). Donald L. Tasto, Ph.D., also conducted a consultative psychological evaluation of Mr. Christensen. In his report dated January 10, 1985, Dr. Tasto stated:

> I think that, *because of his memory problems, concentration difficulties and fatigability, Mr. Christensen is presently unable to hold a job with much responsibility or one that requires much stamina, ability to recall, or intense concentration.* I think it is an unanswered question at this point as to whether he will be able to handle something more demanding in the future. It is quite possible his symptoms will change as he changes his use of medication. *This issue aside, I do not think that Mr. Christensen will ever be able to return to a job with a high degree of stress like he had when working for Sears.* Whether or not his intellectual capabilities return as a result of changing medication usage, I think *his capability to deal with stress has been permanently reduced and he, therefore, must be precluded from any job where stress is more than moderate and periodic.*

(emphasis added). The most recent assessment of residual functional capacity was rendered by Bradley M. Greenblott, M.D. In his report dated February 8, 1985, Dr. Greenblott concluded:

At the present time, Mr. Christensen is clearly totally temporarily disabled from a psychiatric standpoint. *He is unable to tolerate even minimal stress, and can in no way handle competitive employment.* I do not believe that he is capable of re-training programs at the present time. The extent of his depression does not allow for this.

Tr. at 224 (emphasis added).

In rejecting the above findings and conclusions regarding plaintiff's residual functional capacity, the ALJ stated that plaintiff's disability claim was not supported by ". . . the reported clinical findings and laboratory test results." Tr. at 16. Specifically, the ALJ found that the conclusions of Drs. Knutsson and Burr regarding plaintiff's inability to return to his previous work were unsupported by clinical findings which indicated, *inter alia,* that plaintiff's memory was intact, that his intelligence was average, that he exhibited no psychotic symptoms, that he was able to engage in certain leisure activities, and that there were some indications of improvement in his overall mental condition. The ALJ cited no clinical findings, however (and the record reveals none), which indicated that plaintiff was able to engage in any forms of employment which involved even minimal amounts of stress. Rather, the ALJ merely noted that Dr. Burr's report ". . . *does not rule out* other, less stressful forms of substantial gainful activity." Tr. at 17 (emphasis added). The ALJ did not address the findings of Drs. Tasto and Greenblott, and made no findings whatsoever regarding plaintiff's ability to engage in other types of work based on plaintiff's age, education, prior work experience and residual functional capacity.

*   *   *

Plaintiff's motion for summary judgment is three-pronged. First, he argues that inasmuch as the ALJ's decision gave little or no weight to the specific clinical findings of Drs. Knutsson, Burr, Tasto, and Greenblott, quoted above, his determination of non-disability was not supported by substantial evidence. Second, plaintiff contends that the ALJ committed legal error by failing to follow the Secretary's own policy promulgations regarding the evaluation of chronic mental impairments. Finally, plaintiff argues that since the ALJ himself conceded that plaintiff could not return to his former employment, the Secretary bears the burden of proof regarding what specific jobs plaintiff can perform. Plaintiff contends that the Secretary has not met that burden. For the reasons set forth below, the court agrees with plaintiff.

As noted above, substantial evidence means that a finding is supported by "more than a mere scintilla. It means such relevant evidence as a reasonable mind might accept as adequate to support a conclusion."

*   *   *

Applying these principles to the present case, the court concludes that Dr. Ball's findings to the effect that plaintiff's impairments were "not incapacitating" when considered together with the findings of the

four remaining doctors who examined plaintiff and emphatically concluded to the contrary, does not constitute substantial evidence sufficient to support a finding of nondisability.

Plaintiff's second argument is that the ALJ erred both in giving
improper weight to the findings of Drs. Knutsson, Burr, Tasto and
Greenblott, and in failing to follow the Secretary's own policy promulgations regarding the evaluation of chronic mental impairments.

In support of this argument, plaintiff notes that the ALJ evidently
rejected the findings of the aforementioned doctors on the ground that
they were not supported by ". . . the reported clinical findings and
laboratory test results." Plaintiff correctly points out that objective
demonstrability is not the correct standard to be applied in evaluating
evidence of mental disorders. As the court stated in *Lebus v. Harris,*

> Courts have recognized that a psychiatric impairment is not as readily
> amenable to substantiation by objective laboratory testing as is a
> medical impairment and that consequently, the diagnostic techniques
> employed in the field of psychiatry may be somewhat less tangible than
> those in the field of medicine. In general, mental disorders cannot be
> ascertained and verified as are most physical illnesses, for the mind
> cannot be probed by mechanical devices in order to obtain objective
> clinical manifestations of mental illness. A strict reading of the
> statutory requirement that an impairment be 'demonstrable by medi-
> cally acceptable clinical and laboratory diagnostic techniques,' 42
> U.S.C. §§ 423(d)(3), 1382c(a)(3)(C), is inappropriate in the context of
> mental illness. Rather, when mental illness is the basis of a disability
> claim, clinical and laboratory data may consist of the diagnoses and
> observations of professionals trained in the field of psychopathology.
> The report of a psychiatrist should not be rejected simply because of
> the relative imprecision of the psychiatric methodology or the absence
> of substantial documentation, unless there are other reasons to ques-
> tion the diagnostic technique.

526 F.Supp. 56, 60 (N.D.Cal.1981) (extensive citations omitted).

Were the findings of Drs. Knutsson, Burr, Tasto, and Greenblott
properly considered under the *Lebus* standard, plaintiff argues, the ALJ
would have found plaintiff's impairments to be of listed severity under
either the original or the revised criteria. Assuming, *arguendo,* that
plaintiff's impairments were not of listed severity, however, plaintiff
contends that the ALJ failed to follow the Secretary's own policy
promulgations regarding evaluation of mental impairments which are
of less than listed severity. The court agrees with plaintiff.

Social Security Ruling 85–16 ("SSR 85–16"), which became effective
on April 1, 1985, some three weeks prior to the Appeals Council's final
decision in this case, states in pertinent part as follows:

> For impairments of listing severity, inability to perform substantial
> gainful activity (SGA) is presumed from prescribed findings. However,
> with mental impairments of lesser severity, such inability must be
> demonstrated through a detailed assessment of the individual's capaci-

ty to perform and sustain mental activities which are critical to work performance. *Conclusions of ability to engage in SGA are not to be inferred from the fact that the mental disorder is not of listing severity.*

. . .

Reports from psychiatrists and other physicians, psychologists, and other professionals working in the field of mental health should contain the individual's medical history, mental status evaluation, psychological testing, diagnosis, treatment prescribed and response, prognosis, a description of the individual's daily activities, and a medical assessment describing ability to do work-related activities. These *reports may also contain other observations and opinions or conclusions on such matters as the individual's ability to cope with stress, the ability to relate to other people, and the ability to function in a group or work situation.*

Medical documentation can often give clues as to functional limitation. For example, evidence that an individual is markedly withdrawn or seclusive suggests a greatly reduced capacity for close contact and interaction with other people. The conclusion of reduced RFC in this area can then be applied to all steps of vocational assessment. For example, when the vocational assessment establishes that the claimant's past work has been limited to work requiring close contact and interaction with other people, the preceding assessment would indicate that the claimant would be unable to fulfill the requirements of his or her past work. Therefore, the determination of disability in this instance would depend on the individual's capacity for other work.

SSR 85–16 (C.E.1985) (emphasis added).

Upon a review of the record, the court finds that had the evidence of plaintiff's inability to cope with even minimal stress much less competitive employment been evaluated in accordance with the factors listed in SSR 85–16, a finding of inability to engage in past relevant work would have been mandated. Since the ALJ erroneously failed to apply these factors to the evidence before him, his decision must also be set aside on this ground.

Finally, plaintiff argues that when he met his initial burden of establishing his inability to do his previous work as a retail supervisor, the burden shifted to the Secretary to show that he was capable of other types of work, and that the Secretary did not meet this burden. Here again, the court agrees with plaintiff.

In his memorandum of decision, the ALJ found that,

[w]hile the claimant's depressive symptoms might be exacerbated by a return to the level of responsibilities and pressures involved in his most recent work for Sears, he could perform other supervisory, managerial, or even lower level work without the unusually high level of stresses and pressures described in his past work.

Such a generalized finding, however, does not satisfy the requirement, under the law of this Circuit, that the Secretary make specific findings showing that there is other substantial gainful activity that the claimant can perform.   As the Ninth Circuit stated in *Hall v. Secretary of Health, Education & Welfare,*

> [a] general statement that a claimant may engage in "sedentary" work, without testimony by a vocational expert who can identify specific jobs, absent other reliable evidence of the claimant's ability to engage in other occupations, does not satisfy the substantial evidence test.
>
> It is incumbent on the Secretary *at a minimum,* to come forward with specific findings showing that the claimant has the physical *and mental* capacity to perform *specified* jobs, taking into consideration the requirements of the job as well as the claimant's age, education and background.

602 F.2d 1372, 1377 (9th Cir.1979) (emphasis added).

* * *

Since the Secretary has failed to meet this burden, and has not given any reasons for its failure, the court finds that reversal is warranted on this ground as well.

III. Conclusion.

In accordance with the foregoing, * * * plaintiff's motion for summary judgment is granted.

Questions and Comments

1. *Disability benefits programs.*   The Social Security Act provides for two kinds of payments to disabled persons.   Social Security Disability Insurance is a benefit payable to disabled persons who qualify under the Act by reason of coverage earned by tax payments made to the Social Security system during their employment.   An individual who has earned the proper number of quarters of coverage is considered "insured for disability insurance benefits."   If determined to be disabled, his monthly disability insurance benefit will equal the amount to which he would be entitled in old-age benefits if he were 62 years old.   Thus eligibility for and the amount of this benefit payment is based on the claimant's work and earnings history.   See 42 U.S.C. § 423(a)(c).

The Supplemental Security Income program, in contrast, is a benefit available to "aged, blind and disabled individuals" whose income and resources fall below a certain level.   Eligibility is not based on work history but on present level of financial need.   The procedures and criteria for disability determination are the same as those used to determine eligibility for disability insurance.   In addition, the claimant must be a resident of the United States, either as a citizen or as an alien admitted for permanent residence.   See 42 U.S.C. § 1382 et seq.

There are, of course, state programs which may provide benefits to those who become physically or mentally disabled.   For instance, states have workers' compensation laws which typically compensate for injuries or deaths suffered in the course of employment.   The emphasis of these laws, however, is on a finding that the work situation caused the mental or physical disability.   A second category of state benefits which may be available to those incapacitated on mental grounds is state public aid programs. Eligibility generally is predicated on lack of income and resources sufficient to meet basic needs. A person's disability is relevant insofar as it affects his income and resources.

2. *The "objective medical evidence" requirement.* The language in the Social Security Act governing evidence of disability reads as follows:

"Section 423(d)

* * *

(3) For purposes of this subsection, a "physical or mental impairment" is an impairment that results from anatomical, physiological, or psychological abnormalities which are demonstrable by medically acceptable clinical and laboratory diagnostic techniques.

* * *

(5)(A) An individual shall not be considered to be under a disability unless he furnishes such medical and other evidence of the existence thereof as the Secretary may require. An individual's statement as to pain or other symptoms shall not alone be conclusive evidence of disability as defined in this section; there must be medical signs and findings, established by medically acceptable clinical or laboratory diagnostic techniques, which show the existence of a medical impairment that results from anatomical, physiological, or psychological abnormalities which could reasonably be expected to produce the pain or other symptons alleged and which, when considered with all evidence required to be furnished under this paragraph (including statements of the individual or his physician as to the intensity and persistence of such pain or other symptoms which may reasonably be accepted as consistent with the medical signs and findings), would lead to a conclusion that the individual is under a disability. Objective medical evidence of pain or other symptoms established by medically acceptable clinical or laboratory techniques (for example, deteriorating nerve or muscle tissue) must be considered in reaching a conclusion as to whether the individual is under a disability . . . ."

In cases of psychiatric disorders, the questions that arise are: What constitutes "medically acceptable clinical or laboratory diagnostic techniques"? What is the meaning of the phrase "[o]bjective medical evidence of pain and other symptoms . . . must be considered in reaching a conclusion as to whether the individual is under a disability"? It is noteworthy that the court in *Christensen* did not attempt to wrestle with the meaning of this language. Had the issue been confronted, how might or should the court have construed the phrase "objective medical evidence"?

Lebus v. Harris, quoted by the court in the principal case, was decided prior to the enactment of an amendment in 1984, which amended Section 423(d)(5)(A). At the time *Lebus* was decided the operative provisions of the Act read as follows:

"Section 423(d)

* * *

(3) For purposes of this subsection, a "physical or mental impairment" is an impairment that results from anatomical, physiological, or psy-

chological abnormalities which are demonstrable by medically acceptable clinical and laboratory diagnostic techniques.

* * *

(5)(A) An individual shall not be considered to be under a disability unless he furnishes such medical and other evidence of the existence thereof as the Secretary may require."

Did the language added by the 1984 amendment serve at all to clarify the meaning of these provisions? Did the court in *Lebus* and *Christensen* essentially read these evidentiary provisions out of the Act?

3. *Proof of inability to work.* Note that in the principal case, the court found there was conclusive evidence that the claimant was incapable of working in an employment involving even minimal stress, thus precluding his continuation in the managerial position he had occupied. The Act, however, requires not only proof by the claimant that he cannot perform his past work, but also a finding by the SSA that he is not capable of performing "any other kind of substantial gainful work which exists in the national economy." Was there any evidence on this point? On what basis did the court dispose of this issue?

4. *Special problems confronting the mentally handicapped claimant.* Any rule which places the burden on the claimant to make a *prima facie* showing of disability may place particular hardship on those whose disability is ground upon a psychiatric disorder. Such individuals sometimes find it difficult to initiate and sustain a claim or to assert their rights, as noted in *City of New York v. Heckler*, set out at p. 1060, infra. However, some courts have shown an inclination not to distinguish the conditions of the *mentally* handicapped from those of the *physically* handicapped. For instance, in *Tusson v. Bowen*, 675 F.Supp. 1032 (E.D.La.1987), affirmed 847 F.2d 284 (5th Cir.1988), the issue concerned a limitation on the award of *retroactive* benefits to a claimant who had failed, because of a mental disability, to file an earlier claim. The claimant in *Tusson* filed for disability benefits in 1982. Following an initial denial, the Administrative Law Judge to whom the matter had been appealed found Tusson to have been disabled since 1977, or 5 years before his initial application for benefits. In challenging the statutory 12 month limitation on the award of retroactive benefits, the claimant argued that:

"A person suffering from severe mental problems, which prevent him from making applications, should be given the opportunity of having his benefits begin at the same time that the disability began so that he is given equal protection under law as provided others, who although disabled but not to the point that they are unable to file, are capable of making an application with the administration."

In reviewing the claimant's contention that the application of the statutory limitations on the award of retroactive benefits violated his constitutional rights, the court held:

"Even assuming that Tusson's interest in retroactive benefits is cognizable under the Due Process Clause, the twelve-month limitation does not violate due process principles. The loss of retroactive benefits by an individual whose mental impairment prevents a timely application suggests unfairness, but a considered analysis reveals otherwise.

The issue of whether the twelve-month limit on retroactive benefits applies where the failure to file for benefits arises from mental impairment was recently addressed in *Yeiter v. Secretary of Health & Human Services,* 818 F.2d 8 (6th Cir.1987), *cert. denied,* —— U.S. ——, 108 S.Ct. 160, 98 L.Ed.2d 115. In *Yeiter,* the court found that 42 U.S.C. § 423(b) does not violate the Due Process Clause because some person acting in behalf of the mentally impaired person could have filed an application. An application for benefits can be filed not only by the claimant, but also by a guardian, a person responsible for the care of the claimant, or the manager or principle officer of an institution caring for the claimant. 20 C.F.R. § 404.612(c). The court assumed that "[a] person who is mentally incapacitated and totally unable to care for himself or herself will ordinarily be in the care of someone. That person responsible for the claimant's care will have a strong incentive to file for benefits." * * * Ordinarily, a mentally impaired person will have a caretaker of some kind but, of course, that will not always be true. Indeed, in the case at bar, Tusson was not in the care of a guardian or some other person. He was capable of taking care of most of his needs, but relied on family members for special needs.

*   *   *

The fact that *some* mentally impaired persons cannot rely on others to file their application does not render the twelve-month limitation fundamentally unfair, arbitrary, or unreasonable.

> 'Whether wisdom or unwisdom resides in the scheme of benefits set forth in Title II, it is not for us to say. The answer to such inquiries must come from Congress, not the courts. Our concern here, as often, is with power, not with wisdom.' (Citation omitted). Particularly when we deal with a withholding of a noncontractual benefit under a social welfare program such as this, we must recognize that the Due Process Clause can be thought to interpose a bar only if the statute manifests a patently arbitrary classification, utterly lacking in rational justification.

Flemming v. Nestor, 363 U.S. 603, 610–611, 80 S.Ct. 1367, 1373, 4 L.Ed. 2d 1435 (1960). "Congress faces an unusually difficult task in providing for the distribution of benefits under the Social Security Act." *Bowen v. Owens,* 476 U.S. 340, 106 S.Ct. 1881, 1885, 90 L.Ed.2d 316 (1986). In 1958, Congress provided for retroactive payments for a twelve-month period "[t]o avoid penalizing disabled workers who do not timely file applications for disability benefits." S.Rep. No. 2388, 85th Cong., 2d Sess. 4, *reprinted in* 1958 U.S.Code Cong. & Admin.News 4218, 4221–22. Thus, Congress decided to give claimants a year's grace to become aware of and file for benefits. Congress' decision that the grace period should terminate at twelve months is not so arbitrary or irrational as to violate due process.

With respect to Tusson's equal protection claim, a challenged statutory classification is presumed valid if it serves a rational means of furthering a legitimate legislative end. *Mathews v. de Castro,* 429 U.S. 181, 185, 97 S.Ct. 431, 434, 50 L.Ed.2d 389 (1976). The Court notes that the twelve-month limit applies evenhandedly to all claimants; mentally incompetent claimants are not treated differently from other claimants. The legislative purpose for not creating an exception for the mentally impaired is clear. Application of the twelve-month period to all claimants helps to preserve the fiscal integrity of the social security trust fund. Even if the volume of such claims as Tusson's were low enough to allay concerns for financial integrity, an ever-growing corpus of government funds would need to be set aside for late-filers to insure that ample funds would be available when claimed. The Court realizes that some mentally impaired people, who are entitled to disability benefits but who cannot file for themselves or rely on others to do so, may not receive benefits to which they would be entitled upon a timely filing. However, as the Supreme Court has recognized, legislation "does not offend the Constitution simply because [it] 'is not made with mathematical nicety or because in practice it results in some inequality.'" *Mathews,* 97 S.Ct. at 434.

Accordingly, this Court finds no violation of the Equal Protection Clause.

Is the district court's analysis of equal protection as applied to the mentally disabled consistent with that followed by the Supreme Court in *City of Cleburne v. Cleburne Living Center* (a challenge on equal protection grounds to a zoning ordinance which subjected any residence to be used as a group home for the mentally retarded to a special use permit procedure), infra at p. 1098? Does *Cleburne* support the view that some minimal rationality in the legislative scheme, even if it impacts negatively on those suffering from a mental disability, is sufficient to meet equal protection review standards?

B. TERMINATION OF BENEFITS

The Administration set out three years ago to purge the rolls of disabled persons Social Security benefits. It declared that hundreds of thousands had shown medical improvement—without, in many instances, looking at the medical evidence in individual cases. By last spring 491,300 had been deprived of their benefits.

One cruel example among many was what happened to mentally ill people in New York: thousands of them, living on the street or awaiting discharge from hospitals. In what a Federal judge called a "clandestine policy," officials took away their benefits *en masse,* without medical reviews.

All this came to light when the city of New York brought a class action suit on behalf of the victims. A Federal court in New York found their mass removal unlawful and ordered the Government to "promptly reinstate benefits" to many. The Administration then sent them checks but refused to provide Medicare coverage—to people in obvious medical need. That evasion stopped when the court heard about it.

In due course the Administration conceded that it had acted improperly. But it went on arguing that no class action should have been allowed. Instead, it said, each victim should have exhausted his administrative remedies and sued individually—even though many were too ill to know what was happening and none could know about the "clandestine" move against them.

Judge after judge across the United States has condemned practices of that kind. By last spring more than 200,000 of the 491,300 disqualified had been ordered back on the rolls.

The Reagan Administration's answer to the extraordinary wave of adverse judicial decisions was to evade them as far as possible. When a court decided that the rules of disability law had been broken in taking benefits away from John Jones, Mr. Jones was restored to the rolls but the Administration refused to apply the decision to others in the same situation.

The policy reached its extreme in resistance to decisions by the 12 United States Courts of Appeals. The Administration declined to apply the rules as defined by those courts, even within the affected judicial circuit and even when it did not seek review of a decision in the Supreme Court.

This "nonacquiescence," as the Administration politely called its refusal to follow Court of Appeals decisions, aroused much critical comment from judges and lawyers."

Anthony Lewis, *Enough was enough.* New York Times, September 20, 1984, p. 25.

In response to criticism such as that noted in the excerpt above, Congress in 1984 proposed an amendment to the Social Security Act which would have the effect of compelling the Administration to adhere to the procedural requirements of the Act. Even prior to 1984, the Administration's disregard of the Act's procedural requirements had been the subject of numerous court challenges. However, as noted by Lewis, these actions, even though frequently successful, had limited effect because of the Administration's policy of non-acquiescence. The most publicized of these cases challenging the illegal termination of benefits of those disabled on psychiatric grounds was *City of New York v. Heckler,* 578 F.Supp. 1109 (E.D.N.Y.1984). The decision on appeal, set forth below, is instructive of the procedural issues underlying all of these cases.

CITY OF NEW YORK v. HECKLER
United States Court of Appeals, Second Circuit, 1984.
742 F.2d 729.

JON O. NEWMAN, CIRCUIT JUDGE:

The Secretary of Health and Human Services appeals from a judgment of the District Court for the Eastern District of New York (Jack B. Weinstein, Chief Judge) invalidating a procedure used by the Social Security Administration ("SSA") in the determination of original and continuing eligibility of claimants for disability benefits. *City of New York v. Heckler,* 578 F.Supp. 1109 (E.D.N.Y.1984). The ruling affects a class of persons with severe mental illnesses. The class is estimated to include more than 50,000 New York residents. The Secretary raises no challenge on appeal to the District Court's invalidation of the challenged procedure, which has since been abandoned. However, the appeal presents substantial and complicated issues concerning the jurisdiction of the District Court to adjudicate the class members' challenge and to award relief. For reasons that follow, we affirm the judgment of the District Court.

BACKGROUND

The invalidated procedure concerns one aspect of the elaborate process by which people are determined to be eligible for disability benefits under the Social Security Disability Insurance ("DI") program, established by Title II of the Social Security Act ("the Act"), 49 Stat. 622, as amended, 42 U.S.C. § 401 *et seq.* (1982), and the Supplemental Security Income ("SSI") program established by Title XVI of the Act, 76 Stat. 197, as amended, 42 U.S.C. § 1381 et seq. (1982). More specifically, we are concerned with the five-step "sequential evaluation" process adopted by the Secretary to govern determination of initial and continuing eligibility for disability benefits under both DI and SSI programs.

The first step in the sequential process is a decision whether the claimant is engaged in "substantial gainful activity." If so, benefits are denied. 20 C.F.R. §§ 404.1520(a), (b), 416.920(a), (b) (1983). If not, the second step is a decision whether the claimant's medical condition or impairment is "severe." If not, benefits are denied. 20 C.F.R. §§ 404.1520(c), 416.920(c). If the impairment is "severe," the third step is a decision whether the claimant's impairments meet or equal the "Listing of Impairments" set forth in subpart P, app. 1, of the social security regulations, 20 C.F.R. §§ 404.1520(d), 416.920(d). These are impairments acknowledged by the Secretary to be of sufficient severity to preclude gainful employment. If a claimant's condition meets or equals the "listed" impairments, he or she is conclusively presumed to be disabled and entitled to benefits. If the claimant's impairments do not satisfy the "Listing of Impairments," the fourth step is assessment of the individual's "residual functional capacity," *i.e.,* his capacity to engage in basic work activities, and a decision whether the claimant's residual functional capacity permits him to engage in his prior work. If the residual functional capacity is consistent with prior employment, benefits are denied. 20 C.F.R. §§ 404.1520(e), 416.920(e). If not, the fifth and final step is a decision whether a claimant, in light of his residual functional capacity, age, education, and work experience, has the capacity to perform "alternative occupations available in the national economy." *Decker v. Harris,* 647 F.2d 291, 298 (2d Cir.1981); 20 C.F.R. §§ 404.1520(f), 416.920(f). If not, benefits are awarded.

The procedural irregularity challenged in this litigation concerns the fourth step of the sequential evaluation process—the determination

of residual functional capacity. In disregard of the regulatory requirement to conduct an individualized assessment of the residual functional
capacity of each claimant, SSA, informally and without public disclosure, adopted an administrative practice that effectively imposed a
presumption upon the determination of eligibility for DI benefits:
Claimants whose mental impairments were not as severe as those in
the Listing of Impairments were presumed to retain a residual functional capacity sufficient to perform at least unskilled work. This
presumption was conclusive as to most claimants with mental impairments that were "severe" but not "listed." The practical effect of the
presumption was to end the sequential process for most class members
at the third step. The only class members who might progress through
the fourth and fifth steps and receive benefits were those over 50 with
extreme vocational deficiencies and "severe" but unlisted mental impairments. These class members, despite the presumption concerning
residual functional capacity, might be found eligible for benefits by
virtue of the medical-vocational "grid" regulation, 20 C.F.R. subpart P,
app. 2 (1983), but the force of the presumption could still adversely
affect their claims.

   The presumption concerning residual functional capacity was applied throughout the elaborate administrative process by which claims
for initial and continuing disability benefits are determined. The
presumption guided determinations made by the New York State Office
of Disability Determinations, pursuant to its contract with the SSA and
review decisions made at the regional and national levels by SSA
officials. Upon the *de novo* reviews conducted by administrative law
judges, the presumption was not required to be applied, but the District
Court found that ALJ's often relied on determinations of residual
functional capacity that were tainted by use of the presumption earlier
in the review process.

   On February 8, 1983, the City of New York and the New York City
Health and Hospitals Corporation, the Commissioner of the New York
State Department of Social Services, and the Acting Commissioner of
the New York State Office of Mental Health, suing on their own behalf
and as *parens patriae,* and eight named individuals brought this class
action against the Secretary and the Commissioner of SSA on behalf of

> All individuals residing in the State of New York who have applied for
> or received Title II and/or Title XVI benefits on or after April 1, 1980,
> and who have been found by defendants to have a mental impairment
> which is severe . . . and whose applications for benefits have been or
> will be denied or whose benefits have been or will be terminated, on
> the basis of defendants' determination that such persons are capable of
> substantial gainful activity.

Plaintiffs sought declaratory and injunctive relief enjoining the Secretary from continuing to apply the unwritten presumption concerning
residual functional capacity.

The Secretary unsuccessfully resisted class certification on the ground that the District Court lacked jurisdiction over most members of the proposed class.

The District Court rejected the Secretary's jurisdictional contentions. On the merits Chief Judge Weinstein ruled that "from 1978 until at least the early months of 1983" SSA engaged in a covert policy to deny class members an individualized assessment of each claimant's capacity to engage in substantial gainful activity in violation of the strictures of the Social Security Act and regulations enacted thereunder. 578 F.Supp. at 1115. As relief the Court ordered the Secretary (i) to reopen all disability determinations rendered after April 1, 1980, in which disability benefits were denied or terminated, and (ii) to "reinstate benefits of all class members until the claimant's eligibility is properly determined." *Id.* at 1125. These reinstated benefits have been referred to in the litigation as "interim" benefits.

Following the Secretary's motion for a stay pending appeal ＊ ＊ ＊ Chief Judge Weinstein entered an amended judgment modifying the judgment to limit relief to individuals with a "functional psychotic or functional non-psychotic mental impairment which is severe . . ." and to limit interim benefits to recipients whose benefits had been terminated.

On appeal, the Secretary does not challenge the District Court's ruling on the merits, but raises only jurisdictional contentions. ＊ ＊ ＊ The Secretary further contends that mandamus jurisdiction is not available and that the District Court lacked authority to award interim benefits in the absence of an administrative finding of disability.

DISCUSSION

A. Section 405(g) Jurisdiction

[The court held that the District Court had jurisdiction to hear the action and that neither exhaustion of administrative remedies was required nor was a sixty day statute of limitations rule a bar to judicial review.]

B. Mandamus Jurisdiction

[The court held that mandamus jurisdiction might provide an alternate source of jurisdiction as to members of the plaintiff's class.]

C. The Merits and the Remedy

The Secretary has made no claim before the District Court or on appeal that use of the presumption concerning residual functional capacity was lawful. There is thus no dispute that on the merits the class members are entitled to prevail. However, the Secretary challenges on appeal the scope of the District Court's remedial decree, specifically, the reinstatement of benefits for those class members previously determined to be disabled but subsequently terminated from the disability rolls. This reinstatement has the effect of awarding interim benefits to terminated class members until such time as the

(R. & S.) Mental Health, 2d Ed. ACB—36

SSA makes a procedurally correct determination that they are no longer eligible for disability benefits. In the Secretary's view, this award of interim benefits violates the principle of sovereign immunity, which shields the Government from liability for a money judgment in the absence of an express congressional enactment waiving such immunity. We disagree.

The Act authorizes benefit payments following a final decision by the Secretary or a final judgment by a court that a claimant is "entitled" to benefits, 42 U.S.C. § 405(i). The amended judgment provides interim benefits only to those individuals who have previously received a "final decision" from the Secretary that they were "entitled" to disability benefits. New applicants were not awarded interim benefits. Once the District Court properly invalidated the Secretary's termination decisions because of the acknowledged procedural illegality, the Court was clearly entitled to reinstate the earlier favorable final decisions pending lawful redeterminations of each claimant's continuing eligibility. As both the Eighth and Ninth Circuits have held in closely analogous circumstances, the payment of benefits to wrongfully terminated recipients follows a final decision of the Secretary and consequently is consistent with the requirements of section 405(i). *Mental Health Ass'n of Minnesota v. Heckler, supra; Lopez v. Heckler, supra* (preliminary injunction).

We do not construe the recent amendment to section 223 of the Act, Pub.L. No. 97–455, § 2, 96 Stat. 2498 (1983) as indicating a congressional understanding that federal courts lacked remedial power to order the award of interim benefits in appropriate circumstances. That amendment entitles claimants who are challenging a termination decision to continue to receive benefits throughout their administrative appeals. We see no reason to think that Congress, in authorizing interim benefits during administrative appeals, believed that such benefits were not available during pursuit of judicial remedies. The more plausible interpretation is that Congress was anxious to fill a gap and ensure continuity of benefits on the understanding that, after administrative remedies were pursued, courts had adequate authority to continue interim benefits.

More fundamentally, we do not construe section 405(i) as a limitation on a federal court's remedial powers under the Act. While a court's injunctive power must be exercised with caution, respectful of the authority of coordinate branches of Government, where, as here, the award of interim benefits is necessary to make whole individuals harmed by the SSA's failure to abide by the law, federal courts are not without authority to award the necessary relief.

The judgment of the District Court is affirmed.

Questions and Comments

1. *Individual determination v. administrative efficiency.* While the Supreme Court affirmed *City of New York v. Heckler* (see *Bowen v. City of*

New York, 476 U.S. 467, 106 S.Ct. 2022, 90 L.Ed.2d 462 (1986)), the Court has not always favored a construction of the Act which emphasizes individualization over ease of administration. For instance, in *Bowen v. Yuckert,* 482 U.S. 137, 107 S.Ct. 2287, 96 L.Ed.2d 119 (1987), the claimant challenged a review procedure under which the Secretary could deny a claim without reaching some criteria ostensibly required by the Act. The Court held that this truncation of the claims process was both consistent with the original Act and had been expressly approved by Congress in its enactment of amendments to the Act in 1984 "in the interests of reasonable administrative flexibility and efficiency." 482 U.S. at 151, 107 S.Ct. at 2296.

2. *Unique vulnerability of the mentally ill.* To what extent was the outcome of *City of New York* influenced by the fact that the claimants were disabled on psychiatric grounds? The District Court's opinion contains the following statement:

> "The mentally ill are particularly vulnerable to bureaucratic errors. Some do not even understand the communications they receive from SSA. Others are afraid of the system. Even with help from social workers and others, many do not appeal denials or terminations.

> An erroneous termination or denial of benefits to a mentally ill person means more than that he or she will no longer receive benefits. To many it may mean a severe medical setback. [A psychiatrist] testified that one of her patients who had not been hospitalized for fifteen years was hospitalized as a result of the trauma of having benefits cut off. This was not a unique case. Some slip into acute paranoia while others become suicidal."

578 F.Supp. 1109, 1115 (E.D.N.Y.1984).

Does this statement suggest that the procedural errors in applying the presumption of employability works a particular hardship on the mentally ill since they are less able to challenge adverse decisions and, moreover, may be psychologically damaged by an adverse decision?

3. *Quantifying mental illness.* The District Court's opinion took particular aim at the use in psychiatric cases of the Listing of Impairments. The effect of this total reliance on the Listing was to make anyone whose impairment did not meet its criteria ineligible for benefits. As to this reliance, the court cites with approval the conclusions of one psychiatrist that:

> "[T]here is no way you can take the complex of human behaviors recorded in the psychiatric history, or even a summary of a single hospitalization and narrow it down to 17 numbers. That is absolutely ludicrous [sic]. And if you're trying to do it for determination of one's capacity to work, I don't know if it becomes more or less ludicrous [sic]; but its [sic] a silly notion."

578 F.Supp. 1109, 1116 (E.D.N.Y.1984).

Does this mean that the court would disapprove of the use of any quantitative scale to assess mental disability? Is this position defensible?

4. *Reform of the disability determination process.* As noted in *City of New York* and the Lewis article, the SSA refused for more than five years to change its practices and was able to evade Supreme Court review by not

appealing adverse decisions. At the same time, the SSA adopted a practice of applying judicially conforming procedures only to those cases that had been actually litigated. The effect of this practice was to force subsequent claimants to relitigate the same issues repeatedly.

In response to concerns expressed by advocates of the mentally impaired, Congress enacted the Social Security Disability Benefits Reform Act of 1984 (P.L. 98–460, 98 STAT. 1794). The Act required the SSA to revise the criteria for determining the existence of mental impairments and for assessing a mentally impaired claimant's ability to work. Congress intended these revisions to be designed "so as to realistically evaluate the ability of a mentally impaired individual to engage in substantial gainful activity in a competitive environment." House Report No. 98–618, 1984 U.S.Code Cong. & Admin.News 3038, 3052. It also imposed a moratorium on any action by the SSA to suspend the benefits of persons currently receiving benefits on grounds of mental impairments. Finally, the Act required the SSA to reconsider any denial determination, as to persons claiming disability by reason of a mental impairment, made after the date of enactment and before the required revision of procedures.

The House Bill submitted to conference committee also proposed a prohibition against the SSA's policy of non-acquiescence with federal circuit court decisions. The provision, however, was not included in the final version of the Act.

In addition, the Supreme Court recently held that HHS improperly denied Supplemental Security Income (SSI) benefits to disabled children. In *Sullivan v. Zebley*, ___ U.S. ___, 110 S.Ct. 885, 107 L.Ed.2d 967 (1990), the Court found that HHS regulations improperly restricted eligibility for benefits by requiring children's disabilities to meet the Listing of Impairments. The court held that this restriction contravenes the SSI statute, which requires an individualized inquiry to determine whether a child's disability is of "comparable severity" to disabilities which would preclude adult claimants from working. See, 42 U.S.C. § 1382c(a)(3).

Advocates for the disabled have estimated that as many as one million children, including those with Down's syndrome and autism, will now be eligible for SSI benefits as a result of this ruling. See, New York Times, February 21, 1990, p. A20.

5. *Locating potential beneficiaries.* The mentally disabled, because of their disability, may be unable to gain the benefits of legal action taken on their behalf. This is particularly true because a large number of the mentally disabled are among the homeless and cannot be reached at a known address. For instance, as a result of *City of New York v. Heckler,* approximately 14,000 persons were deemed likely to be eligible for back benefits. But by the end of 1987, only 500 of these people had been notified that their cases could be reopened and that, if successful in proving disability under the revised standards, they might be eligible for up to $20,000 in back benefits. The process used to find these potential recipients was described in the New York Times:

Seeking Out Beneficiaries

The notices from the Social Security Administration to former disability beneficiaries in New York are among the first in the nation and are expected to be followed in other states by letters to 200,000 people.

The search in New York began with letters to the last known addresses of the people whose benefits were cut off. In other cases, relatives or others, such as doctors, have been sought out.

But where the usual methods of finding people have been unsuccessful, the search branched out in mid-December to city and private shelters, where so far only 12 people have been found.

'Fragile Members of Society'

Armed with a computer list of names, the caseworkers visit places where homeless people may be and speak with other social workers who may know the people.

"We are dealing with some of the most fragile members of society, so it's not easy to find them and explain everything to them," said Cindy Freidmutter, New York director of the Mental Health Law Project.

Mr. [Dana] Edwards of the Social Security Administration said he could not estimate how many of those on the computer list are homeless.

City officials have contended from the beginning that large numbers of those affected were homeless or would be homeless if their benefits were cut. Ms. Freidmutter said her office was proceeding on the assumption that hundreds are homeless.

New York Times, Jan. 15, 1988, p. 1, p. 32 col. 3.

6. *Disability determination review.* The Act requires determinations of disability to be reviewed by the state agency every three years in order to determine whether recipients are eligible for continued payment of benefits. However, there are two exceptions to this requirement. First, where a disability has been found to be permanent, that determination may be reviewed "at such times as the Secretary determines to be appropriate." Second, the Secretary may waive the three year review requirement for a particular state and instead require the state to review an "appropriate number" of cases. What is the appropriate number of cases depends upon the state's backlog of pending reviews, projected number of new applications, and staffing levels. See 42 U.S.C. § 421(i).

Chapter Twelve

PROTECTION AGAINST DISCRIMINATION

I. ACCESS TO EMPLOYMENT OPPORTUNITIES

The Rehabilitation Act of 1973 provides that "[n]o otherwise qualified individual with handicaps . . . shall, solely by reason of her or his handicap, be excluded from the participation in, be denied the benefits of, or be subjected to discrimination under any program or activity receiving Federal financial assistance or under any program or activity conducted by any Executive agency or by the United States Postal Service. . . ." 29 U.S.C. § 794 (Section 504 of the Act). This broad anti-discrimination provision encompasses protection against employment discrimination by the federal government, federal contractors, and entities that receive federal funds.

A bill now pending in Congress (titled the "Americans with Disabilities Act of 1989"), which is likely to be enacted in 1990, would extend such protection by prohibiting employment discrimination by *any* employer of 15 or more people. The bill would prohibit an employer from discriminating against "a qualified individual with a disability because of [such individual's] disability" in all aspects of employment. S.933, 101st Cong., 1st Sess., § 102(a) (1989). See also, H.R. 2273, 101st Cong., 1st Sess., § 202(a) (companion bill to S. 933). Significantly, S.933 adopts the key substantive protections and language found in the Rehabilitation Act of 1973 and its implementing regulations. In light of the bill's potentially broad impact on employment opportunities for the handicapped, this section examines the legal issues which have arisen under the 1973 law and which are likely to arise in the context of employment in the private sector if Congress enacts into law the new anti-discrimination bill.

A. CONDITIONS GIVING RISE TO COVERAGE UNDER THE REHABILITATION ACT OF 1973

FORRISI v. BOWEN

United States Court of Appeals, Fourth Circuit, 1986.
794 F.2d 931.

WILKINSON, CIRCUIT JUDGE:

The sole question is whether the plaintiff, fired because of his fear of heights, may claim the protection of the Rehabilitation Act of 1973, 29 U.S.C. § 701 *et seq*. We conclude that plaintiff's acrophobia is not a handicap for which he may claim relief from discrimination, and we affirm the summary judgment in favor of defendant.

I.

The Department of Health and Human Services hired Louis P. Forrisi in February 1983 as a utility systems repairer and operator in the Office of Facilities Engineering of the National Institute of Environmental Health Services (NIEHS). The job description requires that the occupant be able to climb stairways and ladders both for emergencies and for routine maintenance. During an introductory tour of the plant at Research Triangle Park, North Carolina, Forrisi told his supervisor that he could not climb to certain heights. Management officials responded that Forrisi therefore could not satisfy the requirements of his job. Forrisi insisted that he could do the necessary work, particularly if the employer would make some adjustments to accommodate his fears. In April 1983, HHS informed Forrisi that it had terminated his appointment because he was "medically unable to perform the full range of the duties of [his] position." Forrisi charged that the decision constituted illegal discrimination against a handicapped person, and, after exhausting the available administrative remedies, brought this lawsuit under § 505 of the Rehabilitation Act of 1973, 29 U.S.C. § 794a.

II.

To succeed in his claim, Forrisi must first establish that he is a handicapped person within reach of the statute. The Rehabilitation Act of 1973, as amended, defines the term "handicapped individual" at 29 U.S.C. § 706(7)(B) as "any person who (i) has a physical or mental impairment which substantially limits one or more of such person's major life activities, (ii) has a record of such an impairment, or (iii) is regarded as having such an impairment." The district court correctly held that plaintiff failed to satisfy this threshold test.

* * *

The inquiry is, of necessity, an individualized one—whether the particular impairment constitutes for the particular person a significant barrier to employment. Relevant to the inquiry are "the number and type of jobs from which the impaired individual is disqualified, the geographical area to which the individual has reasonable access, and the individual's job expectations and training."

The statutory language, requiring a *substantial* limitation of a *major* life activity, emphasizes that the impairment must be a significant one. It was open to Congress to omit these limiting adjectives, but Congress did not do so.

The Rehabilitation Act assures that truly disabled, but genuinely capable, individuals will not face discrimination in employment because of stereotypes about the insurmountability of their handicaps. It would debase this high purpose if the statutory protections available to those truly handicapped could be claimed by anyone whose disability was minor and whose relative severity of impairment was widely shared. Indeed, the very concept of an impairment implies a characteristic that is not commonplace and that poses for the particular individual a more general disadvantage in his or her search for satisfactory employment.

Forrisi does not maintain that his acrophobia substantially limits his major life activities or that he has a history of an impairment that so limits him. To the contrary, he reported in deposition testimony that "My fear of heights never affected my life at all on any job or anything" and that "It never was a problem before I got this job here at NIEHS. It never was a problem."

* * *

Forrisi argues instead that § 706(7)(B)(iii) extends to his situation because, though not in fact a handicapped individual, he was perceived as being so. HHS, he claims, regarded him as having an impairment that substantially limited one of his major life activities. The Equal Employment Opportunity Commission, which is responsible for federal employers' compliance with the Rehabilitation Act, has issued regulations that define "is regarded as having an impairment" to mean

> (1) has a physical or mental impairment that does not substantially limit major life activities but is treated by an employer as constituting such a limitation; (2) has a physical or mental impairment that substantially limits major life activities only as a result of the attitude of an employer toward such impairment; (3) or has none of the impairments defined in (b) of this section but is treated by an employer as having such an impairment.

29 C.F.R. § 1613.702(e). The EEOC has also defined "major life activities" to include "functions, such as caring for one's self, performing

manual tasks, walking, seeing, hearing, and working." 29 C.F.R. § 1613.702(c).

* * *

The statute and regulations both focus our attention on the claim that Forrisi's acrophobia did not substantially limit any of his major life activities but that HHS nevertheless treated the condition as such a handicap on his ability to work. We must identify the degree to which HHS could consider Forrisi's acrophobia to restrict his ability to work without, in the statutory sense, considering the acrophobia to be a substantial limitation in violation of § 706(7)(B)(iii). Forrisi urges a statutory violation on the theory that HHS must have regarded Forrisi as substantially limited in his ability to work when the Department found him unable to perform his job at NIEHS.

Several courts have previously addressed this issue, deciding unanimously that an employer does not necessarily regard an employee as handicapped simply by finding the employee to be incapable of satisfying the singular demands of a particular job.

The statutory reference to a substantial limitation indicates instead that an employer regards an employee as handicapped in his or her ability to work by finding the employee's impairment to foreclose generally the type of employment involved. The court in *E.E. Black, Ltd. v. Marshall*, [497 F.Supp. 1088 (D.Hawaii 1980)] illustrated the conclusion with an example that anticipated Forrisi's predicament as well as his argument. If the Rehabilitation Act extended to all individuals who have been rejected from a particular job because of a perceived inability to perform that job, the court reasoned, the Act would cover an individual with acrophobia "who was offered 10 deputy assistant accountant jobs with a particular company, but was disqualified from one job because it was on the 37th floor." 497 F.Supp. at 1099. The court found that any such interpretation would contravene the exclusive statutory concern for *substantial* limitations, whether genuine or perceived.

We agree both with this theoretical position and with its application to the problem of acrophobia. HHS never doubted Forrisi's ability to work in his chosen occupation of utility systems repair. The Department merely saw him as unable to exercise his acknowledged abilities above certain altitudes in this NIEHS plant.

* * *

Far from being regarded as having a "substantial limitation" in employability, Forrisi was seen as unsuited for one position in one plant—and nothing more.

As one court has noted, adoption of Forrisi's reasoning would imply that anyone who failed to obtain a single job because of a single requirement of employment would become a handicapped individual because the employer would thus be regarding the applicant's failure as a handicap. Such a reading would stand the Act on its head. The Rehabilitation Act seeks to remedy perceived handicaps that, like actual disabilities, extend beyond this isolated mismatch of employer and employee.

The judgment of the district court is

Affirmed.

Questions and Comments

1. *Who is "handicapped" under the act?* As noted in *Forrisi*, the threshold question in a Rehabilitation Act claim is whether the plaintiff is a "handicapped individual" (later changed to "individual with handicaps"), defined as "any person who (i) has a physical or mental impairment which substantially limits one or more of such person's major life activities. . . ." 29 U.S.C. § 706(8)(B). The application of this provision to mental disorders has proven particularly difficult. For instance, should an individual who suffers from acrophobia in that he cannot take an elevator or climb stairs be deemed a "handicapped individual"? Should the answer to this question turn on the availability of some jobs in a particular category for which the individual is qualified which can be performed on the first floor? What if the individual were disqualified from 90% of the jobs in that category because they are normally performed above the first floor?

Note in this connection that the court in *Forrisi* cites *E.E. Black, Ltd. v. Marshall*, 497 F.Supp. 1088 (D.Hawaii 1980), where the court reasoned that the Act would not cover an individual suffering from acrophobia who was offered 10 accounting positions but was disqualified from one job because it was on the 37th floor. But isn't *Forrisi*'s situation distinguishable from that of the hypothetical accountant in that as a maintenance worker he presumably would routinely need to climb stairs and ladders as part of his job?

However, as the subsection which follows indicates, a determination that Forrisi was a "handicapped individual" would not end the inquiry. He still must demonstrate that he is "otherwise qualified" for the job. His impairment might render him not "otherwise qualified" since it is likely to prevent him from carrying out the duties associated with the job.

2. *State employment discrimination laws.* In addition to the federal Rehabilitation Act, a number of states have adopted laws protecting the handicapped from discrimination. Some of these laws apply to narrowly defined classes of disabilities. For instance, in the Michigan Handicappers' Civil Rights Act, the term "handicap" includes "a determinable mental characteristic" which is limited to mental retardation or "a mentally ill restored condition." The Act does not define the term "mentally ill restored." In *Doman v. City of Grosse Pointe Farms*, 170 Mich.App. 536, 428 N.W.2d 708 (1988), the court held that a schizophrenic who was terminated from his public employment was not covered by the Act, since his condition was neither cured nor stabilized by medication at the time he was discharged. Does the Michigan law in effect exclude from its protections persons with incurable or uncontrollable mental illnesses?

In contrast, a North Carolina statute's definition of "handicap" has been narrowly construed to mean "a present, non-correctible loss of function which substantially impairs a person's ability to function normally." *Burgess v. Joseph Schlitz Brewing Co.,* 298 N.C. 520, 528, 259 S.E.2d 248, 253 (1979). Under the statute, a person with such a handicap is entitled to equal state employment opportunities unless his particular disability impairs his ability to perform the particular work involved. Thus, a public university professor who was terminated *after* his mental illness was cured was not a "handicapped person" entitled to coverage under the statute. *Pressman v. University of North Carolina at Charlotte,* 78 N.C.App. 296, 337 S.E.2d 644 (1985).

3. *Pre-employment inquiries as to handicap.* Under a regulation promulgated pursuant to the Rehabilitation Act, a recipient of federal funds "may not make pre-employment inquiry of an applicant as to whether the applicant is a handicapped person or as to the nature or severity of a handicap" but may inquire "into an applicant's ability to perform job related functions." 45 C.F.R. § 84.14(a). (A similar prohibition which applies to federal employers is contained in 29 C.F.R. § 1613.706). This regulation has been construed to prohibit questions of a job applicant designed to elicit whether he has been treated for a mental disorder. *Doe v. Syracuse School District,* 508 F.Supp. 333 (N.D.N.Y.1981). The regulation serves to ensure that an employer will "base the hiring decision on a person's actual job qualifications, rather than on any perceived limitations." Id. at 337.

B. THE "OTHERWISE QUALIFIED" REQUIREMENT

DOE v. REGION 13 MENTAL HEALTH–MENTAL RETARDATION COMMISSION.

United States Court of Appeals, Fifth Circuit, 1983.
704 F.2d 1402.

E. GRADY JOLLY, CIRCUIT JUDGE:

This appeal comes from a grant of judgment notwithstanding the verdict by the court below in favor of the defendants-appellees Region 13 Mental Health–Mental Retardation Commission, d/b/a Gulf Coast Mental Health Center ["GCMHC"] and the Executive Director of GCMHC, Dr. G. Kinsey Stewart, entered against the plaintiff-appellant Jane Doe, a former employee at GCMHC. The case involves an alleged violation of section 504 of the Rehabilitation Act of 1973, 29 U.S.C. § 794.

Because we find that the district court's grant of the J.N.O.V. was proper * * * we affirm.

I.

Region 13 is one of fifteen regional programs authorized by the Mississippi State Legislature in the early 1970's to comply with the National Community Mental Health Centers Act, 42 U.S.C. § 2681, *et seq.,* begun during the Kennedy administration. The program seeks to provide out-patient, in-patient and emergency treatment for persons suffering mental disorders.

* * *

GCMHC is a mental health center operated by Region 13, with its main offices located in Gulfport, Mississippi. GCMHC operates thirteen programs, including programs specifically designed for children. As executive director, Dr. Stewart has general administrative responsibility over the center and its seventy-odd employees. Dr. Stewart has been director of GCMHC since its inception.

GCMHC is funded through a complex mixture of federal, federal-state, state and local financing. The federal funding has been primarily of a block-grant nature, for specific purposes, including a "Children and Youth Grant" which funds staffing of the program for children.

Ms. Doe was reared outside of Mississippi. She obtained an undergraduate psychology degree in an eastern state and in 1977 obtained a graduate degree in psychology also from a university in that state.

Ms. Doe began suffering spells of anxiety, insomnia and depression in 1977. Over a six-to-eight month period she saw a psychiatrist on a weekly basis. The psychiatrist prescribed sleeping pills to help with her problems. At one point in 1977 Ms. Doe took a potentially lethal overdose of the pills and had to be hospitalized for a brief time. Although at trial Ms. Doe did not characterize this incident as an effort to commit suicide, it is capable of being so interpreted.

In June 1978 Ms. Doe applied with GCMHC to work in the Children and Youth Services program. On her application, she stated that her "general health" was "excellent" and that she had no "physical handicap or defect which would prevent a normal performance of duties." Ms. Doe was hired in August 1978 on a probationary basis as a Mental Health Associate with the Child Youth Service program.

By all accounts, Ms. Doe was a superior employee. She maintained a heavy caseload, working at any one time on a one-to-one basis with some thirty out-patient children and adolescents and with their families. She also worked with a local public school and with the local Head Start agency.

According to her immediate supervisor, Ms. Doe "did an excellent job." She carried one of the heaviest caseloads, saw more patients and did a good job as consultant with the local school. Her paper work was prompt and thorough. She had no problems with absenteeism. In February 1979, after an evaluation of her work which found her to be "outstanding," her probationary status was removed and she was given a raise.

Essentially, Ms. Doe continued to do an outstanding job by all objective standards until her termination in November 1979. She worked hard, was diligent and thorough, her patients liked her, and she had no excessive absences from work. She was reevaluated in October 1979, and again was rated "outstanding." She also received another pay raise.

Unfortunately, during the entire term of her employment at GCMHC, Ms. Doe suffered from essentially the same psychological symptomology as she had in 1977. Finding the Mississippi Gulf Coast something of a "culture shock," Ms. Doe continued to experience anxiety and depression after her move there in August 1978. The heat bothered her, the minor day-to-day problems of life bothered her, and she had great difficulties simply in "coping." She was lonely and missed her family and friends in her home state. She had little money, and her apartment was without telephone or furniture.

Her sole source of pleasure and stability was her work. The depression she suffered usually came on the weekends.

In November 1978, three months after moving to her new home and job, Ms. Doe began psychotherapy with a local clinical psychologist, Dr. Joseph Tramontana. Dr. Tramontana was a part-time staff member at GCMHC who maintained a private practice.

Over the course of these weekly, forty-five to fifty-minute sessions, which continued into the summer of 1980, Dr. Tramontana developed the following diagnosis of Ms. Doe. A "depressive neurosis" was the primary psycho-symptomology. She was alone and had a "great deal of difficulty being alone." She suffered from chronic insomnia and frequently resorted to drug/alcohol ingestion to counter that insomnia. She also suffered serious depression as a result of an unsatisfactory relationship with a man.

In stressful situations Ms. Doe employed a "numbers game" as a blocking technique to avoid dealing with the problem. This numbers game essentially involved adding random numbers in her head. Also, she had experienced a plane crash on her way to interview for the job in Mississippi, and for a time had an irrational phobia about planes. In addition, for a time she "day-dreamed" that a monster was chasing her through a cemetery.

Most significantly, Ms. Doe's psychologist was concerned about the possibility of suicide. He considered the incident with the sleeping pills when Ms. Doe was a graduate student to be a serious attempt at suicide.

* * *

Over the course of her therapy with Dr. Tramontana, Ms. Doe made repeated references to suicide as a possible solution to her problems. Dr. Tramontana, believing that Ms. Doe had tried to kill herself once, felt that she continued to consider suicide "a viable alternative" and that she "might do it again."

Ms. Doe's condition, although consistently depressive-neurotic, fluctuated in its severity. Those fluctuations, according to her psychologist, were significant in the late-winter, early-spring of 1979.

In early May 1979, shortly after Ms. Doe had experienced problems with her boyfriend, Dr. Tramontana was leaving for the weekend. Thus left without her principal "support systems," Ms. Doe was anxious about facing the weekend. She did not want Dr. Tramontana to leave and asked for a back-up therapist. Dr. Tramontana suggested Dr.

Leonard Ball, a psychiatrist who was the Medical Director at GCMHC. Dr. Ball talked with her, and she explained her difficulties, telling him that she wanted "the world to stop." Dr. Ball was concerned about her well-being and asked that she meet him at the emergency room at Gulfport Memorial Hospital. Dr. Ball recommended brief hospitalization to see if medication might alleviate her depression. She voluntarily admitted herself to the hospital and stayed for two or three days. She experienced no apparent problems with her work or her caseload as a result of her hospitalization.

The medication did not have any significant ameliorative effect, however, because at the end of May, Ms. Doe was rehospitalized.

* * *

Again, she remained in the hospital for two or three days. During this second hospital stay, Dr. Ball suggested to Ms. Doe that she should consider long-term hospitalization.

Over the course of the summer Ms. Doe remained fairly stable and continued to do a good job. Her immediate supervisor, Dr. Calhoun, while feeling that she was doing good work, was concerned about her obvious anxiety and agitation and recommended to her that she should be seeing someone.

Ms. Doe's anxiety worsened in early August, and she experienced great difficulty sleeping. She hadn't been able to sleep for two or three nights and went to Dr. Ball and asked for medication. He prescribed chloral hydrate, a potent sleeping pill, which she took home but did not take for fear that she could not hear the foster child whom she had taken in and with whom she was living at the time. Again, she couldn't sleep, and she called Dr. Tramontana, explained her problem, and he recommended that she call Dr. Ball. When she saw Dr. Ball at work he recommended that she readmit herself to Gulfport Memorial Hospital. She did so.

During this third hospitalization, which again was brief, Dr. Ball again recommended long-term hospitalization, preferably for one year. Dr. Tramontana did not agree with this suggestion, but thought that more intense psychotherapy was warranted, with more frequent sessions.

No change was made in Ms. Doe's treatment, however; she continued her good work; she continued to be depressed; and she continued her weekly one-hour sessions with Dr. Tramontana. In October she again was rated "outstanding" and given another pay increase.

The culminant event in Ms. Doe's employment occurred in November 1979. Two events precipitated this last crisis—her thirtieth birthday was to occur on November 10 and Dr. Tramontana was going out of town. Ms. Doe made statements to Dr. Tramontana, to her co-workers and to her friends that she would not "see" her thirtieth birthday. She indicated that she was going to kill herself by dropping her hair dryer into the bathtub and electrocuting herself. She indicated that she had made arrangements for her clients to be taken care of, for her foster child to be taken care of, and that she had left her insurance policy where it could be found.

Dr. Tramontana was greatly concerned about Ms. Doe and felt that she was suicidal. Dr. Tramontana informed Ms. Doe's brother through a friend that the brother had the alternative either to institute commitment proceedings or "have her kill herself." The brother thereupon swore out the necessary affidavits to institute Ms. Doe's commitment, and on November 8 at approximately 11:00 p.m., Ms. Doe was taken by police from her home to the psychiatric ward at Gulfport Memorial Hospital. The next day she was "interviewed" by the two on-call doctors for commitment purposes, one of whom happened to be Dr. Ball. Based on the interview, it was determined that Ms. Doe was sufficiently dangerous to herself to warrant further commitment proceedings before the chancery court.

A preliminary hearing was held with testimony as to Ms. Doe's condition from the interviewing doctors and from Ms. Doe. The court felt that Dr. Tramontana was best suited to testify as to Ms. Doe's condition, however, and postponed further hearings until he was able to present testimony to the court. Dr. Tramontana flew back to Gulfport and visited Ms. Doe. He felt that her mood was elevated and that she was no longer suicidal. She promised him that she would be a better patient and that she would allow him to hypnotize her to uncover her past. According to Dr. Tramontana, she "sounded like a completely different person. . . ." He made a tape for the court discussing Ms. Doe's condition and recommended against commitment. Proceedings were dismissed against Ms. Doe, and she was released from the hospital. She returned to work the same day. She reported to her supervisor, Dr. Calhoun, who assured her that nothing had changed.

During this immediate time period, Dr. Ball, who by now was intimately familiar with Ms. Doe's psychopathology, discussed her case with Dr. Stewart, the administrator at GCMHC. In his role as Medical Director at GCMHC, responsible for the medical care provided at the center, Dr. Ball informed Dr. Stewart of Ms. Doe's involuntary hospitalization, of her apparently serious potential for suicide, and of her need, in his opinion, for long-term hospitalization. Dr. Stewart had been aware of Ms. Doe's previous hospitalizations and her ongoing psychiatric problems, but, according to the testimony at trial, this was the first time Dr. Ball had given him the specifics of her case and had indicated the need for long-term treatment. Dr. Ball recommended that Ms. Doe be given the option of taking a leave of absence to "seek another mode of therapy" or that she be terminated. He informed Dr. Stewart that he was concerned about the well-being of Ms. Doe's patients and the impact that her suicide could have on them. Dr. Ball felt that Ms. Doe "was more impaired than the patients she was seeing."

Based on Dr. Ball's recommendation, Dr. Stewart ordered that Ms. Doe not see any more patients. He met with her the day following her return to the center and explained to her his feelings about the situation. According to Ms. Doe, he told her that he was "concerned about funds and public image" and that she could either resign or take a long-term leave for hospitalization with no job upon her "return." According to Dr. Stewart, he told her that she should consider seeking employment elsewhere or take a long-term leave for hospitalization with consideration for rehiring in the future based on her medical status. According to Dr. Stewart, he did not tell her that her job would be phased out.

Ms. Doe considered her options over the Thanksgiving holidays. Upon returning to the clinic after Thanksgiving, she told Dr. Stewart she could not accept his recommendation. She told him that if she were terminated she would go to the local newspaper and reveal how GCMHC treated depressive neurosis. Dr. Stewart thereupon terminated her as an employee.

II.

Ms. Doe filed suit claiming that Dr. Stewart and GCMHC had violated her rights under section 504 of the Rehabilitation Act of 1973, 29 U.S.C. § 794.[2] Ms. Doe sought damages of $12,000 for her lost wages and $100,000 for pain and suffering and for detriment to her future career. She also sought reinstatement and attorneys' fees.

This case was tried before a jury. After trial, in which testimony was received from Ms. Doe, Dr. Tramontana, Dr. Ball, Dr. Stewart, Dr. Calhoun and Dr. Patsy Zakaras, who was program evaluator for the Children's Services Division at GCMHC, the jury found for Ms. Doe and awarded her $25,000 in damages and stated in its verdict that Ms. Doe "should be reinstated." Judgment was entered by the court reflecting that verdict.

Subsequently, the court entertained the defendants' motions for judgment notwithstanding the verdict or, alternatively, for a new trial, and for remittitur of damages. The court ruled that the evidence failed to support the verdict and set aside the verdict.

III.

We note as a preliminary matter that the jurisdictional requirements have been met here. There are essentially two jurisdictional prerequisites in a section 504 case, to wit, that the plaintiff be "handicapped" and that the program in which the plaintiff would be involved be federally funded.

Under 29 U.S.C. § 706(7)(B), a handicapped person is "any person who (i) has a physical or mental impairment which substantially limits one or more of such person's major life activities, (ii) has a record of such an impairment, or (iii) is regarded as having such an impair-

---

2. "No otherwise qualified handicapped individual in the United States, as defined in section 706(6) of this title, shall, solely by reason of his handicap, be excluded from the participation in, be denied the benefits of, or be subjected to discrimination under any program or activity receiving Federal financial assistance."

ment."[5] A mental handicap, such as claimed by Ms. Doe, therefore qualifies under the applicable statute.[6] The parties did not, in fact, contest the issue of whether Ms. Doe was handicapped within the ambit of § 504, and, based on the record, Ms. Doe was so handicapped.

The next jurisdictional prerequisite is that the program itself be federally funded. * * * The plaintiff demonstrated here that the program with which she was involved, the "Children and Youth Services" program, received funds for staffing from the federal government. It therefore appears that the specific program with which Ms. Doe was involved was federally funded.

* * *

IV.

Having found that the plaintiff was "handicapped" within the coverage of the Act, we next turn to the more difficult question under section 504, that is, whether the plaintiff was "otherwise qualified" within the meaning of the Act, or whether the district court correctly found that the evidence produced by the plaintiff did not support the conclusion that she was so qualified.

The Supreme Court in *Southeastern Community College v. Davis,* 442 U.S. 397, 406, 99 S.Ct. 2361, 2367, 60 L.Ed.2d 980 (1979), stated: "An otherwise qualified person is one who is able to meet all of a program's requirements in spite of his handicap." The plaintiff contends that sufficient evidence was presented to the jury to allow a finding that she was "otherwise qualified" and that she therefore was terminated from her employment in violation of the Act. The plaintiff had an exemplary work record. All of the evaluations of her work were highly complimentary of her ability and willingness to undertake a heavy case load. Despite her handicap, her attendance record was acceptable. Her paper work was good. And apparently her interpersonal relationships with other members of the clinic staff were good; no mention was made at trial of any problems with other staff members.

On the other hand, the plaintiff had exhibited serious suicidal tendencies over a long period of time, at least since 1977, when she attempted to commit suicide while in graduate school. The plaintiff had been in fairly intensive psychotherapy with Dr. Tramontana since November of 1978, for approximately a year, and had not shown noticeable improvement. Rather, the situation seemed to be deteriorating, based upon her two hospitalizations in May, her hospitalization in August, and the very serious chain of events in November of 1979 which led to the institution of involuntary commitment proceedings. Her psychotherapist, Dr. Tramontana, considered that she might, in

5. 45 C.F.R. § 84.3(j)(2)(ii) defines "major life activities" as "caring for one's self, performing manual tasks, walking, seeing, hearing, speaking, breathing, learning, and working."

6. The "Catch-22" implicit in virtually all section 504 actions is particularly evi-

dent in this case, that is: Ms. Doe was required to prove her handicap for jurisdictional purposes, but simultaneously required to prove that she was not so handicapped as to be unqualified to perform her job. * * *

fact, kill herself in the early part of November 1979, and Dr. Ball, who was fairly closely involved with her case, also felt that she was suicidal.

According to Dr. Stewart, based upon the recommendation given to him by Dr. Ball, he felt that Ms. Doe was a threat to herself and that it was in the best interests of the patients at GCMHC to terminate her employment or at least to have her take a long-term leave of absence so that she could undergo intense psychiatric therapy on an in-patient basis. All of the doctors who testified as to her condition testified that a therapist who accepts suicide as a reasonable alternative may pass along this bias to his or her patients. Additionally, Dr. Stewart and Dr. Ball testified as to their concern about the effect which a therapist's suicide would have on that therapist's patients.

Dr. Ball made his recommendation that Ms. Doe not be allowed to see patients because of his belief that she might commit suicide. "My concern was her future performance, not her past performance. . . . My clinical impression at the time of the commitment was that she was severely depressed and suicidal. That's what made me concerned regarding her future work performance."

In sum, the plaintiff presented her case to the jury that she was "otherwise qualified" based on her excellent past record at GCMHC. On the other hand, the defendant GCMHC presented its evidence supporting termination of Ms. Doe's employment based on the state of her condition as of November 1979. The hospital argued that although she might have been qualified in the past, her condition had deteriorated to the point where she no longer could be relied upon to be an effective therapist.

Because we find that the evidence overwhelmingly supported Dr. Stewart's action here with regard to Ms. Doe, we find that the district court did correctly grant the judgment notwithstanding the verdict.

We start with the premise that there was no evidence produced of any discriminatory animus against persons with handicaps such as Ms. Doe's. Significant testimony was presented supporting the fact that GCMHC had several employees who suffered from depression and who were undergoing psychiatric counseling. No action was shown to have been taken against these individuals because of their psychiatric problems.

* * *

In determining whether Ms. Doe was "otherwise qualified" under the Act, we believe that, in the absence of any evidence of such discriminatory animus as discussed above, we must analyze the actions by GCMHC to determine whether there was a substantial, reasonable basis for its decision. Then we must apply *Boeing Co. v. Shipman* to determine whether the J.N.O.V. rendered was appropriate under this standard of review.

This standard, crucial to the analysis of employment decisions under section 504, is based on our reading of the Supreme Court's decision in *Southeastern Community College v. Davis.* In *Davis,* the Supreme Court considered whether the defendant college, a state institution receiving federal funds, had acted discriminatorily in denying admission to the plaintiff into the defendant's nursing program because of the hearing handicap suffered by the plaintiff. The court of appeals, in reversing the decision by the district court, had held that under section 504 the plaintiff's application should have been considered without regard to the handicap and that in considering whether she was "otherwise qualified," the college had to limit its inquiry to her academic qualifications.

The Supreme Court, in reversing the court of appeals, held that while section 504 means that mere possession of a handicap is not a permissible ground for "assuming an inability to function in a particular context," 442 U.S. at 405, 99 S.Ct. at 2366, an institution is not required to ignore limitations which result from the handicap. Finding that an institution could reasonably consider the effect of the handicap involved, the Court turned to the particular qualifications of the plaintiff as they bore on the requirements for matriculation at the college. The Court found that the college was justified in its determination that plaintiff would pose a threat to patients' safety if she participated in the clinical phase of the nursing program. Because of her hearing handicap, she could not safely participate in a clinical setting. The Court found that the plaintiff would be very limited insofar as the nursing courses which she could take and the services which she could render as a nurse. Further, the Court found that nothing in the legislative history or in the language of section 504 required affirmative action by a participating program. Thus, the Court held that the community college was not required to supply the "extensive modifications necessary to include" the plaintiff in the nursing program. 442 U.S. at 410, 99 S.Ct. at 2369.

We read this landmark case under section 504 to support a reasonable deference to the decisions made by administrators of federally funded programs so long as no evidence is presented of discriminatory intent with regard to the handicapped person. To repeat, "an otherwise qualified person is one who is able to meet *all* of a program's requirements in spite of his handicap." 442 U.S. at 406, 99 S.Ct. at 2367 (emphasis added). This assumes, of course, that "a program's requirements" are reasonable. 442 U.S. at 414, 99 S.Ct. at 2371.

That we should grant deference to Dr. Stewart's decision in this case is underscored by the nature of the problem which is involved. This is not a case involving whether an employee is able to screw nuts and bolts onto a widget with sufficient speed. No such cut-and-dried factual proof is available when dealing with the "soft science" surrounding the health or affliction of an individual's psyche. Of course we must give weight to an expert's determination where there is no showing that such determination was skewed by unlawful animus.

*   *   *

We believe that in cases of this sort where, as here, there has been no showing of discriminatory animus, and where there is uncontroverted evidence of a chronic, deteriorating situation which is reasonably interpreted to pose a threat to the patients with whom the employee must work, no violation of section 504 could reasonably be found.

* * *

Substantial, rational bases existed for Dr. Stewart's action here. He could not be expected to stand idly by, knowing that Ms. Doe's behavioral disorder might have severe consequences for all concerned. Besides the deleterious effect which suicide or an attempt at suicide would have upon Ms. Doe's patients, there was the question of the ongoing deleterious effect which her continued suicidal ideation was having upon those patients, who were susceptible and suggestible adolescents. Despite the excellent record which Ms. Doe had compiled during her employment at GCMHC, the record fully supported the fact that Dr. Stewart did not act in a discriminatory manner with regard to the termination of her employment. She had been "otherwise qualified," but there was strong and overwhelming evidence, and considered professional opinion, that she was no longer "otherwise qualified."

We therefore conclude that, viewing the evidence under the proper legal standards set forth above, reasonable men could not have differed about the validity of the decision that she was no longer qualified made by Dr. Stewart and by GCMHC, and that the granting of the judgment notwithstanding the verdict was appropriate.

Affirmed.

Questions and Comments

1. *The reasonable accommodation requirement.* Doe v. Region 13 turns on the finding that there was conclusive evidence that Jane Doe was not "otherwise qualified" by reason of her condition. Thus, the statute authorizes an employer to refuse employment to a handicapped individual where the handicap significantly impinges on the capacity of the employee to carry out the normal tasks associated with the employment. The severity of this rule is tempered, however, by a provision in the regulations which defines "qualified handicapped person" as one who "*with reasonable accommodation,* can perform the essential functions of the job in question." (Emphasis added). (Applicable to entities receiving federal funds under 45 C.F.R. § 84.3K and to federal employment by 29 C.F.R. § 1613.702(f)).

The issue of reasonable accommodation was not reached in *Doe v. Region 13* by either the trial or appellate court. Conceivably, the plaintiff could have argued that she *was* "otherwise qualified" despite her depression and suicidal tendencies so long as she was not involved in a therapeutic relationship with patients. For instance, if the Region 13 Mental Health Center had a diagnostic intake unit, could she have argued that she was "otherwise qualified" for a position in diagnostic intake which requires no sustained therapeutic relationship with patients? Would such an assignment have been required as a reasonable accommodation?

Note, in this connection, that the *Doe v. Region 13* opinion cites with approval the conclusion of the court in *Southeastern Community College v. Davis* that "nothing in the legislative history or in the language of Section 504 required *affirmative action* by a participating program." (Emphasis added). While this statement may be technically true if confined to the wording of the 1973 Act itself, the implementing regulations may be seen as requiring some affirmative action as a result of the reasonable accommodation requirement. The scope of the obligations under the reasonable accommodation requirement are considered in the next subsection.

2. *Confidential relationship.* Though the question appears not to have been addressed, the case does raise the issue of breach of confidentiality on the part of Dr. Ball, the psychiatrist medical director of the center where Jane Doe worked. In May 1979, Dr. Tramontana, the psychiatrist who was treating the plaintiff temporarily, referred her to Dr. Ball for treatment. As a result of this referral, Dr. Ball saw the plaintiff, who during the course of the therapeutic session confided the facts of her depression and suicidal impulses.

The following November after having been involved in Jane Doe's treatment, "Dr. Ball, who was by now intimately familiar with Ms. Doe's psychopathology, discussed her case with Dr. Stewart [the Director of the Center]. . . . Dr. Ball informed Dr. Stewart of Ms. Doe's involuntary hospitalization, of her apparently serious potential for suicide, and of her need, in his opinion, for long term hospitalization." At 1406. Was Dr. Ball justified in making these disclosures without Jane Doe's consent? If the disclosures were a violation of Dr. Ball's duty to Ms. Doe, what were Jane Doe's remedies? The obligation imposed by the rules on patient/therapist confidentiality are treated in Chapter Four.

C. EMPLOYER'S DUTY OF REASONABLE ACCOMMODATION

A regulation implementing the Rehabilitation Act of 1973 provides:

(a) An agency shall make reasonable accommodation to the known physical or mental limitations of a qualified handicapped applicant or employee unless the agency can demonstrate that the accommodation would impose an undue hardship on the operation of its program.

(b) Reasonable accommodation may include, but shall not be limited to: (1) Making facilities readily accessible to and usable by handicapped persons, and (2) job restructuring, part-time or modified work schedules, acquisition or modification of equipment or devices, appropriate adjustment or modification of examinations, the provision of readers and interpreters, and other similar actions.

(c) In determining pursuant to paragraph (a) of this section whether an accommodation would impose an undue hardship on the operation of the agency in question, factors to be considered include: (1) The overall size of the agency's program with respect to the number of employees, number and type of facilities and size of budget; (2) the type of agency operation, including the composition and structure of the agency's work force; and (3) the nature and the cost of the accommodation.

29 C.F.R. § 1613.704

(A nearly identical regulation imposes a duty of reasonable accommodation upon entities receiving federal funds. See 45 C.F.R. § 84.12)

The case that follows explores the scope of the obligation under 29 C.F.R. § 1613–704.

SHEA v. TISCH

United States Court of Appeals, First Circuit, 1989.
870 F.2d 786.

PER CURIAM.

Appellant Shea, who worked for the postal service for many years, brought an action against the defendant postmaster general contending he had been discriminated against because of his handicap. Defendant sought summary judgment for either of two independent reasons. First, defendant argued, plaintiff had failed to contact an Equal Employment Opportunity counselor within 30 days of the last alleged act of discrimination as required by 29 C.F.R. § 1613.214(a) (1986) and, second, defendant, as a matter of law, had made a reasonable accommodation of plaintiff's handicap [as required by 29 C.F.R. sec. 1613.704].

The court granted defendant's motion for summary judgment without indicating the basis for its ruling and without any statement of reasons. Plaintiff has appealed. We review the record.

The verified complaint and appended materials, including affidavits and the Equal Employment Opportunity (EEO) case file, indicated that plaintiff, a disabled Vietnam veteran suffering from an anxiety disorder, was hired by the postal service in 1973. He had a good work record through 1981. Thereafter, Shea experienced medically related absences; in April 1985 the postal service attempted to separate him from service on the basis of disability. Plaintiff challenged that decision through the grievance procedure. Dr. Gammon, his clinical psychologist at a veteran's hospital, wrote letters explaining that plaintiff's anxiety was greatly increased by driving in heavy Boston traffic to his duty station, but that if plaintiff were reassigned to a post office within 10 to 15 miles of his Billerica home, his absenteeism would diminish.

The proposed separation was rescinded on December 24, 1985. As a result of negotiations between plaintiff's lawyer and postal officials in April 1986, plaintiff was temporarily assigned to the Stoneham Post Office for one bid cycle. Plaintiff understood that the Stoneham assignment was temporary and that he was supposed to bid on other assignments during the cycle in order to use his seniority rights to obtain a more permanent position near his home.

Positions within a 10 to 15 mile radius of plaintiff's home thereafter became available; plaintiff could have obtained them, given his seniority, but chose not to bid on any. All of the openings, he said, failed to meet his medical needs. Plaintiff was warned that if he refused to bid he would end up being assigned to a less desirable left-over slot, and his stay in Stoneham was extended to three bid cycles, to give him more time to secure a permanent slot. On June 30, 1986, Dr. Gammon wrote a further letter stating that Shea felt that his manager at the Stoneham Post Office was putting a great deal of pressure on Shea to accept a bid. Dr. Gammon thought that for plaintiff to accept a bid which "increases the pressure on him, either by virtue of placing him on a late shift or a split time-off arrangement, [would be] seriously detrimental to his psychological well-being." While some of the jobs available to plaintiff, had he bid, were day shift jobs, they provided for split time off, that is, one weekend day off and one weekday off, rather than the entire weekend (which plaintiff preferred in order to have the same free days as his wife and to decrease the stress he experienced). After three bid cycles had passed without Shea having tendered any bids, he was assigned to the Watertown Post Office on the 11:30 p.m. to 8:00 a.m. shift effective July 5, 1986. On Dr. Gammon's advice, plaintiff did not report for duty.

Although plaintiff had formerly worked in the Boston Management Sectional Center (MSC), his home was located in the Middlesex–Essex MSC. Some of the post offices most proximate to plaintiff's home were in one MSC and some in the other. On the advice of then acting labor relations manager, James Leahy, plaintiff applied in August 1986 to Charles Wilkinson, manager of employee relations in Middlesex–Essex, for a position at the Woburn mail facility. By letter dated September 29, 1986, Wilkinson turned down plaintiff's request, referring, among other things, to plaintiff's poor attendance record.

Plaintiff and his lawyer continued to meet with postal officials through October and November 1986 in an attempt to obtain a posting consistent with what plaintiff believed his medical needs to be. At a November 1986 meeting with William Evans, the manager of labor relations, plaintiff's attorney was informed that no further accommodation would be made.

[The court held that plaintiff's action was not barred by his failure to challenge the initial decision within the statutory thirty day time limit].

*   *   *

II.

We turn, then, to the postal service's argument that it reasonably accommodated plaintiff's handicap. First, it is important to underline what defendant did not argue in moving for summary judgment on the reasonable accommodation issue. Defendant did not dispute plaintiff's contention, supported to some degree by Dr. Gammon's letters, that driving more than 15 miles, working a late night shift, and not being able to spend weekends with his wife were medically contraindicated in view of plaintiff's anxiety disorder.

*   *   *

[I]n moving for summary judgment, defendant argued that it could not have provided plaintiff with the job he desired because to do so would have violated the seniority provisions of the collective bargaining agreement between the service and the American Postal Workers Union. Under that agreement, defendant said, assignments must be bid for and then awarded on the basis of seniority. And defendant cited a number of cases for the proposition that an employer is not required to reassign a handicapped person to a different position, particularly if such a reassignment would violate other employees' rights under a collective bargaining agreement.

Below, plaintiff did not dispute defendant's summary or analysis of the collective bargaining agreement. Indeed, plaintiff did not provide any real response to defendant's argument. Consequently, we must take it as established that to provide plaintiff with the accommodation plaintiff seeks—that is, permanent assignment to a day time, weekday position within 15 miles of his home without competitive bidding and irrespective of seniority—would violate the collective bargaining agreement.

We find *Carter v. Tisch*, 822 F.2d 465 (4th Cir.1987), on which defendant relies, persuasive. In that case, a postal custodian was unable to perform his usual work because of asthma and sought assignment to a permanent light duty position. Reassignment was denied because there were no permanent light duty positions available in the maintenance craft to which plaintiff belonged and, even if there had been one available, plaintiff would not have been eligible for it as the collective bargaining contract required five years prior service, a requirement plaintiff had not met. Plaintiff was discharged.

The question before the court in *Carter* was whether a transfer of the type plaintiff requested was a reasonable accommodation the postal service was required to make. The court concluded it was not. First, the court noted that the Supreme Court had said in dicta that an employer was "not required to find another job for an employee who is not qualified for the job he or she was doing," although he could not "deny an employee alternative employment opportunities reasonably available under the employer's existing policies." *School Board of Nassau County v. Arline*, 480 U.S. 273, 289 n. 19, 107 S.Ct. 1123, 1131 n. 19, 94 L.Ed.2d 307 (1987). The Fourth Circuit read this dicta to mean that an employer is not required to find alternative employment unless he normally does so under his existing policies. In *Carter*, however, the plaintiff was not eligible under the employer's existing policies to obtain the transfer he wanted. The Fourth Circuit next surveyed the existing case law and found the overwhelming weight of authority to be against plaintiff's contention that reassignment was required as a reasonable accommodation. The court then concluded that even if there were a duty to reassign in some cases, "such a duty would not defeat the provisions of a collective bargaining agreement unless it could be shown that the agreement had the effect or the intent of discrimination." *Carter v. Tisch*, 822 F.2d at 469.

To be sure, plaintiff's situation is not identical to the plaintiff's in *Carter*. Unlike the plaintiff in *Carter,* Shea claims he would be capable of doing his usual duties were he able to get to work without being subject to undue stress which adversely affects his work ability. It is the location (and timing) of the duties—not the duties themselves—which pose the problem. But this difference, we think, is not a critical one. The fact remains—as in *Carter*—that plaintiff wants not the position at the East Boston Air Mail Facility he held when his anxiety disorder started to impose additional limitations, but a new position at a different location. To give plaintiff such a new position would violate the collective bargaining rights of other employees, thus drawing a compelling parallel to *Carter.*

* * *

Consequently, we, like the Fourth Circuit, conclude that the postal service was not required to accommodate plaintiff further by placing him in a different position since to do so would violate the rights of other employees under the collective bargaining agreement.

AFFIRMED.

Questions and Comments

1. *Undue hardship on employer.* The employer's duty of reasonable accommodation under the Rehabilitation Act is created by regulation. In the 1989 bill (The Americans With Disabilities Act of 1989) mentioned at the beginning of this section, this duty would be imposed by the statute itself. Under the bill, an employer's failure to "make reasonable accommodations to the known physical or mental limitations" of a qualified handicapped applicant or employee constitutes discrimination, unless to do so would impose an undue hardship. See, S. 933, 101st Cong., 1st Sess., § 102(b)(5) and H.R. 2273, 101st Cong., 1st Sess., § 202(b)(1) (1989). The Senate bill, like the regulation implementing the Rehabilitation Act, sets out factors to be considered in determining whether an accommodation would impose an undue hardship.

2. *Collective bargaining agreements.* In *Shea,* the court rejects the plaintiff's claim for reasonable accommodation on the grounds that to do so would violate the terms of the collective bargaining agreement. Note that the regulations calling for reasonable accommodation set out at the beginning of this section impose the requirement of reasonable accommodation unless the imposition would "impose an undue hardship on the operation of the agency in question". Should any deviation from the terms of a collective bargaining agreement be construed to impose an undue hardship on the employer? If so, why?

3. *Special treatment for alcoholic employees.* Courts generally have held that alcoholism is a handicapping condition for purposes of the Act. The reasonable accommodation requirement has been construed in these cases "to require federal employers to exert substantial affirmative efforts to assist alcoholic employees toward overcoming their handicap before firing them for performance deficiencies related to drinking." *Whitlock v. Donovan,* 598 F.Supp. 126, 131 (D.D.C.1984). In *Whitlock,* the court held

that the alcoholic employee must be offered an unpaid leave of absence to enable him to seek inpatient treatment. The court noted that federal statutes and regulations impose substantial obligations upon federal employers to assist alcoholic employees, including provision of disability retirement benefits (which until 1980 had been denied persons whose disability was "due to vicious habits, intemperance, or willful misconduct.") See, id. at 133.

4. *Compulsive gambling.* At least one court has found a cause of action under the Rehabilitation Act for a compulsive gambler who was dismissed from his federal employment. *Rezza v. United States Department of Justice,* No. 87–6732, memorandum order, May 12, 1988, *motion to reconsider den.,* 698 F.Supp. 586 (E.D.Pa.1988). The plaintiff in *Rezza* was an FBI agent, dismissed from his job for misappropriating government funds and taking an FBI vehicle to gamble in Atlantic City. Despite plaintiff's criminal activity, the court denied the government's motion for summary judgment. Noting that compulsive gambling is a recognized mental disorder, the court found that whether plaintiff was otherwise qualified (i.e., qualified for the job if reasonable accommodations are made) implicated material fact issues. What steps might an agency such as the FBI be required to take to accommodate an employee's compulsive gambling? Might accommodation in this case impose undue hardship on the FBI?

5. *Reasonable accommodation in private sector employment.* The proposed "Americans with Disabilities Act of 1989," extending protection from discrimination to applicants and employees in the private sector, defines "qualified individual with a disability" as "an individual with a disability who, *with or without reasonable accommodation,* can perform the essential functions of the employment position that such individual holds or desires." S.933, 101st Cong., 1st Sess., § 101(7) and H.R. 2273, 101st Cong., 1st Sess., § 201(5) (1989) (emphasis added). The proposed Act imposes a duty of reasonable accommodation in the statute itself, and it defines "qualified individual with a disability" with reference to reasonable accommodation. Thus, the proposed law mandates coverage broader than that of the Rehabilitation Act in that the duty of reasonable accommodation is not one that can be limited, altered or omitted by regulation.

D. SCOPE OF JUDICIAL REMEDIES

Section 505 of the Rehabilitation Act of 1973 (29 U.S.C. § 794a) extends the remedies available under the Civil Rights Act of 1964 to handicapped applicants or employees who allege discrimination in violation of the Act by a federal agency or an entity receiving federal funds.

As to the latter, the Civil Rights Act has been construed to afford a private right of action to persons aggrieved by discriminatory action. In such actions, remedies may include both prospective and retroactive relief, though the award of damages will generally be limited to back pay. See, *Smith v. Robinson,* 468 U.S. 992, 1020 n. 24, 104 S.Ct. 3457, 3472, 82 L.Ed.2d 746 (1984); *Consolidated Rail Corp. v. Darrone,* 465 U.S. 624, 630, 104 S.Ct. 1248, 1252, 79 L.Ed.2d 568 (1984). See also,

Shuttleworth v. Broward County, 649 F.Supp. 35 (S.D.Fla.1986). Moreover, under both the Civil Rights Act and the Rehabilitation Act, the court in its discretion may allow the prevailing party a reasonable attorney's fee. See 42 U.S.C. § 2000e–5(k) and 29 U.S.C. § 794(2)(b).

The Act also requires federal agencies providing funding to ensure that such entities comply with the Act's anti-discrimination policies. To ensure such compliance, an agency may terminate or refuse to grant or continue financial assistance to the entity. See 42 U.S.C. § 2000d–1.

States receive federal financial assistance, and so fall within the scope of the Rehabilitation Act of 1973 and the Civil Rights Act of 1964. However, as a result of various court decisions, states retained their 11th amendment immunity until 1986 when Congress amended the 1966 Civil Rights Act to provide that: "[a] State shall not be immune under the Eleventh Amendment of the Constitution of the United States from suit in Federal court for a violation of section 794 of Title 29 [Section 504 of the Rehabilitation Act] . . . or the provisions of any other Federal statute prohibiting discrimination by recipients of Federal financial assistance." 42 U.S.C. § 2000d–7(a)(1).

Non-judicial remedies are available to persons filing a Section 504 claim against a federal employer. Section 706 of the Civil Rights Act of 1964 authorizes the Equal Employment Opportunity Commission to take administrative action against a federal agency to attempt to secure a "conciliation agreement." If an individual has filed allegations against a federal agency with the EEOC, and the EEOC either dismisses the charge or declines to file a civil action, the individual may thereafter file an action on his own behalf in federal district court. See 42 U.S.C. § 2000e–5. The EEOC, or in certain cases, the Attorney General, also are authorized to file a civil action on behalf of aggrieved individuals.

The proposed "Americans with Disabilities Act of 1989" extends the same remedies to handicapped persons alleging discrimination by private employers, thus extending the EEOC's jurisdiction to include private employers alleged to have discriminated on the basis of disability. The House bill also extends to the handicapped the remedies and procedures available under Section 1981 of the Civil Rights Act. See S.933, 101st Cong., 1st Sess., § 107 and H.R. 2273, 101st Cong., 1st Sess., § 205 (1989).

E. SPECIAL PROBLEMS: AFFIRMATIVE ACTION PROGRAMS

Section 501 of the Rehabilitation Act of 1973 requires each federal agency to promulgate "an affirmative action program plan for the hiring, placement, and advancement of individuals with handicaps. . . ." 29 U.S.C. § 791(b). This affirmative action requirement extends only to federal agencies and not to entities receiving federal funds. The case that follows illustrates some of the issues that may arise from the implementation of these kinds of programs.

ALLEN v. HECKLER

United States Court of Appeals, District of Columbia Circuit, 1985.
780 F.2d 64.

MIKVA, CIRCUIT JUDGE:

This appeal involves a claim under the Rehabilitation Act of 1973. 29 U.S.C. § 701 *et seq.* (1982) ("the Act"). Section 501 of the Act, 29 U.S.C. § 791 (1982), requires each federal executive department to formulate an affirmative action plan that provides adequate career opportunities for handicapped people. The plaintiffs, a class of former patients at St. Elizabeth's, a federal mental hospital, were hired by the Hospital pursuant to one such plan. They now claim that this plan is inadequate because it allows St. Elizabeth's to discriminate against them on the basis of their previous institutionalization.

The district court agreed and granted summary judgment in favor of the plaintiffs. We now affirm the court's finding of discrimination, but vacate and remand for reconsideration of the remedy.

I.

Eleon Allen, the named plaintiff, is a former patient at St. Elizabeth's Hospital, a federal mental institution in Washington, D.C. After his discharge as a patient in 1978, Allen was hired by St. Elizabeth's as a housekeeping aide pursuant to 5 C.F.R. § 213.3102(h) (1984) ("subsection (h)"). Subsection (h) provides that patients who have been discharged from federal mental hospitals may be given special hiring consideration at the institution where they previously received treatment. The key to subsection (h) is that ex-patients are excused from the usual competitive process for obtaining federal employment, and thus are considered "excepted" service employees. Although the former patients must have the necessary skills for the jobs they seek, it is considered "not practical" to subject them to the competitive civil service examination.

Excepted employees, such as the ex-patients here, perform exactly the same work as their "competitive" service counterparts. Their duties and responsibilities are the same, their work is judged by the same standards, and their pay is the same. The excepted workers, however, are given fewer job benefits than competitive employees. Subsection (h) workers may not participate in the civil service retirement program. If they are disciplined or discharged, they do not have the right to an evidentiary hearing before an independent decisionmaker, or the right to appeal to the Merit Systems Protection Board. Excepted workers also have fewer job protections and no "bumping" rights (*i.e.,* no right to take jobs from employees with less seniority) when there is a reduction in work force.

An excepted worker under subsection (h) is free to enter the competitive service at any time by taking the regular civil service exam; the drawback is that the excepted worker must start on the same footing as a first-time applicant. The former patient enjoys no advantage because of his on-the-job experience, nor does he get seniority or other credit for the time spent before conversion toward permanent career status, the federal equivalent of tenure.

Allen and fifty-two other former patients ("plaintiffs") working at St. Elizabeth's sued the Director of the Department of Health and Human Services and the Director of the Office of Personnel Management ("the government") under the Rehabilitation Act. Section 501 of the Act requires that each executive department and agency promulgate an affirmative action plan that provides adequate "hiring, placement, and advancement" opportunities for handicapped people. The plaintiffs contend, and the government does not contest, that they are "handicapped" within the meaning of the Act. Although plaintiffs are no longer institutionalized, the Act recognizes that discrimination also occurs against those who at one time had a disabling condition. The handicap that these people face is the continuing stigma of being a former psychiatric patient; this disability did not disappear upon discharge from the hospital, as the dissent apparently believes. The regulations thus define a handicapped person as, *inter alia,* one who "has a *history* of . . . a mental or physical impairment that substantially limits one or more major life activities."

Plaintiffs claim that granting excepted workers fewer benefits for the same work is discrimination based on their previous medical condition. They argue that subsection (h) violates the Act's affirmative action requirement because it does not provide "adequate" advancement opportunities. The district court (per Judge June Green) agreed and granted summary judgment in favor of the plaintiff class. As a remedy, Judge Green ordered that all subsection (h) employees who had completed two years of satisfactory service must be allowed to convert to competitive status, with full benefits and credits.

The government makes two claims on appeal: first, that subsection (h) does not violate the Act because it does not distinguish among workers on the basis of handicap; second, that the district court's remedy was improper in these circumstances.

II.

There is clearly tension, if not conflict, between the two well-meaning attempts to assist the handicapped at issue in this case. The subsection (h) excepted service program was created by St. Elizabeth's in the 1950s to help recently discharged mental patients return to the work force. Doctors at the Hospital believed that without some special assistance, former patients might be unable to find jobs because of the stigma that follows people who have been institutionalized. By excusing ex-patients from the civil service exam and employing them in familiar surroundings, it was hoped that they would build a good employment record to help them return to the work force when they left the Hospital.

The Rehabilitation Act of 1973 was a more sweeping, statutory attempt to combat all forms of discrimination against the handicapped. Congress made it clear in both the Act and its 1978 amendments, that it viewed discrimination against the handicapped as an evil on a par with racial, sexual, and ethnic discrimination. The Act is a command to remove artificial barriers that prevent handicapped citizens from reaching their full potential. Recognizing the federal government's obligation to be an equal opportunity employer, the Act requires each department and agency to take affirmative steps to hire and promote handicapped workers.

Given this statutory command, subsection (h) clearly falls short of the Act's affirmative action requirement. Giving unequal benefits for equal work is precisely the type of treatment the Act was designed to eliminate. Hiring the excepted workers under a special provision does not justify giving them second-class status once they are on the job.

* * *

Subsection (h) would be less problematic if there were a fair way for former patients to convert from the excepted to the competitive service. But as the trial court found, there is no way for the patients to convert; their only option is to apply, along with all other applicants, for a position as a first-time federal worker. This arrangement gives the workers no seniority credit for time spent in the excepted service. So before a worker can take a step forward to enjoy equal pay for equal work, he must first step back to an entry-level position. Surely the protections of the Rehabilitation Act are not this illusory.

These considerations and the case law reinforce our conclusion that the government may not justify disparate treatment of the handicapped simply because they were beneficiaries of the excepted hiring process. The Act requires that unless there is a legitimate government interest to the contrary, handicapped employees must be treated the same as other workers. We therefore affirm the district court's decision that subsection (h) does not provide adequate opportunities to former mental patients, in violation of § 501 of the Act. Fashioning a remedy for such unequal treatment, however, is more complicated.

III.

The trial court recognized the difficulties in devising a remedy. The relief order has to end the discrimination, and at the same time respect the government's interest in assisting the handicapped. Judge Green's order allowed all subsection (h) employees who have completed two or more years of satisfactory service to convert to career or career-conditional status, which would automatically grant all the benefits and protections of the competitive service. Newly converted workers also would receive seniority credit for their time in the excepted service.

This remedy is modeled after the revised subsections (t) [pertaining to mentally retarded persons] and (u), [pertaining to severely physically handicapped persons] which were amended by Executive Order in 1979. The regulations now allow both physically handicapped and mentally retarded workers with two years of excepted-service experience to convert to competitive status without taking an exam. For some reason, subsection (h) was not amended at the same time.

Although it might seem logical to make subsection (h) conform to the requirements of closely parallel provisions, we have determined that this symmetrical approach is flawed. Such a remedy would impermissibly interfere with a legitimate government interest because it fails to account for work-related differences between former mental patients and other handicapped workers. We therefore remand to the district court for a reconsideration of the remedy.

There is obviously some government interest in distinguishing between handicapped and non-handicapped employees. The existence of the excepted service confirms this: if handicapped employees did not require special consideration, affirmative action goals could be best met by immediately placing excepted workers in the competitive service, with full benefits and protections. But when subsections (t) and (u) were amended, mentally retarded and physically handicapped people were not given full rights instantly; instead they were given a two year "trial" period. If after two years the employee's handicap proves not to be an impediment to satisfactory performance, the government's interest in treating the excepted class differently disappears.

The problem in the current case is that there are continuing differences between former mental patients and other excepted employees. While a mentally retarded or physically handicapped person's condition usually remains constant or changes gradually, a former mental patient's status is more prone to rapid change. A subsection (h) employee may perform perfectly well for several years, and then have recurring problems that require prompt attention, for the sake of both the worker and the employer.

The possibility of recurring problems was recognized by the Second Circuit in *Doe v. New York University,* 666 F.2d 761 (2d Cir.1981), where a former mental patient brought suit under § 504 of the Act, 29 U.S.C. § 794 (1982), to compel her admission to medical school. After her initial hospitalization, plaintiff's symptoms of mental illness lay dormant for almost seven years before reemerging. She was then rehospitalized periodically for several years, but at the time of her suit had gone more than four years without apparent problems. Although there was testimony that plaintiff was cured, the court held that the medical school was entitled to consider the likelihood of a reoccurrence of the illness when evaluating her application.

The government and St. Elizabeth's have a strong interest in maintaining the flexibility to handle these situations as they arise.

* * *

But as anyone familiar with the civil service knows, removing a competitive status employee from his job is a slow and painstaking process. A former patient who is insulated by the competitive-service job protections may experience continuing mental problems, yet the Hospital would be powerless to respond immediately to correct the situation. The ultimate result might well be contrary to the purpose of the Act: St. Elizabeth's might hire only those with a low risk of recurring problems (those least in need of the excepted service program), while those with uncertain diagnoses would be denied the benefits of subsection (h).

On remand, the district court should fashion a remedy that takes account of this interest. Benefits concerning tenure of employment protections should not diminish St. Elizabeth's flexibility to set reasonable rules for granting or denying job tenure to excepted workers, as their condition dictates. We hasten to add, however, that any benefits or protections *un*related to this interest must be granted in full. It is impermissible, for example, to deny subsection (h) workers full pension rights and other financial benefits, since the government has no interest in treating former patients differently in these respects. Even protections against reductions in force should be given without distinction, since they do not affect the Hospital's ability to treat workers according to their individual needs. While the district court is still free to require a two-year delay before granting excepted workers benefits unrelated to the government interest, a *permanent* denial violates the Act; these non work-related benefits must be given to all employees within a reasonable time.

* * *

CONCLUSION

We emphasize the narrowness of our disagreement with the district court. We affirm the finding below that subsection (h) violates § 501 of the Rehabilitation Act. We also agree that at some point excepted workers are entitled to most of the benefits enjoyed by their competitive counterparts. Commendable as the government's initiative in hiring these workers may be, it defeats the clear command of statute and fairness to treat them as inferior employees in benefits and protections afforded to others. Any distinctive treatment must be related to legitimate work-place needs that the government may have.

We therefore vacate the remedy and remand only for a reconsideration of the handicapped workers' entitlement to those benefits relating to job tenure, in light of the government's legitimate interest in preserving flexibility. In all other respects we affirm.

It is so ordered.

FRIEDMAN, CIRCUIT JUDGE, dissenting:

I would reverse the district court's grant of summary judgment in favor of the appellees and direct that court to dismiss their complaint. In my view, St. Elizabeth's Hospital's practice of hiring its former mental patients by appointing them under 5 C.F.R. § 213.3102(h) (1984) (subchapter (h)) to positions in the excepted service without requiring them to meet the standards necessary for appointment in the competitive service, and without their obtaining all the benefits of the competitive service, is consistent with the Rehabilitation Act of 1973, 29 U.S.C. § 701 *et seq.* (1982), and does not improperly discriminate against those employees on the basis of their former institutionalization in the Hospital.

Ordinarily, an individual obtains an executive branch position in the federal civil service by passing a competitive examination that establishes his or her qualifications for the position sought.   After completing a probationary period, an employee thus appointed becomes entitled to the rights and benefits that the civil service system provides. Congress has recognized, however, that there are certain categories of federal positions that should not be subject to the competitive appointment requirements of civil service and therefore has provided for the "excepted service" to cover those positions.   5 U.S.C. § 2107 (1982). Persons appointed to the excepted service do not receive the same rights and benefits as the employees in the competitive service.

In its governing regulations, the Office of Personnel Management has specified a number of positions that are in the excepted service, which may be filled without following the regular procedures for appointment in the classified service.   Two of these categories cover individuals who, because of their handicaps, would not be qualified for initial appointment in the competitive service.   These provisions are 5 C.F.R. §§ 213.3102(t) and (u), which respectively cover "mentally retarded persons" and "severely physically handicapped persons."   Employees in either of these two categories may be converted to competitive status "[u]pon completion of 2 years of satisfactory service under this authority. . . . "

The present case involves subsection (h) of the regulation, which authorizes the appointment at federal mental institutions of former patients of those institutions, who have been discharged and have been certified by medical authority "as recovered sufficiently to be regularly employed but it is believed desirable and in the interest of the persons and the institution that they be employed at the institution."   All of the appellees in this case are in that category.   They were appointed to positions at St. Elizabeth's Hospital without having to meet the competitive civil service requirements that other persons seeking the same position would have had to satisfy.

*   *   *

The differences between subsection (h) and subsections (t) and (u) are substantial.   The latter two subsections deal with persons who are disabled at the time of their appointment and therefore would not qualify for the job under the usual competitive examination procedures. Those individuals are given temporary appointments but, if after two years they have demonstrated their ability to perform the job, they are converted to the competitive status and have the rights and benefits they would have obtained initially had they not been disabled from passing the competitive examination.

Persons given indefinite appointments under subsection (h), on the other hand, are former patients of the mental institution who no longer are disabled at the time of their appointment, but whose well-being favors their employment at the institution with which they are familiar. Some of those individuals might have qualified initially for appointment in the competitive service by taking and passing the usual examination, and any of them could have obtained such competitive permanent positions after appointment by following that course. Indeed, a number of former patients of St. Elizabeth's, originally appointed under subsection (h), have done precisely that and now hold permanent appointments in the classified service with the accompanying rights and benefits. Although the appellees might have obtained a classified position after their appointment by taking and passing the same competitive examination that other nondisqualified persons routinely take, they have not attempted to do so.

The appellees' position is that because they perform the same work as other employees who occupy identical positions in the competitive service, they are entitled to the same benefits the other employees have, and that the denial of those benefits illegally discriminates against them on the basis of their former mental disability. The different treatment of the appellees from the other employees performing the same work, however, results not from the former mental disability of the appellees but from the fact that they were appointed without having to comply with the requirements for the competitive service. In order to achieve the benefits from employment in an environment with which they had become familiar and in which they were comfortable, the government permitted the appellees to obtain their positions without taking and passing the competitive examination that other employees were required to take to obtain the same jobs.

In my view, the government justifiably treated these two categories of employees differently in not giving to the appellees all the civil service protections and benefits of the employees who obtained their positions through the competitive examination process. The difference in the nature of their appointments warranted the different rights and benefits given to each category.

* * *

As a policy matter, the result reached in the present case is commendable. My difficulty with that result is that I do not think it reflects a proper use of judicial power. Congress has given the President broad discretion by regulation to administer the laws regulating government employment and therefore to determine the bases for appointments to positions in the executive branch and to define the rights and benefits of employees so appointed. 5 U.S.C. § 3301 (1982). The President in turn has delegated this authority to the Office of Personnel Management. * * * If the type of appointment under subsection (h) and the rights and benefits of employees appointed under that subsection are to be changed, I think such changes must come from the Office of Personnel Management and not from the courts.

Questions and Comments

1. *Is absolute equality required?* Is the court's reading of the requirement of equality in conditions of employment presumably imposed by Section 501 (requiring federal agencies to adopt affirmative action programs) supported by either the legislative history or the language of the Act? Must an affirmative action requirement necessarily mandate that persons hired through special procedures inaugurated under an affirmative action plan be treated identically to persons hired through normal procedures?

2. *Affirmative action discouraged?* What are the likely long range effects of decisions such as *Allen v. Heckler?* Do decisions such as this, while imposing equality on the conditions of employment, make it more or less likely that agencies will adopt affirmative action programs to employ the handicapped? In answering this question keep in mind that the design and scope of affirmative action programs is not spelled out by the law or regulations but is basically the responsibility of the employing agencies themselves.

3. *Were plaintiffs "otherwise qualified"?* Section 504 of the Act prohibits federal agencies from discriminating against "otherwise qualified" handicapped persons. See 29 U.S.C. § 794. If the *Allen* plaintiffs had brought their suit under Section 504, would it have made any difference if plaintiffs as a class were performing their jobs in a less efficient or slower manner than the competitive service employees? Would such proof have any bearing on the application of the affirmative action requirements which were relied on by the court? With which opinion do you agree?

4. *Disabled v. "recovered" employees.* Note that the dissent places emphasis on the fact that subsections (t) and (u) of the regulations concerning excepted positions cover persons disabled at the time they are hired, but that persons covered by subsection (h) are not disabled at the time they are hired. The dissent claims that for this reason a distinction can be drawn between the treatment of subsection (h) employees and subsection (t) and (u) employees. Is this reasoning compelling? Or do you agree with the majority that subsection (h) employees remain "handicapped" even though they have recovered? If one accepts the majority's conclusion, does this eliminate the difference between subsection (h) employees and the subsection (t) and (u) employees for purposes of applying the affirmative action requirements?

II. ACCESS TO HOUSING

A. CONSTITUTIONAL PROTECTIONS

CITY OF CLEBURNE, TEXAS v. CLEBURNE LIVING CENTER

Supreme Court of the United States, 1985.
473 U.S. 432, 105 S.Ct. 3249, 87 L.Ed.2d 313.

JUSTICE WHITE delivered the opinion of the Court.

A Texas city denied a special use permit for the operation of a group home for the mentally retarded, acting pursuant to a municipal zoning ordinance requiring permits for such homes. The Court of Appeals for the Fifth Circuit held that mental retardation is a "quasi-suspect" classification and that the ordinance violated the Equal Protection Clause because it did not substantially further an important governmental purpose. We hold that a lesser standard of scrutiny is appropriate, but conclude that under that standard the ordinance is invalid as applied in this case.

I

In July 1980, respondent Jan Hannah purchased a building at 201 Featherston Street in the city of Cleburne, Texas, with the intention of leasing it to Cleburne Living Center, Inc. (CLC), for the operation of a group home for the mentally retarded. It was anticipated that the home would house 13 retarded men and women, who would be under the constant supervision of CLC staff members. The house had four bedrooms and two baths, with a half bath to be added. CLC planned to comply with all applicable state and federal regulations.

The city informed CLC that a special use permit would be required for the operation of a group home at the site, and CLC accordingly submitted a permit application. In response to a subsequent inquiry from CLC, the city explained that under the zoning regulations applicable to the site, a special use permit, renewable annually, was required for the construction of "[h]ospitals for the insane or feeble-minded, or alcoholic [*sic*] or drug addicts, or penal or correctional institutions." [3] The city had determined that the proposed group home should be

---

3. The site of the home is in an area zoned "R–3," an "Apartment House District." App. 51. Section 8 of the Cleburne zoning ordinance, in pertinent part, allows the following uses in an R–3 district:

"1. Any use permitted in District R–2.

"2. Apartment houses, or multiple dwellings.

"3. Boarding and lodging houses.

"4. Fraternity or sorority houses and dormitories.

"5. Apartment hotels.

"6. Hospitals, sanitariums, nursing homes or homes for convalescents or aged, *other than for the* insane or *feeble-minded* or alcoholics or drug addicts."

"7. Private clubs or fraternal orders, except those whose chief activity is carried on as a business.

"8. Philanthropic or eleemosynary institutions, other than penal institutions.

"9. Accessory uses customarily incident to any of the above uses. . . ."
Id., at 60–61 (emphasis added).

classified as a "hospital for the feeble-minded." After holding a public hearing on CLC's application, the City Council voted 3 to 1 to deny a special use permit.

CLC then filed suit in Federal District Court against the city and a number of its officials, alleging, *inter alia,* that the zoning ordinance was invalid on its face and as applied because it discriminated against the mentally retarded in violation of the equal protection rights of CLC and its potential residents. The District Court found that "[i]f the potential residents of the Featherston Street home were not mentally retarded, but the home was the same in all other respects, its use would be permitted under the city's zoning ordinance," and that the City Counsel's decision "was motivated primarily by the fact that the residents of the home would be persons who are mentally retarded." Even so, the District Court held the ordinance and its application constitutional. Concluding that no fundamental right was implicated and that mental retardation was neither a suspect nor a quasi-suspect classification, the court employed the minimum level of judicial scrutiny applicable to equal protection claims. The court deemed the ordinance, as written and applied, to be rationally related to the city's legitimate interests in "the legal responsibility of CLC and its residents, . . . the safety and fears of residents in the adjoining neighborhood," and the number of people to be housed in the home.

The Court of Appeals for the Fifth Circuit reversed, determining that mental retardation was a quasi-suspect classification and that it should assess the validity of the ordinance under intermediate-level scrutiny. Because mental retardation was in fact relevant to many legislative actions, strict scrutiny was not appropriate. But in light of the history of "unfair and often grotesque mistreatment" of the retarded, discrimination against them was "likely to reflect deep-seated prejudice." In addition, the mentally retarded lacked political power, and their condition was immutable. The court considered heightened scrutiny to be particularly appropriate in this case, because the city's ordinance withheld a benefit which, although not fundamental, was very important to the mentally retarded. Without group homes, the court stated, the retarded could never hope to integrate themselves into the community. Applying the test that it considered appropriate, the court held that the ordinance was invalid on its face because it did not substantially further any important governmental interests. The Court of Appeals went on to hold that the ordinance was also invalid as applied.

* * *

II

The Equal Protection Clause of the Fourteenth Amendment commands that no State shall "deny to any person within its jurisdiction

Section 16 of the ordinance specifies the uses for which a special use permit is required. These include "[h]ospitals for the insane or feebleminded, or alcoholic [*sic*] or drug addicts, or penal or correctional institutions." * * *

the equal protection of the laws," which is essentially a direction that all persons similarly situated should be treated alike. *Plyler v. Doe,* 457 U.S. 202, 216, 102 S.Ct. 2382, 2394, 72 L.Ed.2d 786 (1982). Section 5 of the Amendment empowers Congress to enforce this mandate, but absent controlling congressional direction, the courts have themselves devised standards for determining the validity of state legislation or other official action that is challenged as denying equal protection. The general rule is that legislation is presumed to be valid and will be sustained if the classification drawn by the statute is rationally related to a legitimate state interest.

* * *

The general rule gives way, however, when a statute classifies by race, alienage, or national origin. These factors are so seldom relevant to the achievement of any legitimate state interest that laws grounded in such considerations are deemed to reflect prejudice and antipathy—a view that those in the burdened class are not as worthy or deserving as others. For these reasons and because such discrimination is unlikely to be soon rectified by legislative means, these laws are subjected to strict scrutiny and will be sustained only if they are suitably tailored to serve a compelling state interest. Similar oversight by the courts is due when state laws impinge on personal rights protected by the Constitution.

Legislative classifications based on gender also call for a heightened standard of review. That factor generally provides no sensible ground for differential treatment. "[W]hat differentiates sex from such nonsuspect statuses as intelligence or physical disability . . . is that the sex characteristic frequently bears no relation to ability to perform or contribute to society." Rather than resting on meaningful considerations, statutes distributing benefits and burdens between the sexes in different ways very likely reflect outmoded notions of the relative capabilities of men and women. A gender classification fails unless it is substantially related to a sufficiently important governmental interest. Because illegitimacy is beyond the individual's control and bears "no relation to the individual's ability to participate in and contribute to society," official discriminations resting on that characteristic are also subject to somewhat heightened review.

* * *

We have declined, however, to extend heightened review to differential treatment based on age. . . .

* * *

III

Against this background, we conclude for several reasons that the Court of Appeals erred in holding mental retardation a quasi-suspect classification calling for a more exacting standard of judicial review than is normally accorded economic and social legislation. First, it is undeniable, and it is not argued otherwise here, that those who are mentally retarded have a reduced ability to cope with and function in the everyday world. Nor are they all cut from the same pattern: as the testimony in this record indicates, they range from those whose disability is not immediately evident to those who must be constantly cared for. They are thus different, immutably so, in relevant respects, and the States' interest in dealing with and providing for them is plainly a legitimate one. How this large and diversified group is to be treated under the law is a difficult and often a technical matter, very much a task for legislators guided by qualified professionals and not by the perhaps ill-informed opinions of the judiciary. Heightened scrutiny inevitably involves substantive judgments about legislative decisions, and we doubt that the predicate for such judicial oversight is present where the classification deals with mental retardation.

Second, the distinctive legislative response, both national and state, to the plight of those who are mentally retarded demonstrates not only that they have unique problems, but also that the lawmakers have been addressing their difficulties in a manner that belies a continuing antipathy or prejudice and a corresponding need for more intrusive oversight by the judiciary.

* * *

Third, the legislative response, which could hardly have occurred and survived without public support, negates any claim that the mentally retarded are politically powerless in the sense that they have no ability to attract the attention of the lawmakers. Any minority can be said to be powerless to assert direct control over the legislature, but if that were a criterion for higher level scrutiny by the courts, much economic and social legislation would now be suspect.

Fourth, if the large and amorphous class of the mentally retarded were deemed quasi-suspect for the reasons given by the Court of Appeals, it would be difficult to find a principled way to distinguish a variety of other groups who have perhaps immutable disabilities setting them off from others, who cannot themselves mandate the desired legislative responses, and who can claim some degree of prejudice from at least part of the public at large. One need mention in this respect only the aging, the disabled, the mentally ill, and the infirm. We are reluctant to set out on that course, and we decline to do so.

Doubtless, there have been and there will continue to be instances of discrimination against the retarded that are in fact invidious, and that are properly subject to judicial correction under constitutional norms. But the appropriate method of reaching such instances is not to create a new quasi-suspect classification and subject all governmental action based on that classification to more searching evaluation. Rather, we should look to the likelihood that governmental action premised on a particular classification is valid as a general matter, not merely to the specifics of the case before us. Because mental retardation is a characteristic that the government may legitimately take into account in a wide range of decisions, and because both State and Federal Governments have recently committed themselves to assisting the retarded, we will not presume that any given legislative action, even one that disadvantages retarded individuals, is rooted in considerations that the Constitution will not tolerate.

Our refusal to recognize the retarded as a quasi-suspect class does not leave them entirely unprotected from invidious discrimination. To withstand equal protection review, legislation that distinguishes between the mentally retarded and others must be rationally related to a legitimate governmental purpose. This standard, we believe, affords government the latitude necessary both to pursue policies designed to assist the retarded in realizing their full potential, and to freely and efficiently engage in activities that burden the retarded in what is essentially an incidental manner. The State may not rely on a classification whose relationship to an asserted goal is so attenuated as to render the distinction arbitrary or irrational.

* * *

IV

We turn to the issue of the validity of the zoning ordinance insofar as it requires a special use permit for homes for the mentally retarded. We inquire first whether requiring a special use permit for the Featherston home in the circumstances here deprives respondents of the equal protection of the laws. If it does, there will be no occasion to decide whether the special use permit provision is facially invalid where the mentally retarded are involved, or to put it another way, whether the city may never insist on a special use permit for a home for the mentally retarded in an R–3 zone. This is the preferred course of adjudication since it enables courts to avoid making unnecessarily broad constitutional judgments.

The constitutional issue is clearly posed. The city does not require a special use permit in an R–3 zone for apartment houses, multiple dwellings, boarding and lodging houses, fraternity or sorority houses, dormitories, apartment hotels, hospitals, sanitariums, nursing homes for convalescents or the aged (other than for the insane or feebleminded or alcoholics or drug addicts), private clubs or fraternal orders, and other specified uses. It does, however, insist on a special permit for the Featherston home, and it does so, as the District Court found, because it would be a facility for the mentally retarded. May the city require the permit for this facility when other care and multiple-dwelling facilities are freely permitted?

It is true, as already pointed out, that the mentally retarded as a group are indeed different from others not sharing their misfortune, and in this respect they may be different from those who would occupy other facilities that would be permitted in an R–3 zone without a special permit. But this difference is largely irrelevant unless the Featherston home and those who would occupy it would threaten legitimate interests of the city in a way that other permitted uses such as boarding houses and hospitals would not. Because in our view the record does not reveal any rational basis for believing that the Featherston home would pose any special threat to the city's legitimate interests, we affirm the judgment below insofar as it holds the ordinance invalid as applied in this case.

The District Court found that the City Council's insistence on the permit rested on several factors. First, the Council was concerned with the negative attitude of the majority of property owners located within 200 feet of the Featherston facility, as well as with the fears of elderly residents of the neighborhood. But mere negative attitudes, or fear, unsubstantiated by factors which are properly cognizable in a zoning proceeding, are not permissible bases for treating a home for the mentally retarded differently from apartment houses, multiple dwellings, and the like.

* * *

Second, the Council had two objections to the location of the facility. It was concerned that the facility was across the street from a junior high school, and it feared that the students might harass the occupants of the Featherston home. But the school itself is attended by about 30 mentally retarded students, and denying a permit based on such vague, undifferentiated fears is again permitting some portion of the community to validate what would otherwise be an equal protection violation. The other objection to the home's location was that it was located on "a five hundred year flood plain." This concern with the possibility of a flood, however, can hardly be based on a distinction between the Featherston home and, for example, nursing homes, homes for convalescents or the aged, or sanitariums or hospitals, any of which could be located on the Featherston site without obtaining a special use permit. The same may be said of another concern of the Council—doubts about the legal responsibility for actions which the mentally retarded might take. If there is no concern about legal responsibility with respect to other uses that would be permitted in the area, such as boarding and fraternity houses, it is difficult to believe that the groups of mildly or moderately mentally retarded individuals who would live at 201 Featherston would present any different or special hazard.

Fourth, the Council was concerned with the size of the home and the number of people that would occupy it. The District Court found, and the Court of Appeals repeated, that "[i]f the potential residents of the Featherston Street home were not mentally retarded, but the home was the same in all other respects, its use would be permitted under the city's zoning ordinance." Given this finding, there would be no restrictions on the number of people who could occupy this home as a boarding house, nursing home, family dwelling, fraternity house, or dormitory. The question is whether it is rational to treat the mentally retarded differently. It is true that they suffer disability not shared by others; but why this difference warrants a density regulation that others need not observe is not at all apparent. At least this record does not clarify how, in this connection, the characteristics of the intended occupants of the Featherston home rationally justify denying to those occupants what would be permitted to groups occupying the same site for different purposes. Those who would live in the Featherston home are the type of individuals who, with supporting staff, satisfy federal and state standards for group housing in the community; and there is no dispute that the home would meet the federal square-footage-per-resident requirement for facilities of this type. In the words of the Court of Appeals, "[t]he City never justifies its apparent view that other people can live under such 'crowded' conditions when mentally retarded persons cannot."

In the courts below the city also urged that the ordinance is aimed at avoiding concentration of population and at lessening congestion of the streets. These concerns obviously fail to explain why apartment houses, fraternity and sorority houses, hospitals and the like, may freely locate in the area without a permit. So, too, the expressed worry about fire hazards, the serenity of the neighborhood, and the avoidance of danger to other residents fail rationally to justify singling out a home such as 201 Featherston for the special use permit, yet imposing no such restrictions on the many other uses freely permitted in the neighborhood.

The short of it is that requiring the permit in this case appears to us to rest on an irrational prejudice against the mentally retarded, including those who would occupy the Featherston facility and who would live under the closely supervised and highly regulated conditions expressly provided for by state and federal law.

The judgment of the Court of Appeals is affirmed insofar as it invalidates the zoning ordinance as applied to the Featherston home. The judgment is otherwise vacated, and the case is remanded.

It is so ordered.

JUSTICE STEVENS, with whom THE CHIEF JUSTICE joins, concurring.

* * *

Every law that places the mentally retarded in a special class is not presumptively irrational. The differences between mentally retarded persons and those with greater mental capacity are obviously relevant to certain legislative decisions. An impartial lawmaker—indeed, even a member of a class of persons defined as mentally retarded—could rationally vote in favor of a law providing funds for special education and special treatment for the mentally retarded. A mentally retarded person could also recognize that he is a member of a class that might need special supervision in some situations, both to protect himself and to protect others. Restrictions on his right to drive cars or to operate hazardous equipment might well seem rational even though they deprived him of employment opportunities and the kind of freedom of travel enjoyed by other citizens. "That a civilized and decent society expects and approves such legislation indicates that governmental consideration of those differences in the vast majority of situations is not only legitimate but also desirable."

Even so, the Court of Appeals correctly observed that through ignorance and prejudice the mentally retarded "have been subjected to a history of unfair and often grotesque mistreatment." 726 F.2d 191, 197 (CA5 1984). The discrimination against the mentally retarded that is at issue in this case is the city's decision to require an annual special use permit before property in an apartment house district may be used as a group home for persons who are mildly retarded. The record convinces me that this permit was required because of the irrational fears of neighboring property owners, rather than for the protection of the mentally retarded persons who would reside in respondent's home.

Although the city argued in the Court of Appeals that legitimate interests of the neighbors justified the restriction, the court unambiguously rejected that argument. *Id.*, at 201. In this Court, the city has argued that the discrimination was really motivated by a desire to protect the mentally retarded from the hazards presented by the neighborhood. Zoning ordinances are not usually justified on any such basis, and in this case, for the reasons explained by the Court, I find that justification wholly unconvincing. I cannot believe that a rational member of this disadvantaged class could ever approve of the discriminatory application of the city's ordinance in this case.

Accordingly, I join the opinion of the Court.

JUSTICE MARSHALL, with whom JUSTICE BRENNAN and JUSTICE BLACKMUN join, concurring in the judgment in part and dissenting in part.

* * *

I share the Court's criticisms of the overly broad lines that Cleburne's zoning ordinance has drawn. But if the ordinance is to be invalidated for its imprecise classifications, it must be pursuant to more powerful scrutiny than the minimal rational-basis test used to review classifications affecting only economic and commercial matters.

* * *

In light of the importance of the interest at stake and the history of discrimination the retarded have suffered, the Equal Protection Clause requires us to do more than review the distinctions drawn by Cleburne's zoning ordinance as if they appeared in a taxing statute or in economic or commercial legislation. The searching scrutiny I would give to restrictions on the ability of the retarded to establish community group homes leads me to conclude that Cleburne's vague generalizations for classifying the "feeble-minded" with drug addicts, alcoholics, and the insane, and excluding them where the elderly, the ill, the boarder, and the transient are allowed, are not substantial or important enough to overcome the suspicion that the ordinance rests on impermissible assumptions or outmoded and perhaps invidious stereotypes.

* * *

In light of the scrutiny that should be applied here, Cleburne's ordinance sweeps too broadly to dispel the suspicion that it rests on a bare desire to treat the retarded as outsiders, pariahs who do not belong in the community. The Court, while disclaiming that special scrutiny is necessary or warranted, reaches the same conclusion. Rather than striking the ordinance down, however, the Court invalidates it merely as applied to respondents. I must dissent from the novel proposition that "the preferred course of adjudication" is to leave standing a legislative Act resting on "irrational prejudice", thereby forcing individuals in the group discriminated against to continue to run the Act's gauntlet.

The Court appears to act out of a belief that the ordinance might be "rational" as applied to some subgroup of the retarded under some circumstances, such as those utterly without the capacity to live in a community, and that the ordinance should not be invalidated *in toto* if it is capable of ever being validly applied. But the issue is not "whether the city may never insist on a special use permit for the mentally retarded in an R–3 zone." The issue is whether the city may require a permit pursuant to a blunderbuss ordinance drafted many years ago to exclude all the "feeble-minded," or whether the city must enact a new ordinance carefully tailored to the exclusion of some well-defined subgroup of retarded people in circumstances in which exclusion might reasonably further legitimate city purposes.

* * *

Invalidating on its face the ordinance's special treatment of the "feebleminded," in contrast, would place the responsibility for tailoring and updating Cleburne's unconstitutional ordinance where it belongs: with the legislative arm of the City of Cleburne. If Cleburne perceives a legitimate need for requiring a certain well-defined subgroup of the retarded to obtain special permits before establishing group homes, Cleburne will, after studying the problem and making the appropriate policy decisions, enact a new, more narrowly tailored ordinance. That ordinance might well look very different from the current one; it might separate group homes (presently treated nowhere in the ordinance) from hospitals, and it might define a narrow subclass of the retarded for whom even group homes could legitimately be excluded. Special treatment of the retarded might be ended altogether. But whatever the contours such an ordinance might take, the city should not be allowed to keep its ordinance on the books intact and thereby shift to the courts the responsibility to confront the complex empirical and policy questions involved in updating statutes affecting the mentally retarded. A legislative solution would yield standards and provide the sort of certainty to retarded applicants and administrative officials that case-by-case judicial rulings cannot provide. Retarded applicants should not have to continue to attempt to surmount Cleburne's vastly overbroad ordinance.

Questions and Comments

1. *Impact of an "invalid as applied" holding.* What is the practical significance of the majority's holding which invalidates the ordinance as applied to the Cleburne Living Center (CLC) but left the regulatory scheme

in place? Are there any circumstances under which the City of Cleburne might legally deny a permit to applicants seeking to establish a group home for the developmentally disabled? For a general analysis of the Cleburne case and a proposal for an alternate approach to the analysis of laws distinguishing on the basis of mental capacity, see Minow, *When Difference Has Its Home: Group Homes For The Mentally Retarded, Equal Protection and Legal Treatment of Difference*, Harv.Civil Rights–Civil Liberties L.Rev., Vol. 22, 1987.

2. *Anti-discrimination legislation.* Congress recently enacted the Fair Housing Amendment Act of 1988 which makes it "unlawful to discriminate in the sale or rental or otherwise make unavailable or deny a dwelling to any buyer or renter because of a handicap." 42 U.S.C. § 3604. Presumably, zoning ordinances of the type adopted by the city of Cleburne could now be challenged on the basis of the Act. The special remedies provided by the Act are discussed in the subsection that follows.

3. *Application of constitutional standard to other forms of discrimination.* Does the majority opinion provide any guidance as to the constitutional status of legislation which has a rational purpose but nonetheless burdens the disadvantaged class? For instance, would it be permissible to require compulsory sterilization of certain classes of the mentally retarded? Such a rule could be and has been defended as a safety protection to both the individual who is retarded and the society at large. See, *Buck v. Bell*, 274 U.S. 200, 207, 47 S.Ct. 584, 585, 71 L.Ed. 1000 (1927) (upholding Virginia's compulsory sterilization law). See also, *Pennsylvania Ass'n for Retarded Children v. Commonwealth*, 343 F.Supp. 279, 294, note 42 (E.D.Pa. 1972) (reviewing state sterilization laws).

The mentally retarded have also been the subject of other restrictions, such as legal prohibitions against marriage. See generally, Linn and Bowers, *The Historical Fallacies Behind Legal Protections of Marriages Involving Mentally Retarded Persons–The External Child Grows Up*, 13 Gonz. L. Rev. 625 (1978) (discussing unsoundness of laws prohibiting mentally retarded persons from marrying). Since both marriage and sterilization statutes deal directly with procreation, constitutional rights in addition to equal protection may come into play. See *Roe v. Wade*, 410 U.S. 113, 93 S.Ct. 705, 35 L.Ed.2d 147 (1973).

B. LEGISLATIVE PROTECTIONS

In its enactment of the Fair Housing Amendments Act of 1988 (P.L. 100–430, 42 U.S.C. § 3601 et seq.), Congress for the first time provided federal protection to the handicapped against discrimination in the rental and sale of housing. Coverage under the Act extends to all sales as well as rentals of multifamily housing. Discriminatory practices include both the outright denial of housing as well as discrimination in the terms and conditions under which property is sold or rented.

Enforcement may be either by private action in court for equitable relief or damages (including punitive) or by an action brought by the Attorney General. The Act also allows the Secretary of Housing and

Urban Development to implement conciliation proceedings either at the federal level or under local agency auspices. Enforcement actions by the Attorney General have to date focused on discriminatory zoning practices. An account of these actions is contained in the following report *:

> In its first lawsuit filed under a new provision of the amended Fair Housing Act, the U.S. Justice Department is accusing the city of Chicago Heights of discriminating against the disabled.
>
> The complaint, filed in June [1989], alleges that this south suburb of Chicago denied a special-use permit for the construction of a 15–bed group home for the mentally retarded because of opposition by neighbors.
>
> A Galesburg, Ill., firm, Residential Facilities Management Specialists Inc. (RFMS), applied for a special-use permit in January. The Chicago Heights City Council voted unanimously to deny the permit on May 1, following hearings by the city's Plan Commission and the Board of Zoning Appeals.
>
> City officials claim that the proposed home would violate local zoning ordinances. However, the suit alleges that the City Council denied the permit based on area residents' fears and prejudices concerning the mentally disabled.
>
> "A large proportion of [the neighbors'] statements indicated, explicitly or by implication, that the speakers' opposition was based on the handicap of the prospective residents of the facility," the suit reads.
>
> The lawsuit seeks an injunction against Chicago Heights to prevent interference of the construction of the proposed RFMS group home. It also requests damages for those persons injured by the city's actions and a civil penalty payable to the United States.
>
> If successful, the lawsuit could open the way for group homes across the nation, homes which have long been opposed because homeowners fear a rise in crime and a drop in property values.
>
>   *   *   *
>
> Although the suit is the first the Justice Department has filed based on disability, it recently won a similar suit based on familial status. In that settlement, Justice obtained $33,000 in damages from a New Jersey town for the victim and the fair housing group that were believed damaged by the discrimination.
>
> There are also several private suits pending in Pennsylvania and one pending in Swansea, Ill., that have been filed under the amendment, according to Beth Pepper of the Mental Health Law Project.

Jacqueline Lee, *Suburb Sued for Unfair Zoning,* American Bar Association Journal, September 1989, p. 40.

It is difficult to predict how the provisions of the 1988 Act will be applied to those disabled on psychiatric grounds. One exception to the amendment's protections is that rental may be denied to a person whose

---

* Reprinted with permission from the September 1989 issue of the *ABA Journal,*   The Lawyer's Magazine, published by the American Bar Association.

tenancy would constitute a direct threat to the health or safety of others or whose tenancy would result in substantial damage to property. 42 U.S.C. § 3604(f)(9). As a result, if a mental affliction is accompanied by aggressive behavior, the Act would countenance denial of tenancy. What remains to be determined by case law is the degree and imminency of danger that the tenant must pose to justify a rejection.

Numerous states have enacted fair housing legislation which provides some degree of protection to the handicapped. Such laws either provide protection *specifically* to the handicapped (see, e.g., Or.Rev.Stat. 659.430), or provide protection against housing discrimination to various minorities, including the handicapped (see, e.g., Mont.Code.Ann. 49–2–305). The scope of protection to the handicapped under the above cited state statutes is substantially similar to that of the federal Act. Both laws prohibit the refusal to sell or lease housing because of the buyer's or renter's handicap. However, the Montana law makes such refusal unlawful "[e]xcept when the distinction is based on reasonable grounds." What might constitute "reasonable grounds" to discriminate against a mentally handicapped person? Might the Montana law countenance denial of tenancy to an individual whose disability makes him dangerous to persons or property, as the federal law appears to do?

*

Index

†